KU-341-599

MTW   0037195

ANATOMIC
PATHOLOGY
BOARD REVIEW

DISCARDED

ANATOMIC PATHOLOGY BOARD REVIEW

SECOND EDITION

Jay H. Lefkowitch, MD

Professor of Clinical Pathology and Cell Biology at the
Columbia University Medical Center
New York, New York

ELSEVIER
SAUNDERS

KMS
£a5·15

THE LIBRARY
ACADEMIC CENTRE
MAIDSTONE HOSPITAL

QZ4

ELSEVIER
SAUNDERS

1600 John F. Kennedy Blvd.
Ste 1800
Philadelphia, PA 19103-2899

ANATOMIC PATHOLOGY BOARD REVIEW, Second Edition   ISBN: 978-1-4557-1140-6

Copyright © 2015, 2006 by Saunders, an imprint of Elsevier Inc. All rights reserved.

No part of this publication may be reproduced or transmitted in any form or by any means, electronic or mechanical, including photocopying, recording, or any information storage and retrieval system, without permission in writing from the publisher. Details on how to seek permission, further information about the Publisher's permissions policies and our arrangements with organizations such as the Copyright Clearance Center and the Copyright Licensing Agency, can be found at our website: www.elsevier.com/permissions.

This book and the individual contributions contained in it are protected under copyright by the Publisher (other than as may be noted herein).

Notices

Knowledge and best practice in this field are constantly changing. As new research and experience broaden our understanding, changes in research methods, professional practices, or medical treatment may become necessary.

Practitioners and researchers must always rely on their own experience and knowledge in evaluating and using any information, methods, compounds, or experiments described herein. In using such information or methods they should be mindful of their own safety and the safety of others, including parties for whom they have a professional responsibility.

With respect to any drug or pharmaceutical products identified, readers are advised to check the most current information provided (i) on procedures featured or (ii) by the manufacturer of each product to be administered, to verify the recommended dose or formula, the method and duration of administration, and contraindications. It is the responsibility of practitioners, relying on their own experience and knowledge of their patients, to make diagnoses, to determine dosages and the best treatment for each individual patient, and to take all appropriate safety precautions.

To the fullest extent of the law, neither the Publisher nor the authors, contributors, or editors, assume any liability for any injury and/or damage to persons or property as a matter of products liability, negligence or otherwise, or from any use or operation of any methods, products, instructions, or ideas contained in the material herein.

Library of Congress Cataloging-in-Publication Data
Anatomic pathology : board review / editor, Jay H. Lefkowitch. – Second edition.
    p. ; cm.
Includes bibliographical references and index.
ISBN 978-1-4557-1140-6 (pbk. : alk. paper)
I. Lefkowitch, Jay H., editor.
[DNLM: 1. Pathology, Clinical–Examination Questions. 2. Anatomy–Examination Questions. QZ 18.2]
RB119
616.07076–dc23

2014009226

Executive Content Strategist: William R. Schmitt
Content Development Specialist: Katy Meert
Publishing Services Manager: Patricia Tannian
Senior Project Manager: Sharon Corell
Senior Book Designer: Lou Forgione

 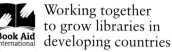

Working together
to grow libraries in
developing countries

www.elsevier.com • www.bookaid.org

Printed in China
Last digit is the print number: 9 8 7 6 5 4 3 2

CONTRIBUTORS

N. Volkan Adsay, MD
Professor of Pathology and Laboratory Medicine, Vice-Chair and Director of Anatomic Pathology, Emory University, Atlanta, Georgia

Aqeel Ahmed, MD
Associate Research Scientist, Herbert Irving Comprehensive Cancer Center, Columbia University Medical Center, New York, New York

Bachir Alobeid, MD
Professor of Pathology and Cell Biology at the Columbia University Medical Center, New York Presbyterian Hospital, New York, New York

Olca Basturk, MD
Assistant Attending Physician, Department of Pathology, Memorial Sloan-Kettering Cancer Center, New York, New York

Alain C. Borczuk, MD
Professor of Pathology and Cell Biology and Vice Chairman of Anatomic Pathology at the Columbia University Medical Center, New York, New York

Jessica M. Comstock, MD
Assistant Professor, University of Utah Department of Pathology, Division of Pediatric Pathology, Salt Lake City, Utah

Vivette D. D'Agati, MD
Professor of Pathology and Cell Biology at the Columbia University Medical Center, New York, New York

Valerie A. Fitzhugh, MD
Assistant Professor of Pathology and Laboratory Medicine, Rutgers, The State University of New Jersey—New Jersey Medical School, Attending Pathologist, Pathology and Laboratory Medicine, University Hospital, Newark, New Jersey

James E. Goldman, MD, PhD
Professor of Pathology and Cell Biology (in Psychiatry), Columbia University, New York, New York

Diane Hamele-Bena, MD
Assistant Professor of Pathology and Cell Biology at the Columbia University Medical Center, New York, New York

Lara R. Harik, MD
Assistant Professor of Pathology and Cell Biology at the Columbia University Medical Center, New York, New York

Debra S. Heller, MD
Professor of Pathology, Rutgers, The State University of New Jersey— New Jersey Medical School, Attending Physician, Pathology and Laboratory Medicine, University Hospital, Newark, New Jersey

Leal C. Herlitz, MD
Associate Professor of Pathology and Cell Biology at the Columbia University Medical Center, New York, New York

Hanina Hibshoosh, MD
Professor of Pathology and Cell Biology at the Columbia University Medical Center, New York, New York

Samer N. Khader, MD
Assistant Professor of Pathology, Associate Director, Cytopathology Fellowship Program, Albert Einstein College of Medicine/Montefiore Medical Center, Bronx, New York

Stephen M. Lagana, MD
Assistant Professor of Pathology and Cell Biology at the Columbia University Medical Center, New York Presbyterian Hospital, New York, New York

John C. Lee, MD
Assistant Professor of Pathology and Laboratory Medicine, Boston University Medical Center, Boston, Massachusetts

Jay H. Lefkowitch, MD
Professor of Clinical Pathology and Cell Biology at the Columbia University Medical Center, New York, New York

Mahesh M. Mansukhani, MD
Associate Professor of Pathology and Cell Biology, Medical Director, CUMC Personalized Genomic Medicine Laboratory, Columbia University Medical Center, New York, New York

Charles C. Marboe, MD
Professor of Pathology and Cell Biology at Columbia University Medical Center, New York Presbyterian Hospital, New York, New York

Glen S. Markowitz, MD
Professor of Pathology and Cell Biology at the Columbia University Medical Center, New York, New York

Lorenzo Memeo, MD
Director of the Pathology Unit, Department of Experimental Oncology, Mediterranean Institute of Oncology, Scientific Director, Iom Ricerca SRL, Catania, Italy

Roger K. Moreira, MD
Senior Associate Consultant and Assistant Professor, Department of Laboratory Medicine and Pathology, Mayo Clinic, Rochester, Minnesota

Jennifer V. Nguyen, MD
Assistant Professor of Clinical Dermatology, Perelman School of Medicine at the University of Pennsylvania, Philadelphia, Pennsylvania

Volker Nickeleit, MD
Professor of Pathology, Director, Division of Nephropathology, Department of Pathology and Laboratory Medicine, The University of North Carolina at Chapel Hill, Chapel Hill, North Carolina

Kathleen M. O'Toole, MD
Professor of Pathology and Cell Biology at the Columbia University Medical Center, New York, New York

May Parisien, MD
Special Lecturer in Clinical Pathology, Columbia University, New York, New York

Karl H. Perzin, MD
Professor Emeritus, Clinical Surgical Pathology, Special Lecturer in Pathology, Columbia University, New York, New York

Fabrizio Remotti, MD
Assistant Professor of Pathology and Cell Biology at the Columbia University Medical Center, New York, New York

Helen Remotti, MD
Professor Emeritus of Pathology and Cell Biology, Special Lecturer, Department of Pathology and Cell Biology, Columbia University, New York, New York

Heidrun Rotterdam, MD
Professor Emeritus of Pathology and Cell Biology, Senior Lecturer, Department of Pathology and Cell Biology, Columbia University Medical Center, New York, New York

Adam I. Rubin, MD
Assistant Professor of Dermatology, Assistant Professor of Dermatology in Pediatrics, Assistant Professor of Dermatology in Pathology and Laboratory Medicine, Hospital of the University of Pennsylvania, The Children's Hospital of Philadelphia, Perelman School of Medicine at the University of Pennsylvania, Philadelphia, Pennsylvania

Suthinee Rutnin, MD
International Dermatopathology Observer, Hospital of the University of Pennsylvania, Philadelphia, Pennsylvania, Clinical Instructor, Division of Dermatology, Faculty of Medicine, Ramathibodi Hospital, Mahidol University, Bangkok, Thailand

Marcela Salomao, MD
Assistant Professor of Pathology and Cell Biology at the Columbia University Medical Center, New York Presbyterian Hospital, New York, New York

Harsharan K. Singh, MD
Professor of Pathology, Director of Electron Microscopy Services, Department of Pathology and Laboratory Medicine, The University of North Carolina at Chapel Hill, Chapel Hill, North Carolina

Jon J. Smith, MD
Forensic Pathologist, Department of Medicine, Ventura County Medical Center, Chief Medical Examiner, Ventura County Medical Examiner Office, Ventura, California

M. Barry Stokes, MD
Associate Professor of Pathology and Cell Biology at the Columbia University Medical Center, New York, New York

Matthias J. Szabolcs, MD
Professor of Clinical Pathology and Cell Biology at the Columbia University Medical Center, New York, New York

Kurenai Tanji, MD, PhD
Professor of Clinical Pathology and Cell Biology (in Neurology), Columbia University, New York, New York

Harsh M. Thaker, MD, PhD
Vice Chair, Department of Pathology, Icahn School of Medicine at Mount Sinai, Mount Sinai Health System, New York, New York

Andrew Turk, MD
Assistant Professor of Pathology and Cell Biology at the Columbia University Medical Center, New York, New York

Efsevia Vakiani, MD, PhD
Assistant Attending Physician, Pathology, Memorial Sloan-Kettering Cancer Center, New York, New York

Julio A. Valentín, MD
Neuropathology Fellow, Columbia University, New York, New York

Xiao-Jun Wei, MD
Assistant Professor of Pathology, New York University Langone Medical Center, New York, New York

Angela J. Yoon, DDS, MPH, MAMSc
John W. Richter Associate, Professor of Oral Pathology in the Faculty of Dental Medicine at the Columbia University Medical Center, New York, New York

PREFACE

This new edition of *Anatomic Pathology Board Review* has been extensively revised and updated and includes many new questions as well as a multifaceted and expanded online version. New contributors have joined the roster of authors, providing considerable expertise in their respective subspecialty areas. The interval between the first and second edition has seen striking advances in genomic and molecular medicine with impact on virtually every facet of diagnostic pathology, and the authors have undertaken due diligence in incorporating those aspects that come to bear on the day-to-day practice of anatomic pathology.

The major goal of the second edition, as in the first, was to provide resident trainees who are preparing for the board examination in anatomic pathology a comprehensive, representative, and amply illustrated set of questions and answers covering the major diagnostic subspecialties in the field. The use of specific immunohistochemical stains, immunofluorescence, *in situ* hybridization, electron microscopy, and molecular diagnostic techniques now constitute routine practice procedures in anatomic pathology, and those elements have been updated and included in the material selected for this textbook. Current references accompany the answers to the questions for readers who wish to further pursue the primary and related published literature. Many Internet search engines are now widely available to trainees for supplemental information.

The diagnostic pathologist in anatomic pathology continues to play a critical role in the clinical care of patients, and we are charged with the considerable task of making accurate and well-considered diagnoses on the patients' behalf. The board examination serves as an instrument to measure breadth of knowledge and standard of care training in anatomic pathology. The collective authors of this second edition have vigorously taken up this charge in assembling their written and illustrative material. We hope that our enthusiasm for our discipline and its inherent quest for understanding the etiopathogenesis and diagnostic features of a wide spectrum of diseases are conveyed in this new edition and that the reader will find it a useful platform for successful completion of the board examination.

Jay H. Lefkowitch

ACKNOWLEDGMENTS

Second editions of medical textbooks are daunting challenges for their authors. Will the new version live up to, or surpass, expectations established with the first edition? Have problems recognized in the first edition been resolved? These and many other substantive issues were taken up by the authors of *Anatomic Pathology Board Review* when the second edition was proposed several years ago, and they have done herculean work to provide major revisions, additions, and updates to the earlier text. Producing both a new print *and* an interactive *online* edition has proved to be a very complex and labor-intensive project, for which I send kudos to all the authors and the creative team at Elsevier. They have collectively spent many, many hours revising and reworking content from the first edition and formatting it according to the needs of the print and online presentation modes. I am sure that I speak for all the authors in saying that we are grateful to many colleagues at our respective institutions, both in our own departments of pathology (not leastwise our residents and fellows) and in our sister clinical departments, for keeping us alerted to current diagnostic issues and instructive teaching cases.

As with the prior edition, I remain indebted to Michael Houston in Elsevier's Edinburgh office, who first suggested bringing out an *Anatomic Pathology Board Review* book. In today's world of publishing in general, and in medical books specifically, Michael continues to be a singular voice of reason and sensibility about the value of the printed word. On the American front, Bill Schmitt at Elsevier, Philadelphia, has been steadfast in his determination to keep this book on its trajectory to publication. The early development stages were under the creative guidance of Gina Donato and Christine Abshire, and more recently the production phase has been overseen by the expert and diligent Katy Meert and Sharon Corell.

Jay H. Lefkowitch

CONTENTS

CHAPTER 1

CARDIAC PATHOLOGY
Stephen M. Lagana and Charles C. Marboe

QUESTIONS

Questions 1-16 refer to a photograph or photomicrograph.

1. The image is from a mass resected from the left atrium of a 65-year-old man. All of the following statements regarding this neoplasm are true EXCEPT:
   a. Most of these lesions arise from the left atrial septum near the fossa ovalis.
   b. Heterologous elements, such as gland formation and extramedullary hematopoiesis, can be found in about 40% of these lesions.
   c. This tumor may be associated with an autosomal dominant syndrome characterized by myxomas, pigmented skin lesions, and endocrine overactivity.
   d. Lesions arising from the right atrium or in young adults are more likely to be associated with a familial syndrome.
   e. Calretinin is expressed in about 75% of these lesions.

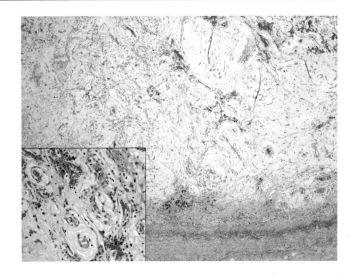

2. A 25-year-old woman with a history of hypothyroidism presented with rapid onset of fulminant congestive heart failure. Echocardiography showed a left ventricular ejection fraction of 15%. Her condition progressed, necessitating cardiac transplantation. A histologic section of the explanted heart is shown. Based on the information given, the MOST likely diagnosis is:
   a. Acute myocardial infarction
   b. Hypertrophic cardiomyopathy
   c. Cardiac sarcoidosis
   d. Idiopathic giant cell myocarditis (IGCM)
   e. Infection with *Trypanosoma cruzi*

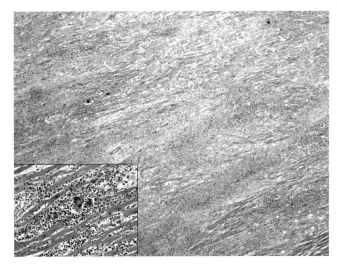

3. Which of the following patients is MOST likely to have this finding?
   a. A 73-year-old man with acute onset of chest pain
   b. A 24-year-old man who recently emigrated from South America
   c. A 12-year-old girl following an episode of pharyngitis
   d. An 80-year-old woman with systemic hypertension
   e. A 20-year-old man who died suddenly

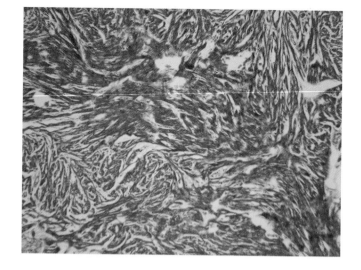

4. Which of the following statements regarding the process shown in the photomicrograph is TRUE?
   a. This process represents the extracellular deposition of an abnormal protein.
   b. This process occurs as a result of acute thrombosis in one of the coronary arteries.
   c. This finding is diagnostic of chronic systemic hypertension.
   d. The causative agent may be coxsackievirus B.
   e. This process occurs most commonly in pediatric patients.

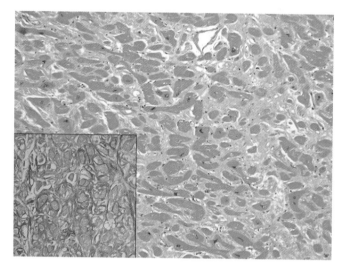

5. A 62-year-old man was killed in an automobile accident. At autopsy, a 0.5-cm lesion was found on the surface of the mitral valve. A histologic section is shown. All of the following statements regarding this lesion are true EXCEPT:
   a. The histogenesis of this lesion is controversial and ranges from neoplastic to a form of organized thrombus that is hamartomatous.
   b. When immersed in water, this lesion resembles a sea anemone.
   c. The papillae are avascular and covered by endothelium, resembling chordae tendineae of Lambl excrescences.
   d. Tumor size is an independent predictor of death or nonfatal embolization.
   e. These lesions resemble Lambl excrescences grossly and histologically.

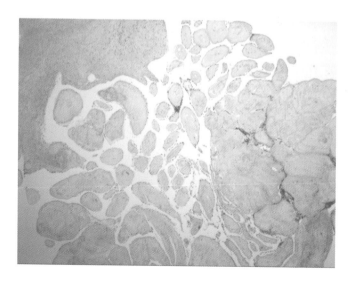

6. A 7-year-old child presented with syncope. An echocardiogram showed a single mass in the ventricular septum bulging into the left ventricle. Grossly, the tumor was white, firm, and well circumscribed. A histologic picture of the tumor with adjacent myocardium and a high-power view of the tumor are shown. All of the following statements regarding this tumor are true EXCEPT:
   a. The tumor will undergo malignant transformation if left untreated.
   b. The tumor is associated with Gorlin syndrome.
   c. The tumor is most commonly found in children.
   d. The tumor cells have a myofibroblastic phenotype.
   e. Calcification and cystic degeneration may occur in these lesions.

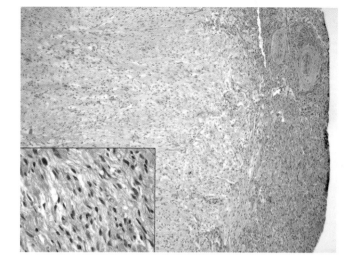

7. The image shows an endomyocardial biopsy specimen from a 53-year-old man who experienced mild chest discomfort and some fatigue. The patient reports that he has been generally healthy. Review of systems elicits a recently treated skin infection and a tooth extraction several weeks ago. He has a peripheral eosinophilia of 5%. Which of the following entities is MOST likely responsible for his symptoms?
   a. Enteroviral infection
   b. Occlusion of the right coronary artery
   c. Hypersensitivity reaction to an antibiotic
   d. Bacterial colonization of a heart valve
   e. Sarcoidosis

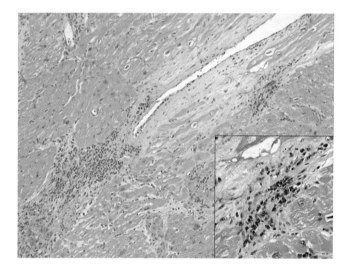

8. The image shows an epicardial coronary artery and vein from a patient who underwent cardiac transplantation 4 years before his death. Which of the following statements regarding the process shown is CORRECT?
   a. High-dose steroids would have reversed this process.
   b. This process is the main cause of death in long-term survivors of cardiac transplantation.
   c. The image shows acute cellular rejection.
   d. These changes are part of the Quilty effect.
   e. Healed panarteritis is the likely diagnosis.

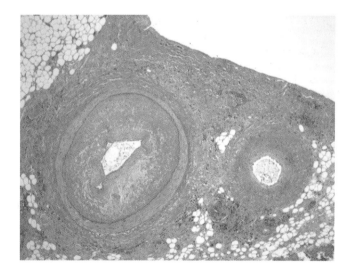

9. The image shows a cardiac biopsy specimen from a 55-year-old man who presented with cardiac arrhythmias and new-onset diabetes mellitus. An echocardiogram showed mild cardiac dysfunction. Which of the following statements is most likely TRUE?

   a. The intramyocyte pigment is an intralysosomal substance that increases in concentration with age.

   b. The patient's disorder is transmitted in an autosomal dominant manner.

   c. The patient's diabetes is unrelated to his cardiac symptoms.

   d. The pathogenesis of the patient's symptoms is due to decreased excretion of iron.

   e. The most common mutation for this disorder is C282Y of the *HFE* gene.

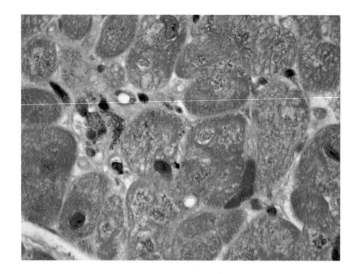

10. A 51-year-old black woman presents with cardiomegaly, heart failure, ventricular arrhythmias, abdominal pain, and constipation. A myocardial biopsy is performed, and the biopsy specimen demonstrates the features in the image. Which of the following statements regarding the patient's diagnosis is MOST accurate?

   a. Although transplantation is associated with rejection, accelerated coronary artery disease, and other issues, recurrence of this condition does not occur in cardiac allografts.

   b. If the patient's heart were transplanted into a different host (with a different immunologic milieu), the disease would resolve, leaving only fibrosis in previously affected regions.

   c. This disease is most commonly diagnosed by the Kveim test.

   d. This patient is likely to have Crohn disease.

   e. It is common to find concentrically laminated intracellular inclusion bodies consisting of calcified proteins in giant cells.

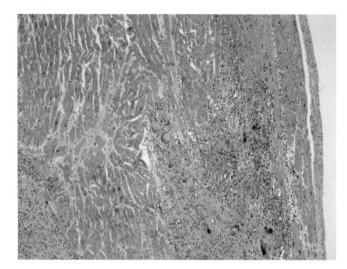

11. A 17-year-old boy has a family history of cardiomyopathy. He has ventricular arrhythmias with left bundle branch block and develops congestive heart failure and dies suddenly. At autopsy, there is thinning of the pulmonary infundibulum with white-yellow tissue replacing the myocardium. A section of the ventricle is shown in the image. Which of the following statements is TRUE?

   a. Half of cases have an autosomal dominant transmission.

   b. The boy had been receiving high-dose steroids.

   c. Involvement of the heart is limited to the right ventricle.

   d. The disease cannot be diagnosed before death or explantation.

   e. The disease is a more common cause of sudden death in the United States than in Italy.

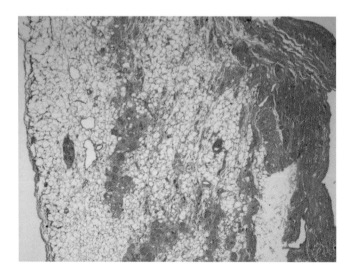

12. A 55-year-old man with a history of shortness of breath over the last few months died at home. An autopsy was performed, which demonstrated only one significant finding—a tumor or tumorlike structure enveloping the heart. The histologic appearance is shown in the image. The pathologist performs immunostaining and finds the tumor to be positive for cytokeratin, WT-1, and cytokeratin 5/6 and strongly positive for D-240. Which of the following statements is TRUE?
    a. This tumor should also express Ber-EP4, MOC-31, and carcinoembryonic antigen (CEA).
    b. The strong D240 staining with this morphologic appearance is suggestive of a lymphangioma or lymphangiosarcoma (depending on features of malignancy).
    c. This finding is likely a benign, reactive proliferation. Another cause should be sought for the patient's death.
    d. This structure is the most common primary pericardial malignant tumor.
    e. This tumor is a common complication of Dressler syndrome.

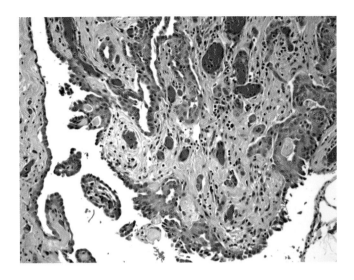

13. A malignant tumor of the heart is discovered at autopsy. After metastatic disease is carefully excluded, a battery of immunohistochemical stains is performed. What is the MOST probable immunophenotype?
    a. Fli-1 positive, CD31 positive, CD34 positive, calretinin negative, S100 negative
    b. Calretinin positive, CD31 positive, CD34 positive, S100 positive
    c. BCL-2 positive, CD99 positive, Fli-1 negative, cytokeratin focal
    d. Cytokeratin positive, cytokeratin 20 positive, CDX-2 positive
    e. S100 positive, HMB-45 positive, tyrosinase positive, CD31 negative

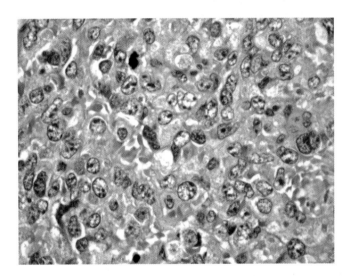

14. A 55-year-old man presents to the hospital 2 weeks after being discharged following an upper gastrointestinal bleed. Shortly after admission, the patient dies. The source of his gastrointestinal bleeding was esophageal varices, which were the result of cirrhosis induced by chronic hepatitis C virus contracted via intravenous drug abuse. The image shows the patient's heart. Which of the following statements about this case is TRUE?

   a. The cause of death was bacterial endocarditis.

   b. The patient appeared to have endocarditis, but because HACEK (*Haemophilus aphrophilus, Actinobacillus actinomycetemcomitans, Cardiobacterium hominis, Eikenella corrodens, Kingella kingae*) endocarditis is so common, it is likely that these bacteria were the cause of his endocarditis, and another factor was more likely the cause of death.

   c. Based on the patient's recent hospital admission, he probably had fungal endocarditis.

   d. The patient's cause of death should be reported as intravenous drug abuse.

   e. Neuropathologic examination is unlikely to demonstrate any findings because patients with this condition rarely develop thromboembolic events.

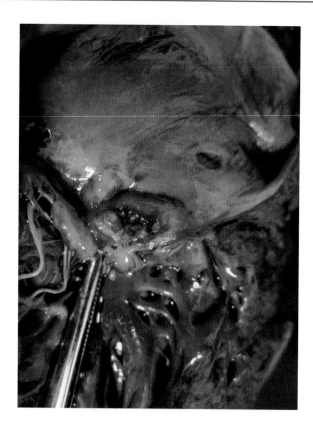

15. What is the BEST description of the clinical importance of these lesions in cardiac allograft biopsy specimens?

   a. When these lesions extend into the myocardium, they mimic rejection, but there is no proven adverse correlation of these lesions with clinical outcome.

   b. All patients with a cardiac allograft form these lesions, and no adverse outcome has been demonstrable.

   c. Of such lesions, 10% to 15% evolve into T-cell lymphoma.

   d. These lesions represent a localized endocardial form of Epstein-Barr virus–related posttransplant lymphoproliferative disease.

   e. Lesions localized to the endocardium have no clinical impact, whereas lesions deep in the myocardium are associated with sudden death.

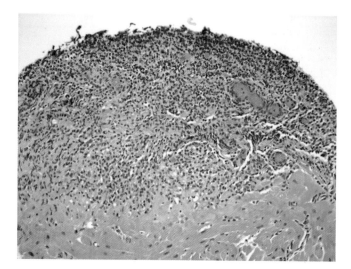

16. Which of the following is MOST likely to be associated with this vegetation?
  a. On histologic examination, there are neutrophils and fungal hyphae and yeast forms.
  b. Severe mitral insufficiency is present.
  c. Symptoms are limited to valve dysfunction.
  d. The patient was in a hypercoagulable state or had disseminated intravascular coagulation (DIC).

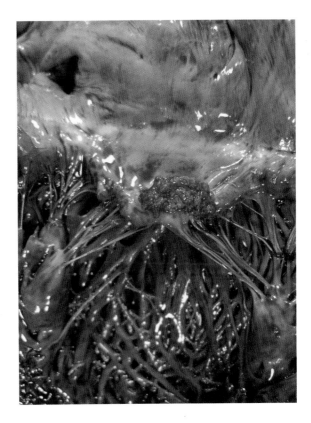

17. A previously healthy, 17-year-old student collapses during a track meet and cannot be revived despite cardiopulmonary resuscitation. Regarding the most likely diagnosis in this scenario, all of the following statements are true EXCEPT:
  a. The student has a hereditary condition, which is the most common cause of sudden cardiac death in young people.
  b. Histologic sections of the cardiac septum show haphazardly arranged and hypertrophied myocytes.
  c. The left ventricle is most likely to show concentric hypertrophy on gross examination.
  d. The most common genetic mutations responsible for this disease involve the beta-myosin heavy chain.
  e. Physiologically, cardiac diastolic dysfunction and left ventricular outflow obstruction can occur.

18. A previously healthy middle-aged man with no significant past medical history reports increasing dyspnea and peripheral edema over the past few months. A chest x-ray shows cardiomegaly and pulmonary edema. An echocardiogram shows four-chamber dilation and a left ventricular ejection fraction of 30%. Coronary angiography shows no significant narrowing of the coronary arteries. His condition progresses over several months, and he dies. The autopsy would MOST likely show:
  a. Dilated cardiomyopathy (DCM)
  b. Healed transmural myocardial infarction
  c. Cardiac amyloidosis
  d. Infective endocarditis
  e. Hypertensive changes

19. All of the following statements regarding congenital heart disease are true EXCEPT:
  a. Septal defects (atrial [ASD] and ventricular [VSD]) account for 50% of congenital cardiac malformations.
  b. Most VSDs require surgical intervention within the first year of life.
  c. Examples of a right-to-left shunt include tetralogy of Fallot and transposition of the great arteries.
  d. Bicuspid aortic valve is a relatively frequent form of congenital heart disease but usually gives rise to clinically important sequelae only after midlife.
  e. When patent ductus arteriosus occurs in isolation and is untreated, it may give rise to severe disease; however, if associated with other cardiac defects, maintaining patency may be crucial for survival of the affected infant.

20. A 58-year-old man experiences a transmural myocardial infarction and dies. Postmortem examination of the infarcted myocardium shows soft, yellow-tan tissue with a hyperemic border. Which of the following would MOST likely be seen microscopically?
  a. Variable wavy fibers at the border of the infarct
  b. Coagulation necrosis with pyknotic nuclei and myocyte hypereosinophilia with marginal contraction band necrosis
  c. A paucicellular area with collagen deposition
  d. Granulation tissue with some inflammation
  e. Dead myofibers and neutrophils with infiltrating macrophages at the edge of the infarct

21. A 35-year-old woman presents with fever and chills. Physical examination reveals a heart murmur, and an echocardiogram shows mitral valve vegetations. On further questioning, she states no previous medical problems but reports that she saw her dentist for a toothache several days ago. Which of the following organisms is LEAST likely to be responsible for her symptoms?
    a. *Actinobacillus actinomycetemcomitans*
    b. *Kingella kingae*
    c. *Haemophilus aphrophilus*
    d. *Staphylococcus epidermidis*
    e. *Eikenella corrodens*

22. A 41-year-old woman with no history of heart disease has begun to experience palpitations over the past few months. On physical examination, she is afebrile and appears comfortable. Auscultation reveals a midsystolic "click." Which of the following is MOST likely to be seen on an echocardiogram?
    a. Aortic stenosis
    b. Mitral stenosis
    c. Mitral valve prolapse (MVP)
    d. Patent ductus arteriosus
    e. Valvular vegetations

23. All of the following statements regarding rheumatic heart disease are true EXCEPT:
    a. "Fish-mouth" deformity of the mitral valve is common.
    b. Commissural fusion of the aortic valve can be present.
    c. Short, thickened chordae tendineae cordis are common.
    d. Viridans streptococci cause rheumatic heart disease.
    e. Rheumatic heart disease is the most common cause of mitral stenosis.

24. A 60-year-old woman presents to the emergency department with shortness of breath. She is found to have intractable arrhythmias and dies shortly after arrival in the emergency department. At autopsy, a 2.4-cm thickened region of the interatrial septum is found. On sectioning, the region has the appearance of fat. Histologic examination demonstrates mature-appearing adipocytes intermixed with large cells with the appearance of myocardial cells. Which of the following statements is TRUE?
    a. This is the typical appearance of a malignant Triton tumor in the heart; sarcoma is the cause of death.
    b. This lesion is likely a lipoma and is unlikely to be the cause of the patient's arrhythmias; fluorescence in situ hybridization (FISH) for MDM2 should be positive, confirming the diagnosis.
    c. This lesion is most likely lipomatous hypertrophy of the interatrial septum, a pseudoneoplasm that can cause arrhythmias and sudden cardiac death.
    d. This lesion is most likely a liposarcoma invading the myocardium; FISH for MDM2 would show deletion, confirming the diagnosis.
    e. Regardless of this lesion, the interatrial septum is not anatomically positioned to cause arrhythmia; this finding is likely incidental, and the cause of death should be investigated further.

25. An autopsy is performed on an 85-year-old man with congestive heart failure secondary to ischemic heart disease. Which of the following vascular changes would NOT be expected in the lungs?
    a. Intimal thickening of arteries and veins
    b. Muscularization of arterioles and venules
    c. Fibrosis of veins and arteries
    d. Increased basement membrane thickness around capillaries
    e. Inflammation of arterial walls with neutrophils, mononuclear cells, and macrophages resulting in areas of necrosis

ANSWERS

1. b. Myxomas are benign tumors that typically arise in the left atrium near the fossa ovalis. This tumor most often occurs sporadically but can be part of a syndrome called Carney complex in a few cases (7%). Patients with this syndrome present with abnormal skin pigmentation, cutaneous and cardiac myxomas, and abnormalities of the endocrine system (adrenal, pituitary, thyroid). Acronyms for this constellation of findings include NAME (nevi, atrial myxoma, ephelides) and LAMB (lentigines, atrial myxoma, blue nevi). Myxomas associated with a familial syndrome are more commonly found in the right atrium. Sporadic tumors occur more often in women with a mean age at presentation of 50 years. A review of patients with Carney complex showed a female predominance (62%), mean age at presentation of 26 years, and multiple tumors in 41% of cases. These findings differ slightly from Carney's report on familial myxomas, which found a male predominance.

   Grossly, myxomas may be mistaken for an atrial thrombus, but in contrast to thrombi, atrial myxomas are usually mobile and attached to the endocardial surface by a stalk. They are typically ball-shaped but can be elongated or papillary. If large enough, myxomas can cause symptoms of mitral valve stenosis. The histologic appearance of myxomas can be variable, but they are usually composed of plump, stellate or spindled cells arranged in cords and primitive-appearing vessels in a loose, myxoid stroma. The stroma often contains hemorrhage or hemosiderin with variable numbers of inflammatory cells. Heterologous elements, such as gland formation and extramedullary hematopoiesis, can be found in only a very few cases (2%). It is important not to confuse a benign myxoma with a metastatic adenocarcinoma. There is no reported prognostic significance of the presence of heterologous elements.

   Myxoma cells stain positively for endothelial markers CD34 and CD31 and are variably positive for S100. Calretinin has been reported positive in 74% to 100% of cases and can be useful to distinguish this lesion from a myxoid thrombus. Tumor cells are negative for cytokeratin, but heterologous glands show positivity. These tumors are curable by resection but tend to recur more often in the familial form.

Acebo E, Val-Bernal JF, Gómez-Roman JJ: Thrombomodulin, calretinin and c-kit (CD117) expression in cardiac myxoma. *Histol Histopathol* 2001;16(4):1031-1036.

Carney JA: Differences between nonfamilial and familial cardiac myxomas. *Am J Surg Pathol* 1985;9(1):53-55.

Edwards A, Bermudez C, Piwonka G, et al: Carney's syndrome: complex myxomas. Report of four cases and a review of the literature. *Cardiovasc Surg* 2002;10(3):264-275.

Terracciano LM, Mhawech P, Suess K, et al: Calretinin as a marker for cardiac myoma. Diagnostic and histogenetic considerations. *Am J Clin Pathol* 2000;114(5):754-759.

2. d. IGCM matches the clinical scenario and the histologic diagnosis shown in the image. IGCM is a severe and rapidly fatal disorder of young, healthy adults who commonly present with congestive heart failure; it affects whites more often than blacks. It has been associated with autoimmune disorders (inflammatory bowel disease, hyperthyroidism, hypothyroidism), but the exact pathogenesis is unknown. The reported rate of death or cardiac transplantation is 89% with a median survival of 5.5 months from the onset of symptoms. Histologic findings include diffuse, geographic myocardial necrosis with a mixed inflammatory infiltrate of lymphocytes, histiocytes, and eosinophils. Multinucleated giant cells in the absence of granulomas are characteristic. IGCM can recur in a transplanted heart despite aggressive immunosuppression.

In contrast to IGCM, cardiac sarcoidosis occurs with approximately equal frequency in blacks and whites and has a longer mean time from onset of symptoms to diagnosis: 5 months for IGCM versus 29 months for cardiac sarcoidosis. Cardiac sarcoidosis is characterized by nonnecrotizing granulomas in a background of fibrous stroma; necrosis is uncommon. Acute myocardial infarction typically occurs in older patients who may have additional risk factors for ischemic heart disease. Giant cells are not a characteristic finding on microscopic examination. Although hypertrophic cardiomyopathy is also a disease of young people, affected individuals usually present with angina, exertional dyspnea, or sudden cardiac death. Myocyte disarray and hypertrophy are the characteristic histologic findings. Infection with *T. cruzi* (Chagas disease) is uncommon in the United States. Histologically, myofibers contain the parasites, and the inflammatory infiltrate typically is composed of neutrophils, lymphocytes, and macrophages with scattered eosinophils.

Cooper LT Jr, Berry GJ, Shabetai R: Idiopathic giant-cell myocarditis—natural history and treatment. Multicenter Giant Cell Myocarditis Study Group Investigators. *N Engl J Med* 1997;336(26):1860-1866.

Okura Y, Dec GW, Hare JM, et al: A clinical and histopathologic comparison of cardiac sarcoidosis and idiopathic giant cell myocarditis. *J Am Coll Cardiol* 2003;41(2):322-329.

3. e. The image shows cardiac myocytes that are hypertrophied and disorganized (myocyte disarray), which are characteristic features of hypertrophic cardiomyopathy (HCM). HCM can be seen at almost any age but is commonly seen in young, otherwise healthy, adults. HCM is caused by 1 of more than 400 mutations in one of several genes that encode sarcomeric proteins; mutations occurring in the gene encoding the beta-myosin heavy chain are most common. There is clinical heterogeneity of this disease; presenting symptoms range from asymptomatic through mild cardiac

disturbances to sudden cardiac death. It has been recommended that first-degree relatives of affected individuals be screened and evaluated according to their risk stratification. The table summarizes the histologic findings in the incorrect answer choices.

Table 1-1 Histologic Findings of Cardiac Diseases

Disease	Characteristic Histologic Findings
Acute myocardial infarction	Myocyte necrosis with influx of inflammatory cells, granulation tissue, or fibrosis, depending on age of infarct
Chagas disease	Dense inflammation with myocyte necrosis and trypanosome amastigotes in myocytes (acute disease)
Acute rheumatic heart disease	Collections of plump macrophages with lymphocytes and plasma cells called Aschoff bodies
Hypertensive heart disease	Myocyte hypertrophy with nuclear enlargement and interstitial fibrosis

Maron BJ, McKenna WJ, Danielson GK, et al; Task Force on Clinical Expert Consensus Documents, American College of Cardiology; Committee for Practice Guidelines, European Society of Cardiology: American College of Cardiology/European Society of Cardiology clinical expert consensus document on hypertrophic cardiomyopathy. A report of the American College of Cardiology Foundation Task Force on Clinical Expert Consensus Documents and the European Society of Cardiology Committee for Practice Guidelines. *J Am Coll Cardiol* 2003;42(9):1687-1713.

4. a. The photomicrograph shows a section of myocardium in which myofibers are surrounded by an amorphous, eosinophilic, extracellular material that is metachromatic with crystal violet stain, consistent with amyloid. Amyloid also can be distinguished with Congo red stain and polarized light. Amyloidosis can be primary, secondary, hereditary, or age-related. Primary and secondary forms are generally related to plasma cell dyscrasias (primary amyloidosis) and inflammatory conditions (secondary amyloidosis). Hereditary forms are due to gene mutations in various proteins. Senile forms can be systemic or localized.

The cardiovascular system is affected most frequently in primary and age-related forms and involves the myocardium, vessels, and valves. In primary amyloidosis, the extracellular protein comprises monoclonal light chains, whereas systemic senile amyloid comprises abnormal transthyretin (prealbumin). Localized senile amyloidosis (isolated atrial amyloidosis) is a common postmortem finding in elderly adults. In this condition, the amyloid is composed of atrial natriuretic peptide. Cardiac amyloidosis is usually associated with restrictive features secondary to poor ventricular compliance. Grossly, the heart is slightly enlarged, and the myocardium is described as stiff, rubbery, or waxy.

Kholová I, Niessen HW: Amyloid in the cardiovascular system: a review. *J Clin Pathol* 2005;58(2):125-133.

5. d. Tumor mobility, not tumor size, is an independent predictor of outcomes. The photomicrograph shows a papillary fibroelastoma (PFE). These benign tumors are the second most common primary cardiac tumor and account for three quarters of all cardiac valvular tumors. PFEs range in size from 2 to 70 mm and are most often located on the aortic valve. They grossly and microscopically resemble Lambl excrescences but differ in their location; PFEs are located on the surface of any heart valve, whereas Lambl excrescences are located most commonly on aortic valve closures. Depending on their location, PFEs can be asymptomatic or cause thromboembolic events. Excision is curative; once excised, these tumors look like a sea anemone if placed in water or saline. Histologically, these tumors are composed of fine, sometimes branching, avascular papillae that are lined by endothelium. Elastic stains highlight the elastic components within the papillae. The exact histogenesis is unknown; different clinical and microscopic features support differing views. According to a more recent review of 725 cases, tumor mobility was an independent predictor of death or nonfatal embolization.

Gowda RM, Khan IA, Nair CK, et al: Cardiac papillary fibroelastoma: a comprehensive analysis of 725 cases. *Am Heart J* 2003;146(3):404-410.

6. a.   The image shows an intramural cardiac fibroma. This lesion is a benign mesenchymal tumor of the heart and is thought to be hamartomatous in nature. In contrast to rhabdomyomas, these tumors generally occur as a single lesion. Grossly, the tumors are well circumscribed, white, and rubbery to firm. The border can be circumscribed or infiltrative. This connective tissue tumor arises from fibroblasts and myofibroblasts and is histologically similar to fibromas elsewhere in the body. The cells are uniform and spindle-shaped surrounded by a variably collagenous matrix that stains blue on Masson trichrome staining. The cells are typically positive for vimentin and smooth muscle actin, consistent with myofibroblastic origin. Muscle-specific markers such as desmin and MyoD1 are negative. Neural elements are not present in this tumor, and tumor cells do not stain for S100 protein. HMB45 positivity is not a feature of fibromas but has been reported in rhabdomyomas.

These tumors are the second most common tumor (or third in some series) in children and have been diagnosed prenatally by ultrasound. Most occur in the ventricular septum or free wall. Symptoms depend on size and location of the tumor. Some tumors are asymptomatic and have been found incidentally at autopsy in older individuals. Cardiac fibromas have been reported in 3% of individuals with Gorlin syndrome (nevoid basal cell carcinoma syndrome). This syndrome is an autosomal dominant disorder characterized by body overgrowth, jaw keratocysts, skeletal abnormalities, and a predisposition to neoplasms. Gorlin syndrome results from a germline mutation in the *PTC* gene on chromosome 9q22.3. The tumors in infants are generally more cellular than tumors of older children or adults and often contain calcifications or areas of cystic degeneration. Although fibromas are benign, they can cause significant morbidity and may be a cause of sudden death in some patients. Good long-term outcomes have been achieved with surgical resection of the tumor even when excision is incomplete. Malignant transformation of benign tumors has not been described. Cardiac transplantation can be performed if the tumor is unresectable.

Cho JM, Danielson GK, Puga FJ, et al: Surgical resection of ventricular cardiac fibromas: early and late results. *Ann Thorac Surg* 2003;76(6):1929-1934.

Vaughan CJ, Veugelers M, Basson CT: Tumors and the heart: molecular genetic advances. *Curr Opin Cardiol* 2001; 16(3):195-200.

Weeks DA, Chase DR, Malott RL, et al: HMB45 staining in angiomyolipoma, cardiac rhabdomyoma, other mesenchymal processes, and tuberous sclerosis-associated brain lesions. *Int J Surg Pathol* 1994;1:191.

7. c.   The most likely diagnosis is hypersensitivity reaction to an antibiotic. Hypersensitivity myocarditis has been linked to many drugs, including antibiotics, anticonvulsants, and antidepressants. The image shows myocardium that is focally infiltrated by eosinophils, lymphocytes, and histiocytes, which are predominantly perivascular and subendocardial but sometimes focally aggregated into poorly formed granulomas. There is little or no myocyte necrosis. Hypersensitivity myocarditis is common in patients undergoing transplantation and has been found in 7% of explanted hearts. This finding is attributed to the multidrug regimen used to sustain patients until a donor is found. Other entities to consider in the differential diagnosis when eosinophilic myocarditis is present include parasitic infection, allergy, hypereosinophilic syndrome, and hematologic malignancies.

Burke AP, Saenger J, Mullick F, et al: Hypersensitivity myocarditis. *Arch Pathol Lab Med* 1991;115(8):764-769.

Gravanis MB, Hertzler GL, Franch RH, et al: Hypersensitivity myocarditis in heart transplant candidates. *J Heart Lung Transplant* 1991;10(5 Pt 1):688-697.

8. b.   The image shows epicardial tissue with cardiac allograft vasculopathy (CAV). In this process, blood vessels demonstrate intimal thickening. CAV is related to coronary artery disease but occurs uniquely in transplant recipients and is an accelerated form of atherosclerosis. Complete obstruction of the vessel lumen can lead to ischemic damage; however, these events may be painless because of a lack of cardiac reinnervation. In contrast to coronary artery disease, CAV shows concentric intimal proliferation, involves intramyocardial vessels, and has few calcifications. Intimal thickening develops in approximately 58% of transplant arteries within the first year, and CAV becomes clinically apparent in 50% of recipients within the first 5 years after transplantation. CAV is the limiting factor for long-term success of cardiac transplantation and in two studies was the main cause of death in long-term survivors. Although medical strategies have been effective in reducing the incidence of graft rejection, there has been little success in reducing the incidence of CAV.

Acute rejection is characterized by an inflammatory infiltrate with or without myocyte damage. The severity of rejection is classified according to the extent, pattern, and type of inflammation and the presence or absence of myocyte necrosis. The Quilty effect is a common finding after transplantation that consists of a dense endocardial collection of lymphocytes. It has no known adverse effect on prognosis. Healed panarteritis may be seen in conjunction with active vasculitis. The inflammatory infiltrates may be mixed (lymphocytes, plasma cells, neutrophils) or lymphocytic. Healed vasculitis shows fibrosis of the media and a fibrous, relatively acellular, intimal proliferative lesion.

Valantine H: Cardiac allograft vasculopathy after heart transplantation: risk factors and management. *J Heart Lung Transplant* 2004;23(5 Suppl):S187-S193.

9. e. The patient in the scenario most likely has hereditary hemochromatosis, but iron overload also can be seen in the setting of thalassemia, multiple blood transfusions, and hemolytic anemia. Hereditary hemochromatosis is a homozygous autosomal recessive disorder resulting from mutations in the *HFE* gene. The most common mutation is C282Y, which is present in 70% to 100% of patients with this diagnosis. The *HFE* gene is responsible for encoding the HFE protein, which is normally expressed in small intestinal cells and is important in the regulation of iron uptake into the cell. The mutant protein results in unregulated uptake of iron regardless of systemic iron content.

The biopsy specimen shows myocytes and interstitial macrophages containing abundant intracellular brown pigment, which would prove to be iron if stained with Prussian blue and is diagnostic of iron overload. It is important not to confuse this pigment with lipofuscin, which is a pigment of granules of undigested material derived from intracellular lipid peroxidation. Lipofuscin granules are more finely granular than hemosiderin and accumulate in the cytoplasm of many cell types over time. However, unless there has been a prior infarct or other myocardial damage, there would not be significant lipofuscin in interstitial macrophages. Iron deposition in the liver, pancreas, heart, pituitary, and skin results in clinical manifestations such as hepatomegaly, diabetes, cardiomyopathy, amenorrhea, and hyperpigmentation. The treatment of hemochromatosis consists of regular phlebotomy. A more recent study showed little correlation between the amount of cardiac iron deposition and systolic dysfunction in patients with hemochromatosis. Of eight patients who showed improved cardiac function with phlebotomy, three had no demonstrable cardiac iron.

Ocel JJ, Edwards WD, Tazelaar HD, et al: Heart and liver disease in 32 patients undergoing biopsy of both organs, with implications for heart or liver transplantation. *Mayo Clin Proc* 2004;79(4):492-501.

10. e. The disease described and shown in the image is cardiac sarcoidosis (granulomas, multinucleated giant cells, fibrosis). The prevalence of cardiac involvement in patients with sarcoidosis depends on the method used for diagnosis (clinical features being the least sensitive) and the population studied. An autopsy series from the 1970s showed cardiac involvement in 27% of patients with sarcoidosis. A more recent U.S. study using a combined clinical and imaging approach found approximately 40% involvement with more than half of patients being asymptomatic.

It is common to find concentrically laminated intracellular inclusion bodies consisting of calcified proteins in giant cells; these are known as Schaumann bodies. Schaumann bodies are found with much higher frequency in sarcoidosis and berylliosis than in infective granulomatous diseases. Asteroid bodies are stellate inclusions that stain with antiubiquitin antibodies. They are less common than Schaumann bodies but do occur frequently. Cardiac involvement is patchy; endomyocardial biopsy establishes the diagnosis in less than 50% of patients, and a negative biopsy result does not exclude the disease. The differential diagnosis for granulomatous myocarditis includes sarcoidosis, infectious causes (tuberculosis and fungal infection), foreign body reaction, and hypersensitivity myocarditis. In sarcoidosis, no organism is identified with acid-fast or silver stains. As noted, Schaumann and asteroid bodies may be seen in sarcoidosis, but other foreign material is not seen. Some cases of hypersensitivity myocarditis have granulomas, but there are also extensive perivascular and interstitial infiltrates of inflammatory cells with numerous eosinophils generally with little myocyte necrosis or interstitial fibrosis unless there is a second, underlying cardiac disease.

The presence of multinucleated, macrophage-derived giant cells brings giant cell myocarditis into the differential diagnosis; the histologic features to distinguish giant cell myocarditis from cardiac sarcoidosis are listed in the table. The clinical distinction is generally straightforward because giant cell myocarditis typically is associated with an abrupt onset of severe heart failure in a previously healthy woman who may have additional autoimmune disease, whereas sarcoidosis is associated with a more indolent and slowly progressive heart failure, frequently with arrhythmias.

Table 1-2 Histologic Features Distinguishing Giant Cell Myocarditis from Cardiac Sarcoidosis

Giant Cell Myocarditis	Cardiac Sarcoidosis
Multinucleated giant cells	Epithelioid granulomas and multinucleated giant cells
Eosinophils are common, neutrophils also found	Eosinophils possible but not particularly characteristic, neutrophils not expected (rule out infection)
Myocardial necrosis	Myocardial fibrosis
Lymphocytes, more commonly CD8$^+$	Lymphocytes, more commonly CD4$^+$

Bragagni G, Brogna R, Franceschetti P, et al: Cardiac involvement in Crohn's disease: echocardiographic study. *J Gastroenterol Hepatol* 2007;22(1):18-22.

Lagana SM, Parwani AV, Nichols LC: Cardiac sarcoidosis: a pathology-focused review. *Arch Pathol Lab Med* 2010;134(7): 1039-1046.

11. a. Approximately half of cases of arrhythmogenic cardiomyopathy are autosomal dominant with at least four genes (ryanodyne receptor, plakoglobin, desmoplakin, and desmin) and at least eight genetic loci involved. Rare autosomal recessive variants occur, such as Naxos disease, which includes palmoplantar keratoderma and woolly hair, and Carvajal syndrome (left ventricular cardiomyopathy). Arrhythmogenic cardiomyopathy typically involves the right ventricle (pulmonary infundibulum, apex, inferior wall) but also may involve the left ventricle and septum. The process of myocyte loss and fatty replacement appears to be acquired, and apoptosis of myocytes and focal lymphocytic infiltrates has been described. The disease is suspected with arrhythmias and cardiomyopathy and may be confirmed with nuclear magnetic resonance imaging (thinned ventricle, diminished contractile function, fatty replacement), echocardiography (dilated right ventricle and outflow tract, diminished ejection fraction), or ventriculography (dilated right ventricular outflow tract).

Diabetes or steroid therapy may be associated with increased amounts of fat in the right ventricle but not with cardiomyopathy or arrhythmias. Arrhythmogenic cardiomyopathy is a rare cause of sudden death in the United States (approximately 3% of sudden deaths) but is an important cause of sudden death in Italy (13% to 20% of all cardiac sudden deaths).

Protonotarios N, Tsatsopoulou A: Naxos disease and Carvajal syndrome: cardiocutaneous disorders that highlight the pathogenesis and broaden the spectrum of arrhythmogenic right ventricular cardiomyopathy. *Cardiovasc Pathol* 2004; 13(4):185-194.

Saffitz JE: Arrhythmogenic cardiomyopathy: advances in diagnosis and disease pathogenesis. *Circulation* 2011;124(15): e390-e392.

12. d. Based on its infiltrative appearance, the tumor shown in the image is not benign. Its architecture, cytology, and immunoprofile all are consistent with malignant mesothelioma, which is associated with a very poor prognosis. Malignant mesothelioma is the most common primary pericardial malignant tumor. D240 staining is characteristically positive in mesothelioma. Although D240 is also positive in tumors of lymphatic histogenesis, these tumors would not be positive for cytokeratins. Malignant mesothelioma is not a common complication of Dressler syndrome, which is a form of pericarditis that typically develops after myocardial infarction. Predisposing factors are not as clear as they are for pleural mesotheliomas, but asbestos may play a role.

Husain AN, Colby TV, Ordóñez NG, et al: Guidelines for pathologic diagnosis of malignant mesothelioma: a consensus statement from the International Mesothelioma Interest Group. *Arch Pathol Lab Med* 2009;133(8):1317-1331.

Ordóñez NG: The immunohistochemical diagnosis of mesothelioma: a comparative study of epithelioid mesothelioma and lung adenocarcinoma. *Am J Surg Pathol* 2003;27(8):1031-1051.

Patel J, Sheppard MN: Primary malignant mesothelioma of the pericardium. *Cardiovasc Pathol* 2011;20(2):107-109.

13. a. Malignant tumors are much less common than benign tumors of the heart, most of which are myxomas. Myxomas have the immunophenotype described in Choice b. However, this question asks for the immunophenotype of the most common primary malignant tumor of the heart, which is angiosarcoma. Angiosarcomas are positive for Fli-1, CD31, CD34, and other endothelial markers. They are also strongly positive for vimentin. They are the most common primary malignant neoplasm of the heart and are most commonly seen in the right atrium. Survival rate is very low. Various other primary sarcomas can be seen in the heart, including rhabdomyosarcoma, osteosarcoma, leiomyosarcoma, and fibrosarcoma, but all occur less frequently than angiosarcoma.

Metastatic tumors are more common than primary malignant tumors in the heart. When encountered, metastatic tumors are most likely to be carcinomas from the lung or breast, hematologic malignancies, or melanomas. Although colorectal metastases occur, they are quite rare and are less common than metastases from the lung or breast.

Metastatic carcinomas are more common than metastatic melanomas in the heart (owing to incidence), but the type of tumor most likely to result in a cardiac metastasis is melanoma.

Glancy DL, Roberts WC: The heart in malignant melanoma. A study of 70 autopsy cases. *Am J Cardiol* 1968;21(4):555-571.

Neragi-Miandoab S, Kim J, Vlahakes GJ: Malignant tumours of the heart: a review of tumour type, diagnosis and therapy. *Clin Oncol (R Coll Radiol)* 2007;19(10):748-756.

Choi PW, Kim CN, Chang SH, et al: Cardiac metastasis from colorectal cancer: a case report. *World J Gastroenterol* 2009; 15(21):2675-2678.

14. d. This question requires you to recognize the pathophysiology of the patient's death and then to understand the difference between cause of death and mechanism of death. The mechanism of death was bacterial endocarditis, but the cause of death was intravenous drug abuse, which caused the patient to become infected with hepatitis C virus, which led to cirrhosis, which caused varices, which bled leading to admission to the hospital where he acquired endocarditis. *Staphylococcus aureus* is the most common cause of both hospital-acquired and community-acquired endocarditis. Coagulase-negative *Staphylococcus* is also a common cause of hospital-acquired endocarditis. *Enterococcus* species are the next most common cause of hospital-acquired endocarditis. In community-acquired endocarditis, viridans streptococci are the second most common cause.

This patient had several risk factors for infective endocarditis, including recent hospital admission and intravenous drug use. Endocarditis is considered to be hospital acquired if it begins within 3 days of admission or within 60 days if the patient had a risk factor for bacteremia. The fact that this patient had mitral valve endocarditis supports the supposition that it is hospital acquired because intravenous drug use more frequently causes right-sided disease. The HACEK organisms are *Haemophilus aphrophilus*, *Actinobacillus actinomycetemcomitans*, *Cardiobacterium hominis*, *Eikenella corrodens*, and *Kingella kingae*.

Haddad SH, Arabi YM, Memish ZA, et al: Nosocomial infective endocarditis in critically ill patients: a report of three cases and review of the literature. *Int J Infect Dis* 2004;8(4):210-216.

Sexton DJ: Epidemiology, risk factors and microbiology of infective endocarditis. In Basow DS (ed): *UpToDate*. Waltham, MA: UpToDate, 2013.

15. a. Although there have been many attempts to correlate nodular endocardial infiltrates with clinical rejection or adverse graft outcome, no correlation has been proved to date. Some groups correlate these lesions with increased risk of cellular rejection on biopsy specimens, but other groups have not found a correlation. Nodular endocardial infiltrates, also known as *Quilty lesions*, named for the Stanford patient in whom they were first recognized, were seen only after the introduction of cyclosporine-based immunosuppression. There is a core of B lymphocytes sometimes with CD21-positive cells and a surrounding rim of T lymphocytes. Immunohistochemical staining may help distinguish these lesions from rejection (which demonstrates predominantly T lymphocytes and macrophages with very few B lymphocytes). Plasma cells and interleukin-2 receptor–positive cells may be present in the lesions, and there is usually a prominent small vessel component.

Of allograft recipients, 40% to 80% form nodular endocardial infiltrates; survival appears similar to survival of allograft recipients who do not form the lesions. There are a few reports of increased coronary artery vasculopathy, microvasculopathy, and coronary intimal thickening (on intravascular ultrasound) in allograft recipients who form Quilty lesions. Numerous reports link Quilty lesions to an increased risk of cellular rejection on biopsy specimens; however, many reports have failed to find an association.

Chu KE, Ho EK, de la Torre L, et al: The relationship of nodular endocardial infiltrates (Quilty lesions) to anti-HLA antibodies, coronary artery disease, and survival following heart transplantation. *Cardiovasc Pathol* 2005;14(4):219-224.
Marboe CC, Billingham ME, Eisen H, et al: Nodular endocardial infiltrates (Quilty lesions) cause significant variability in the diagnosis of ISHLT Grade 2 and 3A rejection in cardiac allograft recipients. *J Heart Lung Transplant* 2005;24(7 Suppl):S219-S226.
Radio SJ, McManus BM, Winters GL, et al: Preferential endocardial residence of B-cells in the "Quilty effect" of human heart allografts: immunohistochemical distinction from rejection. *Mod Pathol* 1991;4(5):654-660.

16. d. Nonbacterial thrombotic endocarditis (NBTE) usually develops on heart valves with no underlying disease. NBTE may manifest with cerebral embolization or emboli in other organs. NBTE may be the result of trauma to valve surfaces by an indwelling catheter. However, NBTE is usually associated with hypercoagulable states or malignancies in which antiphospholipid syndrome develops. Approximately half of NBTE cases are associated with a hypercoagulable state or DIC. The lesions are frequently seen in patients with end-stage malignancy, particularly mucin-producing adenocarcinomas. NBTE may also be seen in AIDS.

The gross appearance of NBTE may be confused with infective endocarditis, but the latter usually has larger lesions, which are friable and red-tan, depending on the degree of organization, and are much more likely to be associated with valve damage. Histologic examination is necessary to rule out infective endocarditis with confidence. The vegetations of NBTE are composed of platelets and fibrin and scattered erythrocytes but do not contain organisms or substantial numbers of neutrophils.

el-Shami K, Griffiths E, Streiff M: Nonbacterial thrombotic endocarditis in cancer patients: pathogenesis, diagnosis, and treatment. *Oncologist* 2007;12(5):518-523.
Lopez JA, Ross RS, Fishbein MC, et al: Nonbacterial thrombotic endocarditis: a review. *Am Heart J* 1987;113(3):773-784.
Steiner I: Nonbacterial thrombotic versus infective endocarditis: a necropsy study of 320 cases. *Cardiovasc Pathol* 1995;4:207.

17. c. The most likely diagnosis in this scenario is HCM. This condition is characterized by asymmetric hypertrophy of the left ventricle that preferentially affects the septum. In contrast, hypertensive hypertrophy is concentric in nature. The hypertrophied myocardium becomes stiffened and results in diastolic dysfunction. In addition, preferential thickening of the septum can impair left ventricular outflow during systole owing to contact of the anterior leaflet of

the mitral valve with the septal wall during ventricular contraction. Fibrous endocardial plaques in the left ventricular outflow tract and mitral valve thickening are common findings on gross examination. Histologic findings include myocyte hypertrophy with haphazard disarray of myofibers. Interstitial fibrosis and arterial abnormalities are also common findings. Affected individuals may complain of angina or exertional dyspnea; however, sudden death is a common presentation.

Although sudden cardiac death is commonly described in the setting of physical activity, it can occur early after waking or during sedentary activity. At least 12 genes encoding sarcomeric proteins, involving thick and thin filaments, with more than 400 mutations have been implicated in the pathogenesis of HCM. Mutations involving the beta-myosin heavy chain are most commonly involved and account for 35% of all cases of HCM. Other common mutations involve genes encoding myosin binding protein C (20%) and cardiac troponin T (15%).

Maron BJ, Kogan J, Proschan MA, et al: Circadian variability in the occurrence of sudden cardiac death in patients with hypertrophic cardiomyopathy. *J Am Coll Cardiol* 1994;23(6):1405-1409.
Maron BJ, McKenna WJ, Danielson GK, et al; Task Force on Clinical Expert Consensus Documents, American College of Cardiology; Committee for Practice Guidelines, European Society of Cardiology: American College of Cardiology/European Society of Cardiology clinical expert consensus document on hypertrophic cardiomyopathy. A report of the American College of Cardiology Foundation Task Force on Clinical Expert Consensus Documents and the European Society of Cardiology Committee for Practice Guidelines. *J Am Coll Cardiol* 2003;42(9):1687-1713.

18. a. The most likely cardiac finding is DCM. This condition is characterized by progressive cardiac dilation with systolic dysfunction. There are many possible associated causes of DCM, including preceding myocarditis (viral), alcohol use, chemotherapeutic agents, and genetic predisposition. With no reported preceding symptoms at presentation, the patient in the scenario probably had a familial form of DCM. Familial cases of DCM usually manifest between 20 and 50 years of age and have been reported most commonly with autosomal dominant inheritance (90%). Other familial cases include cases transmitted by X-linked (5% to 10%), autosomal recessive, and mitochondrial mutations.

The mutations associated with DCM have been identified in genes encoding some of the same sarcomeric proteins affected in hypertrophic cardiomyopathy (e.g., actin, beta-myosin heavy chain, troponin T). However, in contrast to HCM, additional mutations associated with DCM have been found in cytoskeletal, nuclear envelope, and mitochondrial proteins. These mutations show variable penetrance (some are age-dependent) and expression, which leads to a wide range of disease within an affected family.

Cardiac amyloidosis occurs as an isolated form (involving the heart only) in elderly patients or in the setting of systemic amyloidosis secondary to a plasma cell dyscrasia. If cardiac amyloidosis is clinically apparent, it manifests most often with diastolic dysfunction (restrictive cardiomyopathy) because of stiffening of the ventricle secondary to amyloid deposition.

Burkett EL, Hershberger RE: Clinical and genetic issues in familial dilated cardiomyopathy. *J Am Coll Cardiol* 2005;45(7):969-981.

19. b. Isolated VSDs are the most common form of congenital heart disease. Most VSDs (85% to 90%) close spontaneously by 1 year of age, and only defects that are large or associated with other cardiac anomalies require early surgical intervention. VSDs account for approximately 40% of congenital cardiac defects, and ASDs account for approximately 10%; the combined frequency is approximately 50%. Shunting is typically classified as left-to-right (VSD, ASD, and patent ductus arteriosus) or right-to-left (tetralogy of Fallot, transposition of the great arteries, tricuspid atresia). Bicuspid aortic valves are notable for their frequency and late complications. Most often, bicuspid aortic valve is asymptomatic and is detected in childhood only when present with aortic stenosis. Affected individuals remain asymptomatic and usually develop stenosis or incompetence after age 40. Patent ductus arteriosus can be lifesaving in infants with obstructed pulmonary or systemic blood flow and is kept open with prostaglandin E until corrective surgery can be performed.

Hoffman JI, Kaplan S: The incidence of congenital heart disease. *J Am Coll Cardiol* 2002;39(12):1890-1900.

20. e. The gross description of the infarcted area indicates that the insult occurred 3 to 7 days previously. At this age, the infarcted tissue would show dead myofibers and neutrophils with infiltration of macrophages beginning at the edge of the lesion.

Schoen FJ: The heart. In Kumar V, Abbas A, Fausto N (eds): *Robbins and Cotran Pathologic Basis of Disease*, 7th ed. Philadelphia: Saunders, 2005, p 279.

21. d. The clinical description of the patient in the scenario suggests she has infective endocarditis. Several organisms normally found in the oral cavity are notorious for causing this condition and have been referred to as HACEK organisms: *Haemophilus aphrophilus, Actinobacillus actinomycetemcomitans, Cardiobacterium hominis, Eikenella corrodens,* and *Kingella kingae.* HACEK organisms are gram-negative bacilli that grow poorly on media selective for gram-negative organisms (fastidious), require special media or incubation conditions, and are causes of blood culture–negative endocarditis. Although *S. epidermidis* is a cause of infective endocarditis, it is more common in the setting of prosthetic valves.

Mylonakis E, Calderwood SB: Infective endocarditis in adults. *N Engl J Med* 2001;345(18):1318-1330.

22. c. The most likely cause of palpitations and midsystolic click on auscultation in the patient in the scenario is MVP, or myxomatous degeneration of the mitral valve. Affected individuals are most often asymptomatic young women. MVP is diagnosed at routine check-ups.

MVP is characterized by valve leaflets that are redundant and balloon into the left atrium during systole. The chordae are commonly thin and elongated. MVP can predispose affected individuals to various complications including infective endocarditis, thromboembolism, mitral insufficiency, and arrhythmias. Aortic stenosis produces a systolic murmur that is more pronounced in early systole,

whereas mitral stenosis produces a diastolic murmur. The classic condition associated with a continuous murmur is patent ductus arteriosus, which is rarely seen in adults. Valvular vegetations are capable of producing heart murmurs; the murmurs depend on location and degree of damage to the valve.

Schoen FJ: The heart. In Kumar V, Abbas A, Fausto N (eds): *Robbins and Cotran Pathologic Basis of Disease*, 7th ed. Philadelphia: Saunders, 2005, p 279.

23. d. The causative agent of rheumatic heart disease is *Streptococcus pyogenes* (group A or β-hemolytic streptococcus), whereas the viridans streptococci are a common cause of infective endocarditis. The acute phase of rheumatic heart disease can follow an episode of streptococcal pharyngitis and typically manifests as a migratory polyarthritis or carditis. Manifestations of chronic valvular disease can occur many years after the initial insult and are dependent on the affected valve.

Rheumatic heart disease is the most common cause of mitral stenosis. In approximately 65% to 70% of cases, the mitral valve is the only valve affected. The mitral and aortic valves are affected in about 25% of cases. The progressive fibrosis leads to thickening of the valves and chordae. When the mitral leaflets become fused at the commissures, stenosis occurs and imparts a "fish mouth" appearance to the valve. In contrast to calcific aortic stenosis, rheumatic disease results in commissural fusion of the aortic valve.

Mylonakis E, Calderwood SB: Infective endocarditis in adults. *N Engl J Med* 2001;345(18):1318-1330.

24. c. Lipomatous hypertrophy of the interatrial septum is a collection of adipocytes intermixed with myocardial cells (often hypertrophic), which thickens the interatrial septum (usually to >2 cm). This entity has been associated with arrhythmias and sudden cardiac death. The lesion is typically unencapsulated. The adipocytes resemble brown fat and have multiple cytoplasmic vacuoles. There may be associated fibrosis and chronic inflammation.

Lipomatous neoplasms, although rare in the heart, are in the differential diagnosis when fatty lesions are found in the septum. Lipomas are generally encapsulated and do not have many intermixed myocardial cells. Liposarcomas have more hyperchromatic nuclei and more atypia. FISH for MDM2 is very valuable in the distinction of lipomas from well-differentiated liposarcomas (also called *atypical lipomatous tumors*). However, Choices b and d pervert the relationships. MDM2 is amplified in liposarcoma and is not amplified in lipomas. FISH is a highly sensitive and specific discriminator in this context. A malignant Triton tumor is a sarcoma of schwannian derivation with some degree of rhabdomyosarcomatous differentiation (basically a malignant peripheral nerve sheath tumor with rhabdomyosarcomatous elements). It is a very rare tumor seen most commonly in peripheral nerves of patients with neurofibromatosis type 1.

O'Connor S, Recavarren R, Nichols LC, et al: Lipomatous hypertrophy of the interatrial septum: an overview. *Arch Pathol Lab Med* 2006;130(3):397-399.

Stasik CJ, Tawfik O: Malignant peripheral nerve sheath tumor with rhabdomyosarcomatous differentiation (malignant triton tumor). *Arch Pathol Lab Med* 2006;130(12):1878-1881.

Tanas MR, Goldblum JR: Fluorescence in situ hybridization in the diagnosis of soft tissue neoplasms: a review. *Adv Anat Pathol* 2009;16(6):383-391.

25. e. Chronic congestive heart failure is a massive public health burden in the United States. The prevalence has increased dramatically in recent years because of an aging population and better outcomes for acute coronary events. The relationship of primary pulmonary hypertension and the heart is well understood and involves dilation of the right side of the heart (cor pulmonale). Pathologic changes in the lungs are commonly seen at autopsy in patients with left-sided heart failure but are perhaps less commonly discussed outside the autopsy setting. These changes include the following:

- Intimal thickening of the arteries and veins
- Muscularization of the arterioles and venules
- Fibrosis of veins and arteries
- Thickening of alveolar walls with type 2 pneumocyte hyperplasia
- Bronchial smooth muscle hypertrophy
- Increased capillary basement membrane thickness

Inflammation of arterial walls with neutrophils, mononuclear cells, and macrophages resulting in areas of necrosis is found on histologic examination of Wegener granulomatosis. This finding would be unexpected in the clinical scenario described in the question.

Kee K, Naughton MT: Heart failure and the lung. *Circ J* 2010; 74(12):2507-2516.

CHAPTER 2

VASCULAR PATHOLOGY

Volker Nickeleit and Harsharan K. Singh

Questions 1-20 refer to a photo or photomicrograph.

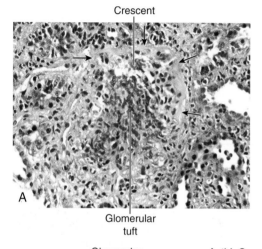

Crescent

Glomerular tuft

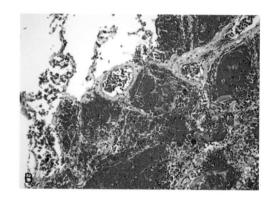

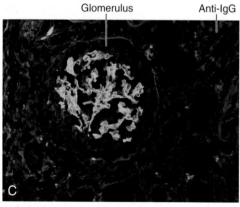

Glomerulus

Anti-IgG

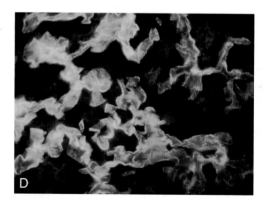

1. Trichrome-stained (panel A) and hematoxylin-eosin-stained (panel B) sections were taken from a 58-year-old white man who presented with acute renal failure and hemoptysis (i.e., pulmonary renal syndrome). Immunofluorescence studies performed on kidney tissue and illustrated in Panels C and D show linear staining along glomerular basement membranes (GBMs) with an antibody directed against IgG. The MOST likely cause is:

a. Anti-GBM disease

b. Malignant hypertension (hypertensive crisis)

c. Antineutrophil cytoplasmic autoantibody (ANCA) disease

d. Polyarteritis nodosa (PAN)

e. Both a and d are correct

2. Hematoxylin- and eosin-stained (top panel) and trichrome-stained (bottom panel) kidney sections were taken from a 78-year-old white woman who presented with acute renal failure and hemoptysis (i.e., pulmonary renal syndrome). Small, interlobular-type arteries (*arrows*) are illustrated. Additional immunofluorescence studies were negative. On physical examination, livedo reticularis was noted on the patient's lower extremities. She also complained of abdominal pain. The MOST likely diagnosis is:
   a. Goodpasture syndrome
   b. Henoch-Schönlein purpura (HSP)
   c. Giant cell arteritis (GCA)
   d. ANCA-associated small vessel vasculitis
   e. Antiphospholipid antibody syndrome (primary or secondary)

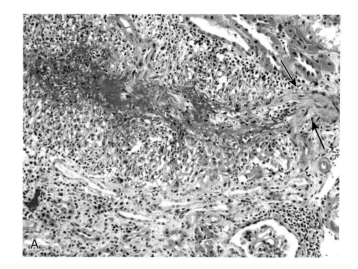

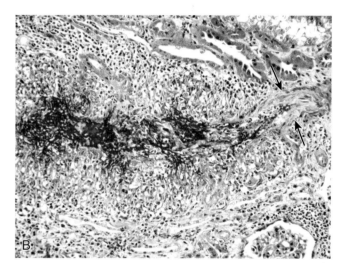

3. A hematoxylin-eosin–stained section demonstrated a severely inflamed large-caliber artery. The MOST likely diagnosis is:
   a. Microscopic polyangiitis
   b. GCA
   c. Granulomatosis with polyangiitis (formerly known as *Wegener granulomatosis*)
   d. Infection (e.g., tuberculosis)
   e. Thrombotic microangiopathy (TMA)

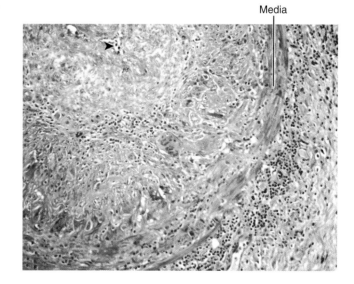

Media

4. A hematoxylin-eosin–stained section was taken from the mesenteric artery of a 31-year-old African American woman with a past history of multiple strokes and myocardial infarcts. The morphologic changes show:
   a. Recent cholesterol emboli
   b. Takayasu arteritis
   c. Severe atherosclerosis with early intimal plaque formation
   d. Typical changes of a remote TMA (late sclerosing stage)
   e. Recanalized thrombus formation

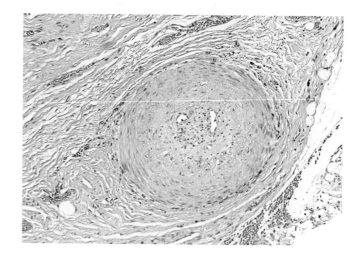

5. Trichrome-stained sections were taken from a kidney biopsy specimen of a 49-year-old African American man who presented with acute renal failure. The changes in the arterioles can be seen in cases of:
   a. Bloody diarrhea associated with renal failure
   b. Malignant hypertension
   c. ADAMTS13 deficiency
   d. Factor H deficiency
   e. All of the above

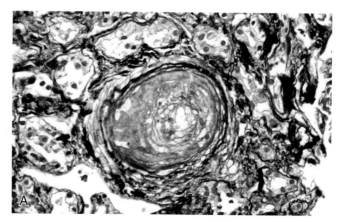

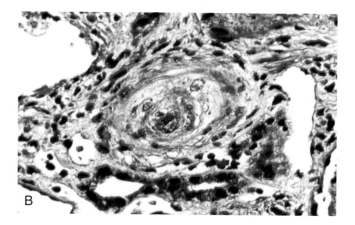

6. The vascular lesions present at the glomerular vascular poles on a kidney needle biopsy specimen represent:
   a. ANCA small vessel vasculitis
   b. Noninflammatory necrotizing vasculopathy (lupus vasculopathy)
   c. True renal vasculitis (seen in lupus)
   d. Severe hyalinosis secondary to hypertension
   e. Amyloidosis

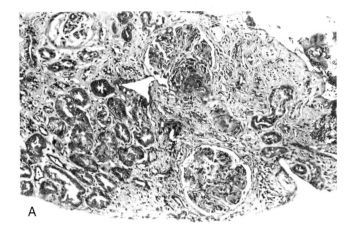

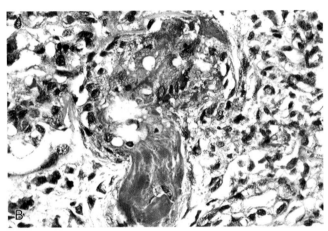

7. Trichrome-stained sections of a medium artery from a kidney transplant were obtained from a 57-year-old white woman. The biopsy was performed 21 days after transplantation because of delayed renal graft function. The intimal changes with fibroelastosis are typically seen in:
   a. Amyloidosis (unexpected donor disease)
   b. Early chronic rejection
   c. Transplant endarteritis
   d. Hypertension
   e. Ischemia-reperfusion injury

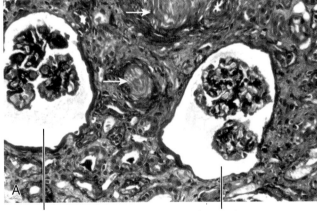

Glomerulus   Glomerulus

Media

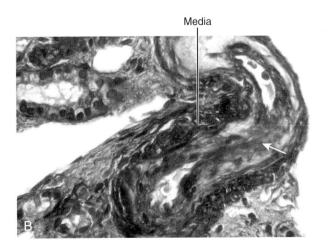

8. An 83-year-old white woman was initially seen by her local physician who had treated her for "nonhealing" skin ulcers of the lower extremities. The patient's history included poorly controlled hypertension, diabetes mellitus, and hyperlipidemia for many years. A kidney biopsy was performed recently for acute renal failure. What does this PAS-stained section of an arteriole show?
   a. Hyalinosis secondary to diabetes mellitus
   b. TMA (likely hypertension induced)
   c. Recanalized thrombus
   d. Small vessel vasculitis (possibly ANCA disease)
   e. Cholesterol emboli

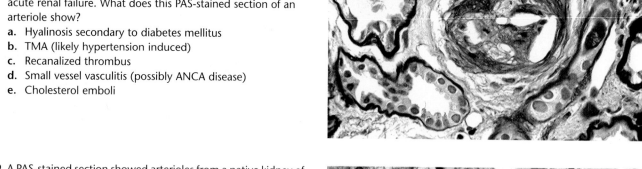

9. A PAS-stained section showed arterioles from a native kidney of a heart transplant recipient (transplant performed 6 years ago). The arterioles demonstrated nodular hyaline deposits. What is the MOST likely diagnosis?
   a. Remote hypertension-induced vasculopathy
   b. Diabetes mellitus
   c. Amyloidosis
   d. Calcineurin inhibitor toxicity (secondary to immunosuppression with cyclosporine or tacrolimus)
   e. Sclerosed ("healed inactive") ANCA small vessel vasculitis

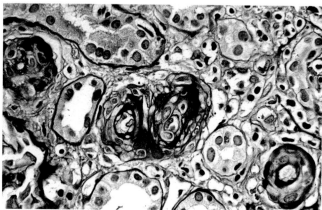

10. The medium arteries shown in hematoxylin-eosin–stained sections were found in a renal allograft biopsy specimen obtained 15 days after transplantation of a cadaveric graft. The intimal inflammation is typically seen in cases of:
    a. Calcineurin inhibitor toxicity (secondary to immunosuppression with cyclosporine or tacrolimus)
    b. Productive cytomegalovirus infection
    c. Polyomavirus nephropathies
    d. Acute rejection with transplant endarteritis
    e. Ischemia-reperfusion injury

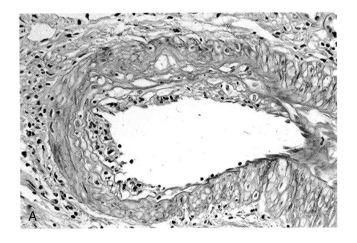

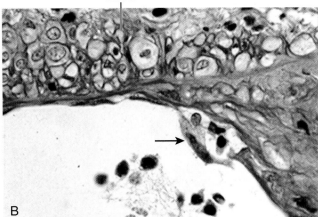

Media

11. A patient lost renal function secondary to ANCA-associated small vessel vasculitis and glomerulonephritis. He had received a renal allograft 6 weeks prior with very good immediate renal function after transplantation. He now presented with acute, rapid deterioration of graft function (no hematuria, no proteinuria, no rash). The lesion illustrated is suggestive of:
    a. Recurrent ANCA-associated small vessel vasculitis
    b. Acute rejection, likely antibody mediated
    c. Ischemia-reperfusion injury and delayed graft function
    d. Sepsis and pyelonephritis
    e. None of the above

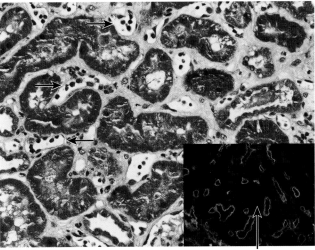

C4d immunofluorescence stain

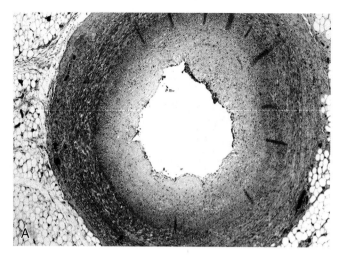

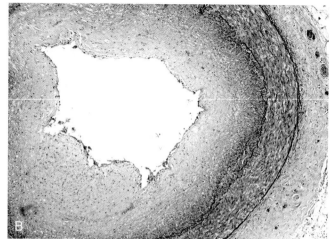

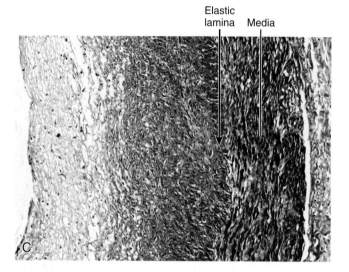

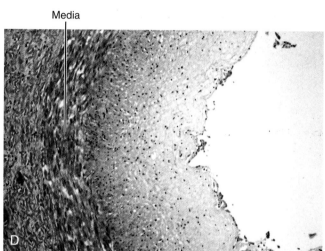

12. A 58-year-old white woman had undergone heart
transplantation 10 years ago. The patient recently presented
with signs of graft dysfunction. Laboratory tests suggested an
acute myocardial infarction. The patient died 2 days after
hospital admission. PAS, trichrome, and elastic stained tissue
sections show representative views of large-caliber coronary
arteries obtained at autopsy. What change is illustrated here?

   a. Sclerosing transplant vasculopathy (chronic vascular
rejection)

   b. Typical intimal fibroelastosis (i.e., atherosclerosis) owing to
hypertension

   c. Calcineurin inhibitor–induced toxicity in the setting of
chronic intense immunosuppression

   d. GCA (sclerosing phase)

   e. Recanalized thrombus formation

13. A 60-year-old woman presented to an emergency department with dyspnea and cyanosis. She related a 1-week history of severe sore throat, nausea, vomiting, arthralgias, and myalgia. Physical examination revealed severe hypotension and a faint blotchy erythema on the lower extremities. Laboratory studies revealed an elevated white blood cell count, no anemia, normal platelet count, normal bleeding times, serum creatinine 2.8 mg/dL, and blood urea nitrogen 25 mg/dL. Throat and blood cultures grew staphylococci that were shown to be methicillin-resistant *Staphylococcus aureus* (MRSA). The patient received intravenous fluids but remained hypotensive and dyspneic. Intravenous antibiotic therapy was administered. The next day, extensive purpura was noted on the patient's extremities, with scattered lesions on the torso. Her platelet count was markedly decreased at 35,000/mm^3, and there was a prolonged bleeding time. A skin biopsy specimen at the margin of the purpura demonstrated hemorrhagic purpura with extravasated red blood cells dissecting between collagen bundles in the dermis and small vessels occluded by thrombi (*arrows* on image). The MOST likely diagnosis is:

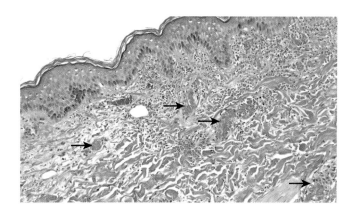

a. Atheroemboli
b. Disseminated intravascular coagulation (DIC)
c. Thrombotic thrombocytopenic purpura (TTP)
d. PAN
e. ANCA-associated small vessel vasculitis

14. A small vessel vasculitis characterized by recurrent episodes of urticaria with underlying leukocytoclastic vasculitis caused by anti-C1q antibodies is BEST classified as:

a. HSP
b. Hypocomplementemic urticarial vasculitis
c. Microscopic polyangiitis
d. PAN

15. This image from a child with cardiac abnormalities and fevers of unknown origin depicts a medium-caliber artery. Small-caliber arteries and arterioles were not involved. Serologic tests were negative for ANCA. The diagnosis is:

a. GCA
b. Pauci-immune ANCA-associated vasculitis
c. Kawasaki disease
d. TMA
e. PAN

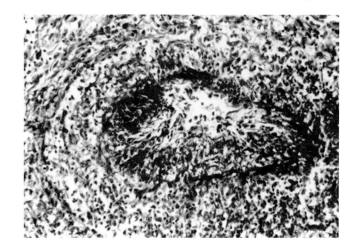

16. Small-caliber arteries in the heart, kidneys, thyroid, and central nervous system demonstrated "thrombi" occluding the vascular lumina as seen in this image from the heart. What disease entity is depicted here?
    a. Cryoglobulinemic vasculitis
    b. A staining artifact of the trichrome stain
    c. TTP
    d. HSP
    e. Lupus vasculopathy

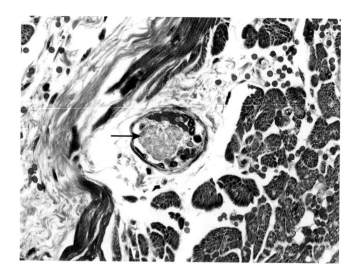

17. A CD62p stain demonstrates intense positivity within the intravascular "thrombi." This staining indicates that the intravascular "thrombi" are:
    a. A staining artifact and not clinically significant
    b. Composed of immune complexes
    c. Composed of platelets
    d. Composed of fibrin

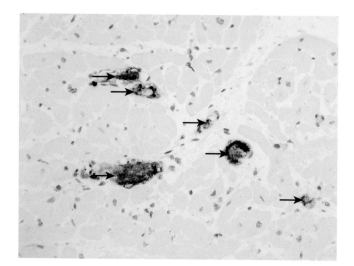

18. A small-caliber artery from a kidney needle biopsy sample demonstrates dense waxy homogeneous deposits in the vessel wall compromising the vascular lumen and without any associated inflammation. A Congo red stain was negative. Immunofluorescence staining depicted monoclonal staining only for kappa light chains in the vessel wall. Electron microscopy examination showed finely granular or powdery electron-dense deposits in the vessel wall. The BEST diagnosis is:
    a. Lupus vasculopathy (noninflammatory necrotizing vasculopathy)
    b. Amyloidosis
    c. Light chain deposition disease
    d. Pauci-immune small vessel vasculitis

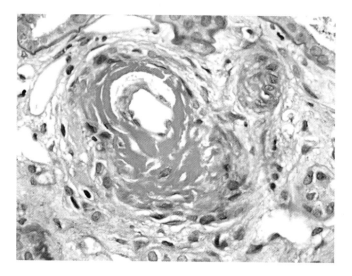

19. The biopsy specimen shown in the image was taken from a 40-year-old African American man who presented with renal dysfunction and had hilar adenopathy on a chest computed tomography (CT) scan. Serologic tests for ANCA were negative. On examination of the renal biopsy specimen, the glomeruli were unremarkable, and there were noncaseating granulomas within the interstitial compartment pushing away and separating the tubules. Immunofluorescence microscopy examination was negative. Immunohistochemical stains for fungal and mycobacterial organisms were negative. What is the MOST likely diagnosis?

   a. Granulomatosis with polyangiitis (formerly known as Wegener granulomatosis)
   b. Sarcoid granulomatous vasculitis
   c. Lupus vasculopathy
   d. Cryoglobulinemic glomerulonephritis

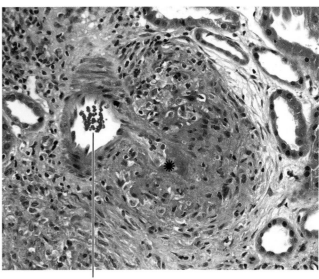

Vessel lumen

20. A 27-year-old man presented with multiple ulcerations on the toes and reported recurrent pain in the feet, worse in the left foot, and recurrent pain and tingling of the hands. The pain occurred most often when he was walking or running, but it sometimes occurred at rest. Physical examination revealed prominent, nodular, erythematous, slightly tender arteries and veins in the left lower extremity and reduced tibial artery pulses on the left but not the right. Reduced flow was detected by Doppler imaging, and angiography showed focal narrowing of arteries and veins. A biopsy specimen of the posterior tibial vein was obtained (see image). This case is MOST representative of which of the following?

   a. Hypertensive atherosclerosis
   b. Thromboangiitis obliterans (Buerger disease)
   c. Antiphospholipid antibody syndrome
   d. GCA

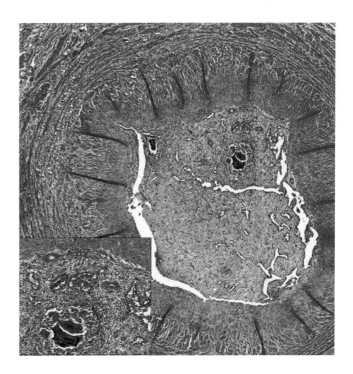

21. What is the MOST common cause of pulmonary-renal syndrome?
    a. Anti-GBM disease
    b. ANCA disease
    c. Immune complex–mediated disease
    d. TMA
    e. PAN

22. Arterial fibrinoid necrosis and TMA can be seen in cases of hypertension. Is this statement TRUE or FALSE?

23. A 4-year-old white boy presents with unexplained high fever, conjunctivitis, reddish tongue, and swollen cervical lymph nodes. Electrocardiogram (ECG) shows changes suggestive of mild myocardial ischemia, and an S_3 gallop is heard on physical examination. A general practitioner makes a diagnosis of "the flu" and sends the child home. What major diagnostic entity should have entered into the differential diagnosis?
    a. Kawasaki disease
    b. GCA
    c. HSP
    d. None of the above

24. Pediatricians use HSP as a synonym for *small vessel vasculitis*, including ANCA-associated cases, occurring in children aged younger than 15 years. Is this statement TRUE or FALSE?

25. A 31-year-old man developed sudden onset of abdominal pain and was admitted to a hospital where a diagnosis of ruptured spleen was made. CT scan of the abdomen demonstrated an enlarged splenic artery and aneurysms in the celiac artery and renal arteries. He underwent splenectomy and partial pancreatectomy with removal of a portion of the splenic artery and adjacent hematoma. Examination of the splenic artery demonstrated a dissecting aneurysm and rupture with mediolysis and dissolution of the muscularis layer. What is the CORRECT diagnosis?
    a. ANCA-associated microscopic polyangiitis
    b. TMA
    c. Segmental mediolytic arteriopathy
    d. Atheroemboli

26. A 31-year-old man developed sudden onset of abdominal pain and was admitted to a hospital where a diagnosis of ruptured spleen was made. CT scan of the abdomen demonstrated an enlarged splenic artery and aneurysms in the celiac artery and renal arteries. He underwent splenectomy and partial pancreatectomy with removal of a portion of the splenic artery and adjacent hematoma. Examination of the splenic artery demonstrated a dissecting aneurysm and rupture with mediolysis and dissolution of the muscularis layer. After the vascular lesion was identified, genetic studies demonstrated a mutation in *COL3A1* gene mutation. Name the disease entity associated with this genetic abnormality, which can be seen in some cases of the disease entity from Question 25.
    a. Vascular Ehlers-Danlos syndrome
    b. Marfan syndrome
    c. Loeys-Dietz syndrome

27. The patient is a 72-year-old African American man with a history of poorly controlled hypertension and diabetes mellitus. He reported recently experiencing fatigue, shortness of breath, back pain, and marked bilateral peripheral edema, and he

noted foamy urine. On admission, the patient presented with severe hypertension. An x-ray of the vertebral column demonstrated small lytic lesions in the lumbar vertebral bodies. Initial laboratory findings showed liver and pancreas enzyme profile within normal limits, red blood cell sedimentation rate and C-reactive protein increased, blood count within normal limits, evidence of mild acute renal failure with serum creatinine of 1.6 mg/dL (previous baseline reading 1.0 mg/dL), no hematuria, and positive proteinuria. Additional serologic data were pending. A renal biopsy was performed. Massive, pale-staining (PAS stain) and amorphous protein deposits were found in vascular walls of small arteries largely replacing medial smooth muscle cells. Glomeruli were less affected but showed mesangial and some segmental peripheral capillary loop expansion by similar pale-staining amorphous protein deposits. What is the MOST likely diagnosis?
    a. Anti-GBM antibody–mediated disease (Goodpasture syndrome)
    b. Amyloidosis
    c. Malignant hypertension–induced injury with features of TMA
    d. End-stage diabetic nephropathy
    e. Small vessel vasculitis, likely ANCA associated

28. The patient is a 72-year-old African American man with a history of poorly controlled hypertension and diabetes mellitus. He reported recently experiencing fatigue, shortness of breath, back pain, and marked bilateral peripheral edema, and he noted foamy urine. On admission, the patient presented with severe hypertension. An x-ray of the vertebral column demonstrated small lytic lesions in the lumbar vertebral bodies. Initial laboratory findings showed liver and pancreas enzyme profile within normal limits, red blood cell sedimentation rate and C-reactive protein increased, blood count within normal limits, evidence of mild acute renal failure with serum creatinine of 1.6 mg/dL (previous baseline reading 1.0 mg/dL), no hematuria, and positive proteinuria. Additional serologic data were pending. A renal biopsy was performed. Massive, pale-staining (PAS stain) and amorphous protein deposits were found in vascular walls of small arteries largely replacing medial smooth muscle cells. Glomeruli were less affected but showed mesangial and some segmental peripheral capillary loop expansion by similar pale-staining amorphous protein deposits. The deposition of massive amyloid deposits in vascular walls can result in:
    a. Hemorrhage
    b. Thrombosis and occlusion
    c. Inflammation and vasculitis
    d. All of the above
    e. None of the above

29. A 60-year-old man presented with a rash and worsening renal function. Palpable purpuric lesions were present on the buttocks and feet, including the soles. There was no clinical history of urticaria. A skin biopsy specimen showed a leukocytoclastic vasculitis. Direct immunofluorescence staining of the biopsy specimen showed granular deposits consisting primarily of IgM and C3 in a vascular pattern in the papillary dermis. Laboratory evaluation revealed anemia and renal insufficiency, with microscopic hematuria and proteinuria in the nephrotic range on urinary examination. Serum complement levels were markedly decreased for C4 and were borderline decreased for C3. Serologic tests for

antistreptolysin O, antinuclear antibody, ANCA, hepatitis C, and cryoglobulins were negative. Rheumatoid factor was elevated. A renal biopsy was performed and demonstrated an immune complex–mediated diffuse proliferative glomerulonephritis, and immunofluorescence studies showed mesangial and focal capillary loop deposits of IgG, C3, and IgM. Examination with electron microscopy revealed small mesangial and subendothelial electron-dense deposits. What is the MOST likely diagnosis?

a. HSP
b. Microscopic polyangiitis
c. Hypocomplementemic urticarial vasculitis
d. Cryoglobulinemic vasculitis

30. A 38-year-old African American woman presented with frank neutropenia and retiform purpura affecting the skin over the ears and zygomatic arch and sparing the trunk and extremities. Serologic tests were positive for antinuclear antibody, lupus anticoagulant, anticardiolipin antibodies, and a very high p-ANCA and c-ANCA titer with a borderline positive MPO-ANCA and PR3-ANCA titer. A skin biopsy specimen at the edge of a purpuric lesion demonstrated intravascular thrombosis with mild surrounding inflammation. The patient was questioned further and admitted to regular use of crack cocaine, which she had used 24 hours before presentation. What is the MOST likely diagnosis?

a. ANCA-associated small vessel vasculitis
b. Cryoglobulinemic vasculitis
c. Vasculopathy associated with levamisole-contaminated cocaine use
d. HSP

ANSWERS

1. a. In this example of anti-GBM disease, the kidney biopsy specimen (Panel A) demonstrates a typical destructive necrotizing glomerulonephritis, often associated with extensive crescent formation. An inflammatory response in the glomeruli is characteristically limited to areas of necrosis, whereas uninvolved glomerular tufts remain unaltered. In most necrotic glomeruli, extensive ruptures of Bowman capsule are seen by trichrome, PAS, or Jones silver staining. The lung biopsy specimen (Panel B) demonstrates diffuse pulmonary hemorrhage with blood-filled alveolar spaces. Goodpasture syndrome refers to the triad of pulmonary (alveolar) hemorrhage, glomerulonephritis of any severity, and anti-GBM antibody production. These circulating antibodies are directed against the NC1 domain of collagen IV in glomerular and alveolar basement membranes. Goodpasture syndrome is associated with high morbidity and mortality rates (owing to exsanguination and suffocation caused by lung hemorrhage). The treatment of choice is plasmapheresis.

Three major categories of small vessel vasculitis can cause pulmonary renal syndrome: anti-GBM disease, ANCA disease, and immune complex–mediated diseases (e.g., systemic lupus erythematosus). Of the small vessel vasculitides, anti-GBM and ANCA disease most often affect the lungs by causing capillaritis, whereas the immune complex–mediated small vessel vasculitides do so rarely. The immunofluorescence features of the various immune complex–mediated diseases allow for their separation from both ANCA and anti-GBM disease. The two disease entities can be distinguished in renal (or lung) biopsy specimens using immunofluorescence microscopy as illustrated in Panels C and D.

Immunofluorescence microscopy is an easily performed laboratory test that can quickly and confidently confirm the diagnosis of anti-GBM disease in the appropriate clinical setting, allowing for immediate treatment. The mere presence of linear staining for IgG along the GBM is not diagnostic for anti-GBM disease. Linear IgG staining may be seen in glomeruli in two other disorders: diabetic glomerulosclerosis and fibrillary glomerulopathy. Clinical and histopathologic findings can be used to distinguish these two disorders from anti-GBM disease.

Immunofluorescence studies can also be performed on lung tissue; however, the interpretation is often problematic. Normal lung tissue can reveal a discontinuous weak staining for IgG along alveolar septa making interpretation difficult.

The diagnosis of anti-GBM antibody disease requires demonstration of anti-GBM antibodies either in the serum or in the kidney. Unless contraindicated, renal biopsy should be performed because the accuracy of serologic assays is variable. In addition, renal biopsy provides important information regarding the activity and chronicity of renal involvement that may help guide therapy.

Jennette JC: Nomenclature and classification of vasculitis: lessons learned from granulomatosis with polyangiitis (Wegener's granulomatosis). *Clin Exp Immunol* 2011;164(Suppl 1):7-10.
Sanders JS, Rutgers A, Stegeman CA, et al: Pulmonary: renal syndrome with a focus on anti-GBM disease. *Semin Respir Crit Care Med* 2011;32(3):328-334.
Tarzi RM, Cook HT, Pusey CD: Crescentic glomerulonephritis: new aspects of pathogenesis. *Semin Nephrol* 2011;31(4):361-368.

2. d. The image illustrates a necrotizing small vessel vasculitis lacking immunoglobulin deposits. These small vessel vasculitides are often associated with a necrotizing and crescentic glomerulonephritis and elevated ANCA titers. High c-ANCA or p-ANCA titers (antibodies directed against proteinase-3 or myeloperoxidase, respectively) can be detected in approximately 90% of patients. In roughly 10% of patients with small vessel vasculitis lacking immune complex deposits, ANCA titers remain within normal limits (see Question 44). If capillaries in the lungs are inflamed simultaneously, patients present with pulmonary renal syndrome.

Vasculitis should be considered in patients who present with systemic symptoms in combination with evidence of single-organ or multiorgan dysfunction. Although neither sensitive nor specific, common complaints and signs of vasculitis include fatigue, weakness, fever, arthralgias, abdominal pain, hypertension, renal insufficiency (with an active urine sediment containing red and white blood cells and occasionally red blood cell casts), and neurologic dysfunction. Certain signs are strongly suggestive of vasculitis, including mononeuritis multiplex, palpable purpura, and combined pulmonary and renal involvement. Abdominal pain in the patient in the scenario is likely another sign of a vasculitis involving the gastrointestinal tract.

To establish a definitive diagnosis of vasculitis, a biopsy specimen should be obtained from the most affected organs or sites. The inflammatory reactions noted in all cases of vasculitides include transmural mononuclear and polymorphonuclear inflammatory cell infiltrates, occasional giant cells, destruction of the internal elastic lamina, and varying degrees of necrosis of the media along with varying degrees of fibrin deposition. Often, adventitial vascular layers are inflamed as well. Based on the inflammatory pattern, vasculitides cannot always be reliably subclassified (with the exception of cases caused by infectious agents, such as *Nocardia* or septic foci).

Criteria for the classification of most of the major forms of vasculitis have been established; they do not include all characteristics of a particular disorder, only the characteristics that help to distinguish the disorder from other vasculitides. The diagnosis of a particular form of vasculitis is virtually always confirmed by tissue biopsy. The Chapel Hill Consensus Conference recommendation on the nomenclature of systemic vasculitides is the most frequently used system for subtyping. This system is primarily based on the caliber of the most inflamed or affected vessels; it additionally incorporates immunofluorescence findings and selected clinical and laboratory parameters. Small vessel vasculitides are changes found in distal vascular branches, including arterioles, capillaries, and venules; medium vessel vasculitis is found in the main muscular arterial segments with multiple medial smooth muscle layers; and large vessel vasculitis is seen in the aorta and its largest branches.

Based on additional findings, small vessel vasculitides (lacking immune complex deposits) can be subtyped further into three groups: (1) *Granulomatosis with polyangiitis* (formerly known as *Wegener granulomatosis*) shows additional granulomatous and necrotizing inflammation of the lungs and nasal sinuses. (2) *Eosinophilic granulomatosis with polyangiitis* (formerly known as *Churg-Strauss syndrome*) is characterized by additional asthma and (blood) eosinophilia. (3) *Microscopic polyangiitis* refers to necrotizing vasculitis affecting small vessels in multiple sites. Small vessel vasculitis may be limited to the kidneys and manifest exclusively with a necrotizing and crescentic glomerulonephritis. Subclassification into the previously listed three major subtypes is not always possible, and many cases may best be categorized as microscopic polyangiitis.

Cases of necrotizing small vessel vasculitides, particularly in older patients in association with elevated ANCA titers, are characterized by the absence (paucity) of immunoglobulins in the inflamed vessel walls. If elevated ANCA titers are not detected, the histopathologist should always consider immune complex–mediated vasculitides, which can be caused by the deposition of IgA (in the setting of HSP), IgG (in the setting of systemic lupus erythematosus), or IgG and IgM (in the setting of cryoglobulinemia). Small vessel vasculitides in the skin may be allergic in nature. The proper diagnostic work-up of inflammatory lesions in small vessels is challenging and requires close clinicopathologic correlation. In equivocal

cases, immunofluorescence microscopy is required specifically to search for the deposition of immunoglobulins in vascular walls.

Jennette JC: Nomenclature and classification of vasculitis: lessons learned from granulomatosis with polyangiitis (Wegener's granulomatosis). *Clin Exp Immunol* 2011;164(Suppl 1):7-10.

Jennette JC: Renal involvement in systemic vasculitis. In Jennette JC, Olson JL, Schwartz MM, et al (eds): *Heptinstall's Pathology of the Kidney*, 5th ed. Philadelphia: Lippincott-Raven, 1998, p 1059.

Watts RA, Scott DG: Recent developments in the classification and assessment of vasculitis. *Best Pract Res Clin Rheumatol* 2009; 23(3):429-443.

3. b. GCA is a granulomatous form of ANCA-negative large vessel vasculitis. It has a predilection for the aorta and its major branches, especially the extracranial arteries. GCA is the most common form of vasculitis in patients older than 50 years of age. A high index of suspicion is essential in making the diagnosis of GCA. The greatest risk factor for developing GCA is aging. The disease almost never occurs before age 50, and its incidence increases steadily thereafter.

Temporal artery biopsy is the gold standard for the diagnosis of GCA. Temporal artery biopsy specimens should undergo full tissue processing, not frozen section alone. On biopsy examination, the inflammatory process, composed of mononuclear cells with a predominance of macrophages and lymphocytes, originates in the media and extends into the intima and adventitia. The minute remnant of the vascular lumen is apparent in the image (*arrow*); note the marked inflammation and edema in the intima and media.

Multinucleated giant cells, either of the Langerhans type or of the foreign body type, are found in about 50% of cases, often adjacent to the fragmented internal elastic lamina. Fibrinoid vascular wall necrosis is infrequently observed, and when present, it is patchy in distribution (compare this case of GCA with the small vessel vasculitis illustrated in the image in Question 2). The presence of extensive fibrinoid necrosis should raise the possibility of another type of systemic ANCA-negative vasculitis found in medium vessels (i.e., PAN).

GCA involves arteries in a segmental fashion. A minimum of a 3-cm-long segment of artery should be obtained for an adequate histologic examination. Samples should ideally be taken from abnormal (indurated and painful) vascular wall segments.

Caspary L: Vasculitides of large vessels. *Vasa* 2011;40(2):89-98.

Meyers AD, Said S: Temporal artery biopsy: concise guidelines for otolaryngologists. *Laryngoscope* 2004;114(11):2056-2059.

Weyand CM, Goronzy JJ: Medium- and large-vessel vasculitis. *N Engl J Med* 2003;349(2):160-169.

4. e. The image shows a remote, completely organized thrombus with typical signs of recanalization. The vessel wall lacks inflammation and necrosis. Antiphospholipid syndrome (APS) is defined as a hypercoagulable state with arterial or venous fibrin thrombus formation caused by high titers of circulating autoantibodies directed against phospholipid and phospholipid-binding protein complexes (i.e., β_2-glycoprotein 1 and phospholipid complexes on platelets and endothelial cells).

APS is classified as *secondary disease* if it is accompanied by other autoimmune disorders (i.e., systemic lupus erythematosus or other connective tissue diseases) and as *primary disease* if it manifests only with a hypercoagulable state. The histologic examination typically shows fibrin thrombi of different ages, sometimes organized with signs of recanalization (e.g., see the case presented in Question 5). Conspicuous inflammation and vascular wall necrosis are lacking.

In APS, venous thrombosis is frequently detected in deep leg veins (55%; *caveat:* pulmonary emboli) as well as in renal, hepatic, and retinal veins. Arterial thrombosis is typically seen in cerebrovascular (50%), coronary (25%), ocular, mesenteric, deep leg, and renal arteries (*caveat:* stroke, myocardial or bowel infarction, ischemia of the lower extremities with skin ulcerations).

Clinical manifestations are variable and can mimic a systemic vasculitis (including livedo reticularis), repeated miscarriages, and cardiac valvular vegetations (Libman-Sacks endocarditis in 4% of patients). In less than 1% of cases, multiple organ sites are affected by thrombosis simultaneously with dramatic clinical consequences and a mortality rate of 50% (termed *catastrophic APS*). APS should always be included in the differential diagnosis in patients presenting with recurrent episodes of thrombosis.

Appenzeller S, Souza FH, Wagner Silva de Souza A, et al: HELLP syndrome and its relationship with antiphospholipid syndrome and antiphospholipid antibodies. *Semin Arthritis Rheum* 2011;41(3):517-523.

Favaloro EJ, Wong RC: Laboratory testing for the antiphospholipid syndrome: making sense of antiphospholipid antibody assays. *Clin Chem Lab Med* 2011;49(3):447-461.

Rodriguez-Garcia JL, Bertolaccini ML, Cuadrado MJ, et al: Clinical manifestations of antiphospholipid syndrome (APS) with and without antiphospholipid antibodies (the so-called "seronegative APS"). *Ann Rheum Dis* 2012;71(2):242-244.

Sangle NA, Smock KJ: Antiphospholipid antibody syndrome. *Arch Pathol Lab Med* 2011;135(9):1092-1096.

Tripodi A, de Groot PG, Pengo V: Antiphospholipid syndrome: laboratory detection, mechanisms of action and treatment. *J Intern Med* 2011;270(2):110-122.

5. e. The trichrome-stained sections show typical acute changes of TMA that can be seen in association with all events listed in Choices a through d. The descriptive term *TMA* characterizes stenosing or thrombotic changes in small vessels (i.e., capillaries, arterioles, prearterioles, and small arteries). Veins and larger arteries with multiple layers of medial smooth muscle cells are characteristically spared. Histologically, the acute phase of TMA is characterized by various changes that can be seen individually or in combination: (1) endothelial cell swelling and mucoid intimal widening with severe narrowing of vascular lumens (see Panel B, accompanied by intimal fibrin deposits in Panel A); (2) intraluminal fibrin thrombi or fragmented red blood cells or both in the intima and media; (3) necrosis of individual endothelial or medial smooth muscle cells; (4) PAS-positive nodular proteinaceous deposits replacing arteriolar smooth muscle cells (blue nodules along the adventitial aspect of the arteriole in Panel B). Fibrin thrombi sometimes may be detected, but they are not essential for establishing the diagnosis of TMA. Thus, the term *thrombotic microangiopathy* is a misnomer. If TMA persists over weeks, affected intimal zones demonstrate increasing sclerosis, often with a layered, so-called onion-skin pattern.

The initial common event in the pathogenesis of all forms of TMA is severe endothelial cell injury that is caused by a wide variety of different agents and results in intimal remodeling. Generally, the pathologist cannot reliably identify the underlying causative agent or event and often can render only a descriptive diagnosis of "TMA."

TMA commonly affects the brain, kidneys, gastrointestinal tract, pancreas, spleen, and adrenal glands, whereas the liver and lungs are generally spared. Typical clinical signs of TMA are thrombocytopenia, hemolytic anemia, fragmented red blood cells (i.e., schistocytes) in peripheral blood smears, and organ dysfunction including seizures or renal failure. Depending on the organ primarily involved (kidney or brain) and the extent of the vascular changes, clinical symptoms may vary considerably from mild to severe.

TMA in adults often primarily affects the brain and is referred to as *TTP*. Children with TMA commonly experience bloody diarrhea, severe renal failure, and hemolysis, and this is referred to as hemolytic uremic syndrome (*HUS*). However, there is vast overlap in clinical symptoms (the same patient may be described as having HUS by a nephrologist and TTP by a hematologist), and the underlying cause of TMA may not be easily discernible.

Table 2-1 Causes of Thrombotic Microangiopathies

Hemolytic Uremic Syndrome (HUS) Predominant

Shiga-like toxin-induced HUS (e.g., *Escherichia coli, Shigella dysenteriae*)—typical HUS cases associated with bloody diarrhea; most types listed here do not manifest with diarrhea

Neuraminidase-induced HUS (e.g., *Streptococcus pneumoniae*)

Other bacterial or viral infections (e.g., typhoid fever, HIV infection, influenza, enterovirus infection)

Iatrogenic HUS
  Drug-induced HUS (e.g., cyclosporine, tacrolimus, mitomycin C, oral contraceptives, quinine)
  Bone marrow transplantation–induced HUS
  Radiation-induced HUS

Scleroderma renal crisis HUS

Familial HUS (e.g., autosomal recessive, autosomal dominant, defects in the complement factor cascade [factor H deficiencies])

Malignant hypertension–induced HUS (malignant nephrosclerosis—*common*)

Idiopathic HUS

Antiphospholipid Syndrome (APS)

Primary and secondary APS with associated HUS

Toxemia of Pregnancy

Preeclampsia

Eclampsia

HELLP syndrome*

Thrombotic Thrombocytopenic Purpura (TTP) Predominant

Familial/recurrent TTP (e.g., defects in or absence of von Willebrand factor [vWF] multimerase/ADAMTS13 deficiencies)

Sporadic TTP (e.g., autoantibodies to vWF multimerase/ADAMTS13)

Drug-induced TTP (e.g., ticlopidine, clopidogrel)

Idiopathic TTP

*Hemolysis, elevated liver enzyme levels, low platelet count.

Dragon-Durey MA, Blanc C, Garnier A, et al: Anti-factor H autoantibody-associated hemolytic uremic syndrome: review of literature of the autoimmune form of HUS. *Semin Thromb Hemost* 2010;36(6):633-640.

Frank C, Werber D, Cramer JP, et al: Epidemic profile of shiga-toxin-producing Escherichia coli O104:H4 outbreak in Germany. *N Engl J Med* 2011;365(19):1771-1780.

Liszewski MK, Atkinson JP: Too much of a good thing at the site of tissue injury: the instructive example of the complement system predisposing to thrombotic microangiopathy. *Hematology Am Soc Hematol Educ Program* 2011;2011:9-14.

Moake JL: Thrombotic microangiopathies. *N Engl J Med* 2002; 347(8):589-600.

6. b. The image illustrates a lupus vasculopathy, descriptively termed a *noninflammatory necrotizing vasculopathy*. Vascular lesions are commonly encountered in lupus nephritis in several morphologically distinct forms. *Vasculopathy* is defined as a noninflammatory lesion initiated by immune complexes as well as secondary to acute or chronic thrombosis resulting from several forms of endothelial injury, including antiphospholipid antibodies. *Vasculitis* is defined as infiltration of the vessel wall (transmural) by leukocytes (mononuclear or polymorphonuclear leukocytes), endothelial damage, segmental or circumferential eosinophilic "fibrinoid" necrosis of the wall with neutrophils, fragmented nuclei, and elastic membrane disruption, features similar to the features seen in small vessel vasculitides (see Question 2).

Immunofluorescence microscopy demonstrates immunoglobulins and complement components along with fibrin in the intima and media indicating a combined injury from immune deposits and intravascular coagulation. Electron microscopy confirms endothelial cell injury or necrosis with luminal granular electron-dense material consisting of abundant immune deposits and insudated plasma proteins including fibrin tactoids. In contrast to ANCA small vessel vasculitis and a true renal vasculitis in lupus, inflammation of the vessel wall is not seen. Lupus vasculopathy is associated with a poor prognosis and is frequently associated with hypertension and a rapidly deteriorating renal course, so it is important to recognize and report to the clinician for patient management and prognostic purposes.

D'Agati V, Jennette JC, Silva FG: *Atlas of Nontumor Pathology: Non-Neoplastic Kidney Diseases*. Washington, DC: American Registry of Pathology, 2005, pp 323-360.

Seshan SV: Lupus vasculopathy and vasculitis: what is the difference and when do they occur? *Pathol Case Rev* 2007; 12(5):214-221.

Seshan SV, Jennette JC: Renal disease in systemic lupus erythematosus with emphasis on classification of lupus glomerulonephritis, advances and implications. *Arch Pathol Lab Med* 2009;133(2):233-248.

7. d. The presence of a hypocellular fibrointimal expansion is characteristic of hypertension-induced changes in arteries. The changes are similar in both native and allograft kidneys. Initially, arterial hypertension results in hypertrophy of the medial smooth muscle cell layer, which is soon accompanied by intimal fibroelastosis. When intimal widening impairs the diffusion of nutrients from the vascular lumen to the media, smooth muscle cells undergo atrophy (as demonstrated here). Typical atherosclerotic plaques, including foam cells and foci of calcification, are generally seen only in the aorta and its major branches of thick muscular arteries; they are uncommon in the distal vasculature.

Two different processes appear to contribute to the development of the vascular lesions:

- A hypertrophic response to chronic hypertension that is manifested by medial hypertrophy and fibroblastic intimal thickening, leading to narrowing of the vascular lumen. This response is initially adaptive by minimizing the degree to which the increase in systemic pressure is transmitted to the arterioles and capillaries.
- The deposition of hyaline-like material (plasma protein constituents, such as inactive C3b, part of the third component of complement) into the damaged, more permeable arteriolar wall.

In renal allograft biopsy specimens, a tissue elastic stain can be extremely helpful in identifying the reduplication of the elastic lamellae seen in cases of hypertension. Chronic vascular rejection (sclerosing transplant vasculopathy) lacks elastic lamellae (see Question 12).

Carretero OA: Vascular remodeling and the kallikrein-kinin system. *J Clin Invest* 2005;115(3):588-591.

Olson J: Hypertension: essential and secondary forms. In Jennette JC, Olson JC, Schwartz MM, et al (eds): *Heptinstall's Pathology of the Kidney*, 5th ed. Philadelphia: Lippincott-Raven, 1998, p 943.

Schulze PC, Lee RT: Oxidative stress and atherosclerosis. *Curr Atheroscler Rep* 2005;7(3):242-248.

8. e. Depending on the original size of the emboli, cholesterol clefts may be found in large or small arteries as well as occasionally in capillaries. Atheroemboli rapidly attract monocytes, which unsuccessfully attempt to phagocytize the embolic material. The atheroemboli stimulate the deposition of collagen resulting in vascular stenosis and occlusion. At a later stage, the clefts are surrounded by fibrous tissue, mononuclear cells, and frequently multinucleated giant cells. Clinical symptoms associated with atheroemboli vary greatly (e.g., livedo reticularis, acute renal failure, hypertension, leg pain, skin ulcerations including black toes, gastrointestinal symptoms, vision loss).

Many cases of atheroembolic disease may not be detected clinically because of the variability of presenting symptoms, especially in cases with multiorgan involvement that can mimic systemic vasculitis. The level of suspicion of atheroemboli should be high in older patients. Atheroembolization also can occur without prior catheterization or manipulation of the aorta. Morphologic features of a recanalized thrombus include prominent intimal remodeling often showing several endothelium-lined spaces that lack the symmetric appearance of cholesterol clefts.

Ben-Horin S, Bardan E, Barshack I, et al: Cholesterol crystal embolization to the digestive system: characterization of a common, yet overlooked presentation of atheroembolism. *Am J Gastroenterol* 2003;98(7):1471-1479.

Donohue KG, Saap L, Falanga V: Cholesterol crystal embolization: an atherosclerotic disease with frequent and varied cutaneous manifestations. *J Eur Acad Dermatol Venereol* 2003;17(5): 504-511.

Fukumoto Y, Tsutsui H, Tsuchihashi M, et al; Cholesterol Embolism Study (CHEST) Investigators: The incidence and risk factors of cholesterol embolization syndrome, a complication of cardiac catheterization: a prospective study. *J Am Coll Cardiol* 2003;42(2):211-216.

9. d. Calcineurin inhibitor–induced toxicity is seen in patients treated with cyclosporine or tacrolimus. These agents are widely used immunosuppressive drugs, and both act via calcineurin inhibition and suppression of interleukin 2. The induced morphologic changes (i.e., structural toxicities) are dose-dependent, are identical for cyclosporine and tacrolimus, and demonstrate great interindividual variations. In some sensitive patients, toxicity may be noted at less than therapeutic drug levels.

Because the highest concentrations of calcineurin inhibitors are administered to suppress the rejection of organ transplants, toxic side effects are common in heart, kidney, lung, and bone marrow allograft recipients. Aside from the arteriolar changes, structural toxicity additionally may be seen in proximal renal tubules demonstrating isometric vacuolation of the cytoplasm (a reversible phenomenon). The most serious toxic side effect of calcineurin inhibitors is a fully developed TMA with clinical signs of HUS. The morphologic appearance of calcineurin inhibitor–induced renal arteriolopathies is typical for toxic side effects, but it is not pathognomonic. Findings must be interpreted in the appropriate clinical context. The differential diagnosis includes (1) hypertension-induced arteriolosclerosis with hyalinosis, (2) diabetic arteriolosclerosis, and (3) amyloidosis.

Burdmann EA, Andoh TF, Yu L, et al: Cyclosporine nephrotoxicity. *Semin Nephrol* 2003;23(5):465-476.

Colvin RB, Nickeleit V: Renal transplant pathology. In Jennette JC, Olson JL, Schwartz MM, et al (eds): *Heptinstall's Pathology of the Kidney,* 6th ed. Philadelphia: Lippincott Williams & Wilkins, 2007, p 1347.

Wilkinson AH, Cohen DJ: Renal failure in the recipients of nonrenal solid organ transplants. *J Am Soc Nephrol* 1999;10(5): 1136-1144.

10. d. Transplant endarteritis characteristically shows infiltration of lymphocytes through the activated endothelial cell layer (see *arrow* in image) into the subendothelial compartment and intima. The media of the vessels is left unaltered. Transplant endarteritis is a common type of acute cellular allograft rejection. According to the Banff scheme of allograft rejection, this lesion falls into category IV, type 2 acute cellular rejection episodes.

We have diagnosed transplant endarteritis from 6 days to 14 years after transplantation. It may be underdiagnosed because of small (inadequate) biopsy samples lacking arteries. The diagnosis of transplant endarteritis is associated with great prognostic and therapeutic significance. Patients usually do not benefit from conventional antirejection therapy with bolus steroids, but rather require potent treatment with antilymphocytic preparations (ATG or OKT3). "Smoldering" or persistent transplant endarteritis results in the activation of myofibroblasts and progressive intimal sclerosis (i.e., sclerosing transplant vasculopathy). Transplant endarteritis is a major risk factor for chronic vascular rejection (see Question 11). Detection of transplant endarteritis permits definitive diagnosis of active or acute rejection.

Colvin RB, Nickeleit V: Renal transplant pathology. In Jennette JC, Olson JL, Schwartz MM, et al (eds): *Heptinstall's Pathology of the Kidney,* 6th ed. Philadelphia: Lippincott Williams & Wilkins, 2007, p 1347.

Haas M, Kraus ES, Samaniego-Picota M, et al: Acute renal allograft rejection with intimal arteritis: histologic predictors of response to therapy and graft survival. *Kidney Int* 2002;61(4): 1516-1526.

Nickeleit V, Vamvakas EC, Pascual M, et al: The prognostic significance of specific arterial lesions in acute renal allograft rejection. *J Am Soc Nephrol* 1998;9(7):1301-1308.

11. b. The prominent peritubular capillary dilation with filling by inflammatory cells indicates a peritubular capillaritis. This peritubular capillaritis along with the positive peritubular capillary C4d deposition seen in the *inset* image is diagnostic of an antibody-mediated acute rejection episode. Circulating donor-specific antibodies, often class I or class II, can induce allograft rejection mainly by injuring the endothelium of glomerular or peritubular capillaries and causing capillary hypercellularity or capillaritis.

Although capillaritis is not pathognomonic for an antibody-mediated rejection process, the clinical presentation in this patient of acute, rapid graft dysfunction early after transplantation in the absence of significant hematuria, which could indicate a recurrent glomerulonephritis, makes rejection most likely. C4d is routinely used in the evaluation of allograft biopsy specimens as a marker for an antibody-mediated rejection episode. The staining pattern in this case is diffuse and strong supporting the suspicion based on light microscopy of an antibody-mediated rejection process.

According to the Banff scheme of allograft rejection, this lesion falls into category II, antibody-mediated rejection. No single histologic feature consistently distinguishes biopsy specimens with acute antibody-mediated rejection. Lesions that favor antibody-mediated rejection compared with pure cellular rejection include neutrophils in peritubular capillaries (capillaritis), fibrinoid necrosis of arteries, glomerulitis, and tissue infarction.

Colvin RB, Nickeleit V: Renal transplant pathology. In Jennette JC, Olson JL, Schwartz MM, et al (eds): *Heptinstall's Pathology of the Kidney,* 6th ed. Philadelphia: Lippincott Williams & Wilkins, 2007, p 1347.

Sis B, Mengel M, Haas M, et al: Banff '09 meeting report: antibody mediated graft deterioration and implementation of Banff working groups. *Am J Transplant* 2010;410(3):464-471.

Solez K, Colvin RB, Racusen LC, et al: Banff 07 classification of renal allograft pathology: updates and future directions. *Am J Transplant* 2008;8(4):753-760.

12. a. Sclerosing transplant vasculopathy (chronic vascular rejection) is defined as rejection-induced arterial intimal thickening secondary to de novo deposition of collagens I and III without associated intimal elastosis. The lumen of arteries is narrowed by concentric or sometimes eccentric intimal fibrosis, which is most pronounced at arterial branching points.

The pattern of intimal fibrosis in cases of chronic vascular rejection displays some distinct, diagnostically helpful features: (1) The lack of elastic lamellae is most characteristic—that is, an absence of marked intimal elastosis best seen in elastic tissue stains (see Panel B and compare with hypertension-induced intimal fibroelastosis illustrated in Panel B for Question 7). Typically, the inner elastic lamina remains intact. (2) The fibrotic intima contains scattered, irregularly arranged myofibroblasts with enlarged "activated" nuclei (a "busy" appearance). (3) The fibrotic intima may contain scattered mononuclear inflammatory cell elements—histiocytes and lymphocytes (see Panel D). (4) Sometimes foam cells are present.

(5) During intimal remodeling, myofibroblasts may occasionally form a new rudimentary media under the endothelial layer. This so-called neo-media formation is very typical for chronic vascular rejection. (6) The endothelial cell nuclei are characteristically enlarged, hyperchromatic, and slightly polymorphic. These histologic features help to establish a specific diagnosis of sclerosing transplant vasculopathy.

Chronic vascular rejection is the scarring stage of early or acute rejection episodes involving the arterial tree (i.e., transplant endarteritis; see Question 10). Persistent "smoldering" transplant endarteritis can evolve into sclerosing transplant vasculopathy within a few weeks.

The case illustrated here represents cardiac allograft vasculopathy, which is a major cause for morbidity and mortality risks after heart transplantation. Intimal sclerosis in the coronary arteries of heart allografts can be aggravated further by hypertension, hyperlipidemia, and diabetes mellitus. Because endomyocardial surveillance biopsies performed after heart transplantation do not include larger arteries (in contrast to renal allograft biopsies), transplant endarteritis and sclerosing transplant vasculopathies in coronary arteries often remain clinically undetected for long periods.

Billingham ME: Chronic rejection in human allografts. In Orosz CG, Sedmak DD, Ferguson RM (eds): *Transplant Vascular Sclerosis.* Austin: Springer Verlag/RG Landes, 1995.

Mihatsch MJ, Nickeleit V, Gudat F: Morphologic criteria of chronic renal allograft rejection. *Transplant Proc* 1999;31(1-2):1295-1297.

Vassalli G, Gallino A, Weis M, et al: Alloimmunity and nonimmunologic risk factors in cardiac allograft vasculopathy. *Eur Heart J* 2003;24(13):1180-1188.

13. b. The presence of purpura, marked thrombocytopenia, and coagulation abnormalities in the setting of sepsis supports a diagnosis of DIC. DIC covers the continuum of events that occur in the coagulation pathway. Initially, there is uncontrolled activation of clotting factors in the blood vessels, causing clotting of blood throughout the whole body. This clotting depletes the body of platelets and coagulation factors and results in a paradoxic increased risk of bleeding (hemorrhaging). Patients with DIC have a loss of balance between the clot-forming activity of thrombin (enzyme that causes blood to clot) and the clot-lysing activity of plasmin (enzyme that dissolves blood clots).

In addition to bleeding, common manifestations of DIC include thromboembolism and dysfunction of the kidneys, liver, lungs, and central nervous system. The diagnosis of DIC is suggested by the history (i.e., presence of sepsis, trauma, malignancy), the clinical presentation with bleeding, moderate to severe thrombocytopenia ($<100,000/\mu L$), and the presence of microangiopathic changes on the peripheral blood smear. DIC is not a specific diagnosis, and its presence always indicates another underlying disease.

Levi M, Schultsz M, van der Poll T: Infection and inflammation as a risk factor for thrombosis. *Semin Thromb Hemost* 2012;38(5):506-514.

Levi M, ten Cate H: Disseminated intravascular coagulation. *N Engl J Med* 1999;341(8):586-592.

Levi M, van der Poll T: Inflammation and coagulation. *Crit Care Med* 2010;38(2 Suppl):S26-S34.

14. b. Hypocomplementemic urticarial vasculitis syndrome is recognized as a specific autoimmune disorder involving 6 or more months of urticaria, with hypocomplementemia, in the presence of various systemic findings. Leukocytoclasis, or fragmentation of leukocytes with nuclear debris, and fibrinoid deposits are important histopathologic findings that represent direct signs of vessel damage. In most patients, immunofluorescence reveals deposits of immunoglobulins, complement, or fibrin around blood vessels. The diagnosis requires the presence of urticaria with leukocytoclastic vasculitis on skin biopsy specimen.

Glomerulonephritis, arthritis, obstructive pulmonary disease, and ocular inflammation are common. Arthralgias or arthritis occurs in 50% to 75% of patients. Gastrointestinal manifestations occur in 35% of patients, including abdominal pain, nausea, vomiting, and diarrhea. Proteinuria or hematuria occurs in 20% to 30% of patients. Glomerular lesions include type I membranoproliferative glomerulonephritis, proliferative glomerulonephritis, and focal necrotizing glomerulonephritis.

IgG autoantibodies to the collagenlike region of C1q (anti-C1q) are usually present and may play a role in pathogenesis. Hypocomplementemia appears to be secondary to classical complement pathway activation with reduced C1, C2, C4, and C3. The pathophysiology is believed to involve the deposition of immune complexes in vessel walls, complement activation, and mast cell degranulation secondary to C3a and C5a with resultant urticaria. Low-titer antinuclear antibodies, rheumatoid factor, lupus anticoagulant, and cryoglobulins may be detected.

Jara LJ, Navarro C, Medina G, et al: Hypocomplementemic urticarial vasculitis syndrome. *Curr Rheumatol Rep* 2009;11(6):410-415.

Kallenberg CG: Anti-C1q autoantibodies. *Autoimmun Rev* 2008;7(8):612-615.

Ozen S: The "other" vasculitis syndromes and kidney involvement. *Pediatr Nephrol* 2010;25(9):1633-1639.

15. c. Kawasaki disease is a vasculitis that affects medium-sized and sometimes small arteries with a predilection for the coronary arteries. The presence of fevers of unknown origin in a child is another important diagnostic clue. GCA affects patients 50 years old and older and is not associated with a predilection for affecting coronary arteries. Although ANCA-associated vasculitis rarely can affect medium vessels, the absence of small vessel involvement in this case would not support this diagnosis. TMA is not characterized by transmural vessel wall inflammation. The classic findings are endothelial injury leading to mucoid swelling and expansion of the endothelium with associated fragmented red blood cells in the vessel wall sometimes accompanied by thrombi in the vessel lumen. The necrotizing vasculitis seen in PAN can mimic Kawasaki disease, but in a child, the diagnosis of Kawasaki disease should always be entertained first over PAN because of the therapeutic differences in treating these entities.

Alexoudi I, Kanakis M, Kapsimali V, et al: Kawasaki disease: current aspects on aetiopathogenesis and therapeutic management. *Autoimmun Rev* 2011;10(9):544-547.

Gerding R: Kawasaki disease: a review. *J Pediatr Health Care* 2011;25(6):379-387.

Takahashi K, Oharaseki T, Yokouchi Y: Pathogenesis of Kawasaki disease. *Clin Exp Immunol* 2011;164(Suppl 1):20-22.

16. c. The diagnosis of TTP is made on clinical grounds from both clinical and laboratory findings. Clinical features required for the diagnosis of TTP are the presence of microangiopathic hemolytic anemia and thrombocytopenia. The presence of both of these features is sufficient to institute plasma exchange therapy. The severity of these abnormalities reflects the extent of the microvascular aggregation of platelets. Fragmented red blood cells (schistocytes) are produced as blood flows through turbulent areas of the microcirculation that are partially occluded by platelet aggregates. This process causes microangiopathic hemolytic anemia. Clinical features that may be present in some patients with TTP but that are not required for a diagnosis include acute renal insufficiency of varying severity, neurologic abnormalities, and fever. Microvascular thrombi occur in most organs in patients with TTP and consist of platelet aggregates with little to no fibrin; there is no perivascular inflammation. Assays for ADAMTS13, the von Willebrand factor (vWF) cleaving protease, and its inhibitor are not always available, and even if available, results may not be known for days, well beyond the time when a decision must be made to institute plasma exchange therapy. In addition, assay techniques for ADAMTS13 are not completely standardized and can yield different or inconsistent results between laboratories.

George JN: Clinical practice. Thrombotic thrombocytopenic purpura. *N Engl J Med* 2006;354(18):1927-1935.
Sadler JE: Von Willebrand factor, ADAMTS13, and thrombotic thrombocytopenic purpura. *Blood* 2008;112(1):11-18.
Tsai HM: Advances in the pathogenesis, diagnosis, and treatment of thrombotic thrombocytopenic purpura. *J Am Soc Nephrol* 2003;14(4):1072-1081.

17. c. In TTP, intravascular platelet aggregation and formation of platelet-rich thrombi impair the microcirculation. Platelet-rich thrombi in the microvasculature lead to the triad of TTP: thrombocytopenia, microangiopathic hemolytic anemia, and fluctuating neurologic dysfunction. Elevated activated platelet aggregates expressing activation marker CD62p are observed in TTP and correlate well with the clinical course of the disease.

The thrombi in TTP consist primarily of vWF and platelets. Advances in recent years have transformed TTP from a mystery to a disease that can be mostly explained based on the deficiency of a metalloprotease, ADAMTS13. In the circulation, endothelial vWF polymer is converted to plasma multimers by ADAMTS13. The physiologic role of ADAMTS13 is to prevent intravascular platelet thrombosis. Deficiency of ADAMTS13 causes vWF-platelet aggregation and formation of thrombi in the arterioles and capillaries characteristic of TTP. The presence of ADAMTS13 inhibitors (e.g., autoantibodies) or genetic mutations in patients with TTP has been repeatedly demonstrated in many studies from different parts of the world.

Levy GG, Nichols WC, Lian EC, et al: Mutations in a member of the ADAMTS gene family cause thrombotic thrombocytopenic purpura. *Nature* 2001;413(6855):488-494.
Tsai HM: Pathophysiology of thrombotic thrombocytopenic purpura. *Int J Hematol* 2010;91(1):1-19.
Tsai HM, Lian EC: Antibodies to von Willebrand factor-cleaving protease in acute thrombotic thrombocytopenic purpura. *N Engl J Med* 1998;339(22):1585-1594.

18. c. Monoclonal immunoglobulin deposition disease (light chain deposition disease) is defined as the deposition of complete or partial monoclonal immunoglobulin components along basement membranes, primarily affecting renal tubules, glomerular capillaries, and arteries. By light microscopy, a nodular expansion of glomerular mesangial regions, similar to Kimmelstiel-Wilson nodules, is most characteristic, seen in 60% of cases. Often, glomeruli are diffusely and globally affected, and the mesangial nodules are of similar sizes. Tubular basement membranes are typically thickened, in particular along nonatrophic tubules. In addition, arterioles and small arteries can show wall hypertrophy and dense waxy deposits. The disease process can spare glomeruli and can be limited to the tubulointerstitial and vascular compartment, reported in 10% to 24% of cases in most series.

The vascular monoclonal immunoglobulin accumulations occasionally can be massive, leading to individual smooth muscle cell necrosis and mimicking vascular amyloid deposits by standard light microscopic examination. By definition, Congo red staining for amyloid is negative. The findings on immunofluorescence microscopy are so characteristic in most cases as to be virtually diagnostic. In vessels, there is basal lamina staining around individual myocytes, producing a "spider web" pattern of positivity in the media. Most cases demonstrate monoclonal kappa light chains (κ:λ ratio 9:1). The detection of monoclonal light chains in the serum or urine increases the probability that a patient has monoclonal immunoglobulin deposition disease, but it does not accurately predict disease.

Lin J, Markowitz GS, Valeri AM, et al: Renal monoclonal immunoglobulin deposition disease: the disease spectrum. *J Am Soc Nephrol* 2001;12(7):1482-1492.
Markowitz GS: Dysproteinemia and the kidney. *Adv Anat Pathol* 2004;11(1):49-63.
Strom EH, Fogazzi GB, Banfi G, et al: Light chain deposition disease of the kidney—morphological aspects in 24 patients. *Virchow Arch* 1994;425(3):271-280.

19. b. Sarcoidosis is a multisystem granulomatous disorder of unknown cause that affects individuals worldwide and is characterized pathologically by the presence of noncaseating granulomas in involved organs. It typically affects young African American adults and initially manifests with one or more of the following abnormalities: bilateral hilar adenopathy, pulmonary reticular opacities, skin lesions, joint lesions, or eye lesions. The presence of noncaseating granulomas encroaching and invading the wall of small blood vessels in the kidney with focal fibrinoid necrosis are features of a granulomatous small vessel vasculitis that can be seen in approximately 5% of patients with sarcoidosis.

Two patterns of vasculopathy in sarcoidosis are described by Churg. In one pattern, granulomas compress and destroy the wall and elastic laminae of blood vessels without necrosis. The second pattern, termed *necrotizing sarcoid granulomatosis*, is characterized by confluent granulomas with variable degrees of necrosis. In the case scenario presented, the absence of glomerular involvement and the negative serologic test results rule out ANCA-associated vasculitis, systemic lupus erythematosus, and related autoimmune diseases.

Negative immunohistochemical stains for fungal and mycobacterial organisms should be performed to rule out an infectious cause for granulomatous interstitial nephritis and vasculitis, especially before instituting therapy with corticosteroids.

Agrawal V, Crisi GM, D'Agati VD, et al: Renal sarcoidosis presenting as acute kidney injury with granulomatous interstitial nephritis and vasculitis. *Am J Kidney Dis* 2012; 59(2):303-308.

Kwong T, Valderrama E, Paley C, et al: Systemic necrotizing vasculitis associated with childhood sarcoidosis. *Semin Arthritis Rheum* 1994;23(6):388-395.

Rosen Y, Moon S, Huang CT, et al: Granulomatous pulmonary angiitis in sarcoidosis. *Arch Pathol Lab Med* 1977;101(4): 170-174.

20. b. Thromboangiitis obliterans (Buerger disease) represents an occlusive inflammatory disorder of medium and small arteries and veins in the distal arms and legs. The disease is more common in Asia, Middle East, and Mediterranean areas. Patients are young, usually between 25 and 40 years of age. The disease is strongly associated with the use of tobacco products. Patients are predominantly young smokers who present with distal extremity ischemia, ischemic digital ulcers, or digital gangrene.

On imaging studies, features suggestive of thromboangiitis obliterans include lack of atherosclerosis, no proximal source for embolism, involvement of small and medium arteries and veins, segmental vascular occlusion, and collateralization around areas of occlusion. A biopsy specimen of a subcutaneous nodule or superficial thrombophlebitis showing typical acute phase changes as illustrated in this case provides a definitive diagnosis. The major diagnostic findings on biopsy include the presence of a vasoocclusive inflammatory thrombus that lacks fibrinoid necrosis and does not involve the vessel wall, with an intact internal elastic lamina.

Mills JL Sr: Buerger's disease in the 21st century: diagnosis, clinical features, and therapy. *Semin Vasc Surg* 2003;16(3):179-189.

Puéchal X, Fiessinger JN: Thromboangiitis obliterans or Buerger's disease: challenges for the rheumatologist. *Rheumatology (Oxford)* 2007;46(2):192-199.

Subhashree AR, Gopalan R, Krishnan KB, et al: Buerger's disease: clinical and histomorphological study. *Indian J Pathol Microbiol* 2006;49(4):540-542.

21. b. Studies of patients with pulmonary renal vasculitic syndrome have shown that ANCA disease accounts for approximately 55% of cases and anti-GBM accounts for 8%, and 25% to 30% of patients with anti-GBM antibodies are also positive for ANCA. The combined clinical presentation of acute glomerulonephritis (hematuria, red blood cell casts, and renal insufficiency) with pulmonary (alveolar) hemorrhage (as manifested by hemoptysis or pulmonary infiltrates) is characteristic of anti-GBM antibodies in Goodpasture syndrome. However, these findings are not diagnostic of anti-GBM antibody disease because they can be seen in many other disorders, such as systemic vasculitis, lupus, and other forms of acute glomerulonephritis.

Jennette JC: Nomenclature and classification of vasculitis: lessons learned from granulomatosis with polyangiitis (Wegener's granulomatosis). *Clin Exp Immunol* 2011;164(Suppl 1):7-10.

Jennings CA, King TE Jr, Tuder R, et al: Diffuse alveolar hemorrhage with underlying isolated, pauciimmune pulmonary capillaritis. *Am J Respir Crit Care Med* 1997; 155(3):1101-1109.

Watts RA, Scott DG: Recent developments in the classification and assessment of vasculitis. *Best Pract Res Clin Rheumatol* 2009; 23(3):429-443.

22. TRUE. Arteriolar fibrinoid necrosis and TMA can be seen in cases of malignant hypertension and are caused by the elevated blood pressure. With increasingly severe hypertension, autoregulation eventually fails, and the increase in pressure in the arterioles and capillaries leads to damage to the vascular wall. Disruption of the vascular endothelium allows plasma constituents (including fibrinoid material) to enter the vascular wall, narrowing or obliterating the vascular lumen. The injury is related to the accumulation of various plasma substances, especially fibrinogen, within the vessel walls owing to the damaged endothelium. Fibrin thrombi also may be seen and result from the release of vWF into the circulation from endothelial cell injury leading to increased adhesion of platelets to the endothelium. It has been suggested that factors other than the level of blood pressure, particularly activation of the renin-angiotensin system, may contribute to the development of fibrinoid necrosis.

Malignant nephrosclerosis leads to acute kidney injury, hematuria, and proteinuria. Renal biopsy reveals fibrinoid necrosis in the arterioles and capillaries, producing histologic changes that are indistinguishable from TMA. Fibrinoid necrosis eventually leads to glomerular ischemia and activation of the renin-angiotensin system, possibly resulting in exacerbation of hypertension.

Frank C, Werber D, Cramer JP, et al; HUS Investigation Team: Epidemic profile of shiga-toxin-producing Escherichia coli O104:H4 outbreak in Germany. *N Engl J Med* 2011;365(19): 1771-1780.

Liszewski MK, Atkinson JP: Too much of a good thing at the site of tissue injury: the instructive example of the complement system predisposing to thrombotic microangiopathy. *Hematology Am Soc Hematol Educ Program* 2011;2011:9-14.

Moake JL: Thrombotic microangiopathies. *N Engl J Med* 2002; 347(8):589-600.

23. a. Kawasaki disease (formerly called *mucocutaneous lymph node syndrome*) is one of the most common cryptogenic vasculitides of childhood (besides HSP caused by IgA deposits). Boys are affected 50% more often than girls. Approximately 90% of cases occur in children younger than 5 years, with an average age of about 2 years. Occurrence beyond late childhood is extremely rare.

Fever is probably the most consistent clinical manifestation of Kawasaki disease, and temperature remains greater than 38.5° C during most of the illness. Bilateral nonexudative conjunctivitis is present in more than 90% of children. Despite the name *mucocutaneous lymph node syndrome*, cervical lymphadenopathy is the least consistent feature of Kawasaki disease, being absent in approximately half of affected patients. When present, it typically involves the anterior cervical lymph node chain. With progression of the disease, mucositis becomes clinically evident. Cracked red lips and a strawberry tongue are characteristic manifestations; the latter is due to sloughing of filiform papillae and denuding of inflamed glossal tissue.

The clinical diagnosis of Kawasaki disease should be considered in *all* children with prolonged unexplained fever, irritability, and laboratory signs of inflammation especially when accompanied by a mucositis. Inflammation in Kawasaki disease often also involves medium arteries, in particular coronary arteries. Arteritis is characterized by segmental mural necrosis with infiltration by polymorphonuclear leukocytes and accumulation of karyorrhectic debris that is much more pronounced than seen with PAN or ANCA-associated vasculitides. Mononuclear leukocytes (i.e., lymphocytes and histiocytes) predominate in older sclerosing lesions. Immunoglobulins are not detected in inflamed vessel walls, and ANCA tests are unrevealing. In Kawasaki disease, pseudoaneurysms can develop secondary to the segmental destruction of arterial walls, typically in coronary arteries. Coronary arteritis can lead to significant morbidity and mortality rates secondary to heart failure, myocardial infarction, and arrhythmias. If left untreated, 25% of patients with Kawasaki disease develop coronary artery aneurysms; this number decreases to approximately 4% with adequate therapy. An expeditious diagnosis is critical to initiate therapy, commonly with aspirin and intravenous immunoglobulin.

According to the Chapel Hill consensus conference definitions, Kawasaki disease is defined as a vasculitis of medium-sized vessels (which also includes PAN). Medium-sized vessel vasculitides are characterized by predominant involvement of main visceral arteries, such as the coronary, hepatic, renal, and mesenteric arteries and their branches. Pulmonary arteries are rarely affected. Immunoglobulins are not detected in the inflamed vessel walls, and ANCA testing typically shows normal titer levels. However, the medium-caliber vessels can potentially be involved by large vessel vasculitides (i.e., granulomatous vasculitides including GCA or Takayasu arteritis) or small vessel vasculitides (i.e., ANCA-associated necrotizing small vessel vasculitides not associated with the deposition of immune complex deposits). Close clinicopathologic correlation is required to establish a definitive diagnosis (including the sex and age of the patient, clinical symptoms, ANCA status).

Brunner J, Feldman BM, Tyrrell PN, et al: Takayasu arteritis in children and adolescents. *Rheumatology (Oxford)* 2010;49(10): 1806-1814.

Gerding R: Kawasaki disease: a review. *J Pediatr Health Care* 2011; 25(6):379-387.

Takahashi K, Oharaseki T, Yokouchi Y: Pathogenesis of Kawasaki disease. *Clin Exp Immunol* 2011;164(Suppl 1):20-22.

24. FALSE. According to the Chapel Hill Consensus Conference, HSP is a distinct variant of small vessel vasculitis that is due to an immune complex (mainly IgA)–mediated vascular inflammatory disease process. ANCA titers are normal in HSP, and so HSP is not a general synonym for all forms of small vessel vasculitides. HSP is most often diagnosed in young children presenting with vasculitis-induced abdominal pain, palpable purpura of the lower extremities, and arthralgias. Many patients also have an IgA-associated glomerulonephritis.

In children, the disease is commonly self-limiting, and the outcome is good. If biopsy specimens are obtained, HSP is characterized in the skin by a leukocytoclastic vasculitis and in the kidneys by a mesangioproliferative glomerulonephritis. Marked vascular wall necrosis or a crescentic glomerulonephritis is typically absent. Immunofluorescence microscopy can show IgA deposits in affected vascular walls and in glomeruli in the mesangial regions.

Brogan P, Eleftheriou D, Dillon M: Small vessel vasculitis. *Pediatr Nephrol* 2010;25(6):1025-1035.

González LM, Janniger CK, Schwartz RA: Pediatric Henoch-Schönlein purpura. *Int J Dermatol* 2009;48(11):1157-1165.

Saulsbury FT: Henoch-Schönlein purpura. *Curr Opin Rheumatol* 2010;22(5):598-602.

25. c. Segmental mediolytic arteriopathy, also called *segmental arterial mediolysis* and *segmental mediolytic arteritis*, is a rare nonatherosclerotic and nonvasculitic arteriopathy of unknown cause. It is characterized by degeneration of the medial layer of the artery wall.

Chan RJ, Goodman TA, Aretz TH, et al: Segmental mediolytic arteriopathy of the splenic and hepatic arteries mimicking systemic necrotizing vasculitis. *Arthritis Rheum* 1998;41(5): 935-938.

Sakata N, Takebayashi S, Shimizu K, et al: A case of segmental mediolytic arteriopathy involving both intracranial and intraabdominal arteries. *Pathol Res Pract* 2002;198(7):493-497; discussion 499-500.

Takagi C, Ashizawa N, Eishi K, et al: Segmental mediolytic arteriopathy involving celiac to splenic and left renal arteries. *Intern Med* 2003;42(9):818-823.

26. a. Vascular Ehlers-Danlos syndrome is an autosomal-dominant connective tissue disorder, which earned its designation as the vascular type because it can manifest with catastrophic arterial, gastrointestinal, or uterine rupture. The diagnosis is confirmed by identification of mutations in the type III procollagen gene. The incidence is estimated at 4 per 1 million. The only congenital abnormalities associated with the cohort were a history of talipes equinovarus and congenital dislocation of the hip.

Marfan syndrome is caused by various mutations in the *FBN1* gene. *FBN1* mutations have been identified in more than 90% of patients with Marfan syndrome. Abnormalities in TGF-β 1 and 2 lead to Loeys-Dietz syndrome, which is a more aggressive vascular disease than Marfan syndrome.

Badawi RA, Brent LH, Feinstein DE: Mimics of vasculitis: vascular Ehlers-Danlos syndrome masquerading as polyarteritis nodosa. *J Rheumatol* 2009;36(8):1845-1847.

Meyer DM, Fry RE, Snyder WH 3rd, et al: Multiple nonatherosclerotic aneurysms unrelated to a clinical syndrome. *Am Surg* 1990;56(9):523-529.

Millar AJ, Gilbert RD, Brown RA, et al: Abdominal aortic aneurysms in children. *J Pediatr Surg* 1996;31(12):1624-1628.

27. b. The finding of massive, pale-staining, and amorphous protein deposits in vascular walls largely replacing medial smooth muscle cells is characteristic of amyloidosis. Amyloidosis comprises a group of diseases characterized by extracellular deposition of β sheet fibrils. In the systemic forms, the amyloid causes progressive organ dysfunction leading to death. More than 20 proteins capable of amyloid formation have been identified, including immunoglobulin light chains in primary systemic amyloidosis (AL), heavy chain (AH), amyloid A in secondary amyloidosis (AA), β_2-microglobulin in dialysis-associated arthropathy (Aβ2M), and amyloid β protein (Aβ) in Alzheimer disease and Down syndrome. There are also hereditary forms that include transthyretin (ATTR), apolipoprotein A-I (AApoAI) and A-II (AApoAII), gelsolin (AGel), lysozyme (ALys), fibrinogen A-alpha chain (AFib), and others. Another amyloidogenic protein is leukocyte chemotactic factor 2 (LECT2).

In Western countries, most cases with systemic or generalized amyloid deposits (involving the kidneys) are due to the deposition of AL-amyloid, mostly secondary to the secretion of abnormal lambda light chains in the setting of a plasmacytoma. This diagnosis is likely in the presented case scenario because the patient showed lytic bone lesions. Although patients with AL amyloidosis have a monoclonal gammopathy, not all patients with renal disease and a monoclonal gammopathy have AL amyloidosis. The clinical manifestations of renal disease vary with the site of involvement. The most common presentation of AL and AA amyloidosis is heavy proteinuria, which is associated with glomerular deposits. Patients with vascular deposits present with slowly progressive chronic kidney disease with less proteinuria secondary to less glomerular involvement.

Nasr SH, Valeri AM, Sethi S, et al: Clinicopathologic correlations in multiple myeloma: a case series of 190 patients with kidney biopsies. *Am J Kidney Dis* 2012;59(6):786-794.

Picken MM: Amyloidosis—where are we now and where are we heading? *Arch Pathol Lab Med* 2010;134(4):545-551.

Sen S, Sarsik B: A proposed histopathologic classification, scoring, and grading system for renal amyloidosis. *Arch Pathol Lab Med* 2010;134(4):532-544.

28. a. Smooth muscle cells and elastic elements of the blood vessel wall are gradually replaced by amyloid deposition potentially leading to blood vessel wall weakening and formation of microaneurysms and subsequent hemorrhage. Periorbital bleeding ("raccoon eyes") and cerebral hemorrhage are the most common manifestations. Instances of pulmonary infarction, diffuse alveolar hemorrhage, and hemoptysis secondary to pulmonary amyloidosis have been described.

Ischemic stroke may be the initial manifestation of amyloidosis. Risk factors for stroke are similar to the risk factors in the general population and include atrial fibrillation, hyperlipidemia, hypertension, and diabetes mellitus. Subcutaneous arteries are often affected in the setting of systemic amyloidosis, and deep subcutaneous abdominal fat aspirates (including Congo red incubations) can be helpful for establishing a diagnosis.

Herrera GA, Joseph L, Gu X, et al: Renal pathologic spectrum in an autopsy series of patients with plasma cell dyscrasia. *Arch Pathol Lab Med* 2004;128(8):875-879.

Markowitz GS: Dysproteinemia and the kidney. *Adv Anat Pathol* 2004;11(1):49-63.

Rocken C, Sletten K: Amyloid in surgical pathology. *Virchows Arch* 2003;443(1):3-16.

29. d. Laboratory findings in this patient that support a diagnosis of cryoglobulinemic vasculitis include hypocomplementemia with low levels of C4 and the presence of rheumatoid factor without antinuclear antibodies. The negative test result for cryoglobulins is puzzling.

HSP typically affects children but occasionally can be seen in adults. Immunofluorescence staining on the skin biopsy specimen did not demonstrate IgA-dominant immune complex deposits, and most cases of HSP show normal complement levels. In most cases, microscopic polyangiitis would demonstrate positive ANCA serologic tests, normal serum complement levels, and a paucity of immune deposition in the skin biopsy specimen. Also, the presence of a diffuse proliferative glomerulonephritis is not seen in microscopic polyangiitis, which in most cases exhibits a necrotizing and crescentic glomerulonephritis. Although the leukocytoclastic vasculitis and immunofluorescence findings of IgG, IgM, and C3 vascular deposits are typically seen (see Question 14), there is no clinical history of urticaria in this patient.

Jennette JC, Falk RJ: Small-vessel vasculitis. *N Engl J Med* 1997; 337(21):1512-1523.

Kay J, McCluskey RT: Case 31-2005. A 60-year-old man with skin lesions and renal insufficiency. *N Engl J Med* 2005;353(15): 1605-1613.

Lamprecht P, Gause A, Gross WL: Cryoglobulinemic vasculitis. *Arthritis Rheum* 1999;42(12):2507-2516.

30. c. A clue to identification of levamisole-contaminated cocaine-induced vasculopathy is discordance between the patterns of ANCA observed by indirect immunofluorescence and the specific antigenic targets observed by enzyme-linked immunosorbent assay (ELISA) testing. Although the combination of purpura and ANCA positivity suggests a diagnosis of microscopic polyangiitis (MPA), several features clearly distinguish this syndrome from MPA. The purpura is retiform and has a distribution (over the ears and zygomatic arch) that is different from the palpable purpura seen in ANCA-associated vasculitis and other small vessel vasculitides. In contrast to patients with MPA, these patients often are neutropenic. The magnitude of the p-ANCA positivity as assessed by immunofluorescence is unusually high for MPA and is discordant with the relatively low levels of antibodies to myeloperoxidase (MPO) detected by ELISA. Finally, despite the presence of ANCAs, the predominant histopathologic finding is small vessel thrombosis rather than classic leukocytoclastic vasculitis. Intravascular thrombosis, neutropenia, and positive serologic tests for various autoantibodies do not support a diagnosis of cryoglobulinemic vasculitis. HSP occurs predominantly in children and is associated with an IgA-dominant leukocytoclastic vasculitis and not small vessel thrombosis. Also, neutropenia is not a feature seen with this lesion.

Graf J, Lynch K, Yeh CL, et al: Purpura, cutaneous necrosis, and antineutrophil cytoplasmic antibodies associated with levamisole-adulterated cocaine. *Arthritis Rheum* 2011;63(12): 3998-4001.

Gulati S, Donato AA: Lupus anticoagulant and ANCA associated thrombotic vasculopathy due to cocaine contaminated with levamisole: a case report and review of the literature. *J Thromb Thrombolysis* 2012;34(1):7-10.

Khan TA, Cuchacovich R, Espinoza LR, et al: Vasculopathy, hematological, and immune abnormalities associated with levamisole-contaminated cocaine use. *Semin Arthritis Rheum* 2011;41(3):445-454.

CHAPTER 3

PULMONARY PATHOLOGY

Alain C. Borczuk

QUESTIONS

Questions 1-18 refer to a photo or photomicrograph.

1. Which is TRUE regarding the process in this image?
   a. An indolent process causing a chronic mass lesion
   b. An angioinvasive process, associated with diabetes mellitus
   c. A low-grade tumor of endothelial origin
   d. A high-grade tumor of adipocytic origin
   e. Provides evidence in support of aspiration pneumonia

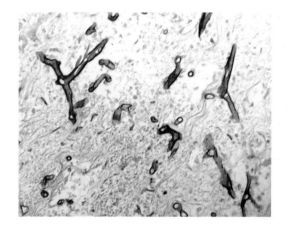

2. These images are from a young woman with pneumothorax and cystic lung disease on computed tomography (CT) scan. Which is TRUE regarding this disease process?
   a. The process is frequently associated with cigarette smoking.
   b. It is a manifestation of acute leukemia called a chloroma or granulocytic sarcoma.
   c. It is associated with an HMB45 positive cell population and in some patients with tuberous sclerosis.
   d. It is progressive and in the majority of cases rapidly results in organ failure requiring transplantation.
   e. It is the result of indolent infection, an acquired macrophage dysfunction.

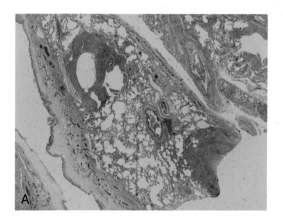

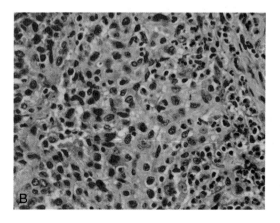

3. The structure in this image is involved in what process?
    a. Bronchiolitis
    b. Lipoid pneumonia
    c. Organizing thrombus
    d. Organizing pneumonia
    e. Vasculitis

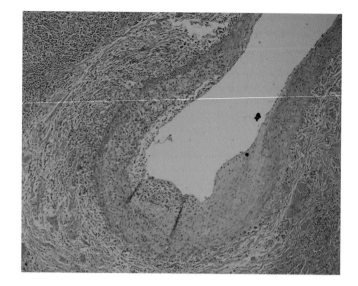

4. Given the histologic appearance of this tumor, which of the following is the MOST likely immunohistochemistry stain on the right?
    a. Smooth muscle actin
    b. Cytokeratin (CK)
    c. CD34
    d. CD117
    e. CD31

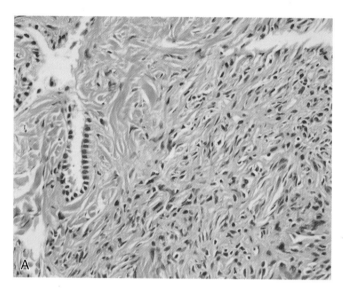

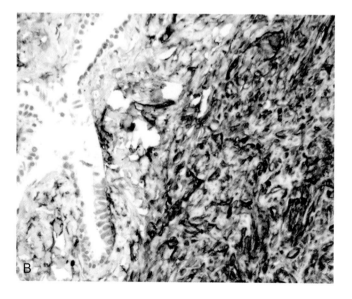

5. Given the distribution of the process in this lung biopsy, what is the MOST likely diagnosis?
   a. Miliary tuberculosis
   b. Extrinsic allergic alveolitis (EAA)
   c. Mesothelioma
   d. Lymphoma
   e. Bronchiectasis

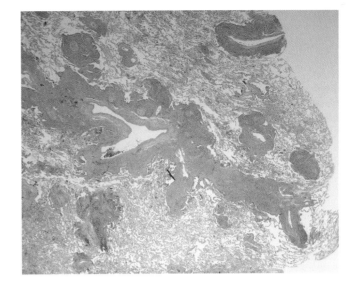

6. Which of the following BEST describes the process shown in this gross image?
   a. It is typically associated with uterine enlargement.
   b. It is typically associated with *Aspergillus*.
   c. It is a high-grade pediatric tumor, with extensive pleural involvement.
   d. It is honeycomb lung and is the typical pattern of usual interstitial pneumonia (UPI).
   e. It is a consolidative type of lung adenocarcinoma.

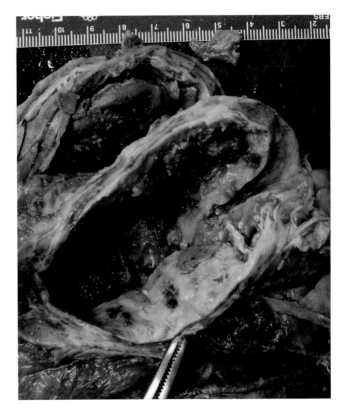

7. A 45-year-old woman presents with worsening dyspnea over 6 months. Which following statement is the BEST diagnosis based on the image of her open lung biopsy?
   a. UPI
   b. Sarcoidosis
   c. Lymphocytic interstitial pneumonia
   d. Nonspecific interstitial pneumonia
   e. Desquamative interstitial pneumonia

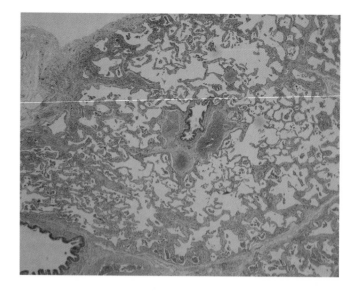

8. In the image, what is the histologic feature shown?
   a. Granuloma
   b. Fibroblastic focus
   c. Organizing pneumonia
   d. Follicular bronchiolitis
   e. Vasculitis

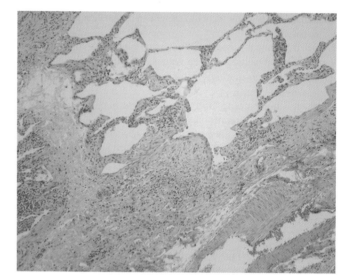

9. This patient had multiple circumscribed fibrotic nodules with the histologic appearance shown. Which statement describes the features of this diagnosis?
   a. It is of epithelial origin and is thyroid transcription factor positive by immunohistochemistry.
   b. It is of dendritic cell origin and is caused by human herpesvirus 8.
   c. It is a myofibroblastic tumor with smooth muscle actin positive cells.
   d. It is of endothelial origin and CD31 positive.
   e. It is a carcinoma of salivary gland origin and is p63 positive.

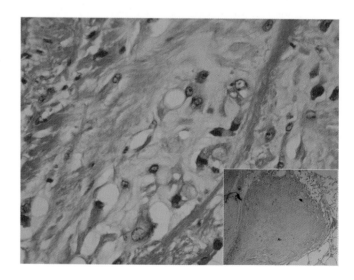

10. Which of the following has NOT been described in association with this histologic finding?
    a. Cirrhosis
    b. Congenital heart disease
    c. Mutation in *BMPR2*
    d. Cigarette smoking
    e. Certain medications, specifically diet pills

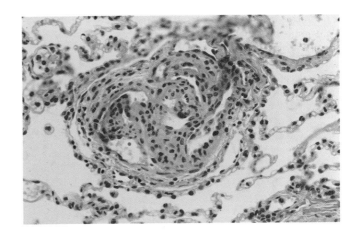

11. This tumor was removed as a 2.2-cm peripheral nodule. Which choice is TRUE regarding the tumor in this photomicrograph?
    a. These tumors are deceptively bland but virtually always reflect metastatic disease to the lungs.
    b. These tumors are chromogranin and synaptophysin positive.
    c. This tumor is metastatic adenocarcinoma from the colon.
    d. Malignancy in these tumors is determined by histologic pattern alone, independent of size and mitotic rate.
    e. This tumor is of meningothelial origin.

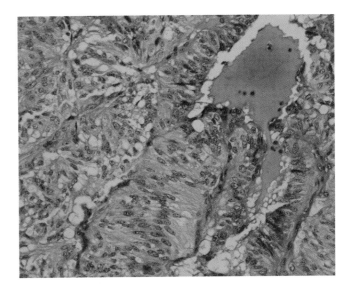

12. Which of the following is a TRUE statement regarding the adenocarcinoma shown in the photomicrograph?
    a. This type of adenocarcinoma is frequently (80% to 90%) associated with mutations in the *KRAS* oncogene.
    b. This type of adenocarcinoma is now considered adenocarcinoma in situ.
    c. This type of adenocarcinoma is associated with EML4-ALK translocations.
    d. Although tumors with epidermal growth factor receptor (EGFR) mutations overall show mutual exclusivity with *KRAS* mutation, EGFR mutated tumors frequently harbor EML4-ALK translocations.
    e. Although rare in the lung, these tumors harbor MECT1-MAML2 translocations.

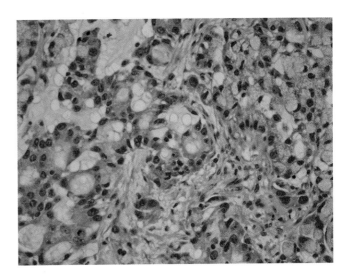

13. Which would be the expected pattern of immunohistochemistry for this malignancy?

   a. Thyroid transcription factor 1 (TTF-1) nuclear reactivity, CK7 positive, and CK20 positive
   b. Strong and diffuse nuclear p63 immunoreactivity, CK5/6 reactivity, and negative TTF-1 reactivity
   c. Weak focal p63 reactivity, TTF-1 nuclear reactivity, CK7 negative
   d. Calretinin positive, CK5/6 positive, WT1 positive, p63 negative
   e. TTF-1 nuclear reactivity, dotlike CK, weak synaptophysin, p63 negative

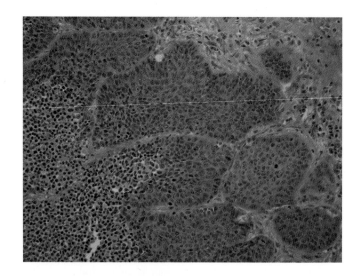

14. Which of these statements is TRUE regarding the process in this image?

   a. This pattern is commonly seen as a metaplastic phenomenon.
   b. This growth pattern is indicative of a primary lung tumor.
   c. These proliferations are the result of mutations in epidermal growth factor receptor.
   d. Like other adenocarcinomas, this histologic diagnosis is associated with CK7 and TTF-1 reactivity, but is negative for CK20.
   e. Cells with this histologic appearance in congenital pulmonary airway malformations are preneoplastic.

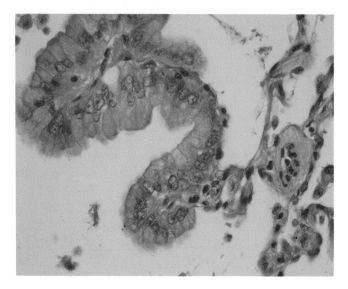

15. Which of the following disease processes will NOT have the histologic appearance shown?
    a. Pigeon breeder's lung
    b. Farmer's lung
    c. Maple bark stripper's disease
    d. Bagassosis
    e. Silo filler's disease

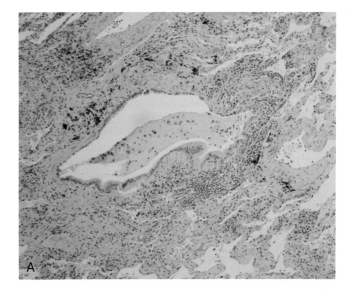

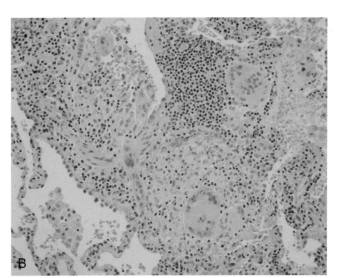

16. A 36-year-old woman has a cystic appearing lung disease on a high-resolution CT scan. The image is a representative field of the biopsy. Of the following list, which would be the MOST helpful immunohistochemistry markers to confirm the diagnosis?
    a. SMA, HMB45
    b. S100, CD1a
    c. CD34, c-kit
    d. S100, Melan A, tyrosinase
    e. CK7 and CK20

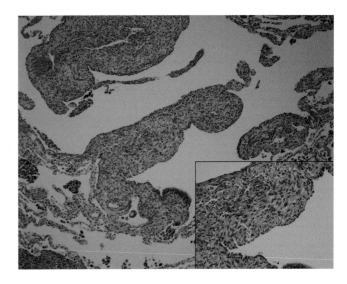

17. A patient has a routine chest x-ray study as part of a physical examination, and is seen to have symmetric hilar lymphadenopathy with mild lung parenchymal abnormalities. A wedge biopsy is performed and a field from that biopsy is shown. Which of the following statements is FALSE regarding this process?

    a. The diagnostic yield of transbronchial biopsy with 4 to 6 pieces is high for this disease.
    b. Special stains for acid-fast bacilli and fungi should be performed and will be negative.
    c. A clinical history of occupational exposures should be obtained.
    d. Pathologically, the process follows lymphatic routes—bronchovascular bundles, pleurae, interlobular septa.
    e. It is generally a self-limiting process and does not progress to lung fibrosis.

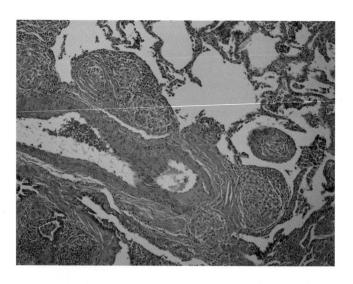

18. Which is TRUE regarding the histologic appearance shown?

    a. It is frequently associated with progressive pulmonary fibrosis.
    b. It is seen in patients with rheumatoid arthritis.
    c. It is a diffuse, nonpatchy disease radiographically.
    d. It is never the cause of a solitary pulmonary nodule.
    e. It is usually the cause of obstructive lung disease.

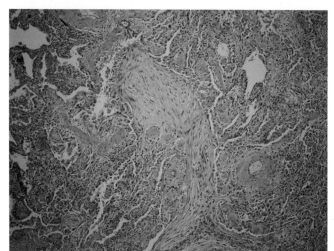

19. Which of the following statements BEST characterizes lymphomatoid granulomatosis?

    a. It is a connective tissue disease causing a vasculitis similar to Wegener granulomatosis and Churg-Strauss syndrome.
    b. It is a B-cell vasculocentric lymphoma, Epstein-Barr virus associated.
    c. It is caused by atypical mycobacteria, but with poorly formed granulomas.
    d. It is a pulmonary reaction to gastrointestinal parasites.
    e. It is a lymphohistiocytic medication reaction with granulomas, associated with sulfa-based medications and anticonvulsants.

20. Which of the following BEST describes pulmonary malakoplakia?

    a. It is granulomatous and most often caused by atypical mycobacteria.
    b. It differs from genitourinary malakoplakia in that Michaelis-Gutmann bodies are absent.
    c. Pulmonary disease can be the result of *Rhodococcus equi* infection.
    d. It is a histiocytic accumulation, and the cells are CD1a positive.
    e. It is not associated with immunosuppression.

21. Which of the following is TRUE regarding rounded atelectasis?

    a. It results from an endobronchial lesion, airway obstruction, and lobar collapse.
    b. Histologically, it represents focal organizing pneumonia.
    c. It occurs in the right middle lobe, anteriorly.
    d. It is seen in patients with asbestos exposure and pleural plaque.
    e. It is associated with tuberous sclerosis.

22. Which of the following represents a CORRECT pairing between parasite and description?

    a. *Strongyloides*—granulomatous and eosinophilic reaction to parasite eggs
    b. *Dirofilaria*—nodular rounded infarct containing nonviable parasite debris
    c. *Paragonimus*—worms pass through lungs without laying eggs causing cough
    d. *Echinococcus*—thin-walled cyst, single layered
    e. *Cryptosporidium*—inside alveolar macrophages

23. Which of the following is TRUE regarding small cell carcinoma?

    a. Most cases show a strong and diffusely membranous pattern of CK staining.
    b. A larger cell population is an unusual finding, seen in less than 5% of cases.

c. Pulmonary small cell carcinoma can be distinguished from small cell carcinomas of other organs by TTF-1 immunoreactivity.

d. The diagnosis is based largely on morphologic appearance, with nuclear molding, salt and pepper chromatin, and high apoptotic/mitotic index.

e. Small cell carcinoma has a poor prognosis because it is chemotherapy resistant.

24. A 50-year-old man has breathing difficulty on exertion and is found to have severe obstructive lung disease. Lung wedge biopsy shows loss of airways, airway occlusion by fibrosis, and airways with fibrosis in their walls. Which of the following statements is of LEAST importance in diagnosing the cause of this process?
    a. The patient had a history of severe adenoviral pneumonia.
    b. The patient received penicillamine therapy for a rheumatologic disease.
    c. The patient has joint disease and a strongly positive rheumatoid factor.
    d. He is a chronic lung transplant patient.
    e. The patient had a history of cigarette and marijuana smoking.

25. Which of the following is TRUE regarding molecular alterations in lung tumors?
    a. Frequent amplifications of the SOX2 gene are seen in mucinous adenocarcinoma.
    b. Amplifications of EGFR do not occur in lung adenocarcinomas that harbor EGFR mutations.
    c. Mutations in β-catenin are associated with well-differentiated fetal type adenocarcinoma.
    d. Mutations in *BRAF* are not seen in cigarette smoking and, therefore, are frequently seen in adenocarcinoma in situ.
    e. Large cell neuroendocrine carcinoma is frequently *KRAS* mutation associated.

26. Which of the following is NOT associated with pulmonary alveolar proteinosis (PAP)?
    a. Infections
    b. Acute inorganic dust exposure

c. Hematologic malignancy
d. Aspiration of mineral oil
e. Experimentally with absence of granulocyte macrophage colony-stimulating factor (GM-CSF)

27. Which of the following is TRUE of pulmonary sclerosing hemangioma?
    a. It is a high-grade endothelial tumor, despite bland histologic findings.
    b. The tumor is typically associated with multiple cutaneous hemangiomas.
    c. The tumor is never associated with multifocality or lymph node involvement.
    d. The growth patterns include papillary, solid, sclerotic, and angiomatoid.
    e. The cells are typically positive for CD31 and CD34, but not D2-40.

28. Which of the following is TRUE of asbestos-related lung disease?
    a. Asbestosis refers to lung fibrosis as associated with ferruginous bodies.
    b. Pleural fibrosis alone can define asbestosis.
    c. Pleural plaques are typically brown from the iron-containing ferruginous bodies.
    d. Asbestos fibers are strongly birefringent on polarized light.
    e. Ferruginous bodies are specific for asbestos exposure.

29. Which statement is TRUE regarding middle lobe syndrome?
    a. It is a congenital lesion, caused by abnormal branching of the middle lobe bronchus.
    b. It is synonymous with sequestration of the lung.
    c. Obstruction of the middle lobe bronchus results in bronchiectasis and inflammation.
    d. It is synonymous with focal organizing pneumonia.
    e. This is a type of adenocarcinoma that causes lobar consolidation that has a predilection for the middle lobe and lingula.

ANSWERS

1. b. Zygomycosis is a rapidly invasive, necrotizing infection, often with angioinvasion. It is associated with acidosis, and is seen in diabetic patients with bouts of diabetic ketoacidosis. Although it is not a common pulmonary infection, when present it is usually acute and angioinvasive and is not the cause of a chronic mass lesion. The structures, because of their branching and empty appearance, can be mistaken for blood vessels, especially on hematoxylin-eosin stain; however, they are not vascular channels and, therefore, are not part of an endothelial neoplasm.

   The structures are fungi, not the vasculature of a myxoid liposarcoma. Some fragmented structures in cases of zygomycosis can resemble foreign material or vegetable matter; however, the regular branching structures are characteristic of fungal hyphae.

   Frater JL, Hall GS, Procop GW: Histologic features of zygomycosis. Emphasis on perineural invasion and fungal morphology. *Arch Pathol Lab Med* 2001;125:375-378.

2. a. Pulmonary Langerhans cell histiocytosis is almost always associated with cigarette smoking, and can be seen in cellular and fibrotic forms. Langerhans cells are positive for S100 and CD1a by immunohistochemistry, and electron microscopy shows characteristic structures known as Birbeck granules. The nodules contain a mixture of smoker's pigmented macrophages, Langerhans cells, and eosinophils. The CT scan findings consist of cystic change, and these cysts can result in pneumothorax.

   Vassallo R, Ryu JH, Colby TV, et al: Pulmonary Langerhans cell histiocytosis. *N Engl J Med* 2000;342:1969-1978.

3. e. The image is an arterial blood vessel with transmural inflammation and segmental necrosis of the wall. Arterial vasculitis in the lung can be secondary to infection, but can be the result of primary vasculitis syndromes, such as Wegener granulomatosis or Churg-Strauss syndrome. Certain connective tissue diseases can also result in

vasculitis. Vasculitis can be associated with geographic necrosis and pulmonary hemorrhage. Polyarteritis nodosa can cause segmental vasculitis, but uncommonly involves the lung.

Bronchiolitis involves bronchioles with inflammation of the wall and peribronchiolar tissue. Lipoid pneumonia is an intraalveolar process characterized by filling with lipid-laden macrophages. The vessel with an organizing thrombus has an intraluminal plug of fibrin and cells or, when resolving, of intimal cells and recanalized channels. Organizing pneumonia is an intrabronchiolar and alveolar duct process characterized by granulation tissue plugs.

Brown K: Pulmonary vasculitis. *Proc Am Thorac Soc* 2006;3:48-57.

4. c.   Solitary fibrous tumors (SFTs) are typically CD34 positive. Immunohistochemistry profile also includes bcl2 and CD99 reactivity, with no reactivity for CK, smooth muscle markers, S100, or CD31. SFTs are usually slow-growing tumors with potential for local spread and with malignant potential. They are generally pleural based and sometimes on a pedicle; however, they can appear to be completely intrapulmonary. Criteria for malignancy include dense cellularity, necrosis, and mitotic rate. Larger tumors are more likely to display these criteria; however, tumors lacking these criteria can recur with invasive growth. The differential diagnosis includes other spindle cell neoplasms. Bland SFTs, especially when they occur posterior and medial, can enter the differential diagnosis of schwannoma (nerve sheath tumors), and cellular SFT with atypia can enter the differential diagnosis with synovial sarcoma, sarcomatoid carcinomas, fibrosarcomas, and fibrous histiocytomas.

England DM, Hochholzer L, McCarthy MJ: Localized benign and malignant fibrous tumors of the pleura. *Am J Surg Pathol* 1989;13:640-658.

5. d.   Lymphoma involves the lung in nodular growth patterns that in the adjacent lung follow lymphatic routes, as in this image. The differential diagnosis of a lung lymphatic pattern includes macrophage disorders, lymphoma, lymphangitic carcinoma, sarcoid, and Kaposi sarcoma. Certain pediatric conditions, including lymphangiectasia and lymphangiomatosis (distinct from lymphangioleiomyomatosis), can also involve lymphatic routes.

Concerning the other answer choices, miliary tuberculosis is characterized by 1- to 2-mm necrotizing granulomas that are distributed randomly throughout the lung parenchyma, the result of hemtogenous spread. EAA is a bronchiolitis and interstitial pneumonia caused by inhalation of a foreign antigen resulting in a type III and type IV hypersensitivity reaction. The pattern is bronchiolar and interstitial. Mesothelioma is a malignant tumor arising from the cells lining the pleural space. It can invade the lung, but often in a "rindlike" growth. This pattern would be distinctly pleural. Bronchiectasis is dilatation of bronchi with massive mucous plugging and is, therefore, airway based.

Leslie KO, Wick MR: *Practical Pulmonary Pathology: A Diagnostic Approach.* Philadelphia: Churchill Livingstone, 2005.

6. b.   The image is that of a chronic dilated cavity with intraluminal necrosis. Although different fungi can cause such a lesion (mycetoma), *Aspergillus* is the most commonly

encountered. Aspergillomas may be the result of colonization of preexisting cavities from other causes, including massively dilated airways of bronchiectasis. They can have areas of epithelial lining, most often with squamous metaplasia. Preexisting disease that may cause cavitary lesions include tuberculosis, treated lung cancer, and bronchiectasis. Aspergillomas contain necrotic debris that is mostly abundant fungal hyphae histologically. Associated hemoptysis may lead to surgical resection. Immunocompromised patients can develop invasive or necrotizing *Aspergillus* infections. *Aspergillus* hyphae are septated, appear uniform in width, and branch at acute angles.

Soubani AO, Chandrasekar PH: Aspergillosis. *Chest* 2002;121: 1988-1999.

7. d.   UPI is most commonly seen in patients over age 50. Histologically, there is irregular scarring throughout the lobule, with peripheral lobular accentuation and spared alveoli at the center of the lobule. Sarcoidosis is characterized by granulomatous inflammation in a lymphatic distribution. Lymphocytic interstitial pneumonia is characterized by dense lymphocytic infiltrates in alveolar walls. Desquamative interstitial pneumonia is characterized by an intraalveolar accumulation of macrophages in addition to interstitial thickening. The best diagnosis is, therefore, nonspecific interstitial pneumonia, which is characterized by a diffuse panlobular, temporally uniform process, which can be cellular/inflammatory or fibrotic but is interstitial, not intraalveolar.

Katzenstein AL, Fiorelli RF: Non-specific interstitial pneumonia. Histologic features and clinical significance. *Am J Surg Pathol* 1994;18:136-147.

8. b.   The image shows a fibroblastic tuft at the interface of scarred and spared lung, consistent with a fibroblastic focus. Fibroblastic foci can be plentiful, although in most cases they are not. They are thought to be the active component of the progressive lung fibrosis of UIP, which is clinically idiopathic pulmonary fibrosis (IPF). The paucity of inflammation is typical of UIP/IPF. This disease does not appear to respond to steroid therapy, and it is likely that complications of steroid therapy outweigh the benefit in these cases. Given the absence of effective therapy, progression to end-stage fibrosis occurs in most patients, leading to a high rate of organ failure requiring transplantation or to death. Fibroblastic proliferations can occur in other interstitial lung diseases. It is the location/distribution and number of fibroblastic foci in conjunction with the absence of inflammation, organizing pneumonia, and granulomas that make the diagnosis of UIP. End-stage or honeycomb lung is the end point of lung fibrosis. In these areas, fibroblastic foci may not be seen. UPI can be part of an idiopathic process, but can be seen in connective tissue disease, some medication reactions, and EAA. Asbestos exposure can lead to lung fibrosis. Lung fibrosis can also occur in Hermansky-Pudlak syndrome, dyskeratosis congenita, and certain surfactant deficiencies. In these syndromes, patients are usually younger than in idiopathic cases with UPI pattern.

Colby TV: Surgical pathology of non-neoplastic lung disease. *Mod Pathol* 2000;13:343-358.

9. d. The tumor shown is an epithelioid hemangioendothelioma. It is typically multifocal and the nodules can be sclerotic, fibrotic, or necrotic. They are endothelial neoplasms and, therefore, they are CD31 positive. This tumor can be seen in lung, liver, and soft tissue and is seen predominantly in women, usually under the age of 50. This is a low-grade endothelial neoplasm when compared to angiosarcomas; however, they are progressive and recurrent despite this more indolent course.

Corrin B, Harrison WJ, Wright DH: The so-called intravascular bronchioloalveolar tumor of lung (low grade sclerosing angiosarcoma). *Diagn Histopathol* 1983;6:229-237.

10. d. There is no clear association between cigarette smoking and plexiform arteriopathy. Cigarette smoking can cause chronic bronchitis, but the pulmonary hypertension in chronic bronchitis is not associated with plexiform arteriopathy. Plexiform lesions are the result of vascular wall injury. Lesions of primary pulmonary arterial hypertension reflect the dilatation and organization associated with this injury. These lesions can be relatively focal in lung biopsies despite the marked overall effect on pulmonary pressure. Familial cases are the result of an autosomal dominant mutation in BMPR2 (bone morphogenic protein receptor 2). The mutation does not result in pulmonary arterial hypertension in all individuals who harbor it. Severe pulmonary hypertension is associated with right-sided heart dilatation and failure. Large pulmonary arteries show atherosclerosis in patients with pulmonary hypertension. Effective treatments for pulmonary hypertension have significantly improved management of this condition and have resulted in improvements in survival. Primary pulmonary arterial hypertension is far more common in women than in men.

Galie N, Hoeper MM, Humbert M, et al: Guidelines for the diagnosis and treatment of pulmonary hypertension. *Eur Respir J* 2009;34:1219-1263.

11. b. This choice accurately describes the staining properties of a carcinoid, whether classic type or spindled. Carcinoid tumors of the lung are classified as typical and atypical. Spindle cell carcinomas are histologic variants that can be either typical or atypical depending on the presence of necrosis and mitotic rates of 2 to 10 mitotic figures in 10 HPFs. Spindle cell carcinoids can be seen in peripheral locations. Carcinoid tumors are low-grade malignancies and have a rate of metastasis of 5% to 15% to regional lymph nodes. A somewhat lower percentage of cases show metastasis to mediastinal nodes. Atypical carcinoids have a far higher rate of nodal metastasis (30%). In addition, 5- and 10-year survival rates in patient with atypical carcinoids are reduced when compared to rates for typical/classic carcinoids. Spindle cell carcinoids evoke a differential diagnosis that includes spindle cell neoplasms such as smooth muscle tumors, melanomas with spindle structure, myofibroblastic tumors, and salivary gland tumors. The stippled nuclear chromatin pattern and bland cellular uniformity are both helpful in this differential diagnosis, as are immunohistochemistry stains. Salivary gland tumors, such as mucoepidermoid carcinoma with intermediate cell predominance, enter the differential diagnosis of classic carcinoids more often than spindle cell carcinoids. The immunohistochemistry profile of CK, synaptophysin, and

chromogranin, usually diffuse and strong, resolves the majority of the cases. In difficult cases, relevant negative immunohistochemistry can include S100, HMB45, smooth muscle actin, desmin, and p63.

Ranchod M, Levine GD: Spindle cell carcinoid tumors of the lung: a clinicopathological study of 35 cases. *Am J Surg Pathol* 1980;4:315-331.

12. c. The echinoderm microtubule-associated proteinlike 4-anaplastic lymphoma receptor tyrosine kinase (EML4-ALK) translocation is a paracentric inversion within the short arm of chromosome 2 resulting in high level activation of the ALK receptor tyrosine kinase activity. It has been subsequently noted that a small percentage (about 5%) of lung adenocarcinomas overall harbor this translocation. Although there are many exceptions to the association, a proportion of adenocarcinomas with the translocation have a cribriform mucinous and signet ring growth pattern. In addition, the patients are younger and are usually nonsmokers or light smokers. The histologic diagnosis, however, is not sufficiently associated with translocation to allow histologic finding to guide selection for translocation testing. The interest in this translocation in part stems from agents known to target the ALK kinase activity. Crizotinib has been shown to have promise in treating high stage patients with these translocation adenocarcinomas. The translocation is mutually exclusive with EGFR and KRAS mutations.

Kwak EL, Bang YJ, Camidge DR, et al: Anaplastic lymphoma kinase inhibition in non small cell lung cancer. *N Engl J Med* 2010;363:1693-1703.
Soda M, Choi YL, Enomoto M, et al: Identification of the transforming EML4ALK fusion gene in nonsmall cell lung cancer. *Nature* 2007;448:561-566.

13. b. Squamous carcinoma is typically positive for nuclear p63 (strong and diffuse) and multifocal CK5/6, and is negative for TTF-1. The CK5/6 can be variable. There are different antibody clones for TTF-1 that give different results in squamous carcinoma; the SPT24 clone is more likely to be positive than the 8G7G1 clone. Solid type adenocarcinoma can enter the differential with squamous carcinoma. Aside from mucicarmine positivity, which is important to include in this staining panel, TTF-1 is positive and p63 should not be diffusely positive in solid type adenocarcinoma. Napsin has also emerged as an immunohistochemistry marker positive in adenocarcinoma. CK7 can be positive in a proportion of lung squamous carcinomas. High-molecular-weight keratin, although frequently positive in squamous cell carcinoma, also reacts with a significant proportion of lung adenocarcinomas, limiting its utility.

This supports a panel approach, combining TTF-1, p63, and CK5/6 to distinguish lung adenocarcinoma from squamous carcinoma.

Rekhtman N, Ang DC, Sima CS, et al: Immunohistochemical algorithm for differentiation of lung adenocarcinoma and squamous cell carcinoma based on large series of whole tissue sections with validation in small specimens. *Mod Pathol* 2011;24:1348-1359.

14. e. Mucinous adenocarcinomas can have a lepidic pattern with extracellular mucin; however, most cases also have stromal alteration and growth patterns of invasive adenocarcinoma. The majority of lepidic pattern mucinous adenocarcinomas harbor oncogenic *KRAS* mutations. The mucinous cells of congenital cystic pulmonary airway malformation, type I, are preneoplastic. This warrants removal of these malformations. Metastatic adenocarcinomas from the pancreas, biliary tree, and gastrointestinal tract can mimic lung primary lepidic mucinous adenocarcinoma. Such tumors can lead to diagnostic problems as the immunohistochemistry profile of lung lepidic mucinous adenocarcinoma can be TTF-1 negative and CK7 and CK20 positive. Nonmucinous adenocarcinoma in situ has the radiologic appearance of ground-glass opacity, but mucinous adenocarcinoma in situ and mucinous adenocarcinomas are more often solid by CT scan.

15. e.   Silo filler's disease will not have the histologic appearance shown. It is the result of a toxic chemical exposure to nitrogen dioxide; this can cause suffocation or acute respiratory distress syndrome (ARDS) and is not immunologically mediated. All of the other answer choices are a cause of chronic hypersensitivity pneumonitis (HP). EAA (chronic HP) is a form of type III/type IV hypersensitivity mediated by IgG and cell-mediated immunity. IgG is the main immunoglobulin of the distal lung. Chronic HP refers to an alveolitis; therefore, the response is a combination of IgG-mediated inflammation with lymphocytes and plasma cells and cell-mediated reaction involving histiocytes. IgE-mediated hypersensitivity can also occur in the lung with eosinophilia; this pattern of hypersensitivity is seen in larger airways in processes such as allergic bronchopulmonary aspergillosis. As noted previously, chronic HP and EAA are synonyms; as an alveolitis the hypersensitivity is an IgG-mediated response. The spectrum of organic antigens that can cause EAA/chronic HP is wide, although birds, molds, and bacteria are frequent culprits. More recently, cases of hypersensitivity to nontuberculous mycobacteria have been reported in sources of contaminated water ("hot tub lung").

Chronic HP without fibrosis responds to steroid therapy and avoidance of the offending antigen if it can be identified. Unfortunately, some cases can lead to severe lung fibrosis and such cases do not have a favorable response. In some instances, this leads to end-stage lung fibrosis mimicking UPI.

Certain medications such as methotrexate can mimic HP. Because this is not an inhaled antigen, such cases do not have the prominent bronchiolitis of EAA/chronic HP.

Coleman A, Colby TV: Histologic diagnosis of extrinsic allergic alveolitis. *Am J Surg Pathol* 1988;12:514-518.

16. a.   SMA, HMB45 markers are positive in the spindled cells of lymphangioleiomyomatosis. S100, CD1a markers are positive in Langerhans cells. Although Langerhans cell histiocytosis can cause cystic lung disease, the lesions are usually nodular or fibrotic and the cells histiocytic. CD34, c-kit is a profile for gastrointestinal stromal tumor. S100, Melan A, tyrosinase is a profile for malignant melanoma. Although this enters the differential diagnosis of HMB45 positive cells, the overall picture of cystic lung disease is not that of malignant melanoma. CK7 and CK20 are used in the assessment of adenocarcinomas to help determine the primary site and, therefore, plays no role in this case.

Taylor JR, Ryu J, Colby TV, Raffin TA: Lymphangioleiomyomatosis. Clinical course in 32 patients. *N Engl J Med* 1990;323:1254-1260.

17. e.   Although it is true that sarcoidosis can resolve spontaneously, as well as with therapy, a subset of cases will not and do progress to end-stage fibrosis, resulting in organ failure. Sarcoidosis is an idiopathic disease characterized by nonnecrotizing granulomas. Although typically involving mediastinal lymph nodes and the lung, sarcoidosis can be a systemic process. Cardiac involvement, central nervous system involvement, skin involvement, and ocular involvement are well described. The yield on transbronchial biopsy is excellent in pulmonary sarcoid, and especially high if an airway abnormality is seen during bronchoscopy. Four to six negative biopsy fragments have a high negative predictive value. Ruling out sarcoidosis remains one of the major nonneoplastic uses of transbronchial biopsy. When open-lung biopsies are performed, sarcoidal granulomas are observed to follow lymphatic routes. Sarcoidosis can be nodular. Vascular involvement can be seen as well, especially in areas of confluent granulomas. A variety of inclusions can be seen in granulomatous disease, including sarcoidosis. These inclusions are not sufficiently specific to attribute a granulomatous process to sarcoidosis. However, calcium oxalate, asteroid bodies (stellate), Schaumann bodies (concentric lamellated bodies), and least frequently Hamazaki-Wesenberg bodies (minute oval bodies) can be seen. Their recognition is important as cautionary advice to not mistake them for yeast forms.

Travis WD, Colby TV, Koss MN, et al: Non-neoplastic Disorders of the Lower Respiratory Tract. Washington, DC: AFIP, 2002.

18. b.   Organizing pneumonia can be seen in patients with rheumatoid arthritis.

Whether idiopathic or of known cause the process does not usually lead to permanent scarring and, therefore, does not lead to progressive pulmonary fibrosis. Cases of organizing pneumonia in which a clinical cause is not identified is called cryptogenic organizing pneumonia (COP). Patients with COP have either normal pulmonary function or a restrictive defect. COP is often multifocal but patchy, with normal lobules adjacent to involved lobules. This pattern is manifested radiologically by patchy consolidation, sometimes peribronchial nodularity or patchy ground-glass opacity. Organizing pneumonia can sometimes be seen as a solitary nodule. In that setting, it is called focal or localized organizing pneumonia. Some cases of localized organizing pneumonia are resected as solitary pulmonary nodules because they are in the clinical differential diagnosis of lung cancer. Patients with COP usually respond well to corticosteroids; some patients develop persistent disease or recurrent disease. Causes of organizing pneumonia are numerous, including collagen vascular disease, previous infection, adjacent to mass lesions, and associated with other causes of bronchiolitis.

Epler GR, Colby TV, McLoud TC, et al: Bronchiolitis obliterans organizing pneumonia. *N Engl J Med* 1985;312:152-158.

19. b. Lymphomatoid granulomatosis is an Epstein-Barr virus–positive pulmonary lymphoma of B-cell origin. Lymphomatoid granulomatosis is a nodular pulmonary process characterized by vasculocentric necrotic nodules. These nodules contain a lymphoid infiltrate that can be demonstrated to invade vascular walls. The vessels can often show lifting of endothelium by the invading lymphocytes. The vascular invasion, necrosis, and, sometimes, lymphocyte atypia all suggest a malignant process. Despite the name, true granulomas are not generally seen in this condition. In addition to the lung, skin and the central nervous system can be involved.

Nicholson AG, Wotherspoon AC, Diss TC, et al: Lymphomatoid granulomatosis: evidence that some cases represent Epstein Barr virus associated B cell lymphoma. *Histopathology* 1996;29:317-324.

20. c. Pulmonary disease can be the result of *Rhodococcus equi* infection, although other organisms including *Escherichia coli* can also cause pulmonary malakoplakia. Malakoplakia is an accumulation of histiocytes that form large areas of consolidation and even masses. Within these histiocyte-rich areas are concentric bodies that contain calcium and iron, known as Michaelis-Gutmann bodies. Patients with pulmonary malakoplakia are frequently immunosuppressed; it is associated with AIDS. Atypical mycobacterial infection can cause histiocytic accumulation, but not Michaelis-Gutmann bodies of malakoplakia. Histiocytic disorders that involve the lung can include Langerhans cell histiocytosis, Rosai-Dorfman disease, and Erdheim-Chester disease. In addition, xanthogranulomatous inflammation can occur in chronic infection and associated with bronchiectasis. Although Whipple disease is not common in the lung, these macrophage accumulations are very similar to those of malakoplakia. Malakoplakia remains distinguished by the Michaelis-Gutmann bodies.

Kwon KY, Colby TV: Rhodococcus equi pneumonia and pulmonary malakoplakia in acquired immunodeficiency syndrome. Pathologic features. *Arch Pathol Lab Med* 1994;118:744-748.

21. d. Rounded atelectasis represents a nonneoplastic mass lesion in the lung, occurring posteriorly in the lower lobes. It is the result of an adhesion that forms between a parietal pleural plaque and the visceral pleura of the lung. The adhesion causes progressive fibrosis and retraction. The retraction entraps and folds a portion of lung, and the result is a mass. Such a mass can be recognized as rounded atelectasis clinically. The radiologic "comet tail" sign reflects airways and vessels curving into the folded lung and when recognized identifies the lesion as nonneoplastic. If an attempt is made at resection, the mass unfolds/reinflates when the pleural adhesions are lysed and the mass seemingly disappears. The parietal pleural plaque in these patients is often the result of asbestos exposure. The histologic examination of the lung tissue, if resected, is largely unremarkable with the exception of the identification of localized visceral pleural fibrosis.

Hillerdal G: Rounded atelectasis. Clinical experience with 74 patients. *Chest* 1989;95:836-841.

22. b. Dirofilariasis is caused by the dog heartworm. Humans are not the definitive hosts, and the disease is seen in dogs and other animals. When humans are infected, the immature worm reaches the right ventricle but dies, embolizing fragments into the lung. This causes nodular infarcts that may contain eosinophils. Cross sections of dead worms can be seen within vascular lumina. *Strongyloides* passes through the lung during its life cycle. Larval forms are seen in the lung and can cause hemorrhage and neutrophilic inflammation. Eggs are not laid in the lung but in the gastrointestinal tract. *Paragonimus* worms are found in the lung, and they lay egg-filled cysts that can rupture in the lung. Although this infection is seen in Asia, North American paragonimiasis also exists and can cause pulmonary and pleural disease. Ingestion of fresh water soft-shelled crabs/crayfish that are undercooked is the source of the disease. Echinococcal cysts are relatively thick walled and multilamellated. Echinococcal infection results from the ingestion of poorly cooked meat from sheep and cows. These infections are often hepatic, but can be pulmonary as well. Cryptosporidia are found on and in airway epithelial cells, seeming to sit on the surface of the cell but in fact residing within a paracytophorous vacuole.

Travis WD, Colby TV, Koss MN, et al: Non-neoplastic disorders of the lower respiratory tract. In *Armed Forces Institute of Pathology Atlas of Non-tumor Pathology*. Washington, DC: American Registry of Pathology, 2002.

23. d. Small cell carcinoma is an undifferentiated carcinoma that has demonstrable neuroendocrine differentiation by immunohistochemistry or electron microscopy; however, a significant number of morphologically small cell carcinomas have very weak or absent synaptophysin and chromogranin immunoreactivity. The biologic behavior of morphologically small cell carcinomas with immunohistochemically positive neuroendocrine markers is no different from that in carcinomas in which these markers cannot be demonstrated. TTF-1 is positive in lung adenocarcinomas and small cell carcinomas; however, TTF-1 is also positive in extrapulmonary small cell carcinomas. The biologic behavior of small cell carcinoma is of an aggressive neoplasm that is frequently metastatic at the time of presentation. It is true that small cell carcinoma is associated with poor prognosis, but these tumors are sensitive to chemotherapy. Unfortunately, chemotherapy is not curative and the high frequency of metastatic disease contributes to the poor outcome. The morphologic features of small cell carcinoma include salt and pepper chromatin, nuclear molding, scant cytoplasm, and high numbers of apoptotic and mitotic figures. It has been recognized that small cell carcinoma can have a histologically larger cell population, and this has been incorporated into lung carcinoma classifications under a variety of terminologies. This larger cell population has been identified in a significant proportion of cases, more than 20%; biologic behavior does not appear to be altered by this finding. When any amount of squamous cell carcinoma or adenocarcinoma is present in a small cell carcinoma, the designation of combined small cell carcinoma is used. For cases of small cell carcinoma that contain at least 10% of a large cell neuroendocrine carcinoma component, the designation of combined small cell carcinoma is used as well.

Nicholson SA, Beasley MB, Brambilla E, et al: Small cell lung carcinoma (SCLC): a clinicopathologic study of 100 cases with surgical specimens. *Am J Surg Pathol* 2002;26:1184-1197.

24. e. Although smoking can lead to airways disease, including chronic bronchitis, emphysema, and respiratory bronchiolitis, it does not appear to progress to obliterative/constrictive bronchiolitis. Obliterative or constrictive bronchiolitis results in airways that are completely obliterated, with eventual replacement of the lumen by fibrous tissue. This form of lung disease involves the airway, but can be deceptively subtle. Alveolar changes are often minimal and not all airways show easily identifiable changes. In addition to complete fibrous obliteration, airways can show inflammation and fibroblastic proliferation in their walls. The result is severe obstructive lung disease. Constrictive bronchiolitis is not common, but has specific associations. Infections such as adenovirus that can cause bronchiolitis can result in fibrosis later. Additional causes of connective tissue diseases can include rheumatoid arthritis and medication reactions from penicillamine. Lung transplant patients develop obliterative bronchiolitis with increasing time after transplantation. Other causes include fume exposures; some cases remain idiopathic. Diffuse pulmonary neuroendocrine cell hyperplasia can result in severe obstruction similar to that of obliterative bronchiolitis. Neuroendocrine cell hyperplasia is more often asymptomatic than symptomatic.

Colby TV: Bronchiolitis, pathologic considerations. *Med J Clin Pathol* 1998;109:101-109.

25. c. Mutations in β-catenin are infrequent in lung cancer, but are seen in well-differentiated fetal type adenocarcinoma. Small cell carcinomas and large cell neuroendocrine carcinomas are p53 mutated at a high rate, but not *EGFR* or *KRAS* mutated. Adenocarcinomas can have *KRAS* mutations, *EGFR* mutations, *ALK* translocations, or *BRAF* mutations. These are not seen in the same tumor. Mutations in *PI3KCA* are seen at low rates, but can be seen in conjunction with other mutations. Squamous cell carcinomas have amplifications in chromosome 3q that involve the *SOX2* gene and in some cases p63. Mucinous adenocarcinomas (formerly mucinous bronchioloalveolar carcinoma) are often *KRAS* mutated.

Travis WD, Brambilla E, Noguchi M, et al: International association for the study of lung cancer/American Thoracic Society/European Respiratory Society international multidisciplinary classification of lung adenocarcinoma. *J Thorac Oncol* 2011;6:244-285.

26. d. Aspiration of mineral oil results in lipoid pneumonia, not PAP.

PAP can be primary and idiopathic, or can be associated with silica exposure, aluminum exposure, hematologic malignancy, immunodeficiency, or infection. Proteinosislike areas can be seen adjacent to lung cancers. Alveolar proteinosis is associated with loss of stimulation of macrophages by GM-CSF. This was described experimentally in mice, but may be related to anti-GM-CSF antibody in humans. A classic alveolar filling pattern is seen on a CT scan called the "crazy paving" pattern. The intraalveolar material is characteristically granular and PAS positive.

Khan A, Agarwal R: Pulmonary alveolar proteinosis. *Respir Care* 2011;56:1016-1028.

27. d. There are four typical patterns in sclerosing hemangiomas—papillary, solid, sclerotic, and angiomatoid. They are not always all present in the same tumor. Sclerosing hemangiomas are perhaps better called pneumocytomas as the cells are more likely related to pneumocytes at different stages of maturation. As a result, the lesional cells are CK positive in lining areas and diffusely TTF-1 positive. The tumors are generally benign, although rare cases have been shown to have lymph node metastasis. These metastases do not appear to affect prognosis.

Devouassoux-Shisheboran M, Hayashi T, Linnoila RI, et al: A clinicopathologic study of 100 cases of pulmonary sclerosing hemangioma with immunohistochemical studies: TTF1 is expressed in both round and surface cells, suggesting an origin from primitive respiratory epithelium. *Am J Surg Pathol* 2000;24:906-916.

28. a. Asbestos exposure results in pleural fibrosis, pleural plaque formation, lung fibrosis, and mesothelioma. Asbestosis refers to the lung fibrosis caused by asbestos exposure.

Ferruginous bodies are iron-encrusted fibers. These bodies are seen in a variety of particle/fiber exposures. When the fiber is proved to be asbestos, these asbestos bodies provide evidence of asbestos exposure. The fibers of asbestos are nonpolarizing. Pleural plaques are typically parietal pleural and are thick, white, and sometimes nodular. Although visceral pleural fibrosis can be seen in asbestos exposure, a diffuse rindlike thickening of visceral pleura is suspicious for malignant mesothelioma. Pleural plaques are densely collagenized and often have a "basket weave" growth pattern.

Leslie Ko, Wick MR: *Practical Pulmonary Pathology*. Philadelphia: Churchill Livingstone, 2005.

29. c. Middle lobe syndrome is caused by chronic obstruction resulting in bronchiectasis, organizing pneumonia, mucostasis, and very often lymphoid hyperplasia with follicular bronchiolitis. The obstruction is the result of the susceptibility of the middle lobe and lingular bronchus to compression. In children it occurs in chronic airways disease and can be related to mucous impaction or foreign body aspiration. In adults, the cause of compression can be hilar lymphadenopathy, although precise causes cannot always be determined. The cause can be an intrinsic obstructionlike tumor or extrinsic compression. Broncholiths have also been reported. Granulomatous inflammation has been reported in some cases. Resection may be needed to avoid chronic bouts of pneumonia.

Kwon KY, Myers JL, Swensen SJ, Colby TV: Middle lobe syndrome: a clinicopathological study of 21 patients. *Hum Pathol* 1995;26:302-307.

CHAPTER 4

GASTROINTESTINAL PATHOLOGY

Efsevia Vakiani, Roger K. Moreira, and Helen Remotti

QUESTIONS

Questions 1-30 refer to a photo or photomicrograph.

1. A 19-year-old college student presents with a 2-week history of diarrhea and abdominal pain. Choose the CORRECT diagnosis and MOST likely site of biopsy.
   a. *Entamoeba histolytica* infection/colonic biopsy
   b. Strongyloidiasis/small intestinal biopsy
   c. *Giardia lamblia* infection/small intestinal biopsy
   d. *Cryptosporidium parvum* infection/gastric biopsy
   e. Microsporida infection/small intestinal biopsy

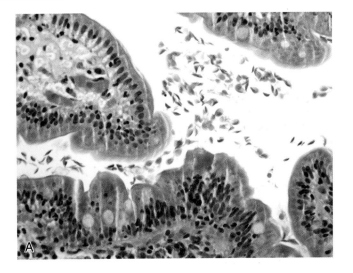

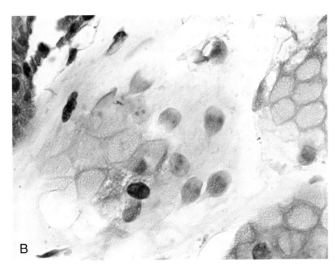

2. A 38-year-old HIV-positive patient presents with diarrhea. Colonic biopsy is shown. Which of the following alternatives is INCORRECT regarding this patient's diagnosis?

  a. This condition is most commonly described in association with HIV, but has been reported in a variety of clinical settings, including as an incidental finding.

  b. Clinical significance is unclear in most settings, but some studies have shown response to antibiotic therapy.

  c. The condition is caused by bacteria belonging to the *Campylobacter* genus.

  d. Colonic mucosa usually has a normal appearance on endoscopic or gross examination.

  e. Special stains (including Warthin-Starry or Steiner) usually suffice to confirm the diagnosis.

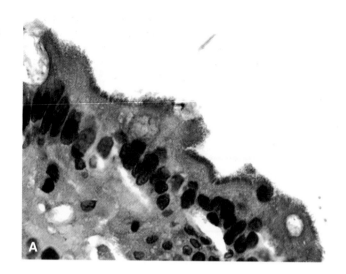

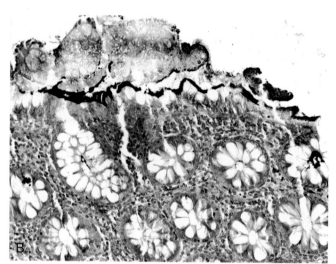

3. The esophageal biopsy shown is from a lesion in the lower esophagus of a 65-year-old man who complained of dysphagia. The following are risk factors for this lesion EXCEPT:

  a. Tobacco smoking

  b. Heavy alcohol consumption

  c. Food high in nitrosamines

  d. Consumption of burning-hot beverages

  e. Long-standing reflux esophagitis

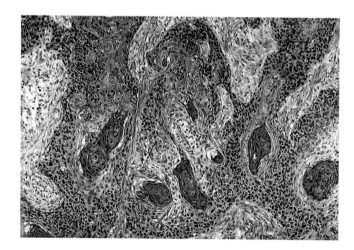

4. The biopsy shown was taken from the lower esophagus of a 56-year-old man with long-standing reflux symptoms. Tongues of salmon-pink mucosa were identified endoscopically extending several centimeters into the esophagus. Which of the following alternatives is INCORRECT regarding this patient's diagnosis?

a. Long-standing gastroesophageal reflux is thought to be an etiologic factor.

b. Endoscopic correlation is required for diagnosis.

c. This finding is associated with an increased risk for adenocarcinoma.

d. In the United States, presence of goblet cells is a required component for the histopathologic characterization of this condition.

e. The extent/length of this change in the absence of dysplasia directly correlates with the risk of developing esophageal adenocarcinoma.

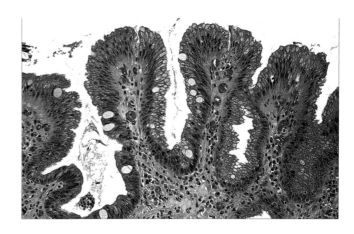

5. A 10-year-old boy with a history of allergic conditions presents with dysphagia. Previous antireflux treatment was unsuccessful. Esophageal biopsy is shown. Which of the following statements is INCORRECT about this diagnosis?

a. Current definition includes 15 or more eosinophils/HPF (high-power field) and exclusion of esophageal reflux.

b. Typical endoscopic features include a "ringed," or "feline," esophagus (resembling the appearance of a trachea) as well as vertical furrows.

c. Esophageal strictures represent a common complication.

d. Similarly to reflux disease, the distal esophagus is primarily affected.

e. Very high concentration of eosinophils with a superficial distribution and presence of eosinophilic microabscesses are clues to the diagnosis.

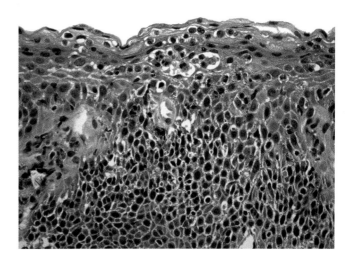

6. A 73-year-old woman with pernicious anemia was found to have several gastric polyps ranging from 1 mm to 5 mm. The image shown is from the largest polyp.

Choose the CORRECT statement about the gastric tumor shown in the image:

a. G-cell hyperplasia is a common precursor lesion.

b. They are often seen in the setting of *H. pylori*-associated atrophic gastritis.

c. In autoimmune atrophic gastritis, they are usually associated with hyperchlorhydria and hypergastrinemia.

d. Multifocal carcinoids are frequent in the setting of autoimmune atrophic gastritis.

e. Sporadic carcinoids in general have a better prognosis than hypergastrinemia-associated carcinoids.

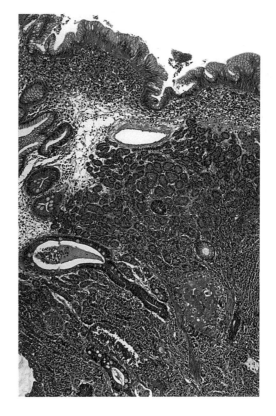

7. This photomicrograph shows one of several gastric polyps found in a 38-year-old man. These polyps may occur in a syndrome associated with all of the following EXCEPT:

a. Autosomal dominantly inherited hamartomatous polyposis syndrome of the gastrointestinal (GI) tract

b. Increased risk of breast cancer

c. Germline mutations in the *LKB1* (*STK11*) gene

d. Focal dysplasia identified in the majority of syndromic polyps

e. Increased risk of Sertoli cell tumors of the testis

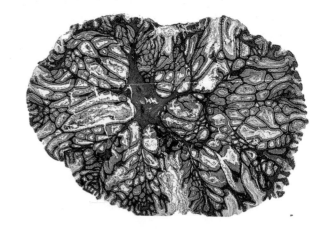

8. A 62-year-old man presented with upper GI tract bleeding. This photomicrograph is from a 6.5-cm submucosal mass identified in the stomach. The spindle cells are CD117 positive, desmin negative, and S100 negative. All of the following statements are true EXCEPT:

a. The most common site for this tumor is the stomach.

b. This tumor may occur in association with pulmonary chondroma and extraadrenal paraganglioma, almost exclusively in young women (Carney's triad).

c. Germline mutations in *KIT* are associated with these tumors in familial cases.

d. Gain of function mutations in *KIT* or platelet-derived growth factor receptor (PDGFR) may occur in this tumor.

e. The use of imatinib mesylate (Gleevec/STI-571) is ineffective in treating tumors with *KIT* mutations involving the regulatory site, but effective in treating tumors with *KIT* mutations involving the enzymatic site.

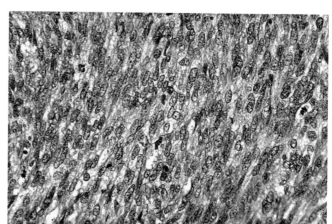

9. This photomicrograph is from a submucosal 3-cm gastric mass found in a 56-year-old man. The neoplastic cells are positive for smooth muscle actin, and negative for desmin, chromogranin, S100, and CD117 (*KIT*). The MOST likely diagnosis is:

a. Gastrointestinal stromal tumor (GIST), CD117-negative variant

b. Glomus tumor

c. Angiomyolipoma

d. Granular cell tumor (GCT)

e. Leiomyoma

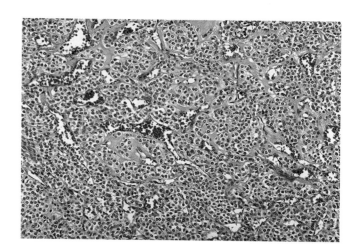

10. A 56-year-old HIV-positive man presented with epigastric pain and upper GI tract bleeding. On upper GI endoscopy, several small red nodules were identified in the stomach. The biopsy of one of these nodules is shown here. The spindle cells are immunoreactive for CD31 and LANA (latent nuclear antigen). Which of the following statements is true?

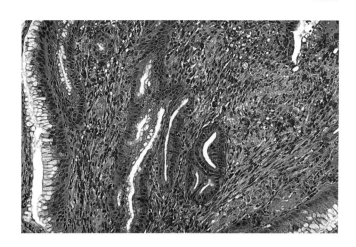

   a. Histopathologic clues to this diagnosis includes the presence of slitlike vascular spaces containing red blood cells, intracellular hyaline globules, and atypical cytologic features, resembling high-grade angiosarcomas.
   b. Epstein-Barr virus is thought to play a major role in the pathogenesis of this disease.
   c. Immunoreactivity for LANA is not specific for this lesion and may be seen in a range of mesenchymal lesions, including spindle cell hemangioma, dermatofibrosarcoma protuberans, and pyogenic granuloma.
   d. GI involvement is common in the classic form of the disease.
   e. GI tract involvement may occur without cutaneous involvement.

11. Regarding the disease shown in the figure, which of the following alternatives is INCORRECT?
   a. Characteristic histologic findings include chronic inflammation and neutrophilic infiltrate of gastric glands (chronic active gastritis [CAG]).
   b. Lymphoid follicles with germinal centers in the lamina propria may be present.
   c. Immunohistochemistry and special stains, such as Giemsa and Warthin-Starry, may be helpful in identifying organisms.
   d. The organism can be eradicated with antibiotic therapy in approximately 50% of cases.
   e. Clinical features are variable and include no symptoms, mild dyspepsia, and upper GI tract bleeding.

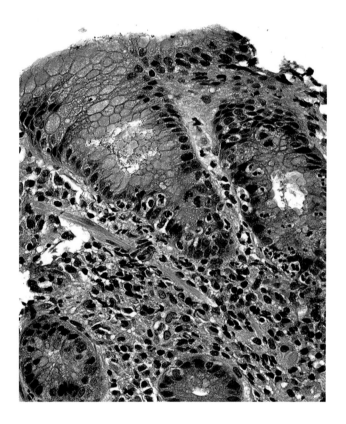

12. This gastric biopsy was obtained from a 50-year-old man who presented with epigastric pain. This pattern of injury is associated with all of the following EXCEPT:
    a. Heavy use of nonsteroidal antiinflammatory drugs (NSAIDs), particularly aspirin
    b. Moderate alcohol consumption
    c. Chronic *H. pylori* infection
    d. Ischemia and shock
    e. Bile reflux

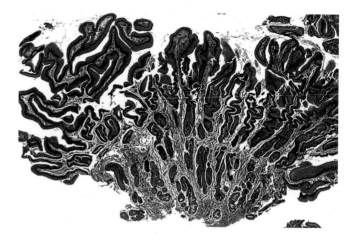

13. The lesion shown was found in the ileum of a 44-year-old woman who complained of abdominal pain. All of the following are true regarding this lesion EXCEPT:
    a. The majority of patients have symptomatic crampy lower quadrant pain or hematochezia.
    b. Terminal ileal involvement may mimic cancer, Crohn disease, ischemia, or *Yersinia* infection.
    c. The most common sites of involvement in the GI tract are rectosigmoid colon, appendix, and small intestine.
    d. The stromal component of this lesion is CD10 positive.
    e. The glandular and stromal components of the lesion are positive for estrogen receptors and progesterone receptors.

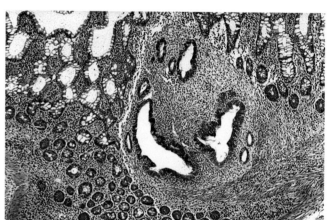

14. A 27-year-old college student presents with diarrhea, abdominal pain, and weight loss. An upper endoscopy with biopsy is perfomed and histologic findings are shown. All of the following statements are true about this condition, EXCEPT:
    a. Anti–tissue transglutaminase (tTG) antibody is currently considered the most sensitive and specific serologic test.
    b. Intraepithelial lymphocytosis in duodenal biopsies is a highly specific finding.
    c. Patients test positive for DQ2 or DQ8 human leukocyte antigen (HLA).
    d. The majority of intraepithelial lymphocytes are CD8 positive.
    e. The histopathologic findings overlap with those seen in tropical sprue.

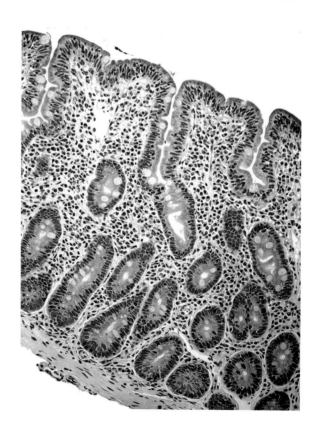

15. These photomicrographs are from a nodule found in the ileum of a 56-year-old man who presented with intermittent crampy abdominal pain. Which of the following is TRUE regarding this neoplasm:
    a. Ileal tumors are less aggressive than duodenal tumors.
    b. These tumors are strongly associated with multiple endocrine neoplasia type 1 (MEN1).
    c. Multiple nodules are seen in 25% to 30% of the cases.
    d. The majority of patients with midgut tumors clinically present with carcinoid syndrome.
    e. The majority of the tumors are smaller than 1 cm.

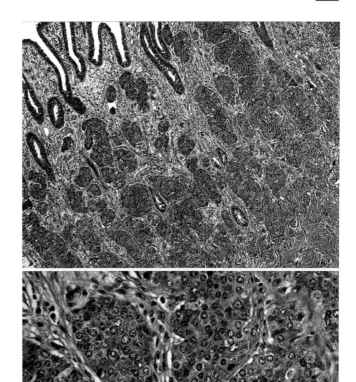

16. The gross and microscopic images shown are from the appendix of a 60-year-old woman who presented with symptoms of acute appendicitis. All of the following statements regarding this lesion are true EXCEPT:
    a. It may clinically first present as an ovarian neoplasm.
    b. It is the most common appendiceal neoplasm.
    c. It may be associated with colonic neoplasms.
    d. It may present with complications of pseudomyxoma peritonei (PMP).
    e. It should be sampled extensively to rule out malignancy.

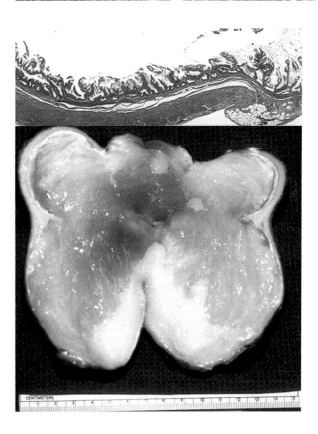

17. The lesion shown in this photomicrograph was discovered incidentally in the appendectomy specimen from a 25-year-old woman. The MOST likely diagnosis is:
    a. Mucinous neoplasm
    b. Lymphoma
    c. Neuroendocrine tumor (NET)/carcinoid
    d. Leiomyoma
    e. GI stromal tumor

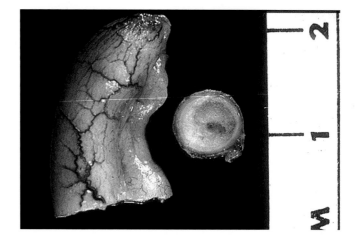

18. The lesion shown is from a 22-year-old woman with bloody diarrhea and crampy abdominal pain. Endoscopy revealed pancolitis. The term that BEST describes this lesion is:
    a. Pseudopolyp
    b. Hyperplastic polyp
    c. Dysplasia-associated lesion/mass (DALM)
    d. Tubular adenoma
    e. Inflammatory fibroid polyp.

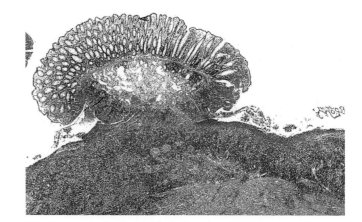

19. A 45-year-old man with a 15-year history of inflammatory bowel disease (IBD) presented with acute abdominal pain. Numerous polyps were identified throughout his colon. The gross and microscopic images shown here are representative of:
    a. Pseudopolyposis
    b. Filiform (postinflammatory) polyposis
    c. Colitis cystica profunda
    d. Hyperplastic polyposis
    e. Hamartomatous polyposis

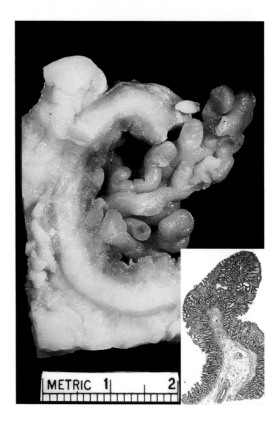

20. A 19-year-old man presented with abdominal pain and bloody
diarrhea. Representative images of the ascending colon are
shown. The MOST likely diagnosis is:
  a. Sarcoidosis
  b. Crohn colitis
  c. Ulcerative colitis
  d. Shigella colitis
  e. *Clostridium difficile* colitis.

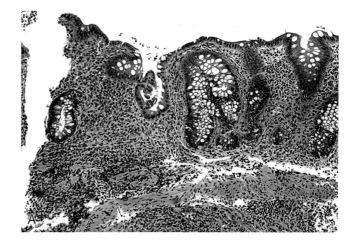

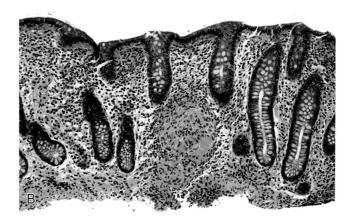

21. The two images shown are from the colon of a patient with
idiopathic IBD. All of the following statements are true EXCEPT:
  a. This is a chronic relapsing disorder.
  b. *CARD15/NOD2* gene mutations may be associated with this
  condition.
  c. Perinuclear antineutrophil cytoplasmic antibodies (ANCA)
  is positive in the majority of patients with this condition.
  d. Fistula tracts are complications of this condition.
  e. This condition may affect any portion of the GI tract.

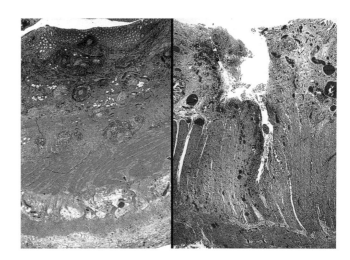

22. The photomicrograph shown is from the ascending colon. The LEAST likely diagnosis is:
   a. *C. difficile* colitis
   b. Ischemic colitis
   c. Ulcerative colitis
   d. Enterohemorrhagic *Escherichia coli* colitis
   e. Neonatal necrotizing enterocolitis

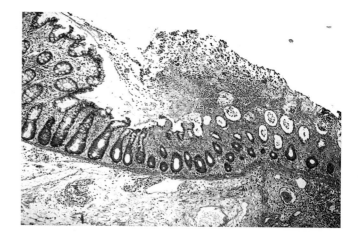

23. The following image is from a colectomy specimen of a 25-year-old woman. All the following regarding this syndrome are true EXCEPT:
   a. The pattern of inheritance is autosomal dominant.
   b. It is associated with a germline mutation of a tumor suppressor gene that is a negative regulator of the Wnt signaling pathway.
   c. Gardner syndrome is a variant that includes epidermoid cysts, osteomas, and desmoid tumors.
   d. Turcot syndrome is a variant that is associated with medulloblastoma.
   e. The majority of colorectal carcinomas (CRCs) developing in this setting have microsatellite instability.

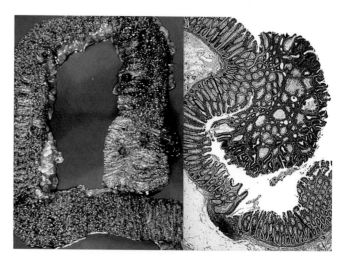

24. This biopsy is from a small nodule found in the rectum of a 60-year-old woman who underwent screening colonoscopy. Which of the following statements regarding this lesion is TRUE:
   a. The 5-year survival rate is poor (<20%).
   b. It is always benign.
   c. It is often small (<1 cm).
   d. It is often associated with the carcinoid syndrome.
   e. The neoplastic cells are PSA (prostate-specific antigen) positive.

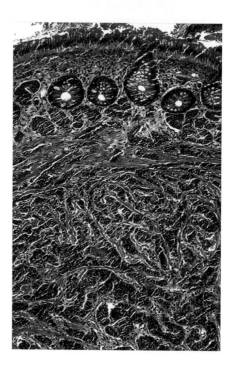

25. The biopsy shown is from the anal area of a 67-year-old man. All of the following are true regarding this lesion EXCEPT:
   a. It may be associated with a synchronous or metachronous carcinoma of the rectum.
   b. Pruritus is a common presenting complaint.
   c. The typical gross appearance of this lesion is an erythematous eczematoid plaque.
   d. The differential diagnosis includes pagetoid Bowen disease and melanoma.
   e. It is associated with HPV.

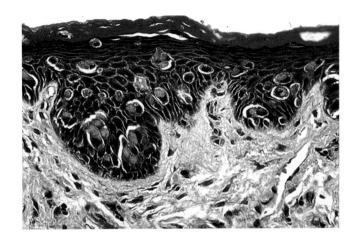

26. This biopsy was obtained from the anal canal of a 35-year-old man. All of the following statements are true regarding this lesion EXCEPT:
   a. Immunocompromised patients are at greater risk.
   b. It is often associated with HPV genotypes 16 and 18, and less commonly with genotypes 6 and 11.
   c. It is often discovered incidentally in minor surgical specimens removed for benign conditions, such as hemorrhoids.
   d. Female patients are at increased risk of developing vulvar or cervical squamous carcinoma.
   e. It is rarely multicentric.

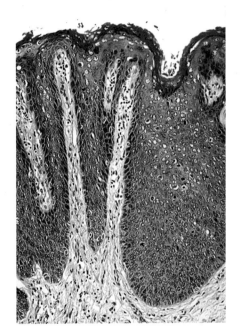

27. A 25-year-old woman with multiple colonic polyps underwent colectomy. The gross and microscopic images shown are from a representative polyp. All of the following are true EXCEPT:
   a. Patients with this polyposis syndrome are at increased risk for developing CRC, greater than 50% by age 60.
   b. Germline mutations in the *SMAD4/DPC4* tumor suppressor gene are associated with a subset of patients with this syndrome.
   c. This syndrome is an autosomal dominant disorder.
   d. Polyps in this syndrome are always restricted to the large intestine.
   e. Polyps in this syndrome may show areas of dysplasia.

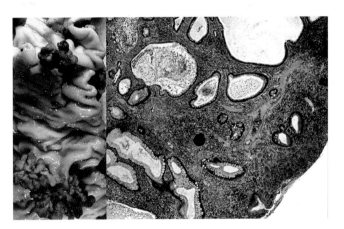

28. A 67-year-old woman presents with chronic diarrhea. A colonic biopsy is shown. Which of the following alternatives is CORRECT regarding this patient's diagnosis?

  a. This disease is equally common in men and women.

  b. Endoscopic abnormalities are common and range from mild erythema to extensive ulceration.

  c. All histologic findings are relatively nonspecific and can also be seen in IBD infections and ishemic injury.

  d. Long-standing disease is associated with an increased risk of colonic adenocarcinoma.

  e. Findings are often more prominent in the right and transverse colon than in the left colon.

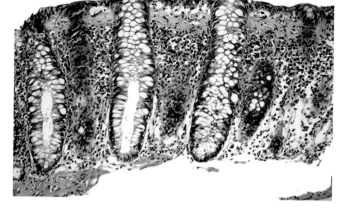

29. A 1-cm nodule of the lower esophagus is incidentally found on endoscopic examination. Histologic findings of the lesion are depicted in the image following. All the following statements regarding this diagnosis are correct EXCEPT:

  a. Tumor cells are thought to derive from Schwann cells and express S100 protein.

  b. The tumor is benign in the vast majority of cases, but malignant examples have been described.

  c. The overlying squamous epithelium may show changes that can be mistaken for SCC.

  d. The lesion is associated with MEN syndromes.

  e. The tongue and the esophagus are the most frequent sites for this lesion.

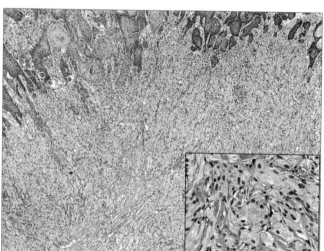

30. Which of the following statements is INCORRECT regarding the type of polyp shown:

  a. The diagnosis of this type of polyp is based primarily on architectural rather than cytologic features.

  b. Histologic features include crypt dilatation extending to the muscularis mucosa, "horizontal" growth pattern of the bottom of dilated crypts, and abnormal (or asymmetric) proliferation.

  c. Patients should not be considered to be at increased risk for subsequent development of colonic adenocarcinomas and surveillance is not currently recommended.

  d. These polyps are typically right-sided, sessile, and relatively large (often 1 cm or larger).

  e. These polyps often harbor *BRAF*-activating mutations and are considered precursors to microsatellite unstable (MSI-high) adenocarcinomas.

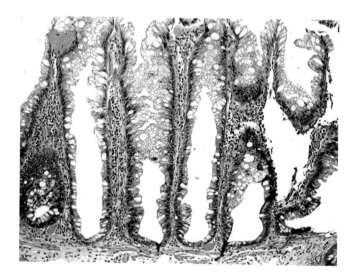

31. All of the following are associated with hereditary nonpolyposis colorectal cancer (HNPCC) syndrome EXCEPT:
    a. Carcinomas with DNA microsatellite instability
    b. Carcinomas with increased numbers of tumor infiltrating lymphocytes
    c. Proximally located large serrated polyps
    d. Proximally located mucinous colon adenocarcinomas
    e. Proximally located poorly differentiated colon adenocarcinomas

32. Which of the following syndromes is an inherited hamartomatous polyposis syndrome:
    a. Cowden syndrome
    b. Peutz-Jeghers syndrome (PJS)
    c. Familial juvenile polyposis syndrome
    d. Bannayan-Ruvalcaba-Riley syndrome
    e. All of the above

33. Which of the following molecular changes are common in the colorectal adenoma-carcinoma sequence:
    a. Mutations in the *APC* gene
    b. Mutations in the *KRAS* gene
    c. Loss of heterozygosity at 18q21
    d. Mutations of the TP53 gene
    e. All of the above

ANSWERS

1. c. *Giardia* infections most commonly occur through contact with contaminated water. *Giardia* is the most common cause of epidemic waterborne diarrhea. It is prevalent in children in developing countries, although the majority of such infections are asymptomatic. If symptomatic, usually symptoms consist of vomiting and diarrhea. Organisms identified on GI biopsies are motile trophozoites, which are slightly larger than an enterocyte nucleus (measuring up to 15 μm) and typically show a pear-shaped configuration with two round nuclei when seen in the correct orientation ("owl's eyes"). When numerous parasites are present within the lumen of the bowel, a pattern resembling "falling leaves" may be seen. Associated histologic abnormalities are variable, but include intraepithelial lymphocytosis, nonspecific chronic inflammation, eosinophils, and villous atrophy. Associated findings are most commonly minimal or absent. Patients with common variable immunodeficiency, hypogammaglobulinemia, and selective IgA deficiency are at increased risk for giardiasis and may develop chronic infection.

Handousa AE, El Shazly AM, Rizk H, et al: The histopathology of human giardiasis. *J Egypt Soc Parasitol* 2003;33(3):875-886.

Koot BG, ten Kate FJ, Juffrie M, et al: Does Giardia lamblia cause villous atrophy in children?: a retrospective cohort study of the histological abnormalities in giardiasis. *J Pediatr Gastroenterol Nutr* 2009;49(3):304-308.

Oberhuber G, Kastner N, Stolte M: Giardiasis: a histologic analysis of 567 cases. *Scand J Gastroenterol* 1997;32(1):48-51.

2. c. Intestinal spirochetosis is a noninvasive infection by spirochetes, most commonly *Brachyspira pilosicoli*, and *Brachyspira aalborgi*, which proliferate along the colonic epithelial surface. Although thought to represent an incidental finding in some cases, spirochetosis has been associated with diarrhea, anal discharge, and abdominal pain in immunosuppressed individuals, especially in the setting of HIV/AIDS (definite cause-effect relationship still uncertain because of the concomitant infections and other confounding factors in these cases).

The prevalence is 2% to 16% in Western countries but significantly higher in developing countries. It is most commonly seen in homosexual men with HIV/AIDS. Gross/endoscopic appearance of the mucosa is usually normal. This infection must be suspected and a "fringed," basophilic line is seen along the apical border of colonocytes (including colonocytes within crypts). Organisms along the epithelial surface are highlighted by silver stains (Warthin-Starry and Steinter stains). Alcial blue pH 2.5 and PAS stains can also be used, although Gram stain usually fails to highlight these organisms.

Koteish A, Kannangai R, Abraham SC, Torbenson M: Colonic spirochetosis in children and adults. *Am J Clin Pathol* 2003;120(6):828-832.

Carr NJ: The histological features of intestinal spirochetosis in a series of 113 patients. *Int J Surg Pathol* 2010;18(2):144-148.

Palejwala AA, Evans R, Campbell F: Spirochetes can colonize colorectal adenomatous epithelium. *Histopathology* 2000;37(3):284-285.

3. e. Although long-standing reflux esophagitis is a risk factor for developing Barrett esophagus (BE) and adenocarcinoma of the esophagus, it is not a significant risk factor for developing SCC. The pathogenesis of SCC is multifactorial and varies significantly among different regions in the world. Consumption of food rich in nitrates and nitrosamines is a risk factor in high-prevalence areas (e.g., China). Other known risk factors include tobacco smoke, alcohol, and various vitamin deficiencies (e.g., vitamin A, vitamin C, thiamine, and riboflavin). Predisposing conditions include achalasia, strictures associated with hot beverage burns, acid or lye ingestion, and Plummer-Vinson syndrome. Esophageal SSC invades both horizontally and vertically through the esophageal wall and may involve contiguous organs, such as the trachea, aorta, and pericardium. Regional lymph node metastasis is present in approximately 60% of patients at the time of diagnosis, and the presence of lymph node metastasis correlates with depth of invasion (<5% for intramucosal carcinomas and up to 45% for submucosal carcinomas). The most common molecular alterations of esophageal SCC include loss of p53, p16, and Rb. In biopsy specimens, distinguishing between in situ neoplasia (dysplasia) and invasive SCC may be difficult. Squamous dysplasia has smooth-edged papillations connected to the surface epithelium and lacks single-cell infiltration, discontinuous irregular clusters of cells, and a desmoplastic stroma. Invasive SCC must also be distinguished from nonneoplastic lesions, such as pseudoepitheliomatous hyperplasia. Pseudoepitheliomatous hyperplasia does not show

significant nuclear pleomorphism, loss of polarity, or overlapping of nuclei and always reveals a connection to the surface epithelium.

Ribiero U, Posner MC, Safatle-Ribiero AV, et al: Risk factors for squamous cell carcinoma of the oesophagus. *Br J Surg* 1996;83:1174-1183.

Rubio CA, Liu FS, Zhao HZ: Histological classification of intraepithelial neoplasias and microinvasive squamous carcinoma of the esophagus. *Am J Surg Pathol* 1989;13:685-690.

Eguchi T, Nakanishi Y, Shimoda T, et al: Histopathological criteria for additional treatment after endoscopic mucosal resection for esophageal cancer: analysis of 464 surgically resected cases. *Mod Pathol* 2006;19:475-480.

4. e. The length of the nondysplastic metaplastic epithelium does not correlate directly with the risk of developing carcinoma. When dysplasia is present, however, the extent of the dysplasia correlates with the risk of developing adenocarcinoma. BE is characterized by the presence of salmon-colored mucosa in the tubular esophagus. Traditionally, BE is separated into long-segment, short-segment, and ultra-short-segment types, depending on the length (>3 cm, 1 to 3 cm, or <1 cm, respectively) of involved esophageal mucosa. Although in the United States the presence of intestinal metaplasia with discrete goblet cells in the tubular esophagus is required for diagnosing BE, different criteria may be used by British and Japanese colleagues in which cardiac-type or intestinal-type columnar epithelium may support the diagnosis of BE provided that the endoscopic impression is consistent with BE. An alternative classification system has been proposed that would utilize the term BE to refer to columnar metaplasia of the esophagus and subclassify as either with or without goblet cells. The development of adenocarcinoma in BE follows a metaplasia-dysplasia-carcinoma sequence, characterized by the accumulation of multiple genetic and epigenetic alterations. The most common genetic alterations in BE involve inactivation of the p16 *INK4A/CDKN* tumor suppressor gene (chromosome 9p21) or loss or mutations of the p53 tumor suppressor gene (chromosome 17p13). The overall cancer risk of patients with BE, but without dysplasia, is approximately 2%. The risk of either having or developing cancer in patients with high-grade dysplasia ranges from 16% to 59%.

Buttar NS, Wang KK, Sebo TJ, et al: Extent of high-grade dysplasia in Barrett's esophagus correlates with risk of adenocarcinoma. *Gastroenterology* 2001;120(7):1630-1639.

Reid BJ: p53 and neoplastic progression in Barrett's esophagus. *Am J Gastroenterol* 2001;96(5):1321-1323.

Wang KK, Sampliner RE; Practice Parameters Committee of the American College of Gastroenterology: Updated guidelines 2008 for the diagnosis, surveillance and therapy of Barrett's esophagus. *Am J Gastroenterol* 2008;103(3):788-797.

5. d. Eosinophilic esophagitis (EE) affects primarily, but not exclusively, children and young adults. Increased intraepithelial eosinophils (≥ 15/HPFs) and exclusion of esophageal reflux represent diagnostic criteria. Endoscopic features include multiple mucosal rings/webs (i.e., "feline," "ringed," or corrugated esophagus), vertical lines/furrows, white punctate exudates, and strictures. Histologic features overlap significantly with reflux esophagitis. Features that favor EE over reflux esophagitis include markedly increased eosinophils, similar mucosal eosinophilia throughout the esophagus, gradient of eosinophilia within the mucosa (more severe toward the surface), and eosinophilic microabscesses (clusters of eosinophils) near the surface. Nonspecific changes that often accompany the previous findings include basal cell hyperplasia, spongiosis, and reactive epithelial changes. When other parts of the GI tract are involved by eosinophilia, a diagnosis of eosinophilic gastroenteritis should be rendered.

Collins MH: Histopathologic features of eosinophilic esophagitis. *Gastrointest Endosc Clin North Am* 2008;18(1):59-71.

Dellon ES: Approach to diagnosis of eosinophilic esophagitis. *Gastroenterol Hepatol* (NY) 2011;7(11):742-744.

Furuta GT, Liacouras CA, Collins MH, et al: Eosinophilic esophagitis in children and adults: a systematic review and consensus recommendations for diagnosis and treatment. *Gastroenterology* 2007;133(4):1342-1363.

6. d. Autoimmune atrophic gastritis is associated with autoantibody against parietal cells and is characterized (in its late stages) by complete loss of oxyntic glands, mucosal atrophy, and presence of metaplastic epithelium, including intestinal metaplasia and pseudopyloric gland metaplasia. The massive destruction of parietal cells seen in autoimmune atrophic gastritis results in the markedly decreased production of HCl, which in turn leads to compensatory hyperproduction of gastrin by antral G cells. Enterochromaffin-like (ECL) cells in the gastric body and fundus, under chronic stimulation by increased gastrin levels, undergo hyperplasia, which can present in two patterns: (1) linear hyperplasia, whereby gastric glands are lined by a contiguous layer of endocrine cells, and (2) nodular hyperplasia, in which small nests of endocrine cells are seen.

The entire spectrum of ECL-cell growth from hyperplasia to neoplasia has been observed in chronic atrophic gastritis and in MEN1-associated with Zollinger-Ellison syndrome. When the nodules increase in size to greater than 0.5 mm or invade submucosa, the lesion is classified as a carcinoid. In the setting of chronic atrophic gastritis, carcinoids smaller than 1 cm and fewer than three to five in number can be endoscopically removed and have an excellent prognosis. If the carcinoid is larger than 1 cm or more than five lesions are present, antrectomy may be considered (to remove the source of gastrin) and local excision of the fundic lesions is recommended.

Modlin IM, Kidd M, Lye KD: Biology and management of gastric carcinoid tumours: a review. *Eur J Surg* 2002;168:669-683.

Solcia E, Fiocca R, Villani L, et al: Hyperplastic, dysplastic, and neoplastic enterochromaffin-like-cell proliferations of the gastric mucosa: classification and histogenesis. *Am J Surg Pathol* 1995;19(Suppl 1):S1-S7.

7. d. The polyp shows typical features of a hamartomatous Peutz-Jeghers polyp with a distinctive arborizing pattern of smooth muscle that is derived from the underlying muscularis mucosae. Polyps in PJS most often occur in the small intestine, but may also occur in the stomach (as in this example) and colon. Wherever located, Peutz-Jeghers polyps contain a central core of smooth muscle that shows treelike branching. PJS is an autosomal dominantly inherited hamartomatous polyposis syndrome of the GI tract. Polyps in PJS most often occur in the small intestine, but may also occur in the stomach (as in this example) and colon. Criteria for the syndrome include: (1) three or more histologically confirmed Peutz-Jeghers polyps; or (2) any number of Peutz-Jeghers polyps in a patient with a family history of PJS; or (3) characteristic, prominent, mucocutaneous pigmentation with a family history of PJS; or (4) any number of Peutz-Jeghers polyps and characteristic, prominent, mucocutaneous pigmentation. Although patients with Peutz-Jeghers polyposis are at increased risk of developing adenocarcinoma of the GI tract, most of the carcinomas that arise in the GI tract are not directly arising within the Peutz-Jeghers polyps. Not only do patients with PJS have an increased risk of GI carcinoma (including gastric, small intestinal, and colonic carcinoma) but they are also at increased risk for developing breast carcinoma and pancreatic carcinoma, as well as less common tumors, such as sex cord tumors with annular tubules (SCTAT) of the ovary, adenoma malignum of the uterine cervix, and Sertoli cell tumors of the testis. The histologic distinction of gastric polyps in PJS patients versus other hamartomatous or hyperplastic gastric polyps without the context of clinical history of these syndromes is difficult and unreliable, even with adherence to a set of morphologic criteria. In the small intestine and large intestine, the characteristic histologic features of the arborizing delicate smooth muscle core within the Peutz-Jegher polyp are more pronounced.

Lam-Himlin D, Park JY, Cornish TC, et al: Morphologic characterization of syndromic gastric polyps. *Am J Surg Pathol* 2010;34(11):1656-1662.

Latchford AR, Phillips RK: Gastrointestinal polyps and cancer in Peutz-Jeghers syndrome: clinical aspects. *Fam Cancer* 2011; 10(3):455-461. Review.

Lim W, Hearle N, Shah B, et al: Further observations on LKB1/STK11 status and cancer risk in Peutz-Jeghers' syndrome. *Br J Cancer* 2003;89:308-313.

8. e. GISTs are the most common mesenchymal tumor in the GI tract. GIST is most common in the stomach (60%) and small intestine (30%), but can occur anywhere in the GI tract and the intraabdominal soft tissues (mesentery, omentum). GISTs are usually sporadic lesions; however, some GISTs may occur in association with familial syndromes, such as those associated with *KIT* germline mutations. The Carney triad, which affects young women, includes three types of tumors: GIST, pulmonary chondromas, and extraadrenal paragangliomas. Germline mutations in *KIT* are associated with GIST. Other tumors that may be associated with *KIT* germline mutations include melanomas and mast cell neoplasms. The most common mutations detected are *KIT* activating mutations leading to ligand-independent constitutive activation of the *KIT* receptor. A subset of GIST negative for *KIT* mutations has shown PDGFR activating mutations. The therapeutic use of Gleevec (imatinib mesylate), a tyrosine kinase inhibitor, has been of great utility in treating GISTs. *KIT* activating mutations comprise two groups: the regulatory site type and the enzymatic site type. The regulatory type of mutation is conserved at the imatinib binding site, so the drug can bind and effectively inhibit the mutated *KIT*. The enzymatic site mutation has a structurally changed binding site, resulting in drug resistance.

DeMatteo RP, Gold JS, Saran L, et al: Tumor mitotic rate, size, and location independently predict recurrence after resection of primary gastrointestinal stromal tumor (GIST). *Cancer* 2008;112:608-615.

Miettinen M, Lasota J: Histopathology of gastrointestinal stromal tumor. *J Surg Oncol* 2011;104(8):865-873.

Miettinen M, Lasota J: Gastrointestinal stromal tumors: pathology and prognosis at different sites. *Sem Diagn Pathol* 2006;23:70-83.

9. b. Glomus tumors are composed of modified smooth muscle cells that represent a counterpart of the perivascular glomus body. Glomus tumors most commonly occur in the peripheral soft tissues of the distal extremities. In the GI tract the vast majority involve the stomach. They are characterized by a proliferation of sharply demarcated, uniform cells, often arranged around prominent dilated hemangiopericytoma-like vascular spaces. The tumor cells are round with a centrally located, uniform nucleus and pale to clear cytoplasm. Mitotic activity is typically low (fewer than five mitoses per 50 HPFs). Frequently, the mucosa overlying the tumor ulcerates leading to bleeding, which is a common initial symptom. Glomus tumors can also be found incidentally. Most are small, with an average size of 2 to 3 cm. There is a strong female predilection (female-male ratio > 2:1) with median age 55 years. They are generally considered benign, although rare cases of metastasizing gastric glomus tumors have been reported. They are immunoreactive for smooth muscle actin, and are negative for desmin, CD117, chromogranin, and S100.

Miettinen M, Paal E, Lasota J, Sobin LH: Gastrointestinal glomus tumors: a clinicopathologic, immunohistochemical, and molecular genetic study of 32 cases. *Am J Surg Pathol* 2002;26: 301-311.

10. e. Four forms of Kaposi sarcoma (KS) are described: (1) classic form, an indolent, primarily cutaneous disease typically affecting older men of Mediterranean ancestry; (2) endemic form, primarily affecting HIV-negative children in Africa; (3) iatrogenic form, affecting organ transplantation patients on immunosuppressive therapy; and (4) HIV-associated cases. Visceral involvement, including the GI tract, occurs in only a minority of patients. The GI tract is one of the most common sites of visceral involvement of HIV-associated Kaposi sarcoma. Human herpesvirus-8 (HHV-8) is thought to play a major role in all forms of KS. Histologically, KS is characterized by a proliferation of relatively bland spindle to epithelioid cells forming slitlike spaces containing red blood cells. Eosinophilic, PAS-positive hyaline inclusions may be seen within tumor cells. The histopathologic findings of KS may be extremely subtle, particularly on endoscopic biopsy specimens. The monoclonal antibody to human herpesvirus-8 LANA is a highly sensitive and specific marker of HHV-8 infection in paraffin-embedded tissue sections of Kaposi sarcoma. Other spindle cell lesions, such as spindle cell hemangioma, dermatofibrosarcoma protuberans, and pyogenic granuloma, are LANA negative.

Antman K, Chang Y: Kaposi's sarcoma. *N Engl J Med* 2000;342:1027-1038.

Hammock L, Reisenauer A, Wang W, et al: Latency-associated nuclear antigen expression and human herpesvirus-8 polymerase chain reaction in the evaluation of Kaposi sarcoma and other vascular tumors in HIV-positive patients. *Mod Pathol* 2005;18:463-468.

Mesri EA, Cesarman E, Boshoff C: Kaposi's sarcoma and its associated herpesvirus. *Nat Rev Cancer* 2010; 10:707-719.

11. d. Triple drug regimen is used to treat *H. pylori* infection and typically consists of a proton pump inhibitor, clarithromycin, and either amoxicillin or metronidazole. Successful eradication is achieved in approximately 90% of patients. CAG is caused by *H. pylori* in the vast majority of cases. *H. pylori*-negative CAG is often due to treated or partially treated disease (i.e., use of broad-spectrum antibiotics for unrelated infections), in which case the number of organisms may decrease significantly. Numerous special stains may be useful in highlighting the organism against the background of surface and glandular mucus. These stains include Giemsa, Diff-Quik, Warthin-Starry, and alcian yellow. Immunohistochemistry, however, shows superior sensitivity and specificity and is currently considered the method of choice for *H. pylori* detection. *H. pylori* infection is associated with numerous conditions, including peptic ulcer disease, marginal zone B-cell lymphoma, multifocal atrophic gastritis, and gastric adenocarcinoma. Another *Helicobacter* species (*H. heilmanii*) may also cause disease in humans, often presenting with milder inflammation compared to *H. pylori* infection. The latter organisms can be distinguished from *H. pylori* by their larger size and more obvious corkscrew appearance. *H. heilmanii* is generally transmitted to humans by domestic pets and is thought to be associated with lesser risk for gastric cancer and lymphoma compared to *H. pylori*.

Non-*Helicobacter* organisms are sometimes seen within gastric mucin and should not be confused with *H. pylori*. These are usually cocci and can be distinguished by their shape. One possible pitfall is that, following treatment, *H. pylori* may assume a coccoid form and immunohistochemistry may be needed for a correct diagnosis. *H. pylori* bacteria produce urease, which breaks down urea into ammonia and carbon dioxide. This is a key reaction used in detecting *H. pylori* by the CLO test or by the breath test.

Amieva MR, et al: Host-bacterial interactions in Helicobacter pylori infection. *Gastroenterology* 2008;134(1):306-323.

Anim JT, et al: Assessment of different methods for staining Helicobacter pylori in endoscopic gastric biopsies. *Acta Histochem* 2000;102(2):129-137.

Warren JR, et al: Gastric pathology associated with Helicobacter pylori. *Gastroenterol Clin North Am* 2000;29(3):705-751.

12. c. *H. pylori* gastritis is a CAG with increased chronic inflammation in the lamina propria, often with lymphoid aggregates, and varying degrees of acute inflammation. Reactive gastropathy, in contrast, is a pattern of injury characterized by vascular congestion with only minimal chronic inflammation, reactive foveolar hyperplasia, and fibromuscular hyperplasia in the lamina propria. Reactive gastropathy changes may be associated with a variety of different causes, including NSAIDs, alcohol, chemotherapeutic drugs, heavy smoking, uremia, severe stress (e.g., trauma, burns, and surgery), ischemia/shock, and bile reflux. The most common endoscopic abnormality in reactive gastropathy is the presence of erythema or intramucosal hemorrhage, varying from petechiae to large ecchymoses.

Laine L: Nonsteroidal anti-inflammatory drug gastropathy. *Gastrointest Endosc Clin North Am* 1996;6:489-504.

Sobala GM, O'Connor HJ, Dewar EP, et al: Bile reflux and intestinal metaplasia in gastric mucosa. *J Clin Pathol* 1993;46:235-240.

13. a. Intestinal endometriosis is usually asymptomatic. It affects 15% to 37% of patients with pelvic endometriosis and clinically can mimic several conditions, including Crohn disease, ischemia, acute infection, and carcinoma. The most common sites include rectosigmoid colon, appendix, and small intestine. When symptomatic, patients commonly present with obstructive symptoms secondary to adhesions. Less frequently patients may present with crampy abdominal pain and GI bleeding. Symptoms are often associated with the onset of menses. Grossly, endometriosis is usually found on the serosal surface, but may involve any layer of the bowel wall. Microscopically, there are endometrial glands or stroma that may be associated with hemorrhage or hemosiderin-laden macrophages. Endometrial glands and stromal cells are immunoreactive for estrogen and progesterone receptors. Endometrial stromal cells are also CD10 positive.

Cappell MS, Friedman D, Mikhail N: Endometriosis of the terminal ileum simulating the clinical, roentgenographic, and surgical findings in Crohn's disease. *Am J Gastroenterol* 1991;86:1057-1062.

Yantiss RK, Clement PB, Young RH: Endometriosis of the intestinal tract: a study of 44 cases of a disease that may cause diverse challenges in clinical and pathologic evaluation. *Am J Surg Pathol* 2001;25:445-454.

14. b. Histopathologic features of celiac disease include intraepithelial lymphocytosis (characteristically showing a "tip-heavy" distribution), and variable architectural abnormalities, including villous atrophy (ranging from none to total) with variable crypt hyperplasia and expansion of the lamina propria by chronic inflammatory cells, especially plasma cells. None of the preceding findings, however, are specific for celiac disease and clinical correlation is required to establish this diagnosis. IgA anti-tTG (tissue transglutaminase) testing has now become the serologic test of choice for evaluation of celiac disease, largely replacing the more labor-intensive (although similarly accurate) antiendomysium antibody for initial testing. Genetic testing for HLA-DQ2 and HLA-DQ8 is utilized in selected cases as part of the clinical evaluation of celiac disease. HLA-DQ2 is present in approximately 95% of patients with celiac disease and most of the remaining 5% are positive for HLA-DQ8. Although positive DQ2/DQ8 testing is not diagnostic of celiac disease (present in approximately one third of the Caucasian population), absence of these haplotypes virtually excludes celiac disease. In typical cases of celiac disease, intraepithelial lymphocytes are $CD3^+/CD8^+$. Abnormal lymphocyte populations (with $CD3^+/CD8^-$ phenotype) may be seen in cases of refractory celiac disease and these patients are at increased risk for development of enteropathy-associated T-cell lymphoma. Most or all features of celiac disease, including intraepithelial lymphocytosis and variable amount of villous atrophy, may be present in cases of tropical sprue. Correlation with clinical (i.e., traveling to tropical regions) and laboratory findings (negative celiac disease work-up) are generally required to establish this diagnosis.

The prevalence of celiac disease is higher in patients with Down syndrome and diabetes mellitus than in the general population. Patients with celiac disease (also known as gluten-sensitive enteropathy) are at risk for developing enteropathy-associated T-cell lymphoma.

Di Sabatino A, Corazza GR: Coeliac disease. *Lancet* 2009;373 (9673):1480-1493.

Kagnoff MF: Overview and pathogenesis of celiac disease. *Gastroenterology* 2005;128(4 Suppl 1):S10-18.

Oberhuber G, Granditsch G, Vogelsang H: The histopathology of celiac disease: time for a standardized report scheme for pathologists. *Eur J Gastroenterol Hepatol* 1999;11(10):1185-1194.

15. c. Most clinically apparent midgut NETs are larger than 2 cm and show transmural invasion with metastasis at the time of diagnosis; however, metastasis and death from NET may also occur with tumors smaller than 1 cm. Five-year survival rates for localized NET approach 65%; however, in patients with distant spread, survival rates fall to 20% to 30%. Predictors of poor prognosis include distant metastasis, presence of the carcinoid syndrome.

The small intestine is the most frequent site of GI NET, accounting for approximately 30% of all GI NETs. The middle to distal ileum is the most common site, but they may also arise in the jejunum and proximal ileum, in Meckel diverticulum, and even in duplication cysts.

Tumors that infiltrate the muscle are often associated with hypertrophy of the muscle, possibly related to cytokine production by the tumor and sclerosis of the serosa. The combination of muscle hypertrophy and sclerosis may lead to obstructive symptoms and kinking of intestinal loops. Local lymph nodes are usually involved early in the course of the disease. In fact, tumor growth within lymph nodes may exceed that of the primary tumor. The lymph nodes may become matted by fibrosis. Hematogenous spread to the liver is common. Massive growth of hepatic metastases may occur even in the presence of a small primary tumor. Despite lymph node and hepatic metastases, the prognosis of patients with small intestinal NET is much better than for adenocarcinoma. The 5-year survival rate in patients with distant metastasis approaches 40%, which compares favorably with the 5-year survival rate of stage-matched adenocarcinoma (5%). Long-term survival is possible in patients with hepatic metastasis. Serotonin produced by the NET undergoes high first-pass metabolism in the liver. In patients with metastasis to the liver, circulating serotonin levels rise and the carcinoid syndrome may develop. Carcinoid syndrome occurs in 8% of patients with small intestinal NET. Elevated urinary 5-HIAA levels are diagnostic; circulating serotonin (5-HT) may also be measured.

Yantiss RK, Odze RD, Farraye FA, Rosenberg AE: Solitary versus multiple carcinoid tumors of the ileum: a clinical and pathologic review of 68 cases. *Am J Surg Pathol* 2003;27:811-817.

Burke AP, Thomas RM, Elsayed AM, Sobin LH: Carcinoids of the jejunum and ileum: an immunohistochemical and clinicopathologic study of 167 cases. *Cancer* 1997;79:1086-1093.

Oberg K: Neuroendocrine tumors of the gastrointestinal tract: recent advances in molecular genetics, diagnosis, and treatment. *Curr Opin Oncol* 2005;17:386-391.

16. b. Primary mucinous appendiceal tumors are found in less than 2% of appendix resections. These tumors characteristically cause cystic dilatation of the appendix owing to accumulation of copious gelatinous material in the lumen. Mucinous appendiceal neoplasms display a circumferential growth pattern with a variable papillary architecture. The tumor cells often contain abundant cytoplasmic mucin and with mildly enlarged nuclei that are basally located with minimal cytologic atypia. PMP is a term used to describe mucinous ascites or mucin deposits within the peritoneal cavity. PMP consists of organizing pools of mucin within peritoneal fat or on the serosal surfaces of the viscera, which contain variable numbers of neoplastic epithelial cells. Most cases reflect dissemination of an appendiceal mucinous neoplasm, in which case mucin pools that contain scant strips and clusters of low-grade neoplastic epithelial cells are typical. Cytologic grade should be specified when classifying PMP into low-grade mucinous carcinoma peritonei and high-grade mucinous carcinoma peritonei. Bradley and colleagues found that low-grade mucinous carcinoma peritonei was associated with a significantly better 5-year survival rate (63%) than was high-grade mucinous carcinoma peritonei (38%). Treatment for a mucinous adenoma that has not ruptured and that is confined to the appendix is appendectomy. Treatment of mucinous tumors that have spread extensively into the abdomen, resulting in PMP, includes cytoreduction (debulking) surgery to remove mucin and tumor implants in the abdominal cavity followed by intraoperative peritoneal chemotherapy. In cases in which high-grade or poorly differentiated carcinoma is present, treatment includes systemic chemotherapy. The American Joint Committee on Cancer staging guidelines assign tumor (T) stage for appendiceal mucinous neoplasms similar to those used for colonic adenocarcinoma, with the exception that T4a denotes both serosal involvement and extra-appendiceal disease limited to the right lower quadrant. Mucinous deposits beyond the right lower quadrant (PMP) are considered to represent metastatic disease and are denoted as M1a.

Bradley RF, Stewart JH, Russell GB, et al: Pseudomyxoma peritonei of appendiceal origin: a clinicopathologic analysis of 101 patients uniformly treated at a single institution, with literature review. *Am J Surg Pathol* 2006;30(5):551-559.

Panarelli NC, Yantiss RK: Mucinous neoplasms of the appendix and peritoneum. *Arch Pathol Lab Med* 2011;135(10):1261-1268.

Edge SB, Byrd DR, Compton CC, et al (eds): *AJCC Cancer Staging Manual,* 7th ed. New York: Springer, 2010, pp 133-141.

17. c. Appendiceal neuroendocrine tumors occur with an incidence of 2 million to 3 million per year, with a 2:1 female-male ratio. Most appendiceal neuroendocrine tumors are diagnosed incidentally during appendectomy; (1% of appendectomies), they are not related to a specific clinical presentation. The diagnosis is associated with, but not related to, acute appendicitis. Most tumors are located at the tip of the appendix (60% to 75%) and do not induce obstruction. Immunohistochemical analysis with chromogranin A and synaptophysin antibodies helps to confirm the diagnosis. Prognosis is related to the size of the tumor, and a maximal diameter larger than 2 cm is the most important parameter for prognosis. Another parameter related to prognosis is the presence and extent of mesoappendiceal invasion (>3 mm). The surgical margins of the appendectomy specimen (R0/R1) must be reported clearly. If the resection margin is positive for a tumor, a right hemicolectomy is generally required. Goblet cell carcinoids are considered to represent a separate clinicopathologic entity, distinct from classic appendiceal NETs and adenocarcinomas, with an uncertain histogenesis. They are more aggressive than classic NETs and require a different diagnostic and therapeutic approach.

Klöppel G, Perren A, Heitz PU: The gastroenteropancreatic neuroendocrine cell system and its tumors: the WHO classification. *Ann N Y Acad Sci* 2004;1014:13-27.

Deschamps L, Couvelard A: Endocrine tumors of the appendix: a pathologic review. *Arch Path Lab Med* 2010;134(6):871-875.

18. a. Several different types of polyps may be seen in ulcerative colitis. Some are true neoplasms, but others are a result of the inflammatory process. In cases of extensive ulceration there may be only scattered islands of relatively normal mucosa; upon endoscopy the ulcerated surface is perceived as the "baseline" mucosa and the islands of normal mucosa as polyps (pseudopolyposis of the colon). Pseudopolyps as defined previously often coexist with inflammatory polyps in patients with IBD. Inflammatory polyps consist of inflamed mucosa and/or granulation tissue that project above the level of the surrounding mucosa. As the extensive ulcerations heal and the epithelium regenerates there may be formation of filiform polyps (also referred to as postinflammatory polyps) that are composed of elongated projections of almost normal mucosa and submucosa. Patients with IBD can also have hyperplastic polyps that are similar to those that arise sporadically in the absence of an inflammatory background. Polypoid lesions showing cytologic dysplasia present unique challenges. Some of these lesions are similar to sporadic adenomas and can be removed completely endoscopically. In contrast DALMs are irregular, raised polypoid lesions without a defined stalk that are difficult to manage endoscopically and are an indication for colectomy. The distinction between sporadic adenoma and DALM is often difficult based solely on histologic examination, though in DALMs dysplasia may be seen at any location in the crypts and one might see a mixture of benign and dysplastic crypts at the surface of the polyp. Additional features favoring a DALM are young age at diagnosis and the presence of the polyp in an area of the colon that is affected by the inflammatory process.

Odze RD, Brien T, Brown CA, et al: Molecular alterations in chronic ulcerative colitis-associated and sporadic hyperplastic polyps: a comparative analysis. *Am J Gastroenterol* 2002;97(5):1235-1242.

Torres C, Antonioli D, Odze RD: Polypoid dysplasia and adenomas in inflammatory bowel disease: a clinical, pathologic, and follow-up study of 89 polyps from 59 patients. *Am J Surg Pathol* 1998;22(3):275-284.

19. b. Filiform polyposis is a rare form of GI polyposis. The polyps are often long and thin, hence the name of this condition. The term postinflammatory polyposis, which reflects the pathogenesis of these lesions, has also been proposed and used by some authors.

Filiform polyps can occasionally coalesce forming a mass, a condition that has been termed giant filiform polyposis and can mimic carcinoma. Histologically, the elongated projections are lined by normal colonic mucosa. They are thought to arise as a result of long-standing inflammation with alternating periods of healing. Given their proposed pathogenesis it is not surprising that they are most commonly seen in patients with IBD. They have also been reported in association with other inflammatory conditions, such as intestinal tuberculosis (TB). Rare reports of filiform polyposis also exist in patients without IBD or another recognizable inflammatory condition suggesting that, at least in some cases, the pathogenesis of these polyps might not be due to a postinflammatory reparative process. Filiform polyposis is not an indication for surgical resection by itself. It can, however, cause intestinal obstruction or bleeding necessitating surgical intervention.

Rozenbajgier C, Ruck P, Jenss H, Kaiserling E: Filiform polyposis: a case report describing clinical, morphological, and immunohistochemical findings. *Clin Investig* 1992;70(6):520-528.

Oakley GJ 3rd, Schraut WH, Peel R, Krasinskas A: Diffuse filiform polyposis with unique histology mimicking familial adenomatous polyposis in a patient without inflammatory bowel disease. *Arch Pathol Lab Med* 2007;131(12):1821-1824.

20. b. Biopsies from patients with Crohn disease often show varying degrees of active inflammation and chronic inflammatory changes, such as architectural distortion and basal cell plasmacytosis. Noncaseating granulomas are seen in approximately 50% of resection specimens and 30% of biopsies. The presence of granulomas in the bowel is not specific for Crohn disease, although the latter is the most common cause in the Western world. Granulomas may also be seen in certain immunodeficiency disorders, such as chronic granulomatous disease and common variable immunodeficiency, and sarcoidosis, as well as in several infections.

TB can mimic Crohn disease and in areas where it is an endemic differentiating between the two entities can be especially challenging. Histologic features that favor TB are caseation and large confluent granulomas larger than 0.4 mm. Chronic granulomatous disease is a rare genetic immunodeficiency disorder in which phagocytes are unable to kill certain bacteria and fungi as a result of reduced production of superoxide and hydrogen peroxide. Involvement of the GI tract is seen in up to 50% of patients. Sarcoidosis affects the GI tract in less than 5% of cases. When it affects the colon and terminal ileum it can mimic Crohn disease by producing moderate fibrosis and narrowing of the terminal ileum. It does not cause fistulas and there is usually a lack of mucosal architectural distortion and acute inflammation.

Pulimood AB, Amarapurkar DN, Ghoshal U, et al: Differentiation of Crohn's disease from intestinal tuberculosis in India in 2010. *World J Gastroenterol* 2011;17(4):433-443.

Marks DJ, Miyagi K, Rahman FZ, et al: Inflammatory bowel disease in CGD reproduces the clinicopathological features of Crohn's disease. *Am J Gastroenterol* 2009;104(1):117-124.

Daniels JA, Lederman HM, Maitra A, Montgomery EA: Gastrointestinal tract pathology in patients with common variable immunodeficiency (CVID): a clinicopathologic study and review. *Am J Surg Pathol* 2007;31(12):1800-1812.

21. c. Crohn disease is a chronic idiopathic IBD with an annual incidence of 5 to 10 per 100,000 inhabitants in Western countries. Its incidence has been increasing over the last three decades. Crohn disease has a multifactorial cause in which genetic and environmental factors interact to produce the immunological background for the diseases. Many genes have been associated with Crohn disease, one of the best studied being the *CARD15/NOD2* gene, which is located on chromosome 16 and contains caspase recruitment domains (CARDs). The CARD15/NOD2 protein serves as an intracellular receptor for bacterial products in monocytes, and transduces signals leading to nuclear factor-κB activation.

Immunologic biomarkers have been used as biomarker panels in IBD, including Crohn disease. The most common ones are ANCA and anti-*Saccharomyces cerevisiae* antibodies (ASCAs). ASCAs bind mannose sequences in phosphopeptidomannan located in the cell wall of *S. cerevisiae* (baker's/brewer's yeast). They are found in 39% to 76% of patients with Crohn disease, up to 15% of patients with ulcerative colitis, and 5% of healthy control subjects. ANCAs are found in a variety of immune conditions, such as Wegener granulomatosis and rheumatoid arthritis, as well as in ulcerative colitis. Perinuclear ANCA (pANCA) is found in 20% to 85% of ulcerative colitis patients and 2% to 28% of Crohn disease patients. Of note, a positive ASCA has also been seen in patients with Behçet disease, celiac disease, autoimmune hepatitis, and primary biliary cirrhosis. ANCA positivity can be found in other forms of colitis, such as eosinophilic and collagenous colitis.

Grossly, patients with Crohn disease have a thickened bowel wall with strictures, fistula tract formation, and fat wrapping. The disease involves the ileum in the majority of patients (approximately 80%) and tends to spare the rectum. Inflammation throughout the bowel typically shows skip areas, although unusual cases of Crohn disease with continuous inflammation are described. Bowel resections for Crohn disease show significant mural changes. There is typically transmural inflammation, which may be associated with fissuring ulcers that extend into the muscularis propria. Neuronal and smooth muscle hypertrophy within the submucosa and muscularis propria are also common. In addition, vascular changes in the form of endothelial injury, intimal proliferation, and thrombosis may be observed.

Cho JH: Significant role of genetics in IBD: the NOD2 gene. *Rev Gastroenterol Disord* 2003;3(Suppl 1):S18-S22.
Sandborn WJ: Serologic markers in inflammatory bowel disease: state of the art. *Rev Gastroenterol Disord* 2004;4:167-174.

22. c. The infection most typically associated with pseudomembrane formation is *C. difficile*. *C. difficile* infection is associated with prior antibiotic exposure and can range in severity from mild diarrhea to fulminant disease with toxic megacolon or perforation. Endoscopically, there usually are yellow plaques (pseudomembranes) that are more prominent on the left colon. Classic histologic findings are the "volcano" lesions with ballooned crypts giving rise to pseudomembranes, consisting of fibrin, mucin, and neutrophils. *C. difficile* infection can occur in patients with IBD. In fact, patients with IBD may be at a disproportionately higher risk for acquiring *C. difficile* infection compared to non-IBD patients. *C. difficile* infection may precipitate an IBD flare, although in some cases it might be an innocent bystander.

Histologic features similar to those seen in *C. difficile* colitis, such as pseudomembrane formation, mucosal necrosis, and hemorrhage, may be seen in other infections as well as in ischemic colitis and neonatal necrotizing enterocolitis. Ischemic colitis can also show pseudomembranes with mucosal necrosis and hemorrhage in the lamina propria. Hyalinization of the lamina propria is commonly seen along with the presence of atrophic and withered crypts showing regenerative changes. These latter findings favor the diagnosis of ischemic colitis. Ischemic injury can be secondary to a number of insults, including occlusion of a major vessel, infection, and drugs. Enterohemorrhagic *E. coli* can cause bloody diarrhea with severe abdominal cramping. The histologic findings are similar to those seen in ischemic colitis, because the colitis is presumed to be secondary to the numerous fibrin thrombi that develop during the infection.

Griffin PM, Olmstead LC, Petras RE: Escherichia coli O157:H7-associated colitis. A clinical and histological study of 11 cases. *Gastroenterology* 1990;99(1):142-149.
Nguyen GC, Kaplan GG, Harris ML, Brant SR: A national survey of the prevalence and impact of Clostridium difficile infection among hospitalized inflammatory bowel disease patients. *Am J Gastroenterol* 2008;103(6):1443-1450.

23. e. Familial adenomatous polyposis (FAP) is the most common polyposis syndrome that has a prevalence of 1 in 5000 to 7000 people. It is characterized by hundreds to thousands of adenomas that can progress to adenocarcinoma. Patients with FAP have a 100% risk of colorectal cancer, and therefore patients must undergo prophylactic total colectomy.

In contrast to FAP, attenuated FAP (AFAP) is characterized by fewer than 100 adenomas. Development of adenocarcinoma is not inevitable; however, the risk is significant, estimated to be up to 69%. FAP and AFAP are associated with important extracolonic manifestations. Duodenal, ampullary, and periampullary adenomas occur in more than 90% of patients and up to 10% of patients develop duodenal adenocarcinoma by the age of 60. Gastric fundic gland polyps are also common in FAP/AFAP patients and frequently show low-grade dysplasia. Progression to carcinoma has been reported, but it is rare. Additional extracolonic cancers in FAP patients include follicular and papillary thyroid cancers, which may precede the development of polyposis in some patients. Hepatoblastoma has been reported in children. In Turcot syndrome FAP patients show central nervous system tumors. These are usually medulloblastomas and less commonly gliomas. Patients with Gardner syndrome show desmoids, osteomas, supernumerary teeth, epidermoid cysts, congenital hyperplasia of the retinal epithelium, and/or adrenal adenomas. The gene mutated in FAP and AFAP is adenomatous polyposis coli (APC), which is located on chromosome 5q21. It is a tumor suppressor gene that inhibits Wnt signaling. Specific mutations in the *APC* gene are associated with distinctive phenotypes. For example, mutations between codons 463 and 1444 are associated with congenital hyperplasia of the retinal epithelium, but mutations between codons 1310 and 2011 are associated with desmoid tumors.

Fodde R: The APC gene in colorectal cancer. *Eur J Cancer* 2002;38: 867-871.

Wehrli BM, Weiss SW, Yandow S, Coffin CM: Gardner-associated fibromas (GAF) in young patients: a distinct fibrous lesion that identifies unsuspected Gardner syndrome and risk for fibromatosis. *Am J Surg Pathol* 2001;25:645-651.

24. c. According to the World Health Organization (WHO) 2010 classification NETs of the GI tract should be classified as (1) well-differentiated NET, low grade (G1); (2) well-differentiated NET, intermediate grade (G2); and (3) neuroendocrine carcinoma (G3). The term carcinoid corresponds to the low-grade well-differentiated NET. Grading is based upon mitotic count and Ki67 proliferation index with G1 tumors showing less than 2 mitoses per 10 HPFs or 2% or less Ki67 index, G2 tumors showing 2 to 20 mitoses per 10 HPFs or 3% to 20% Ki67 index, and G3 tumors showing more than 20 mitoses in 10 HPFs or more than 20% Ki67 index. NETs have historically been classified by their embryologic origin: foregut (including the respiratory tract, thymus, stomach, and pancreas), midgut (including the small intestine, appendix, and right colon), and hindgut (including the transverse, descending, sigmoid colon, and rectum). The most common site for carcinoids in the GI tract is the small bowel, followed by the appendix and rectum. Rectal carcinoids are more common in Asian and African American populations, are often small (<1 cm), and are found incidentally. Pathologic features that have been associated with metastasis and poor prognosis include increased tumor size, muscularis invasion, lymphovascular invasion, and increased mitotic rate. The neoplastic cells in rectal carcinoids are positive for synaptophysin, chromogranin, and neuron-specific enolase. Rectal carcinoids are PAP (prostatic acid phosphatase) positive but negative for PSA. The latter is helpful in distinguishing these lesions from prostatic adenocarcinoma.

Modlin IM, Sandor A: An analysis of 8305 cases of carcinoid tumors. *Cancer* 1997;79:813-829.

Azumi N, Traweek ST, Battifora H: Prostatic acid phosphatase in carcinoid tumors. Immunohistochemical and immunoblot studies. *Am J Surg Pathol* 1991;15:785-790.

Fahy BN, Tang LH, Klimstra D, et al: Carcinoid of the rectum risk stratification (CaRRs): a strategy for preoperative outcome assessment. *Ann Surg Oncol* 2007;14(5):1735-1743.

25. e. Paget disease of the anus occurs predominantly in elderly patients without a gender predilection. Patients usually present with a raised, red area in the anal canal or perianal skin. Histologically Paget disease is characterized by an intraepidermal proliferation of large neoplastic cells with vacuolated cytoplasm. The neoplastic cells may be found in clusters, especially at the base of the epithelium, or as discrete cells. The neoplastic cells in Paget disease contain intracytoplasmic mucin and are positive with diastase-PAS and alcian blue. These special stains can help distinguish Paget disease from other neoplastic lesions, such as melanoma and squamous cell dysplasia/carcinoma. Immunohistochemical stains can also help in establishing the diagnosis. The neoplastic cells in Paget disease are negative for melanoma and squamous markers. They are positive for carcinoembryonic antigen (CEA), epithelial membrane antigen (EMA), and, usually, CK7. In classical Paget disease without an underlying adenocarcinoma the neoplastic cells show sweat gland differentiation and are GCDFP15 positive and CK20 negative. In cases due to a primary anal adenocarcinoma the cells are GCDFP15 negative and variably CK20 positive. Cases associated with a colorectal adenocarcinoma are CK20 positive and GCDFP15 negative and may be CK7 negative. The treatment of Paget disease associated with an underlying adenocarcinoma is secondary to the treatment of the primary tumor. In cases where there is no underlying carcinoma, the treatment consists of wide local excision, which is unfortunately associated with a significant risk for recurrence.

Goldblum JR, Hart WR: Perianal Paget's disease: a histologic and immunohistochemical study of 11 cases with and without associated rectal adenocarcinoma. *Am J Surg Pathol* 1998;22: 170-179.

Battles OE, Page DL, Johnson JE: Cytokeratins, CEA, and mucin histochemistry in the diagnosis and characterization of extramammary Paget's disease. *Am J Clin Pathol* 1997;108:6-12.

26. e. Anal intraepithelial neoplasia (AIN) is a precursor lesion to anal SCC, similar to its cervical counterpart; however, rates of progression to cancer seem to be substantially lower than they are for cervical precancerous lesions. Risk factors for anal SCC include HIV infection, HPV infection (especially persistent infection with a high-risk HPV genotype), heavy cigarette smoking, immunosuppression, and radiation. In HIV-positive patients the risk for AIN increases as the CD4 count decreases and the HIV RNA viral load increases. AIN is classified into three groups based on the degree of atypia. AIN I shows mild dysplasia, AIN II shows moderate dysplasia, and AIN III shows severe dysplasia. In cases with mild dysplasia dysmaturation and mitoses are seen in the lower third of the epithelium. In cases with moderate dysplasia dysmaturation and mitoses involve the lower two thirds of the epithelium, but in cases with severe dysplasia they involve the entire epithelial thickness. In a two-tier system, AIN I is considered low-grade dysplasia, and AIN II and III are considered high grade. Immunohistochemical stains for HPV antigens and/or detection of HPV DNA by in situ hybridization or polymerase chain reaction (PCR) may be used although they are not required for histologic diagnosis. Immunohistochemistry is much less sensitive than molecular methods. Distinction of AIN from reactive atypia or immature metaplastic epithelium can be challenging. Immunostaining with p16 and Ki67 can be helpful in this context. Overexpression of p16 (strong, diffuse nuclear and cytoplasmic staining) and increased Ki67 staining (>50% of mucosal thickness) favor the diagnosis of dysplasia; p16 has higher specificity as increased Ki67 may be seen in some inflammatory and hyperplastic lesions. A lesion with histologic features similar to AIN III in the perianal skin is referred to as Bowen disease.

Frisch M, Fenger C, van den Brule AJ, et al: Variants of squamous cell carcinoma of the anal canal and perianal skin and their relation to human papillomaviruses. *Cancer Res* 1999;59: 753-757.

Pirog EC, Quint KD, Yantiss RK: P16/CDKN2A and Ki-67 enhance the detection of anal intraepithelial neoplasia and condyloma and correlate with human papillomavirus detection by polymerase chain reaction. *Am J Surg Pathol* 2010;34(10):1449-1455.

27. d. Juvenile polyps are usually solitary and not associated with a polyposis syndrome. Sporadic/isolated juvenile polyps are the most common type of colonic polyp in children, but they also occur frequently in adults. Juvenile polyposis syndrome is characterized by multiple polyps in the colorectum ranging in number from three to several hundred. Polyps can also be found in the stomach and small intestine. In juvenile polyposis coli the polyps are predominantly located in the colon. Small intestinal polyps, if present, are few. In generalized juvenile polyposis polyps are found through the GI tract. In rare cases, there may be multiple gastric polyps in the absence of colonic polyps (familial gastric juvenile polyposis). Juvenile polyposis of infancy presents in infants with polyps in the stomach, small intestine, and colon. Infants present with diarrhea, protein-losing enteropathy, bleeding, and intussusception and usually die within the first 2 years of life. Histologically, juvenile polyps show dilated glands often filled with neutrophils and inspissated mucin. The lamina propria is edematous and expanded by inflammatory cells. Strands of muscle fibers may be present. Approximately 60% of patients with juvenile polyposis syndrome have a germline mutation in the *SMAD4* or *BMPR1A* genes. Both genes are involved in the BMP/TGF-β signaling pathway. The majority of mutations are point mutations or small deletions, although some cases show large deletions of one or more exons. Juvenile polyposis syndrome is associated with an increased risk of GI cancer. The risk of colon cancer has been reported to be 68% by the age of 60, though a more recent study found a risk of 39%. Gastric and small bowel carcinomas are estimated to occur at approximately one fifth the frequency of CRC. Pancreatic carcinoma has also been reported in patients with juvenile polyposis syndrome.

Lam-Himlin D, Park JY, Cornish TC, et al: Morphologic characterization of syndromic gastric polyps. *Am J Surg Pathol* 2010;34(11):1656-1662.

Brosens LA, van Hattem A, Hylind LM, et al: Risk of colorectal cancer in juvenile polyposis. *Gut* 2007;56(7):965-967.

Hizawa K, Iida M, Yao T, et al: Juvenile polyposis of the stomach: clinicopathological features and its malignant potential. *J Clin Pathol* 1997;50(9):771-774.

28. e. Collagenous colitis is a form of microscopic colitis that generally affects middle-aged and elderly women, who present with chronic diarrhea. Contrary to IBD, colonocoscopic examination is normal in patients with microscopic colitis. Thickening of the subepithelial collagen table (minimum of 15 μm, normal = 5 to 7 μm) is a hallmark feature of collagenous colitis. Care must be taken to avoid overinterpretation of tangentially cut surface epithelium and underlying collagen, which may appear thickened. When abnormally thick, the subepithelial collagen often shows an irregular, basket weave–like interface where the underlying lamina propria and subepithelial capillary vessels are frequently surrounded by collagen—a useful diagnostic feature. In addition to a thickened collagen table, various degrees of epithelial injury, with nuclear irregularity, loss of mucin, intraepithelial lymphocytes, and focal neutrophilic infiltrate are often present. The surface epithelium is commonly stripped off from the underlying thick collagen table and is also a useful diagnostic feature. Crypt architecture should be normal. Lymphocytic colitis and collagenous colitis have been proposed to be related. Both have an identical chronic inflammatory pattern and are distinguished only by the presence of a thickened collagen layer in collagenous colitis. Collagen deposition in collagenous colitis may be patchy, and commonly more pronounced in the right colon. In addition, patients may show change from one to the other on sequential biopsies. Spontaneous remissions and relapses are common. Treatment usually starts with prescription antiinflammatory medications, such as mesalamine (Rowasa or Canasa) and sulfasalazine (Azulfidine). Steroids, including budesonide (Entocort) and prednisone, may be used to control a sudden attack of diarrhea. Immunosuppressive agents, such as azathioprine (Imuran), may be needed in unresponsive cases.

Tagkalidis P, Bhathal P, Gibson P: Microscopic colitis. *J Gastroenterol Hepatol* 2002;17:236-248.

Chetty R, Govender D: Lymphocytic and collagenous colitis: an overview of so-called microscopic colitis. *Nat Rev Gastroenterol Hepatol* 2012;21;9(4):209-218.

29. d. Granular cell tumor (GCT) is a relatively common, benign tumor of Schwann/neuroectodermal origin, most commonly seen in the tongue and esophagus, but it may occur in any location within the luminal GI tract. Morphologically, GCTs are characterized by sheets or nests of pink cells with small nuclei and abundant, granular, eosinophilic cytoplasm. GCTs are positive for S100 and PAS-diastase. Pseudoepitheliomatous hyperplasia of the overlying squamous epithelium occurs in approximately half of the cases and, when exuberant, may mimic SCC on biopsies. Differential diagnosis includes rhabdomyoma, melanoma, and histiocytic proliferations.

Johnston J, Helwig EB: Granular cell tumors of the gastrointestinal tract and perianal region: a study of 74 cases. *Dig Dis Sci* 1981; 26(9):807-816.

Fanburg-Smith JC, Meis-Kindblom JM, Fante R, Kindblom LG: Malignant granular cell tumor of soft tissue: diagnostic criteria and clinocopathologic correlation. *Am J Surg Pathol* 1998;22(7): 779-794.

Lack EE, Worsham GF, Callihan MD, et al: Granular cell tumor: a clinicopathologic study of 110 patients. *J Surg Oncol* 1980;13(4): 301-316.

30. c. Sessile serrated adenomas (SSAs) or sessile serrated polyps (SSPs) are most commonly seen in the right colon and are generally large (>0.5-1.0 cm) and flat. This picture is in contrast with that seen for hyperplastic polyps, which are usually left-sided, small (<0.5 cm), and more obviously polypoid. The diagnosis of SSA relies on the recognition of architectural features, which includes epithelial serration, crypt dilatation extending to the muscularis mucosa, and horizontal growth (sometimes forming "L-shaped" or "inverted T-shaped" crypts). Abnormal proliferation is also a described feature, which is characterized by upward migration of epithelial mitosis, often in an asymmetric manner (higher on one side of the crypt).

SSAs are associated with the so-called "serrated pathway" of colorectal neoplasia, which lacks the *APC/KRAS/P53* mutations or chromosomal instability seen in most colorectal carcinomas, but instead show *BRAF* mutations and CpG island methylator phenotype (CIMP), leading to CRCs with microsatellite instability (approximately 10% to 15% of colon cancers). Cytologic dysplasia (either low grade or high grade), although not required for diagnosis, may be seen as SSAs progress. Recent studies indicate that patients diagnosed with SSAs are at risk for subsequent CRCs and should probably be followed at least as aggressively as patients with conventional adenomas.

Snover DC, Jass JR, Fenoglio-Preiser C, Batts KP: Serrated polyps of the large intestine: a morphologic and molecular review of an evolving concept. *Am J Clin Pathol* 2005;124(3):380-391.

Noffsinger AE: Serrated polyps and colorectal cancer: new pathway to malignancy. *Annu Rev Pathol* 2009;4:343-364.

Lu FI, van Niekerk de W, Owen D, et al: Longitudinal outcome study of sessile serrated adenoma of the colorectum: an increased risk for subsequent right-sided colorectal carcinoma. *Am J Surg Pathol* 2010;34(7):927-934.

31. c. Patients with hereditary nonpolyposis colon cancer (HNPCC) syndrome have a germline mutation in a mismatch repair gene. The majority of mutations are in the *MLH1* and *MSH2* genes and approximately 10% of patients show mutations in the *MSH6* and *PMS2* genes.

Patients with HNPCC develop microsatellite unstable tumors. Testing for microsatellite instability can be performed using a PCR or immunohistochemical staining for MLH1, MSH2, MSH6, and PMS2. In vivo MLH1 forms a heterodimer with PMS2, but MSH2 forms a heterodimer with MSH6. As a result when MLH1 expression is lost, PMS2 expression is also lost because PMS2 is unstable in the absence of the heterodimer. Similarly, when MSH2 expression is lost, so is MSH6 expression. Of note, loss of PMS2 and MSH6 due to defects in these genes is not accompanied by loss in MLH1 and MSH2 because of the heterodimer configuration. Colon adenocarcinomas in HNPCC patients arise in conventional adenomas that may show mutations in *KRAS*. In contrast, *BRAF* mutations are almost never found in HNPCC-associated carcinomas. In contrast to HNPCC-associated tumors, sporadic colon cancers showing microsatellite instability are characterized by hypermethylation of the MLH1 promoter and *BRAF* mutations. *BRAF* mutations are also found in sessile serrated polyps (adenomas) that are thought to be precursors to some sporadic microsatellite unstable tumors.

Shia J, Ellis NA, Paty PB, et al: Value of histopathology in predicting microsatellite instability in hereditary nonpolyposis colorectal cancer and sporadic colorectal cancer. *Am J Surg Pathol* 2003;27(11):1407-1417.

Shia J, Klimstra DS, Nafa K, et al: Value of immunohistochemical detection of DNA mismatch repair proteins in predicting germline mutation in hereditary colorectal neoplasms. *Am J Surg Pathol* 2005;29(1):96-104.

McGivern A, Wynter CV, Whitehall VL, et al: Promoter hypermethylation frequency and BRAF mutations distinguish hereditary non-polyposis colon cancer from sporadic MSI-H colon cancer. *Fam Cancer* 2004;3(2):101-107.

32. e. Hamartomatous polyps are characterized by an overgrowth of cells native to the area in which they normally occur and can contain cellular components from any of the three germinal layers forming the intestines. The hamartomatous syndromes occur at approximately one tenth the frequency of the adenomatous syndromes and account for less than 1% of colorectal cancer in North America. Nonetheless, identification of affected families is important for screening and management. The most common of the hamartomatous syndromes is familial juvenile polyposis, which has an estimated incidence of 1 per 100,000 births. This disorder shows an autosomal dominant pattern of inheritance and patients show germline mutations in the *SMAD4* gene or in the *BMPR1A* gene. Cowden syndrome and Bannayan-Ruvalcaba-Riley syndrome are characterized by germline mutations in the *PTEN* tumor suppressor gene. Other inherited hamartomatous polyposis syndromes not listed previously are basal cell nevus syndrome, MEN syndrome 2B, and neurofibromatosis 1.

Schreibman IR, Baker M, Amos C, McGarrity TJ: The hamartomatous polyposis syndromes: a clinical and molecular review. *Am J Gastroenterol* 2005;100:476-490.

Eng C: PTEN: one gene, many syndromes. *Hum Mutat* 2003;22(3):183-198.

Calva-Cerqueira D, Chinnathambi S, Pechman B, et al: The rate of germline mutations and large deletions of SMAD4 and BMPR1A in juvenile polyposis. *Clin Genet* 2009;75(1):79-85.

33. e. Colorectal tumorigenesis proceeds through well-defined clinicopathologic stages that are associated with specific molecular events. The initiating event is a somatic mutation in a gene inactivating the APC/β-catenin pathway. Mutations that constitutively activate the KRAS/BRAF/MAPK pathway promote tumor growth and adenoma formation, but subsequent waves of clonal expansion driven by genes controlling other pathways, such as the TP53 and TGFβ pathways, lead to the transition from adenoma to CRC. In the majority of CRCs the progression of adenoma to carcinoma is also associated with chromosomal instability, most notably gains in chromosomes 8q, 13q, and 20q and losses of the 1p, 8p, 17p, and 18q chromosomal regions (so-called chromosomal instability pathway). Approximately 15% of CRCs do not show chromosomal instability and these develop through the microsatellite instability pathway. These tumors are characterized by early mutations in *BRAF* and CpG island hypermethylation. Loss of heterozygosity at 18q21 is thought to be a late event in the adenoma to carcinoma progression and results in the loss of the tumor suppressor gene, *SMAD4*. CRCs showing loss of heterozygosity at 18q21 have been shown to have a worse prognosis. Mutations in the *KRAS* gene have become very important in routine clinical practice because of the use of epidermal growth factor receptor (EGFR) inhibitors in the treatment of metastatic CRC. These drugs have been shown to be ineffective in tumors that harbor *KRAS* mutations and for this reason testing of advanced CRC for *KRAS* mutations is now required prior to treatment with EGFR inhibitors.

Jass JR: Pathogenesis of colorectal cancer. *Surg Clin North Am* 2002;82:891-904.

Watanabe T, Wu TT, Catalano PJ, et al: Molecular predictors of survival after adjuvant chemotherapy for colon cancer. *N Engl J Med* 2001;344(16):1196-1206.

Plesec TP, Hunt JL: KRAS mutation testing in colorectal cancer. *Adv Anat Pathol* 2009;16(4):196-203.

CHAPTER 5

PANCREAS PATHOLOGY

Olca Basturk and N. Volkan Adsay

QUESTIONS

All questions in this chapter refer to a photograph or photomicrograph.

1. A 38-year-old man with a history of primary sclerosing cholangitis underwent resection of a solid pancreatic mass. Macroscopically, the head of the pancreas appeared fibrotic. The specimen was submitted entirely for microscopic examination and showed relatively uniform findings throughout, which are illustrated in this picture. Which of the following serum tests would have helped to confirm the diagnosis in this patient?
   a. Carcinoembryonic antigen (CEA)
   b. CA19.9
   c. IgG4
   d. CA125
   e. α-Fetoprotein (AFP)

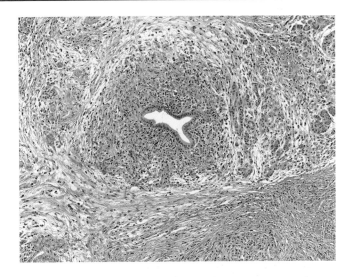

2. A 63-year-old male patient presented with recent-onset diabetes mellitus, back pain, jaundice, and a 25-pound weight loss in the past 4 months. The tumor resected was firm and displayed the characteristics shown in this picture. The tumor cells in this case are MOST likely to be diffusely positive for:
   a. Chromogranin
   b. Cytokeratin 7 (CK7)
   c. Trypsin
   d. Cytokeratin 20 (CK20)
   e. β-Catenin

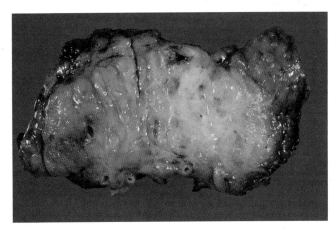

3. A 68-year-old man presented with rapid weight loss and a 6-cm relatively well demarcated solid pancreatic tumor with hemorrhagic areas. The tumor appeared to be arising from a mucinous cystic neoplasm. The microscopic findings of this tumor are shown here. All of the following statements for this tumor type are correct EXCEPT:

   a. This malignant tumor is considered to be of epithelial origin.
   b. Some examples can be admixed with ordinary ductal adenocarcinomas (DAs).
   c. Multinucleated giant cells in this tumor express keratin.
   d. Multinucleated giant cells in this tumor express CD68.
   e. The malignant cells in this tumor type are the smaller, atypical mononuclear cells in the background rather than the multinucleated giant cells.

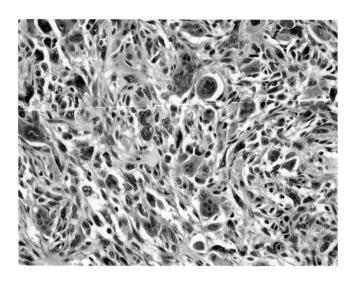

4. A 48-year-old woman presented with abdominal pain and was found to have a cystic tumor in the tail of the pancreas on computed tomography (CT) scan. The cyst contained thick mucinous fluid. Which of the following would be MOST likely valid for this tumor?

   a. Overall 5-year survival rate for this tumor is less than 5%.
   b. Lymph node metastasis is common.
   c. This lesion is most commonly seen in childhood.
   d. Serologic examination of the aspirate may have been helpful in the preoperative differential diagnosis.
   e. One section per centimeter of this lesion is regarded as adequate sampling for the diagnosis.

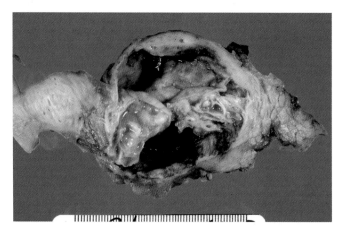

5. A 63-year-old woman was found to have a 13-cm mass in the tail of the pancreas during a work-up for gastrointestinal (GI) bleeding, which later proved to be due to an independent gastric ulcer related to aspirin ingestion. The tumor was resected and the cut surface of the tumor is shown here. All of the following regarding this tumor type are correct EXCEPT:

   a. It is almost always benign.
   b. It is slightly more common in women.
   c. It may be as large as 25 to 30 cm.
   d. It is characterized by abundant mucin production.
   e. It has almost no potential for recurrence.

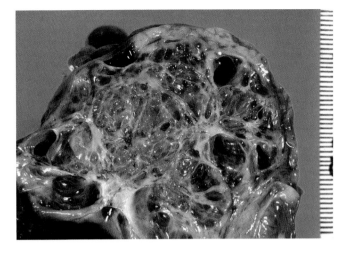

6. A 31-year-old woman recently developed abdominal pain and was found to have a 7-cm mass in the head of the pancreas that was radiologically cystic. There was no history of pancreatitis. There was also a 1.5-cm nodule in the liver. Both the pancreatic and liver fine needle aspirations (FNAs) showed a tumor composed of relatively uniform cells with nuclear grooves. Preoperative cyst fluid aspiration showed no CEA activity; amylase and lipase were also negative. The tumor was resected and macroscopic features of this tumor are shown here. All of the following statements for this tumor type would be correct EXCEPT:

   a. Cystic component of this tumor has a mucinous lining.
   b. Microscopic projections into the adjacent pancreas are common.
   c. Metastatic tumor in the peritoneum or liver may be present in approximately 15% of the cases.
   d. Even patients with metastasis often have a protracted clinical course.
   e. Histologic features are not very reliable in predicting outcome.

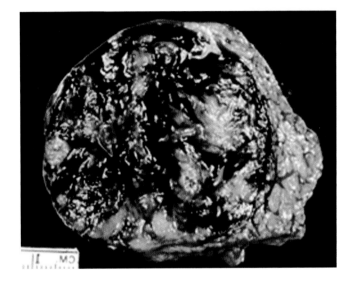

7. A tumor in a 35-year-old woman's pancreas showed the microscopic features in this figure. Which of the following is NOT a typical finding for this tumor type?

   a. Cystic areas
   b. Zones of foamy macrophages
   c. Hyaline globules
   d. Consistent progesterone receptor and abnormal β-catenin expression
   e. Consistent keratin and chromogranin expression

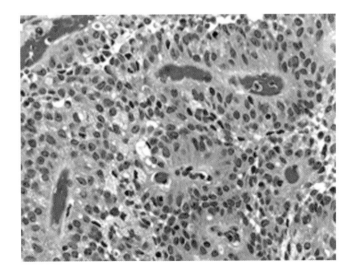

8. A 52-year-old woman presented with a papular skin rash with eczematous psoriasiform appearance and bulla formation. During work-up, she was found to have normochromic, normocytic anemia, glossitis, and mild diabetes mellitus. CT scan revealed a 7-cm mass in the body of the pancreas, which is shown in the photograph. Which of the following is TRUE for this tumor?

   a. From 50% to 70% are metastatic at the time of diagnosis.

   b. Severe persistent hyperinsulinemic hypoglycemia is very common.

   c. Multiple gastric ulcers are typical.

   d. Most examples of this tumor type are smaller than 1 cm.

   e. Severe watery diarrhea with hypokalemia and achloryhdria is also characteristic.

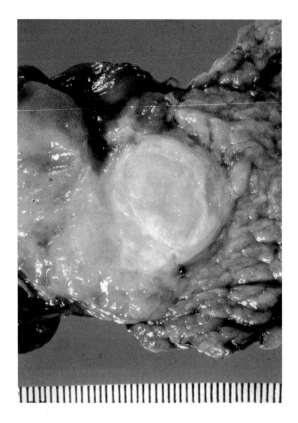

9. Which of the following is MOST helpful in grading the tumor type illustrated in this photograph, and predicting its metastatic potential?

   a. Microvessel density

   b. Vascular or perineural invasion

   c. Immunohistochemical profile for hormones

   d. Size and mitotic count

   e. Aneuploidy and genetic instability

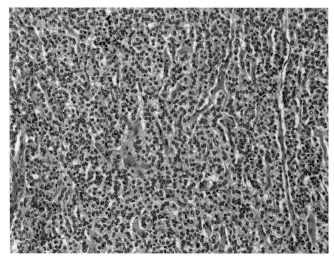

10. A 60-year-old man presented with abdominal pain and weight loss. He also complained of polyarthralgia. On physical examination he was found to have multiple small subcutaneous nodules in his arms and abdomen. One of these nodules was examined microscopically and showed fat necrosis. Serum lipase level was elevated. Abdominal CT scan showed a 12-cm solid pancreatic mass, which was fleshy and had necrotic areas. There were also multiple nodules in the liver. The photomicrograph is from the pancreatic tumor. Which one of the following would be expected to be positive in this tumor?

   a. Trypsin

   b. Diffuse and strong chromogranin expression

   c. *KRAS* mutation

   d. CEA

   e. Areas with glandular patterns and mucin

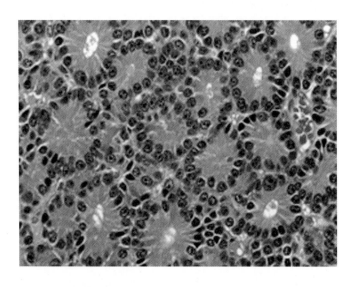

11. A 4-year-old child was found to have a large tumor in the liver and a separate mass in the pancreas. All of the following statements regarding this tumor type are correct EXCEPT:

   a. Serum AFP is elevated in some cases.

   b. Pancreatic acinar differentiation is common.

   c. Some are associated with Beckwith-Wiedemann and familial adenomatous polyposis syndromes.

   d. Pancreatic ductal differentiation may be seen.

   e. It is curable in most cases.

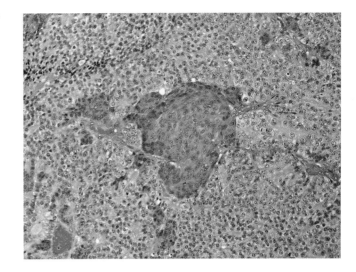

12. A 68-year-old man with a history of pancreatitis presented with abdominal pain. Endoscopic examination showed mucin extrusion from ampulla of Vater, and radiograms showed marked dilatation of the ducts in the head of the pancreas. In the pancreaticoduodenectomy specimen, the ducts not only were dilated but also contained irregularly distributed feathery granulations as well as well-circumscribed soft, tan friable nodules focally filling the ducts, a segment of which is illustrated here. All of the following statements about this tumor type are correct EXCEPT:

   a. It is seen predominantly in elderly patients.

   b. It is more common in the head of the pancreas.

   c. Papillary nodules in dilated ducts may be prominent.

   d. Invasive carcinoma is present in a third of the cases.

   e. The 5-year survival rate is below 5%.

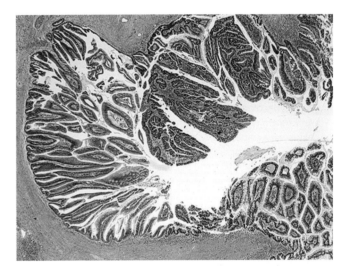

13. A 65-year-old man was brought to the emergency room with multiple abdominal injuries inflicted by a sharp instrument that ruptured the spleen. During splenectomy, for technical reasons, a portion of distal pancreas was also resected. The pancreas was grossly unremarkable; however, some of the ducts showed the changes illustrated in this figure. Which of the following is CORRCT for this type of lesion?

   a. These changes are uncommon; they are present in less than 1% of the population.

   b. Total pancreatectomy is indicated, especially if these changes involve multiple ducts.

   c. Mutation in codon-12 of *KRAS* oncogene is detectable in such lesions.

   d. These changes are much more common in younger patients.

   e. These lesions typically measure larger than 1 cm.

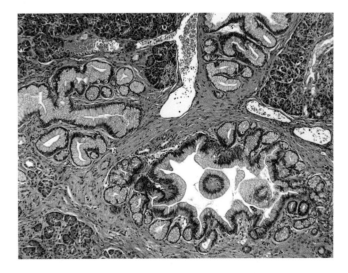

14. This 58-year-old otherwise healthy woman presented with GI bleeding and was found to have a polypoid and focally ulcerated mass in the third portion of the duodenum, away from the ampulla of Vater. Grossly identified polypoid areas corresponded to a villous adenoma, and at the base of the ulcer, a small focus of invasive tumor shown in the figure was identified. Which of the following combination of immunohistochemical markers does this tumor MOST likely express?

    a. TTF-1 and napsin A
    b. CK20 and CDX2
    c. Chromogranin and synaptophysin
    d. Trypsin and lipase
    e. CK7 and MUC1

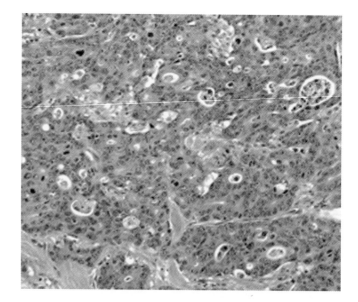

15. This 58-year-old smoker with a history of pancreatitis and the chief complaints of weakness and a 30-pound weight loss in the last 3 months presented to her primary physician who felt bilateral pelvic masses in examination, and referred the patient to a gynecologist. Serum CA19-9 level was markedly elevated and serum CA125 level was slightly high. Radiograms and exploratory laparotomy showed bilateral ovarian cystic masses (4 and 6 cm, respectively), omental nodules, multiple liver nodules, numerous small peritoneal nodules, and a 6-cm mass in the head of the pancreas. Biopsy of the omental nodule is shown. All of the following statements about this tumor type are correct EXCEPT:

    a. The 5-year survival rate is below 5%.
    b. Mutation in *KRAS* oncogene is common.
    c. It can be familial.
    d. Rare cases may be associated with *BRCA* mutation.
    e. It is a very uncommon tumor.

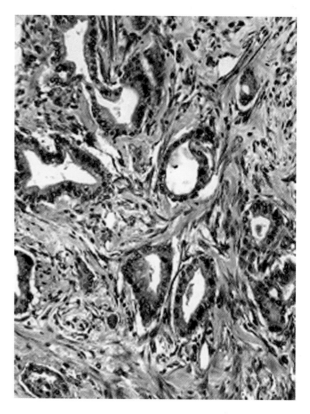

16. All of the following statements about the tumor type depicted in the figure are correct EXCEPT:
    a. This tumor is seen almost exclusively in perimenopausal women.
    b. It does not communicate with the pancreatic ductal system.
    c. It is invariably benign.
    d. The stromal cells express progesterone receptor.
    e. A coexisting ovarian tumor is very uncommon.

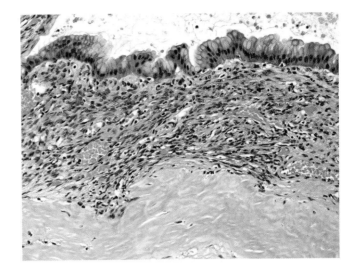

17. All of the following statements about the tumor type depicted in the figure are correct EXCEPT:
    a. Malignant transformation is very uncommon in this tumor type.
    b. Some may be associated with *vHL* gene abnormalities.
    c. PAS is positive in the cytoplasm.
    d. Aspirate of this lesion commonly shows very high CEA levels.
    e. This tumor is presumed to originate in centroacinar cells.

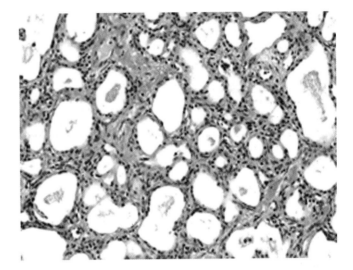

18. A patient with longstanding chronic pancreatitis underwent pancreatic resection for intractable pain. The pancreas was diffusely firm and fibrotic appearing, and no discrete nodules were identified. One of the sections showed the findings depicted. Which of the following is CORRECT?
    a. This process typically causes diabetes mellitus in such patients.
    b. Immunohistochemically these cells would express only one hormone type.
    c. This finding is common in patients with chronic pancreatitis.
    d. If these findings were detected at the margin, further resection would be necessary.
    e. This process is referred to as acinar cell dysplasia.

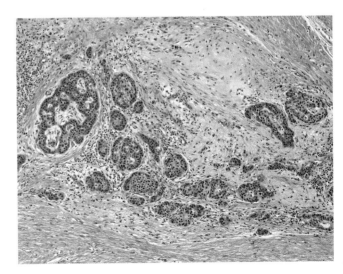

19. A 68-year-old woman presented with a 9-cm tumor in the head of the pancreas, which was biopsied. Which of the following is CORRECT for the tumor type depicted in this figure?
  a. It is most likely a metastasis from the breast.
  b. These tumors are commonly associated with intraductal papillary mucinous neoplasia.
  c. Prognosis of this tumor is significantly worse than that of ordinary ductal carcinoma.
  d. Tumors composed predominantly of this pattern are usually very small.
  e. This tumor is the most common type found in the pancreas.

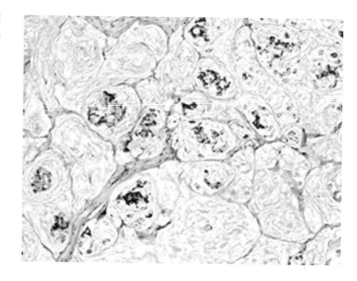

20. A 45-year-old woman was found to have a partially cystic and partially solid tumor in the tail of the pancreas. The tumor was resected. What would be the BEST diagnosis for this tumor among the possibilities provided here?
  a. Serous cystadenoma
  b. Intraductal papillary mucinous neoplasm (IPMN) with low-grade dysplasia
  c. Metastatic ovarian clear-cell adenocarcinoma in the pancreas
  d. Colloid carcinoma
  e. Sugar tumor

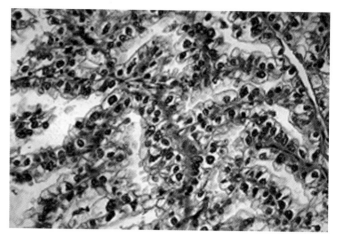

ANSWERS

1. c. This is a typical picture of autoimmune pancreatitis type 1 (so-called lymphoplasmacytic sclerosing type). It should be kept in mind, however, that any solid mass in the pancreas is a ductal adenocarcinoma (DA) unless proved otherwise, and this diagnosis can be excluded only with very careful and thorough microscopic examination of the specimen. There are some findings in the history of this patient that should have raised eyebrows. Pancreatic DA occurs at a mean age of 63, and is rather uncommon in patients in their early 40s or younger. Autoimmune history, especially primary sclerosing cholangitis and Sjögren syndrome, which are detected in approximately a fourth of the patients with autoimmune pancreatitis, is also suggestive of this diagnosis. The microscopic findings here are characteristic of autoimmune pancreatitis type 1 showing benign ducts surrounded by duct-centric lymphoplasmacytic inflammation and expansion of periductal space with sclerosis. Periphlebitis is also quite characteristic and frank vasculitis may be seen. Some examples have interstitial storiform fibroblastic proliferation admixed with lymphoplasmacytic infiltrates. In fact, many examples of autoimmune pancreatitis had been called "inflammatory pseudotumor" in the past. Immunohistologically, IgG4-positive plasma cells, a minimum of 10/HPF (high-power field), is also of diagnostic help; proposed cut-off ranges from 10 to 30 depending on the study. Some are even advocating greater than 50 cells/HPF. Along with the clinical history, these findings are diagnostic for autoimmune pancreatitis, type 1, provided that DA is carefully excluded by thorough examination. Serum IgG4 level is typically elevated in patients with autoimmune pancreatitis, type 1 (usually >135 mg/dL), and can be crucial in preoperative diagnosis of autoimmune pancreatitis. Serum CA19-9, CEA, and CA125 are typically increased in ductal neoplasia; however, these (especially CA19-9) may also be elevated in chronic pancreatitis. Of note, autoimmune pancreatitis type 2 is distinguished from type 1 by the presence of intraepithelial neutrophils and occasionally eosinophils (granulocytic epithelial lesions [GELs]), especially in intralobular ducts. In this type, phlebitis is not a common pattern. IgG4-positive plasma cell infiltration may be mild and serum IgG4 levels may be normal.

Adsay NV, Basturk O, Thirabanjasak D: Diagnostic features and differential diagnosis of autoimmune pancreatitis. *Semin Diagn Pathol* 2005;22(4):309-317.
Klöppel G, Sipos B, Zamboni G, et al: Autoimmune pancreatitis: histo- and immunopathological features. *J Gastroenterol* 2007;42(Suppl 18):28-31.

Zhang L, Chari S, Smyrk TC, et al: Autoimmune pancreatitis (AIP) type 1 and type 2: an international consensus study on histopathologic diagnostic criteria. *Pancreas* 2011;40(8): (1172-1179.

2. b. More than 85% of solid, ill-defined, scirrhous (scarlike) tumors in the pancreas as illustrated here will prove to be DA. This patient presented with the typical symptoms and signs of DA: jaundice (due to invasion into the common bile duct), rapid weight loss, and abdominal pain or back pain. Diabetes mellitus, especially of recent onset, is also often present in the history of patients with DA. The presence of diabetes may raise the question of a hormone-secreting neuroendocrine tumor (NET); however, pancreatic neuroendocrine tumors (PanNETs) seldom cause jaundice (because of their slower and more expansive growth), and back pain or rapid weight loss are also very uncommon. Also, macroscopically, NETs are fleshier and form well-delineated tumors rather than the scirrhous appearance of adenocarcinoma. Pancreatic DAs typically show diffuse CK7 and mucin-related glycoproteins and oncoproteins (CA19-9, CEA, B72.3, MUC1, MUC5AC, DUPAN2) expression. CK20 is often focal. Loss of DPC4 (SMAD4) is also a finding strongly in favor of adenocarcinoma, provided that in-built controls are working properly. Diffuse positivity for chromogranin is characteristic of NETs, trypsin of acinar neoplasia, and nuclear β-catenin is of solid-pseudopapillary neoplasms or pancreatoblastoma.

Hruban RH, Pitman MB, Klimstra DS: Tumors of the pancreas. In Silverberg SG (ed): *AFIP Atlas of Tumor Pathology,* 4th ed. Washington, DC: ARP Press, 2007.

Klimstra DS, Adsay NV: Tumors of the pancreas. In Odze RD, Goldblum JR (eds): *Surgical Pathology of the GI Tract, Liver, Biliary Tract, and Pancreas,* 3rd ed. St. Louis: Elsevier, 2014.

3. c. This is a typical example of "osteoclast-like giant cell carcinoma (OGCC)," which is essentially an undifferentiated (sarcomatoid) carcinoma with osteoclast-like giant cells. It is fairly uncommon; however, it appears to be much more common in the pancreas and biliary tract than anywhere else in the body, especially the examples with abundant osteoclast-like giant cells. Grossly, OGCC is often more circumscribed than ordinary DA; however, some examples have an ordinary DA component or arise in association with a mucinous cystic neoplasm (MCN). The neoplastic elements are usually moderately to markedly atypical, discohesive, and somewhat epithelioid in shape. A variable number of osteoclast-like giant cells, with multiple nuclei showing no or only mild atypia, are typically scattered randomly among the neoplastic elements. A component of mononuclear histiocytic cells is also present. The multinucleated giant cells in OGCC show all the characteristic morphologic features of osteoclastic giant cells, express histiocytic markers such as CD68, as well as CD45, but not keratins, and are not to be confused with pleomorphic carcinoma cells. *KRAS* gene mutations are present in more than 90% of these neoplasms. In addition, when there is an associated epithelial neoplastic component, identical *KRAS* gene mutations are found in both undifferentiated and epithelial components. It is not known how and why so many osteoclast-like giant cells appear in these undifferentiated (sarcomatoid) carcinomas. Of note, osteoclast-like giant cells may also be seen in sarcomatoid mesotheliomas, sarcomatoid melanomas, and sarcomatoid carcinomas of other organs, but this degree is unusual.

Westra WH, Sturm P, Drillenburg P, et al: KRAS oncogene mutations in osteoclast-like giant cell tumors of the pancreas and liver: genetic evidence to support origin from the duct epithelium. *Am J Surg Pathol* 1998;22:1247-1254.

Hruban RH, Pitman MB, Klimstra DS: Tumors of the pancreas. In Silverberg SG (ed): *AFIP Atlas of Tumor Pathology,* 4th ed. Washington, DC: ARP Press, 2007.

Klimstra DS and Adsay NV: Tumors of the pancreas. In Odze RD, Goldblum JR (eds): *Surgical Pathology of the GI Tract, Liver, Biliary Tract, and Pancreas,* 3rd ed. St. Louis: Elsevier, 2014.

4. d. Cystic lesions in the pancreas constitute approximately 10% of pancreatic tumors. This tumor is an example of what is referred to as a megacystic type of lesion. It is a multilocular cyst with a few individual loculi, and each locule is on the order of centimeters. The main differential diagnosis is between a pseudocyst and an MCN. This tumor was in fact a mucinous cystadenocarcinoma, and the multilocular septate nature of the lesion as well as its location within the pancreas (rather than in peripancreatic tissue) suggests the likelihood of an MCN. Pseudocysts contain granular debris rather than mucin; they are peripancreatic and unilocular. Preoperative cyst fluid analysis may have been helpful in differentiating the two. Pseudocysts often contain high enzyme levels (amylase, lipase, etc.), whereas MCNs often have high mucin-related antigen levels, such as CEA. Regardless of the diagnosis, however, cystic lesions in the pancreas are relatively indolent tumors. Even in MCNs, which are most likely among the cystic tumors to metastasize, the incidence of lymph node metastasis is less than 10%. On the other hand, MCNs may harbor in situ or invasive carcinoma, which may be very focal and invisible to the naked eye; therefore, extensive sampling of these tumors is required. In fact, some authors advocate total examination of these tumors, because the prognosis changes significantly if there is carcinoma. Cystic tumors of any kind seldom occur in children.

Zamboni G, Scarpa A, Bogina G, et al: Mucinous cystic tumors of the pancreas: clinicopathological features, prognosis, and relationship to other mucinous cystic tumors. *Am J Surg Pathol* 1999;23:410-422.

Basturk O, Coban I, Adsay NV: Cystic neoplasms of the pancreas. *Arch Pathol Lab Med* 2009;133(3):423-438.

5. d. This is a typical example of serous (microcystic) cystadenoma. The microcystic appearance is so specific and characteristic that it has become synonymous with this tumor type. There are innumerable small cysts, most of which measure within a few millimeters, although a few loculi may become larger. The tumor has the characteristic spongelike appearance. It is well circumscribed. A central stellate scar is also evident in many cases. Although the content of microcystic adenoma appears shiny, it is actually serous. No mucin production is seen in these tumors. Serous cystadenomas are more common in women (male/female ratio = 1:3) and occur and involve the head and body/tail of the pancreas at about the same frequency. The mean age is in the 60s. They have a well-established association with von Hippel-Lindau (vHL) syndrome and the *vHL* gene and chromosome 10q alterations have been reported in 40%. These tumors may become very large, measuring up to 25 to 30 cm. Serous cystadenomas are invariably benign tumors, with no recurrence potential; only a few case reports of a malignant counterpart of this tumor were presented in the literature. Many are detected incidentally during work-up for other conditions, as was the case in this example.

Compton CC: Serous cystic tumors of the pancreas. *Semin Diagn Pathol* 2000;17:43-56.

Basturk O, Adsay NV: Pathology of pancreas. In Cheng L, Bostwick DG (eds): *Essentials of Anatomic Pathology,* 3rd ed. New York: Springer, 2011.

Zhu H, Qin L, Zhong M, et al: Carcinoma ex microcystic adenoma of the pancreas: a report of a novel form of malignancy in serous neoplasms. *Am J Surg Pathol* 2001;36(2):305-310.

6. a. The combination of clinical, cyst fluid and macroscopic findings in this patient is characteristic of solid pseudopapillary neoplasm (SPN), previously known as papillary-cystic or solid and cystic tumor. This tumor occurs most commonly in young women (female/male ratio = 9:1 and mean age = 30). The young age of the patient and the lack of CEA in cyst fluid speak against mucinous cystic tumors. Grossly, SPN is characterized by solid and cystic components in which the cystic component represents a degenerative phenomenon and is devoid of a lining, mucinous or otherwise. Although often deceptively well circumscribed, as seen in this example, SPN commonly sends microscopic projections into the adjacent pancreas in which native acini and islets may be entrapped, and may lead to diagnostic difficulty. More than 85% of the patients are cured by complete excision. In 10% to 15%, however, there is metastasis to the peritoneum or the liver. Even patients with metastasis often follow a protracted clinical course. Only a few fatalities have been attributed to this tumor type.

Klimstra DS, Wenig BM, Heffess CS: Solid-pseudopapillary tumor of the pancreas: a typically cystic tumor of low malignant potential. *Semin Diagn Pathol* 2000;17:66-81.

Chetty R, Serra S: Membrane loss and aberrant nuclear localization of E-cadherin are consistent features of solid pseudopapillary tumour of the pancreas. An immunohistochemical study using two antibodies recognizing different domains of the E-cadherin molecule. *Histopathology* 2008;52:325-330.

Basturk O, Coban I, Adsay NV: Cystic neoplasms of the pancreas. *Arch Pathol Lab Med* 2009;133(3):423-438.

7. e. This is a typical example of SPN of the pancreas (see also Question 6). It is characterized by relatively uniform, cytologically bland cells with round to ovoid nuclei. Distinctive pseudopapillary pattern, which is a degenerative phenomenon causing the disappearance of the cells away from the vasculature, creates an ependymoma-like appearance, diagnostic of SPN. Nuclear grooves, hyaline globules, and zones of macrophages are other common characteristic findings. Cystic changes are also so common that SPN was previously referred to as a solid and cystic tumor. The lineage and differentiation of SPN are not known; it does not show ductal, acinar, or neuroendocrine differentiation; however, this feature can be used as a benefit in the differential diagnosis, especially from neuroendocrine neoplasia. SPN shows consistent (diffuse and strong) labeling with vimentin, progesterone receptors, CD10, and α_1-antitrypsin. Inhibin and estrogen receptors are less

consistent, and keratins are often focal and weak. So-called neuroendocrine markers neuron-specific enolase (NSE), synaptophysin, and CD56 are almost always positive; however, chromogranin, the most specific endocrine marker, is mostly negative or very focally/weakly positive. More importantly, Wnt-signaling pathway alterations with abnormal nuclear accumulation of β-catenin, overexpression of cyclin D1, and loss of membranous E-cadherin expression with/without relocalization to nucleus are typical.

Tiemann K, Heitling U, Kosmahl M, et al: Solid pseudopapillary neoplasms of the pancreas shows an interruption of the Wnt-signaling pathway and expresses gene products of 11q. *Mod Pathol* 2007;20:955-960.

Serra S, Chetty R: Revision 2: an immunohistochemical approach and evaluation of solid pseudopapillary tumour of the pancreas. *J Clin Pathol* 2008;61:1153-1159.

Kim MJ, Jang SJ, Yu E: Loss of E-cadherin and cytoplasmic-nuclear expression of beta-catenin are the most useful immunoprofiles in the diagnosis of solid-pseudopapillary neoplasm of the pancreas. *Hum Pathol* 2008;39:251-258.

8. a. This is the typical appearance of a PanNET: solid, relatively fleshy, homogeneous mass that is well demarcated. Approximately half of the PanNETs are functional, and the hormone they secrete may lead to a specific set of symptoms and signs. The clinical picture described in this question (skin rash, normochromic/normocytic anemia, glossitis, and mild diabetes mellitus) is characteristic of *glucagonoma*. Severe persistent hypoglycemia due to inappropriate secretion of insulin is typical of *insulinoma* (most common functional PanNET, represents 40% of all functional PanNETs, and approximately 5% of insulinomas arises in patients with MEN1 [multiple endocrine neoplasia] syndrome). Multiple gastric ulcers are typical of *gastrinoma*. Severe watery diarrhea with hypokalemia and achloryhdria is typical of VIPoma (a tumor that produces vasoactive intestinal peptide). The clinical syndrome of *somatostatinoma* is rather nonspecific. The type of hormone produced also correlates somewhat with the biology of the tumor. Most insulinomas behave in a benign fashion, but that is because most insulinomas are also small (>70% are less than 1 cm) at the time of diagnosis, presumably due to early detection of the symptoms. In contrast, most glucagonomas are larger (mean size = 7.5 cm) and metastatic (70%) at the time of diagnosis, partially due to the more subtle nature of the symptoms it creates. Immunohistochemical markers do not correlate with the functionality status and, therefore, are not routinely used in this distinction.

Hruban RH, Pitman MB, Klimstra DS: Tumors of the pancreas. In Silverberg SG (ed): *AFIP Atlas of Tumor Pathology,* 4th ed. Washington, DC: ARP Press, 2007.

Klimstra DS, Modlin IR, Adsay NV, et al: Pathology reporting of neuroendocrine tumors: application of the Delphic consensus process to the development of a minimum pathology data set. *Am J Surg Pathol* 2010;34(3):300-313.

Klimstra DS, Arnold R, Capella C, et al: Neuroendocrine neoplasms of the pancreas. In Bosman FT, Carneiro F, Hruban RH, Theise ND (eds): *WHO Classification of Tumors of the Digestive Systems.* Geneva: WHO Press, 2010, pp 13-14, 322-326.

9. d. This is a typical example of a PanNET characterized by round, uniform cells with a fair amount of cytoplasm and neuroendocrine (salt and pepper) chromatin. PanNETs exhibit a spectrum of malignant behavior. Many of the parameters listed in the answers including size, mitotic count/Ki67 index, vascular or perineural invasion, hormonal status (glucagonoma >>insulinoma), aneuploidy, and genetic instability have been found to be associated with higher metastatic potential; however, size, which is a part of the staging system (*stage 1: tumor limited to the pancreas, ≤2 cm in greatest dimension; **stage 2:** tumor limited to the pancreas, >2 cm in greatest dimension; **stage 3:** tumor extends beyond the pancreas but without involvement of the celiac axis or the superior mesenteric artery; **stage 4:** tumor involves the celiac axis or the superior mesenteric artery*) and *mitotic count*/Ki67 index, which is a part of the grading system (**grade 1:** *mitotic count <2/10 HPF and/or ≤2% Ki67 index;* **grade 2:** *mitotic count 2-20/10 HPF and/or 3% to 20% Ki67 index;* **grade 3:** *mitotic count >20/10 HPF and/or >20% Ki67 index*) have been proved to have the best prognostic value. The role of microvessel density is debatable. Nuclear pleomorphism often reflects a degenerative phenomenon (referred to as endocrine atypia, which is not uncommon in NETs of any site) and does not necessarily imply higher-grade tumors. Most PanNETs are either low-grade (grade 1) or intermediate-grade (grade 2) well-differentiated tumors. In the current (2010) WHO classification, all pancreatic "high-grade neuroendocrine carcinomas" (NECs) are now included under the grade 3 category; however, preliminary studies have shown that the grade 3 category includes two distinct entities: (1) a highly proliferative group of well-differentiated NETs; and (2) the small cell and large cell NECs (true poorly differentiated NECs). The first group appears to have a significantly more protracted clinical course but less dramatic response to platinum-based chemotherapy compared to true poorly differentiated NECs. It is also the impression of many pathologists that the true poorly differentiated NECs usually have a very high Ki67 labeling index, well above the 20% threshold (typically above 50%) that defines a neuroendocrine neoplasm to be high grade (WHO 2010).

Klimstra DS, Arnold R, Capella C, et al: Neuroendocrine neoplasms of the pancreas. In Bosman FT, Carneiro F, Hruban RH, Theise ND (eds): *WHO Classification of Tumors of the Digestive Systems.* Geneva: WHO Press, 2010, pp 13-14, 322-326.

Adsay V: Ki67 labeling index in neuroendocrine tumors of the gastrointestinal and pancreatobiliary tract: to count or not to count is not the question, but rather how to count. *Am J Surg Pathol* 2012;36(12):1743-1746.

Basturk O, Yang Z, Tang LH, et al: Increased (> 20%) Ki67 proliferation index in morphologically well differentiated pancreatic neuroendocrine tumors (PanNETs) correlates with decreased overall survival (abstract). *Mod Pathol* 2013;26:423A.

10. a. This is a typical example of acinar cell carcinoma (ACC). The tumor forms sheets of relatively uniform, round, large cells with a single prominent nucleolus. Rosettelike acinar formations may also be seen (as illustrated here). ACCs often have a distinctive chromophilia; they either appear basophilic overall, or some examples may have acidophilic granules. History of enzyme hypersecretion syndrome is also typical (lipase causing subcutaneous fat necrosis, and proteases causing polyathralgia); however, it is seen in only 10% to 15%. Many ACCs are metastatic to the liver at the time of diagnosis. The mean age of the patients is about 60.

The tumors can be large (mean size = 10 cm). They are typically fleshy (reflecting the cellularity of this stroma-poor tumor) and have areas of necrosis. Immunohistochemically, ACCs express trypsin (most reliable), chymotrypsin, and lipase. Endocrine markers, such as chromogranin, sometimes highlight scattered endocrine cells or zones of endocrine differentiation that may be seen in ACCs; however, diffuse strong chromogranin expression is not a feature. *KRAS* mutation is a characteristic finding in ductal neoplasia, detected in more than 90% of DA, so much so that it is regarded as a ductal marker. It is generally not seen in nonductal tumors, and ACCs lack *KRAS* mutation. CEA expression, glandular formation, and mucin are also markers of ductal differentiation and generally not seen in nonductal tumors.

Klimstra DS, Heffess CS, Oertel JE, et al: Acinar cell carcinoma of the pancreas. A clinicopathologic study of 28 cases. *Am J Surg Pathol* 1992;16:815-837.

Klimstra DS: Non-ductal neoplasms of the pancreas. *Mod Pathol* 2007;20(Suppl 1):S94-112.

La Rosa S, Adsay V, Albarello L, et al: Clinicopathologic study of 62 acinar cell carcinomas of the pancreas: insights into the morphology and immunophenotype and search for prognostic markers. *Am J Surg Pathol* 2012;36(12):1782-1795.

11. e. This tumor shows typical features of pancreatoblastoma, including sheets of nondescript round cells with moderate amount of cytoplasm, and scattered squamoid corpuscles (small distinct clusters of plump to elongated cells forming meningothelium-like whorls). These squamoid corpuscles are pathognomonic for pancreatoblastoma. They often have nuclear pseudoinclusions. Pancreatoblastomas are very uncommon. They typically occur in early childhood (mean age = 4) with a second peak in the mid-30s. They are more common in Asians. Elevated AFP may occur in some cases. Rare cases occur in association with Beckwith-Wiedemann or familial adenomatous polyposis syndromes. The tumors are often large (7 to 18 cm), well demarcated, solid, and multilobulated, with yellow-tan cut surfaces. They show multiphenotypic differentiation including acinar (most consistent), ductal, and endocrine with corresponding immunostaining patterns. Abnormal (nuclear/cytoplasmic) immunolabeling for β-catenin and overexpression of cyclin D1, more strikingly in squamoid corpuscles, is important. Unlike other childhood tumors, the cure rate is fairly low for pancreatoblastomas, with a 5-year survival rate below 25%.

Klimstra DS, Wenig BM, Adair CF, et al: Pancreatoblastoma. A clinicopathologic study and review of the literature. *Am J Surg Pathol* 1995;19:1371-1389.

Hruban RH, Adsay NV: Molecular classification of neoplasms of the pancreas. *Hum Pathol* 2009;40(5):612-623.

12. e. This tumor is a typical example of intraductal papillary mucinous neoplasm (IPMN), which is characterized by cystic dilatation of pancreatic ducts lined by mucinous epithelium that forms papillary nodules. IPMNs are seen predominantly in elderly patients (median age at diagnosis of about 68 years), are slightly more common in men, and occur predominantly in the head of the organ (for this reason the mucin produced by these tumors often exudes from the ampulla of Vater). Many patients have a history of pancreatitis. IPMNs show a spectrum of neoplastic change, ranging from low-grade dysplasia to high-grade dysplasia (carcinoma in situ [CIS]), not only from case to case, but in a given case as well. In approximately 35% of the patients, there is an associated invasive carcinoma of either colloid (mucinous) or tubular (similar to ordinary DA) type. The carcinoma in IPMNs may be invisible grossly, and therefore extensive, if not total, sampling is warranted. Overall, the 5-year survival rate of IPMNs (including both noninvasive and invasive forms) is approximately 75%, although cases with invasive carcinoma have a significantly lower survival rate.

Adsay NV, Merati K, Basturk O, et al: Pathologically and biologically distinct types of epithelium in intraductal papillary mucinous neoplasms: delineation of an "intestinal" pathway of carcinogenesis in the pancreas. *Am J Surg Pathol* 2004;28(7): 839-848.

Hruban RH, Takaori K, Klimstra DS, et al: An illustrated consensus on the classification of pancreatic intraepithelial neoplasia and intraductal papillary mucinous neoplasms. *Am J Surg Pathol* 2004;28:977-987.

Tanaka M, Fernández-del Castillo C, Adsay V, et al: International consensus guidelines 2012 for the management of IPMN and MCN of the pancreas. International Association of Pancreatology. *Pancreatology* 2012;12(3):183-197.

13. c. The changes illustrated in this figure represent pancreatic intraepithelial neoplasia (PanIN). By definition, PanINs are not grossly detectable, and they typically measure less than 0.5 cm. In contrast, IPMNs represent grossly and clinically detectable forms of dysplasia that typically measure larger than 1 cm. Like IPMNs, PanINs show a spectrum of neoplastic changes. Those that used to be called mucinous hypertrophy or mucinous metaplasia are regarded as PanIN-1A. These types were included in the PanIN category because mutation in codon-12 of *KRAS* oncogene, which is characteristic of DAs, can be detected in such lesions. Grading of PanINs can be summarized as follows:

- **1A:** well-polarized mucinous cells with perfect polarity and no atypia (what used to be called mucinous metaplasia or mucinous hypertrophy; which is illustrated in this question)
- **1B:** same cells in IA forming papillary projections
- **2:** mild disorganization, nuclear enlargement, hyperchromatism; mild nuclear pleomorphism; some cells dyspolarized to the apical aspect of the epithelium
- **3** (also includes CIS): significant loss of cell polarity and marked cytologic atypia; high nucleus/cytoplasm (N/C) ratio; tufting and detached epithelial cell clusters; necrosis; mitoses

PanINs 1 and 2 are common incidental findings in pancreatectomies performed for any type of disease (neoplastic or nonneoplastic), they can be multifocal, and they are estimated to be present in approximately 50% of the population over the age of 50. For this reason, the current approach is that low-grade PanINs do not require any further therapy, and they do not have to be mentioned in the surgical disease reports. PanIN-3, on the other hand, is rarely detected in the absence of invasive adenocarcinoma. It is regarded as a clinically significant process and should be duly reported.

Hruban RH, Adsay NV, Albores-Saavedra J, et al: Pancreatic intraepithelial neoplasia: a new nomenclature and classification system for pancreatic duct lesions. *Am J Surg Pathol* 2001;25:579-586.

Hruban RH, Takaori K, Klimstra DS, et al: An illustrated consensus on the classification of pancreatic intraepithelial neoplasia and intraductal papillary mucinous neoplasms. *Am J Surg Pathol* 2004;28:977-987.

14. b. Both the clinical and pathologic findings in this case are those of an intestinal-type adenocarcinoma arising in the duodenum, rather than a pancreatobiliary type carcinoma, which is more common in the ampulla-pancreatobiliary region. The presence of duodenal adenoma indicates that the tumor is indeed arising from the duodenum. GI bleeding is also less common in pancreatic adenocarcinomas unless they ulcerate into the duodenum, whereas many duodenal carcinomas present with bleeding. The morphologic features of this tumor are also typical of intestinal adenocarcinoma. The basophilic tumor cells have elongated, cigar-shaped nuclei. Luminal necrosis is also characteristic. Immunohistochemically, intestinal adenocarcinomas show diffuse CK20 and focal or diffuse CDX2 (nuclear) and MUC2 labeling, while MUC1 and MUC5AC are often negative. Pancreatobiliary adenocarcinomas show the opposite of this profile. TTF-1 is a marker of pulmonary carcinomas; chromogranin and synaptophysin of NETs; and trypsin and lipase of ACC.

Adsay NV: Tumors of major and minor ampulla. In Odze RD, Goldblum JR (eds): *Surgical Pathology of the GI Tract, Liver, Biliary Tract, and Pancreas*, 3rd ed. St. Louis: Elsevier (in press).

15. e. This patient has widely spread carcinoma and intraabdominal carcinomatosis. The presence of a separate mass in the pancreas and the morphologic findings showing widely separated small tubules lined by a single layer of dyspolarized cuboidal cells and abundant desmoplastic stroma are characteristic of pancreatobiliary adenocarcinoma. Eventually abdominal carcinomatosis and liver metastasis occur in the course of many pancreas cancer cases. In fact, pancreatobiliary adenocarcinoma is regarded as the most common source of "carcinoma of unknown primary." A 5-year survival rate of this tumor type is below 5% even in the cases that are diagnosed at an earlier stage. Approximately 30,000 Americans die of this disease every year, and it is the fourth most common cause of cancer deaths. Pancreatitis (especially the hereditary form) and smoking are regarded as risk factors. Based on the clinical findings, the main differential in this case is with ovarian carcinoma, and in fact, elevation of CA19-9 and CA125 can be seen in both tumors. In addition to the morphologic findings, other findings also speak against an ovarian primary tumor, including bilaterality of the ovarian lesions, and their relatively smaller size. Often the metastatic pancreatic adenocarcinoma in the ovary becomes cystic and deceptively benign-appearing; misdiagnosis as primary mucinous borderline tumor is common. Pancreatic adenocarcinomas typically have mutation in codon-12 of *KRAS* oncogene, and it is one of the *BRCA*-related cancers (although only 7% of pancreas cancer cases are presumed to have *BRCA* mutations).

Hruban RH, Pitman MB, Klimstra DS: Tumors of the pancreas. In Silverberg SG (ed): *AFIP Atlas of Tumor Pathology*, 4th ed. Washington, DC: ARP Press, 2007.

Basturk O, Adsay NV: Pathology of pancreas. In Cheng L, Bostwick DG (eds): *Essentials of Anatomic Pathology*, 3rd ed. New York: Springer, 2011.

Klimstra DS, Adsay NV: Tumors of the pancreas. In Odze RD, Goldblum JR (eds): *Surgical Pathology of the GI Tract, Liver, Biliary Tract, and Pancreas*, 3rd ed. St. Louis: Elsevier, 2014.

16. c. This is a typical example of pancreatic MCN revealing the characteristic ovarian-type stroma, which is specific for this tumor type and has all the characteristics of ovarian stroma, including expression of hormone receptors (estrogen and progesterone receptors) and muscular markers (actin, desmin, and others). Even luteal type cells and hyalinized nodules can be seen. The vast majority of MCNs occur in perimenopausal women (>95% of the patients are women and mean age = 48), and in the body or tail of the pancreas. The lesions do not communicate with the ducts. Similar to IPMNs, MCNs show a spectrum of neoplastic change, ranging from low-grade dysplasia to invasive carcinoma (up to one third of the cases have an associated invasive carcinoma); therefore these tumors ought to be examined carefully. If the possibility of carcinoma is ruled out confidently by extensive, if not total, sampling of the tumor, and the cysts are lined by bland mucinous cells, then the case is classified as "mucinous cystic neoplasm with low-grade dysplasia." These lesions tend to be small (<3 cm) and less complex (devoid of papillary nodules), and typically behave as benign tumors. In contrast, MCNs with invasion are often fatal. A coexisting ovarian tumor is very uncommon and should raise the possibility of metastasis to the ovary.

Zamboni G, Scarpa A, Bogina G, et al: Mucinous cystic tumors of the pancreas: clinicopathological features, prognosis, and relationship to other mucinous cystic tumors. *Am J Surg Pathol* 1999;23:410-422.
Tanaka M, Fernández-del Castillo C, Adsay V, et al: International consensus guidelines 2012 for the management of IPMN and MCN of the pancreas. International Association of Pancreatology. *Pancreatology* 2012;12(3):183-197.

17. d. This is a typical example of serous cystadenoma (microcystic adenoma and "glycogen-rich adenoma" are synonyms). See also Question 5. Serous cystadenomas are invariably benign tumors, with only a handful of cases reported in the literature as malignant. The cytologic features shown here are highly characteristic and are displayed with fidelity in almost every case. The cells have glycogen-rich cytoplasm that is positive for PAS and centrally located, with small and round nuclei with homogenous chromatin pattern. Cytoplasmic borders are often distinct. This tumor is considered to originate from centroacinar cells and does not show any mucin production. Accordingly, CEA level in the aspirate fluid is usually low, which is sometimes helpful in the preoperative differential from mucinous tumors. Pancreatic cysts that occur in patients with the vHL syndrome are highly similar morphologically to serous cystadenomas apart from the localized (solitary tumor-forming) nature of the latter.

Compton CC: Serous cystic tumors of the pancreas. *Semin Diagn Pathol* 2000;17:43-56.
Basturk O, Adsay NV: Pathology of pancreas. In Cheng L, Bostwick DG (eds): *Essentials of Anatomic Pathology*, 3rd ed. New York: Springer, 2011.
Zhu H, Qin L, Zhong M, et al: Carcinoma *ex* microcystic adenoma of the pancreas: a report of a novel form of malignancy in serous neoplasms. *Am J Surg Pathol* 2001;36(2):305-310.

18. c. This process is composed of numerous islets of Langerhans. The cells have round nuclei and abundant pale cytoplasm, characteristic of islet cells. Foci of islet aggregation (so-called "islet cell hyperplasia") such as this one are fairly common in chronic pancreatitis. Chronic pancreatitis is characterized by acinar atrophy (disappearance of acinar lobules) and emergence interstitial fibrosis. During this process, islets are well preserved, and may even appear hyperplastic, forming microscopic nodules seen in this example; however, there are no data demonstrating that the total endocrine cell mass is increased and this is not associated with any specific clinical symptom such as diabetes, and does not require specific therapy. Rarely, these nodules may be difficult to distinguish from a small PanNET. In such cases, absence of clinical and gross findings is helpful, and immunohistochemistry typically shows a multihormone pattern similar to those of normal islets, unlike in PanNETs where the distribution of different endocrine cell types in islets is often deranged. Acinar cell dysplasia is the term applied for micronodules of atypical acinar cells within acinar lobules.

Klöppel G: Chronic pancreatitis of alcoholic and nonalcoholic origin. *Semin Diagn Pathol* 2004;21(4):227-236.
Adsay NV, Basturk O, Klimstra DS, et al: Pancreatic pseudotumors: non-neoplastic solid lesions of the pancreas that clinically mimic pancreas cancer. *Semin Diagn Pathol* 2004; 21(4):260-267.
Klöppel G, Adsay NV: Chronic pancreatitis and the differential diagnosis versus pancreatic cancer. *Arch Pathol Lab Med* 2009;133(3):382-387.

19. b. This is a typical example of colloid (mucinous noncystic) carcinoma, characterized by mucin lakes with scanty carcinoma cells floating in them. Although colloid carcinoma has been well characterized in the breast, it was recognized relatively recently in the pancreas, and had been mostly categorized with ordinary carcinomas previously. Colloid carcinomas in the pancreas are very uncommon, but those that occur are usually primary tumors, and are commonly associated with IPMNs of this organ. Studies indicate that the prognosis of this tumor is better than that of ordinary DA. These tumors occur in the elderly and usually are larger but at a lower stage than conventional carcinomas at the time of presentation.

Adsay NV, Pierson C, Sarkar F, et al: Colloid (mucinous noncystic) carcinoma of the pancreas. *Am J Surg Pathol* 2001;25:26-42.
Adsay NV, Merati K, Nassar H, et al: Pathogenesis of colloid (pure mucinous) carcinoma of exocrine organs: coupling of gel-forming mucin (MUC2) production with altered cell polarity and abnormal cell-stroma interaction may be the key factor in the morphogenesis and indolent behavior of colloid carcinoma in the breast and pancreas. *Am J Surg Pathol* 2003; 27(5):571-578.

20. c. As in any other organ, secondary tumors, although rare, ought to be considered in the differential diagnosis of pancreatic tumors. This tumor is a metastatic ovarian clear cell adenocarcinoma in the pancreas. Serous cystadenomas do have clear cytoplasm but this degree of nuclear atypia is never seen in serous adenomas, and if present, should raise the possibility of serous cystadenocarcinomas (not provided among the answers). IPMN with low-grade dysplasia is composed of tall, columnar mucinous cells in which the mucin in the cytoplasm is overtly evident. Furthermore, this degree of atypia would not be seen in "low-grade dysplasia." Colloid carcinoma is characterized by mucin lakes and scanty carcinoma cells floating in these lakes. Sugar tumor, which is regarded in the category of perivascular epithelioid cell tumors (PEComas) or angiomyolipomas, typically do not show papillary architecture or the degree of nuclear atypia seen here. Also, they have granular cytoplasm at least in some of the cells.

Adsay NV, Andea A, Basturk O, et al: Secondary tumors of the pancreas: an analysis of a surgical and autopsy database and review of the literature. *Virchows Arch* 2004; 444:527-535.

CHAPTER 6

LIVER PATHOLOGY

Jay H. Lefkowitch

QUESTIONS

Questions 1-31 in this chapter refer to a photograph or photomicrograph.

1. An 18-year-old woman underwent liver transplantation because of cirrhosis secondary to autoimmune hepatitis (AIH). She developed serum liver function test abnormalities 2 months after transplantation, and a liver biopsy was performed. One representative portal tract is shown in the image. The CORRECT diagnosis is:
   a. Recurrent autoimmune hepatitis
   b. Transition to another autoimmune disease, primary biliary cirrhosis (PBC)
   c. Acute rejection
   d. Chronic rejection
   e. Posttransplant lymphoproliferative disease

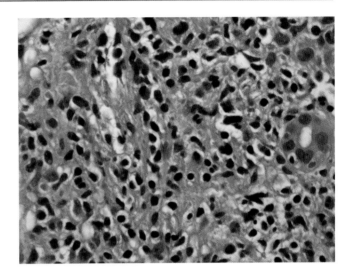

2. The image shows a liver biopsy specimen stained with PAS with diastase digestion. All of the following statements about this patient's liver disease are correct EXCEPT:
   a. This disorder has been referred to as a *serpinopathy*.
   b. The intracellular inclusions are typical of α_1-antitrypsin (AAT).
   c. The patient's serum AAT phenotype is most likely PiMM.
   d. The presentation of this disease in neonates or infants includes giant cell hepatitis and paucity of intrahepatic bile ducts.
   e. The spectrum of related disease in adults includes chronic hepatitis, cirrhosis, liver cell dysplasia, and hepatocellular carcinoma (HCC).

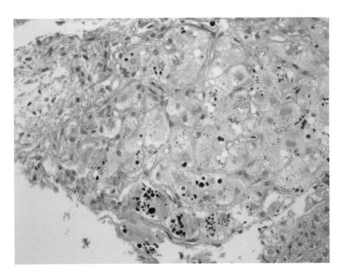

3. A 22-year-old woman had been followed for 2 years because of increased serum aminotransferases (aspartate aminotransferase [AST] and alanine aminotransferase [ALT]). A liver biopsy was performed. Based on the features seen in the periportal specimen shown in the image, the pathologist attributed the cause of her chronic hepatitis to:
   a. AIH
   b. Hepatitis B virus (HBV)
   c. Hepatitis C virus (HCV)
   d. Alcohol
   e. Wilson disease

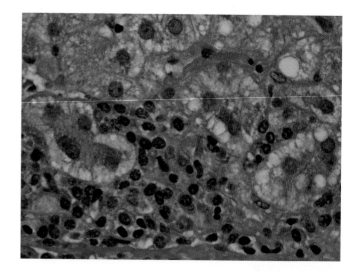

4. A 60-year-old man underwent an open cholecystectomy. During the procedure, the surgeon noted a 1-cm white nodule on the capsular surface of the liver and sent a piece for frozen section. Based on the features shown on medium power in the image, the pathologist's diagnosis should be:
   a. Metastatic adenocarcinoma
   b. von Meyenburg complex (bile duct malformation)
   c. Bile duct adenoma
   d. Biliary cystadenofibroma
   e. Normal peribiliary glands

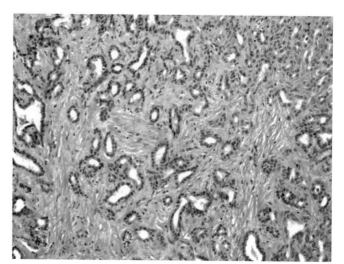

5. Which of the following findings would MOST likely be present in a patient with the liver biopsy changes shown in the image?
   a. Antimitochondrial antibodies
   b. Marked elevation (10-fold to 20-fold) of serum aminotransferases AST and ALT
   c. Perinuclear antineutrophilic cytoplasmic antibody (p-ANCA)
   d. Antinuclear and anti–smooth muscle antibodies
   e. IgG antibody to hepatitis A virus (HAV)

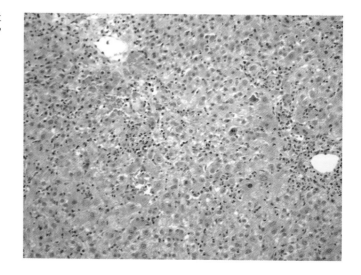

6. The postmortem section of liver shown in the image was
   MOST likely from a patient whose terminal course was
   characterized by:
   a. Sepsis
   b. Fulminant viral hepatitis
   c. Choledocholithiasis
   d. Drug hepatotoxicity
   e. Widely disseminated melanoma

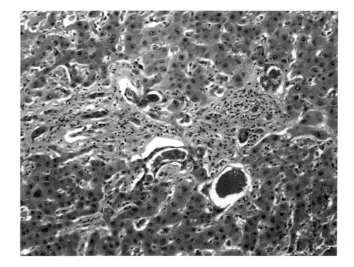

7. The MOST likely diagnosis in a patient with the portal tract
   features shown in the image would be:
   a. Acute hepatitis B
   b. Chronic hepatitis C
   c. Non-Hodgkin lymphoma
   d. AIH
   e. PBC

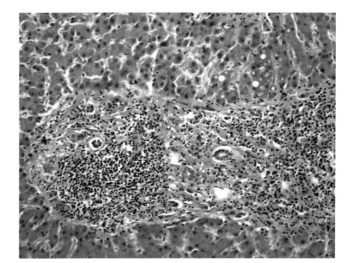

8. The liver biopsy specimen shown in the image was obtained
   from a 35-year-old man with chronically elevated serum
   alkaline phosphatase levels three to four times normal. Which of
   the following conditions is MOST likely present in this patient?
   a. Chronic hepatitis C
   b. AIH
   c. Ulcerative colitis
   d. Long-term acetaminophen use
   e. Congenital web of the inferior vena cava

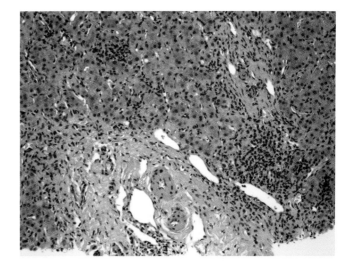

9. A pathologist is asked to review a liver biopsy specimen for a medicolegal case. The major changes in the biopsy specimen are shown in the image, with the centrilobular vein and perivenular area at center and at right and a minimally inflamed portal tract seen at left. According to the attorney for the plaintiff, a critical clinical investigation was omitted in the care of this patient because of a misinterpretation of the biopsy findings. Which clinical investigation would have been indicated based on the biopsy changes?

a. Obtain the phenotype for ATT
b. Cholangiography
c. Doppler ultrasound of the inferior vena cava and hepatic veins
d. Obtain a serum test for antinuclear antibodies
e. Obtain serologic tests for hepatitis B and hepatitis C

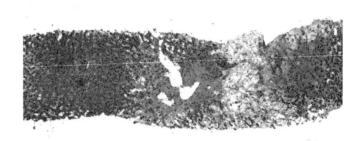

10. A 28-year-old woman who was taking oral contraceptives had a liver mass detected on ultrasound. The partial hepatectomy specimen shown in the image demonstrates the mass in cross section with several distinctive gross features. Based on the gross appearance, this lesion is MOST likely:

a. Liver cell adenoma (hepatocellular adenoma)
b. Biliary cystadenofibroma
c. Focal nodular hyperplasia (FNH)
d. Metastasis
e. Bile duct adenoma

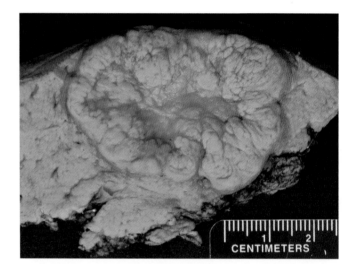

11. A liver biopsy was performed in the work-up of a 30-year-old woman with prolonged elevations of serum total bilirubin and alkaline phosphatase and normal aminotransferases. Based on the portal tract features seen in her liver biopsy specimen as shown in the image, the BEST diagnosis is:

a. PBC
b. Chronic hepatitis
c. Pericholangitis
d. Primary sclerosing cholangitis (PSC)
e. Idiopathic portal hypertension

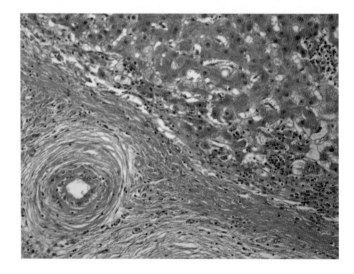

12. The liver biopsy specimen shown in the image is MOST likely to come from which of the following patients?
    a. A 63-year-old woman with severe bronchopneumonia and sepsis
    b. A 42-year-old HIV-positive patient receiving highly active antiretroviral therapy (HAART)
    c. A 58-year-old morbidly obese man
    d. A 60-year-old former intravenous drug user with chronic hepatitis C
    e. A 50-year-old woman who received a liver transplant 3 weeks earlier for end-stage PBC

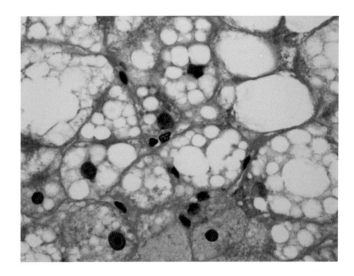

13. A liver biopsy was performed during the work-up of a 40-year-old woman with fourfold elevation of serum alkaline phosphatase and hepatosplenomegaly. The specimen shown in the image is representative of changes seen elsewhere in the needle biopsy specimen. Based on these features, the BEST diagnosis is:
    a. Sarcoidosis
    b. Tuberculosis
    c. PBC
    d. Drug hepatotoxicity
    e. Brucellosis

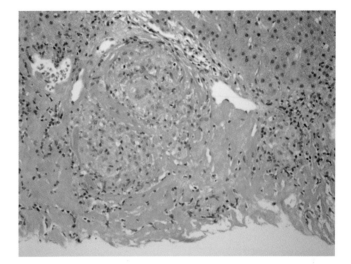

14. The image shows a Prussian blue iron stain of a liver biopsy specimen. A portal tract is seen at right with a bile duct and portal vein. Based on the cellular distribution of hemosiderin seen here, the pathologist should diagnose:
    a. Classic *HFE* hereditary hemochromatosis
    b. Excessive oral iron ingestion
    c. Multiple prior transfusions for many years
    d. Hemodialysis for recent onset of renal failure 3 months ago
    e. Chronic hepatitis C with secondary iron overload

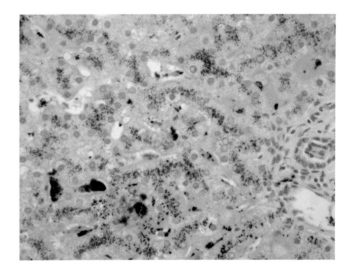

15. A 30-year-old woman complained of right upper quadrant pain of several months' duration. Computed tomography (CT) scan demonstrated a 5-cm subcapsular mass in the right lobe of the liver. A biopsy was performed, and the specimen is shown in the image. This tumor is known to be associated with which of the following?
    a. K-*ras* activation
    b. *P53* mutations
    c. *Jagged-1* mutations
    d. *HNF-1α* mutations
    e. *c-myc* mutations

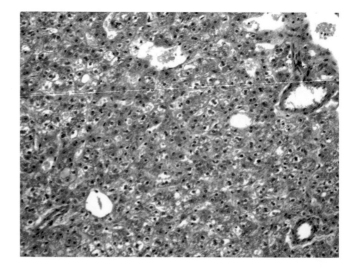

16. A 2-year-old boy was found to have a mass occupying the entire right lobe of the liver. A frozen section was requested, and the permanent section of the tissue resected is shown in the image. The CORRECT diagnosis is:
    a. Hepatoblastoma
    b. HCC
    c. Mesenchymal hamartoma
    d. von Meyenburg complex
    e. Malignant mixed tumor

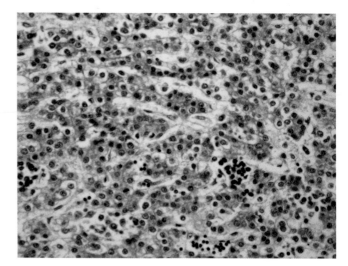

17. The slide presented in the image shows an immunostain of a CT-guided liver biopsy specimen from a 5-cm tumor in a 56-year-old man with chronic hepatitis C and cirrhosis. Serum α-fetoprotein was markedly elevated, and HCC was suspected. Which of the following immunostain methods was used?
    a. Polyclonal carcinoembryonic antigen (CEA)
    b. Cytokeratin 7
    c. Cytokeratin 20
    d. α-Fetoprotein
    e. Hepatocyte paraffin 1 (HepPar1)

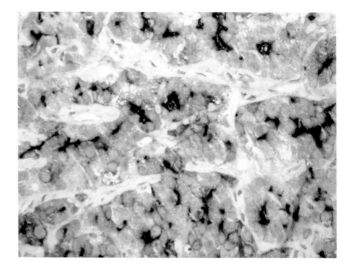

18. A surgeon had to reoperate 3 days after a cadaveric liver transplantation because of a problem with biliary anastomosis. After successfully completing the surgical revision, a liver biopsy was performed. The centrilobular region is shown in the image (central vein at bottom left). The hepatocellular changes demonstrated should be attributed to:

a. Preservation injury (ischemia-perfusion injury)
b. Steatohepatitis of the donor liver
c. Humoral (hyperacute) rejection
d. Acute rejection
e. Primary graft nonfunction

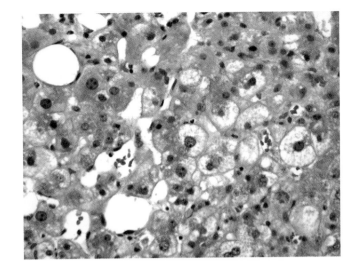

19. The histologic section of liver shown in the image was taken from an explanted liver specimen from a patient with acute liver failure. Which of the following conditions is LEAST likely to have resulted in the pathologic features seen in the image (short arrows indicate portal veins, long arrows indicate central veins)?

a. Ferrous sulfate toxicity
b. Ischemia
c. Mushroom poisoning (*Amanita* spp.)
d. Carbon tetrachloride
e. Halothane

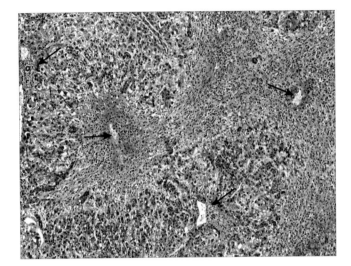

20. A 24-year-old man is known to have had multiple episodes of jaundice since childhood, each one resolving without medical therapy. Liver function tests were normal in between episodes. During a recent bout of jaundice, a liver biopsy is performed; the parenchymal changes are shown in the image. Based on the clinical information and the biopsy features, the MOST likely diagnosis is:

a. PSC
b. Chronic granulomatous disease with intermittent sepsis
c. Choledochal cyst
d. Alagille syndrome
e. Benign recurrent intrahepatic cholestasis (BRIC)

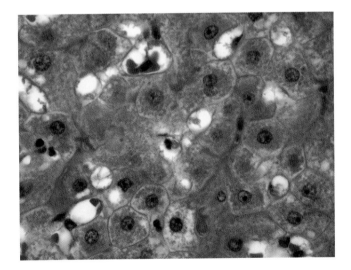

21. The abnormalities demonstrated in the portal tract shown in the image are LEAST likely to be seen in:
    a. Hepatic venous outflow obstruction
    b. Chronic hepatitis C
    c. Acute rejection after liver transplantation
    d. PBC
    e. Drug hepatotoxicity

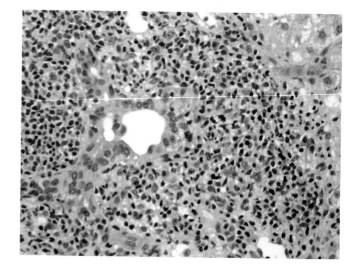

22. The photomicrograph in the image shows a core needle biopsy specimen of a solitary liver mass in a 30-year-old woman with negative serologic tests for hepatitis B and C and AIH. Which of the following is the MOST likely diagnosis?
    a. Reactive portal tract changes resulting from an adjacent neoplasm not sampled in the biopsy specimen
    b. Liver cell adenoma (hepatocellular adenoma)
    c. FNH
    d. Bile duct adenoma
    e. Ductal plate malformation (von Meyenburg complex)

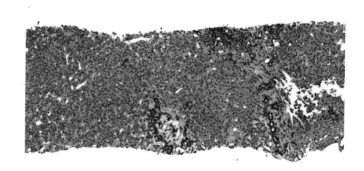

23. A 58-year-old woman underwent a liver biopsy to evaluate abnormal liver function tests. Hepatitis B and C virologic studies were negative. Based on the liver biopsy features shown in the image, the cause of this patient's liver disease may have been directly related to all of the following EXCEPT:
    a. Obesity
    b. Diabetes
    c. Hyperlipidemia
    d. Metabolic syndrome
    e. AIH

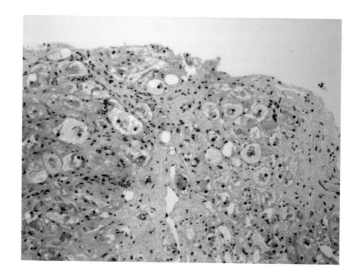

24. A patient underwent liver biopsy for grading and staging of chronic hepatitis C. One portal tract, shown in the image, appeared different from the others. The pathologist reviewing this case identified the CORRECT diagnosis as:

a. Large bile duct obstruction
b. von Meyenburg complex
c. Caroli disease
d. Isolated ductular hyperplasia
e. Fibrosing cholestatic hepatitis

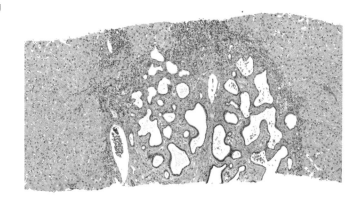

25. The liver biopsy specimen in the image was stained with the Victoria blue method, and the periportal regions throughout the sample showed changes similar to those seen in the image. This type of staining would MOST likely be seen in which of the following diseases?

a. Chronic hepatitis B
b. PSC
c. Cardiac hepatopathy
d. Stage 1 or 2 PBC
e. AAT deficiency

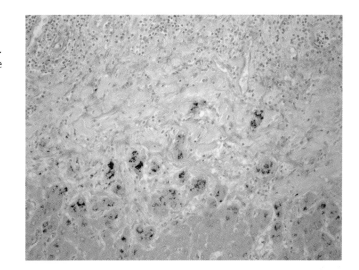

26. The liver biopsy specimen shown in the image was obtained from a 67-year-old man with a history of 2 years of abnormal liver function tests. Given the histopathologic pattern of damage demonstrated in the specimen, which of the following tests would MOST likely be positive?

a. p-ANCA
b. Antimitochondrial antibodies
c. Antibodies to hepatitis B surface antigen (anti-HBs)
d. Antinuclear antibodies
e. IgG antibodies to HAV

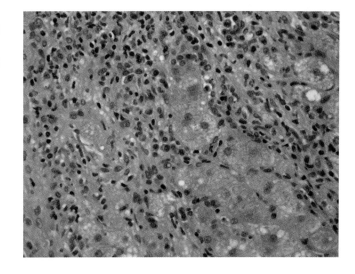

27. A 14-year-old girl who presented to the pediatrician with a protuberant abdomen was found to have hepatomegaly and elevated serum aminotransferases in the range of 200 to 300 IU/L (normal, <40 IU/L). A liver biopsy was ordered to determine the cause of the hepatomegaly and abnormal liver function tests. Based on the histopathologic features seen in the image, which of the following additional serum tests would the pediatrician MOST likely order?
    a. IgG antibody to HAV
    b. p-ANCA
    c. Hemoglobin A_{1c} (HbA$_{1c}$)
    d. HCV RNA
    e. Sphingomyelinase activity

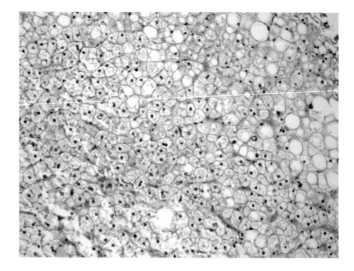

28. A patient with a liver biopsy specimen that shows the cytoplasmic changes seen in the image MOST likely has a history of:
    a. AIH
    b. Alcohol abuse
    c. PBC
    d. Chronic hepatitis C
    e. Chronic hepatitis B

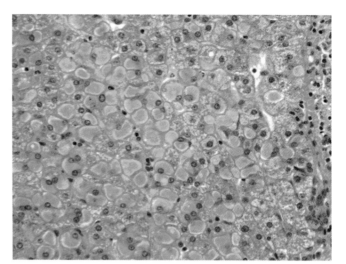

29. A 53-year-old man with known chronic hepatitis C underwent a liver biopsy. If the field shown in the specimen in the image is representative of changes elsewhere in the biopsy specimen, the appropriate grade and stage of disease are:
    a. Grade 1, stage 1
    b. Grade 2, stage 2
    c. Grade 2, stage 3
    d. Grade 2, stage 4
    e. Grade 3, stage 4

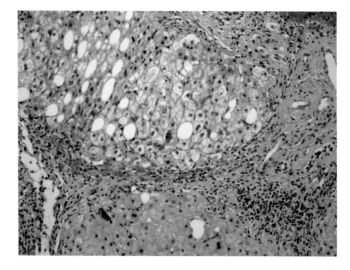

30. A patient presented with thrombocytopenia, splenomegaly, and portal hypertension of uncertain origin. A liver biopsy was performed, and a specimen is shown in the image. Based on the changes seen, the pathogenesis of this lesion and the patient's portal hypertension is thought to be:
    a. Scarring after severe hepatitis (posthepatitic cirrhosis)
    b. Fibrosis secondary to activation of hepatic stellate cells (HSCs)
    c. Variations between hypoperfused and hyperperfused regions of liver parenchyma with a resultant vigorous response in the form of regenerative hyperplasia
    d. Repeated chronic necroinflammation followed by cirrhosis
    e. Prolonged biliary obstruction

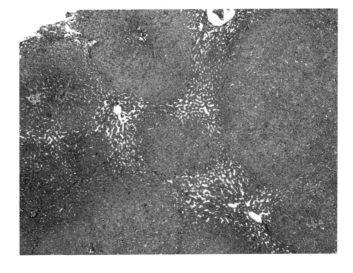

31. A 58-year-old man underwent a liver biopsy because of abnormal serum liver function tests and increasing bilirubin 8 months after liver transplantation for cirrhosis resulting from chronic hepatitis C. Based on the changes in the photomicrograph shown in the image, which of the following conditions is MOST likely responsible for the liver dysfunction?
    a. Acute cellular rejection
    b. Chronic ductopenic rejection
    c. Mild recurrent chronic hepatitis C
    d. Fibrosing cholestatic hepatitis C
    e. Cytomegalovirus (CMV) hepatitis

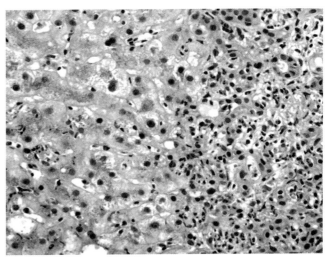

32. Wilson disease is due to mutations in which gene?
    a. Ceruloplasmin
    b. Copper-binding protein
    c. *Murr-1*
    d. *ATP7B*
    e. *MDR3*

33. Alagille syndrome is BEST defined as:
    a. Nonsyndromic paucity of bile ducts
    b. Paucity of bile ducts associated with various facial, vertebral, cardiac, and ophthalmologic abnormalities
    c. Progressive familial intrahepatic cholestasis
    d. Idiopathic adulthood ductopenia
    e. BRIC

34. In which of the following conditions are fibroobliterative lesions found?
    a. Chronic venous outflow obstruction
    b. PSC
    c. PBC

    d. Nonalcoholic fatty liver disease (NAFLD)
    e. Schistosomiasis

35. The MOST important pathologic feature on a liver biopsy specimen to establish the diagnosis of extrahepatic biliary atresia in a neonate is the presence of:
    a. Cholestasis
    b. Chronic portal inflammation
    c. Cirrhosis
    d. Ductular reaction
    e. Paucity of interlobular bile ducts

36. MOST cases of hereditary hemochromatosis in which there is excessive iron storage in hepatocytes leading to portal fibrosis or cirrhosis are known to be due to which of the following?
    a. *HFE* gene mutation
    b. Ferroportin-1 gene mutation
    c. Hepcidin gene mutation
    d. Aceruloplasminemia
    e. Transferrin receptor-2 gene mutation

37. Which of the following statements regarding Mallory-Denk bodies (MDBs) is NOT correct?
    a. MDBs can be stained immunohistochemically with antibodies to ubiquitin.
    b. MDBs are seen in both alcoholic and nonalcoholic steatohepatitis.
    c. MDBs contain cytokeratin 8 and cytokeratin 18.
    d. Copper overload in Wilson disease induces a constituent of MDBs, p62, which is an adapter protein involved in cell rescue from oxidative stress.
    e. MDBs contain degenerated mitochondria.

38. Microabscesses found in a liver biopsy specimen after liver transplantation are diagnostic of:
    a. Herpes hepatitis
    b. Biliary anastomotic stricture
    c. Sepsis
    d. Recurrent HCV infection
    e. CMV hepatitis

39. The hepatic cell responsible for MOST forms of hepatic fibrosis is the:
    a. Hepatocyte
    b. Kupffer cell
    c. Pit cell
    d. Stellate cell
    e. Portal tract fibroblast

40. When an overlap syndrome arises in patients with liver disease, this specifically refers to overlap between:
    a. Acute hepatitis and chronic hepatitis
    b. AIH and PBC or PSC
    c. AIH and systemic lupus erythematosus (SLE)
    d. Chronic hepatitis and cirrhosis
    e. Chronic hepatitis stage 3 and stage 4

41. Which one of the following stains in the panel routiunely used for liver biopsy evaluation is MOST useful for the diagnosis of HCC?
    a. Reticulin
    b. Trichrome
    c. PAS
    d. Diastase-treated PAS
    e. Iron

42. The term *pipestem fibrosis* specifically refers to a lesion seen in:
    a. Incomplete septal cirrhosis
    b. Hemochromatosis
    c. Schistosomiasis
    d. Idiopathic portal hypertension
    e. Chronic hepatitis

43. The major hepatic change associated with preeclampsia is:
    a. Microvesicular steatosis
    b. Centrilobular necrosis
    c. Arteritis affecting portal tract arterioles
    d. Fibrin in portal tract vessels and periportal sinusoids
    e. Peliosis hepatis

44. All of the following statements concerning HCC are true EXCEPT:
    a. Small cell dysplasia (small cell change) is currently favored over large cell dysplasia (large cell change) as the more likely direct precursor of carcinoma.

    b. The fibrolamellar variant typically occurs in young patients with chronic hepatitis B or hepatitis C or other well-recognized risk factors for carcinoma.
    c. Histologic subtypes include microtrabecular, acinar (adenoid), clear cell, and giant cell.
    d. This tumor may develop in noncirrhotic liver.
    e. Tumors closely resembling HCC (even with bile formation), termed *hepatoid carcinomas*, have been described in the stomach, ovary, pancreas, and other organs.

45. Fibrin ring granulomas of the liver have been MOST closely associated with which of the following conditions?
    a. Tuberculosis
    b. Q fever (*Coxiella burnetii* infection)
    c. Drug hepatotoxicity
    d. Sarcoidosis
    e. PBC

46. Cholangiocarcinoma is an important sequela of:
    a. PBC
    b. PSC
    c. Chronic hepatitis C
    d. AIH
    e. Schistosomiasis

47. Graft-versus-host disease (GVHD) affecting the liver typically targets:
    a. Central veins
    b. Intrahepatic bile ducts
    c. Arterioles
    d. Subcapsular region
    e. Hilar lymph nodes

48. A 60-year-old woman was found to have three liver masses, the largest measuring 5 cm × 4 cm × 8 cm. CT-guided biopsy of the largest mass showed extensive sclerosis, numerous signet ring cells, and vacuoles resembling lipid, with occlusion of portal and hepatic vein branches. Many areas strongly suggested adenocarcinoma, but mucicarmine and cytokeratin immunostains were negative. The MOST likely diagnosis is:
    a. Angiomyolipoma
    b. Combined HCC and cholangiocarcinoma
    c. Epithelioid hemangioendothelioma
    d. Fibrolamellar carcinoma
    e. Desmoplastic nested small cell tumor

49. All of the following are well-recognized hepatic findings associated with parenteral nutrition EXCEPT:
    a. Steatosis
    b. Steatohepatitis.
    c. Ductular reaction
    d. Cholestasis
    e. HCC

50. Which of the following is LEAST likely to be associated with a significant ductular reaction?
    a. PBC
    b. PSC
    c. Chronic hepatitis B
    d. Large bile duct obstruction owing to gallstones
    e. Massive hepatic necrosis

ANSWERS

1. c. During the first year after liver transplantation, acute cellular rejection is the most common cause of liver dysfunction and is the most common liver allograft lesion encountered by the pathologist. The classic triad of changes seen in acute rejection includes (1) an inflammatory infiltrate predominated by lymphocytes but often, helpfully, accompanied by numerous eosinophils and occasionally other effector cells; (2) bile duct damage; and (3) portal vein endotheliitis, which is not always present and often recedes quickly when immunosuppression is administered. AIH usually recurs at a later time frame than 2 months and should be supported histologically by evidence of active interface hepatitis with lymphoplasmacytic infiltration. In more severe cases of acute rejection, evidence of endotheliitis is found involving the central veins (central perivenulitis) and sometimes involving sinusoids as well.

Banff schema for grading liver allograft rejection: an international consensus document. *Hepatology* 1997;25(3):658-663.

Nagral A, Ben-Ari Z, Dhillon AP, Burroughs AK: Eosinophils in acute cellular rejection in liver allografts. *Liver Transpl Surg* 1998;4(5):355-362.

2. c. Serum isoelectric focusing is used to establish the diagnosis of AAT phenotype. A normal subject has PiMM and normal serum levels of this enzyme. AAT deficiency is associated with the Z allele, which may be present in the homozygous (PiZZ) or heterozygous (PiMZ, PiSZ) state. AAT deficiency should be considered in the differential diagnosis of liver disease in patients of all ages, particularly in the work-up of chronic hepatitis with or without cirrhosis of uncertain cause. Diastase PAS stain should be part of the routine special stain regimen for assessment of liver tissue (including biopsy, explant, and postmortem specimens). AAT deficiency is an autosomal codominant disease resulting from a mutation in the *SERPINA1* gene on the long arm of chromosome 14. Although more than 120 different AAT alleles are recognized, the Z allele is the most common (95% of cases of clinically recognized AAT deficiency) and results in a single amino acid substitution of lysine for glutamic acid at position 342. Diastase PAS is the diagnostic special stain for AAT deficiency; diastase PAS stain demonstrates purple-stained globules of varying size (representing the mutated AAT gene product within distended endoplasmic reticulum cisternae) within periportal hepatocytes. In homozygous (PiZZ) cases with numerous globules, the globules are also frequently evident on hematoxylin-eosin and trichrome stains. The exact mechanism whereby retention of intrahepatocellular AAT globules causes the varying morphologic forms of liver disease at different ages is controversial. Immunostaining for AAT in the diagnosis of AAT deficiency should show a targetoid appearance of the retained intrahepatocellular globules, with a relatively pale or nonstaining center and more concentrated positive brown staining around the circumference of each globule.

Bals R: Alpha-1-antitrypsin deficiency. *Best Pract Res Clin Gastroenterol* 2010;24(5):629-633.

Carrell RW, Lomas DA: Alpha₁-antitrypsin deficiency— a model for conformational diseases. *N Engl J Med* 2002; 346(1):45-53.

Silverman EK, Sandhaus RA: Clinical practice. Alpha1-antitrypsin deficiency. *N Engl J Med* 2009;360(26):2749-2757.

Stoller JK, Aboussouan LS: A review of α₁-antitrypsin deficiency. *Am J Respir Crit Care Med* 2012;185(3):246-259.

3. a. The liver biopsy specimen shows characteristic features of autoimmune chronic hepatitis, including active interface hepatitis, abundant plasma cells within the inflammatory infiltrate, and periportal regenerative liver cell rosettes. Type 1 AIH most often manifests in young adults (women are affected more than men) with positive serum antinuclear antibody or anti–smooth muscle antibody. Type 2 AIH is predominantly a disorder of children who have positive serum anti–liver-kidney microsomal antibody. Type 3 AIH is seen in adults with anti–soluble liver antigen antibodies. Simplified criteria for AIH by Hennes et al. include scores of 0, 1, or 2 for liver biopsy results: no diagnostic features (score of 0), compatible lymphocytic portal inflammation (score of 1), and lymphoplasmacytic interface hepatitis with regenerative rosettes (score of 2). The histologic component is added to several other parameters (including autoantibody test results) to provide an overall diagnostic score. The histologic differential diagnosis of periportal interface hepatitis with admixed lymphocytes and plasma cells includes the major causes of chronic hepatitis, including chronic hepatitis B and hepatitis C, drug-induced liver injury (e.g., minocycline hepatitis), AIH, and two metabolic disorders (ATT deficiency and Wilson disease).

Hennes EM, Zeniya M, Czaja AJ, et al: Simplified diagnostic criteria for autoimmune hepatitis. *Hepatology* 2008;48(1):169-176.

Manns MP, Czaja AJ, Gotham JD, et al: Diagnosis and management of autoimmune hepatitis. *Hepatology* 2010; 51(6):2193-2213.

4. c. The lesion is a bile duct adenoma. The chief histologic features of bile duct adenoma are medium-sized, regular bile duct structures (without nuclear pleomorphism or prominent nucleoli) embedded in a densely hyalinized fibrous stroma. Lymphoid aggregates are often present where the fibrous tissue of the bile duct adenoma interfaces with the nonlesional liver parenchyma. Bile duct adenomas are currently thought to be a type of pyloric gland metaplasia of the peribiliary glands of the liver, with immunopositivity for MUC6 and MUC5AC and positivity for variable degrees of acid mucin. Bile duct adenoma is part of the histologic differential diagnosis of white or tan capsular nodules of the liver that may be found incidentally at the time of surgery. In addition to bile duct adenoma, the differential histologic diagnoses include focal fibrosis, metastasis, healed granuloma, von Meyenburg complex, FNH, hemangioma, and arteriovenous malformation.

Bhathal PS, Hughes NR, Goodman ZD: The so-called bile duct adenoma is a peribiliary gland hamartoma. *Am J Surg Pathol* 1998;20(7):858-864.

Hughes NR, Goodman ZD, Bhathal PS: An immunohistochemical profile of the so-called bile duct adenoma. Clues to pathogenesis. *Am J Surg Pathol* 2010;34(9):1312-1318.

5. b. Acute hepatitis of viral or drug origin often shows moderate to marked elevation of serum aminotransferases owing to the diffuse damage and cell death of affected hepatocytes, with release of cytosolic AST and ALT. The presence of antimitochondrial antibodies is diagnostic in PBC. The p-ANCA serum test is most often positive in PSC. Antinuclear and anti–smooth muscle antibodies are positive in AIH, which is most often characterized by portal and periportal lymphoplasmacytic inflammation and interface hepatitis, not by the features of a diffuse acute hepatitis. If the diagnosis was acute hepatitis A, the serum would be positive for IgM antibody to HAV. The major causes of acute hepatitis include hepatitis viruses (A through E) and drugs (usually idiosyncratic or unpredictable agents); alternative, herbal, and recreational agents should be considered. Histologic determination of the cause is often difficult. Helpful additional features favoring drug-induced liver injury include abundant eosinophils, bile duct damage, granulomas, and otherwise atypical histologic features for acute hepatitis. AIH may rarely appear on histologic examination as acute hepatitis. Features that may raise suspicion for autoimmune liver disease include prominence of central perivenulitis (inflammation and liver cell dropout around central veins, with inflammation, prominently lymphocytes and plasma cells), plasma cell prominence within the portal and periportal inflammatory infiltrates, and the presence of bridging necrosis (central-to-portal bridging necrosis).

Acute and chronic hepatitis revisited. Review by an international group. *Lancet* 1977;2(8024):914-919.

Stickel F, Kessebohm K, Weimann R, et al: Review of liver injury associated with dietary supplements. *Liver Int* 2011;31(5): 595-605.

6. a. Bile ductular cholestasis (inspissated bile concretions within proliferated periportal bile ductular structures) is pathognomonic for sepsis. In fulminant hepatitis, activation of periportal progenitor cells frequently occurs to produce numerous periportal proliferating bile ductules (neocholangiolar proliferation), but they typically do not contain inspissated bile. In acute large bile duct obstruction, the trio of changes characteristically present in the portal tract includes edema, proliferation of bile ductules (without inspissated bile), and a mild neutrophil infiltrate. An exception is a liver biopsy specimen obtained within the first few months of life in cases of extrahepatic biliary atresia, when the presence of inspissated bile within periportal bile ductular structures is helpful in establishing the diagnosis of biliary atresia. Cholestasis in drug hepatotoxicity usually manifests as centrilobular hepatocellular or bile canalicular bile stasis and not bile ductular cholestasis. The brown pigment seen in the liver section in the image is bile, not melanin, and it is present within bile ductular structures (not within tumor cells).

Geier A, Fickert P, Trauner M: Mechanisms of disease: mechanisms and clinical implications of cholestasis in sepsis. *Nat Clin Pract Gastroenterol Hepatol* 2006;3(10):574-585.

Kosters A, Karpen SJ: The role of inflammation in cholestasis: clinical and basic aspects. *Semin Liver Dis* 2010;30(2):185-194.

Lefkowitch JH: Bile ductular cholestasis: an ominous histopathologic sign related to sepsis and "cholangitis lenta." *Hum Pathol* 1982;13(1):19-24.

7. b. The most common cause of portal tract lymphoid aggregates in liver biopsy and other histologic specimens is chronic hepatitis C. The lymphoid aggregate should be identified by its well-circumscribed, dense nature, which separates it from adjacent chronic inflammation that typically accompanies the lesion (in chronic hepatitis and in chronic cholestatic disorders such as PBC and PSC). The lymphoid aggregate is often present near the interlobular bile duct or encloses the duct. The immune cells within the lymphoid aggregate (and within lymphoid follicles with germinal centers, which are also sometimes seen in chronic hepatitis C) have a heterogeneity and arrangement similar to lymph nodes, based on immunohistochemical staining results (see Mosnier et al.). The portal lymphoid aggregates seen in chronic cholestatic diseases usually form at the site of previous bile duct destruction (PBC) and near ducts affected by periductal "onion-skin" fibrosis or sometimes within the dense periductal fibrosis where ducts have become atrophic and disappear (PSC).

Mosnier JF, Degott C, Marcellin P, et al: The intraportal lymphoid nodule and its environment in chronic active hepatitis C: an immunohistochemical study. *Hepatology* 1993;17(3):366-371.

Scheuer PJ, Ashrafzadeh P, Sherlock S, et al: The pathology of hepatitis C. *Hepatology* 1992;15(4):567-571.

Scheuer PJ, Davies SE, Dhillon AP: Histopathological aspects of viral hepatitis. *J Viral Hepat* 1996;3(6):277-283.

8. c. The image shows a portal tract with two prominent cross-sectional cuts through a hepatic arteriole with no accompanying bile duct (ductopenia). Periportal lymphocytic interface hepatitis also is seen. Because most patients with PSC have underlying inflammatory bowel disease, and ulcerative colitis is much more common than Crohn disease, ulcerative colitis is the correct choice. Although the presence of chronic portal inflammation and interface hepatitis superficially is compatible with chronic hepatitis of several causes, the absence of native bile ducts should focus attention on a chronic biliary tract disease, such as PSC. Bile ducts are not characteristically destroyed in AIH, and the duct loss in the photomicrograph shown in the image is not consistent with a diagnosis of AIH. Acetaminophen liver injury is centrilobular and is not known to produce ductopenia. Congenital web of the inferior vena cava is a cause of venous outflow obstruction, producing centrilobular congestion with or without fibrosis.

Deshpande V, Sainani NI, Chung RT, et al: IgG4-associated cholangitis: a comparative histological and immunophenotypic study with primary sclerosing cholangitis on liver biopsy material. *Mod Pathol* 2009;22(10):1287-1295.

Gotthardt D, Chahoud F, Sauer P: Primary sclerosing cholangitis: diagnostic and therapeutic problems. *Dig Dis* 2011;29(Suppl 1): 41-45.

9. c. The needle biopsy specimen shown in the image demonstrates two centrilobular regions with marked congestion and neighboring sinusoidal dilatation, which are the two chief histologic hallmarks of venous outflow obstruction. The periportal liver parenchyma in the left side of the biopsy core specimen appears thickened and nodular (owing to periportal regenerative hyperplasia in the face of narrowing and progressive atrophy of centrilobular hepatocyte plates secondary to congestive compression). Doppler ultrasound of the inferior vena cava and hepatic veins would be appropriate to assess whether or not the hepatic veins and inferior vena cava are patent or are obstructed and to determine better where the block in venous outflow is. The investigations listed in the other answer choices are not relevant to this disease. With chronicity, venous outflow obstruction is associated not only with centrilobular congestion and sinusoidal dilatation but also with narrowing and atrophy of liver cell plates, perivenular or perisinusoidal fibrosis ("cardiac sclerosis"), and compensatory regenerative hyperplasia of periportal hepatocytes (from which nodular regenerative hyperplasia [NRH] may evolve). The differential diagnosis of liver biopsy changes of venous outflow obstruction includes hepatic vein or inferior vena cava thrombosis or tumor invasion (e.g., HCC, renal cell carcinoma), Budd-Chiari syndrome, constrictive pericarditis, and right-sided or left-sided cardiac failure. Pathologists should also be aware that the classic centrilobular changes of hepatic venous outflow obstruction occasionally may be accompanied by portal tract features that mimic biliary disease (i.e., ductular reaction, portal and periportal fibrosis) in the absence of biliary obstruction (see Kakar et al.).

DeLeve LD, Valla DC, Garcia-Tsao G; American Association for the Study of Liver Diseases: vascular disorders of the liver. *Hepatology* 2009;49(5):1729-1764.

Kakar S, Batts KP, Poterucha JJ, et al: Histologic changes mimicking biliary disease in liver biopsies with venous outflow impairment. *Mod Pathol* 2004;17(7):874-878.

10. c. FNH is a mass composed of cirrhosislike nodules with a central, sometimes radiating scar. FNH is a reactive hyperplasia of hepatocytes, fibrous tissue, and bile ductular structures resulting from hyperperfusion from a centrally (or sometimes eccentrically) located arterial malformation. Microscopy features include cirrhosislike nodules of hepatocytes growing in thickened plates, a central scar with an abnormal artery or artery branches that often show eccentric muscular hypertrophy, and proliferating bile ductular structures (derivatives of activated progenitor cells) within or adjacent to the scar. FNH is the second most common benign liver tumor after hemangioma. FNH is mostly polyclonal, consistent with a hyperplastic (nonneoplastic) lesion resulting from vascular hyperperfusion. FNH may develop as a secondary process in various vascular disorders in which combinations of venous outflow obstruction and atrophy and residual adjacent perfusion result in lesions nearly identical to the de novo lesion. Examples include FNH that develops in Budd-Chiari syndrome and FNH in the liver allograft after liver transplantation as described by Ra et al. Liver cell adenomas usually are homogeneous, orange-tan, well-circumscribed or encapsulated masses without regions of nodularity or central scar. The multiple cystic spaces of biliary cystadenofibroma, a rare lesion, are not seen here. Metastatic tumors typically are more homogeneous and diffusely fibrotic (owing to reactive desmoplasia). Bile duct adenomas are usually smaller in size than the FNH shown in the image and show a homogeneous white-tan gross appearance, without nodularity or a central scar.

Nguyen BN, Fléjou JF, Terris B, et al: Focal nodular hyperplasia of the liver: a comprehensive pathologic study of 305 lesions and recognition of new histologic forms. *Am J Surg Pathol* 1999;23(12):1441-1454.

Ra SH, Kaplan JB, Lassman CR: Focal nodular hyperplasia after orthotopic liver transplantation. *Liver Transpl* 2010;16(1): 98-103.

Rebouissou S, Bioulac-Sage P, Zucman-Rossi J: Molecular pathogenesis of focal nodular hyperplasia and hepatocellular adenoma. *J Hepatol* 2008;48(1):163-170.

11. d. The portal tract shown in the image contains a bile duct with "onion-skin" periductal fibrosis, the diagnostic lesion of PSC. The adjacent periportal hepatocytes are swollen (pseudoxanthomatous change) as a result of bile salt retention. The diagnostic lesion of PBC is nonsuppurative (i.e., lymphoplasmacytic) destructive cholangitis, not periductal fibrosis. Although there is a mild chronic inflammatory infiltrate in the portal tract shown in the image, periductal fibrosis is not an expected finding in chronic hepatitis. Pericholangitis was thought to represent a specific disease entity of inflammation near bile ducts in individuals with inflammatory bowel disease before recognition that most such cases represented PSC. The term *pericholangitis* was discarded more than 2 decades ago and should no longer be used. Periductal fibrosis is not a feature seen in idiopathic portal hypertension; varying degrees of portal and periportal fibrosis, often subtle and sometimes with loss or compression of portal vein branches, as well as regions of neighboring hyperplastic liver cell plates are the main features of idiopathic portal hypertension.

Chapman R, Cullen S: Etiopathogenesis of primary sclerosing cholangitis. *World J Gastroenterol* 2008;14(21):3350-3359.

Pollheimer MJ, Halilbasic E, Fickert P, et al: Pathogenesis of primary sclerosing cholangitis. *Best Pract Res Clin Gastroenterol* 2011;25(6):727-739.

Silveira MG, Lindor KD: Primary sclerosing cholangitis. *Can J Gastroenterol* 2008;22(8):689-698.

12. b. The high-power view of the liver biopsy specimen shows predominance of microvesicular (small droplet) steatosis within the hepatocytes and a few large lipid vacuoles. Of the answer choices, this liver biopsy specimen is most likely to come from a 42-year-old, HIV-positive patient receiving HAART. The nucleoside reverse transcriptase inhibitor group of agents in HAART consists of several drugs that may cause mitochondrial injury and resultant microvesicular steatosis. Microvesicular (small droplet) steatosis is defined as the accumulation of many small lipid vacuoles within the cytoplasm of hepatocytes surrounding a centrally located nucleus. The histologic differential diagnosis of microvesicular steatosis includes inherited and acquired conditions and exposures to hepatotoxic agents that cause serious impairment of mitochondrial beta oxidation of fatty acids. Examples of drugs that may result in microvesicular steatosis include valproic acid, nucleoside reverse transcriptase inhibitors, and tetracycline and its derivatives. Microvesicular steatosis may be associated with liver failure, hypoglycemia, and encephalopathy. The classic trio of conditions associated with microvesicular steatosis includes Reye syndrome, acute fatty liver of pregnancy (third trimester), and tetracycline toxicity. Oil red O staining of frozen liver biopsy material is occasionally necessary for exclusion of acute fatty liver of pregnancy to confirm this diagnosis. The use of terms such as *macrosteatosis* and *microsteatosis* should be avoided because they represent a bowdlerization of the appropriate terms *macrovesicular steatosis* and *microvesicular steatosis*.

Table 6-1 Differential Diagnosis of Steatosis

Macrovesicular Steatosis	Microvesicular Steatosis
Ethanol	Antiretroviral agents
Obesity	Acute fatty liver of pregnancy
Diabetes	Reye syndrome
Hyperlipidemia	Tetracycline toxicity
Metabolic syndrome/insulin resistance	Alcoholic foamy degeneration
Corticosteroid therapy	Valproic acid toxicity

Burt AD, Mutton A, Day CP: Diagnosis and interpretation of steatosis and steatohepatitis. *Semin Diagn Pathol* 1998;15(4): 246-258.

Labbe G, Pessayre D, Fromenty B: Drug-induced liver injury through mitochondrial dysfunction: mechanisms and detection during preclinical safety studies. *Fundam Clin Pharmacol* 2008;22(4):335-353.

Núñez M: Clinical syndromes and consequences of antiretroviral-related hepatotoxicity. *Hepatology* 2010;52(3):1143-1155.

13. a. When granulomas are seen in a liver biopsy specimen, the major differential diagnosis includes five conditions: sarcoidosis, tuberculosis, PBC, drug hepatotoxicity, and schistosomiasis. In tuberculosis, hepatic granulomas are usually randomly located, without a predilection for portal tracts or periportal regions. When granulomas develop in PBC, they are usually directly adjacent to florid bile duct lesions. Clustered, multiple granulomas are not associated with PBC. Granulomas associated with drug-induced liver injury may be located anywhere in the hepatic lobules, may sometimes contain eosinophils, and do not have a predilection for portal or periportal regions or for clustering. Hepatic granulomas seen in brucellosis are usually randomly located within the lobular parenchyma. Sarcoidosis is the favored diagnosis in this case scenario. Involvement of the liver by sarcoidosis in its most histopathologically characteristic pattern shows clustering of portal and periportal granulomas, as is seen in the photomicrograph shown in the image. The granulomas seen in sarcoidosis may have specific histopathologic features depending on the type of associated damage they produce in the liver parenchyma. Devaney et al. described categories of sarcoid-related liver disease, including *hepatitic* (associated with variable chronic portal and periportal inflammation that may mimic chronic hepatitis), *biliary* (wherein portal tracts show changes of bile duct obstruction or of bile duct loss resembling PBC), and *vascular* (wherein the granulomas impact on portal tract vascular structures). Sarcoidosis may lead to destruction of interlobular bile ducts and a clinical syndrome resembling PBC; sarcoidosis also may rarely result in cirrhosis and extensive confluent regions of fibrosis in the liver.

Devaney K, Goodman ZD, Epstein MS, et al: Hepatic sarcoidosis. Clinicopathologic features in 100 patients. *Am J Surg Pathol* 1993;17(12):1272-1280.

Ishak KG: Sarcoidosis of the liver and bile ducts. *Mayo Clin Proc* 1998;73(5):467-472.

14. c. The Prussian blue iron stain in the image demonstrates moderate to marked (grade 3 of 4) hemosiderosis of periportal hepatocytes (the portal tract is seen at the right).

There is also clumped hemosiderin within sinusoidal Kupffer cells. This distribution of iron overload involving both Kupffer cells and hepatocytes is consistent with secondary (acquired) iron overload that developed in a patient with prolonged transfusion therapy. Classic hemochromatosis, even in the late, cirrhotic stage, shows very little iron overload of Kupffer cells and affects predominantly parenchymal cells (i.e., hepatocytes). Portal macrophages and sinusoidal Kupffer cells are the predominant sites for iron overload with oral iron ingestion, and the lack of significant iron-laden macrophages in the portal tract at right makes this an incorrect choice. Hemodialysis is among the chief causes of Kupffer cell hemosiderosis (the other causes are hemolysis and transfusions), but a brief, several-month course of dialysis would not likely contribute to the marked Kupffer cell and hepatocellular iron overload seen in the image. Iron overload in chronic hepatitis C, with or without cirrhosis, is usually minimal or mild (in contrast to the present case scenario) and may be in Kupffer cells, hepatocytes, or both.

Deugnier Y, Turlin B: Pathology of hepatic iron overload. *Semin Liver Dis* 2011;31(3):260-271.

Pietrangelo A: Hereditary hemochromatosis: pathogenesis, diagnosis, and treatment. *Gastroenterology* 2010;139(2): 393-408.

15. d. The mass lesion shown in the image is composed of benign-appearing hepatocytes arranged in thickened plates with interspersed isolated blood vessels, including small venules and arterioles. The absence of normal lobular architecture, portal tracts, and bile ducts is consistent with the features of hepatocellular adenoma (liver cell adenoma). Hepatocellular adenomas have been assessed for histologic-genomic correlates, and the most common category of adenomas (accounting for about 35%) is steatotic *HNF-1α* mutation liver cell adenoma. Hepatocellular adenomas are currently subclassified into four groups based on genomic classification: type 1, *HNF-1α* mutations, with large droplet steatosis and without atypia; type 2, β-catenin mutations, with atypia and features that may transition to HCC; type 3, interleukin 6 ST mutations, including inflammatory or telangiectatic adenoma; and type 4, no known mutation, with no specific features. The routine histologic evaluation to confirm a diagnosis of hepatocellular adenoma (and to distinguish it from carcinoma) should include hematoxylin-eosin stain, reticulin (which should show preserved reticulin framework throughout, in contrast to the "paucireticulin" pattern seen in HCC), and possibly CD34 (should show limited expression near pseudoportal tracts). Other immunostains can be added, such as the trio of glypican-3, glutamine synthetase, and heat shock protein 70 (which all should be negative) and various other stains to specify adenoma subtype. Children and young adults with multiple adenomas (adenomatosis is defined as ≥10 adenomas) and diabetes are very likely to have *HNF-1α* mutation and maturity-onset diabetes of the young type 3. Adenomas with suspicious features for the development of or transition to HCC (nuclear atypia, pseudoglandular growth, increased mitotic activity, focal loss of reticulin) and harboring β-catenin mutations should demonstrate glutamine synthetase expression and nuclear overexpression of β-catenin on immunohistochemical staining. K-*ras* activation and *c-myc* mutations are seen in cholangiocarcinoma, *P53* mutations are seen in HCC, and *Jagged-1* mutations are identified in many biliary tract disorders, particularly Alagille syndrome (syndromic paucity of intrahepatic bile ducts).

Bioulac-Sage P, Balabaud C, Zucman-Rossi J: Subtype classification of hepatocellular adenoma. *Dig Surg* 2010;27(1):39-45.
Bioulac-Sage P, Cubel G, Balabaud C, et al: Revisiting the pathology of resected benign hepatocellular nodules using new immunohistochemical markers. *Semin Liver Dis* 2011;31(1): 91-103.

16. a. The patient's age and the histologic features of this tumor are characteristic of hepatoblastoma, including the "light-dark" pattern of thickened cords of neoplastic hepatocytes and the accompanying foci of extramedullary hematopoiesis. Hepatoblastoma is the most common malignant liver tumor in the first 5 years of life. Hepatoblastoma is classified into the broad categories of epithelial and mixed epithelial-mesenchymal types. Epithelial hepatoblastoma includes fetal epithelial and embryonal epithelial types, which may be combined. The fetal type demonstrates thickened cords and sheets of incompletely differentiated fetal hepatoblasts with clear (glycogen and lipid-rich) or granular cytoplasm. The embryonal type demonstrates a higher nucleus-to-cytoplasm ratio, less cytoplasm, more basophilia, and focal glandular or ductlike structures. Both subtypes may have intrasinusoidal foci of extramedullary hematopoiesis, although this is more common in the fetal epithelial type. When mesenchymal elements are intermixed in hepatoblastoma, these may include chondroid-containing and osteoid-containing foci. The incorrect answer choices are tumors with different histologic appearance than shown in the image. HCC in children usually occurs in children older than 2 years and shows discohesive microtrabeculae of tumor (and no significant extramedullary hematopoiesis as a rule). Mesenchymal hamartoma of childhood is grossly distinctive because there are numerous, grossly enlarged cystic spaces (abnormal and dilated lymphatics) amid proliferations of islands of benign-appearing hepatocytes and numerous bile ductular structures. The von Meyenburg complex refers to a benign lesion derived from a ductal plate malformation and consists of bile duct–type epithelium (not hepatocyte-derived or hepatoblast-derived neoplasm similar to hepatoblastoma). Malignant mixed tumor has a pleomorphic histology.

Finegold MJ, Egler RA, Goss JA, et al: Liver tumors: pediatric population. *Liver Transpl* 2008;14(11):1545-1556.
Hadzic N, Finegold MJ: Liver neoplasia in children. *Clin Liver Dis* 2011;15(2):443-462, vii-x.

17. a. Polyclonal CEA immunostain shows the characteristic canalicular and apical staining at the surfaces of neoplastic cells in HCC (as well as normal bile canaliculi). When a liver specimen demonstrates a malignant neoplasm, the classic set of immunostains to be ordered first to distinguish between metastatic carcinoma versus primary HCC includes cytokeratin 7+cytokeratin 20+HepPar1+polyclonal CEA (or, alternatively, CD10 in place of polyclonal CEA). HCCs stain negatively with cytokeratin 7 and cytokeratin 20 in most cases. α-Fetoprotein staining is positive in 75% or less of HCCs, and the pattern is cytoplasmic, not apical and membranous as seen in the present case. If the HCC is only

moderately differentiated or poorly differentiated, HepPar1 immunostaining may be negative, and in that case an alternative trio including glypican-3, glutamine synthetase, and heat shock protein 70 should be ordered. Arginase-1 is an additional immunohistochemical marker of hepatocytes and hepatocellular neoplasms.

Kakar S, Gown AM, Goodman ZD, et al: Best practices in diagnostic immunohistochemistry: hepatocellular carcinoma versus metastatic neoplasms. *Arch Pathol Lab Med* 2007;131(11):1648-1654.
Shifizadeh N, Ferrell LD, Kakar S: Utility and limitations of glypican-3 expression for the diagnosis of hepatocellular carcinoma at both ends of the differentiation spectrum. *Mod Pathol* 2008;21(8):1011-1018.
Yan BC, Gong C, Song J, et al: Arginase-1. A new immunohistochemical marker of hepatocytes and hepatocellular neoplasms. *Am J Surg Pathol* 2010;34(8): 1147-1154.

18. a. The hepatocellular changes seen in the image should be attributed to preservation injury (ischemia-perfusion injury). Because of reduced blood supply of the devascularized donor liver and transportation from distant sites on iced physiologic (University of Wisconsin or variant) solution, hepatocytes in acinar zone 3 (centrilobular region), which are vulnerable to hypoperfusion, have developed leaky membranes with resultant fluid entry and ballooning. Another preservation injury seen in the 7 to 10 days after liver transplantation is centrilobular cholestasis ("functional bile flow impairment"), in which there is impaired bile transport across canaliculi in centrilobular regions. Scattered perivenular apoptotic bodies or hepatocytes showing coagulative necrosis should always be sought (to determine the extent, if any, of preservation injury) in an early posttransplantation biopsy specimen (i.e., within several days of transplant) or in a "time 0" liver allograft biopsy specimen obtained when vascular anastomoses have been completed. If damage to centrilobular hepatocytes is limited to ballooning (without significant coagulative necrosis), the lesion usually resolves within approximately 1 week. A band of subcapsular hemorrhagic necrosis may be another type of preservation injury evident in a posttransplant liver biopsy specimen, but this injury usually has no negative sequelae.

Adeyi O, Fischer SE, Guindi M: Liver allograft pathology: approach to interpretation of needle biopsies with clinicopathological correlation. *J Clin Pathol* 2010;63(1):47-74.
Kukan M, Haddad PS: Role of hepatocytes and bile duct cells in preservation-reperfusion injury of liver grafts. *Liver Transpl* 2001;7(5):381-400.

19. a. Ferrous sulfate toxicity is least likely to have resulted in the pathologic features seen here. Acetaminophen (*N*-acetyl-*p*-aminophenol) is metabolized by centrilobular hepatocyte CYP2E1 to the toxic metabolite *N*-acetyl-*p*-benzoquinone imine (NAPQI). In cases of overdose that deplete cellular stores of glutathione, NAPQI produces extensive damage to hepatocellular (and mitochondrial) proteins, resulting in centrilobular coagulative necrosis. Centrilobular necrosis may be caused by other specific drugs and toxins (e.g., carbon tetrachloride, halothane, mushroom poisoning) and by ischemia/hypoperfusion. The lobular (acinar) distribution of necrosis is helpful in determining the cause. Periportal necrosis is typical of phosphorus poisoning and ferrous sulfate, whereas midzonal necrosis is attributed to heat stroke and Dengue virus infection. The differential diagnoses for centrilobular necrosis have already been mentioned. Acetaminophen toxicity is a cause of acute liver failure with a specific therapeutic modality—administration of *N*-acetylcysteine for repletion of cellular glutathione stores. Hepatotoxicity at lower doses than doses typical of suicidal gestures may be seen in alcoholics or individuals with chronic alcohol ingestion or after inadvertent excessive dosing for therapeutic reasons. Routine stains are usually sufficient to demonstrate the chief pathologic changes in acetaminophen toxicity, but immunostain for CD68 may be useful in further highlighting the role of macrophages (both indigenous Kupffer cells and newly recruited macrophages) in cytokine release and phagocytosis in the centrilobular regions.

Jaeschke H, Williams CD, Ramachandran A, et al: Acetaminophen hepatotoxicity and repair: the role of sterile inflammation and innate immunity. *Liver Int* 2012;32(1):8-20.

Williams CD, Antoine DJ, Shaw PJ, et al: Role of the Nalp3 inflammasome in acetaminophen-induced sterile inflammation and liver injury. *Toxicol Appl Pharmacol* 2011;252(3):289-297.

20. e. Bland bile canalicular cholestasis characterizes BRIC, in which the function of the familial intrahepatic cholestasis 1 bile transport protein on the bile canaliculus is periodically impaired. No residual histologic damage is evident following episodes of jaundice. Although cholestasis is likely to be present when major bile ducts in PSC are obstructed, there should be accompanying diagnostic portal tract changes (e.g., periductal "onion-skin" fibrosis, fibroobliterative cholangitis). There may be bland cholestasis during periods of sepsis as a result of endotoxin-mediated inhibition of the bile salt export pump, but in chronic granulomatous disease there are also typically many prominent foamy Kupffer cells and portal macrophages with tan pigmentation, the result of repeated phagocytosis of microbial organisms. The histologic picture of choledochal cyst should include not only cholestasis but also portal tract changes of large bile duct obstruction (i.e., edema, ductular reaction, scattered neutrophils). In Alagille syndrome, the history of clinical jaundice would be prominent from birth and the neonatal period, and other syndromic effects would be apparent (e.g., abnormal vertebrae, cardiac anomalies).

Beauséjour Y, Alvarez F, Beaulieu M, et al: Of two new ABCB11 mutations responsible for type 2 benign recurrent intrahepatic cholestasis in a French-Canadian family. *Can J Gastroenterol* 2011;25(6):311-314.

Finegold MJ: Common diagnostic problems in pediatric liver pathology. *Clin Liver Dis* 2002;6(2):421-454.

Müllenbach R, Lammert F: An update on genetic analysis of cholestatic liver diseases: digging deeper. *Dig Dis* 2011;29(1):72-77.

21. a. A moderate infiltrate of lymphocytes and plasma cells surrounds a damaged bile duct within the portal tract shown in the image. The bile duct damage consists of multiple lumina, nuclear stratification and pleomorphism, and intraepithelial inflammation. This may occur in any of the conditions listed in the answer choices *except* hepatic venous outflow obstruction.

Scheuer PJ: Ludwig symposium on biliary disorders—part II. Pathologic features and evolution of primary biliary cirrhosis and primary sclerosing cholangitis. *Mayo Clin Proc* 1998;73(2):179-183.

22. c. FNH lesions studied by needle biopsy definitely require knowledge of the clinical setting (and a statement that the biopsy specimen represents a mass lesion). Without this information, the portal tract changes are highly suggestive of biliary tract obstruction. The irregular fibrous septa that emanate from the central fibrous scar of FNH are typically accompanied by activated progenitor cells in the form of proliferated bile ductules. The watery, mucinous stroma of the portal tract–like scars has a slightly different appearance from the characteristic edematous portal tract stroma of simple large bile duct obstruction. In the latter, neutrophils are usually much more prominent than in FNH.

Bioulac-Sage P, Cubel G, Balabaud C, et al: Revisiting the pathology of resected benign hepatocellular nodules using new immunohistochemical markers. *Semin Liver Dis* 2011;31(1):91-103.

Makhlouf HR, Abdul-Al HM, Goodman ZD: Diagnosis of focal nodular hyperplasia of the liver by needle biopsy. *Hum Pathol* 2005;36(11):1210-1216.

23. e. AIH typically produces portal and periportal lymphoplasmacytic inflammation and interface hepatitis, not the centrilobular steatohepatitis that is seen in the image. This question stresses the importance of recognizing fatty liver disease (large droplet or macrovesicular steatosis) and its complications. Steatohepatitis is a complication of large droplet (macrovesicular) steatosis and includes a constellation of histologic changes, including steatosis, hepatocyte ballooning, intracellular MDBs, inflammation (lymphocytes, neutrophils, or admixtures), and a network of perivenular and pericellular or perisinusoidal "chicken-wire" fibrosis. Depending on the individual case, the entire spectrum of pathologic features may not be present. NAFLD is currently considered the hepatic manifestation of metabolic syndrome. NAFLD is a spectrum of liver disease encompassing macrovesicular steatosis through steatohepatitis to cirrhosis and, potentially, HCC. MDBs (formerly known as Mallory bodies) are clumped, strandlike eosinophilic filamentous cytoplasmic inclusions. They are composed of keratins 8 and 18, which are produced in excess, cross-linked and misfolded, and subsequently ubiquitinated. MDBs form under conditions of hepatocyte stress, including oxidative stress present in alcoholic fatty liver disease and NAFLD. *Alcoholic fatty liver disease* and *nonalcoholic fatty liver disease* are standard terms. When steatohepatitis develops secondary to alcohol use and secondary to obesity, diabetes, and insulin resistance (i.e., risk factors for NAFLD), the terms *alcoholic steatohepatitis* and *nonalcoholic steatohepatitis* are used, respectively. Histologic differentiation between alcoholic steatohepatitis and nonalcoholic steatohepatitis is not usually possible.

Diehl AM, Goodman ZA, Ishak KG: Alcohollike liver disease in nonalcoholics. A clinical and histologic comparison with alcohol-induced liver injury. *Gastroenterology* 1988;95(4):1056-1062.

Kleiner DE, Brunt EM: Nonalcoholic fatty liver disease: pathologic patterns and biopsy evaluation in clinical research. *Semin Liver Dis* 2012;32(1):3-13.

Yeh MM, Brunt EM: Pathology of nonalcoholic fatty liver disease. *Am J Clin Pathol* 2007;128(5):837-847.

24. b. The pathologist reviewing this case correctly diagnosed von Meyenburg complex (bile duct malformation; ductal plate malformation). The abnormal bile duct structures with dilatation and irregular contours are characteristic of von Meyenburg complexes, which arise from abnormal remodeling of the embryonic bile duct plate. These malformations are common findings in needle biopsy, explant, and postmortem liver specimens. Grossly, bile duct malformations are white nodules, 1 to 2 mm in diameter, located at or directly beneath the liver capsule. The gross appearance is similar to bile duct adenoma (see Question 4), which is the major histologic differential diagnosis of small benign nodules composed of bile duct structures. Other conditions grouped in the category of ductal plate malformation diseases (also termed *fibropolycystic diseases*) include Caroli disease, congenital hepatic fibrosis, multiple microhamartomas, and polycystic liver disease. In large bile duct obstruction, it is unusual to see dilated bile ducts on a liver biopsy specimen (even with mechanical obstruction), and the native bile ducts even when dilated do not have the irregular contours of the bile duct malformation. The affected bile duct structures in Caroli disease show marked dilatation of several centimeters, are visible radiologically, and predispose to acute cholangitis. Fibrosing cholestatic hepatitis is a severe disorder related to marked liver damage from HCV, typically seen after liver (or other organ) transplantation as a result of the immunosuppressed state. This disorder combines marked parenchymal cholestasis with prominent periportal ductular reaction (proliferation of bile ductular structures derived from activated periportal progenitor or stem cells) and periportal fibrosis. Isolated ductular hyperplasia is a rare hyperplasia of interlobular bile ducts that was reported in one series of patients with abnormal serum liver function tests without any known cause. The affected ducts are not dilated and do not resemble bile duct malformations.

Desmet VJ: Ductal plates in hepatic ductular reactions. Hypothesis and implications. III. Implications for liver pathology. *Virchows Arch* 2011;458(3):271-279.

Jørgensen MJ: The ductal plate malformation. *Acta Pathol Microbiol Scand Suppl* 1977;(257):1-87.

Strazzabosco M, Fabris L: Development of the bile ducts: essentials for the clinical hepatologist. *J Hepatol* 2012;56(5):1159-1170.

25. b. This type of staining with Victoria blue stain would most likely be seen in PSC. There is impaired egress of bile (including the copper in bile) from the liver in late, chronic cholestatic disorders including PSC and PBC, resulting in periportal copper overload. There is resultant upregulation of synthesis of an intralysosomal metallothionein protein (i.e., copper-binding protein, stainable with Victoria blue stain), which sequesters copper and decreases the likelihood of hepatocellular damage from copper retention. Among the other answer choices, only PBC is associated with hepatic copper overload. However, significant copper overload that is associated with significant periportal copper-binding protein staining on Victoria blue stain is not seen until the late stages (i.e., stage 3 or 4) of PBC.

Lefkowitch JH: Special stains in diagnostic liver pathology. *Semin Diagn Pathol* 2006;23(3-4):190-198.

Sumithran E, Looi LM: Copper-binding protein in liver cells. *Hum Pathol* 1985;16(7):677-682.

26. d. Given the histopathologic pattern of damage seen in the image, antinuclear antibodies would most likely be positive. Antinuclear antibodies or anti–smooth muscle antibodies are an important diagnostic feature of AIH. The presence of lymphoplasmacytic interface hepatitis is another important diagnostic feature of AIH. p-ANCA is typically positive in patients with PSC or ulcerative colitis. Antimitochondrial antibodies are typically positive in PBC, in which the diagnostic histopathologic lesion is damage to interlobular bile ducts ("florid bile duct lesion"). The presence of positive serum anti-HBs indicates either immunization against HBV infection or immunity from prior infection. The liver should not show evidence of chronic hepatitis. IgG antibodies to HAV indicate previous HAV infection; a patient would not have chronic liver disease related to a previous HAV infection.

Goodman ZD: Grading and staging systems for inflammation and fibrosis in chronic liver diseases. *J Hepatol* 2007;47(4):598-607.

Ishak KG: Chronic hepatitis: morphology and nomenclature. *Mod Pathol* 1994;7(6):690-713.

Washington MK: Autoimmune liver disease: overlap and outliers. *Mod Pathol* 2007;20(Suppl 1):S15-S30.

27. c. The pediatrician would most likely order HbA_{1c} tests. Marked hepatocellular glycogenosis and glycogenated periportal hepatocyte nuclei are important histologic features of poorly controlled diabetes, and the combination of hepatomegaly, poor glycemic control, elevated HbA_{1c}, and hepatic glycogenosis corresponds to Mauriac syndrome, described by Mauriac in 1930. Serum liver tests and liver size usually return to normal with improvement in glycemic control. Use of PAS and diastase-pretreated PAS stains may help confirm the cause of hepatocyte swelling as due to glycogenosis. The histologic differential diagnosis in this case is glycogen storage disease. However, the patient in the case scenario would most likely already have been diagnosed with a glycogen storage disease by age 14. Nonetheless, except for type IV glycogen storage disease (with ground-glass polyglucosan cytoplasmic inclusions), the plant cell–like membrane accentuation (owing to compression of hepatocyte organelles to the periphery of the cell by the excess glycogen granules), pallor, and swelling seen in glycogenic hepatopathy resemble the changes in glycogen storage disease.

Mahesh S, Karp RJ, Castells S, et al: Mauriac syndrome in a 3-year-old boy. *Endocr Pract* 2007;13(1):63-66.

Mauriac P: Gros ventre, hepatomegalie, troubles de las croissance chez les enfants diabetiques traits depuis plusieurs annes par l'insuline. *Gax Hebd Med Bordeaux* 1930;26:402-410.

Torbenson M, Chen YY, Brunt E, et al: Glycogenic hepatopathy. An underrecognized hepatic complication of diabetes mellitus. *Am J Surg Pathol* 2006;30(4):508-513.

28. e. The patient most likely has a history of chronic hepatitis B. Ground-glass inclusions represent intrahepatocellular HBsAg, which is produced in variable numbers of hepatocytes in chronic hepatitis B with or without cirrhosis. Cytoplasmic ground-glass inclusions of HBsAg can be confirmed by specific immunoperoxidase staining; this should always be accompanied by immunostaining for hepatitis B core antigen (HBcAg) to evaluate the tissue evidence of active viral replication. When many hepatocyte nuclei show positive staining for HBcAg or there is also accompanying cytoplasmic staining, active viral replication is present. Patients with these findings often have high levels of serum HBV DNA and are positive for hepatitis B early antigen (HBeAg); HBeAg is another indicator of ongoing active viral replication. The differential diagnosis of ground-glass hepatocellular inclusions includes cyanamide alcohol aversion therapy, glycogen or abnormal glycogen inclusions (polyglucosan bodies) in type IV glycogen storage disease or in patients treated with polypharmacy after liver transplantation, Lafora disease (myoclonic epilepsy), and fibrinogen storage disease. If specific antibody to HBsAg and orcein or Victoria blue stains are negative in a biopsy specimen with ground-glass inclusions, other stains such as colloidal iron and PAS may be helpful in diagnosis. Colloidal iron and PAS stains are usually positive in the ground-glass inclusions on biopsy specimens from patients with Lafora disease or posttransplant polypharmacy.

Ishak KG: Chronic hepatitis: morphology and nomenclature. *Mod Pathol* 1994;7(6):690-713.

Lefkowitch JH, Lobritto SJ, Brown RS Jr, et al: Ground-glass, polyglucosan-like hepatocellular inclusions: a "new" diagnostic entity. *Gastroenterology* 2006;131(3):713-718.

Vázquez JJ: Ground glass hepatocytes: light and electron microscopy. Characterization of the different types. *Histol Histopathol* 1990;5(3):379-386.

29. d. The presence of cirrhosis with two regenerative nodules qualifies as stage 4, whereas the mild, focal interface hepatitis at lower right is indicative of mild necroinflammatory activity (grade 2). Grading and staging chronic hepatitis should be based on the worst necroinflammatory activity and architectural change present in the specimen. Several scoring systems are available for grading and staging chronic hepatitis, including the Scheuer and Batts-Ludwig methods (both use 4-point scores for grade and stage) and the modified Knodell (Ishak) score, which incorporates a 6-point staging score. Adoption of a specific scoring system for chronic hepatitis should serve as a practicable one for the pathologist and should be widely understood by the clinical team at the institution where it is being used. Clinical research studies may require the use of specific scoring systems to provide data, but the scoring system used in day-to-day disease practice at a given institution may be different. Trichrome and reticulin stains are important for establishing the stage of architectural change in chronic hepatitis.

Goodman ZD: Grading and staging systems for inflammation and fibrosis in chronic liver diseases. *J Hepatol* 2007;47(4):598-607.

Ishak K, Baptista A, Bianchi L, et al: Histological grading and staging of chronic hepatitis. *J Hepatol* 1995;22(6):696-699.

30. c. Based on the changes seen in the image, the pathogenesis of this lesion and the patient's portal hypertension is thought to be variations between hypoperfused and hyperperfused regions of liver parenchyma with a resultant vigorous response in the form of regenerative hyperplasia. This is the unifying concept behind the pathogenesis of NRH. NRH is a cause of noncirrhotic portal hypertension and is multifactorial in cause. NRH may be associated with underlying connective tissue disorders, previous or current use of chemotherapeutic agents (e.g., 6-mercaptopurine,

oxaliplatin), myeloproliferative disorders, and other conditions (including chronic cardiac failure). Wedge biopsies are preferable to needle biopsies to establish a definitive diagnosis of NRH because needle biopsy may not demonstrate the parenchymal nodules well. Because NRH shows neither significant fibrosis nor cirrhosis, Choices a, b, and d are incorrect. With regard to prolonged biliary obstruction, there would be prominent portal or periportal fibrosis associated with ductular reaction.

Reshamwala PA, Kleiner DE, Heller T: Nodular regenerative hyperplasia: not all nodules are created equal. *Hepatology* 2006;44(1):7-14.

31. d. Fibrosing cholestatic hepatitis is a posttransplantation complication resulting from overimmunosuppression of a patient who underwent liver (or other organ) transplantation for HCV-related disease. The effect of overimmunosuppression is to heighten recurrent hepatocyte infection with HCV, which leads to marked cholestasis and likely impaired hepatocyte replication and regeneration (triggering a prominent activation of progenitor cells to form proliferating bile ductular structures, termed the *ductular reaction*). The main features in the image, marked parenchymal cholestasis and portal and periportal bile ductular proliferation, are not features of acute rejection. Ductular reaction is very prominent in the image; this is not a significant feature of chronic ductopenic rejection. Mild recurrent chronic hepatitis C should look very similar to the native disease before transplantation, characterized by mild portal lymphocytic infiltrates with a few scattered plasma cells and occasional periportal foci of interface hepatitis. These changes are not seen in the image. A presentation of CMV hepatitis at 8 months is very late (it usually peaks at approximately 1 month after transplantation). CMV hepatitis after transplantation often demonstrates characteristic intranuclear and intracytoplasmic viral inclusions or microabscesses, or both. Other changes that may be seen include granulomas and occasionally a diffuse acute hepatitis (but not usually with the prominent ductular reaction seen in the image).

Davies SE, Portmann BC, O'Grady JG, et al: Hepatic histological findings after transplantation for chronic hepatitis B virus infection, including a unique pattern of fibrosing cholestatic hepatitis. *Hepatology* 1991;13(1):150-157.

Heneghan MA, Sylvestre PB: Cholestatic diseases of liver transplantation. *Semin Gastrointest Dis* 2001;12(2):133-147.

Xiao SY, Lu L, Wang HL: Fibrosing cholestatic hepatitis: clinicopathologic spectrum, diagnosis and pathogenesis. *Int J Clin Exp Pathol* 2008;1(5):396-402.

32. d. Wilson disease is due to mutations in the gene for *ATP7B*. This gene encodes a copper-transporting ATPase located in the trans-Golgi network of the liver; mutations in this gene lead to the accumulation of copper in hepatocytes in Wilson disease. The mutation in Wilson disease results in copper overload in hepatocytes. The gene for ceruloplasmin and the gene for copper-binding protein are not altered in Wilson disease. *Murr-1* mutations have been found in the Bedlington terrier animal model of copper overload but not in human Wilson disease. Mutations in the multidrug resistance 3 (*MDR3*) gene for a phospholipid bile salt export pump of the canalicular membrane are seen in progressive familial intrahepatic cholestasis type 3.

Roberts EA, Schilsky ML; American Association for Study of Liver Diseases (AASLD): Diagnosis and treatment of Wilson disease: an update. *Hepatology* 2008;47(6):2089-2111.

Rosencrantz R, Schilsky M: Wilson disease: pathogenesis and clinical considerations in diagnosis and treatment. *Semin Liver Dis* 2011;31(3):245-259.

33. b. Alagille syndrome is best defined as paucity of bile ducts associated with various facial, vertebral, cardiac, and ophthalmologic abnormalities. It is a genetic disorder that is due to mutation of the *JAG1* gene (Jagged-1 protein), which results in a paucity of intrahepatic bile ducts manifesting as neonatal jaundice, in association with cardiac defects (chiefly peripheral pulmonary stenosis) and vertebral and facial anomalies. Alagille syndrome is one of the major differential diagnoses of neonatal jaundice. The differential diagnosis also includes extrahepatic biliary atresia, neonatal hepatitis, bile salt transporter mutations, and metabolic diseases. Parenchymal cholestasis and loss of interlobular bile ducts in portal tracts (with maintenance of hepatic artery branches) are the chief histologic features of Alagille syndrome. Cirrhosis develops in only approximately 15% of patients with Alagille syndrome. Immunostaining with antibody to cytokeratin 7 or cytokeratin 19 is helpful in assessing the presence of or decrease in interlobular bile ducts. Cytokeratin 7 or cytokeratin 19 immunostaining also is diagnostically useful for confirmation of a well-developed ductular reaction in one of the alternative differential diagnoses of neonatal jaundice, extrahepatic biliary atresia.

Desmet VJ: Ductal plates in hepatic ductular reactions. Hypothesis and implications. III. Implications for liver pathology. *Virchows Arch* 2011;458(3):271-279.

Turnpenny PD, Ellard S: Alagille syndrome: pathogenesis, diagnosis and management. *Eur J Hum Genet* 2012;20(3):251-257.

34. b. Fibroobliterative lesions (also known as fibroobliterative cholangitis) are the end result of circumferential fibrous ablation of interlobular bile ducts in PSC. This term is specific to PSC and does not apply to the entities in other answer choices. PSC is a chronic inflammatory and fibrosing disorder involving the extrahepatic and intrahepatic bile ducts, frequently in association with underlying inflammatory bowel disease (chiefly ulcerative colitis). The characteristic histologic feature of PSC is periductal, concentric "onion-skin" fibrosis. Progression of PSC may result in obliteration of ducts entirely, resulting in ovoid, intraportal fibroobliterative scars (or fibroobliterative lesions). Serum test for p-ANCA is elevated in approximately 80% of patients with PSC. The diagnosis of PSC is best established radiologically using either magnetic resonance cholangiopancreatography or endoscopic retrograde cholangiopancreatography to demonstrate the characteristic beading and strictures of the biliary tree.

Demetris AJ: Distinguishing between recurrent primary sclerosing cholangitis and chronic rejection. *Liver Transpl* 2006;12(11 Suppl 2):S68-S72.

Scheuer PJ: Ludwig symposium on biliary disorders—part II. Pathologic features and evolution of primary biliary cirrhosis and primary sclerosing cholangitis. *Mayo Clin Proc* 1998;73(2):179-183.

35. d. Proliferation of bile ductular structures (ductular reaction) is the pathognomonic diagnostic feature for extrahepatic biliary atresia on a liver biopsy specimen. Other diagnostic features of extrahepatic biliary atresia on a liver biopsy specimen are portal and periportal fibrosis and inspissated bile within periportal bile ductular structures. Various nondiagnostic changes are seen in the liver in cases of extrahepatic biliary atresia, including extramedullary hematopoiesis, giant cells (multinucleated hepatocytes), and chronic portal inflammation, but none of these is specific for extrahepatic biliary atresia. Clinical data play a significant role in interpretation in evaluating neonatal jaundice and cholestasis, particularly in cases in which a liver biopsy specimen shows changes that are otherwise diagnostic for biliary atresia (i.e., there is a prominent ductular reaction and possibly fibrosis present). Both total parenteral nutrition and ATT liver disease may closely resemble changes seen in biliary atresia, which should be kept in mind when interpreting a neonatal biopsy specimen. Choices a, b, and c do not provide specificity for biliary atresia. Loss of interlobular bile ducts *is* one of the differential diagnoses of neonatal cholestasis, but in contrast to biliary atresia, few proliferating bile ductules are noted, and native ducts are diminished in number.

Russo P, Magee JC, Boitnott J, et al: Design and validation of the biliary atresia research consortium histologic assessment system for cholestasis in infancy. *Clin Gastroenterol Hepatol* 2011;9(4):357-362.

36. a. Greater than 85% to 95% of cases of hereditary hemochromatosis result from the *C282Y/C82Y* homozygous *HFE* gene mutation. Ferroportin-1 gene mutation represents type 4 hereditary hemochromatosis, a non-*HFE* and much less common (<5%) form of hereditary hemochromatosis. Mutation of the *HAMP* gene for hepcidin results in type 2B hereditary hemochromatosis, an uncommon form of hereditary (non-*HFE*) hemochromatosis. Aceruloplasminemia can also produce iron overload in hepatocytes and Kupffer cells because of the key role of ceruloplasmin in mediating iron egress from cells. Transferrin receptor-2 gene mutation represents type 3 hereditary hemochromatosis, a non-*HFE* hemochromatosis, which accounts for a minority of individuals with hereditary hemochromatosis (compared with the majority who have classic *HFE* hemochromatosis).

Pietrangelo A: Hereditary hemochromatosis: pathogenesis, diagnosis, and treatment. *Gastroenterology* 2010;139(2):393-408.

Pietrangelo A, Caleffi A, Corradinii E: Non-HFE hepatic iron overload. *Semin Liver Dis* 2011;31(3):302-318.

37. e. MDBs are filamentous and composed of abnormal keratins; they do not contain degenerated mitochondria. MDBs are intracytoplasmic inclusions within hepatocytes that develop in pathobiologic processes associated with cell stress, chiefly oxidative stress (e.g., macrovesicular steatosis) and copper overload (e.g., Wilson disease, chronic cholestasis). As abnormal cytoplasmic inclusions, MDBs are scheduled for degradation and are ubiquitinated, which can be advantageous to their identification in histologic liver sections by using specific immunoperoxidase staining with antibodies to ubiquitin. MDBs contain cytokeratin 8 and cytokeratin 18, which are produced in excess in the affected hepatocytes that experience stress. These keratins become abnormally cross-linked, misfolded, and bound to another constituent (p62) and are ubiquitinated. MDBs are a histologic feature of steatohepatitis and are seen in both alcoholic and nonalcoholic steatohepatitis. MDBs often elicit neutrophil chemotaxis so that hepatocytes with MDBs (or extruded MDBs) appear histologically to have neutrophil "satellitosis" surrounding them.

Strnad P, Zatloukal K, Stumptner C, et al: Mallory-Denk bodies: lessons from keratin-containing hepatic inclusion bodies. *Biochim Biophys Acta* 2008;1782(12):764-774.

Zatloukal K, French SW, Stumptner C, et al: From Mallory to Mallory-Denk bodies: what, how and why? *Exp Cell Res* 2007;313(10):2033-2049.

38. e. Microabscesses found in a liver biopsy specimen obtained after liver transplantation are diagnostic of CMV hepatitis. Herpes hepatitis in the immunosuppressed host leads to broad, irregular "geographic" zones of confluent necrosis in which viral inclusions are often evident (without microabscesses). A biliary stricture leads to large bile duct obstructive features, which are typically a combination of lobular cholestasis (within bile canaliculi and hepatocytes) plus the portal trio of changes (edema, ductular reaction, and neutrophil infiltrate). The chief manifestations of sepsis in the liver include centrilobular cholestasis and bile ductular cholestasis. Recurrence of HCV in the liver is manifested early (i.e., within the first few months) by lobular apoptotic bodies and variable necroinflammatory foci (containing lymphocytes, not neutrophils) and later by chronic lymphoplasmacytic portal inflammation with or without interface hepatitis.

Bosch W, Heckman MG, Pungpapong S, et al: Association of cytomegalovirus infection and disease with recurrent hepatitis C after liver transplantation. *Transplantation* 2012;93(7): 723-728.

Lefkowitch JH: Diagnostic issues in liver transplantation pathology. *Clin Liver Dis* 2002;6(2):555-570, ix.

van Hoek B, de Rooij BJ, Verspaget HW: Risk factors for infection after liver transplantation. *Best Pract Res Clin Gastroenterol* 2012;26(1):61-72.

39. d. HSCs, also known as Ito cells, are the major collagen-synthesizing cells in liver disease. Their normal function is to store vitamin A. Kupffer cells are predominantly phagocytic and cytokine-secreting cells. Hepatic pit cells are natural killer lymphocytes within the sinusoidal lumina, and their primary function is tumor cell surveillance. Data support the portal tract fibroblast or myofibroblast as a contributor to hepatic fibrosis, but most hepatic scars result from stellate cell collagen production.

Hernandez-Gea V, Friedman SL: Pathogenesis of liver fibrosis. *Annu Rev Pathol* 2011;6:425-456.

Lee UE, Friedman SL: Mechanisms of hepatic fibrogenesis. *Best Pract Res Clin Gastroenterol* 2011;25(2):195-206.

40. b. Although some cases of AIH are seen in association with SLE, the term *overlap syndrome* does not refer to this. *Overlap syndrome* specifically refers to overlap between AIH and PBC or PSC. These overlap syndromes are clinical and sometimes pathologic problem cases chiefly because of a variant pattern of serum autoantibody expression, type of serum liver function test abnormalities, or both. The pathologist should consider AIH-PBC and AIH-PSC overlap syndromes

to be unusual hepatic disorders that are outliers. The diagnosis of overlap syndrome likely reflects a current clinical or pathologic inability to distinguish certain patients with liver disease who lie at the extremes of these disorders. The diagnosis of a true overlap syndrome may affect therapeutic management. Because the main histologic feature of AIH is interface hepatitis, questions of possible histologic overlap arise when there is excessive interface hepatitis in a case in which damaged bile ducts are found (i.e., PBC) or there is periductal "onion-skin" fibrosis (i.e., PSC). Sometimes the combined presence of disorders signals a transition from one to the other, such as PBC to AIH-PBC overlap syndrome (see Twaddell et al.).

Carpenter HA, Czaja AJ: The role of histologic evaluation in the diagnosis and management of autoimmune hepatitis and its variants. *Clin Liver Dis* 2002;6(3):685-705.

Czaja AJ: Difficult treatment decision in autoimmune hepatitis. *World J Gastroenterol* 2010;16(8):934-947.

Twaddell WS, Lefkowitch J, Berk PD: Evolution from primary biliary cirrhosis to primary biliary cirrhosis/autoimmune hepatitis overlap syndrome. *Semin Liver Dis* 2008;28(1):128-134.

Washington MK: Autoimmune liver disease: overlap and outliers. *Mod Pathol* 2007;20(Suppl 1):S15-S30.

41. a. Reticulin stain is part of the routine special stain panel of liver stains ordered in the work-up of liver diseases. Reticulin stain not only demonstrates the underlying microscopic architecture (including portal tract and sinusoidal collagen distributions and liver cell plate thickness) but also is useful in identifying regenerative hyperplasia, regions of developing parenchymal nodularity, and cirrhosis. In HCC, the tumor has a "paucireticulin" pattern, which is diagnostically useful in distinguishing carcinoma from underlying normal liver tissue and from liver cell adenoma, both of which show a preserved reticulin pattern. In cases in which reticulin stain does not show a paucireticulin pattern but HCC is still suspected, immunostains (including CD34, glypican-3, glutamine synthetase, and heat shock protein 70) may provide additional help in establishing a correct diagnosis.

Lefkowitch JH: Special stains in diagnostic liver pathology. *Semin Diagn Pathol* 2006;23(3-4):190-198.

42. c. In schistosomal infection, ova within portal vein branches elicit granuloma formation and eventual thickening and tortuosity of the veins with surrounding portal fibrosis, termed *clay pipestem fibrosis* or *Symmers fibrosis*. Narrowing of the portal veins by this fibrosis may produce a presinusoidal form of intrahepatic portal hypertension.

Andrade ZA, Peixoto E, Guerret S, et al: Hepatic connective tissue changes in hepatosplenic schistosomiasis. *Hum Pathol* 1992;23(5):566-573.

43. d. The characteristic pathologic change seen in preeclampsia includes fibrin within portal tract vessels and periportal sinusoids. In more severe cases, periportal necrosis, hemorrhage, or rupture of the liver may occur. When interpreting a liver biopsy specimen, a pathologist should be aware that there are four relatively rare hepatic conditions unique to pregnancy. HELLP syndrome (*h*emolysis, *e*levated *l*iver enzymes, and *l*ow *p*latelets) may show overlapping disease with preeclampsia/eclampsia. Details of the four rare hepatic conditions unique to pregnancy are presented in the table.

Table 6-2 Liver Disease Unique to Pregnancy

Disease	Pathologic Features
Acute fatty liver of pregnancy	Microvesicular fat Occasionally lymphocytes
Intrahepatic cholestasis of pregnancy	Bile canalicular cholestasis (perivenular)
Preeclampsia	Fibrin in portal vessels and sinusoids Periportal necrosis if severe
HELLP syndrome (*hemolysis, elevated liver enzymes, and low platelets*)	Nonspecific inflammation Glycogenated hepatocyte nuclei Periportal fibrin and necrosis

Schutt VA, Minuk GY: Liver diseases unique to pregnancy. *Best Pract Res Clin Gastroenterol* 2007;21(5):771-792.
Wakim-Fleming J, Zein NN: The liver in pregnancy: disease vs. benign changes. *Cleve Clin J Med* 2005;72(8):713-721.

44. b. HCC is preceded in at least three fourths of cases by cirrhosis related chiefly to chronic hepatitis B and hepatitis C, alcohol abuse, hemochromatosis, and ATT deficiency. Histologically, HCCs demonstrate various patterns, including microtrabecular, pseudoacinar (glandular), clear cell, and giant cell types. Liver biopsy specimens obtained from individuals with known risk factors for HCC may demonstrate preneoplastic changes referred to as large cell dysplasia (large cell change) and small cell dysplasia (small cell change). Small cell dysplasia is thought to be a direct precursor of HCC, whereas gene mutations and other changes are associated with both forms of dysplasia. Fibrolamellar HCC is a unique type of HCC because it most often affects young individuals *without* known risk factors for HCC. This variant has an improved prognosis compared with standard HCC because of its potential resectability or survival following transplantation. The histologic features of fibrolamellar HCC, including the fibrous lamellae in parallel arrangement between plump, eosinophilic, mitochondria-rich malignant hepatocytes with "pale body" (fibrinogen) cytoplasmic inclusions, are distinctive. Large cell dysplasia (large cell change) is the longest known lesion associated with increased risk of HCC. It is characterized by large hepatocytes with atypical nuclei showing hyperchromatism, pleomorphism, multinucleation, and prominent and sometimes multiple nucleoli.

Lee RG, Tsamandas AC, Demetris AJ: Large cell change (liver cell dysplasia) and hepatocellular carcinoma in cirrhosis: matched case-control study, pathological analysis, and pathogenetic hypothesis. *Hepatology* 1997;26(6):1415-1422.
Park YN: Update on precursor and early lesions of hepatocellular carcinomas. Arch Pathol Lab Med 2011;135:704-715.
Torbenson M: Review of the clinicopathologic features of fibrolamellar carcinoma. *Adv Anat Pathol* 2007;14(3):217-223.

45. b. Fibrin ring granulomas (also called "donut granulomas") are lobular granulomas that are distinguished from other types of granulomas by their central, seemingly empty space (a lipid vacuole) surrounded by strands of fibrin with outer lymphocytes and macrophages. Fibrin ring granulomas are chiefly formed as a result of infections, the most frequent association being with Q fever (*C. burnetii*

infection). The histologic differential diagnosis of fibrin ring granulomas includes CMV, *Leishmania* spp., HAV infection, and allopurinol toxicity. These granulomas have been considered a nonspecific reaction, chiefly to infections. Fibrin ring granulomas are typically located within the lobular parenchyma and are not within portal tracts. Their central empty hole and surrounding strands of fibrin are histologically distinct from sarcoid granulomas, which are usually fibrosing and often clustered adjacent to portal tracts, and drug-related granulomas, which lack the central vacuole and sometimes contain eosinophils.

Khanlari B, Bodmer M, Terracciano L, et al: Hepatitis with fibrin-ring granulomas. *Infection* 2008;36(4):381-383.
Marazuela M, Moreno A, Yebra M, et al: Hepatic fibrin-ring granulomas: a clinicopathologic study of 23 patients. *Hum Pathol* 1991;22(6):607-613.
Murphy E, Griffiths MR, Hunter JA, et al: Fibrin-ring granulomas: a non-specific reaction to liver injury? *Histopathology* 1991;19(1):91-93.

46. b. Cholangiocarcinoma is an important sequela of PSC. Patients with PSC involving the major extrahepatic ducts are at risk of developing cholangiocarcinoma. This risk is apparently not true of intrahepatic, small duct PSC alone. HCC is the chief malignancy that arises (infrequently) in late-stage PBC, late AIH, and late chronic hepatitis C. However, fewer patients with chronic hepatitis C may also develop cholangiocarcinoma. HCC may rarely develop in late schistosomiasis, although there is also coinfection with hepatitis B and hepatitis C in certain endemic areas, which may add further risk.

Bangarulingam SY, Bjornsson E, Enders F, et al: Long-term outcomes of positive fluorescence in situ hybridization tests in primary sclerosing cholangitis. *Hepatology* 2010;51(1):174-180.
Barr Fritcher EG, Kipp BR, Voss JS, et al: Primary sclerosing cholangitis patients with serial polysomy fluorescence in situ hybridization results are at increased risk of cholangiocarcinoma. *Am J Gastroenterol* 2011;106(11):2023-2028.
Boberg KM, Lind GE: Primary sclerosing cholangitis and malignancy. *Best Pract Res Clin Gastroenterol* 2011;25(6):753-764.

47. b. GVHD affecting the liver typically targets intrahepatic bile ducts. Typical liver biopsy assessment should evaluate dysmorphism of the interlobular bile ducts, including attenuation and elongation of the entire length of the bile duct, altered nuclear polarity with attenuation of the nuclear profiles, and intraepithelial lymphocytes.

Saunders MD, Shulman HM, Murakami CS, et al: Bile duct apoptosis and cholestasis resembling acute graft-versus-host disease after autologous hematopoietic cell transplantation. *Am J Surg Pathol* 2000;24(7):1004-1008.
Strasser SI, Shulman HM, Flowers ME, et al: Chronic graft-versus-host disease of the liver: presentation as an acute hepatitis. *Hepatology* 2000;32(6):1265-1271.

48. c. The histologic features described are "textbook" features of epithelioid hemangioendothelioma. Immunostains to demonstrate endothelium (CD31, CD34) are also diagnostically important. Angiomyolipoma shows a different combination of features. Although the histologic description might be compatible with combined HCC and cholangiocarcinoma, the absence of cytokeratins and mucin make this diagnosis exceedingly unlikely. Fibrolamellar carcinomas have parallel-arranged fibrous lamellae and nests or islands of plump eosinophilic hepatocytes with "pale bodies" containing fibrinogen inclusions. Desmoplastic nested small cell tumor is a rare, slowly aggressive childhood malignancy.

Makhlouf HR, Ishak KG, Goodman ZD: Epithelioid hemangioendothelioma of the liver: a clinicopathologic study of 137 cases. *Cancer* 1999;85(3):562-582.

Mistry AM, Gorden DL, Busler JF, et al: Diagnostic and therapeutic challenges in hepatic epithelioid hemangioendothelioma. *J Gastrointest Cancer* 2012;43(4):521-525.

49. e. HCC is not described as a complication of parenteral nutrition. Parenteral nutrition–induced liver disease may occur in neonates, children, and adults. The histopathologic findings are age-related in that cholestasis and ductular reaction with fibrosis or cirrhosis are more prominent in neonates and children, whereas fatty liver and steatohepatitis and steatosis are seen more often in adults. In neonates and children with suspected parenteral nutrition–related liver disease, the diagnostic histopathologic features include cholestasis, a prominent ductular reaction (proliferation of bile ductular structures), and, over many months or more of administration, progressive fibrosis that may eventuate in cirrhosis. Parenteral nutrition–related liver injury in adults may include large droplet steatosis and steatohepatitis. Steatohepatitis secondary to parenteral nutrition resembles and should be included among the causes of nonalcoholic steatohepatitis. When cholestasis and ductular reaction (with or without portal or periportal fibrosis) are encountered in neonates, the major histologic differential diagnosis includes extrahepatic biliary atresia (if age and other clinical findings are consistent), large bile duct obstruction (e.g., choledochal cyst), and total parenteral nutrition (if a history of total parenteral nutrition administration is present).

Peyret B, Collardeau S, Touzet S, et al: Prevalence of liver complications in children receiving long-term parenteral nutrition. *Eur J Clin Nutr* 2011;65(6):741-749.

Quigley EM, Marsh MN, Shaffer JL, et al: Hepatobiliary complications of total parenteral nutrition. *Gastroenterology* 1993;104(1):286-301.

Zambrano E, El-Hennawy M, Ehrenkranz RA, et al: Total parenteral nutrition induced liver pathology: an autopsy series of 24 newborn cases. *Pediatr Dev Pathol* 2004;7(5):425-423.

50. c. Unless interface hepatitis is particularly marked in a case of chronic hepatitis B, there is only limited activation of periportal progenitor cells to produce any visible ductular reaction. Stage 2 of PBC is specifically designated and characterized by ductular reaction. Because extrahepatic bile ducts are typically involved in PSC, the portal tracts often show ductular reaction. Major mechanical obstruction of large bile ducts is a typical stimulus for the proliferation of bile ductular structures (ductular reaction) at the edges of portal tracts 24 to 48 hours after the obstruction. Massive hepatic necrosis is a severe type of acute hepatitis (i.e., fulminant hepatitis) that destroys so much liver parenchyma that hepatocyte division to replace the necrotic liver is insufficient for function, and there is usually a vigorous periportal ductular reaction ("neocholangiolar proliferation") evident (regardless of the cause of massive hepatic necrosis).

Gouw AS, Clouston AD, Theise ND: Ductular reactions in human liver: diversity at the interface. *Hepatology* 2011;54(5):1853-1863.

Roskams T, Desmet V: Ductular reaction and its diagnostic significance. *Semin Diagn Pathol* 1998;15(4):259-269.

Roskams T, Katoonizadeh A, Komuta M: Hepatic progenitor cells: an update. *Clin Liver Dis* 2010;14(4):705-718.

CHAPTER 7

SALIVARY GLAND PATHOLOGY

Andrew Turk and Karl H. Perzin

QUESTIONS

Question 1-26 refer to a photograph or photomicrograph.

1. This photograph shows the edge of a well-circumscribed
   parotid neoplasm. The lesion shows the histologic features
   of which one of the following entities?
   a. Pleomorphic adenoma
   b. Monomorphic adenoma
   c. Adenoid cystic carcinoma
   d. Polymorphous low-grade adenocarcinoma (PLGA)
   e. Mucoepidermoid carcinoma (MEC)

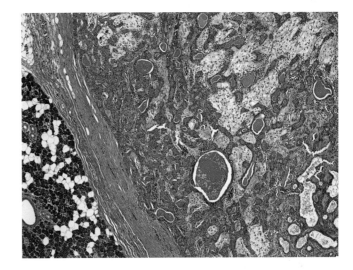

2. In this illustration, multiple well-circumscribed tumor nodules
   lie in a dense fibrous stroma adjacent to skeletal muscle. Which
   one of the following options represents the BEST diagnosis?
   a. Primary pleomorphic adenoma
   b. Recurrent pleomorphic adenoma
   c. Primary monomorphic adenoma
   d. Recurrent monomorphic adenoma
   e. Carcinoma ex pleomorphic adenoma

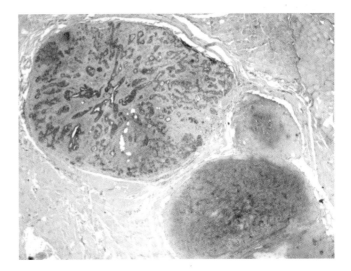

3. A subtotal parotidectomy specimen contained a firm, well-circumscribed, tan/gray lesion. The illustration shows the histologic features of this tumor. Which one of the following options represents the MOST likely diagnosis?
   a. Pleomorphic adenoma
   b. Myoepithelioma
   c. Basal cell adenoma
   d. Adenoid cystic carcinoma
   e. PLGA

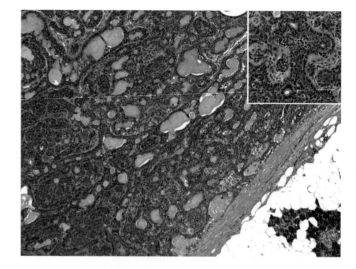

4. A well-circumscribed tumor measuring 3 cm in greatest dimension was resected by subtotal parotidectomy. The cut surface of the lesion was tan/brown and exuded sticky mucinous material. Careful examination revealed several small cysts. The photograph shows the histologic appearance of the tumor. Which one of the following options represents the CORRECT diagnosis?
   a. Pleomorphic adenoma
   b. Basal cell adenoma
   c. Warthin tumor (papillary cystadenoma lymphomatosum)
   d. Lymphoepithelial cyst
   e. Oncocytoma

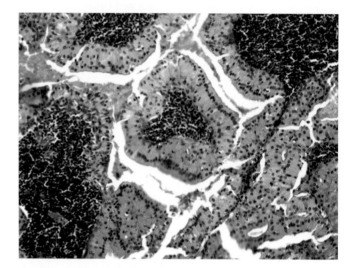

5. A 56-year-old woman with difficulty swallowing underwent incisional biopsy of a palatal tumor. Which one of the following options corresponds to the MOST likely diagnosis?
   a. Pleomorphic adenoma
   b. MEC
   c. Adenoid cystic carcinoma
   d. PLGA
   e. Sialometaplasia

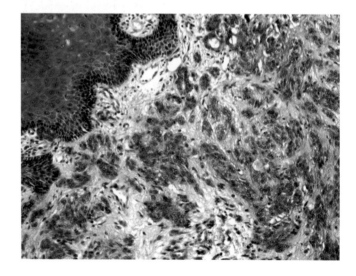

6. A subtotal parotidectomy specimen contained a moderately circumscribed tumor measuring 3 cm in greatest dimension. Histologic examination of the lesion showed nests of relatively uniform cells, with invasive growth into adjacent nonneoplastic tissue. Some lesional cells contained intracytoplasmic material that stained positively with mucicarmine and PAS stains. Which one of the following options represents the CORRECT diagnosis?
   a. PLGA
   b. Adenoid cystic carcinoma
   c. MEC
   d. Carcinoma ex pleomorphic adenoma
   e. Acinic cell carcinoma

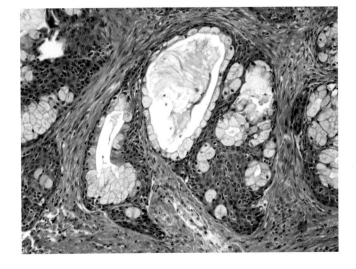

7. A 56-year-old patient underwent incisional biopsy of a 2-cm palatal mass. Which one of the following options represents the MOST likely diagnosis?
   a. Pleomorphic adenoma
   b. Carcinoma ex pleomorphic adenoma
   c. PLGA
   d. Adenoid cystic carcinoma
   e. MEC

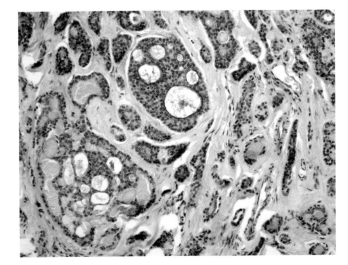

8. A 28-year-old man underwent subtotal parotidectomy for removal of a 2-cm lesion. Grossly, the lesion appeared well circumscribed and gray. Histologic and immunohistochemical examination showed reactive lymphoid tissue with scattered nests and cords of round to ovoid epithelial cells, occasionally forming small tubules, as shown in the illustration. Which one of the following options represents the MOST likely diagnosis?
   a. Metastatic carcinoma
   b. Warthin tumor
   c. Sjögren disease
   d. Lymphoepithelial lesion
   e. Chronic sialadenitis

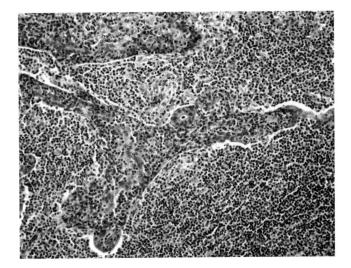

9. A 48-year-old woman had painful swelling of her submandibular gland due to sialolithiasis. She underwent resection of the gland. No tumor was grossly evident. Given the histologic features shown, which one of the following options represents the MOST likely diagnosis?
   a. Pleomorphic adenoma
   b. Lymphoepithelial lesion
   c. Squamous cell carcinoma
   d. MEC
   e. Sialometaplasia

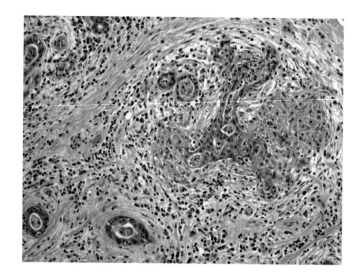

10. Which of the following statements regarding adenoid cystic carcinoma is FALSE?
    a. Adenoid cystic carcinoma is the most common malignant neoplasm of the minor salivary glands.
    b. Positive immunohistochemical staining for c-kit would definitively establish the diagnosis of adenoid cystic carcinoma.
    c. Molecular analyses have demonstrated the translocation t(6;9) (q22 to 23;p23 to 24), which creates the chimeric *MYB-NFIB* fusion gene, in 25% to 50% of adenoid cystic carcinoma cases.
    d. Well-defined patterns of this tumor include tubular, cribriform, and solid patterns.
    e. The finding of squamous or sebaceous elements in a salivary gland tumor with cribriform architecture would suggest a diagnosis of cribriform basal cell adenoma; adenoid cystic carcinoma rarely contains metaplastic elements.

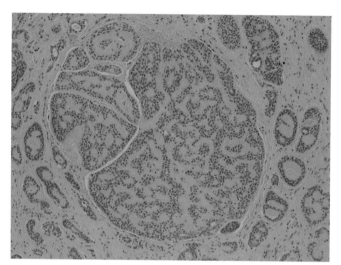

11. Which of the following statements regarding adenoid cystic carcinoma is TRUE?
    a. Adenoid cystic carcinoma involves the minor salivary glands more frequently than the major salivary glands.
    b. By definition, cases with a tubular component that comprises more than 30% of the tumor are considered high grade.
    c. Squamous differentiation is a characteristic finding in adenoid cystic carcinoma.
    d. Chemotherapy is generally more effective than radiation in the management of this disease.
    e. Lymph node involvement is seen in most cases of adenoid cystic carcinoma.

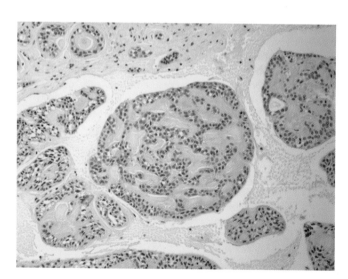

12. The photograph shows a high-grade mucoepidermoid carcinoma (MEC), and the inset shows the tumor's robust Ki-67 immunohistochemical staining. Multiple different grading systems for MEC have been proposed. Although these different systems are distinct, they also share considerable overlap. Which of the following features is LEAST consistent with a high-grade/grade III MEC?
    a. Pronounced nuclear atypia/anaplasia
    b. Intracystic component greater than 25%
    c. More than four mitoses per 10 high-power fields
    d. Perineural invasion
    e. Necrosis

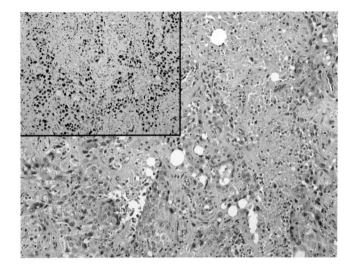

13. Which of the following chromosomal aberrations is considered a defining feature of mammary analogue secretory carcinoma (MASC)?
    a. t(11;19) (q21;p13), which creates the chimeric *CRTC1-MAML2* fusion gene
    b. t(12;15) (p13;q25), which creates the *ETV6-NTRK3* chimeric gene
    c. t(12;22) (q21;q12), which creates the chimeric *EWSR1-ATF1* fusion gene
    d. 8q12 alterations, involving the gene *PLAG1*
    e. 17q21.1 amplification, involving the gene *ERBB2*

14. Which of the following tumors is LEAST likely to demonstrate the same chromosomal aberration as MASC?
    a. Congenital fibrosarcoma
    b. Myxoid/round cell liposarcoma
    c. Cellular mesoblastic nephroma
    d. Secretory breast carcinoma
    e. Acute myeloid leukemia

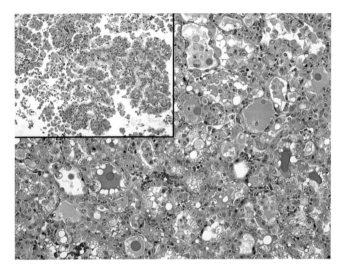

15. The illustration displays a representative focus of a lip biopsy from a 63-year-old woman. The biopsy material shows one aggregate of 50 or more chronic inflammatory cells per 4 mm^2 of minor salivary glandular tissue. This finding corresponds to which of the following Chisholm grades?
    a. 0
    b. 1
    c. 2
    d. 3
    e. 4

16. Which one of the following connective tissue disorders is MOST frequently comorbid with Sjögren disease?
    a. Rheumatoid arthritis
    b. Polymyositis
    c. Polyarteritis nodosa
    d. Progressive systemic sclerosis (scleroderma)
    e. Systemic lupus erythematosus

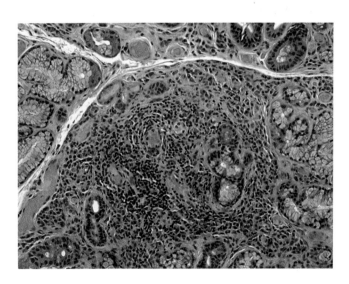

17. A 29-year-old woman underwent resection of an intranasal mass. Histologic examination of the lesion resulted in a diagnosis of pleomorphic adenoma. Foci of squamous metaplasia were evident in the tumor, as shown in the photograph. Which one of the following lesions is LEAST likely to display squamous metaplasia?

    a. Basal cell adenoma
    b. Pleomorphic adenoma
    c. Basal cell adenocarcinoma
    d. Epithelial-myoepithelial carcinoma
    e. Adenoid cystic carcinoma

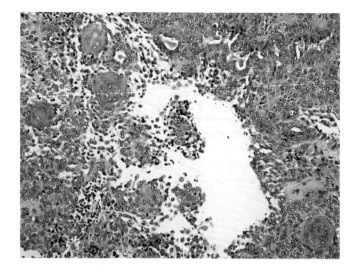

18. The photograph displays normal serous salivary glandular tissue. Which one of the following options CORRECTLY identifies the structures indicated by the yellow and red arrows?

    a. Yellow: striated duct; red: intercalated duct
    b. Yellow: intercalated duct; red: striated duct
    c. Yellow: intercalated duct; red: interlobular duct
    d. Yellow: intralobular duct; red: striated duct
    e. Yellow: striated duct; red: intralobular duct

19. In the epithelial cells lining the structures indicated by the yellow and red arrows, which one of the following immunohistochemical markers is MOST likely to show strongly positive staining?

    a. p63
    b. CAM 5.2
    c. CK5/6
    d. CK14
    e. CK34βE12

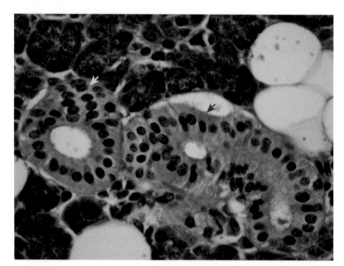

20. A 62-year-old woman underwent resection of a parotid tumor. A representative histologic image is shown. Elsewhere, the tumor displayed an invasive growth pattern. Which one of the following lesions BEST corresponds to the histologic features shown in the photograph?

    a. Basal cell adenocarcinoma
    b. Adenoid cystic carcinoma
    c. Low-grade salivary duct carcinoma
    d. MASC
    e. Epithelial-myoepithelial carcinoma

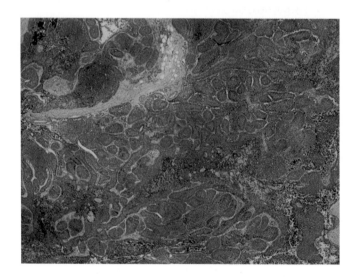

21. A 35-year-old woman complained of tender swelling of the left side of her face. Additional studies led to identification of a left parotid tumor, and she subsequently underwent parotidectomy. Histologic examination resulted in diagnosis of acinic cell carcinoma; immunohistochemical stains were performed in order to exclude the possibility of MASC. Of the following immunohistochemical stains, which one is LEAST likely to facilitate differentiation between acinic cell carcinoma and MASC?
    a. GCDFP-15
    b. HER2
    c. MUC1
    d. BRST-2
    e. Mammaglobin

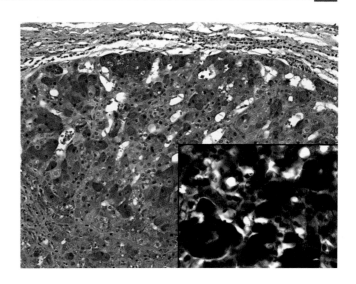

22. According to the 2005 World Health Organization classification, acinic cell carcinoma represents a "low-risk" malignancy. Which one of the following tumors also belongs within this category, rather than the "high-risk" category?
    a. Sebaceous carcinoma
    b. Epithelial-myoepithelial carcinoma
    c. Adenoid cystic carcinoma
    d. Mucinous adenocarcinoma
    e. Carcinosarcoma

23. A 65-year-old woman underwent resection of a tumor arising in the right side of her hard palate. Histologic examination led to a diagnosis of PLGA. Which one of the following features would be LEAST consistent with this diagnosis?
    a. "Sweeping" or "whorling" arrangements of tumor cells along the periphery of the lesion
    b. Cells with myoepithelial features
    c. Entrapment/incorporation (rather than obliteration/effacement) of uninvolved, nonneoplastic seromucinous glands
    d. Single-file arrangements of tumor cells (formerly described as "Indian filing")
    e. Cells with ovoid vesicular nuclei

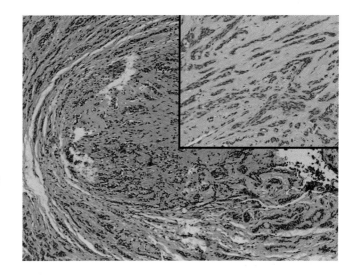

24. Positive immunohistochemical staining for c-kit may occur in cases of PLGA. Which of the following head and neck tumors also display(s) positive c-kit staining?
    a. Adenoid cystic carcinoma
    b. Epithelial-myoepithelial carcinoma
    c. Basal cell adenocarcinoma
    d. Sinonasal melanoma
    e. All of the above

25. PLGA can share significant morphologic overlap with adenoid cystic carcinoma. Which one of the following immunohistochemical stains is LEAST likely to be diagnostically useful, in terms of differentiating PLGA from adenoid cystic carcinoma?
    a. S100
    b. Epithelial membrane antigen (EMA)
    c. Carcinoembryonic antigen (CEA)
    d. Ki67
    e. c-kit

26. Which of the following chromosomal aberrations has been demonstrated in 40% to 80% of MEC cases?
   a. t(11;19) (q21;p13), which creates the chimeric *CRTC1-MAML2* fusion gene
   b. t(12;15) (p13;q25), which creates the *ETV6-NTRK3* chimeric gene
   c. t(12;22) (q21;q12), which creates the chimeric *EWSR1-ATF1* fusion gene
   d. 8q12 alterations, involving the gene *PLAG1*
   e. 17q21.1 amplification, involving the gene *ERBB2*

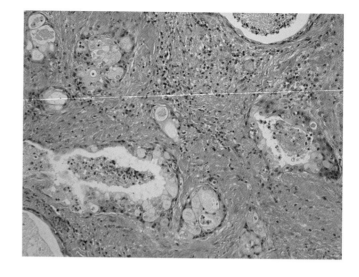

27. Which one of the following statements concerning normal salivary gland histology is INCORRECT?
   a. The acini in the parotid gland contain both serous and mucous cells.
   b. Sebaceous cells represent a normal finding in parotid gland acini.
   c. The acini in the submandibular gland contain mostly serous cells, as well as occasional small clusters of mucous cells.
   d. The acini in the sublingual gland contain mostly mucous cells.
   e. The acini in minor salivary glands of the oral cavity contain variable combinations of serous and mucous cells.

28. Which one of the following lesions is the MOST common salivary gland tumor?
   a. Basal cell adenoma
   b. Pleomorphic adenoma
   c. Warthin tumor (papillary cystadenoma lymphomatosum)
   d. MEC
   e. Adenoid cystic carcinoma

29. According to series that include both major and minor salivary glands, which one of the following lesions is the MOST common malignant salivary gland tumor?
   a. MEC
   b. Adenoid cystic carcinoma
   c. Acinic cell carcinoma
   d. Carcinoma ex pleomorphic adenoma
   e. Salivary duct carcinoma

30. Which one of the following salivary gland tumors is MOST likely to show perineural invasion?
   a. MEC
   b. Adenoid cystic carcinoma
   c. Acinic cell carcinoma
   d. Carcinoma ex pleomorphic adenoma
   e. PLGA

ANSWERS

1. a. The combination of epithelial cells arranged in trabecular and tubular structures, together with myoepithelial cells in a myxoid background, is consistent with pleomorphic adenoma. Carcinoma ex pleomorphic adenoma would show a similar biphasic composition, but this tumor would also display frankly malignant features. Monomorphic adenoma shares morphologic similarities with pleomorphic adenoma, but the former lacks myxoid areas. Myoepithelioma (monomorphic adenoma composed exclusively of myoepithelial cells) is usually highly cellular, and lacks myxoid/chondroid tissue. These tumors show positive immunohistochemical staining for cytokeratin and smooth muscle actin. Adenoid cystic carcinoma, PLGA, and MEC would show invasive growth (unlike the present case).

Dardick I (ed): *Salivary Gland Tumor Pathology.* New York: Igaku-Shoin, 1996.
Ellis GL, Auclair PL: *Atlas of Tumor Pathology—Tumors of the Salivary Glands,* Fascicle 17, 3rd series. Washington, DC: Armed Forces Institute of Pathology, 1996.

Huvos AG, Paulino AFG: Salivary glands. In Mills SE, Carter D, Greenson JK, et al (eds): *Sternberg's Diagnostic Surgical Pathology,* 4th ed. Philadelphia: Lippincott Williams & Wilkins, 2004, pp 933-962.
Rosai J: Major and minor salivary glands. In Rosai J (ed): *Rosai and Ackerman's Surgical Pathology,* 9th ed. Vol. 1, Chaps. 9 and 10. St. Louis: Mosby, 2004, pp 873-916.

2. b. Lesional cells may become implanted within the operative site during surgical resection of pleomorphic adenoma. This phenomenon sometimes leads to development of multiple tumor nodules within residual (unresected) salivary gland tissue, as well as within scar tissue associated with the operative procedure. Recurrences occur more frequently following pleomorphic adenoma with prominent myxoid/chondroid elements, perhaps because this type of tissue sticks more readily to surgical instruments. Recurrent pleomorphic adenoma may become apparent months or years following the initial resection. Surgical resection of recurrent pleomorphic adenoma may be complicated by entrapment of the facial nerve (or other structures) in scar tissue from the initial resection, or by the presence of unapparent nodules in addition to those that are evident clinically. The nodules of recurrent pleomorphic adenoma are usually well circumscribed, and show variable proportions of epithelial and myoepithelial features, as in primary pleomorphic adenoma. Each nodule should be examined histologically, because these nodules may give rise to carcinoma. If carcinoma is present in one or more nodule(s) of recurrent pleomorphic adenoma, the lesion may behave in a malignant manner, despite apparent circumscription of the nodule(s). This phenomenon possibly results from the multifocal distribution of recurrent lesions, which provides the tumor widespread access to lymphatics and veins.

Dardick I (ed): *Salivary Gland Tumor Pathology.* New York: Igaku-Shoin, 1996.

Ellis GL, Auclair PL: *Atlas of Tumor Pathology—Tumors of the Salivary Glands,* Fascicle 17, 3rd series. Washington, DC: Armed Forces Institute of Pathology, 1996.

Huvos AG, Paulino AFG: Salivary glands. In Mills SE, Carter D, Greenson JK, et al (eds): *Sternberg's Diagnostic Surgical Pathology,* 4th ed. Philadelphia: Lippincott Williams & Wilkins, 2004, pp 933-962.

Rosai J: Major and minor salivary glands. In Rosai J (ed): *Rosai and Ackerman's Surgical Pathology,* 9th ed. Vol. 1, Chaps. 9 and 10. St. Louis: Mosby, 2004, pp 873-916.

3. c. Multiple types of basal cell adenoma have been described and include the solid, membranous, tubular, trabecular, and tubulotrabecular types. In some examples of basal cell adenoma, some areas lack the characteristically prominent basal cell layer. These cases may be difficult to distinguish from pleomorphic adenoma. Some lesions diagnosed as basal cell adenoma show areas with prominent myoepithelial cells. Accordingly, basal cell adenoma may sometimes share morphologic overlap with myoepithelioma. Unlike the various types of basal cell adenoma, malignant tumors such as PLGA, MEC, and adenoid cystic carcinoma show evidence of invasive growth. When present, interlacing trabecular structures (as seen in this case) may provide a clue to the diagnosis of basal cell adenoma. Structures such as these are usually evident only in benign salivary gland tumors, and are generally inconsistent with a diagnosis of adenoid cystic carcinoma or PLGA.

Dardick I (ed): *Salivary Gland Tumor Pathology.* New York: Igaku-Shoin, 1996.

Ellis GL, Auclair PL: *Atlas of Tumor Pathology—Tumors of the Salivary Glands,* Fascicle 17, 3rd series, Washington, DC: Armed Forces Institute of Pathology, 1996.

Huvos AG, Paulino AFG: Salivary glands. In Mills SE, Carter D, Greenson JK, et al (eds): *Sternberg's Diagnostic Surgical Pathology,* 4th ed. Philadelphia: Lippincott Williams & Wilkins, 2004, pp 933-962.

Rosai J: Major and minor salivary glands. In Rosai J (ed): *Rosai and Ackerman's Surgical Pathology,* 9th ed. Vol. 1, Chaps. 9 and 10. St. Louis: Mosby, 2004, pp 873-916.

4. c. The parotid gland normally contains several intraparotid lymph nodes. Intraparotid and periparotid lymph nodes may contain ectopic salivary gland tissue. Warthin tumor arises within intraparotid (and occasionally periparotid) lymph nodes, apparently within ectopic glandular tissue. The lymphoid component of Warthin tumor derives from the lymphoid tissue of these nodes. This lymphoid tissue is normal or reactive, rather than neoplastic. The epithelial/glandular component of Warthin tumor is neoplastic. This component may occupy all or only part of the node in which the tumor arises. Warthin tumor is frequently multifocal. Consequently, parotid glands with grossly evident Warthin tumors often contain additional, clinically inapparent Warthin tumors. In some cases of Warthin tumor resected by unilateral parotidectomy, patients develop Warthin tumors in the contralateral parotid gland several years later. Warthin tumor occurs most commonly in men over 50 years of age. In terms of its natural progression when the lesion remains untreated, some cases (especially large tumors) undergo infarction. Rare cases of poorly differentiated carcinoma arising within Warthin tumors have been reported.

Dardick I (ed): *Salivary Gland Tumor Pathology.* New York: Igaku-Shoin, 1996.

Ellis GL, Auclair PL: *Atlas of Tumor Pathology—Tumors of the Salivary Glands,* Fascicle 17, 3rd series. Washington, DC: Armed Forces Institute of Pathology, 1996.

Huvos AG, Paulino AFG: Salivary glands. In Mills SE, Carter D, Greenson JK, et al (eds): *Sternberg's Diagnostic Surgical Pathology,* 4th ed. Philadelphia: Lippincott Williams & Wilkins, 2004, pp 933-962.

Rosai J: Major and minor salivary glands. In Rosai J (ed): *Rosai and Ackerman's Surgical Pathology,* 9th ed. Vol. 1, Chaps. 9 and 10. St. Louis: Mosby, 2004, pp 873-916.

5. d. In terms of its architecture, PLGA comprises cellular nests of variable size and shape. In most cases, the nests are relatively small, but larger, more lobulated structures are occasionally observed. The stroma between these nests may be hyalinized or myxoid, but lacks myoepithelial cell proliferation. In terms of its cytology, PLGA consists of relatively bland cells with slightly basophilic, round to spindly nuclei. Some cases of adenoid cystic carcinoma show nested architecture focally, and thereby share architectural overlap with PLGA. The cells of adenoid cystic carcinoma usually show more mitotic activity, nuclear pleomorphism, and hyperchromasia, compared to PLGA. Additionally, cellular nests in adenoid cystic carcinoma are usually larger, and situated in denser, more fibrous stroma, relative to this case. This case shows focal extracellular mucin within nests of epithelial cells. MEC, by contrast, should display intracellular mucin (in goblet cells), with or without extracellular mucin. Sialometaplasia generally shows nests of reactive epithelial cells within preexisting salivary gland tissue. This condition does not display the invasive features of this case.

Dardick I (ed): *Salivary Gland Tumor Pathology.* New York: Igaku-Shoin, 1996.

Ellis GL, Auclair PL: *Atlas of Tumor Pathology—Tumors of the Salivary Glands,* Fascicle 17, 3rd series. Washington, DC: Armed Forces Institute of Pathology, 1996.

Huvos AG, Paulino AFG: Salivary glands. In Mills SE, Carter D, Greenson JK, et al (eds): *Sternberg's Diagnostic Surgical Pathology,* 4th ed. Philadelphia: Lippincott Williams & Wilkins, 2004, pp 933-962.

Rosai J: Major and minor salivary glands. In Rosai J (ed): *Rosai and Ackerman's Surgical Pathology,* 9th ed. Vol. 1, Chaps. 9 and 10. St. Louis: Mosby, 2004, pp 873-916.

6. c. MEC consists of irregular cellular nests that show invasive growth into adjacent nonneoplastic tissue. The lesion contains variable proportions of three cell types: epidermoid/squamoid cells, goblet cells, and intermediate/basaloid cells. Squamous metaplasia and keratinization may be present. Mitotic activity ranges from rare to brisk. The degree of differentiation of MEC is directly proportional to the amount of goblet cells, and inversely proportional to the amount of intermediate/basaloid cells. Well-differentiated cases show abundant goblet cells, whereas goblet cells are rare in poorly differentiated tumors. Carcinoma ex pleomorphic adenoma usually manifests as poorly differentiated adenocarcinoma, which may be histologically similar to poorly differentiated MEC. In carcinoma ex pleomorphic adenoma, adequate sampling should demonstrate a relationship between the carcinoma and a preexisting pleomorphic adenoma. Likewise, some cases of poorly differentiated MEC may require generous sampling in order to demonstrate recognizable areas of better differentiated tumor. Goblet cells are not a feature of PLGA or adenoid cystic carcinoma. Acinic cell carcinoma may contain cells with intracytoplasmic vacuoles, which may show positive PAS staining. These vacuoles contain secretory granules rather than mucin, and are not stained by mucicarmine.

Dardick I (ed): *Salivary Gland Tumor Pathology.* New York: Igaku-Shoin, 1996.

Ellis GL, Auclair PL: *Atlas of Tumor Pathology—Tumors of the Salivary Glands,* Fascicle 17, 3rd series. Washington, DC: Armed Forces Institute of Pathology, 1996.

Huvos AG, Paulino AFG: Salivary glands. In Mills SE, Carter D, Greenson JK, et al (eds): *Sternberg's Diagnostic Surgical Pathology,* 4th ed. Philadelphia: Lippincott Williams & Wilkins, 2004, pp 933-962.

Rosai J: Major and minor salivary glands. In Rosai J (ed): *Rosai and Ackerman's Surgical Pathology,* 9th ed. Vol. 1, Chaps. 9 and 10. St. Louis: Mosby, 2004, pp 873-916.

7. d. Adenoid cystic carcinoma may show variable architecture, including tubular, cribriform, and solid patterns. This lesion generally contains at least some cribriform nests, although small biopsy specimens may lack these areas. Adenoid cystic carcinoma typically displays stromal hyalinization, which represents thickening of the basement membrane. The hyalinized fibrous stroma of adenoid cystic carcinoma, as shown in this case, differs from the myxoid stroma that characterizes pleomorphic adenoma. Stromal hyalinization also occurs in PLGA, but the latter differs from adenoid cystic carcinoma in terms of its cytology. The lesional cells of adenoid cystic carcinoma demonstrate dense hyperchromatic nuclei, unlike the other tumors listed among the answer choices (particularly PLGA, which characteristically displays a relatively light chromatin pattern). The lesional cells of adenoid cystic carcinoma should not contain intracytoplasmic mucin, which is typical of MEC. Carcinoma ex pleomorphic adenoma usually manifests as poorly differentiated adenocarcinoma, although it may rarely resemble adenoid cystic carcinoma. In carcinoma ex pleomorphic adenoma, adequate sampling should demonstrate a relationship between the carcinoma and a preexisting pleomorphic adenoma.

Dardick I (ed): *Salivary Gland Tumor Pathology.* New York: Igaku-Shoin,1996.

Ellis GL, Auclair PL: *Atlas of Tumor Pathology—Tumors of the Salivary Glands,* Fascicle 17, 3rd series. Washington, DC: Armed Forces Institute of Pathology, 1996.

Huvos AG, Paulino AFG: Salivary glands. In Mills SE, Carter D, Greenson JK, et al (eds): *Sternberg's Diagnostic Surgical Pathology,* 4th ed. Philadelphia: Lippincott Williams & Wilkins, 2004, pp 933-962.

Rosai J: Major and minor salivary glands. In Rosai J (ed): *Rosai and Ackerman's Surgical Pathology,* 9th ed. Vol. 1, Chaps. 9 and 10. St. Louis: Mosby, 2004, pp 873-916.

8. d. Lymphoepithelial lesions, which comprise nests of reactive epithelioid cells ("epithelial-myoepithelial islands") associated with lymphoid hyperplasia, represent one subset of several inflammatory lesions that involve salivary glands. Lymphoepithelial lesions occur within intraparotid and periparotid lymph nodes, as well as within salivary and lacrimal gland parenchyma. These lesions represent hyperplastic phenomena, rather than neoplasia. Salivary acini and ducts are sometimes present within intraparotid and periparotid lymph nodes. In lymphoepithelial lesions that occur within these lymph nodes, epithelial-myoepithelial islands represent proliferation of ectopic salivary tissue. Additionally, lymphoepithelial lesions sometimes result from viral infections (particularly HIV infection) that lead to lymphoid hyperplasia within intraparotid/periparotid lymph nodes. Chronic sialadenitis represents another inflammatory lesion that involves salivary glands. Its histologic features include multifocal, variable (but usually light) infiltration of salivary tissue by lymphocytes and plasma cells. The epithelium of large ducts may show reactive changes in this context. Chronic sialadenitis usually results from duct obstruction, frequently secondary to sialolithiasis. This phenomenon (chronic sialadenitis caused by duct obstruction due to sialolithiasis) occurs most commonly in the submandibular gland, probably because the gland is inferior to the oral cavity, into which the submandibular duct drains.

Dardick I (ed): *Salivary Gland Tumor Pathology.* New York: Igaku-Shoin, 1996.

Ellis GL, Auclair PL: *Atlas of Tumor Pathology—Tumors of the Salivary Glands,* Fascicle 17, 3rd series. Washington, DC: Armed Forces Institute of Pathology, 1996.

Huvos AG, Paulino AFG: Salivary glands. In Mills SE, Carter D, Greenson JK, et al (eds): *Sternberg's Diagnostic Surgical Pathology,* 4th ed. Philadelphia: Lippincott Williams & Wilkins, 2004, pp 933-962.

Rosai J: Major and minor salivary glands. In Rosai J (ed): *Rosai and Ackerman's Surgical Pathology,* 9th ed. Vol. 1, Chaps. 9 and 10. St. Louis: Mosby, 2004, pp 873-916.

9. e. Sialometaplasia refers to reactive proliferation of epithelial and myoepithelial cells that results from injury to salivary gland tissue. The inciting injury may be inflammation (as in this case), radiation, biopsy, or another traumatic process. Establishment of this diagnosis may be particularly difficult when sialometaplasia occurs following biopsy or incomplete resection of a neoplasm. Histologically, sialometaplasia manifests as proliferation of round to spindly cells in acini or intercalated ducts, usually at the interface between damaged tissue and adjacent unaffected tissue. The glandular tissue in which sialometaplasia occurs generally maintains its lobulated architecture. By contrast, malignant tumors do not generally display the lobulated, branching architecture of the native glandular tissue. Benign lesions, such as basal cell adenoma, may show branching patterns. In sialometaplasia, the proliferative cells are generally uniform in contour, and show little pleomorphism or mitotic activity. By contrast, neoplastic epithelial and myoepithelial cells usually show greater irregularity in size and shape.

Dardick I (ed): *Salivary Gland Tumor Pathology.* New York: Igaku-Shoin, 1996.

Ellis GL, Auclair PL: *Atlas of Tumor Pathology—Tumors of the Salivary Glands,* Fascicle 17, 3rd series. Washington, DC: Armed Forces Institute of Pathology, 1996.

Huvos AG, Paulino AFG: Salivary glands. In Mills SE, Carter D, Greenson JK, et al (eds): *Sternberg's Diagnostic Surgical Pathology,* 4th ed. Philadelphia: Lippincott Williams & Wilkins, 2004, pp 933-962.

Rosai J: Major and minor salivary glands. In Rosai J (ed): *Rosai and Ackerman's Surgical Pathology,* 9th ed. Vol. 1, Chaps. 9 and 10. St. Louis: Mosby, 2004, pp 873-916.

10. b. and 11. a. Adenoid cystic carcinoma occurs most frequently in the fifth to the seventh decades, and has a female-male ratio of approximately 3:2. Adenoid cystic carcinoma represents approximately 10% of malignant salivary gland neoplasms and is the most common malignant neoplasm of the minor salivary glands. Approximately 60% of cases involve the minor salivary glands. The palate is the most frequent site of minor salivary gland involvement (17% of cases). Approximately 40% of cases involve the major salivary glands. The parotid gland is the most frequently involved major salivary gland (21% of cases). The tumor is biphasic, consisting of ductal and myoepithelial cells, and shows tubular, cribriform, and solid growth patterns. Tumors with a solid component that composes more than 30% of the tumor are considered high grade. This disease is characterized by slow but relentless progression, with a 5-year survival rate of approximately 80%, 10-year survival rate of approximately 50%, and 15-year survival rate of less than 15%. Lymph node involvement has been reported to range from 5% to 25% of cases. Studies have demonstrated a role for radiation in the management of microscopic residual disease, and a limited role in the management of recurrent or metastatic disease. The value of chemotherapy remains to be proven.

El-Naggar AK, Huvos AG: Adenoid cystic carcinoma. In Barnes L, Eveson JW, Reichart P, Sidransky D (eds): *World Health Organization Classification of Tumours: Pathology and Genetics of Head and Neck Tumours.* Lyon: IARC Press, 2005, pp 221-222.

Szanto PA, Luna MA, Tortoledo ME, White RA: Histologic grading of adenoid cystic carcinoma of the salivary glands. *Cancer* 1984;54:1062-1069.

van der Wal JE, Snow GB, Karim AB, van der Waal I: Intraoral adenoid cystic carcinoma: the role of postoperative radiotherapy in local control. *Head Neck* 1989;11:497-499.

12. b. Multiple different grading systems for MEC have been proposed. Although these different systems are distinct, they also share considerable overlap. MEC is graded as low, intermediate, or high grade (Goode et al.) or grade I, II, or III (Brandwein et al.). The grading systems proposed by Goode et al. and by Brandwein et al. both incorporate the following as features of high-grade/grade III lesions: pronounced nuclear atypia/anaplasia, intracystic

component less than 25% (Brandwein et al.) or less than 20% (Goode et al.), more than 4 mitoses per 10 high-power fields, perineural invasion, and necrosis. The grading system proposed by Brandwein et al. also incorporates the following as features of grade III lesions: tumor front consisting of invasive small nests and islands, lymphatic or vascular invasion, and bony invasion.

Brandwein MS, Ivanov K, Wallace DI, et al: Mucoepidermoid carcinoma a clinicopathologic study of 80 patients with special reference to histological grading. *Am J Surg Pathol* 2001;25:835-845.

Goode RK, Auclair PL, Ellis GL: Mucoepidermoid carcinoma of the major salivary glands. Clinical and histopahol99ic analysis of 234 cases with evaluation of grading criteria. *Cancer* 1998;82:1217-1224.

Goode RK, El-Naggar AK: Mucoepidermoid carcinoma. In Barnes L, Eveson JW, Reichart P, Sidransky D (eds): *World Health Organization Classification of Tumours: Pathology and Genetics of Head and Neck Tumours.* Lyon: IARC Press, 2005, pp 219-220.

13. b. and 14. b. MASC occurs mainly in the parotid gland. This tumor typically displays microcystic, papillary, and tubular patterns. Microcystic architecture predominates in most cases. The translocation t(12;15) (p13;q25), which creates the *ETV6-NTRK3* chimeric gene, is considered a defining feature of MASC. The translocation t(11;19) (q21;p13), which creates the chimeric *CRTC1-MAML2* fusion gene, has been demonstrated in 40% to 80% of MEC cases. The translocation t(12;22) (q21;q12), which creates the chimeric *EWSR1-ATF1* fusion gene, has been demonstrated in approximately 80% of hyalinizing clear cell carcinoma cases. 8q12 alterations, involving the gene *PLAG1*, have been demonstrated in 25% to 30% of pleomorphic adenomas. 17q21.1 amplification, involving the gene *ERBB2*, has been demonstrated in approximately 40% of salivary duct carcinomas.

Bhaijee F, Pepper DJ, Pitman KT, Bell D: New developments in the molecular pathogenesis of head and neck tumors: a review of tumor-specific fusion oncogenes in mucoepidermoid carcinoma, adenoid cystic carcinoma, and NUT midline carcinoma. *Ann Diagn Pathol* 2011; 15:69-77.

Seethala RR: Histologic grading and prognostic biomarkers in salivary gland carcinomas. *Adv Anat Pathol* 2011;18:29-45.

Skálová A, Vanecek T, Sima R, et al: Mammary analogue secretory carcinoma of salivary glands, containing the *ETV6-NTRK3* fusion gene: a hitherto undescribed salivary gland tumor entity. *Am J Surg Pathol* 2010;34(5):599-608.

15. d. and 16. a. Sjögren disease results from chronic inflammation of the salivary and lacrimal glands, which leads to dryness of the mouth (xerostomia) and eye (keratoconjunctivitis sicca), as well as salivary or lacrimal gland enlargement in a proportion of cases. In approximately 50% to 60% of cases, patients may have a concomitant connective tissue disorder, usually rheumatoid arthritis. Polymyositis, polyarteritis nodosa, progressive systemic sclerosis (scleroderma), and systemic lupus erythematosus also occur in association with Sjögren disease. The term "sicca complex" refers to cases of Sjögren disease without comorbid connective tissue disease. Sjögren disease is more common among female patients. The histologic features of Sjögren disease include chronic inflammatory infiltration of salivary gland tissue, disappearance of acini, and hyperplasia of the cells that line intraglandular ducts. The histologic grading system devised by Chisholm and Mason (1968) refers to the number of chronic inflammatory foci (defined as ≥ 50 lymphocytes, plasma cells, and/or histiocytes) per 4 mm^2 of minor salivary glandular tissue. A grade of 0 indicates absence of inflammation; 1 indicates slight infiltration; 2 indicates moderate infiltration (less than one focus); 3 indicates one focus; and 4 indicates more than one focus. At least one focus of chronic inflammatory cells (≥ 50 lymphocytes, plasma cells, or histiocytes) per 4 mm^2 of minor salivary glandular tissue (i.e., Chisholm grade of 3 or 4) is a consistent finding among patients with Sjögren disease.

Chisholm DM, Mason DK: Labial salivary gland biopsy in Sjogren's disease. *J Clin Pathol* 1968;21:656-660.

Greenspan JS, Daniels TE, Talal N, Sylvester RA: The histopathology of Sjogren's syndrome in labial salivary gland biopsies. *Oral Surg Oral Med Oral Pathol* 1974;37(2):217-229.

17. e. Different types of metaplasia (e.g., squamous and sebaceous) sometimes occur in various salivary gland tumors. Pleomorphic adenoma sometimes displays squamous metaplasia, as in this case. Basal cell adenoma and basal cell adenocarcinoma can show squamous (as well as sebaceous) elements. Squamous and sebaceous differentiation have been described in epithelial-myoepithelial carcinoma. Squamous differentiation does not usually occur in adenoid cystic carcinoma. This generality is sometimes useful in terms of differentiating adenoid cystic carcinoma from various mimics.

Chiosea SI, Peel R, Barnes EL, Seethala RR: Salivary type tumors seen in consultation. *Virchows Arch* 2009;454:457-466.

Eveson JW, Kusafuka K, Stenman G, Nagao T: Pleomorphic adenoma. In Barnes L, Eveson JW, Reichart P, Sidransky D (eds): *Pathology and Genetics of Head and Neck Tumours. World Health Organization Classification of Tumours.* Lyon: IARC Press, 2005, pp 254-258.

18. b. and 19. b. Salivary gland acini secrete their proteinaceous or mucous products into intercalated ducts, which drain into intralobular/striated ducts, which in turn drain into interlobular ducts. The acini in the parotid gland comprise serous secretory cells only. The acini in the submandibular gland contain mostly serous cells, as well as occasional small clusters of mucous cells. The acini in the sublingual gland contain mostly mucous cells. The acini in minor salivary glands of the oral cavity contain variable combinations of serous and mucous cells. Ductal (and acinar) epithelial cells show strongly positive immunohistochemical staining for low-molecular-weight keratins, such as CAM 5.2, CK7, and CK19. Immunohistochemical staining for high-molecular-weight keratins, such as CK5/6, CK14, and CK34βE12, is generally negative (or focally positive). Immunohistochemical staining for p63 is negative.

Myoepithelial cells are present in acini and intercalated ducts. These cells stain positively for p63 and high-molecular-weight keratins, such as CK5/6, CK14, and CK34βE12. Immunohistochemical staining for low-molecular-weight keratins, such as CAM 5.2, CK7, and

CK19, is weakly positive. Basal cells are present in intralobular/striated ducts and interlobular ducts. These cells stain positively for p63 and high-molecular-weight keratins, such as CK5/6, CK14, and CK34βE12. Immunohistochemical staining for low-molecular-weight keratins, such as CAM 5.2, CK7, and CK19, is negative (or weakly positive).

Eveson JW, Auclair P, Gnepp DR, El-Naggar AK: Tumours of the salivary glands: introduction. In Barnes L, Eveson JW, Reichart P, Sidransky D (eds): *Pathology and Genetics of Head and Neck Tumours. World Health Organization Classification of Tumours.* Lyon: IARC Press, 2005, pp 212-215.

20. a. Salivary gland malignancies may share considerable morphologic overlap. Recognition of features that characterize specific lesions is consequently important. Basal cell adenocarcinoma characteristically shows prominent palisading within nests of lesional cells. This finding may help distinguish basal cell adenocarcinoma from mimics, such as epithelial-myoepithelial carcinoma. Basal cell adenocarcinoma sometimes shows small collections of matrix material within nests of tumor cells. This finding may help distinguish basal cell adenocarcinoma from mimics, such as adenoid cystic carcinoma. Within cribriform areas of adenoid cystic carcinoma, pseudocysts contain either mucoid basophilic material (glycosaminoglycans) or hyaline eosinophilic material (reduplicated basal lamina). These pseudocysts are generally distinguishable from the small collections of matrix material that sometimes appear in basal cell adenocarcinoma. Basal cell adenocarcinoma commonly shows partial circumscription/encapsulation, unlike adenoid cystic carcinoma, which characteristically demonstrates extensively invasive growth.

Chiosea SI, Peel R, Barnes EL, Seethala RR: Salivary type tumors seen in consultation. *Virchows Arch* 2009;454:457-466.

Ellis G: Basal cell adenocarcinoma. In Barnes L, Eveson JW, Reichart P, Sidransky D (eds): *Pathology and Genetics of Head and Neck Tumours. World Health Organization Classification of Tumours.* Lyon: IARC Press, 2005, pp 229-230.

Ward BK, Seethala RR, Barnes EL, Lai SY: Basal cell adenocarcinoma of a hard palate minor salivary gland: case report and review of the literature. *Head Neck Oncol* 2009; 1:41-44.

21. b. and 22. b. Staining for GCDFP-15, MUC1, BRST-2, and mammaglobin is usually positive in MASC, and negative in acinic cell carcinoma. Neither acinic cell carcinoma nor MASC is likely to stain positively for HER2. MASC sometimes shows positive mucicarmine staining within intraluminal spaces; this finding is more characteristic of MASC than acinic cell carcinoma. According to the 2005 World Health Organization classification, the following tumors represent "low-risk" malignancies: acinic cell carcinoma, low-grade MEC, epithelial-myoepithelial carcinoma, PLGA, clear cell carcinoma, basal cell adenocarcinoma, low-grade salivary duct carcinoma, myoepithelial carcinoma, oncocytic carcinoma, and sialoblastoma.

The following tumors represent "high-risk" malignancies: sebaceous carcinoma, high-grade MEC, adenoid cystic carcinoma, mucinous adenocarcinoma, squamous cell carcinoma, small cell adenocarcinoma, large cell carcinoma, lymphoepithelial carcinoma, and carcinosarcoma.

Eveson JW, Auclair P, Gnepp DR, El-Naggar AK: Tumours of the salivary glands: introduction. In Barnes L, Eveson JW, Reichart P, Sidransky D (eds): *Pathology and Genetics of Head and Neck Tumours. World Health Organization Classification of Tumours.* Lyon: IARC Press, 2005, pp 212-215.

Ellis G, Simpson RHW: Acinic cell carcinoma. In Barnes L, Eveson JW, Reichart P, Sidransky D (eds): *Pathology and Genetics of Head and Neck Tumours. World Health Organization Classification of Tumours.* Lyon: IARC Press, 2005, pp 216-218.

Griffith C, Seethala R, Chiosea SI: Mammary analogue secretory carcinoma: a new twist to the diagnostic dilemma of zymogen granule poor acinic cell carcinoma. *Virchows Arch* 2011;459:117-118.

23. b., 24. e., and 25. c. PLGA, as its name implies, can show various growth patterns, including tubular, cribriform, solid, and papillary architecture. Classical histologic features of PLGA include "sweeping" or "whorling" arrangements of cells along the lesion's periphery, entrapment/incorporation (rather than obliteration/effacement) of uninvolved, nonneoplastic seromucinous glands, single-file arrangements of tumor cells, and ovoid vesicular nuclei. PLGA consists of cells that resemble ductal (rather than myoepithelial) cells. In PLGA, S100 and EMA staining is diffusely positive, CEA staining is variable, and c-kit staining is weakly positive. In adenoid cystic carcinoma, S100 staining is variable, EMA and CEA staining is typically localized to ductal lumina, and c-kit staining is strongly positive.

Castle JT, Thompson LDR, Frommett RA, et al: Polymorphous low grade adenocarcinoma: a clinicopathologic study of 164 cases. *Cancer* 1999;86:207-219.

Gnepp DR, Chen JC, Warren C: Polymorphous low-grade adenocarcinoma of minor salivary gland. *Am J Surg Pathol* 1988;12:461-468.

Seethala RR, Johnson JT, Barnes EL, Myers EN: Polymorphous low-grade adenocarcinoma: the University of Pittsburgh experience. *Arch Otolaryngol Head Neck Surg* 2010; 136:385-392.

26. a. The translocation t(11;19) (q21;p13), which creates the chimeric *CRTC1-MAML2* fusion gene, has been demonstrated in 40% to 80% of MEC cases. The translocation t(12;15) (p13;q25), which creates the *ETV6-NTRK3* chimeric gene, is considered a defining feature of MASC. The translocation t(12;22) (q21;q12), which creates the chimeric *EWSR1-ATF1* fusion gene, has been demonstrated in approximately 80% of hyalinizing clear cell carcinoma cases. 8q12 alterations, involving the gene *PLAG1*, have been demonstrated in 25% to 30% of pleomorphic adenoma cases. 17q21.1 amplification, involving the gene *ERBB2*, has been demonstrated in approximately 40% of salivary duct carcinoma cases.

Bhaijee F, Pepper DJ, Pitman KT, Bell D: New developments in the molecular pathogenesis of head and neck tumors: a review of tumor-specific fusion oncogenes in mucoepidermoid carcinoma, adenoid cystic carcinoma, and NUT midline carcinoma. *Ann Diagn Pathol* 2011; 15:69-77.

Goode RK, El-Naggar AK: Mucoepidermoid carcinoma. In Barnes L, Eveson JW, Reichart P, Sidransky D (eds): *World*

Health Organization Classification of Tumours: Pathology and Genetics of Head and Neck Tumours. Lyon: IARC Press, 2005, 219-220.

Seethala RR: Histologic grading and prognostic biomarkers in salivary gland carcinomas. *Adv Anat Pathol* 2011; 18:29-45.

27. a. The acini in the parotid gland comprise serous secretory cells only. Parotid gland acini may also contain rare sebaceous cells. The acini in the submandibular gland contain mostly serous cells, as well as occasional small clusters of mucous cells. The acini in the sublingual gland contain mostly mucous cells. The acini in minor salivary glands of the oral cavity contain variable combinations of serous and mucous cells.

Dardick I (ed): *Salivary Gland Tumor Pathology.* New York: Igaku-Shoin, 1996.

Ellis GL, Auclair PL: *Atlas of Tumor Pathology—Tumors of the Salivary Glands,* Fascicle 17, 3rd series. Washington, DC: Armed Forces Institute of Pathology, 1996.

Huvos AG, Paulino AFG: Salivary glands. In Mills SE, Carter D, Greenson JK, et al (eds): *Sternberg's Diagnostic Surgical Pathology,* 4th ed. Philadelphia: Lippincott Williams & Wilkins, 2004, pp 933-962.

Rosai J: Major and minor salivary glands. In Rosai J (ed): *Rosai and Ackerman's Surgical Pathology,* 9th ed. Vol. 1, Chaps. 9 and 10. St. Louis: Mosby, 2004, pp 873-916.

28. b. and 29. a. Various series report different frequencies of different salivary gland tumor types. Pleomorphic adenoma is the most common salivary gland tumor. Approximately 65% to 75% of salivary gland tumors are benign. In series that include both major and minor salivary glands, MEC is the most common malignant salivary gland tumor overall. MEC is by far the most common malignant tumor of the parotid gland. Different series list either MEC or adenoid cystic carcinoma as the most common carcinoma of oral cavity minor salivary glands. Most series identify adenoid cystic carcinoma as the most common malignancy of the submandibular gland, sublingual gland, lacrimal gland, and salivary glands of the nasal cavity and paranasal sinuses. Primary tumors of tracheal salivary glands are rare. Of these, adenoid cystic carcinoma is the most common.

Dardick I (ed): *Salivary Gland Tumor Pathology.* New York: Igaku-Shoin, 1996.

Ellis GL, Auclair PL: *Atlas of Tumor Pathology—Tumors of the Salivary Glands,* Fascicle 17, 3rd series. Washington, DC: Armed Forces Institute of Pathology, 1996.

Huvos AG, Paulino AFG: Salivary glands. In Mills SE, Carter D, Greenson JK, et al (eds): *Sternberg's Diagnostic Surgical Pathology,* 4th ed. Philadelphia: Lippincott Williams & Wilkins, 2004, pp 933-962.

Rosai J: Major and minor salivary glands. In Rosai J (ed): *Rosai and Ackerman's Surgical Pathology,* 9th ed. Vol. 1, Chaps. 9 and 10. St. Louis: Mosby, 2004, pp 873-916.

30. b. Adenoid cystic carcinoma frequently shows perineural invasion, which may be extensive. Intraoperative examination of the facial nerve is occasionally warranted during parotidectomy performed for resection of adenoid cystic carcinoma. Low-grade MEC does not generally demonstrate perineural invasion, although high-grade lesions sometimes involve nerves. PLGA and carcinoma ex pleomorphic adenoma may involve nerves, but this feature does not represent a hallmark of these lesions, as it does in cases of adenoid cystic carcinoma. Acinic cell carcinoma generally does not involve nerves.

Dardick I (ed): *Salivary Gland Tumor Pathology.* New York: Igaku-Shoin, 1996.

Ellis GL, Auclair PL: *Atlas of Tumor Pathology—Tumors of the Salivary Glands,* Fascicle 17, 3rd series. Washington, DC: Armed Forces Institute of Pathology, 1996.

Huvos AG, Paulino AFG: Salivary glands. In Mills SE, Carter D, Greenson JK, et al (eds): *Sternberg's Diagnostic Surgical Pathology,* 4th ed. Philadelphia: Lippincott Williams & Wilkins, 2004, pp 933-962.

Rosai J: Major and minor salivary glands. In Rosai J (ed): *Rosai and Ackerman's Surgical Pathology,* 9th ed. Vol. 1, Chaps. 9 and 10. St. Louis: Mosby, 2004, pp 873-916.

CHAPTER 8

RENAL PATHOLOGY

Leal C. Herlitz, M. Barry Stokes, Vivette D. D'Agati, and Glen S. Markowitz

QUESTIONS

Questions 1-35 refer to a photo or photomicrograph.

1. An 18-year-old African American man presents with full nephrotic syndrome. The image shows the light microscopy findings. Immunofluorescence showed focal glomerular positivity for IgM and C3 only. Electron microscopy showed complete foot process effacement and no detectable electron-dense deposits. What is the BEST diagnosis?
   a. Minimal change disease (MCD)
   b. Membranous glomerulopathy
   c. Crescentic glomerulonephritis
   d. Collapsing focal segmental glomerulosclerosis (FSGS)
   e. Membranoproliferative glomerulonephritis (MPGN)

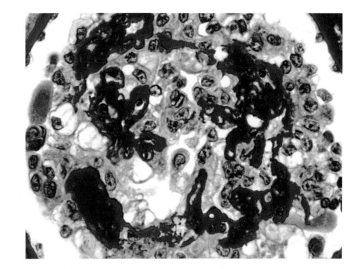

2. A 33-year-old white woman with a known history of systemic lupus erythematosus has creatinine 1.9 mg/dL, 24-hour urine protein 5 g/day, hematuria, positive antinuclear antibody (ANA), positive anti-DNA antibody, and depressed serum complement levels. Sampling for light microscopy reveals 12 glomeruli, all of which appear similar to the one shown in the image. Immunofluorescence reveals deposits that stain 3+ for IgG, 2+ for IgA, 3+ for C3, 2+ for C1q, 3+ for kappa light chain, and 3+ for lambda light chain. Electron microscopy revealed mesangial and subendothelial deposits. What is the BEST diagnosis?
   a. Lupus nephritis (LN) class II
   b. LN class III
   c. LN class IV
   d. LN class V
   e. Lupus anticoagulant syndrome

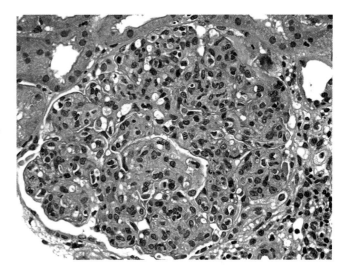

3. A 46-year-old white man presents with full nephrotic syndrome. The ultrastructural findings are shown in the image. This condition may occur secondary to all of the following EXCEPT:
a. Colonic carcinoma
b. Wegener granulomatosis
c. Hepatitis B virus (HBV) infection
d. Treatment with gold or penicillamine
e. Systemic lupus erythematosus

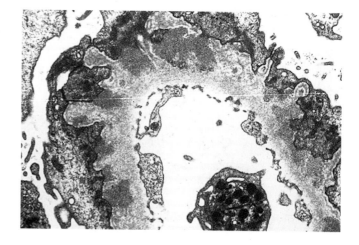

4. The light microscopy finding depicted in the image is commonly seen in which of the following conditions?
a. Microscopic polyangiitis
b. Autosomal dominant polycystic kidney disease (ADPKD)
c. Benign hypertensive arterionephrosclerosis
d. Scleroderma
e. Amyloidosis

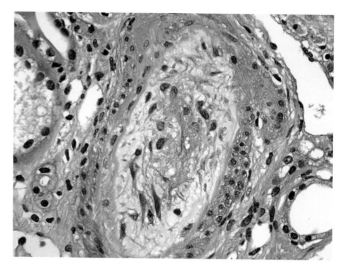

5. Light microscopy reveals 12 glomeruli that appear histologically unremarkable. Immunofluorescence is negative for all immune reactants (immunoglobulins and complement components) studied. The electron microscopy findings are shown in the image. What is the MOST likely clinical history to accompany this biopsy specimen?
a. An adult with microscopic hematuria, low-grade proteinuria, and normal renal function
b. An adult with gross hematuria, nephrotic syndrome, and acute renal failure
c. A child with fever, rash, and eosinophilia
d. A child with abrupt onset of full nephrotic syndrome
e. A child with gross hematuria, low-grade proteinuria, and depressed serum complement levels

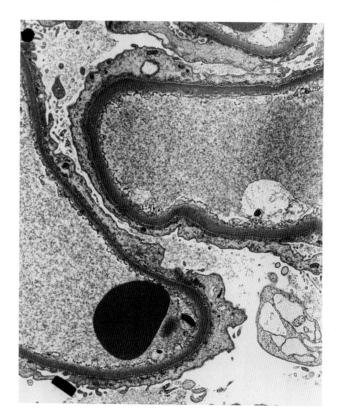

6. A renal transplant recipient develops an increase in serum creatinine from 1.4 mg/dL to 1.9 mg/dL at 2 months after transplantation. What is the diagnosis?
   a. Cyclosporine toxicity
   b. Acute cellular rejection
   c. BK polyomavirus infection
   d. Acute antibody-mediated rejection (AAMR)
   e. Acute tubular necrosis (ATN)

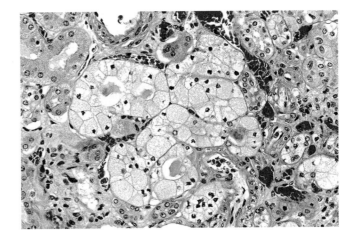

7. A renal transplant recipient develops acute renal failure with an increase in serum creatinine from 1.4 mg/dL to 3.0 mg/dL at 1 month after transplantation. Immunofluorescence staining for C4d is shown in the image. What is the MOST likely diagnosis?
   a. Tacrolimus (Prograf) toxicity
   b. Acute cellular rejection
   c. BK polyomavirus infection
   d. AAMR
   e. Hyperacute rejection

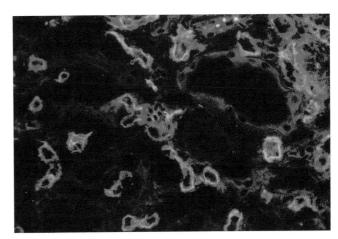

8. A 28-year-old man develops acute renal failure and hemoptysis. Light microscopy reveals a diffuse necrotizing and crescentic glomerulonephritis. Immunofluorescence staining for IgG is shown in the image. What is the BEST diagnosis?
   a. Wegener granulomatosis
   b. Goodpasture syndrome
   c. LN with pulmonary vasculitis
   d. Churg-Strauss syndrome
   e. Microscopic polyangiitis

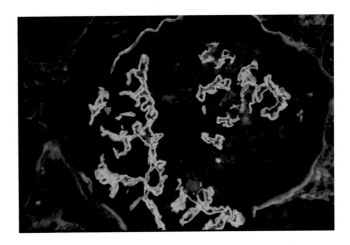

9. A 46-year-old woman presents with acute renal failure, leukocyturia, eosinophilia, and a rash; there is no significant proteinuria or hematuria. Which of the following might have led to the development of this condition?
   a. Recent cardiac catheterization
   b. Recent streptococcal pharyngitis
   c. Recent treatment with a β-lactam antibiotic
   d. Recent HBV infection
   e. Recent heart failure with resultant ischemic injury to the kidney

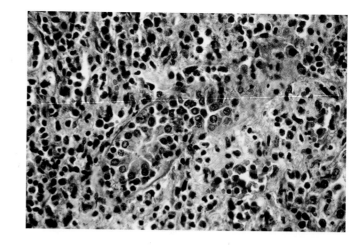

10. The complication of nephrotic syndrome depicted in the image is MOST commonly seen in association with which renal disease?
    a. IgA nephropathy
    b. FSGS
    c. Membranous nephropathy
    d. Diabetic glomerulosclerosis
    e. Renal amyloidosis

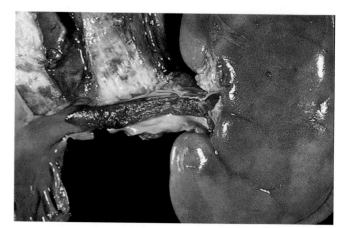

11. A 73-year-old white man develops acute renal failure with an increase in creatinine from 1.2 mg/dL to 5.6 mg/dL. Work-up reveals anemia, hypercalcemia, and hypogammaglobulinemia. The renal biopsy specimen is shown in the image. The BEST diagnosis is:
    a. Urate nephropathy
    b. Myeloma cast nephropathy
    c. Acute vasculitis
    d. Renal atheroembolization
    e. Ethylene glycol intoxication

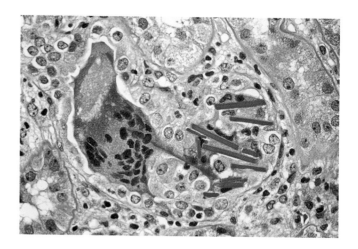

12. A 72-year-old man presents with microscopic hematuria, red blood cell (RBC) casts, and an increase in creatinine from 1.2 mg/dL to 4.5 mg/dL over 6 weeks. A representative glomerulus is shown in the image. Immunofluorescence staining was negative for IgG, IgM, IgA, C3, and kappa and lambda light chains. No deposits were seen on ultrastructural evaluation. Which of the following serologic tests is MOST likely to be positive?

a. ANA
b. Anti-GBM (glomerular basement membrane) antibody
c. Rheumatoid factor
d. Antihistone antibody
e. Antineutrophilic cytoplasmic antibody (ANCA)

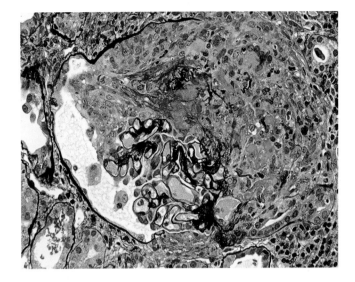

13. A renal transplant recipient develops acute renal failure with an increase in serum creatinine from 1.4 mg/dL to 2.0 mg/dL 3 weeks after transplantation. What is the MOST likely diagnosis?

a. Tacrolimus (Prograf) toxicity
b. Acute T cell–mediated rejection
c. BK polyomavirus infection
d. AAMR
e. Hyperacute rejection

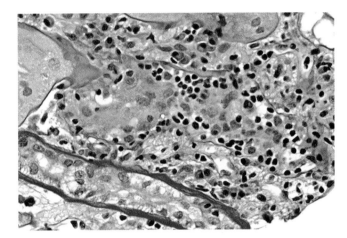

14. The image is from a patient with acute renal failure. What is the MOST likely corresponding clinical history?

a. Gross and microscopic hematuria, recent streptococcal infection, depressed serum complement levels
b. Florid nephrotic syndrome with severe edema and 24-hour urine protein of 19 g/day
c. Recent exposure to a large amount of nonsteroidal antiinflammatory drugs (NSAIDs)
d. Recent ingestion of ethylene glycol (antifreeze)
e. Recent cardiac catheterization in an elderly patient with severe atherosclerosis

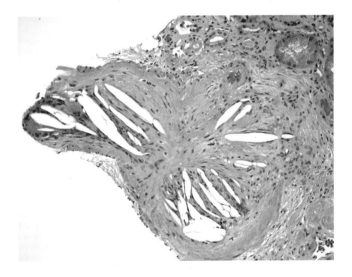

15. A 37-year-old woman with a history of hepatitis C virus (HCV) infection develops a purpuric rash, hematuria, and proteinuria. Depressed C3 and C4 complement levels are noted. Immunofluorescence reveals global mesangial and intracapillary deposits that stain positively for IgM (3+), IgG (1+), C3 (2+), and kappa (3+) and lambda (1+) light chains. The light microscopy findings are shown in the image. Which of the following blood tests would be the MOST likely to be positive?

  a. ANCA

  b. Serum cryoglobulins

  c. ANA

  d. Anti-DNA antibody

  e. Hepatitis B surface antigen

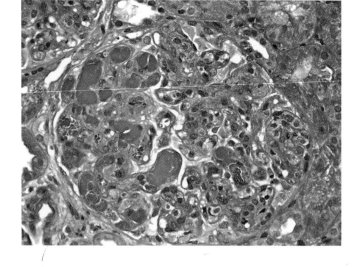

16. A 22-year-old man has a history of sensorineural hearing loss, longstanding microscopic hematuria, low-grade proteinuria, and normal renal function. What is the diagnosis?

  a. Fabry disease

  b. Denys-Drash syndrome

  c. Thin basement membrane disease

  d. IgA nephropathy

  e. Alport syndrome

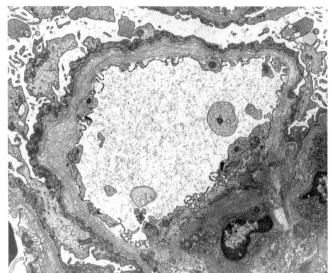

17. A 77-year-old man presents with nephrotic syndrome, normal renal function, and negative serologic tests. Immunofluorescence and electron microscopy are unavailable. Based on the light microscopy findings shown in the image, the BEST diagnosis is:

  a. MPGN

  b. Membranous glomerulopathy

  c. MCD

  d. Diffuse diabetic glomerulosclerosis

  e. Amyloidosis

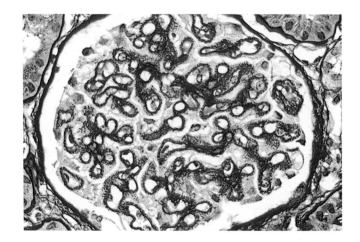

18. A 56-year-old man develops acute renal failure. The diagnostic renal biopsy findings are shown in the image. Immunofluorescence and electron microscopy are noncontributory. All of the following might have led to the development of this condition EXCEPT:

   a. Renal hypoperfusion secondary to cardiogenic shock or heart failure

   b. Renal hypoperfusion secondary to trauma with severe blood loss

   c. Arsenic exposure

   d. Aminoglycoside antibiotic exposure

   e. Wegener granulomatosis

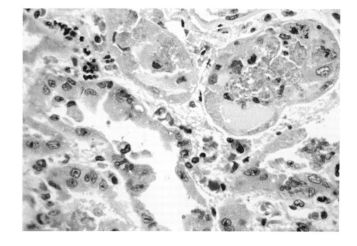

19. A 26-year-old man is found to have new-onset hypertension. Subsequent evaluation reveals the disease depicted in the image. Ultrasound reveals similar findings in the patient's 54-year-old mother. Which of the following statements about this disease is TRUE?

   a. The disease has an X-linked pattern of inheritance.

   b. Most patients have cerebral berry aneurysms.

   c. Hepatic cysts are rarely seen.

   d. Clinical manifestations include hypertension, renal insufficiency, and flank pain.

   e. The disease is typically unilateral.

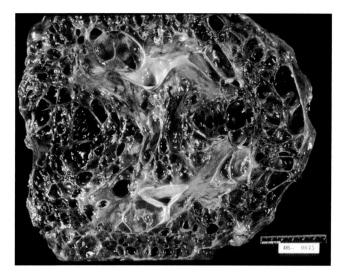

20. The ultrastructural finding seen in the electron micrograph in the image is MOST characteristic of which of the following diagnoses?

   a. LN

   b. Acute postinfectious glomerulonephritis (APIGN)

   c. MPGN

   d. Diabetic glomerulosclerosis

   e. IgA nephropathy

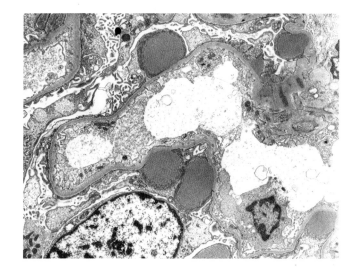

21. A 44-year-old woman is found to have microscopic hematuria. Work-up reveals minimal proteinuria, normal renal function, and negative serologic tests. There is no family history of renal disease. No tissue is available for light microscopy or immunofluorescence. The ultrastructural findings are diagnostic of:

  a. Fabry disease

  b. MCD

  c. Thin basement membrane nephropathy (TBMN)

  d. Alport syndrome

  e. IgA nephropathy

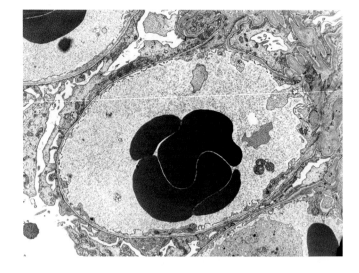

22. The light microscopy finding seen in the glomerulus with Jones methenamine silver stain is MOST characteristic of which of the following diseases?

  a. Membranous nephropathy

  b. MCD

  c. MPGN

  d. APIGN

  e. Amyloidosis

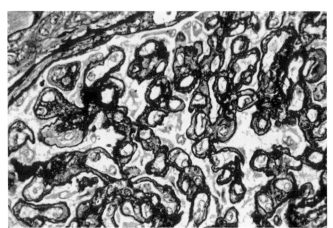

23. A 17-year-old boy presents with proteinuria, hematuria, and depressed C3 complement level. The ultrastructural findings are shown in the image. The BEST diagnosis is:

  a. APIGN

  b. Diabetic glomerulosclerosis

  c. MPGN type I

  d. Dense deposit disease (MPGN type II)

  e. IgA nephropathy

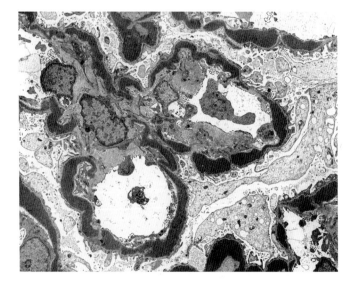

24. A 32-year-old man with a history of coronary artery disease and multiple angiokeratomas in a bathing suit distribution has proteinuria and mild renal insufficiency. The inclusion demonstrated in the image is located in a visceral epithelial cell. What is the diagnosis?
    a. Fabry disease
    b. Gaucher disease
    c. Sickle cell anemia
    d. Alport syndrome
    e. Denys-Drash syndrome

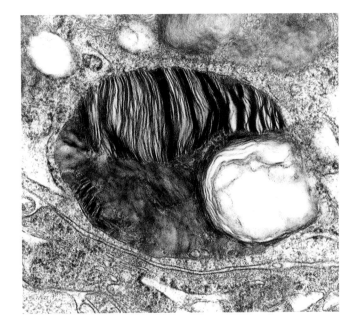

25. The findings in the electron micrograph are MOST typical of which of the following diseases?
    a. Dense deposit disease
    b. Membranous nephropathy
    c. APIGN
    d. Fibrillary glomerulonephritis
    e. IgA nephropathy

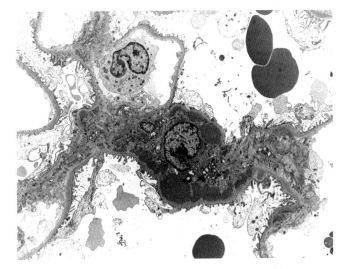

26. A 24-year-old white man presents with gross hematuria and is found to have new onset of hypertension, edema, and acute renal failure. Laboratory evaluation reveals serum creatinine 2.2 mg/dL, 24-hour urine protein 2.5 g/day, and an active urine sediment with numerous dysmorphic RBCs. Serologic testing shows negative ANA, decreased C3, normal C4, and negative antineutrophilic cytoplasmic antibodies. A renal biopsy is performed. Immunofluorescence shows granular global mesangial and glomerular capillary wall staining of 3+ intensity for C3 and 2+ for IgG, without positive staining for IgM, IgA, or C1q. What is the MOST likely diagnosis?
    a. Seronegative LN
    b. Pauciimmune necrotizing and crescentic glomerulonephritis
    c. Dense deposit disease
    d. APIGN
    e. Fibrillary glomerulonephritis

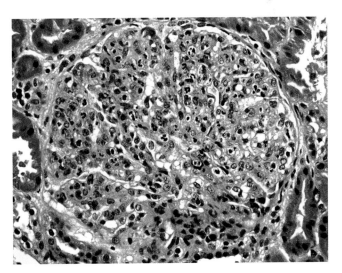

27. The electron micrograph depicted in the image demonstrates fibrils with a mean diameter of 10 nm. Which of the following clinical presentations is MOST likely to accompany this biopsy specimen?

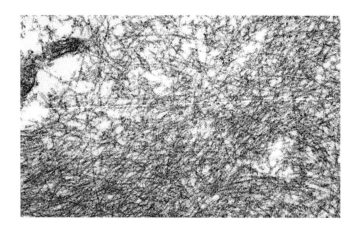

   a. A 60-year-old man with proteinuria 2 g/day and urine microscopy showing 20 to 30 dysmorphic RBCs per high-power field with occasional RBC casts

   b. A 70-year-old woman with a history of poorly controlled hypertension and slowly progressive renal insufficiency over the last 5 years; current serum creatinine is 2.5 mg/dL, and urinalysis shows trace protein; serum and urine protein electrophoresis are unrevealing

   c. A 10-year-old boy with longstanding microscopic hematuria, hearing loss, and a history of renal disease on the maternal side of the family

   d. A 10-year-old boy with sudden onset of full nephrotic syndrome

   e. An 80-year-old woman with creatinine 1.4 mg/dL, 24-hour urine protein 4 g/day, edema, serum albumin 3.3 g/dL, and IgG-lambda spike on serum protein electrophoresis

28. A 1-week-old boy is discovered to have a palpable right flank mass. Renal ultrasound reveals a multicystic mass in the location of the right kidney. The mass is composed of a mixture of echogenic parenchyma and cysts of varying size. The left kidney appears normal on ultrasound. The abnormal kidney is removed, and the renal parenchyma is found to be largely replaced by numerous cysts of varying sizes. A representative section of a noncystic portion of parenchyma is shown in the image. What is the MOST likely diagnosis?

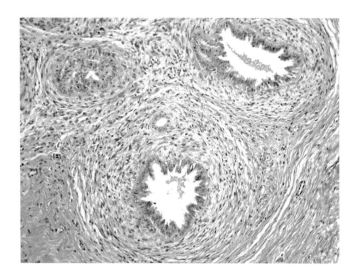

   a. ADPKD

   b. Autosomal recessive polycystic kidney disease (ARPKD)

   c. Cystic renal dysplasia

   d. Nephronophthisis

   e. Alport syndrome

29. A 45-year-old man with end-stage renal disease secondary to Alport syndrome presents with an increase in creatinine from 1.4 mg/dL to 2.2 mg/dL 8 months after unrelated renal transplantation. The patient's immunosuppressive medications include tacrolimus and mycophenolate mofetil. A biopsy of the renal allograft is performed. The finding in the image is MOST characteristic of which of the following processes?

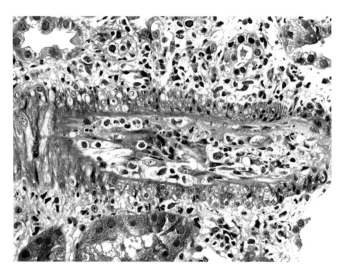

   a. Acute cellular rejection

   b. AAMR

   c. Recurrent Alport syndrome

   d. Acute tacrolimus toxicity

   e. BK polyomavirus nephropathy

30. A 55-year-old white woman presents with abrupt onset of full nephrotic syndrome. The image shows a representative glomerulus. Immunofluorescence was negative. Electron microscopy confirmed the absence of deposits and revealed complete foot process effacement. What is the BEST diagnosis?
   a. MCD
   b. Focal proliferative LN (LN class III)
   c. FSGS, collapsing variant
   d. Membranous glomerulopathy
   e. FSGS, tip lesion variant

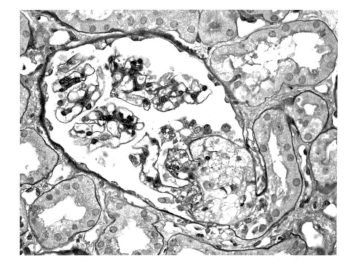

31. Which of the following conditions is the MOST likely cause of the changes seen in this glomerulus?
   a. HIV infection
   b. HCV infection
   c. Multiple myeloma
   d. Systemic lupus erythematosus
   e. Diabetes mellitus

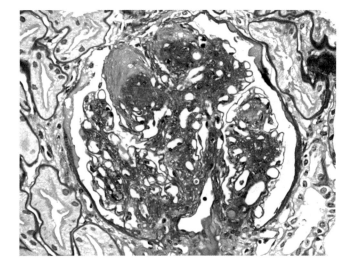

32. A 60-year-old woman presents with fever, flank pain, cloudy urine, and difficulty voiding. The patient has a serum creatinine of 0.7 mg/dL. The histologic appearance of this biopsy specimen is BEST explained by:
   a. Acute pyelonephritis
   b. Allergic interstitial nephritis resulting from a recently started medication
   c. Systemic lupus erythematosus
   d. ATN
   e. Chronic pyelonephritis

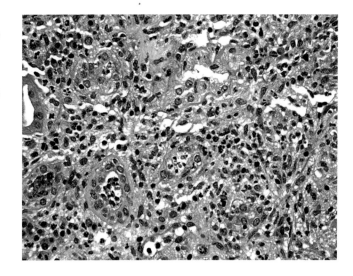

33. A 67-year-old white man with a past medical history of autoimmune pancreatitis is found to have an increase in creatinine from 1.1 mg/dL to 2.3 mg/dL over 1 year. Abdominal computed tomography (CT) scan reveals ill-defined bilateral renal masses. A biopsy of one of the masslike areas is performed. No definitive mass is identified histologically, but areas of dense sclerosis (shown in the image) are intermixed with areas of severe inflammation comprising numerous plasma cells and lymphocytes. Immunofluorescence reveals granular tubular basement membrane deposits that stain for IgG, C3, and kappa and lambda light chains. Which of the following immunohistochemical stains would be MOST helpful in establishing the diagnosis?

  a. IgG4
  b. CD138
  c. Desmin
  d. Cytokeratin AE1/AE3
  e. Serum amyloid A (AA)

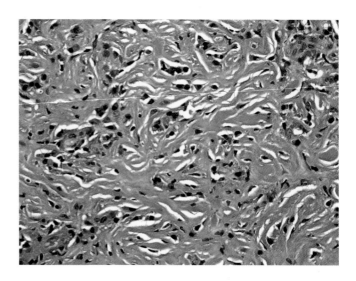

34. Which of the following conditions would feature the ultrastructural findings shown in the image?

  a. Antiphospholipid antibody syndrome
  b. MPGN type 1
  c. Hemolytic uremic syndrome (HUS)
  d. Alport syndrome
  e. Choices a and c

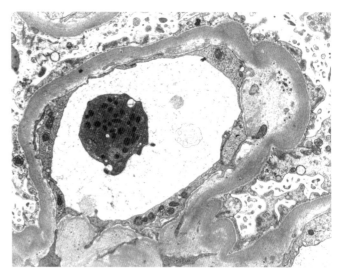

35. A 34-year-old African American man is found to have renal insufficiency and nephrotic range proteinuria on routine evaluation. A renal biopsy is performed and reveals the glomerular lesion shown in the image. Which of the following statements is TRUE?

  a. Variations in the apolipoprotein L1 (*APOL1*) gene have more recently been identified as risk factors for the development of this lesion in African American patients.
  b. The glomerular endothelial cell is the primary target of injury in this condition.
  c. Electron microscopy is likely to reveal granular immune type, electron-dense deposits.
  d. Urinalysis and urine microscopy show many RBCs with RBC casts.
  e. This condition almost never recurs in an allograft after renal transplantation.

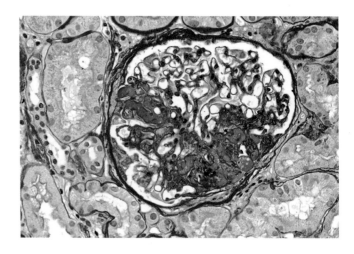

36. All of the following conditions can lead to the development of AA amyloidosis EXCEPT:

  a. Multiple myeloma
  b. Tuberculosis
  c. Intravenous drug abuse with skin popping
  d. Familial Mediterranean fever
  e. Rheumatoid arthritis

37. The components of Henoch-Schonlein purpura (HSP) include all of the following EXCEPT:

  a. Vasculitis of the skin
  b. Arthralgias
  c. Abdominal pain
  d. Nephritis with glomerular deposits of IgA
  e. Thrombocytopenia

38. Which of the following findings is NOT associated with chronic pyelonephritis?
    a. Thyroid-type tubular atrophy
    b. Acute onset of back pain, fever, and pyuria
    c. Broad U-shaped cortical scars
    d. Blunting of papillae and calyceal deformity
    e. Insidious onset of renal insufficiency and low-grade proteinuria

39. Which of the following statements about HUS is FALSE?
    a. HUS can follow a gastrointestinal infection with *Shigella* or *Escherichia coli* O157:H7.
    b. HUS causes immune complex deposition in the glomeruli, leading to postinfectious glomerulonephritis.
    c. HUS is more common in children than adults.
    d. Outbreaks of HUS have been linked to the consumption of undercooked hamburger meat.
    e. The clinical presentation of HUS may include anemia and thrombocytopenia.

40. Which of the following patterns of renal disease may result from treatment with NSAIDs?
    a. MCD
    b. Acute interstitial nephritis (AIN)
    c. ATN
    d. Crescentic glomerulonephritis
    e. a, b, and c

41. Which of the following statements about nephrotic syndrome is TRUE?
    a. The most common cause of nephrotic syndrome in adults is IgA nephropathy.
    b. The most common cause of nephrotic syndrome in African American adults is FSGS.
    c. The most common cause of nephrotic syndrome in children is membranous glomerulopathy.
    d. The most common cause of nephrotic syndrome in adults is MCD
    e. a and d

42. Which of the following conditions is associated with papillary necrosis?
    a. Sickle cell disease
    b. Wegener granulomatosis
    c. Analgesic abuse
    d. Polycystic kidney disease
    e. a and c

43. Alport syndrome results from mutations in the gene for which of the following proteins?
    a. Phospholipase A_2 receptor
    b. Factor H
    c. Apolipoprotein L1
    d. Type IV collagen
    e. α-Galactosidase A

44. What is the MOST common cause of AIN?
    a. Sarcoidosis
    b. Infection
    c. Pharmacologic agents
    d. Schönlein-Henoch purpura
    e. IgG4-related tubulointerstitial nephritis

45. Which of the following statements is CORRECT regarding secondary causes of glomerular disease?
    a. HIV infection is most commonly associated with membranous glomerulopathy.
    b. Among glomerular diseases, NSAIDs are most commonly associated with FSGS.
    c. Rheumatoid arthritis is most commonly associated with MCD.
    d. Carcinomas are most commonly associated with membranous glomerulopathy.
    e. HCV infection is most commonly associated with collapsing FSGS.

46. A 10-year-old girl presents with lower extremity vasculitis. Laboratory evaluation reveals 24-hour urine protein 2 g/day, microscopic hematuria with rare RBC casts, normal serum complement levels, negative ANA, and creatinine 0.5 mg/dL. She has a history of recent arthralgias and intermittent abdominal pain. Renal biopsy reveals a mesangial proliferative glomerulonephritis with mesangial immune deposits that stain dominantly for IgA. What is the BEST diagnosis for this patient?
    a. Microscopic polyangiitis
    b. Churg-Strauss syndrome
    c. Systemic lupus erythematosus
    d. Henoch-Schonlein purpura (HSP)
    e. IgA nephropathy

47. Which of the following statements about dysproteinemia-related renal disease is TRUE?
    a. The fibrils in light chain amyloidosis have a greater diameter than the fibrils seen in fibrillary glomerulonephritis.
    b. Light chain deposition disease is more commonly associated with light chains of the kappa isotype.
    c. Light chain amyloidosis is more commonly associated with light chains of the kappa isotype.
    d. Myeloma cast nephropathy is more commonly associated with light chains of the lambda isotype.
    e. Light chain deposition disease is a glomerular lesion that does not involve tubules or blood vessels of the kidney.

48. Antibodies against M-type phospholipase A_2 receptor (PLA2R) are central to the pathogenesis of which of the following conditions?
    a. Primary membranous nephropathy
    b. Membranous nephropathy secondary to chronic HBV infection
    c. Membranous nephropathy secondary to malignancy
    d. Pauciimmune necrotizing and crescentic glomerulonephritis
    e. Primary and secondary forms of membranous nephropathy

49. Which of the following statements about IgA nephropathy is TRUE?
    a. The defining feature of IgA nephropathy is mesangial deposits that stain dominantly for either IgA or IgG.
    b. IgA nephropathy is most common in Asian patients and is rare in African American patients.
    c. Patients with IgA nephropathy typically present with nephrotic syndrome and a bland urine sediment (i.e., no evidence of hematuria).
    d. Extraglomerular immune deposits involving tubular basement membranes and arterioles are a common feature of IgA nephropathy.
    e. Hypocomplementemia is a characteristic feature of IgA nephropathy.

50. Which of the following statements about ADPKD is TRUE?
    a. ADPKD is a rare hereditary disorder in the United States, far less common than cystic fibrosis or sickle cell disease.
    b. Renal cyst formation in ADPKD does not occur until adulthood.
    c. Most cases of ADPKD are caused by defects in either polycystin-1 (*PKD1*) or polycystin-2 (*PKD2*).
    d. Extrarenal disease is not a feature of ADPKD.
    e. ARPKD is more common than ADPKD.

ANSWERS

1. d. The findings of global wrinkling and retraction of the GBM with swelling and hyperplasia of overlying visceral epithelial cells are diagnostic of the collapsing variant of FSGS. In MCD, glomeruli appear normal on standard light microscopy. In membranous glomerulopathy, findings on light microscopy include GBM thickening with spike formation. Crescentic glomerulonephritis results from glomerular inflammation leading to GBM rupture and extracapillary proliferation of spindle-shaped epithelial cells and mononuclear leukocytes between Bowman capsule and the glomerular tuft. MPGN is a diffuse proliferative pattern of glomerulonephritis characterized by segmental to global GBM duplication with cellular interposition.

D'Agati VD: The spectrum of focal segmental glomerulosclerosis: new insights. *Curr Opin Nephrol Hypertens* 2008;17(3):271-281.

2. c. LN class IV is characterized by endocapillary proliferation involving at least 50% of glomeruli. LN class IV is further subdivided based on whether the endocapillary proliferation is segmental (LN IV-S) or global (LN IV-G). In the image, endocapillary proliferation is present globally, consistent with LN IV-G. LN class II is characterized by solely mesangial proliferation. LN class III is characterized by endocapillary proliferation involving less than 50% of glomeruli. The endocapillary proliferation is typically segmental in distribution and is usually accompanied by mesangial proliferation. LN class V is characterized by membranous changes including subepithelial deposits typically accompanied by intervening GBM spikes. Mesangial proliferation may be present. Endocapillary proliferation is not a feature of class V LN; if this finding is present, an additional diagnosis (i.e., LN class III or LN class IV) is likely. Lupus anticoagulant syndrome is characterized by renal biopsy findings of thrombotic microangiopathy (TMA) involving glomeruli and blood vessels. Immune deposits are not present, and significant cellular proliferation is not typically identified. A characteristic feature is the presence of fibrin thrombi.

Markowitz GS, D'Agati VD: Classification of lupus nephritis. *Curr Opin Nephrol Hypertens* 2009;18(3):220-225.

3. b. The characteristic renal biopsy finding in Wegener granulomatosis is a pauciimmune necrotizing and crescentic glomerulonephritis. Malignancy is one of the four main categories of secondary causes of membranous nephropathy. The most common malignancies are of gastrointestinal, pulmonary, or prostatic origin. Infection is one of the four main categories of secondary causes of membranous nephropathy. The most common infections associated with membranous nephropathy are hepatitis B and C viruses. Drug-induced disease is one of the four main categories of secondary causes of membranous nephropathy, and two of the most common therapeutic agents implicated in this condition are gold and penicillamine. The most common secondary cause of membranous nephropathy is systemic lupus erythematosus (i.e., membranous LN, or LN class V). Additional autoimmune or collagen vascular diseases associated with membranous glomerulopathy include Sjögren syndrome, rheumatoid arthritis, and mixed connective tissue disease.

Beck LH Jr, Salant DJ: Membranous nephropathy: recent travels and new roads ahead. *Kidney Int* 2010;77(9):765-770.

Markowitz GS: Membranous glomerulopathy: emphasis on secondary forms and disease variants. *Adv Anat Pathol* 2001; 8(3):119-125.

4. d. Mucoid intimal edema is a characteristic feature of thrombotic microangiopathies, a group of conditions that target the glomeruli and blood vessels of the kidney. Thrombotic microangiopathies comprise diverse entities that share a common pathomechanism of endothelial injury and intravascular coagulation. Clinical features include microangiopathic hemolytic anemia (i.e., with fragmented RBCs [schistocytes] on peripheral blood smear) and thrombocytopenia. Renal involvement includes acute renal failure. The differential diagnosis of a TMA pattern of renal injury includes HUS, thrombotic thrombocytopenic purpura, malignant hypertension, scleroderma renal disease, antiphospholipid or anticardiolipin antibody syndrome, preeclampsia, and hereditary and drug-induced forms of disease. All of these conditions may exhibit glomerular endothelial swelling, intracapillary fibrin thrombi, congestion, double contours of the GBM, mesangial interposition, and mesangiolysis (dissolution of mesangial matrix). Blood vessels exhibit fibrin thrombi and onion-skin mucoid intimal edema.

Moake JL: Thrombotic microangiopathies. *N Engl J Med* 2002; 347(8):589-600.

5. d. MCD is the most common cause of nephrotic syndrome in children and often is abrupt in onset. The main pathologic abnormality in MCD is extensive foot process effacement. Electron-dense deposits are absent, and GBM abnormalities are not seen. Most children with MCD have normal renal function, normal serum complement levels, and no evidence of hematuria. The disease is highly responsive to steroid therapy, although the course may be remitting and relapsing in a few patients. MCD is also a common cause of nephrotic syndrome in adults. In older adults, the florid nephrotic syndrome that characterizes MCD may be associated with acute renal failure.

Eddy AA, Symons JM: Nephrotic syndrome in childhood. *Lancet* 2003;362(9384):629-639.

6. a. Isometric tubular vacuolization is a characteristic histologic pattern of acute calcineurin inhibitor nephrotoxicity. The vacuoles affect proximal tubules and appear clear with hematoxylin-eosin and trichrome stains. The term *isometric* refers to the fact that the vacuoles tend to be of uniform size. The calcineurin inhibitors (cyclosporine and tacrolimus) are the mainstay of modern immunosuppressive protocols to prevent allograft rejection. Isometric tubular vacuolization is an acute, potentially reversible cause of renal allograft dysfunction. Other patterns of calcineurin inhibitor nephrotoxicity include hyaline arteriolopathy, "striped" fibrosis with tubular atrophy, and TMA.

Nankivell BJ, Borrows RJ, Fung CL, et al: Calcineurin inhibitor nephrotoxicity: longitudinal assessment by protocol histology. *Transplantation* 2004;78(4):557-565.

7. d. C4d staining of peritubular capillaries is a defining feature of AAMR. AAMR is caused by de novo formation of antibodies against donor antigens expressed on endothelial cells (usually HLA class I or II). Criteria for the clinicopathologic diagnosis of AAMR include (1) documentation of donor-specific antibodies in recipient serum; (2) positive immunostaining for C4d in the distribution of peritubular capillaries; and (3) morphologic evidence of acute tissue injury, most commonly neutrophil or monocytes margination in peritubular capillaries. Immunoglobulins and other complement components (e.g., C1 and C3) are not typically detectable in AAMR. C4d is a breakdown product of the fourth component of complement (C4) and has the unique feature of covalently binding to tissue and serving as a durable marker of complement activation. The presence of C4d in the distribution of peritubular (interstitial) capillaries is a sensitive marker of recent AAMR.

Solez K, Colvin RB, Racusen LC, et al: Banff 07 classification of renal allograft pathology: updates and future directions. *Am J Transplant* 2008;8(4):753-760.

8. b. Crescentic glomerulonephritis is a pattern of glomerular injury that can be divided into three major etiologic categories based on immunofluorescence findings: granular positivity, linear positivity, and minimal to absent positivity (pauciimmune). In crescentic glomerulonephritis with granular positivity and immune complex–mediated disease, antigen-antibody immune complexes deposit within the glomerulus, leading to cellular proliferation, leukocyte infiltration, and crescent formation. Granular deposits of immunoglobulins and complement are detected by immunofluorescence. Examples include crescentic forms of LN, MPGN, postinfectious glomerulonephritis, and IgA nephropathy. In crescentic glomerulonephritis with linear positivity in GBM for IgG (i.e., anti-GBM disease), the cause is circulating anti-GBM antibodies with specificity for type IV collagen, a structural component of the GBM. In a subset of patients with anti-GBM disease, the antibodies cross-react with type IV collagen in alveolar basement membranes, leading to pulmonary hemorrhage. When anti-GBM disease involves both the kidneys and the lungs, the condition is known as Goodpasture syndrome. Crescentic glomerulonephritis with minimal or no positivity and pauciimmune crescentic glomerulonephritis is the most common form of crescentic glomerulonephritis occurring in adults and is defined by its lack of

significant glomerular antigen-antibody deposition. Most cases are associated with ANCA seropositivity. Examples include Wegener granulomatosis, microscopic polyangiitis, Churg-Strauss syndrome, and renal-limited pauciimmune crescentic glomerulonephritis.

Jennette JC: Rapidly progressive crescentic glomerulonephritis. *Kidney Int* 2003;63(3):1164-1177.

9. c. The finding of interstitial eosinophils strongly favors an allergic or drug-induced cause of AIN. Interstitial nephritis may occur as an adverse reaction to many therapeutic agents, most commonly antibiotics (e.g., sulfonamides, penicillin), diuretics (furosemide, thiazides), proton pump inhibitors, and NSAIDs. The pathogenesis of allergic or drug-induced AIN involves a cell-mediated hypersensitivity reaction to the drug. Acute renal failure usually begins 1 to 2 weeks after drug exposure and is often accompanied by fever, eosinophilia, and a skin rash. Renal manifestations include acute renal failure, sterile pyuria (including urinary eosinophils), and mild proteinuria. Renal function often returns to normal within several weeks after withdrawal of the offending agent. Steroids may be used to achieve a more rapid and complete resolution of renal dysfunction.

Praga M, González E: Acute interstitial nephritis. *Kidney Int* 2010;77(11):956-961.

10. c. Among patients with nephrotic syndrome, patients with membranous glomerulopathy and a serum albumin less than 2.0 g/dL are at the highest risk for the development of renal vein thrombosis (RVT). Hypercoagulability is a well-known complication of nephrotic syndrome, resulting from increased hepatic production of fibrinogen and coagulation factors in response to hypoalbuminemia. Urinary losses of antithrombin III secondary to increased glomerular permeability make the renal vein particularly vulnerable to thrombosis. It is unclear why patients with membranous glomerulopathy are at greatest risk for RVT. Patients with MCD, FSGS, and amyloidosis have a much smaller risk of RVT. Embolization of deep vein thrombosis and RVT to the lung may occur with grave consequences. Patients with these conditions are often treated with oral anticoagulation.

Glassock RJ: Prophylactic anticoagulation in nephrotic syndrome: a clinical conundrum. *J Am Soc Nephrol* 2007;18(8): 2221-2225.

11. b. The light microscopy findings in myeloma cast nephropathy (also known as light-chain cast nephropathy) include distinctive tubular casts and widespread tubular injury. The casts have a hard, crystalline appearance with sharp, angulated contours. They typically stain brightly eosinophilic with hematoxylin-eosin and stain pale or negative with PAS. The casts form predominantly in distal tubular segments. A very helpful diagnostic feature is the presence of multinucleated giant cells surrounding the cast material. Immunofluorescence microscopy demonstrates intense staining of the casts for either kappa or lambda light chain. Staining for the reciprocal light chain is typically weak to negative. Many patients also have Bence Jones proteinuria with free light chains in the urine and an abnormal ratio of free kappa and lambda light chains in the blood. Myeloma cast nephropathy is the most common pattern of renal involvement in patients with multiple myeloma, and patients usually present with acute renal failure.

Urate nephropathy produces clear crystals, primarily in the medulla, typically surrounded by a granulomatous response. Urate granulomas are often an incidental finding in patients with hyperuricemia or gout and do not cause acute renal failure. Urate crystals are better preserved in alcohol-fixed specimens, where they can produce birefringence when polarized. Acute vasculitis is associated with crescentic glomerulonephritis and arteritis. Renal atheroembolization is associated with clear needle-shaped defects in arteries and arterioles, corresponding to cholesterol emboli that have dissolved in processing, often surrounded by inflammatory cells, including giant cells in some cases. Ethylene glycol intoxication produces acute renal failure secondary to acute oxalate crystal deposition in tubules, resulting in ATN with vacuolar epithelial degeneration. In formalin-fixed tissue, oxalate crystals, in contrast to urate crystals or myeloma casts, are birefringent under polarized light.

Iványi B: Frequency of light chain deposition nephropathy relative to renal amyloidosis and Bence Jones cast nephropathy in a necropsy study of patients with myeloma. *Arch Pathol Lab Med* 1990;114(9):986-987.

12. e. ANCA seropositivity is associated with pauciimmune necrotizing and crescentic glomerulonephritis, which is the entity depicted in the image. At least 80% of patients with pauciimmune crescentic glomerulonephritis test seropositive for ANCA. The pathogenesis of pauciimmune crescentic glomerulonephritis involves ANCA-mediated neutrophil activation, causing neutrophil degranulation on endothelial surfaces and leading to vasculitis and crescentic glomerulonephritis. ANA is associated with LN, which contains immune complex deposits. Anti-GBM antibody is associated with anti-GBM disease and linear immunofluorescence staining of the GBM for IgG and C3. Rheumatoid factor is most commonly positive in rheumatoid arthritis but is also positive in mixed cryoglobulinemic glomerulonephritis, an entity associated with glomerular deposits that contain IgM, IgG, C3, and kappa and lambda light chains. Antihistone antibody is associated with drug-induced lupus.

Jennette JC: Rapidly progressive crescentic glomerulonephritis. *Kidney Int* 2003;63(3):1164-1177.

13. b. In a renal allograft, the finding of interstitial inflammation that extends across tubular basement membranes to produce extensive tubulitis is diagnostic of acute T cell–mediated rejection. Interstitial inflammation, tubulitis, and endarteritis are the hallmarks of acute T cell–mediated rejection. It is a cell-mediated immune response mounted by the recipient to donor-specific antigens (predominantly class I and II human leukocyte antigens [HLAs]) and is an important cause of allograft dysfunction in the first 6 months after transplantation. If untreated, it can lead to irreversible graft failure. Acute T cell–mediated rejection can be seen at any time in the life of the allograft, including more than 10 years after transplantation. Acute T cell–mediated

rejection may coexist with AAMR, which is characterized by deposition of circulating donor-specific anti-HLA antibodies.

Solez K, Colvin RB, Racusen LC, et al: Banff 07 classification of renal allograft pathology: updates and future directions. *Am J Transplant* 2008;8(4):753-760.

14. e. Renal atheroembolic disease results from dislodging of atheromatous plaques in the aorta or main renal artery and their embolization distally into intrarenal arteries or arterioles. Giant cells, monocytes, and fibrin often accumulate around the atheroemboli. At a later time, reactive myointimal proliferation occurs. This condition is most commonly seen in elderly patients with extensive atherosclerosis. In many cases, there is a recent history of vascular instrumentation, most commonly cardiac catheterization. Other cases follow cardiac surgery or recent anticoagulation. A significant minority of cases occur spontaneously. Risk factors for atheroembolic disease include atherosclerotic cardiovascular disease, baseline renal insufficiency, anticoagulation, and recent endovascular procedures. Embolization often affects other organs, such as the skin, gastrointestinal tract, and brain, giving rise to protean clinical features.

Scolari F, Ravani P: Atheroembolic renal disease. *Lancet* 2010; 375(9726):1650-1660.

15. b. HCV infection is associated with MPGN, cryoglobulinemic glomerulonephritis (which frequently has overlapping findings with MPGN), and membranous nephropathy. In HCV-associated cryoglobulinemic glomerulonephritis, light microscopy typically reveals diffuse proliferative glomerulonephritis with large intracapillary deposits that occlude capillary lumina. The deposits are eosinophilic on hematoxylin-eosin stain and red on trichrome stain. Similar-appearing deposits may be seen in intrarenal arteries or arterioles, where they can produce a cryoglobulinemic vasculitis. Immunofluorescence staining reflects the composition of the cryoglobulin in the circulation. In HCV-associated cryoglobulinemic glomerulonephritis, the cryoglobulin is mixed (type 2), usually consisting of monoclonal IgM and kappa light chains complexed to polyclonal IgG. The deposits typically stain dominantly for IgM and kappa chains, with less intense staining for IgG and lambda light chains. Staining for complement components C3 and C1 also is typically present. In the skin, cryoglobulinemic vasculitis manifests as a palpable purpuric rash.

Beddhu S, Bastacky S, Johnson JP: The clinical and morphologic spectrum of renal cryoglobulinemia. *Medicine (Baltimore)* 2002;81(5):398-409.

16. e. The lamellated, "basket-weave" appearance of the GBM is characteristic of Alport syndrome, which is a hereditary condition caused by defective synthesis of type IV collagen in GBMs. Most cases are X-linked and result from mutation in *COL4A5*, the gene encoding the alpha-5 subunit of collagen IV, and the most severely affected patients are male. Female carriers of the X-linked form of Alport syndrome may have benign asymptomatic hematuria or slowly progressive renal insufficiency. Patients with Alport syndrome frequently have sensorineural hearing loss because the same collagen chain is distributed in the cochlea. Most affected patients present with hematuria in childhood, with progressive development of proteinuria and renal failure in adulthood. Immunohistochemical staining for collagen IV alpha-3 and alpha-5 subunits in the kidney and skin is reduced in a significant percentage of patients with Alport syndrome. This finding is not always seen, but when present, it confirms the diagnosis.

Bekheirnia MR, Reed B, Gregory MC, et al: Genotype-phenotype correlation in X-linked Alport syndrome. *J Am Soc Nephrol* 2010;21(5):876-883.
Haas M: Alport syndrome and thin glomerular basement membrane nephropathy: a practical approach to diagnosis. *Arch Pathol Lab Med* 2009;133(2):224-232.

17. b. GBM thickening with spike formation is characteristic of membranous nephropathy. MPGN is characterized by GBM duplication, mesangial cell interposition, and subendothelial electron-dense deposits. GBM thickening with spike formation is characteristic of membranous nephropathy. Glomeruli appear normal by light microscopy in MCD. No GBM thickening or spikes are seen. Diffuse diabetic glomerulosclerosis is characterized by mesangial sclerosis and thickening of GBM and tubular basement membrane, but GBM spikes and deposits are not seen. Amyloidosis is characterized by amorphous eosinophilic deposits that expand the mesangial matrix and can thicken the GBM. Well-developed GBM spikes, as seen in the image, are not a feature of amyloidosis.

Beck LH Jr, Salant DJ: Membranous nephropathy: recent travels and new roads ahead. *Kidney Int* 2010;77(9):765-770.

18. e. The findings of tubular simplification, loss of brush border, and sloughing of necrotic epithelial cells into the tubular lumen are diagnostic of ATN. ATN can be subdivided into two main pathogenic categories: ischemic and toxic. Ischemic ATN occurs in the setting of severe hypotension or shock, such as secondary to acute blood loss, heart failure, or sepsis. Pathologic changes may be subtle in ischemic ATN. Toxic ATN follows exposure to various toxins, including heavy metals (mercury, lead, gold, arsenic, bismuth, chromium, uranium), organic solvents (carbon tetrachloride, chloroform, methyl alcohols, glycols), antibiotics (aminoglycosides, polymyxin), anesthetics (methoxyflurane), physical agents (radiation), diagnostic agents (contrast media), pigments (hemoglobin, myoglobin), and osmotic agents (mannitol). Toxic ATN typically demonstrates more severe pathologic changes than ischemic ATN. ATN is the most common cause of acute renal failure. It is particularly common in hospitalized patients, reflecting the high prevalence of cardiovascular disease and frequent exposure to nephrotoxic agents. Most patients with ATN eventually recover renal function, although many require hemodialysis for days or weeks until the tubules can regenerate.

Rosen S, Stillman IE: Acute tubular necrosis is a syndrome of physiologic and pathologic dissociation. *J Am Soc Nephrol* 2008;19(5):871-875.

19. d. ADPKD is one of the most common human heritable diseases, affecting approximately 1:500 to 1:1000 individuals. The disease is characterized by bilateral renal cyst formation, leading to massively enlarged kidneys. Initial clinical manifestations of ADPKD typically are seen between 20 and 40 years of age and include renal insufficiency, hypertension, hematuria, and renal colic. The disease is slowly progressive, and most patients develop end-stage renal disease. Patients with ADPKD account for 8% to 10% of all patients with end-stage renal disease in the United States. In ADPKD, the kidneys are markedly enlarged (8 kg and 40 cm in length). The expanded renal parenchyma comprises a massive aggregate of cysts lined by flattened-to-cuboidal epithelium.

The most common extrarenal manifestations of ADPKD are hepatic cysts, which are seen in 50% of patients. Although polycystic liver disease may cause pain, it is not associated with functional impairment. Other complications of ADPKD reflect the expression of polycystin in vascular smooth muscle. Cardiac valve abnormalities, in particular, mitral valve prolapse, occur in 25% of patients. Intracranial berry aneurysms are the most catastrophic complication of ADPKD, affecting 5% to 8% of patients. Mutations in the genes *PKD1* (located on chromosome 16) and *PKD2* (located on chromosome 4) are responsible for 85% and 13% of cases of ADPKD, respectively. The gene products, polycystin-1 and polycystin-2, are proteins that regulate renal epithelial cell proliferation and differentiation. The mechanism of cyst formation requires an inherited (autosomal dominant) mutation of one allele and the development of a somatic mutation (second hit) in the second allele.

Bonsib SM: Renal cystic diseases and renal neoplasms: a mini-review. *Clin J Am Soc Nephrol* 2009;4(12):1998-2007.

20. b. Subepithelial "hump-shaped" deposits are a distinctive, characteristic feature of APIGN. Subepithelial deposits are seen mainly in two conditions: APIGN and membranous nephropathy. In membranous nephropathy, the subepithelial deposits are uniform and are typically separated by GBM spikes. The subepithelial deposits of APIGN appear larger, are less numerous, have a "hump-shaped" appearance, and are not associated with intervening spikes. On light microscopy, APIGN typically manifests a diffuse proliferative glomerulonephritis with numerous infiltrating neutrophils. Immunofluorescence shows the deposits of APIGN stain dominantly or codominantly for C3, with weaker and more variable staining for IgG. APIGN is classically associated with group A streptococcal infection in children; most children recover completely. In adults, APIGN may be associated with an immunocompromised state (e.g., diabetes mellitus, AIDS, alcoholism). Streptococcal and staphylococcal infections are equally prevalent. There is a higher rate of permanent renal injury following APIGN in adults, particularly in patients with diabetes mellitus.

Nasr SH, Markowitz GS, Stokes MB, et al: Acute postinfectious glomerulonephritis in the modern era: experience with 86 adults and review of the literature. *Medicine (Baltimore)* 2008;87(1):21-32.

21. c. The finding of diffuse GBM thinning, in the absence of GBM lamellation, is diagnostic of TBMN. The clinical presentation of microscopic hematuria, in the absence of significant proteinuria or renal insufficiency, is most commonly encountered in the following three renal conditions: TBMN, hereditary nephritis (i.e., Alport syndrome), and IgA nephropathy. Before a patient with microscopic hematuria undergoes renal biopsy, possible urologic causes for hematuria must be excluded. The glomeruli in TBMN usually appear unremarkable on light microscopy. The normal GBM thickness averages approximately 320 nm in women and 350 nm in men. Diagnostic criteria for TBMN are diffuse GBM thinning, with mean thickness less than 225 nm in women and less than 250 nm in men. The main clinical finding in TBMN is isolated microscopic hematuria. Many patients have a family history of isolated hematuria with autosomal dominant transmission. TBMN results from a heterozygous mutation in either *COL4A3* or *COL4A4*; these genes encode the alpha-3 (*COL4A3*) and alpha-4 (*COL4A4*) chains of collagen IV. TBMN is a nonprogressive condition that is often referred to clinically as *benign essential hematuria*.

Haas M: Alport syndrome and thin glomerular basement membrane nephropathy: a practical approach to diagnosis. *Arch Pathol Lab Med* 2009;133(2):224-232.

22. c. MPGN is a pattern of glomerular disease characterized by duplication of the GBM ("double contours") and mesangial cell interposition between the duplicated layers. Mesangial and subendothelial immune deposits are present in most cases. Primary MPGN is more commonly seen in children. Some cases are related to persistent activation of the alternative complement pathway. Secondary forms of MPGN are more common in adults, and the most frequent cause is HCV infection. Other secondary causes include autoimmune connective tissue disease (e.g., lupus), HBV infection, and dysproteinemia. Clinically, MPGN is characterized by nephrotic syndrome, hematuria, hypocomplementemia, and renal insufficiency in some cases.

Sethi S, Fervenza FC, Zhang Y, et al: Proliferative glomerulonephritis secondary to dysfunction of the alternative pathway of complement. *Clin J Am Soc Nephrol* 2011;6(5): 1009-1017.

23. d. Dense deposit disease is characterized by broad, fusiform, or ribbonlike intramembranous dense deposits that thicken and replace the lamina densa of the GBM. Similar dense deposits may be seen within the mesangial matrix, Bowman capsule, and tubular basement membrane. The deposits in dense deposit disease stain solely for C3 on immunofluorescence. Dense deposit disease is most common in children and young adults and usually manifests with proteinuria, hematuria, and depressed serum C3 complement level. Many patients with dense deposit disease have a circulating C3 nephritic factor, an autoantibody to the C3 convertase that continually activates complement through the alternative pathway. Dense deposit disease was formerly known as MPGN type II, but it is now recognized that most cases do *not* show a membranoproliferative pattern of injury, and so the name *dense deposit disease* is preferred.

Nasr SH, Valeri AM, Appel GB, et al: Dense deposit disease: clinicopathologic study of 32 pediatric and adult patients. *Clin J Am Soc Nephrol* 2009;4(1):22-32.

24. a. The image shows a zebra body, which is the characteristic intracytoplasmic osmiophilic, lamellated, myelinlike inclusion seen in Fabry disease. In the kidney, zebra bodies are commonly identified in visceral epithelial cells, endothelial cells, and tubular epithelial cells. The visceral epithelial cells have a foamy, vacuolated appearance on light microscopy. Fabry disease is an X-linked lysosomal storage disorder resulting from α-galactosidase A deficiency. The enzymatic defect leads to progressive accumulation of neutral glycosphingolipids (predominantly globotriaosylceramide). Affected males usually present in childhood with acroparesthesias, angiokeratomas, hypohidrosis, and corneal and lenticular opacities. With advancing age, there is progressive renal, cardiac, and cerebrovascular disease. Renal failure usually develops in the fourth or fifth decade. Heterozygous females may manifest symptoms owing to skewed lyonization. Glycosphingolipid deposits accumulate in many cell types, including vascular endothelial cells, cardiomyocytes, and renal epithelial cells. Fabry disease is diagnosed by demonstrating absent α-galactosidase A in peripheral blood leukocytes and confirmed by genetic testing. Heterozygotes display reduced α-galactosidase A levels. Enzyme replacement therapy may help ameliorate symptoms.

Ramaswami U, Najafian B, Schieppati A, et al: Assessment of renal pathology and dysfunction in children with Fabry disease. *Clin J Am Soc Nephrol* 2010;5(2):365-370.

25. e. Mesangial deposits are the hallmark of IgA nephropathy and are seen in all cases. Typically, the deposits aggregate at the edges of the mesangium (paramesangial region). Some cases of IgA nephropathy may demonstrate subendothelial or subepithelial deposits. The diagnosis of IgA nephropathy requires dominant or codominant immunofluorescence staining for IgA. Patients with IgA nephropathy typically have microscopic hematuria, low-grade proteinuria, and normal renal function. Transient gross hematuria may occur simultaneously with an upper respiratory tract infection ("synpharyngitic gross hematuria"). Serum ANA and complement levels are normal. End-stage renal disease occurs in approximately 30% of patients with IgA nephropathy. IgA nephropathy is the most common glomerular disease worldwide and is particularly common in Asian patients.

Glassock RJ: The pathogenesis of IgA nephropathy. *Curr Opin Nephrol Hypertens* 2011;20(2):153-160.

26. d. The clinical presentation of acute nephritic syndrome with hypocomplementemia is classic for APIGN. Histologically, APIGN is most often an exudative (neutrophil-rich) diffuse proliferative glomerulonephritis, as seen in the image. Immunofluorescence is typically dominant for C3 and is often accompanied by staining for IgG. Seronegative LN is very rare; although it can manifest as a diffuse proliferative glomerulonephritis on light microscopy, the diagnosis requires immune deposits that stain dominantly or codominantly for IgG. Pauciimmune necrotizing and crescentic glomerulonephritis is by definition "pauciimmune" and should not show more than +/– to 1+ staining for immunoglobulins or complement. Additionally, antineutrophilic cytoplasmic antibodies are present in most

patients with this condition. Although dense deposit disease can manifest as a proliferative glomerulonephritis with hypocomplementemia and strong C3 staining, the presence of 2+ positivity for IgG would be unusual for dense deposit disease. APIGN is a more common condition than dense deposit disease and is more typically associated with exudative features (i.e., neutrophils infiltrating glomeruli). Fibrillary glomerulonephritis is IgG dominant or codominant by immunofluorescence, is not associated with hypocomplementemia, rarely exhibits exudative features, and is mainly seen in older adults.

Nasr SH, Markowitz GS, Stokes MB, et al: Acute postinfectious glomerulonephritis in the modern era: experience with 86 adults and review of the literature. *Medicine (Baltimore)* 2008; 87(1):21-32.

27. e. The most likely clinical presentation would be an 80-year-old woman with creatinine 1.4 mg/dL, 24-hour urine protein 4 g/day, edema, serum albumin 3.3 g/dL, and IgG-lambda spike on serum protein electrophoresis. Most cases of amyloidosis seen in the United States are amyloid light chain (AL) amyloidosis, and this condition is typically seen in older patients with plasma cell dyscrasias who present with nephrotic syndrome and renal insufficiency. The presence of dysmorphic RBCs and RBC casts in the urine sediment is typical of acute glomerulonephritis, as can be seen in IgA nephropathy. Amyloidosis is usually associated with a bland urine sediment that is devoid of RBC casts. The clinical presentation described in Choice c is typical of Alport syndrome. Alport syndrome shows lamellation and splitting of the GBM on electron microscopy, a distinctly different appearance from the fibrillar deposits shown in the image. The clinical presentation described in Choice D is typical of MCD. Although amyloidosis often manifests with full nephrotic syndrome, it is rare in children.

Picken MM: Amyloidosis—where are we now and where are we heading? *Arch Pathol Lab Med* 2010;134(4):545-551.
von Hutten H, Mihatsch M, Lobeck H, et al: Prevalence and origin of amyloid in kidney biopsies. *Am J Surg Pathol* 2009;33(8): 1198-1205.

28. c. The image demonstrates mesenchymal cuffing, a characteristic histologic feature of cystic renal dysplasia. Renal dysplasia can be cystic or noncystic and unilateral or bilateral. ADPKD is primarily a disease of adulthood, is characterized by bilateral renal involvement, and is only rarely clinically apparent in children. ARPKD is characterized by bilateral rather than unilateral disease. The finding of mesenchymal cuffing is not typically seen in ARPKD. Nephronophthisis is a common hereditary form of progressive renal disease in children. Pathologic findings include marked thickening and thinning of tubular basement membrane and an irregular branching tubular architecture. Occasional medullary and cortical tubular cysts are seen, but the kidneys are not typically enlarged. Alport syndrome is characterized by GBM lamellation producing a "basket-weave" appearance. Cyst formation is not a feature of Alport syndrome.

Kissane JM: Renal cysts in pediatric patients. *Pediatr Nephrol* 1990;4(1):69-77.
Matsell DG: Renal dysplasia: new approaches to an old problem. *Am J Kidney Dis* 1998;32(4):535-543.

29. a. The lesion shown in the image is endovasculitis and is typical of the vascular lesions seen in acute T cell–mediated rejection. Vascular lesions can be seen in acute T cell–mediated rejection, AAMR, and calcineurin inhibitor (tacrolimus) toxicity. Differentiating these vascular lesions is essential to guiding therapy. Acute T cell–mediated rejection is graded by the Banff criteria and is divided into three main categories. Grade 1 rejection is characterized by interstitial inflammation and tubulitis. Grade 2 rejection is characterized by vessel wall inflammation (i.e., endovasculitis). Grade 3 rejection is characterized by more severe vessel wall inflammation with evidence of transmural or necrotizing arteritis. The vascular lesions seen in grade 3 acute T cell–mediated rejection are also seen in severe AAMR. In the latter condition, C4d staining is identified in peritubular capillaries. BK polyomavirus nephropathy is characterized by similar findings of interstitial inflammation and tubulitis and is a well-known mimic of acute T cell–mediated rejection. However, BK polyomavirus nephropathy is not associated with endovasculitis. The calcineurin inhibitors (cyclosporine and tacrolimus) are the mainstay of modern immunosuppressive protocols to prevent allograft rejection. Patterns of calcineurin inhibitor nephrotoxicity include isometric tubular vacuolization, hyaline arteriolopathy, "striped" fibrosis with tubular atrophy, and TMA.

Solez K, Colvin RB, Racusen LC, et al: Banff 07 classification of renal allograft pathology: updates and future directions. *Am J Transplant* 2008;8(4):753-760.

30. e. The image is diagnostic of FSGS, tip lesion variant. By definition, the tip lesion variant is a lesion of FSGS that projects into or is confluent with the initial segment of the proximal tubule. There are multiple subtypes of FSGS, including the collapsing variant, the cellular variant, the tip lesion variant, the perihilar variant, and FSGS not otherwise specified (FSGS NOS). Among the subtypes of FSGS, the tip lesion variant is associated with the best prognosis. Most patients with the tip lesion variant of FSGS present with abrupt onset of full nephrotic syndrome. In contrast to FSGS NOS and the collapsing variant of FSGS, the tip lesion variant is more common in white patients. In the tip lesion variant of FSGS, electron microscopy typically reveals extensive foot process effacement.

Stokes MB, Markowitz GS, Lin J, et al: Glomerular tip lesion: a distinct entity within the minimal change disease/focal segmental glomerulosclerosis spectrum. *Kidney Int* 2004; 65(5):1690-1702.

31. e. Diabetic nephropathy is the leading cause of end-stage renal disease in the United States and is seen in patients with type 1 or type 2 diabetes mellitus. Nodular diabetic glomerulosclerosis, which is shown in the image, is characterized by nodular mesangial sclerosis (Kimmelstiel-Wilson nodules) and thickening of glomerular and tubular basement membranes. HIV infection is mainly associated with collapsing FSGS. HCV infection is associated with MPGN and cryoglobulinemic glomerulonephritis. Less common associations include membranous nephropathy and fibrillary glomerulonephritis. HCV infection is not associated with nodular mesangial sclerosis. Myeloma can cause a diverse array of renal lesions, including light chain deposition disease, amyloidosis, and light chain cast nephropathy. On light microscopy, nodular mesangial sclerosis in light chain deposition disease can resemble the nodular mesangial sclerosis in nodular diabetic glomerulosclerosis. The two entities are easily distinguished by immunofluorescence and electron microscopy. LN is a proliferative form of glomerulonephritis and is not characterized by nodular mesangial sclerosis.

Tervaert TW, Mooyaart AL, Amann K, et al: Pathologic classification of diabetic nephropathy. *J Am Soc Nephrol* 2010; 21(4):556-563.

Wirta O, Helin H, Mustonen J, et al: Renal findings and glomerular pathology in diabetic subjects. *Nephron* 2000;84(3):236-242.

32. a.   The histologic findings of a neutrophil-rich interstitial infiltrate with neutrophil casts as well as the clinical history are most compatible with acute pyelonephritis. Acute pyelonephritis is an acute suppurative infection of the kidney and renal pelvis associated with urinary tract infection. Greater than 85% of infections are due to gram-negative bacilli, most commonly *E. coli*. The most common pathway of renal infection is ascension of bacteria up the urinary stream from the bladder. Organisms reach the bladder most commonly in the setting of obstruction to urinary flow (e.g., prostatic hypertrophy, lower urinary tract tumor, pregnancy, incomplete voiding of the bladder owing to neurogenic bladder in patients with diabetes), urethral instrumentation (e.g., catheterization, cystoscopy), and vesicoureteral reflux (particularly prevalent in infants and young children with pyelonephritis). The alternative, less frequent pathway of renal infection is via the hematogenous route, typically occurring in patients with bacteremia or a source of septic emboli (e.g., endocarditis). Histologic findings in acute bacterial pyelonephritis include neutrophil-rich interstitial inflammation with neutrophilic tubulitis and intratubular neutrophil casts. Clinically, patients with acute pyelonephritis present with fever, flank pain, and dysuria. The diagnosis is usually made on clinical grounds with urinalysis and urine culture, and renal biopsy is generally not required.

Hill GS: Renal infection. In Hill GS (ed): *Uropathology*. New York: Churchill Livingstone, 1989, pp 333-429.

33. a.   An IgG4 stain would highlight the presence of many IgG4+ plasma cells. The presence of numerous IgG4+ cells (often defined as >50 cells/high-power field) is typical of IgG4 immune complex tubulointerstitial nephritis, which is the renal manifestation of IgG4-related sclerosing disease. The most common systemic manifestation of IgG4-related sclerosing disease is autoimmune pancreatitis. Staining for CD138 would confirm the presence of numerous plasma cells but would not point to a specific diagnosis. Staining for desmin is useful to confirm myocyte differentiation but is not helpful in diagnosing IgG4-related sclerosing disease. Staining for cytokeratin is useful to identify epithelial differentiation. This stain is not helpful in diagnosing IgG4-related sclerosing disease. Although AA is an acellular eosinophilic material that can accumulate in the interstitium, it is not typically associated with prominent inflammation. Autoimmune pancreatitis is not a feature of AA amyloidosis.

Bateman AC, Deheragoda MG: IgG4-related systemic sclerosing disease—an emerging and under-diagnosed condition. *Histopathology* 2009;55(4):373-383.

Cornell LD, Chicano SL, Deshpande V, et al: Pseudotumors due to IgG4 immune-complex tubulointerstitial nephritis associated with autoimmune pancreatocentric disease. *Am J Surg Pathol* 2007;31(10):1586-1597.

34. e.   TMAs comprise diverse entities that share a common pathomechanism of endothelial injury and intravascular coagulation. The differential diagnosis of a TMA pattern of renal injury includes HUS, thrombotic thrombocytopenic purpura, malignant hypertension, scleroderma renal disease, antiphospholipid or anticardiolipin antibody syndrome, preeclampsia, and hereditary and drug-induced forms of disease. Glomerular findings of TMA include endothelial swelling, intracapillary fibrin thrombi, RBC congestion, double contours of the GBM, mesangial interposition, mesangiolysis (dissolution of mesangial matrix), and subendothelial electron-lucent material ("fluff"). Acute vascular findings of TMA include fibrin thrombi, mucoid intimal edema, and fibrinoid necrosis. Chronic vascular changes of TMA include fibrous intimal hyperplasia, which may have a concentric "onion-skin" pattern. When TMA exhibits prominent duplication of the GBM with mesangial interposition, the findings may appear similar to MPGN. MPGN is an immune complex–mediated glomerulonephritis with ultrastructural findings of mesangial and subendothelial electron-dense deposits. In contrast, TMA is characterized by subendothelial electron-lucent "fluff."

Nochy D, Daufas E, Droz D, et al: The intrarenal vascular lesions associated with primary antiphospholipid syndrome. *J Am Soc Nephrol* 1999;10(3):507-518.

35. a.   In black patients of African descent, *APOL1* G1 and G2 haplotypes were under strong selection pressure because carriers had the ability to lyse subspecies of trypanosomes, the parasite that causes sleeping sickness. Analogous to sickle cell trait and malaria, heterozygotes gain protection from the parasite. Homozygotes, although resistant to parasitic infection, have a significantly increased risk of developing FSGS and end-stage renal disease. The mechanism by which the *APOL1* gene acts on podocytes to cause FSGS is unknown.

FSGS is a pattern of glomerular injury in which sclerosis initially affects a subset of glomeruli (i.e., focal) and involves a portion of the glomerular tuft (i.e., segmental). Podocyte injury is a feature common to all types of FSGS. Podocyte injury leads to effacement of podocyte foot processes, which are critical to the integrity of the glomerular filtration barrier. Patients with end-stage renal disease as a result of primary FSGS who undergo renal transplantation have a significant rate of recurrent disease in the allograft (40%). FSGS recurrence can be seen within hours after transplantation; this provides evidence that in some patients a circulating permeability factor is responsible for podocyte injury. In early recurrence, plasmapheresis to remove the circulating factor may induce remission. A classification of FSGS into five histologic variants has been proposed. The image in this question demonstrates FSGS NOS. The other variants are perihilar FSGS (most of the lesions of FSGS are located at the glomerular vascular pole), cellular FSGS (characterized by expansile "cellular" lesions typically containing foam cells and leukocytes), glomerular tip lesion (defined by the location of FSGS lesions at the tubular pole of glomeruli), and collapsing FSGS (showing implosive glomerular tuft collapse with hyperplasia and hypertrophy of overlying epithelial cells).

D'Agati VD, Fogo AB, Bruikn JA, et al: Pathologic classification of focal segmental glomerulosclerosis: a working proposal. *Am J Kidney Dis* 2004;43(2):368-382.

D'Agati VD, Kaskel FJ, Falk RJ: Focal segmental glomerulosclerosis. *N Engl J Med* 2011;365(25):2398-2411.

Genovese G, Friedman DJ, Ross MD, et al: Association of trypanolytic ApoL1 variants with kidney disease in African Americans. *Science* 2010;329(5993):841-845.

36. a. Plasma cell dyscrasias are associated with AL amyloidosis, also termed *primary amyloidosis*, which is composed of a monoclonal immunoglobulin. AA amyloidosis, also termed *secondary amyloidosis*, is derived from serum AA, an acute phase reactant protein synthesized by the liver. AA amyloidosis develops in patients with chronic inflammatory disorders of autoimmune or infectious cause. Associated underlying conditions include rheumatoid arthritis (the most common), psoriasis, ankylosing spondylitis, tuberculosis, Crohn disease, chronic draining infections (i.e., chronic osteomyelitis, bronchiectasis), intravenous drug abuse with skin popping, and familial Mediterranean fever. Immunostains for the precursor proteins (serum AA and kappa and lambda light chains) are extremely useful in renal amyloidosis to distinguish AA amyloidosis from AL amyloidosis, which collectively constitute greater than 95% of cases of renal amyloidosis.

Picken MM: Amyloidosis—where are we now and where are we heading? *Arch Pathol Lab Med* 2010;134(4):545-551.

37. e. The platelet count is typically normal in HSP. HSP is most common in children but can occur in patients of all ages. HSP usually manifests as a syndrome of purpura (predominantly involving the lower extremities), arthralgias, abdominal pain, and hematuria. Hematuria may be accompanied by proteinuria or renal insufficiency or both. Renal biopsy usually reveals a proliferative glomerulonephritis (mesangial proliferative, focal proliferative, or crescentic) with dominant immune staining for IgA. HSP often is considered a systemic form of IgA nephropathy, and the renal biopsy findings and renal clinical manifestations are similar in the two conditions. Renal outcomes in children are generally good, with preserved kidney function in most cases. In adults, heavy proteinuria, elevated serum creatinine, and hypertension are associated with worse outcomes. Biopsy of the purpuric skin lesions in HSP reveals leukocytoclastic vasculitis with vessel wall deposits of IgA.

Chang WL, Yang YH, Wang LC, et al: Renal manifestations in Henoch-Schönlein purpura: a 10-year clinical study. *Pediatr Nephrol* 2005;20(9):1269-1272.

38. b. The typical clinical presentation of chronic pyelonephritis is insidious development of renal insufficiency with low-grade proteinuria. In contrast, acute pyelonephritis has a more dramatic presentation, which includes flank pain, fever, and pyuria. Chronic pyelonephritis is caused by chronic parenchymal infection of the kidney (usually by bacterial organisms) resulting in chronic inflammation and scarring of the renal cortex, calyces, and pelvis. It is often associated with chronic urinary obstruction and vesicoureteral reflux. Urine cultures are frequently negative for microorganisms despite ongoing chronic inflammation. Grossly, the kidneys are shrunken and irregularly deformed, with broad, flat, U-shaped scars. There is often evidence of previous ascending infection in the form of papillary blunting and calyceal deformity. Microscopically, there is disproportionate damage to tubules and interstitium, with relative sparing of glomeruli. Tubules are extensively atrophied, and many are filled with colloid casts (a pattern termed *thyroidization*). Periglomerular fibrosis and thickening of Bowman capsule are common. In chronic pyelonephritis, tubular dysfunction may manifest as polyuria and nocturia owing to loss of the ability to concentrate urine.

Alpers CE: The kidney. In Kumar V, Abbas AK, Fausto N (eds): *Robbins and Cotran Pathologic Basis of Disease*, 8th ed. Philadelphia: Saunders, 2010, pp 939-944.

39. b. HUS is classified into two main categories based on the presence or absence of a diarrheal prodrome. The classic form of HUS is more common in children and is usually associated with bloody diarrhea resulting from infectious gastroenteritis. The most common agents are *E. coli* strain O157:H7 and *Shigella dysenteriae*. Owing to the infectious origin of HUS, epidemics may be traced to a single contaminated source of water or food (i.e., undercooked meat). *E. coli* O157:H7 produces a Shiga-like toxin that particularly targets endothelial cells, leading to endothelial injury and microthrombosis. In the atypical or "diarrhea-negative" form of HUS, most patients have no prodromal symptoms and no clear precipitating factors. This group comprises familial forms of HUS, including patients with deficiency in the vWF cleaving protease. Other patients may have an autoantibody to this protease. Other patients have dysregulation of the alternative complement pathway, owing to either genetic defects or inhibitory autoantibodies, notably to factor H, factor I, or membrane cofactor protein. Clinical outcomes are less favorable in atypical HUS, with a more insidious onset of disease, greater likelihood of relapse, and increased risk of progression to end-stage renal disease. Pathologic findings in both forms of HUS demonstrate TMA, which is characterized by fibrin thrombi in glomeruli and small blood vessels, arterial mucoid intimal edema, GBM double contours, and mesangiolysis. Immune complex deposition is not seen. Recurrent disease in renal allograft is a significant problem for patients with atypical HUS. Patients with HUS present with acute renal failure, anemia, and thrombocytopenia. Treatment of HUS consists of supportive care and plasma exchange.

Noris M, Caprioli J, Bresin E, et al: Relative role of genetic complement abnormalities in sporadic and familial aHUS and their impact on clinical phenotype. *Clin J Am Soc Nephrol* 2010;5(10):1844-1859.

40. e. NSAIDs are widely used agents in the treatment of pain and inflammation that act by inhibiting cyclooxygenase, the enzyme that converts arachidonic acid to prostaglandins prostacyclin and thromboxane. Prostaglandin-mediated vasodilatation plays an important autoregulatory role in the maintenance of renal perfusion. In the setting of reduced renal perfusion secondary to heart failure or volume depletion, NSAIDs can attenuate prostaglandin-mediated vasodilatation and precipitate hemodynamically mediated acute renal failure, which histologically resembles ischemic ATN. NSAIDs are commonly implicated agents in the development of AIN. Other patterns of renal disease seen after treatment with NSAIDs include MCD, rare cases of membranous nephropathy, and papillary necrosis (i.e., analgesic nephropathy).

Harirforoosh S, Jamali F: Renal adverse effects of non-steroidal anti-inflammatory drugs. *Expert Opin Drug Saf* 2009;8(6): 669-681.

41. b. The most common cause of nephrotic syndrome varies depending on age and ethnic group. The most common cause of primary nephrotic syndrome in children is MCD. Sources differ with respect to whether the most common cause of nephrotic syndrome in nondiabetic adults is membranous nephropathy or FSGS. FSGS is the most common cause of nephrotic syndrome in African American adults. Patients with IgA nephropathy typically present with hematuria and subnephrotic proteinuria; full nephrotic syndrome is unusual in IgA nephropathy.

Haas M, Meehan SM, Karrison TG, et al: Changing etiologies of unexplained adult nephrotic syndrome: a comparison of renal biopsy findings from 1976-1979 and 1995-1997. *Am J Kidney Dis* 1997;30(5):621-631.

42. e. Necrosis of the renal papilla (papillary necrosis) is a condition that occurs mainly in one of four clinical settings: obstructive pyelonephritis, diabetic nephropathy, sickle cell anemia, and analgesic abuse. The pathogenesis of papillary necrosis in diabetic nephropathy probably involves a combination of ischemia (owing to frequently severe small vessel disease) and infection. In sickle cell anemia, papillary necrosis is caused by repeated sickling of erythrocytes in the vasa recta renis with resulting medullary ischemia. Analgesic abuse (consumption of large quantities of analgesics over years) frequently leads to chronic interstitial nephritis and papillary necrosis. Papillary damage is thought to result from combined direct toxic effects of phenacetin metabolites on tubular cells with aspirin-induced or NSAID-induced inhibition of prostaglandin synthesis. The latter predisposes to ischemia by reduction in medullary synthesis of vasodilatory prostaglandins.

Brix AE: Renal papillary necrosis. *Toxicol Pathol* 2002;30(6): 672-674.

43. e. Antibodies against phospholipase A_2 receptor are linked to the development of primary membranous nephropathy. Factor H mutations are seen in disorders of the alternative complement pathway, including dense deposit disease and C3 glomerulopathy. The association between apolipoprotein L1 mutations and the development of FSGS has been documented more recently. Fabry disease results from mutations in α-galactosidase, a lysosomal hydrolase.

Alport syndrome results from mutations in the alpha-3, alpha-4, and alpha-5 subunits of type IV collagen. Alport syndrome is a hereditary condition caused by defective synthesis of type IV collagen in GBMs. The alpha-3, alpha-4, and alpha-5 subunits of type IV collagen combine to form a triple helical protomer, which is a critical structural component of the GBM. Mutations in any one of these subunits can produce Alport syndrome.

The alpha-3 and alpha-4 subunits are encoded on chromosome 2, whereas the alpha-5 subunit is encoded on the X chromosome. Because these genes are located on both autosomes and sex chromosomes, Alport syndrome can show autosomal recessive, autosomal dominant, or X-linked inheritance patterns. Mutations in the alpha-5 subunit of type IV collagen underlie 85% of cases of Alport syndrome. As a result, most cases of Alport syndrome are transmitted in an X-linked manner and affect males. Female carriers of the X-linked form of Alport syndrome may have benign asymptomatic hematuria or slowly progressive renal insufficiency. Approximately 15% of cases of Alport syndrome result from mutations in the alpha-3 and alpha-4 subunits of type IV collagen and exhibit an autosomal (mainly autosomal recessive) pattern of inheritance. Most patients with Alport syndrome present with hematuria in childhood, followed by progressive development of proteinuria and renal failure in adulthood.

Hudson BG, Tryggvason K, Sundaramoorthy M, et al: Alport's syndrome, Goodpasture's syndrome and type IV collagen. *N Engl J Med* 2003;348(25):2543-2556.

44. c. The most common cause of AIN is drug-induced disease, which accounts for 70% of cases. The pharmacologic agents that are most frequently implicated in AIN are antibiotics, NSAIDs, and proton pump inhibitors. Additional causes of AIN include infection (bacteria, fungi, and viruses), systemic, presumed autoimmune processes (e.g., Sjögren syndrome, systemic lupus erythematosus, Wegener granulomatosis), tubulointerstitial nephritis with uveitis syndrome, sarcoidosis, IgG4-related tubulointerstitial nephritis, and idiopathic forms of disease. Patients with AIN typically present with renal dysfunction, leukocyturia, and subnephrotic proteinuria. The pathogenesis of drug-induced AIN likely involves a type IV (delayed-type) hypersensitivity response.

Baker RJ, Pusey CD: The changing profile of acute tubulointerstitial nephritis. *Nephrol Dial Transplant* 2004; 19(1):8-11.
Perazella MA, Markowitz GS: Drug-induced acute interstitial nephritis. *Nat Rev Nephrol* 2010;6(8):461-470.

45. d. Carcinomas are most commonly associated with membranous glomerulopathy. Malignancy should be excluded in adult patients with newly diagnosed membranous glomerulopathy. Membranous glomerulopathy is mainly associated with carcinomas of the lung, breast, prostate, and gastrointestinal tract. Other secondary causes of membranous glomerulopathy include autoimmune systemic diseases (i.e., systemic lupus erythematosus), infection (i.e., HBV, HCV), and exposure to certain pharmaceutical agents (i.e., gold, penicillamine). The most common secondary cause of collapsing FSGS is HIV infection. Less frequent associations include parvovirus B19 and drug-induced forms of disease related to treatment with pamidronate or interferon-α, interferon-β, or interferon-γ. Secondary causes of MCD include therapeutic agents (i.e., NSAIDs, lithium, interferon), Hodgkin lymphoma, and rarely allergic reactions (i.e., bee stings). Causes of AA amyloidosis include autoimmune inflammatory conditions (i.e., rheumatoid arthritis, juvenile rheumatoid arthritis, ankylosing spondylitis, Crohn disease), chronic infections (i.e., tuberculosis, chronic osteomyelitis, bronchiectasis, chronic infection in intravenous drug users who resort to skin popping), and familial Mediterranean fever.

Lefaucheur C, Stengel B, Nochy D, et al: Membranous nephropathy and cancer: epidemiologic evidence and determinants of high-risk cancer association. *Kidney Int* 2006;70(8):1510-1517.

46. d. HSP has been described as a systemic form of IgA nephropathy. In addition to renal biopsy findings that resemble IgA nephropathy, systemic manifestations are present, the most common of which are purpura, arthralgias, and abdominal pain. Microscopic polyangiitis is associated with pauciimmune necrotizing and crescentic glomerulonephritis, an entity in which immune deposits typically are not seen. Churg-Strauss syndrome is associated with pauciimmune necrotizing and crescentic glomerulonephritis, an entity in which immune deposits typically are not seen. LN is characterized by immune deposits that stain dominantly for IgG. Although the biopsy findings would meet criteria for IgA nephropathy, HSP is a better answer based on the clinical history.

Davin JC: Henoch-Schonlein purpura nephritis: pathophysiology, treatment, and future strategy. Clin J Am Soc Nephrol 2011; 6(3):679-689.

47. b. The particular amino acid sequence of a monoclonal light chain dictates its biochemical properties, which determine the propensity of the light chain to form light chain amyloidosis, light chain deposition disease, or light chain cast nephropathy (i.e., myeloma cast nephropathy). The lambda light chain isotype is seen in most cases of primary amyloidosis. In contrast, the kappa isotype predominates in myeloma cast nephropathy and light chain deposition disease. In approximately 90% of cases of light chain deposition disease, the deposits stain solely for kappa light chain. A monoclonal lambda light chain is responsible for the remaining 10%. By definition, Congo red staining for amyloid is negative. In approximately 75% of cases of light chain amyloidosis, the deposits stain for lambda light chain. A monoclonal kappa light chain is responsible for the remaining 25%. By definition, Congo red staining reveals apple green birefringence when viewed under polarized light. Myeloma cast nephropathy or light chain cast nephropathy is the most common pattern of renal involvement in patients with multiple myeloma, and the usual manifestation is acute renal failure. The light microscopy findings in myeloma cast nephropathy include distinctive tubular casts and widespread tubular injury. Immunofluorescence microscopy demonstrates intense staining of the casts for either kappa or lambda light chain; staining for the reciprocal light chain is typically weak or negative. Kappa staining is seen in most cases.

Markowitz GS: Dysproteinemia and the kidney. *Adv Anat Pathol* 2004;11(1):49-63.
Solomon A, Weiss DT, Kattine AA: Nephrotoxic potential of Bence Jones proteins. *N Engl J Med* 1991;324(26):1845-1851.

48. a. Approximately 75% of cases of membranous nephropathy represent primary (idiopathic) disease. Secondary forms of membranous nephropathy are seen with autoimmune or collagen vascular disease (i.e., systemic lupus erythematosus, rheumatoid arthritis), drugs (i.e., gold, penicillamine, rarely NSAIDs), infection (mainly HBV or HCV), and malignancy (mainly carcinomas, including prostatic, pulmonary, and gastrointestinal neoplasms). The classic animal model of membranous nephropathy is the Heymann nephritis model produced by immunizing rats with fractionated renal cortex enriched in proximal tubular brush border. The immunogenic component of the fractionated renal cortex is Gp330 (megalin), which is present on rat proximal tubular brush border and podocyte foot processes. Gp330 is *not* present on human podocytes and is not the causative antigen of membranous nephropathy in humans. The search for the human "Heymann antigen" was ongoing until recently. Antibodies against a conformation-dependent epitope of the M-type PLA2R have been demonstrated in the serum of approximately 75% of patients with primary membranous nephropathy and are present within the subepithelial deposits. PLA2R appears to be the human equivalent of the "Heymann antigen." Anti-PLA2R antibodies are not present in patients with secondary forms of membranous nephropathy.

Beck LH, Boneigo RG, Lambeau G, et al: M-type phospholipase A$_2$ receptor as target antigen in idiopathic membranous nephropathy. *N Engl J Med* 2009;361(1):11-21.

49. b. IgA nephropathy is the most common glomerular disease worldwide and is particularly common in Asian patients. Mesangial deposits that stain dominantly for IgA are the defining feature of IgA nephropathy. IgG and IgM may be present, but the intensity of staining for IgA is greatest. The most common clinical feature of IgA nephropathy is microscopic hematuria. Proteinuria is typically present, but full nephrotic syndrome is seen in only a few patients. Extraglomerular deposits, for instance, involving tubular basement membranes and arterioles, are a common feature of LN but are not typically encountered in IgA nephropathy. Most patients with IgA nephropathy have normal serum complement levels throughout the course of disease. In contrast, hypocomplementemia is commonly encountered in APIGN, LN, and MPGN.

Glassock RJ: The pathogenesis of IgA nephropathy. *Curr Opin Nephrol Hypertens* 2011;20(2):153-160.
Tumlin JA, Madaio MP, Hennigar R: Idiopathic IgA nephropathy: pathogenesis, histopathology, and therapeutic options. *Clin J Am Soc Nephrol* 2007;2(5):1054-1061.

50. c. Mutations in *PKD1* are responsible for approximately 85% of cases of ADPKD, whereas *PKD2* mutations account for approximately 13% of cases. ADPKD is a common hereditary disease with a significantly higher incidence than cystic fibrosis or sickle cell disease. Although formerly known as "adult polycystic kidney disease," it is now recognized that ADPKD can become clinically evident at any time from infancy to adulthood. Extrarenal manifestations of ADPKD include hepatic cysts, pancreatic cysts, cerebral berry aneurysms, and cardiac valve abnormalities such as mitral valve prolapse. ARPKD is far less common than ADPKD, with an incidence of approximately 1:20,000 births. In contrast, the incidence of ADPKD is 1:500 to 1:1000 births.

Calvet JP, Grantham JJ: The genetics and physiology of polycystic kidney disease. *Semin Nephrol* 2001;21(2):107-123.

Gabow PA: Autosomal dominant polycystic kidney disease. *N Engl J Med* 1993;329(5):332-342.

Ong AC, Harris PC: Molecular pathogenesis of ADPKD: the polycystin complex gets complex. *Kidney Int* 2005;67(4): 1234-1247.

CHAPTER 9

GENITOURINARY PATHOLOGY

Lara R. Harik and Kathleen M. O'Toole

$\mathbf{Q}$*UESTIONS*

Questions 1-24 in this chapter refer to a photo or photomicrograph.

1. A 55-year-old woman is incidentally discovered to have a 5-cm mahogany brown mass in the upper pole of her right kidney. Which of the following statements about this tumor is FALSE?
   a. It is characterized by loss of chromosomes Y and 1.
   b. Infiltration of the surrounding fat can occur and does not alter prognosis.
   c. Vascular involvement increases the likelihood of metastatic disease.
   d. It is associated with Birt-Hogg-Dubé syndrome.
   e. It is slightly more common in males.

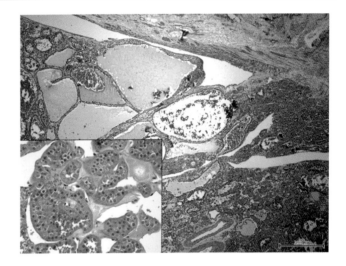

2. The diagnosis for the lesion depicted in this needle core biopsy of the prostate in a 65-year-old man with elevated serum prostate-specific antigen (PSA) is:
   a. High-grade prostatic intraepithelial neoplasia (HGPIN)
   b. Ductal prostatic adenocarcinoma
   c. Intraductal prostatic adenocarcinoma
   d. Seminal vesicle epithelium
   e. Invasive rectal adenocarcinoma involving the prostate

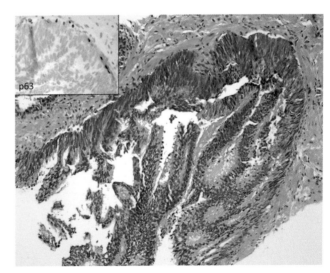

3. A 63-year-old man presents to the urologist with hematuria and is found to have a bladder mass on cystoscopy. A representative H&E stain from the biopsy of the mass is attached. Which statement about this entity is TRUE?

   a. It is not associated with in situ urothelial carcinoma.

   b. It is characterized by a low rate of lymph node metastases.

   c. It is frequently associated with advanced stage at presentation.

   d. It is characterized by a single nest of cells in each space or lacunae.

   e. It is associated with hypertension and elevated serum catecholamines.

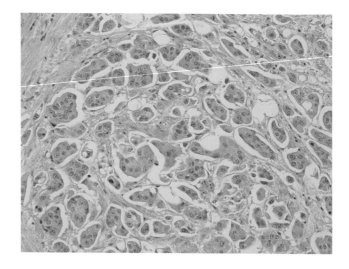

4. A 65-year-old man with an itchy red rash on his right hemiscrotum underwent a biopsy, which is represented in the accompanying photograph. The following are true about this lesion EXCEPT:

   a. Is human papillomavirus (HPV) associated

   b. Can be primary or secondary

   c. Is positive for cytokeratin 7 (CK7)

   d. Is positive for mucins

   e. Can be positive for Her2/neu

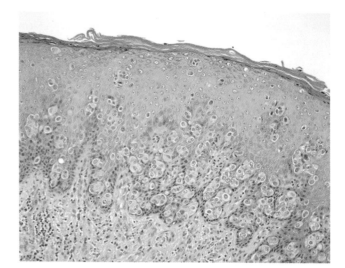

5. A 2-year-old male patient was discovered to have a renal mass while having a physical examination, and subsequently on imaging he had enlarged ipsilateral renal hilar lymph nodes and bone lesions. The mass is represented in the accompanying image. The genetic abnormality seen in this tumor is:

   a. Translocation involving the *MITF/TFE* family of genes

   b. Translocation t(10;17)

   c. Translocation t(12;15)

   d. N-myc amplification

   e. None of the above

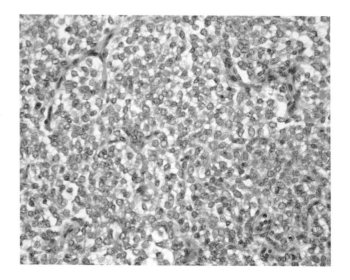

6. A 65-year-old man presents with flank pain and is found to have a right renal mass. The tumor in the image represents a nice example of:

a. Wilms tumor

b. Angiomyolipoma

c. Cellular mesoblastic nephroma

d. Mixed epithelial and stromal tumor

e. Sarcomatoid carcinoma

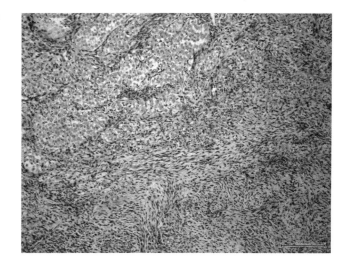

7. A 57-year-old man presents for evaluation of hematuria and is found to have several erythematous lesions in the trigone. Which of the following is the LEAST likely risk factor for the bladder lesion represented in the accompanying image?

a. High-fat diets

b. Radiotherapy to the pelvic region

c. Tobacco smoking

d. Naphthylamine exposure

e. Cyclophosphamide therapy

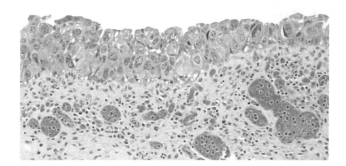

8. A 2.5-year-old female patient was found to have a left-sided suprarenal abdominal mass. Which of the following statements regarding this mass is FALSE?

a. The patient has a biallelic inactivation of *hSNF5/INI1*.

b. The patient has an elevated urine level of vanillylmandelic acid (VMA) and homovanillic acid (HVA).

c. These tumors arise from the sympathetic system.

d. The patient could have systemic hypertension.

e. It is associated with Hirschsprung disease.

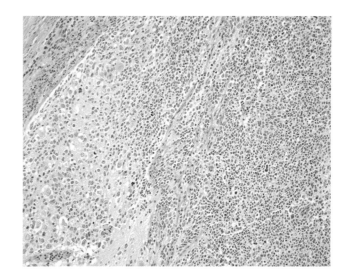

9. A 70-year-old man presents with gross hematuria and a bladder dome mass, represented in the accompanying image. Which immunohistochemical panel favors an adenocarcinoma arising in the bladder versus local extension of a colonic primary?
   a. CK7 negative, CK20 positive, CDX2 positive, β-catenin positive (nuclear)
   b. CK7 positive, CK20 positive, CDX2 positive, β-catenin positive (nuclear)
   c. CK7 positive, CK20 positive, CDX2 positive, p63 negative
   d. CK7 positive, CK20 positive, CDX2 positive, β-catenin positive (cytoplasmic)
   e. None of the above

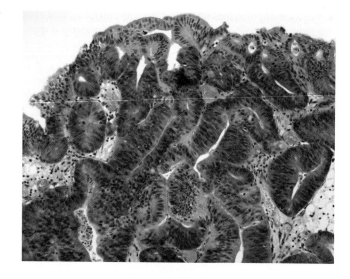

10. This photograph shows the cut surface of a kidney. Which disease is pictured?
    a. Autosomal recessive polycystic kidney disease
    b. Medullary cystic disease
    c. Autosomal dominant polycystic kidney disease
    d. Multilocular cystic nephroma
    e. Cystic renal dysplasia

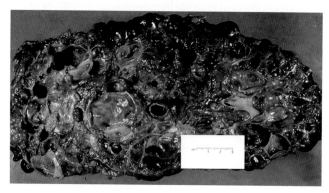

11. This lesion was encountered on transurethral resection of the prostate (TURP). Which of the following is the MOST useful stain expressed by the proliferating cells?
    a. High-molecular-weight keratin (HMWK)
    b. PSA
    c. α-Methylacyl-CoA racemase (AMACR)/P504S
    d. CK7
    e. CK20

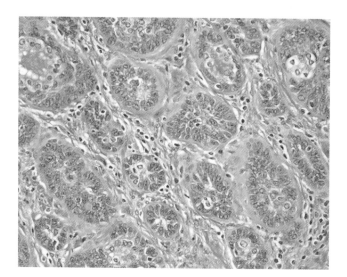

12. This photomicrograph depicts a section of a testicular mass in a healthy 39-year-old man. Which stain is MOST useful in making the correct diagnosis?
    a. CD68
    b. Epithelial membrane antigen (EMA)
    c. CK
    d. Ziehl-Neelsen (acid-fast bacilli)
    e. c-kit (CD117)

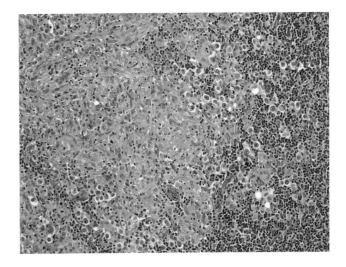

13. This image illustrates a needle biopsy of the prostate in a 78-year-old man with a PSA of 1.2 ng/mL. The CORRECT diagnosis is:
    a. Poorly differentiated adenocarcinoma
    b. Malignant lymphoma
    c. Carcinoma with neuroendocrine features
    d. Basal cell carcinoma
    e. Undifferentiated small cell carcinoma

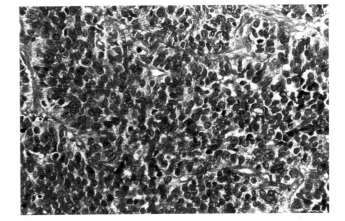

14. A cystoscopic examination of a 62-year-old man, who presented with gross hematuria, identified a 2.0-cm mass in the bladder wall. A partial cystectomy was performed. The histologic findings are seen here. The neoplastic cells are LIKELY to be strongly and diffusely immunoreactive for which of the following?
    a. Pancytokeratin
    b. Chromogranin A
    c. HMB-45
    d. S100 protein
    e. None of the above

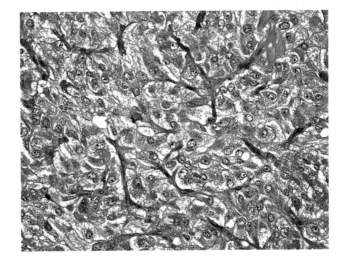

15. This section depicts a biopsy of one of several liver masses in a 21-year-old man with a testicular mass. All of the following statements about this tumor are true EXCEPT:
    a. Most patients present with symptoms related to metastasis.
    b. It occurs in prepubescent boys.
    c. The primary tumor in the testis is often small and may be "burned out."
    d. Metastasis is preferentially, but not exclusively, via the hematogenous route.
    e. Patients with this tumor may present with thyrotoxicosis.

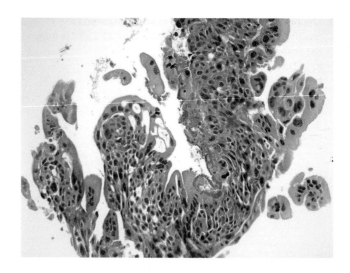

16. This image depicts a section from a prostate biopsy of a 67-year-old man with a PSA value of 0.2 ng/mL. The CORRECT diagnosis is:
    a. Adenocarcinoma
    b. Radiation effect
    c. Androgen ablation effect
    d. Seminal vesicle tissue
    e. Cryotherapy effect

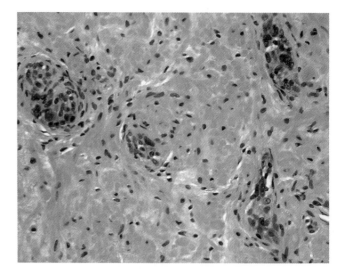

17. This image illustrates a renal mass in a 65-year-old man. Which chromosomal abnormality is MOST often associated with this lesion?
    a. Trisomy 7
    b. TFE-3 translocation
    c. Loss of chromosome 1 and/or the Y chromosome
    d. Loss of short arm of chromosome 3
    e. None of the above

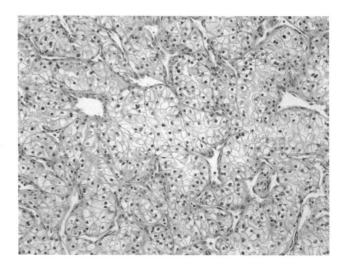

18. This picture shows a renal tumor in a 22-year-old man who presented with back pain. The kidney contained a centrally located brown to tan mass that involved the parenchyma and hilar fat. The diagnosis is:
a. Medullary carcinoma
b. Wilms tumor
c. Sarcomatoid carcinoma
d. Chromophobe carcinoma
e. Clear cell sarcoma

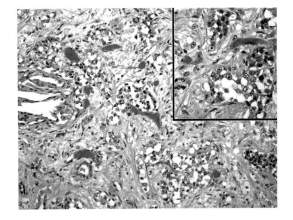

19. All of the following are true about the renal tumor shown in this photomicrograph EXCEPT:
a. The cells contain numerous mitochondria.
b. Focal cytologic atypia characterized by smudgy enlarged hyperchromatic nuclei can occur but does not affect prognosis.
c. The tumor can occur in the setting of Birt-Hogg-Dubé syndrome.
d. The most frequent genetic change is loss of chromosomes 1 and Y.
e. The tumor is derived from cells of the proximal convoluted tubule.

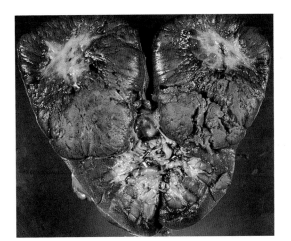

20. Which of the following immunohistochemical stains is MOST useful in the differential diagnosis of the lesion illustrated in this picture?
a. PSA
b. HMWK
c. AMACR
d. Prostatic acid phosphatase (PAP)
e. CK20

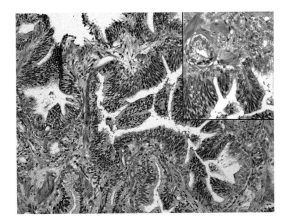

21. A 57-year-old man, who presented with gross hematuria, underwent a cystoscopy. A polypoid mass was noted in the prostatic urethra, and resected. A representative field is depicted in this image. What is the diagnosis?
a. Prostatic ductal (endometrioid) carcinoma
b. Nephrogenic adenoma
c. Hyperplastic prostatic polyp
d. Papillary urothelial carcinoma, low grade
e. Caruncle

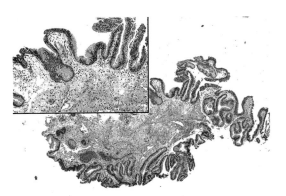

22. This picture demonstrates the nephrectomy specimen of a 2-month-old boy, who had a large, palpable abdominal mass. All of the following statements are true about this tumor EXCEPT:
    a. This is the most common renal neoplasm in infants less than 3 months old.
    b. The tumor typically has infiltrating edges, and interdigitates with, and incorporates, renal parenchyma.
    c. The tumor is associated with polyhydramnios.
    d. The tumor displays a t(12;15)(p13;q25) chromosome translocation.
    e. Widespread metastases are common.

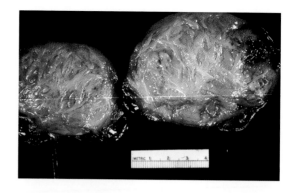

23. A 68-year-old man presented to his physician with hematuria and symptoms of urinary retention. The patient's digital rectal examination was remarkable for an enlarged prostate, and his serum PSA level was moderately elevated. The image shows a representative field of the patient's TURP. The CORRECT diagnosis is:
    a. Squamous cell carcinoma of prostatic urethra
    b. Squamous cell carcinoma of the prostate
    c. Radiated prostate
    d. Infarct of the prostate
    e. Benign hyperplasia of the prostate

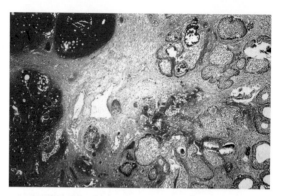

24. An 18-year-old pregnant woman suffered from preeclampsia and HELLP (hemolytic anemia, elevated liver enzymes, and low platelets) syndrome, which led to the termination of her pregnancy. Her medical history was remarkable for systemic hypertension since age 14. She was also noted to have an enhancing renal mass on computed tomographic examination of her abdomen with intravenous contrast material. She then underwent a radical nephrectomy. The photomicrographs are obtained from the removed kidney. Which statement is NOT correct?
    a. The overwhelming majority of these tumors are benign lesions.
    b. Most patients have hypertension, hypoaldosteronism, and hypokalemia.
    c. The cells of almost all described tumors express renin and the majority of tumors are vimentin positive, as well as focally α-smooth muscle actin positive.
    d. Tumor resection is curative, and usually ceases the patient's hypertension.
    e. Ultrastructural study reveals characteristic membrane-bound rhomboid crystals.

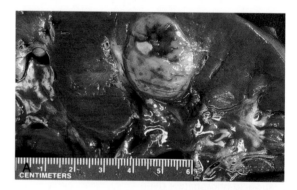

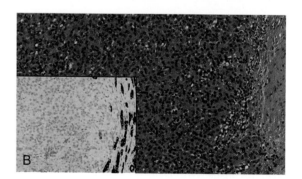

25. A 56-year-old woman presented to her physician complaining of urinary frequency, urgency, and pain. She was referred to a urologist, who performed a urine culture, a cystoscopic examination, and a bladder biopsy. The urologist concluded that the patient had interstitial cystitis. Which of the following statements is TRUE?
    a. The bladder biopsy showed increased numbers of eosinophils in all bladder layers, including lamina propria and muscularis propria.
    b. This condition has an infectious cause.
    c. The diagnosis is one of exclusion.
    d. The bladder biopsy shows a characteristic perivascular infiltrate of plasma cells.
    e. These patients typically have an increased bladder capacity.

26. The following are true of granulosa cell tumor, juvenile type, EXCEPT:
    a. Positive for CK
    b. Associated with X/XY mosaicism
    c. Congenital
    d. Mitotically active
    e. Associated with isochromosome 12p

27. All of the following are true in von Hippel-Lindau (vHL) syndrome patients EXCEPT:
    a. It is associated with pancreatic islet cell tumors.
    b. It is inherited in an autosomal recessive manner with age-dependent penetrance.
    c. Renal tumors occur at a younger age group than sporadic renal cell carcinoma and can be bilateral and multifocal.
    d. It is associated with the presence of retinal and central nervous system hemangioblastoma.
    e. It is characterized by mutations in the vHL gene located on the short arm of chromosome 3.

28. Klinefelter syndrome is characterized by all of the following EXCEPT:
    a. A karyotype of 47XXY
    b. Elevated serum follicle-stimulating hormone (FSH) and luteinizing hormone (LH) levels
    c. Increased risk of germ cell tumors
    d. Increased risk of breast carcinoma
    e. Sclerosis of the seminiferous tubules and Leydig cell nodules

29. Immunohistochemical markers can be useful in establishing the diagnosis of a metastatic prostatic adenocarcinoma. Which of the following statements is TRUE?
    a. Racemase positivity can be used to establish a primary prostatic origin.
    b. PSA is expressed in equal proportions in well-differentiated and poorly differentiated prostatic adenocarcinoma.
    c. PSA is a prostate-specific marker that is not expressed in other carcinomas.
    d. Polyclonal PSA is equally specific and more sensitive than monoclonal PSA.
    e. None of the above

30. All of the following are poor prognostic indicators in neuroblastoma, EXCEPT:
    a. MYCN amplification
    b. A mitosis-karyorrhexis index (MKI) of more than 200
    c. Age at diagnosis of more than 2 years
    d. 1 p deletion in children younger than 1 year of age
    e. A serum ferritin level of less than 150 ng/mL

31. TMPRSS2-ERG gene rearrangement has been recently described in prostate adenocarcinoma. The following statements are true, EXCEPT:
    a. The TMPRSS2-ERG rearrangement is reported to be present in approximately half of primary prostate tumors, detected by PSA screening, and treated with radical prostatectomy.
    b. The TMPRSS2-ERG gene rearrangement is a functional rearrangement that produces an aberrant androgen-regulated expression of the ERG protein.
    c. The TMPRSS2 gene is located on the short arm of chromosome 21, and the ERG gene is located on the long arm of chromosome 21.
    d. The impact of the TMPRSS2-ERG gene rearrangement on prognosis is still controversial.
    e. TMPRSS2-ERG gene rearrangement might be associated with prostate cancer progression.

32. Which of the following is NOT a feature of adrenocortical carcinoma?
    a. A mitotic rate of more than 5 per 50 high-power fields
    b. The presence of less than 25% of clear cells
    c. A slight female predominance
    d. Necrosis
    e. Absence of symptoms of hormone overproduction

33. A 65-year-old man with a previous history of flat urothelial carcinoma in situ presents to the urologist for follow-up after bacillus Calmette-Guérin (BCG) therapy. Follow-up cytologic finding was equivocal and the urologist performed a fluorescence in situ hybridization (FISH) study on his urine. Which of the following statements regarding this FISH study is FALSE?
    a. The test is FDA (Food and Drug Administration) approved for patients with a family history of bladder carcinoma.
    b. The FISH test includes probes for chromosome 3, 7, 17, and 9p21.
    c. The test is FDA approved for follow-up of patients with a history of urothelial carcinoma.
    d. Low-grade papillary tumors usually demonstrate homozygous 9p21 loss.
    e. The test is FDA approved for patients with hematuria.

34. A 72-year-old man with a history of prostatic adenocarcinoma presents with a bladder mass. Which of the following findings is diagnostic of urothelial carcinoma?
    a. The presence of a monotonous population of malignant cells with prominent nucleoli
    b. Negative PSA immunostain
    c. Negative CK7 and CK20 immunohistochemical stains
    d. Positive p63 and HMWK
    e. Squamous differentiation

35. In the clinical scenario of a renal mass, PAX-8 immunostain is usually positive in the following EXCEPT:
    a. Conventional clear cell renal cell carcinoma
    b. Wilms tumor
    c. Renal oncocytoma
    d. Urothelial carcinoma
    e. Collecting duct carcinoma

36. Which of the following is NOT a risk factor for the development of squamous cell carcinoma of the bladder?
    a. Schistosoma infection
    b. Bladder stones

c. Keratinizing squamous metaplasia of the urothelium

d. Indwelling catheter

e. Nonkeratinizing squamous metaplasia of the bladder trigone

37. All of the following statements are true about prostatic ductal adenocarcinoma (endometrioid) EXCEPT:
    a. This carcinoma is derived from müllerian remnants in the prostatic utricle.
    b. Serum levels of PSA are elevated only minimally or not at all.
    c. The neoplastic cells show immunoreactivity for PSA.
    d. Patients often present with hematuria, and the clinical differential diagnosis includes urothelial carcinoma.
    e. The exophytic component of these tumors is composed of tall columnar cells arranged in complex papillary formations.

38. Which of the following profiles is the typical immunophenotype for embryonal carcinoma of the testis?
    a. PLAP positive, CK positive, EMA negative, OCT3/4 negative, and CD30 negative
    b. PLAP negative, CK positive, EMA negative, OCT3/4 negative, and CD30 positive
    c. PLAP positive, CK positive, EMA negative, OCT3/4 positive, and CD30 positive
    d. PLAP negative, CK negative, EMA positive, OCT3/4 negative, and CD30 negative
    e. None of the above

39. Which of the following primary testicular neoplasms is NOT considered to be a teratoma?
    a. Dermoid cyst
    b. Carcinoid tumor
    c. PNET (primitive neuroectodermal tumor)
    d. Epidermoid cyst
    e. Diffuse embryoma

40. Which specific testicular neoplasm is associated with Carney syndrome?
    a. Sclerosing Sertoli cell tumor
    b. Large cell calcifying Sertoli cell tumor
    c. Granulosa cell tumor
    d. Sertoli-Leydig cell tumor
    e. Gonadal stromal fibroma

41. Which of the following renal neoplasms is often associated with polycythemia?
    a. Nephroblastoma (Wilms tumor)
    b. Metanephric adenoma
    c. Oncocytoma
    d. Clear cell sarcoma
    e. Rhabdoid tumor

42. Which of the following microscopic features is considered diagnostic of unfavorable histologic finding in a Wilms tumor?
    a. Predominance of blastemal element
    b. Presence of diffuse anaplasia
    c. Presence of a rhabdomyomatous stromal component
    d. Presence of perilobar nephrogenic rests
    e. All of the above

43. Metastatic carcinoma to the penis from another primary site is uncommon. Which of the following primary sites is the MOST common source of metastasis to the penis?
    a. Testis
    b. Kidney

c. Lung

d. Prostate

e. Rectum

44. Which is the MOST common malignant paratesticular tumor of childhood?
    a. Liposarcoma
    b. Sarcoma botryoides
    c. Malignant fibrous histiocytoma
    d. Alveolar rhabdomyosarcoma
    e. Spindle cell variant of embryonal rhabdomyosarcoma

45. Which histologic variant of penile squamous cell carcinoma is the MOST aggressive?
    a. Verrucous carcinoma
    b. Basaloid carcinoma
    c. Condylomatous carcinoma
    d. Papillary carcinoma
    e. Bowenoid carcinoma

46. Malignant melanoma rarely occurs primarily in the urinary tract. At which site is primary malignant melanoma MOST common?
    a. Bladder trigone
    b. Bladder neck
    c. Urethral mucosa
    d. Kidney
    e. None of the above

47. Which is the MOST common testicular germ cell tumor in the prepubertal age group?
    a. Malignant mixed germ cell tumor
    b. Mature teratoma
    c. Embryonal carcinoma
    d. Yolk sac tumor
    e. Sertoli cell tumor

48. The finding of which of the following components in a testicular germ cell tumor results in a poorer prognosis?
    a. PNET
    b. Syncytiotrophoblastic giant cells
    c. Skeletal muscle differentiation
    d. Immature glial tissue
    e. Cytotrophoblastic cells

49. Which is the MOST frequent testicular tumor occurring in patients with dysgenetic gonads or an intersex syndrome?
    a. Gonadal sex-cord stromal tumor
    b. Stromal fibroma
    c. Granulosa cell tumor, adult type
    d. Polyembryoma
    e. Gondoblastoma

50. Which of the following histologic subtypes of prostate carcinoma is positive for PSA?
    a. Signet ring carcinoma
    b. Mucinous carcinoma
    c. Adenocarcinoma with paneth-cell-like neuroendocrine differentiation
    d. Ductal adenocarcinoma
    e. All of the above

Answers

1. c. Oncocytomas are benign renal tumors characterized by a mahogany brown gross appearance, often with a central scar. A small percentage of oncoctyomas exhibit worrisome histologic features, such as perinephric fat infiltration and vascular invasion; however, despite these findings, oncocytomas maintain an excellent prognosis and are considered benign tumors. Histologically they show oncocytic cytoplasm with small round nuclei and nucleoli, characteristic of oncocytes. Immunohistochemically, they show rare cell positivity for CK7, a feature that distinguishes them from the eosinophilic variant of chromophobe renal cell carcinoma. On electron microscopy, numerous mitochondria are present in the cytoplasm with lamellar cristae.

Amin MB, Crotty TB, Tickoo SK, Farrow GM: Renal oncocytoma: a reappraisal of morphologic features with clinicopathologic findings in 80 cases. *Am J Surg Pathol* 1997;21(1):1-12.

Carvalho JC, Wasco MJ, Kunju LP, et al: Cluster analysis of immunohistochemical profiles delineates CK7, vimentin, S100A1 and C-kit (CD117) as an optimal panel in the differential diagnosis of renal oncocytoma from its mimics. *Histopathology* 2011;58(2):169-179.

2. c. This is an example of intraductal carcinoma, characterized by complex cribriforming architecture and marked nuclear pleomorphism. The lesion depicted in the accompanying photomicrograph is architecturally more complex than HGPIN. The accompanying p63 immunostain highlights the intraductal nature with preservation of the surrounding basal cells. Ductal adenocarcinoma is an invasive adenocarcinoma and is characterized by an infiltrative architecture and the absence of a basal cell layer. Seminal vesicle epithelium usually shows coarse golden brown pigment and an orderly arborizing and branching architecture. Nuclear pleomorphism can be present but is often degenerative in quality. Invasive rectal adenocarcinoma is characterized by infiltrating irregular glandular structures, composed of columnar cells with pencil-shaped nuclei and accompanied by extensive "dirty" necrosis.

Guo CC, Epstein JI: Intraductal carcinoma of the prostate on needle biopsy: histologic features and clinical significance. *Mod Pathol* 2006;19(12):1528-1535. Epub 2006 Sep 15.

Robinson BD, Epstein JI: Intraductal carcinoma of the prostate without invasive carcinoma on needle biopsy: emphasis on radical prostatectomy findings. *J Urol* 2010;184(4):1328-1333. Epub 2010 Aug 17.

3. c. Micropapillary variant of invasive urothelial carcinoma is associated with a high pathologic stage and has a propensity for lymph node metastases due to the presence of a high rate of lymphovascular invasion. The classical morphologic features that prompt the diagnosis of invasive micropapillary carcinoma include nuclear pleomorphism, small tumor nests devoid of fibrovascular cores, back-to-back retraction spaces, multiple small nests within a space or lacunae, ring forms or intracytoplasmic vacuolization, and reverse polarity of the nuclei. The highly aggressive behavior attributed to this subtype of urothelial carcinoma has led some institutions to aggressively treat with radical cystectomy irrespective of the presence or absence of documented muscularis propria invasion. Therefore, it is important to use strict criteria for the diagnosis of micropapillary carcinoma. Unfortunately, the morphologic spectrum of micropapillary carcinoma is not well established yet. The noninvasive counterpart of micropapillary carcinoma exists and is characterized by filiform projections into the lumen of neoplastic cells without fibrovascular cores. The significance of this subtype of noninvasive urothelial carcinoma is controversial and published studies supporting, as well as negating, an aggressive behavior can be found. Because of the lack of consensus on the prognostic significance of such a diagnosis, and the presence of a highly aggressive behavior associated with the invasive form of micropapillary carcinoma, surgical reports should clearly state whether the micropapillary component is invasive or noninvasive.

Amin MB, Ro JY, el-Sharkawy T, et al: Micropapillary variant of transitional cell carcinoma of the urinary bladder. Histologic pattern resembling ovarian papillary serous carcinoma. *Am J Surg Pathol* 1994;18(12):1224-1232.

Sangoi AR, Beck AH, Amin MB, et al: Interobserver reproducibility in the diagnosis of invasive micropapillary carcinoma of the urinary tract among urologic pathologists. *Am J Surg Pathol* 2010;34(9):1367-1376.

Watts KE, Hansel DE: Emerging concepts in micropapillary urothelial carcinoma. *Adv Anat Pathol* 2010;17(3):182-186.

4. a. There is no known association between extramammary Paget disease (EM-PD) and HPV. EM-PD involving the male genitalia, usually penile or scrotal, is classified as primary or secondary. Primary Paget disease arises either as an epidermal lesion, which could extend along adnexal structures and have the possibility of invading into the underlying dermis, or in association with an underlying sweat gland carcinoma. Secondary Paget disease represents involvement of the epidermis by an adjacent carcinoma, which in those locations usually originates from the urethra or bladder. Immunohistochemically they can stain positive for EMA, CEA, CK19, CK7, and GCDFP15. Her2/neu gene amplification can be present and might be of importance therapeutically.

Liegl B, Leibl S, Gogg-Kamerer M, et al: Mammary and extramammary Paget's disease: an immunohistochemical study of 83 cases. *Histopathology* 2007;50(4):439-447.

Mitsudo S, Nakanishi I, Koss LG: Paget's disease of the penis and adjacent skin: its association with fatal sweat gland carcinoma. *Arch Pathol Lab Med* 1981;105(10):518-520.

Tanskanen M, Jahkola T, Asko-Seljavaara S, et al: HER2 oncogene amplification in extramammary Paget's disease. *Histopathology* 2003;42(6):575-579.

Zhang N, Gong K, Zhang X, et al: Extramammary Paget's disease of scrotum—report of 25 cases and literature review. *Urol Oncol* 2010;28(1):28-33. Epub 2008 Sep 21.

5. b. Clear cell sarcoma is composed of sheets of neoplastic cells with indistinct cell borders, vesicular nuclei, and inconspicuous nucleoli, separated by a "chicken-wire" network of delicate vessels. Recently, a new translocation, the t(10;17), was discovered in clear cell sarcoma. This finding could be useful diagnostically, and possibly therapeutically, through future targeted drug therapy. The MITF/TFE family of genes is involved in translocation-associated renal cell carcinoma, and is not present in clear cell sarcoma. Histologically, translocation-associated renal cell carcinomas have large bulbous clear cytoplasm and a variable architecture, including papillary projections. Clear cell sarcoma, interestingly, gets its name due to the clear spaces surrounding the cells that are filled with mucopolysaccharides, rather than a clear cytoplasm. t(12;15) is seen in the cellular variant of mesoblastic nephroma. The cellular variant of mesoblastic nephroma can look epithelioid and mimic clear cell sarcoma; however, the chicken-wire vasculature of clear cell sarcoma, as well as the enlarged lymph nodes and bone lesions, reflective of the aggressive nature of clear cell sarcoma, give away the correct diagnosis. N-myc amplification is present in neuroblastoma and imparts a poor prognosis.

Argani P, Perlman EJ, Breslow NE, et al: Clear cell sarcoma of the kidney: a review of 351 cases from the National Wilms Tumor Study Group Pathology Center. *Am J Surg Pathol* 2000;24(1):4-18.

O'Meara E, Stack D, Lee CH, et al: Characterization of the chromosomal translocation t(10;17)(q22;p13) in clear cell sarcoma of kidney. *J Pathol* 2012;227(1):72-80. Epub 2012 Feb 17.

6. e. The figure shows a dual population: the first population consists of epithelioid cells with eosinophilic cytoplasm, high Fuhrman nuclear grade, and rhabdoid features suggestive of a high-grade renal cell carcinoma. This component is intermixed with a population of spindle cells arranged in fascicles and intimately associated with the epithelioid component, compatible with sarcomatoid renal cell carcinoma. Any subtype of renal cell carcinoma can give rise to sarcomatoid carcinoma. It is diagnostically satisfying to be able to demonstrate areas of transition between the epithelial and the sarcomatoid components.

Cheville JC, Lohse CM, Zincke H, et al: Sarcomatoid renal cell carcinoma: an examination of underlying histologic subtype and an analysis of associations with patient outcome. *Am J Surg Pathol* 2004;28(4):435-441.

de Peralta-Venturina M, Moch H, Amin M, et al: Sarcomatoid differentiation in renal cell carcinoma: a study of 101 cases. *Am J Surg Pathol* 2001;25(3):275-284.

7. a. Although some studies suggest that diets rich in fat cause bladder carcinoma, this causal relationship has not been unequivocally established like the other risk factors enumerated next. The bladder lies in the field of irradiation during treatment for prostatic or cervical carcinoma. Radiotherapy is a known risk factor for bladder carcinoma. Smoking is a common risk factor for many types of carcinoma, and has a strong association with urothelial carcinoma. Chemical occupational exposure to aromatic amines, including benzidines and naphthylamines, is associated with the development of bladder carcinoma, as is *Schistosoma hematobium* infection, which is primarily associated with squamous cell carcinoma and urothelial carcinoma. In addition, cyclophosphamide therapy is associated with a higher risk of developing urothelial carcinoma.

Johansson SL, Cohen SM: Epidemiology and etiology of bladder cancer. *Semin Surg Oncol* 1997;13(5):291-298.

Kaufman DS, Shipley WU, Feldman AS: Bladder cancer. *Lancet* 2009;374(9685):239-249. Epub 2009 Jun 10.

8. a. Biallelic inactivation of *hSNF5/INI1* is a molecular alteration that is seen in rhabdoid tumors of the kidney, which are histologically distinct from neuroblastoma. This image represents a section from this adrenal mass in a 2.5-year-old girl showing a neuroblastoma with varying degrees of maturation, present side by side. The neuroblastoma on the left is a differentiating stroma-poor neuroblastoma with abundant neuropil, and extensive ganglionic differentiation, which should provide the clue to the diagnosis. The component on the right features relatively little neuropil and is compatible with a poorly differentiated neuroblastoma.

Shimada H, Ambros IM, Dehner LP, et al: Terminology and morphologic criteria of neuroblastic tumors: recommendations by the International Neuroblastoma Pathology Committee. *Cancer* 1999;86(2):349-363.

Shimada H, Ambros IM, Dehner LP, et al: The International Neuroblastoma Pathology Classification (the Shimada system). *Cancer* 1999;86(2):364-372.

9. d. CK7 positive, CK20 positive, CDX2 positive, and β-catenin positive (cytoplasmic) immunoprofile is compatible with a bladder primary site. β-Catenin usually shows nuclear expression in colonic adenocarcinoma and is negative or shows cytoplasmic expression in bladder primary tumors. CK7 negative, CK20 positive, CDX2 positive, and β-catenin positive (nuclear) is more typical of colonic adenocarcinoma. CK7 positive, CK20 positive, CDX2 positive, and β-catenin positive (nuclear): Can also be seen in colonic adenocarcinoma, although CK7 positivity is unusual and present in a small percentage of colonic adenocarcinoma. Double expression of CK7 and CK20 is more commonly seen in urothelial primaries; however, the nuclear β-catenin stain favors a colonic adenocarcinoma. CK7 positive, CK20 positive, CDX2 positive, and p63 negative does not distinguish between a colonic versus a bladder enteric type adenocarcinoma; p63 negativity does not favor a colonic primary site, and the remaining positive stains can be seen in both types of adenocarcinoma.

Wang HL, Lu DW, Yerian LM, et al: Immunohistochemical distinction between primary adenocarcinoma of the bladder and secondary colorectal adenocarcinoma. *Am J Surg Pathol* 2001;25(11):1380-1387.

Zaghloul MS, Nouh A, Nazmy M, et al: Long-term results of primary adenocarcinoma of the urinary bladder: a report on 192 patients. *Urol Oncol* 2006;24(1):13-20.

10. c. This is the classic appearance of autosomal dominant polycystic kidney disease, formerly referred to as "adult polycystic kidney disease." The kidney is enlarged, often massively so, but retains a reniform shape. The cysts range in size from a fraction of a millimeter to several centimeters. Microdissection studies have demonstrated that the cysts arise in all parts of the nephron; this has been confirmed by lectin binding studies. In a given kidney, only about 20% of the nephrons are involved, and the kidneys increase in size owing to enlargement of the cysts, rather than development of new cysts. Autosomal dominant polycystic kidney disease is the most common cystic renal disease and the most common genetically transmitted disease. It is the third to fourth leading cause of end-stage renal disease, and patients with this disease make up 5% to 10% of dialysis patients. The disease is mostly caused by mutations in *PKD1* on chromosome 16p13.3. Most of the remaining cases have mutations in *PKD2* on chromosome 4q21, and in general show delayed onset of presentation and a slightly milder course. The disease is also associated with polycystic liver disease, intracranial berry aneurysms, and subarachnoid hemorrhage, as well as cardiac valve abnormalities. Autosomal recessive polycystic kidney disease affects neonates. The kidneys are massively enlarged. The cysts correspond to dilated collecting ducts, and have a distinctive linear radiating appearance. In medullary cystic disease, the kidneys are usually small, and the cysts are confined to the medulla. Cystic nephroma is a neoplasm consisting of a cystic mass growing in an otherwise unremarkable kidney. Cystic renal dysplasia usually has a "bunch of grapes" appearance.

D'Agati V, Trudel M: Lectin characterization of cystogenesis in the SBM transgenic model of polycystic kidney disease. *J Am Soc Nephrol* 1992;3:975-983.

11. a. Basal cells of the prostate express HMWK and p63, and therefore HMWK is the most useful stain to make the correct diagnosis. Rare residual luminal cells are the clue to the diagnosis. Basal cell hyperplasia is a benign proliferation of basal cells that can be seen in 10% of the prostates. It is seen usually as part of benign prostatic hyperplasia (BPH) of the transition zone, and can be especially prominent in chronically inflamed prostates. It is defined by the presence of more than one layer of basal cells. Several patterns of basal cell hyperplasia can be seen and are defined as usual basal cell hyperplasia, atypical basal cell hyperplasia, atrophy-associated basal cell hyperplasia, and adenoid cysticlike hyperplasia. Atypical basal cell hyperplasia is defined as basal cell hyperplasia with prominent nucleoli. Atrophy-associated basal cell hyperplasia is seen following therapy for prostatic adenocarcinoma, particularly hormonal therapy. Adenoid cysticlike hyperplasia is a very rare form of hyperplasia characterized by a cribriform architecture, resembling adenoid cystic carcinoma.

Cleary KR, Choi HY, Ayala AG: Basal cell hyperplasia of the prostate. *Am J Clin Pathol* 1983;80(6):850-854.

Hosler GA, Epstein JI: Basal cell hyperplasia: an unusual diagnostic dilemma on prostate needle biopsies. *Hum Pathol* 2005;36(5): 480-485.

12. e. Seminoma cells show strong positive staining for c-kit (CD117). Therefore, of the choices listed here, c-kit is the most useful stain in making the correct diagnosis. The histiocytes will be positive for CD68; however, this finding provides no useful information toward the diagnosis. Seminoma cells do not stain for EMA. Although seminoma cells may show focal, weak, often dotlike staining for CK, the staining is far less impressive than the staining for c-kit. A negative CK would not exclude the diagnosis of seminoma. Ziehl-Neelsen is a stain for acid-fast bacilli. No matter the findings, this stain would not lead to the diagnosis. Nonneoplastic granulomatous masses, infectious and noninfectious, do occur in the testis. Generous sampling of such masses is critical, because brisk granulomatous inflammation can obscure the neoplastic seminoma cells. Seminoma constitutes 50% of germ cell tumors in patients around the age of 40. Patients with seminoma present at a slightly older age than patients with mixed germ cell tumors. Serum PLAP can be elevated, and minimal elevation

of serum β-human chorionic gonadotropin (hCG) can be present, owing to production by the scattered syncytiotrophoblastic cells, commonly seen in seminoma. It is important to distinguish seminomatous versus nonseminomatous tumors because of the extreme sensitivity of seminoma to radiation treatment and chemotherapy. The prognosis of seminomatous tumors depends on the stage at presentation. They usually have a good prognosis with cure rates above 95%.

Natali PG, Nicotra MR, Sures I, et al: Expression of c-kit receptor in normal and transformed human nonlymphoid tissues. *Cancer Res* 1992;52:6139-6143.

13. e. This is an undifferentiated small cell carcinoma. Small cell carcinoma of the prostate is characterized by sheets of small cells with high nucleus-to-cytoplasm ratio, imparting a low-power bluish look. Nuclear molding is seen and the chromatin is usually granular. Necrosis and mitoses are readily seen. Poorly differentiated prostatic adenocarcinoma is usually a mixture of Gleason grades 4 and 5, and although it could have necrosis and mitoses, they are not usually as extensive as in small cell carcinoma. In addition, as is typical, the PSA level in this patient is not elevated, unlike a big percentage of poorly differentiated prostatic adenocarcinomas that express PSA. Lymphoma comes in the differential diagnosis when the tumors are sheetlike and are discohesive. The features of the tumor in this photomicrograph support an epithelial malignancy. In practice, this differential diagnosis can be resolved through immunohistochemical stains for hematopoietic and epithelial markers, although one should keep in mind that pancytokeratin shows a dotlike pattern in small cell carcinoma, compared to the diffuse pattern in poorly differentiated adenocarcinoma of the prostate. Many prostatic adenocarcinomas, especially poorly differentiated adenocarcinomas, show positive staining for neuroendocrine markers. These tumors should be distinguished from classic undifferentiated small cell carcinoma because of therapeutic differences. Basal cell carcinomas of the prostate are extremely rare and are characterized by sharply outlined nests of basal cells. These tumors are PSA negative, but the cells do express the antigens typical of prostatic basal cells, most commonly p63 and HMWK.

Wang W, Epstein JI: Small cell carcinoma of the prostate. A morphologic and immunohistochemical study of 95 cases. *Am J Surg Pathol* 2008;32(1):65-71.

Yao JL, Madeb R, Bourne P, et al: Small cell carcinoma of the prostate: an immunohistochemical study. *Am J Surg Pathol* 2006;30(6):705-712.

14. b. This image shows an example of a paraganglioma, which is strongly and diffusely positive for neuroendocrine markers including chromogranin. Paragangliomas are negative for CK, although rare reports of CK positivity have been reported. The neoplastic cells are negative for HMB45. HMB45 is positive in melanocytic tumors, as well as perivascular epithelioid cell tumors (PEComas). Scattered cells show positive staining for S100 protein; these are the sustentacular cells, which are an integral part of the tumor. Paragangliomas of the bladder are rare tumors, which usually occur in young adult women. The clinical symptoms include hypertension and hematuria. Histologically they are composed of large polygonal cells with eosinophilic granular cytoplasm, arranged in nests of cells with surrounding vasculature referred to as Zellballen pattern. There is often marked variability in nuclear size; however, mitotic figures and necrosis are not seen in the majority of cases. Although these tumors behave mainly in a benign fashion, they could have an infiltrative growth pattern, and usually involve the muscular wall. Clues to the true nature include the prominent vascularity and the abundant cytoplasm. Similar to pheochromocytoma of the adrenal gland, there are no reliable histologic markers to determine benignity versus malignancy except proof of metastases. Studies have suggested that a pathologic stage of T3 or greater is associated with a higher rate of recurrence or metastases. Because paragangliomas of the bladder are treated with conservative local excision, it is critical not to overdiagnose a paraganglioma as an invasive carcinoma.

Cheng L, Leibovich BC, Cheville JC, et al: Paraganglioma of the urinary bladder: can biologic potential be predicted? *Cancer* 2000;88:844-852.
Somasundar P, Krouse R, Hostetter R, et al: Paragangliomas— a decade of clinical experience. *J Surg Oncol* 2000;74:286-290.

15. b. This photomicrograph depicts choriocarcinoma; note the two cell types (syncytiotrophoblasts intermingled with cytotrophoblasts). Presenting symptoms are often related to metastatic tumor and include local symptoms, such as bleeding and gynecomastia, due to production of β-hCG. The primary tumor in the testis is often small and may go unnoticed. Spontaneous regression of germ cell tumors is a well-known phenomenon that could occur in the setting of germ cell tumors of the testes. The histologic findings are the presence of a distinct scar, characterized by fibrosis with increased vascularity, lymphoplasmacytic inflammation, and calcification. The neoplastic cells have a tropism for blood vessels and, thus, enter the vascular system early in tumor development. Thyrotoxicosis can be a presenting symptom and is thought to be due to cross-reactivity of hCG with thyroid-stimulating hormone (TSH). Choriocarcinoma does not occur in the prepubertal testis. The only two germ cell tumors in that age group are yolk sac tumor and teratoma.

Goodarzi MO, Van Herle AJ: Thyrotoxicosis in a male patient associated with excess human chorionic gonadotropin production by germ cell tumor. *Thyroid* 2000;10:611-619.
Ulbright TM: Germ cell neoplasms of the testis. *Am J Surg Pathol* 1993;17(11):1075-1091.

16. b. This is the characteristic appearance of radiated prostate. The stroma is fibrotic. The epithelial component is involuted and fairly inconspicuous. The branching ductal structures have a basal cell layer and luminal cell layer. The cells can be highly atypical. Characteristically, their nuclei are large, with degenerative atypia and maintained normal nucleus-to-cytoplasm ratio. Against the diagnosis of adenocarcinoma are the lack of an infiltrative pattern and the presence of a basal cell layer. Androgen ablation results in a more atrophic appearance of the epithelial cells, with the presence of decreased cytoplasm, which has a clear quality. This field does not have the typical architecture of seminal vesicle tissue, and the typical golden brown lipofuscin pigment is absent. Following cryotherapy, the epithelial component is essentially eradicated, and the stroma has an elastotic or necrotic appearance.

Bostwick DG, Egbert BM, Fajardo LF: Radiation injury of the normal and neoplastic prostate. *Am J Surg Pathol* 1982;6(6): 541-551.
Magi-Galluzzi C, Sanderson H, Epstein JI: Atypia in nonneoplastic prostate glands after radiotherapy for prostate cancer: duration of atypia and relation to type of radiotherapy. *Am J Surg Pathol* 2003;27(2):206-212.

17. d. This image shows clear cell renal cell carcinoma (conventional), which is composed of nests of clear cells surrounded by a delicate branching fibrovascular network. The most consistent chromosomal abnormality in clear cell renal cell carcinoma is the loss of the short arm of chromosome 3. Loss of chromosome 1 and the Y chromosome are features of renal oncocytoma and chromophobe renal cell carcinoma. Trisomy 7 and 17 are associated with papillary renal cell carcinoma, and TFE3 translocations are associated with translocation associated renal cell carcinoma.

Amin MB, Tamboli P, Javidan J, et al: Prognostic impact of histologic subtyping of adult renal epithelial neoplasms: an experience of 405 cases. *Am J Surg Pathol* 2002;26(3): 281-291.
Nese N, Paner GP, Mallin K, et al: Renal cell carcinoma: assessment of key pathologic prognostic parameters and patient characteristics in 47,909 cases using the National Cancer Data Base. *Ann Diagn Pathol* 2009;13(1):1-8. Epub 2008 Dec 12.
Tickoo SK, Gopalan A: Pathologic features of renal cortical tumors. *Urol Clin North Am* 2008;35(4):551-561.

18. a. This image represents renal medullary carcinoma. The microcystic or reticular growth pattern and fibromyxoid stroma are characteristic features. The cells are cytologically atypical (i.e., pleomorphic, with hyperchromatic nuclei) and are arranged in solid nests and cords. Renal medullary carcinoma is thought to arise from the distal portion of the collecting duct, and may have a relationship to collecting duct carcinoma. Renal medullary carcinoma is an uncommon highly aggressive carcinoma usually seen in young patients with the sickle cell trait. The age at presentation is between 5 and 39 years old, and it is more common in males. Most patients have metastatic disease at the time of presentation. It arises in the medulla and can show several architectural patterns histologically including solid, reticular, cribriform, and tubular. It is usually accompanied by a marked inflammatory infiltrate and a characteristic desmoplastic reaction. The differential diagnosis includes urothelial carcinoma arising from the renal pelvis. The presence of urothelial carcinoma in situ favors urothelial carcinoma; however, on needle core biopsy, a panel of immunohistochemical stains, including PAX-2, PAX-8, p63, and HMWK, is helpful. PAX-2 and PAX-8 are positive in renal cell carcinoma, including collecting duct and medullary carcinomas, whereas urothelial carcinoma is typically positive for p63 and HMWK. In addition, the presence of divergent differentiation, such as squamous differentiation, supports a urothelial carcinoma.

Adsay NV, deRoux SJ, Sakr W, Grignon D: Cancer as a marker of genetic medical disease: an unusual case of medullary carcinoma of the kidney. *Am J Surg Pathol* 1998;22:260-264.
Davis CJ Jr, Mostofi FK, Sesterhenn IA: Renal medullary carcinoma. The seventh sickle cell nephropathy. *Am J Surg Pathol* 1995;19(1):1-11.

19. e. This is a renal oncocytoma. Cells with granular oncocytic cytoplasm usually have a large number of mitochondria. Renal oncocytoma can have focal degenerative atypia characterized by hyperchromasia and pleomorphism, as well as smudgy chromatin. These nuclear changes are thought to be related to anoxia, and have no impact on tumor behavior. Rare cases of renal oncocytoma are familial and arise in association with the Birt-Hogg-Dubé syndrome. Renal oncocytomas are frequently associated with loss of chromosomes 1 and Y. Lectin studies have demonstrated that renal oncocytoma is derived from intercalated cells of the renal cortical collecting duct, the same cells thought to give rise to chromophobe renal cell carcinoma.

Amin MB, Crotty TB, Tickoo SK, Farrow GM: Renal oncocytoma: a reappraisal of morphologic features with clinicopathologic findings in 80 cases. *Am J Surg Pathol* 1997;21(1):1-12.

20. b. This image shows an example of "budding" HGPIN. Basal cells distinguish HGPIN from prostatic adenocarcinoma, and HMWK is a marker of basal cells, in addition to p63 and CK5/6. Budding HGPIN will often show a positive basal cell layer in the large glands and rare basal cells in the surrounding small glands. The luminal cells of HGPIN are immunophenotypically indistinguishable from invasive prostatic adenocarcinoma, and stains for PSA, AMACR, and PAP are positive in both entities, but CK20 is usually negative in both.

Kronz JD, Shaikh AA, Epstein JI. High-grade prostatic intraepithelial neoplasia with adjacent small atypical glands on prostate biopsy. *Hum Pathol* 2001;32(4):389-395.

McNeal JE, Villers A, Redwine EA, et al: Microcarcinoma in the prostate: its association with duct-acinar dysplasia. *Hum Pathol* 1991;22(7):644-652.

21. c. The image shows the characteristic features of a hyperplastic prostatic polyp. Prostatic polyps are polypoid/papillary projections into the urethra lined predominantly by prostatic epithelium, although they can be mixed with urothelial mucosa. Differentiation from prostatic ductal adenocarcinoma requires recognition of the bland cytologic features in the polyp. Also, the prostatic glands in the hyperplastic polyp will retain their basal cell layer, which can be stained by p63 and HMWK immunohistochemical stains. Nephrogenic adenoma or metaplasia can be polypoid or papillary, but is usually lined by cuboidal to flat epithelium, unlike prostatic polyp, which is lined by predominantly prostatic epithelium with two cell layers. Low-grade papillary urothelial carcinoma is characterized by a disorganized urothelial lining with moderate cytologic atypia, scattered mitotic activity, and punctate necrosis. Caruncles are polypoid reactive lesions that can occur in the urethra in postmenopausal women and are lined by hyperplastic urothelium, which can exhibit squamous metaplasia. The urothelium is underlined by an inflamed fibrotic and vascular stroma.

Remick DG Jr, Kumar NB: Benign polyps with prostatic-type epithelium of the urethra and the urinary bladder. A suggestion of histogenesis based on histologic and immunohistochemical studies. *Am J Surg Pathol* 1984;8(11):833-839.

22. e. The image illustrates the classic gross appearance of a mesoblastic nephroma, which is the most common renal neoplasm diagnosed in the first 3 months of life. There are two variants of mesoblastic nephroma. The "classic" mesoblastic nephroma has a gross appearance similar to a leiomyoma. In contrast, the "cellular" mesoblastic neophroma is soft and friable and frequently has areas of hemorrhage, necrosis, and cystic change. Both variants have an infiltrative growth pattern and interdigitate with, and incorporate within them, adjacent renal parenchyma, resulting in entrapped islands, which can mimic an epithelial component of the tumor. Recent cytogenetic studies have demonstrated a chromosomal translocation in cellular mesoblastic nephroma that is identical to the chromosomal translocation in infantile fibrosarcoma of various sites. Many patients are found to have polyhydramnios in prenatal sonography, because this is a tumor of early infancy. In spite of the histologic features, the majority of cellular mesoblastic nephromas are cured by nephrectomy and do not recur or metastasize.

van den Heuvel-Eibrink MM, Grundy P, Graf N, et al: Characteristics and survival of 750 children diagnosed with a renal tumor in the first seven months of life: a collaborative study by the SIOP/GPOH/SFOP, NWTSG, and UKCCSG Wilms tumor study groups. *Pediatr Blood Cancer* 2008; 50(6):1130-1134.

23. d. The image represents an infarct of the prostate. Notice the orderly arrangement of the glands in distinct lobules. Recent infarcts typically show coagulative necrosis, as seen on the far left. With healing, the prostatic glands show squamous metaplasia. The lower right corner shows prostatic glands with an outer basal layer, and early squamous metaplasia. Established squamous metaplasia is seen in the central portion of the image. Prostatic infarcts generally occur in markedly enlarged prostates that show BPH, and are due to ischemia in dependent areas of the prostate. The changes seen here are not part of BPH, but are superimposed on it. These changes are not the usual effect of radiation. Radiation results in general atrophy of the prostate with conservation of the general architecture. The glands appear angulated. The degenerative atypia and nucleomegaly attributed to radiotherapy in other organs is also present in the irradiated prostate.

Brawn PN, Foster DM, Jay DW, et al: Characteristics of prostatic infarcts and their effect on serum prostate-specific antigen and prostatic acid phosphatase. *Urology* 1994;44(1):71-75.

Milord RA, Kahane H, Epstein JI: Infarct of the prostate gland: experience on needle biopsy specimens. *Am J Surg Pathol* 2000;24(10):1378-1384.

24. b. The gross photomicrograph shows a well-outlined lesion in the renal medulla with small foci of necrosis (Panel A). The microscopic picture (Panel B) demonstrates a highly cellular tumor composed of nests of epithelioid, round and monomorphic tumor cells embedded in a dense meshwork of vascular channels. These features, along with the information of the clinical vignette, are typical of a juxtaglomerular apparatus (JGA) tumor. The patients typically present with medically uncontrollable hypertension, due to hypersecretion of renin, with subsequent *hyper*aldosteronism and hypokalemia; hence, answer b is physiologically implausible and incorrect. These tumors are usually benign, and only a rare metastasizing tumor is on record. The bland architectural features, such as the lack of invasion and a well-circumscribed, pushing tumor margin, and the cytologic features of these tumors, such as the lack of pleomorphism and substantial mitotic activity, are consistent with their benign biologic behavior. Therefore, answer a is a correct statement. The tumor cells of JGA tumor are thought to originate from juxtaglomerular cells, the naturally renin-producing and rennin-secreting cells of the kidney. This is underscored by the cytoplasmic accumulation of proto-renin crystals in membrane-bound vesicles, which have a characteristic rhomboid shape on electron microscopic examination. Accordingly, answer e is an acceptable statement. In a series of elegant transplantation experiments in mice, Sequeira Lopez et al. demonstrated evidence for a common origin of juxtaglomerular cells, smooth muscle cells, and endothelial cells from the metanephric mesenchyme. This consistently explains the focal staining for renin, SMA (sequential multiple analysis), and CD34 in at least a subset of tumors. The immunoprofile outlined in answer c supports the diagnosis. It is important to note that the demonstration of renin by immunohistochemistry is not entirely specific to JGA, as several other tumors may be positive, for example, renal cell carcinoma, Wilms tumor, and sarcomas, among others. Treatment for benign JGA tumor is resection, which usually leads to prompt or gradual cessation of systemic hypertension and hypokalemia; for that reason, answer d is true.

Kim HJ, Kim CH, Choi YJ, et al: Juxtaglomerular cell tumor of kidney with CD34 and CD117 immunoreactivity: report of 5 cases. *Arch Pathol Lab Med* 2006;130(5):707-711.
McVicar M, Carman C, Chandra M, et al: Hypertension secondary to renin-secreting juxtaglomerular cell tumor: case report and review of 38 cases. *Pediatr Nephrol* 1993;7(4):404-412.
Sequeira Lopez ML, Pentz ES, Robert B, et al: Embryonic origin and lineage of juxtaglomerular cells. *Am J Physiol Renal Physiol* 2001;281:F345-F356.

25. c. Interstitial cystitis is an uncommon and controversial inflammatory process that generally involves the bladder of middle-aged women. The cause is unknown, but may be autoimmune. The diagnosis is generally one of exclusion, following elimination of other possible causes, including infection and neoplasm. The symptoms tend to be severe and disabling, due to the markedly diminished bladder capacity in this group of patients. There are no pathognomonic histologic features; however, the presence of increased numbers of intramural mast cells has been reported as an association.

Gillenwater JY, Wein AJ: Summary of the National Institute of Arthritis, Diabetes, Digestive and Kidney Diseases Workshop on Interstitial Cystitis, National Institutes of Health, Bethesda, Maryland, Aug. 28-29, 1987. *J Urol* 1988;140(1):203-206.
Rosamilia A, Igawa Y, Higashi S: Pathology of interstitial cystitis. *Int J Urol* 2003;10(Suppl):S11-15.

26. e. Juvenile granulosa cell tumor is not associated with i12p, which is usually seen in adult mixed germ cell tumors. Granulosa cell tumor, juvenile type, is a benign sex cord stromal tumor that occurs in infancy and can be congenital. Grossly it has a variable solid and cystic appearance and ranges in color from yellow to white. Histologically it is composed of alternating solid and cystic areas or follicular pattern. The follicles range from small to large and usually have mucicarminophilic secretions. The solid areas can be sheets of cells or irregular clusters. The tumoral cells have abundant clear to eosinophilic cytoplasm. Nuclear pleomorphism and hyperchromasia are present in a few of the cases. Mitotic figures are usually seen and can be numerous. The most important distinction is from pediatric yolk sac tumors. Juvenile granulosa cell tumor is the most common testicular neoplasm before the age of 6 months and yolk sac tumor is the most common thereafter. Infants can have a physiologic elevation of serum α-fetoprotein (AFP) that can contribute to the confusion and misdiagnosis. It is important to keep in mind the variable patterns usually seen in yolk sac tumor and the characteristic follicular pattern seen in juvenile granulosa cell tumor. A panel of immunohistochemical markers can be helpful and should include CK, AFP, and inhibin. Yolk sac tumors are positive for CK (diffuse) and AFP, but granulosa cell tumors are positive for inhibin and can be positive for CK.

Perez-Atayde AR, Joste N, Mulhern H: Juvenile granulosa cell tumor of the infantile testis. Evidence of a dual epithelial-smooth muscle differentiation. *Am J Surg Pathol* 1996;20(1):72-79.
Young RH: Sex cord-stromal tumors of the ovary and testis: their similarities and differences with consideration of selected problems. *Mod Pathol* 2005;18(Suppl 2):S81-98.

27. b. It is an autosomal *dominant* inherited syndrome with age-dependent penetrance. The vHL syndrome is characterized by retinal and central nervous system hemangioblastomas, clear cell renal cell carcinomas, visceral cysts, and adrenal and extraadrenal pheochromocytomas. In addition, it can be associated with pancreatic neuroendocrine tumors and endolymphatic sac tumors. Tumors arise through biallelic inactivation of the *vHL* tumor suppressor gene located on chromosome 3p25. Patients with vHL syndrome have a 70% risk of developing renal tumors in their lifetime. Kidneys of vHL syndrome patients usually show multiple foci of clear cell renal cell carcinoma, including microscopic foci of carcinoma, as well as renal cysts that are thought to also be neoplastic. The treatment for renal tumors in vHL syndrome patients is a delicate balance between preserving renal function and minimizing the risk of metastases from the multiple and bilateral renal tumors brewing in the kidney.

Maher ER, Neumann HP, Richard S: Von Hippel-Lindau disease: a clinical and scientific review. *Eur J Hum Genet* 2011;19(6):617-623. Epub 2011 Mar 9.
Poston CD, Jaffe GS, Lubensky IA, et al: Characterization of the renal pathology of a familial form of renal cell carcinoma associated with von Hippel-Lindau disease: clinical and molecular genetic implications. *J Urol* 1995;153(1):22-26.
Wagner JR, Linehan WM: Molecular genetics of renal cell carcinoma. *Semin Urol Oncol* 1996;14(4):244-249.

28. c. Klinefelter syndrome does not predispose to an increased risk of germ cell neoplasia, such as the increased risk seen in undescended testes. Rare reports of germ cell tumors arising in the testes of Klinefelter syndrome patients have been reported. Klinefelter syndrome patients are characterized by tall habitus, abnormal body proportions, and small and firm testes. They have a decrease in pubic and facial hair and a large percentage have gynecomastia. They have decreased spermatogenesis, can either be azoospermic or oligospermic, and frequently have problems of infertility. The histologic changes in the testes of Klinefelter syndrome patients include tubular hyalinization, a decrease or absence of germ cells in nonhyalinized tubules when present, and Leydig cell hyperplasia.

Wikström AM, Dunkel L: Klinefelter syndrome. *Best Pract Res Clin Endocrinol Metab* 2011;25(2):239-250.

29. d. Studies have shown a higher rate of PSA positivity in poorly differentiated prostatic adenocarcinoma when using a polyclonal versus a monoclonal antibody. Well-differentiated to moderately differentiated adenocarcinomas have a high rate of PSA expression with either antibody. PSA positivity decreases in poorly differentiated carcinoma and it can even be absent in a small percentage of cases. PSA and prostate-specific acid phosphatase (PSAP) can be expressed in some breast and salivary gland carcinomas, although they are considered highly specific markers. Racemase (AMACR, P504S) positivity is not useful to establish a prostatic origin because it is expressed in multiple other tumor types, such as renal, lung, colorectal, and breast, among others; however, it is useful in distinguishing benign prostatic glands from HGPIN and prostatic adenocarcinoma. It is usually highly expressed in HGPIN and adenocarcinoma.

Hameed O, Humphrey PA: Immunohistochemistry in diagnostic surgical pathology of the prostate. *Semin Diagn Pathol* 2005; 22(1):88-104.

Varma M, Jasani B: Diagnostic utility of immunohistochemistry in morphologically difficult prostate cancer: review of current literature. *Histopathology* 2005;47(1):1-16.

30. e. An increased serum ferritin (>150 ng/mL) is associated with a worse prognosis in neuroblastoma. Neuroblastoma is a neoplasm of the sympathetic nervous system, occurring more commonly in the abdomen, in both adrenal, and extraadrenal sites, with a slight predominance of adrenal tumors. They are the most common solid tumors in children, excluding central nervous system tumors. Neuroblastoma often produce catecholamines, which can be tested for in the urine; elevated levels of their derivatives, such as HVA or VMA, should prompt more extensive testing for neuroblastoma. Grossly they range from gray to yellow and could have areas of hemorrhage, necrosis, cystic change, and calcification in larger tumors. Histologically, neuroblastoma is divided into three categories based on the level of differentiation: (1) undifferentiated, (2) poorly differentiated, and (3) differentiating. The classification depends on the presence or absence of neuropil and ganglion cells. They are composed of sheets of small cells with little cytoplasm and hyperchromatic nuclei. Homer Wright rosettes can be present and often provide the clue. Immunohistochemically they stain for neuron-specific enolase (NSE), synaptophysin, and chromogranin, and can be positive for neurofilament protein. The differential diagnosis of neuroblastoma includes all small round blue cell tumors that occur in children; however, of note is the difficulty in separating neuroblastoma from Ewing

sarcoma/PNET. EWRS1 break-apart rearrangement probe FISH studies are useful to exclude PNET/Ewing sarcoma when necessary.

Ikeda H, Iehara T, Tsuchida Y, et al: Experience with International Neuroblastoma Staging System and Pathology Classification. *Br J Cancer* 2002;86:1110-1116.

Shimada H, Ambros IM, Dehner LP, et al: Terminology and morphologic criteria of neuroblastic tumors: recommendations by the International Neuroblastoma Pathology Committee. *Cancer* 1999;86(2):349-363.

Shimada H, Ambros IM, Dehner LP, et al: The International Neuroblastoma Pathology Classification (the Shimada system). *Cancer* 1999;86(2):364-372.

31. c. Both *TMPRSS2* and the *ERG* gene are located on the long arm of chromosome 21, and the most frequent method of the *TMPRSS2-ERG* gene rearrangement is through interstitial deletion. The percentage of primary prostatic adenocarcinoma with *TMPRSS2-ERG* gene rearrangements is variable across the literature depending on the patient population studied and the referral bias of the institution involved; however, the rearrangement is thought to occur in approximately half of primary prostatic adenocarcinoma discovered on routine PSA serum level screening and treated with radical prostatectomy. The *TMPRSS2* gene is regulated through androgens. The *TMPRSS2-ERG* gene rearrangement results in overexpression of *ERG*, labeling it as a functional rearrangement. Although the majority of studies seem to associate the *TMPRSS2-ERG* gene rearrangement with a worse prognosis, other studies show no associations or an association with a better outcome. In addition, some studies implicate increased copy number of the *TMPRSS2-ERG* locus to be associated with a worse prognosis, irrespective of whether there is a rearrangement. Additional data to clarify the association are needed.

Gopalan A, Leversha MA, Satagopan JM, et al: TMPRSS2-ERG gene fusion is not associated with outcome in patients treated by prostatectomy. *Cancer Res* 2009;69(4):1400-1406. Epub 2009 Feb 3.

Tomlins SA, Bjartell A, Chinnaiyan AM, et al: ETS gene fusions in prostate cancer: from discovery to daily clinical practice. *Eur Urol* 2009;56(2):275-286. Epub 2009 Apr 24.

Toubaji A, Albadine R, Meeker AK, et al: Increased gene copy number of ERG on chromosome 21 but not TMPRSS2-ERG fusion predicts outcome in prostatic adenocarcinomas. *Mod Pathol* 2011;24(11):1511-1520. Epub 2011 Jul 8.

32. e. Cushing syndrome and sex hormone overproduction are more commonly seen in adrenocortical carcinoma than in adrenocortical adenoma. Several systems have been proposed to determine malignancy in adrenocortical tumors; the recurrent theme is that several criteria are taken into consideration and are assigned points, which are then summed up in a point-based system to determine the malignant potential. An elevated mitotic count is one of the features seen in adrenocortical carcinoma. The presence of less than 25% of the clear cell component is a recurrent feature present in both the Weiss system and the modification of Weiss system, and seems to be associated with a malignant behavior. Of course, this criterion does not apply for the oncocytic adrenocortical neoplasms, which have their own risk stratification system. Although conflicting studies are present, it is generally accepted that adrenocortical carcinoma is more common in women. The presence of tumoral necrosis is one of the features seen in malignant adrenocortical neoplasms.

Aubert S, Wacrenier A, Leroy X, et al: Weiss system revisited: a clinicopathologic and immunohistochemical study of 49 adrenocortical tumors. *Am J Surg Pathol* 2002;26(12): 1612-1619.

Weiss LM, Medeiros LJ, Vickery AL Jr: Pathologic features of prognostic significance in adrenocortical carcinoma. *Am J Surg Pathol* 1989;13(3):202-206.

33. a. FISH is not FDA approved for patients with a family history of bladder carcinoma. The test is, however, FDA approved for follow-up of patients with a history of urothelial carcinoma and patients presenting with gross or microscopic hematuria. Positive FISH results can precede histologic results of recurrence in patients with a previous history of bladder carcinoma; approximately 40% of patients with previous history of bladder carcinoma, positive FISH results, and negative biopsy/cytologic specimens, developed recurrence on follow-up. FISH testing for four of the molecular alterations commonly seen in urothelial carcinoma, is helpful, when performed in patients with a previous history of urothelial carcinoma or a high clinical suspicion of a urothelial neoplasm. It provides added benefit in patients with equivocal cytologic specimens. The most commonly detected chromosomal alteration using this test is polysomy of the corresponding chromosomes. Currently available FISH studies are a useful adjunct to routine cytologic and histologic examinations when used in a high prevalence patient population, and should be interpreted by individuals with the proper training and experience.

Halling KC, Kipp BR: Bladder cancer detection using FISH (UroVysion assay). *Adv Anat Pathol* 2008;15(5):279-286.

34. d. Urothelial carcinoma is usually positive for HMWK and nuclear expression of p63. These markers are positive in the basal cells of normal prostatic glands, which are lost in prostatic adenocarcinoma. Poorly differentiated prostatic adenocarcinoma presents as sheets of cells with possible glandular formation or cribriforming. The cells are relatively monotonous, with the characteristic prominent nucleolus, which is the hallmark of prostatic adenocarcinoma. Urothelial carcinoma is usually more pleomorphic and heterogeneous. Positive expression of PSA or PSAP is very helpful in establishing prostatic origin; however, poorly differentiated prostatic adenocarcinoma can be negative, and negative PSA immunostain does not exclude prostatic adenocarcinoma. Prostatic adenocarcinoma can be negative for both CK7 and CK20. Urothelial carcinoma is usually positive for CK7 and can also be positive for CK20. Squamous differentiation is more common in urothelial carcinoma; however, it can also be seen in prostatic adenocarcinoma, particularly in recurrent adenocarcinoma posttreatment.

Chuang AY, DeMarzo AM, Veltri RW, et al: Immunohistochemical differentiation of high-grade prostate carcinoma from urothelial carcinoma. *Am J Surg Pathol* 2007;31(8):1246-1255.

McKenney JK, Amin MB: The role of immunohistochemistry in the diagnosis of urinary bladder neoplasms. *Semin Diagn Pathol* 2005;22(1):69-87.

35. d. PAX-8 immunostain is positive in all subtypes of renal cell carcinoma, Wilms tumor, and collecting duct carcinoma. Renal oncocytoma has also been reported to be positive for PAX-8, and hence, PAX-8 cannot be used in the differential diagnosis between renal oncocytoma and the oncocytic variant of chromophobe renal cell carcinoma. Urothelial carcinoma is usually negative for PAX-8, although some studies have reported a small percentage of cases of renal urothelial carcinoma that are positive for PAX-8. In general, the assumption is that urothelial carcinoma is negative for PAX-8 and this could be helpful in the distinction of collecting duct carcinoma from urothelial carcinoma.

Ordóñez NG: Value of PAX 8 immunostaining in tumor diagnosis: a review and update. *Adv Anat Pathol* 2012;19(3):140-151.

36. e. Nonkeratinizing squamous metaplasia, vaginal subtype, is a common form of metaplasia, occurring more frequently in women than men. It is commonly seen in the trigone and bladder neck and is not considered as an abnormal finding. Keratinizing squamous metaplasia, unlike nonkeratinizing squamous metaplasia, is an abnormal finding that arises due to chronic irritation and can be associated with either concurrent or subsequent development of squamous cell carcinoma. Schistosomal infection, bladder calculi, and indwelling catheters are all known causes of such chronic irritation.

Lagwinski N, Thomas A, Stephenson AJ, et al: Squamous cell carcinoma of the bladder: a clinicopathologic analysis of 45 cases. *Am J Surg Pathol* 2007;31(12):1777-1787.

Rundle JS, Hart AJ, McGeorge A, et al: Squamous cell carcinoma of bladder. A review of 114 patients. *Br J Urol* 1982;54(5):522-526.

Wiener DP, Koss LG, Sablay B, Freed SZ: The prevalence and significance of Brunn's nests, cystitis cystica and squamous metaplasia in normal bladders. *J Urol* 1979;122:317-321.

37. a. Ductal adenocarcinoma is a histologically distinctive neoplasm. When first described, its histologic appearance led to the hypothesis that this variant of prostate carcinoma arises from müllerian remnants and might, therefore, be estrogen dependent. Subsequent studies have disproved this notion and established that the tumor is derived from large prostatic ducts, which are immunoreactive for PSA. The serum levels of PSA may be elevated, but often only modestly. The carcinoma when centrally or periurethrally located frequently presents with hematuria because it forms exophytic projections into the urethra. The hallmark of the diagnosis of ductal adenocarcinoma is the presence of tall columnar cells and papillary projections.

Epstein JI: Prostatic ductal adenocarcinoma: a mini review. *Med Princ Pract* 2010;19(1):82-85. Epub 2009 Dec 9.

Lee TK, Miller JS, Epstein JI: Rare histological patterns of prostatic ductal adenocarcinoma. *Pathology* 2010;42(4):319-324.

38. c. Characteristically, embryonal carcinomas of the testis are strongly positive for pancytokeratin, OCT3/4, and CD30, but negative for EMA. They show variable staining for PLAP, which can be positive. Embryonal carcinoma is mostly seen as a component of a mixed germ cell tumor and usually occurs in an age range 10 years younger than that associated with seminoma. Embryonal carcinoma has a propensity to invade lymphovascular channels.

Histologically it is characterized by pleomorphic overlapping cells with vesicular chromatin and prominent nucleoli, growing in a papillary or solid architecture. It is usually associated with necrosis and increased mitotic activity.

Jones TD, Ulbright TM, Eble JN, et al: OCT4 staining in testicular tumors: a sensitive and specific marker for seminoma and embryonal carcinoma. *Am J Surg Pathol* 2004;28(7): 935-940.

Moul JW, McCarthy WF, Fernandez EB, Sesterhenn IA: Percentage of embryonal carcinoma and of vascular invasion predicts pathological stage in clinical stage I nonseminomatous testicular cancer. *Cancer Res* 1994;54(2):362-364.

39. e. In the testis, dermoid cysts, carcinoid tumors, PNETs, and epidermoid cysts are all considered to be monodermal variants of teratoma. Dermoid and epidermoid cysts have a benign clinical course; extensive or complete sectioning is required to ensure that no other germ cell elements are present. Diffuse embryoma is a distinctive mixed germ cell neoplasm composed of a mixture of embryonal carcinoma and yolk sac tumor; therefore, it is not considered a teratoma.

Ulbright TM, Hattab EM, Zhang S, et al: Primitive neuroectodermal tumors in patients with testicular germ cell tumors usually resemble pediatric-type central nervous system embryonal neoplasms and lack chromosome 22 rearrangements. *Mod Pathol* 2010;23(7):972-980. Epub 2010 Mar 26.

Ulbright TM, Srigley JR: Dermoid cyst of the testis: a study of five postpubertal cases, including a pilomatrixomalike variant, with evidence supporting its separate classification from mature testicular teratoma. *Am J Surg Pathol* 2001;25(6):788-793.

Wang WP, Guo C, Berney DM, et al: Primary carcinoid tumors of the testis: a clinicopathologic study of 29 cases. *Am J Surg Pathol* 2010;34(4):519-524.

40. b. Large cell calcifying Sertoli cell tumor is a unique variant of Sertoli cell tumor that is seen as part of Carney syndrome, a complex clinical syndrome. It can also be seen in Peutz-Jeghers syndrome. Other elements of Carney syndrome include myxomas of skin, soft tissue, and heart; myxoid fibroadenomas; cutaneous blue nevi; pituitary adenomas; and melanocytic schwannomas, among others. Large cell calcifying Sertoli cell tumor occurs in young males and is composed of sheets or cords of cells, with ample eosinophilic cytoplasm, present in a fibromyxoid stromal background. Foci of calcification are often present. They are positive immunohistochemically for inhibin, S100, and EMA, and can be positive for desmin and CK. They usually follow a benign clinical course in the absence of malignant histologic features.

Stratakis CA, Kirschner LS, Carney JA: Clinical and molecular features of the Carney complex: diagnostic criteria and recommendations for patient evaluation. *J Clin Endocrinol Metab* 2001;86:4041-4046.

Washecka R, Dresner MI, Honda SA: Testicular tumors in Carney's complex. *J Urol* 2002;167(3):1299-1302.

41. b. Metanephric adenoma is a renal neoplasm that occurs across all age groups including young children. Up to 12% of patients with metanephric adenoma have polycythemia as a paraneoplastic syndrome. Grossly, metanephric adenoma presents as a well-circumscribed, unencapsulated, homogeneous mass that is usually tan to yellow in color.

Histologically, they are composed of acini, tubules, and papillary structures formed by small cells with little cytoplasm. They could contain calcifications. Metanephric adenomas are benign tumors that should be distinguished from type 1 papillary renal cell carcinoma. An immunohistochemical panel could be helpful, including WT1 and CD57 (positive in metanephric adenoma) and CK7 and AMACR (diffusely positive in papillary renal cell carcinoma). In children, the differential diagnosis includes Wilms tumor; however, Wilms tumor is usually triphasic and expresses the three components (blastemal, epithelial, and stromal) and shows nuclear atypia and mitotic activity. In addition, molecular studies to look for WT1 and WT2 gene alterations can be helpful. Metanephric adenoma has been linked to a tumor suppressor gene on chromosome 2p13.

Davis CJ Jr, Barton JH, Sesterhenn IA, Mostofi FK: Metanephric adenoma. Clinicopathological study of fifty patients. *Am J Surg Pathol* 1995;19(10):1101-1114.

Pesti T, Sükösd F, Jones EC, Kovacs G: Mapping a tumor suppressor gene to chromosome 2p13 in metanephric adenoma by microsatellite allelotyping. *Hum Pathol* 2001;32(1):101-104.

42. b. Anaplasia in Wilms tumors is defined as the presence of cells with markedly enlarged nuclei, defined as threefold increase in nuclear size, compared with those of the majority of the cells, and the presence of multipolar or polyploid mitotic figures. When the anaplastic cells are not confined to one or more discrete sites within the primary tumor, and/or are present in invasive foci or in extrarenal sites, this is considered as diffuse anaplasia and an unfavorable histology. Each of the other three features may be seen in Wilms tumor. The predominance or even exclusivity of blastema, heterologous stromal elements including skeletal muscle cells, and nephrogenic rests do not justify the classification in the unfavorable histologic group.

Beckwith JB, Palmer NF: Histopathology and prognosis of Wilms tumors: results from the First National Wilms' Tumor Study. *Cancer* 1978;41(5):1937-1948.

Davidoff AM: Wilms' tumor. *Curr Opin Pediatr* 2009;21(3): 357-364.

Faria P, Beckwith JB, Mishra K, et al: Focal versus diffuse anaplasia in Wilms tumor—new definitions with prognostic significance: a report from the National Wilms Tumor Study Group. *Am J Surg Pathol* 1996;20(8):909-920.

43. d. In spite of the rich vascularity of the penis, it is a rare site for metastatic carcinoma. All of the carcinomas listed have been reported to metastasize to the penis; however, genitourinary tumors, particularly of prostatic and urinary bladder origin, are the most common primary site for tumors metastasizing to the penis. In the penis, most metastases are within the vascular channels of the erectile tissues of the penis. This is usually manifested as multiple painless subcutaneous nodules. Rarely, malignant priapism can occur. The distinction between metastatic urothelial carcinoma of the urinary bladder and primary penile urethral carcinoma can be difficult. Demonstration of in situ urothelial carcinoma at the site in the penile urethra can be a helpful clue that it is a primary carcinoma.

Chaux A, Amin M, Cubilla AL, Young RH: Metastatic tumors to the penis: a report of 17 cases and review of the literature. *Int J Surg Pathol* 2011;19(5):597-606. Epub 2010 Jan 14.

44. e. The spindle variant of embryonal rhabdomyosarcoma is a histologically distinct subtype of embryonal rhabdomyosarcoma, and is the most common malignant tumor of the paratesticular region in childhood. It has a better prognosis than other subtypes of embryonal rhabdomyosarcoma. These tumors have a firm consistency on palpation, owing to the presence of collagenous stroma. The tumor cells are arranged in sharply outlined bundles and fascicles, and sometimes have a leiomyosarcomatous appearance. In the majority of cases, microscopic foci of more conventional myxoid type embryonal rhabdomyosarcoma are present. Liposarcoma and malignant fibrous histiocytoma are the most frequently encountered malignant tumors of the spermatic cord in adults. Sarcoma botryoides is a variant of embryonal rhabdomyosarcoma. This is a tumor of the pediatric age group, and does occur in the urogenital tract; however, this variant occurs in areas with mucosal surfaces, including the urinary bladder, urethra, and vagina. Alveolar rhabdomyosarcoma is a histologically and cytogenetically distinctive type of rhabdomyosarcoma that occurs most often in children and adolescents. Although alveolar rhabdomyosarcoma has been reported in the genitourinary tract, it is extremely uncommon. It usually carries a worse prognosis.

Reeves HM, MacLennan GT: Paratesticular rhabdomyosarcoma. *J Urol* 2009;182(4):1578-1579. Epub 2009 Aug 15.

Stewart LH, Lioe TF, Johnston SR: Thirty-year review of intrascrotal rhabdomyosarcoma. *Br J Urol* 1991;68(4):418-420.

Sugita Y, Clarnette TD, Cooke-Yarborough C, et al: Testicular and paratesticular tumours in children: 30 years' experience. *Aust N Z J Surg* 1999;69(7):505-508.

45. b. The basaloid variant of squamous cell carcinoma is the most aggressive variant of those listed. It is usually high grade and deeply infiltrating, with a high likelihood of metastatic disease at the time of presentation. Microscopically it is characterized with nests of small cells exhibiting a high nucleus-to-cytoplasm ratio, often showing central necrosis. Pure verrucous carcinoma is a well-differentiated, exophytic carcinoma that has an excellent prognosis. It is characterized microscopically with acanthotic papillae and broad invasive fronds surrounded with chronic inflammation. Condylomatous ("warty") carcinoma is a well-differentiated to moderately differentiated subtype of carcinoma. It is characterized by squamous papillae with marked koilocytic change. When high grade or deeply invasive, they can metastasize to regional lymph nodes. Papillary carcinoma of the penis is a well-differentiated, slowly growing carcinoma. Microscopically, it is characterized by acanthotic papillae overlying an infiltrative base. Bowenoid carcinoma is a variant of squamous cell carcinoma in situ and, as such, has no metastatic potential.

Cubilla AL, Reuter VE, Gregoire L, et al: Basaloid squamous cell carcinoma: a distinctive human papilloma virus-related penile neoplasm: a report of 20 cases. *Am J Surg Pathol* 1998;22:755-761.

Cubilla AL, Reuter V, Velazquez E, et al: Histologic classification of penile carcinoma and its relation to outcome in 61 patients with primary resection. *Int J Surg Pathol* 2001;9:111-120.

46. c. Most melanomas affecting the urinary tract are metastatic. Primary malignant melanomas of the urinary tract are rare and are diagnosed after exclusion of metastatic disease. Primary urethral melanomas have been described in men and women. Demonstration of an associated in situ component favors it to be primary at this site; however, this can be difficult, because urethral melanomas are often large and ulcerated at the time of presentation. Urethral melanomas are aggressive tumors, which metastasize widely; metastases to inguinal and pelvic lymph nodes, as well as hematogenous metastases to liver, lungs, and brain, are not uncommon. Histologically malignant melanoma of the urethra shares the same histologic spectrum as the more common cutaneous melanoma. The main differential diagnosis could be EM-PD; however, immunohistochemical demonstration of S100 and HMB45, which are negative in Paget disease, are helpful in establishing the diagnosis.

Oliva E, Quinn TR, Amin MB, et al: Primary malignant melanoma of the urethra: a clinicopathologic analysis of 15 cases. *Am J Surg Pathol* 2000;24:785-796.

Sánchez-Ortiz R, Huang SF, Tamboli P, et al: Melanoma of the penis, scrotum and male urethra: a 40-year single institution experience. *J Urol* 2005;173(6):1958-1965.

47. d. There are essentially only two variants of germ cell tumor that occur in the testes of prepubertal boys: yolk sac tumor and teratoma. The former accounts for approximately 60% of testicular germ cell tumors in this age group; the remainder are teratomas. Mixed germ cell tumors, embryonal carcinomas, and seminomas do not occur in the prepubertal testes. Although Sertoli cell tumors do occur in this age group, they are not germ cell tumors.

Agarwal PK, Palmer JS: Testicular and paratesticular neoplasms in prepubertal males. *J Urol* 2006;176(3):875-881.

Oottamasathien S, Thomas JC, Adams MC, et al: Testicular tumours in children: a single-institutional experience. *BJU Int* 2007;99(5):1123-1126.

Ulbright TM: Gonadal teratomas: a review and speculation. *Adv Anat Pathol* 2004;11(1):10-23.

48. a. Clinical stage 1 patients with a PNET component have a higher rate of relapse. Pure testicular PNET is a very infrequent finding, and is considered a monodermal teratoma. It is more commonly seen in the setting of a germ cell tumor as a secondary malignant transformation, usually associated with a teratomatous component, although even in this setting, it is also quite rare. Histologically, the same spectrum of patterns seen in peripheral PNET/Ewing sarcoma of other sites can be seen; however, gonadal PNETs tend to be more often similar to central nervous system tumors of the embryonic type, seen in the pediatric population. Immunohistochemically, FLI-1 and CD99 positivity are frequently seen, with variable expression of CD57, synaptophysin, neuron-specific enolase (NSE), and chromogranin A. Gonadal PNETs lack chromosome 22 rearrangements seen in peripheral Ewing/PNETs. The presence of a secondary malignant transformation arising from a testicular germ cell tumor, such as PNET or rhabdomyosarcoma, generally depicts a worse prognosis. Patients with PNETs confined to the primary testicular germ cell tumor have a better prognosis than patients with PNETs arising in metastatic sites, which tend to have a dismal prognosis.

Michael H, Hull MT, Ulbright TM, et al: Primitive neuroectodermal tumors arising in testicular germ cell neoplasms. *Am J Surg Pathol* 1997;21(8):896-904.

Ulbright TM, Hattab EM, Zhang S, et al: Primitive neuroectodermal tumors in patients with testicular germ cell tumors usually resemble pediatric-type central nervous system embryonal neoplasms and lack chromosome 22 rearrangements. *Mod Pathol* 2010;23(7):972-980. Epub 2010 Mar 26.

49. e. Gonadoblastoma is a tumor composed of a mixture of germ cells and sex cord cells. The most frequently encountered combination consists of seminoma cells and Sertoli cells. Gonadoblastoma is considered an in situ neoplasm, and has an excellent prognosis; however, it can be associated with a malignant neoplasm, especially seminoma, and the prognosis would then depend on the prognosis of the malignant neoplasm. About 80% of patients with gonadoblastoma are phenotypic females, and 20% are phenotypic males. Genetically all patients have the Y chromosome and are a mixture of 46XY and X/XY mosaicism. They have persistence of the müllerian duct–derived structures.

Ng SB, Yong MH, Knight LA, et al: Gonadoblastoma-associated mixed germ cell tumour in 46,XY complete gonadal dysgenesis (Swyer syndrome): analysis of Y chromosomal genotype and OCT3/4 and TSPY expression profile. *Histopathology* 2008; 52(5):644-646. Epub 2008 Feb 23.

Scully RE: Gonadoblastoma. A review of 74 cases. *Cancer* 1970;25:1340-1356.

50. e. All of the choices are prostate carcinoma variants of prostatic epithelial origin. Although the extent and intensity of immunohistochemical staining for PSA may vary, each of those subtypes has at least focal positive staining.

Hameed O, Humphrey PA: Immunohistochemistry in diagnostic surgical pathology of the prostate. *Semin Diagn Pathol* 2005; 22(1):88-104.

Hammerich KH, Ayala GE, Wheeler TM: Application of immunohistochemistry to the genitourinary system (prostate, urinary bladder, testis, and kidney). *Arch Pathol Lab Med* 2008;132(3):432-440.

CHAPTER 10

GYNECOLOGIC PATHOLOGY

Valerie A. Fitzhugh and Debra S. Heller

QUESTIONS

All questions in this chapter refer to a photo or photomicrograph.

1. This ovarian lesion represents:
    a. Struma ovarii
    b. Carcinoid tumor
    c. Endometrioid adenocarcinoma
    d. Clear cell carcinoma
    e. Endometriosis

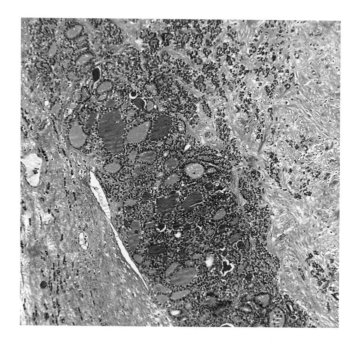

2. The uterine lesion demonstrated is:
    a. Heterologous malignant mixed müllerian tumor
    b. Homologous malignant mixed müllerian tumor
    c. Adenosarcoma
    d. Grade 3 endometrial carcinoma
    e. Endometrial stromal sarcoma

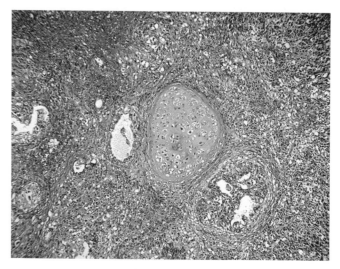

3. This placental lesion is MOST often treated by:
   a. Observation
   b. Evacuation of the uterus and follow-up visit in 6 months
   c. Radiation therapy
   d. Evacuation of the uterus and chemotherapy
   e. Evacuation of the uterus and performance of serial β-hCG (human chorionic gonadotropin) titers

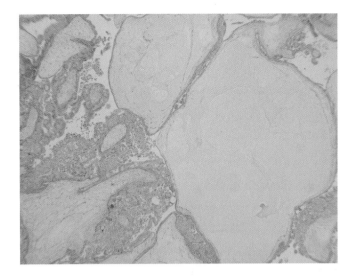

4. This vulvar lesion shows the following immunohistochemical profile: cytokeratin 7 positive, cytokeratin 20 negative, carcinoembryonic antigen (CEA) positive, gross cystic disease fluid protein 15 (GCDFP-15) positive, HMB45 negative, uroplakin III negative. The MOST likely diagnosis is:
   a. Extramammary Paget disease of vulva
   b. Pagetoid spread of urothelial carcinoma
   c. Pagetoid spread of rectal adenocarcinoma
   d. Melanoma
   e. None of the above

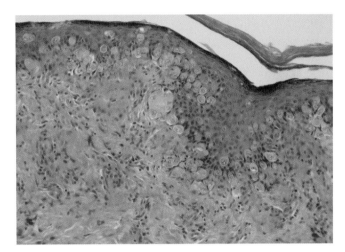

5. The lesion shown in the image was present in sections of the cervix taken from a hysterectomy performed for uterine prolapse. This patient needs:
   a. Exploratory laparotomy and staging
   b. Chemotherapy
   c. Radiation therapy
   d. All of the above
   e. None of the above

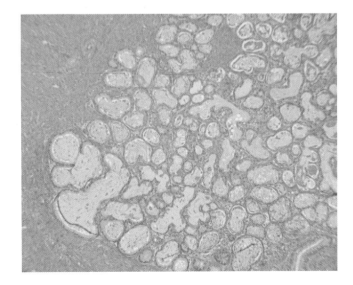

6. This endometrial neoplasm is:
   a. Carcinosarcoma of the uterus
   b. Grade 3 (poorly differentiated) endometrial adenocarcinoma
   c. Grade 2 (moderately differentiated) endometrial adenocarcinoma
   d. Grade 1 (well differentiated) endometrial adenocarcinoma
   e. Complex hyperplasia

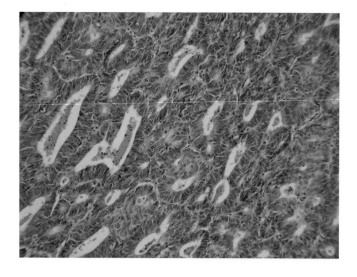

7. This ovarian neoplasm was excised. Which of the following statements is TRUE?
   a. The lesion will not metastasize.
   b. If not excised, a dysgerminoma may develop.
   c. The patient may carry a Y chromosome.
   d. None of the above
   e. All of the above

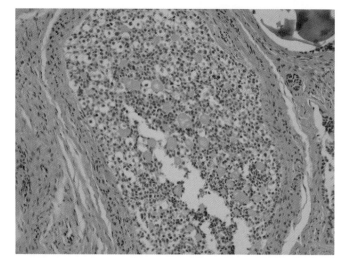

8. This vulvar lesion is a:
   a. Schwannoma
   b. Melanoma
   c. Granular cell tumor
   d. Granulosa cell tumor
   e. Yolk sac tumor

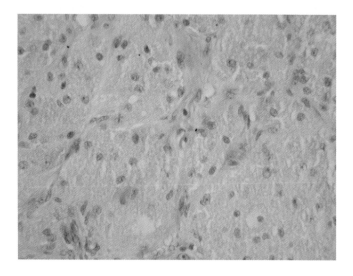

9. This ovarian lesion is recognizable by the distinctive structures shown, which are consistent with:
a. Schiller-Duval bodies
b. Embryoid bodies
c. Arias-Stella change
d. Call-Exner bodies

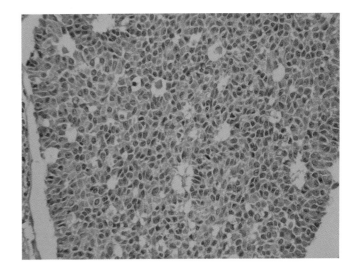

10. The ovarian lesion seen in the image usually does not result in death. The most reliable diagnostic feature distinguishing it from the more aggressive neoplasm arising from this tissue type is:
a. Cancer antigen 125 (CA 125) level
b. Lack of stromal invasion
c. Psammoma bodies
d. It is almost never seen outside the ovary.
e. It is almost never bilateral.

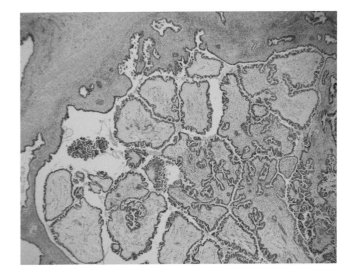

11. A 71-year-old woman underwent a vulvar biopsy. The pathologic finding is seen here. The following may be said about this patient:
a. This patient is likely to have experienced severe pruritus.
b. The patient is most likely African American.
c. The patient probably experienced postmenopausal bleeding.
d. The patient is at no increased risk of developing a vulvar carcinoma.

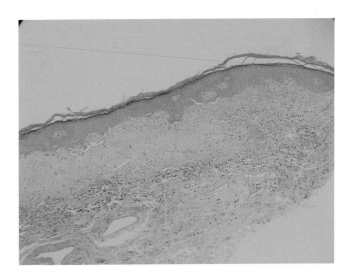

12. The BEST diagnosis for this vaginal biopsy specimen is:
    a. Squamous metaplasia
    b. Condyloma acuminatum
    c. Vaginal intraepithelial neoplasia
    d. Bartholin duct cyst
    e. Adenosis

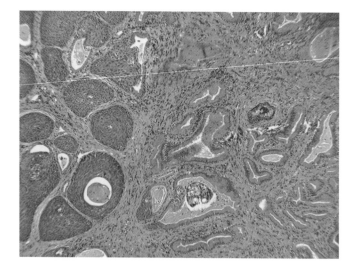

13. A 26-year-old woman underwent endometrial curettage. The image shows a representative field of the curettings. The following may be concluded with certainty:
    a. The patient has an endometrial malignancy.
    b. The patient has endometrial hyperplasia.
    c. The patient was pregnant 6 months ago.
    d. The patient has a very recent or current pregnancy.
    e. The patient has an ectopic pregnancy.

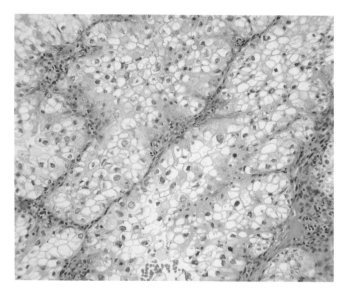

14. This ovarian neoplasm is a:
    a. Thecoma
    b. Fibroma
    c. Brenner tumor
    d. Leiomyoma
    e. Krukenberg tumor

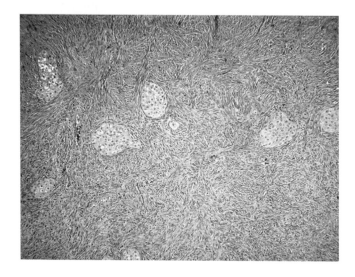

15. The MOST common origin of an ovarian lesion with these features is:
   a. Breast carcinoma
   b. Carcinoma of gastrointestinal origin
   c. Lung carcinoma
   d. Melanoma
   e. Cervical carcinoma

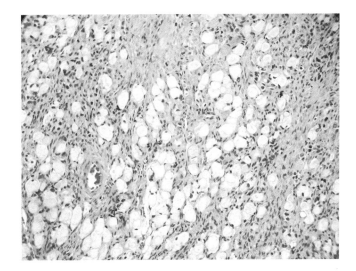

16. The lesion shown in the image was from a vulvar biopsy. All of the following answer choices correspond to this lesion EXCEPT:
   a. Usually occurs in older patients more often than basaloid and warty vulvar intraepithelial neoplasia (VIN)
   b. Is associated with human papillomavirus (HPV)
   c. Is more likely than basaloid or warty VIN to progress to invasion
   d. May go unrecognized on histologic examination, particularly in a superficial biopsy specimen

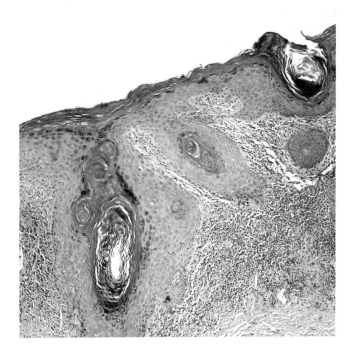

17. A 15-year-old girl presented with a multilobular polypoid mass that is protruding out of the vagina. The histologic appearance is shown. The MOST likely diagnosis is:

a. Sarcoma botryoides of the cervix
b. Yolk sac tumor of the vagina
c. Sarcoma botryoides of the vagina
d. Condyloma acuminatum
e. Condyloma latum

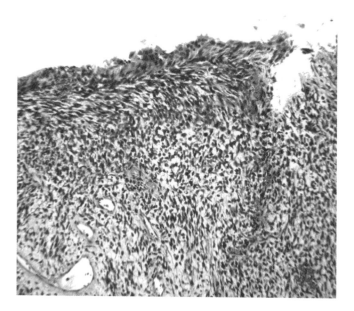

18. An endometrial biopsy specimen shows secretory endometrium and evidence of cells similar to the ones noted in the image. Which of the following statements is TRUE?

a. Dating of this endometrium is reliable.
b. The patient is pregnant.
c. The patient has an intrauterine contraceptive device (IUD).
d. The patient has chronic endometritis.
e. There is increased risk of malignancy.

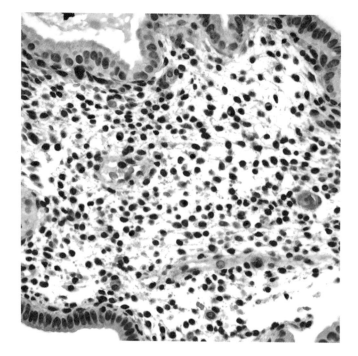

19. All of the following lesions are reliably diagnosed by
    endometrial curettage EXCEPT the one depicted in the image.
    The image corresponds to which of the following diagnoses?
    a. Low-grade endometrial stromal sarcoma
    b. Endometrial hyperplasia
    c. Endometrial carcinoma
    d. Hydatidiform mole
    e. Malignant mixed müllerian tumor

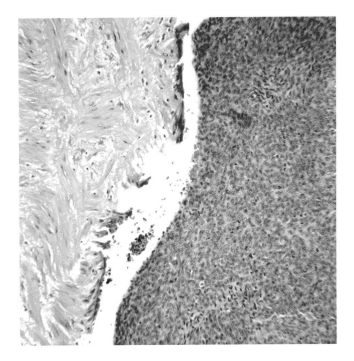

20. The uterine lesion shown in the image:
    a. Has histologically malignant glands in a benign stroma
    b. Has histologically benign glands in a benign stroma
    c. Has histologically malignant glands in a malignant stroma
    d. Has histologically benign glands in a malignant stroma

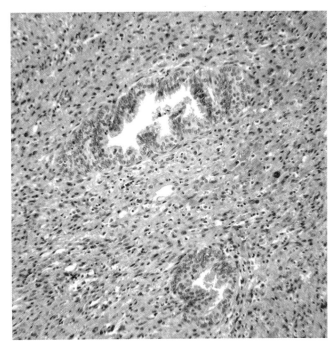

21. All of the following lesions are associated with tubal ectopic pregnancy EXCEPT the one shown in the image. The depicted lesion corresponds to:
  a. Salpingitis isthmica nodosa
  b. Chlamydial infection
  c. Follicular salpingitis
  d. IUD
  e. Adenomatoid tumor of the fallopian tube

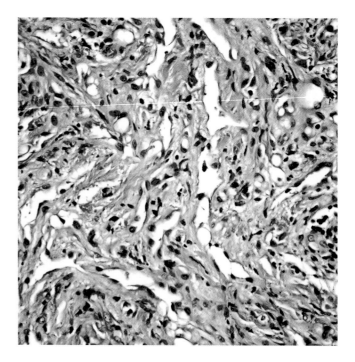

22. A 17-year-old girl presents with the mass shown in the image. The tumor is MOST likely:
  a. Of epithelial origin
  b. Of stromal origin
  c. Of germ cell origin
  d. Metastatic
  e. None of the above

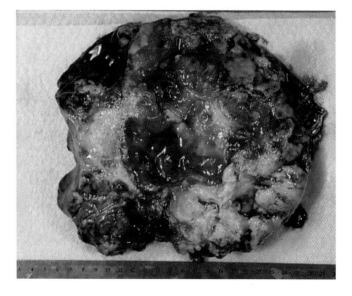

23. A 16-year-old patient has an ovarian cyst resected. Histologic sections of the cyst reveal foci similar to the one shown in the image. How is this lesion graded?

   a. The amount of immature neuroepithelium

   b. The amount of immature cartilage

   c. The amount of mature tissue

   d. The spectrum of mature tissue types

   e. The spectrum of immature tissue types

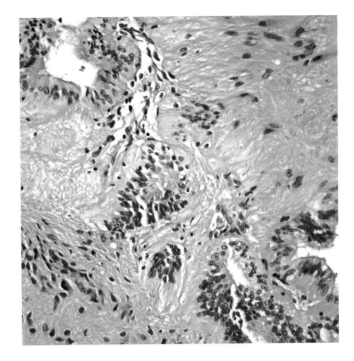

24. A 65-year-old woman presents with the lesion shown in the image and an adnexal mass. The differential diagnosis of the adnexal mass includes all of the following EXCEPT:

   a. Granulosa cell tumor

   b. Fibrothecoma

   c. Steroid cell tumor

   d. Luteoma

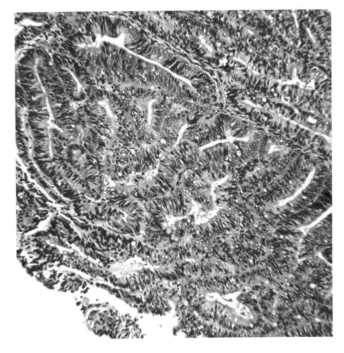

25. All of the following statements about the lesion in the image are true EXCEPT:
    a. The lesions are usually triploid.
    b. The lesions tend to have a higher risk of progression to gestational trophoblastic neoplasia.
    c. The lesions show more pronounced trophoblastic proliferation.
    d. The lesions may be inadvertently diagnosed as missed abortions by both the clinician and the pathologist.

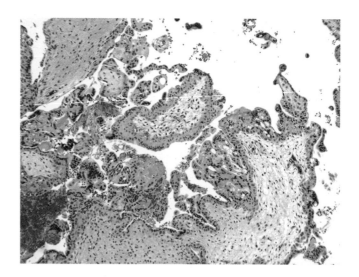

26. A 14-year-old girl presents with vaginal bleeding. Her mother is concerned that the bleeding is distinct from her menses. Colposcopic examination reveals a friable mass along the lateral upper vaginal wall. The results of the biopsy are shown. All of the following statements about this lesion are true EXCEPT:
    a. The immunohistochemical profile of this neoplasm includes positivity for cytokeratin 7, CEA, cytokeratin 34βE12, CA 125, and CAM 5.2.
    b. All cases are linked to perinatal exposure of diethylstilbestrol (DES).
    c. The diagnosis is very rare in patients younger than 12 years and older than 30 years.
    d. Ultrastructurally, these tumors resemble the endometrial and ovarian counterparts seen in older women.
    e. Histologically, there are tubules and cysts lined by clear cells. Solid and papillary areas may be identified. Where tubules are present, hobnail cells protrude into the glandular lumina.

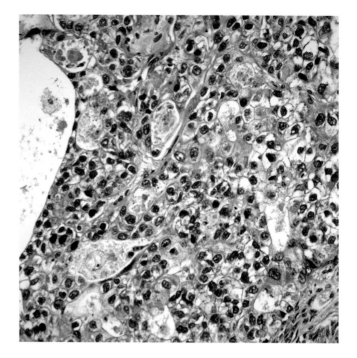

27. A 19-year-old woman is concerned about the presence of new facial hair that she did not previously have. She has also noticed changes in her breasts, and her periods have become irregular. An ovarian mass was identified after an appropriate work-up and was excised. All of the following statements about the lesion in the image are true EXCEPT:
    a. Peutz-Jeghers syndrome is associated with this tumor.
    b. A lipid-rich variant exists, also called folliculoma lipidique.
    c. The lesion is most commonly unilateral.
    d. Epithelial membrane antigen (EMA) would be positive in this tumor.
    e. These tumors can be functional and cause signs of hyperestrinism, virilization, and rarely a combination of both.

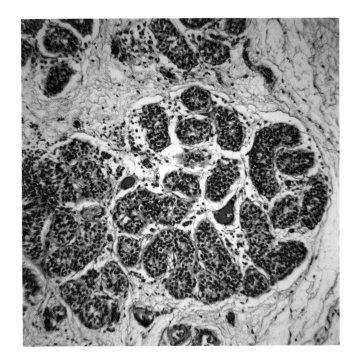

28. A 66-year-old woman presents with complaints of abdominal pain and increasing abdominal girth. An oophorectomy is performed 2 months later. The histologic finding is shown in the image. What is the BEST diagnosis?
    a. Endometrioid adenocarcinoma
    b. Granulosa cell tumor
    c. Krukenberg tumor
    d. Endometriosis
    e. Endometrioid borderline tumor

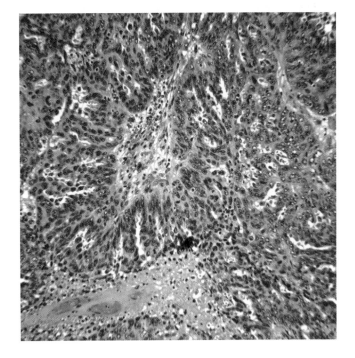

29. A 14-year-old girl presents with abdominal pain and a large pelvic mass. The mass was removed, and the representative histologic result is shown. Which of the following statements is TRUE about this lesion?
    a. This is one of the least common ovarian tumors in children and adolescents.
    b. A testicular counterpart for this tumor does not exist.
    c. Granulomas identified within this tumor are a result of concurrent tuberculosis infection.
    d. This lesion never has a precursor lesion.
    e. Placenta-like alkaline phosphatase (PLAP) is strongly positive in this tumor.

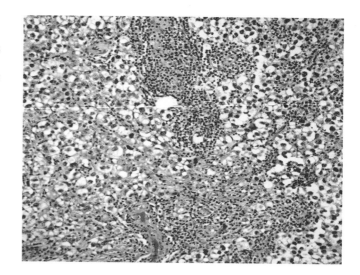

30. A 52-year-old woman presents with a complaint of increasing abdominal girth. Her uterus is found to be 28 weeks' gestation size, and a hysterectomy is performed. An intramural lesion is identified in the uterine fundus. The histologic finding is shown. Which of the following is MOST important in making the diagnosis?
    a. Coagulative necrosis
    b. Mitotic activity
    c. Pleomorphism
    d. Cellularity
    e. Multiple lesions

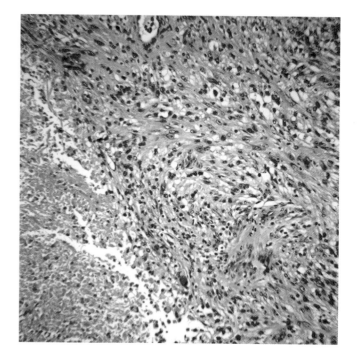

31. A 28-year-old woman presents for cone biopsy after an abnormal Papanicolaou (Pap) smear confirmed by colposcopy. Her histologic finding is shown. Which of the following HPV types is MOST likely to be detected in this patient?
   a. HPV 45
   b. HPV 6
   c. HPV 18
   d. HPV 33
   e. HPV 11

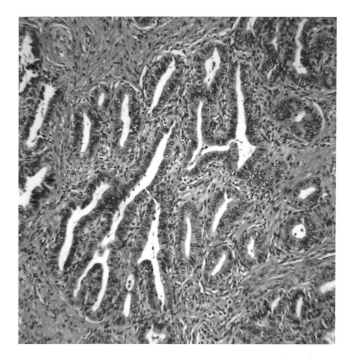

32. A 44-year-old HIV-positive woman presents with vaginal bleeding. Speculum examination reveals a large, fungating mass, and a biopsy is performed. The histologic finding is shown. Which of the following is LEAST likely to correlate with this diagnosis?
   a. The patient likely had abnormal Pap smears in the past.
   b. The patient is unlikely to have ever had a diagnosis of VIN.
   c. The patient experienced postcoital bleeding.
   d. The patient has been exposed to HPV 16.
   e. The tumor would stain immunohistochemically for cytokeratin 5/6 and p63.

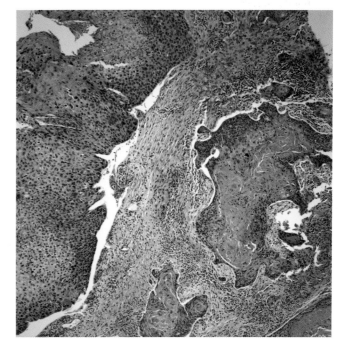

33. A woman brings her 12-year-old daughter to the pediatrician because of concern of lesions on the child's vulva. A biopsy is performed, and the histologic finding is shown. What is your diagnosis?
 a. Herpes
 b. Molluscum contagiosum
 c. Syphilis
 d. Condyloma acuminatum
 e. Granuloma inguinale

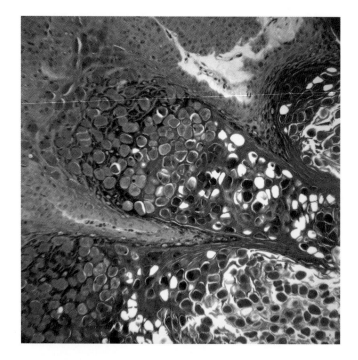

34. A 33-year-old woman presents with amenorrhea that has lasted since the end of her uneventful term pregnancy 13 months earlier. Her β-hCG level is 122 IU/L. She states she has completed having children, and so a hysterectomy is performed. A large mass is identified on the hysterectomy section. What is your diagnosis?
 a. Complete hydatidiform mole
 b. Choriocarcinoma
 c. Placental site trophoblastic tumor
 d. Partial hydatidiform mole
 e. Placental site nodule

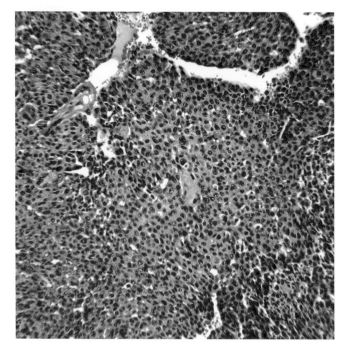

35. A 36-year-old woman reports two missed periods and has reason to believe she is pregnant. Her β-hCG levels are elevated for gestational age. Ultrasound examination does not reveal a uterine gestational sac. Salpingectomy is performed, and the histologic finding is shown. All of the following statements regarding this entity are true EXCEPT:

  a. An identifiable embryo may have been present at the time of gross examination.

  b. The lesion is most commonly identified in the ampulla.

  c. An important differential diagnostic consideration is missed abortion.

  d. Endometriosis is a risk factor for this lesion.

  e. There is no association with chronic salpingitis or pelvic inflammatory disease (PID).

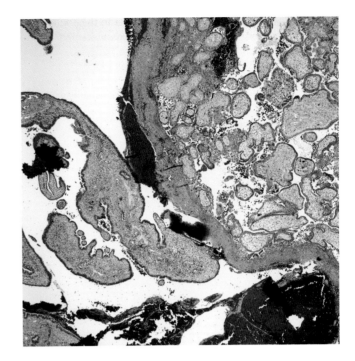

36. A 42-year-old G2P2 (gravida 2, para 2) woman presents with abdominal pain and vaginal bleeding. She delivered her second child 13 months earlier. Radiologic examination demonstrated a mass within the uterine fundus. A hysterectomy was performed, and the histologic finding is shown. Which of the following statements about the lesion is CORRECT?

  a. The multinucleate giant cell would stain strongly for human placental lactogen (hPL) and weakly for β-hCG.

  b. The lesion would be negative for cytokeratin.

  c. If enough sections are submitted, chorionic villi will be identified in the specimen.

  d. Tumor stroma and vessels are prominent within the specimen.

  e. Rarely, the diagnosis has been made in a placenta immediately following pregnancy.

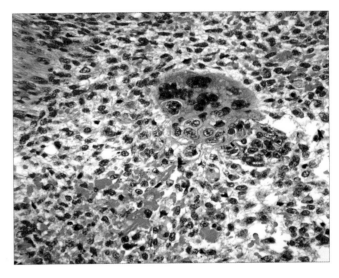

37. A 67-year-old woman presents with increasing abdominal pain. Pelvic examination reveals a large mass. Staging radiology demonstrates disease limited to the pelvis. A total abdominal hysterectomy with bilateral salpingo-oophorectomy is performed, and a lesion of the right ovary is discovered. The histologic finding is shown. What is your diagnosis?
   a. Metastatic neuroendocrine carcinoma
   b. Pulmonary-type small cell carcinoma
   c. Endometrioid adenocarcinoma
   d. Dysgerminoma
   e. Serous carcinoma

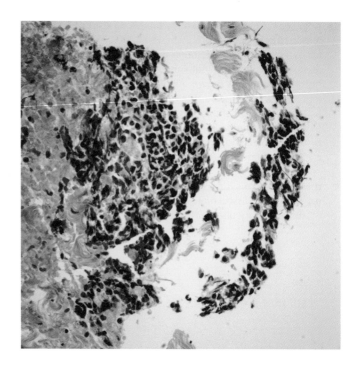

38. A 21-year-old woman presents in labor. She has had no prenatal care. As the patient is set up to deliver, several ulcerated lesions are identified on her vulva. A biopsy of a lesion is performed, and a frozen section is requested. All of the following are features of her lesion EXCEPT:
   a. Molding
   b. Cowdry type B inclusions
   c. Multinucleation
   d. Margination of chromatin
   e. Cowdry type A inclusions

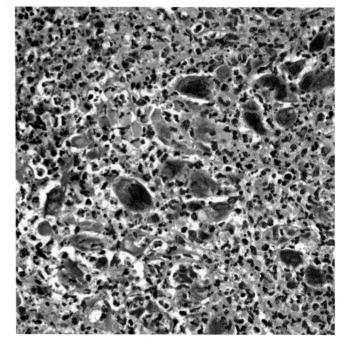

39. Which of the following lesions is the MOST common malignancy associated with the lesion in the image?
    a. Squamous cell carcinoma
    b. Papillary thyroid carcinoma
    c. Rhabdomyosarcoma
    d. Osteosarcoma
    e. Melanoma

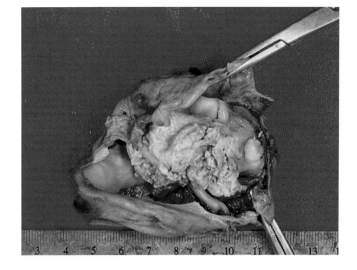

40. A 71-year-old woman complains of vaginal bleeding and vaginal fullness. Speculum examination reveals a mass protruding through the cervix into the upper vagina. A biopsy is performed, which leads to a total abdominal hysterectomy with bilateral salpingo-oophorectomy. All of the following statements about this lesion are likely true EXCEPT:
    a. The patient likely experienced pelvic pain.
    b. Histologic examination reveals carcinomatous and sarcomatous elements.
    c. The lesion is far more common in premenopausal women than in postmenopausal women.
    d. Deep myometrial invasion is common in this lesion.
    e. The malignant epithelial element is most commonly of glandular origin.

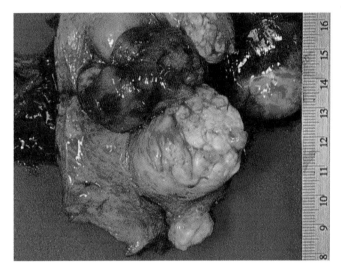

41. A 44-year-old woman presents with abdominal pain. Imaging demonstrates a right ovarian mass. Oophorectomy is performed, and the histologic finding is shown. From which of the following lesions did this MOST likely arise?
    a. Serous carcinoma
    b. Serous cystadenoma
    c. Mucinous cystadenoma
    d. Struma ovarii
    e. Brenner tumor

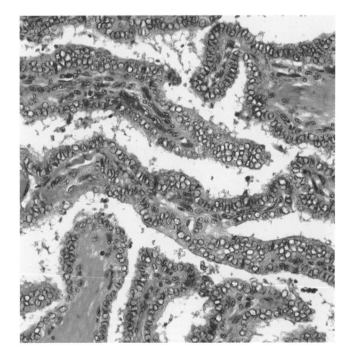

42. After an abnormal Pap smear, a 38-year-old woman undergoes a cervical biopsy. The histologic finding is demonstrated in the image. Which of the following is the MOST common HPV to be implicated in this lesion?
   a. HPV 33
   b. HPV 45
   c. HPV 31
   d. HPV 18
   e. HPV 16

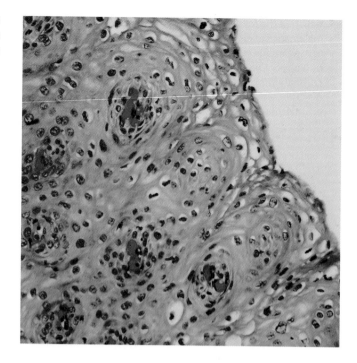

43. A 27-year-old woman returns home after a vacation in Malawi, where she had gone swimming in local waters. She notices several patches on her vulva and makes an emergency appointment to see her gynecologist. A biopsy is performed. What is your diagnosis?
   a. *Histoplasma capsulatum*
   b. *Schistosoma* spp.
   c. *Coccidioides immitis*
   d. *Cryptococcus neoformans*
   e. *Blastomyces dermatiditis*

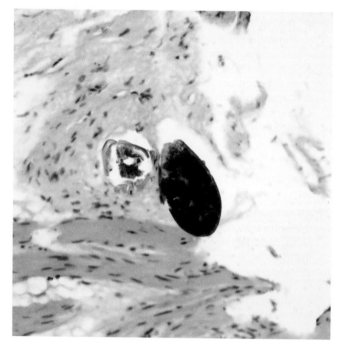

44. A 69-year-old woman presents for a routine gynecologic examination. A 3-cm vulvar mass is identified, and a biopsy is performed. What is your diagnosis?
   a. Poorly differentiated squamous cell carcinoma
   b. Diffuse large B-cell lymphoma
   c. Merkel cell carcinoma
   d. Basal cell carcinoma
   e. Differentiated VIN

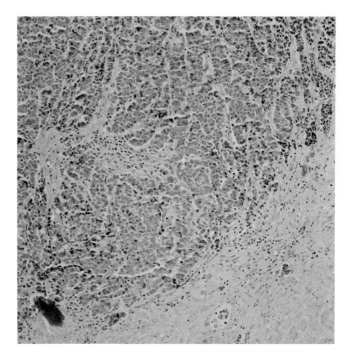

45. A 33-year-old woman has a large vulvar mass that has made it difficult for her to sit comfortably. Surgery is performed. The histologic finding is shown. All of the following statements about this lesion are true EXCEPT:
   a. Close attention to surgical margins is essential when confronted with this neoplasm.
   b. The lesion is locally aggressive, and metastasis is common.
   c. The lesion occurs most commonly in the reproductive years.
   d. The lesion is of low to moderate cellularity.
   e. HGMA2 immunohistochemistry is positive in 50% of cases.

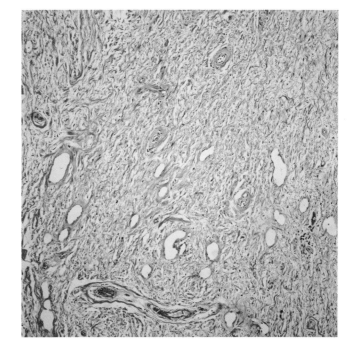

46. A 46-year-old HIV-positive woman complains of abdominal fullness. Imaging reveals a left ovarian mass. Surgery is performed, and the histologic findings led to the special stain shown. All of the following statements about this entity are true EXCEPT:

a. It is not difficult to differentiate this lesion from ovarian neoplasia preoperatively.

b. CA 125 levels may have been elevated in this patient.

c. Similar findings may be seen in adolescent patients.

d. The lesion may be a cause of infertility.

e. The patient's HIV status increased her risk for developing this condition.

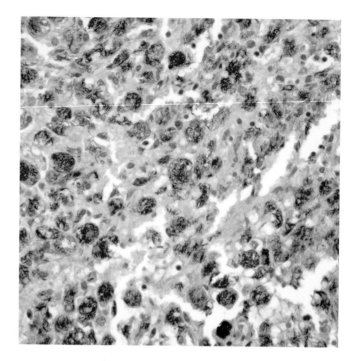

47. A 69-year-old woman presents with postmenopausal bleeding. An in-office endometrial biopsy is performed, and the results lead to hysterectomy. The histologic finding is shown. All of the following statements about this lesion are true EXCEPT:

a. Increased Ki-67 activity in this lesion portends a poor prognosis.

b. Increased p53 activity is never seen in this entity.

c. Low p21 activity portends a poor prognosis even in low-grade lesions.

d. Microsatellite instability is identified in about 25% of these cases.

e. High survivin expression is a marker of poor prognosis in this entity.

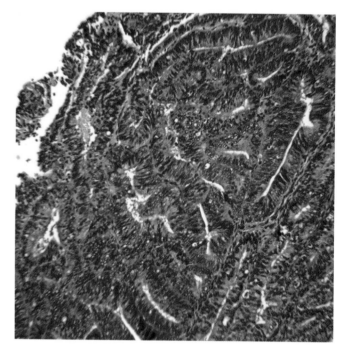

48. A 15-year-old girl presents with a 6-month history of abdominal pain. She is found to have a right ovarian mass. The gross specimen and one of the histologic findings are shown. Which of the following chromosomes is MOST likely to be seen on analysis of this lesion?

   a. 6
   b. 8
   c. 16
   d. X
   e. 12

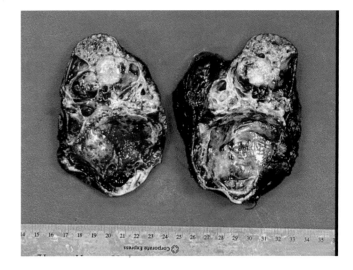

49. An 18-year-old woman recently underwent left oophorectomy. The histologic finding of one component of the tumor is shown. You would expect all of the following immunohistochemical markers to be positive in this lesion EXCEPT:

   a. CD30
   b. Alpha-fetoprotein (AFP)
   c. OCT4
   d. D2-40
   e. CD117

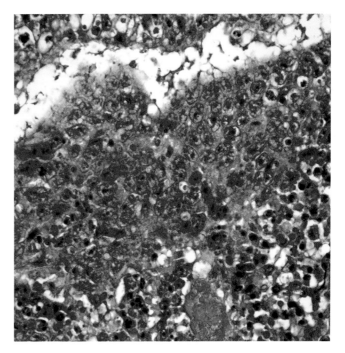

50. A 28-year-old woman undergoes a cervical biopsy after a Pap smear diagnosis of atypical glandular cells of undetermined significance. The histologic finding is shown. What is the diagnosis?
   a. Endocervical adenocarcinoma in situ
   b. Endometrioid endometrial adenocarcinoma
   c. Microglandular hyperplasia
   d. Tubal metaplasia
   e. Squamous metaplasia

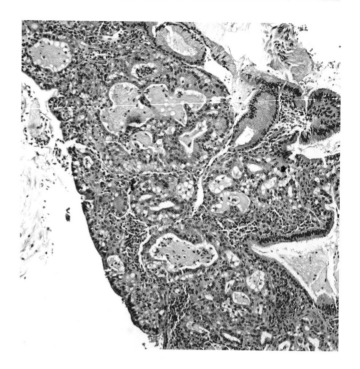

51. All of the following are histologic variants of the tumor shown EXCEPT:
   a. Embryonal
   b. Endodermal sinus
   c. Hepatoid
   d. Reticular
   e. Polyvesicular vitelline

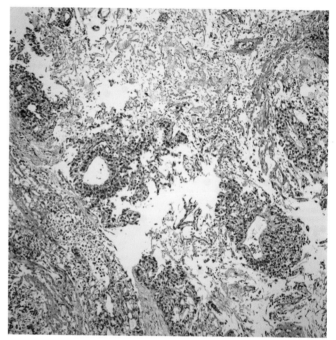

ANSWERS

1. a. This ovarian lesion represents struma ovarii, which is a specialized teratoma that is predominately composed of thyroid tissue. It is usually not a difficult diagnosis. However, unusual forms, such as cystic struma ovarii and malignant struma ovarii, have been described.

   Histologically, insular carcinoid tumors often resemble carcinoids of the gastrointestinal tract. They are distinguished by nests of cells with the classic neuroendocrine "salt and pepper" pattern of nuclear chromatin. Mitotic activity is uncommon. Trabecular carcinoid tumors more closely resemble colorectal carcinoids, which are characterized by cords of cells, two to three cells thick, again with the classic "salt and pepper" nuclear pattern. No thyroid tissue is present.

   Endometrioid adenocarcinoma most closely resembles endometrial carcinoma of the uterine corpus. Although struma ovarii can rarely demonstrate histologic malignancy, this feature is not represented in the image. Clear cell carcinoma is characterized by a predominance of clear cells in a diffuse, papillary, trabecular, or tubulocystic pattern. To confirm endometriosis histologically, the presence of both endometrial glandular epithelium and endometrial stroma is necessary.

Devaney K, Snyder R, Norris HJ, et al: Proliferative and histologically malignant struma ovarii: a clinicopathologic study of 54 cases. *Int J Gynecol Pathol* 1993;12(4):333-343.

Szyfelbein WM, Young RH, Scully RE: Struma ovarii simulating ovarian tumors of other types: a report of 30 cases. *Am J Surg Pathol* 1995;19(1):21-29.

Szyfelbein WM, Young RH, Scully RE: Cystic struma ovarii: a frequently unrecognized tumor. A report of 40 cases. *Am J Surg Pathol* 1994;18(8):785-788.

2. a. The uterine lesion demonstrated is a heterologous malignant mixed müllerian tumor. The lesion contains malignant epithelial and mesenchymal elements. The mesenchymal element, in this case, cartilage, is not native to the uterine corpus and indicates heterologous differentiation.

Homologous malignant mixed müllerian tumors also contain malignant epithelial and mesenchymal elements. However, the mesenchymal elements in homologous tumors are of tissue types that would normally arise in the uterine corpus, such as smooth muscle or endometrial stroma. Adenosarcoma is considered a tumor of mixed origin. However, the epithelial component of the tumor is composed of benign glands. Only the mesenchymal portion of the tumor is malignant. Grade 3 endometrial carcinoma is composed of malignant glandular elements with varying amounts of solid areas contained within a benign stroma; this is not depicted in the image. Endometrial stromal sarcoma comes in two varieties—a low-grade sarcoma and a high-grade, undifferentiated sarcoma. These lesions are composed of oblong, round, or spindled cells only. No epithelial component is identified within the neoplasm.

Kempson RL, Hendrickson MR: Smooth muscle, endometrial stromal, and mixed Müllerian tumors of the uterus. *Mod Pathol* 2000;13(3):328-342.

Silverberg SG, Major FJ, Blessing JA, et al: Carcinosarcoma (malignant mixed mesodermal tumor) of the uterus. A Gynecologic Oncology Group pathologic study of 203 cases. *Int J Gynecol Pathol* 1990;9(1):1-19.

3. e. Hydatidiform moles are treated by evacuation of the uterus with follow-up serial β-hCG titers. If β-hCG titers plateau or increase, gestational trophoblastic neoplasia is diagnosed, and the patient receives chemotherapy. High-risk and low-risk gestational trophoblastic neoplasms are diagnosed on the basis of various clinical features, and several staging and scoring systems are in use. Often the diagnosis of gestational trophoblastic neoplasia is a clinical one, and only uncommonly does the pathologist receive tissue to confirm it.

Hancock BW: Staging and classification of gestational trophoblastic disease. *Best Pract Res Clin Obstet Gynecol* 2003; 17(6):869-883.

Soper JT, Mutch DG, Schink JC; American College of Obstetricians and Gynecologists: Diagnosis and treatment of gestational trophoblastic neoplasia: ACOG Practice Bulletin No. 537. *Gynecol Oncol* 2004;93(3):575-585.

4. a. The most likely diagnosis is extramammary Paget disease of the vulva, which stains strongly and diffusely positive for cytokeratin 7 and CEA. It is also often positive for GCDFP-15. Staining for cytokeratin 20 is occasionally positive. Staining for uroplakin III and HMB45 is negative.

Conventional urothelial carcinoma would stain positively for cytokeratin 7, cytokeratin 20, and uroplakin III. Staining for CEA is variable. Staining for HMB45 and GCDFP-15 is consistently negative. Rectal adenocarcinomas most commonly stain strongly positive for cytokeratin 20 and CEA. Rare cells may demonstrate cytokeratin 7 positivity. Staining for GCDFP-15, HMB45, and uroplakin III is expected to be negative. With the given panel, HMB45 would be the only positive stain with melanoma. All the other stains listed would be negative.

Brown HM, Wilkinson EJ: Uroplakin-III to distinguish primary vulvar Paget disease from Paget disease secondary to urothelial carcinoma. *Hum Pathol* 2002;33(5):545-548.

Schned L, Mount SL: Unusual neoplasms of the vulva. *Diagn Histopathol* 2010;16:517-525.

5. e. The lesion in the image is an example of endocervical tunnel clusters. These lesions are one of many benign mimics of endocervical adenocarcinoma. There are two histologic patterns. One demonstrates dilated spaces filled with mucin, similar to nabothian cysts; however, the outline of the glands is scalloped, resulting in an appearance of fusion rather than that of a single space. The other histologic pattern is characterized by lobular groups of small acini or tubules lined by flattened epithelium. Various incidental findings in the cervix, such as microglandular hyperplasia, Arias-Stella reaction, endocervical glandular hyperplasia, and mesonephric rests, represent other benign findings that should not be confused with endocervical adenocarcinoma. With the exception of florid microglandular hyperplasia, p53 staining is seen only in neoplastic lesions of the endocervix, making this a useful marker in distinguishing benign mimics from true endocervical adenocarcinoma.

The pathogenesis of endocervical tunnel clusters is unclear. It was originally hypothesized that their presence was due to the involution of endocervical glands that had become hyperplastic as a response to the hormonal changes of pregnancy. The lesion has since been identified in women who have never been pregnant, indicating that other causative factors are likely implicated. The common mixture of the two types of tunnel clusters, referred to as type A and type B; the lobulated architecture; and the absence of desmoplasia and deep invasion all are helpful histologic clues in the diagnosis of these structures. Endocervical tunnel clusters are completely benign lesions, and patients do not require any further intervention.

Cina SJ, Richardson MS, Austin RM, et al: Immunohistochemical staining for Ki-67 antigen, carcinoembryonic antigen, and p53 in the differential diagnosis of glandular lesions of the cervix. *Mod Pathol* 1997;10(3):176-180.

Nucci MR: Symposium part III: tumor-like glandular lesions of the uterine cervix. *Int J Gynecol Pathol* 2002;21(4):347-359.

Young RH, Clement PB: Pseudoneoplastic glandular lesions of the uterine cervix. *Semin Diagn Pathol* 1991;8(4):234-249.

6. d. The endometrial neoplasm depicted in the image is grade 1 (well differentiated) endometrial adenocarcinoma. The histologic grade of endometrial carcinoma is an important predictor of both the depth of myometrial invasion of the tumor and the likelihood of regional lymph node metastasis. Grade 3 adenocarcinomas are much more likely to demonstrate deep invasion of the myometrium and paraaortic and pelvic lymph node metastases than grade 1 adenocarcinomas.

The histologic grading system of usual endometrial carcinomas is as follows: Grade 1 tumors demonstrate less than 5% solid (nonsquamous) component. Grade 2 tumors demonstrate 5% to 50% solid component. Grade 3 tumors demonstrate greater than 50% solid component. Grade 1 and grade 2 tumors with nuclear atypia inappropriate for the architectural grade are upgraded by one grade.

Although the grade of adenocarcinoma assigned at the time of biopsy often determines the surgical planning of the patient, the grade of the tumor may change at the time of the definitive surgery because of sampling error. This possibility increases the importance of intraoperative consultations in determining the next step for the patient. The concordance rate for high-grade carcinomas is significantly higher compared with well-differentiated carcinomas.

Some endometrial carcinomas are selected out of the histologic grading system, mainly owing to prognosis. Serous carcinomas and clear cell carcinomas of the uterus are high grade by definition because of the poor prognosis associated with them. Secretory carcinoma is a low-grade carcinoma with an excellent clinical outcome. This tumor is also selected out of the grading system and is by definition grade 1.

Heller DS, Drosinos S, Westhoff C: Accuracy of tumor grade assigned at initial endometrial sampling. *Int J Gynecol Obstet* 1994;47(3):301-302.

Mitchard J, Hirschowitz L: Concordance of FIGO grade of endometrial carcinoma in biopsy and hysterectomy specimens. *Histopathology* 2003;42(4):372-378.

7. e. This lesion is a gonadoblastoma. The most common histologic finding of gonadoblastoma is large cellular nests separated by fibrous stroma. The nests are a mixture of germ cells and sex cord cells, most commonly resembling immature Sertoli cells. Mitotic activity is present but is rare. The admixed germ and sex cord cells surround circular deposits of eosinophilic basement membrane material. The fibrous stroma surrounding the nests often contains cells resembling Leydig cells and dystrophic calcification. Gonadoblastomas are most often seen in the context of mixed gonadal dysgenesis, in which patients may carry Y chromosome material. Although gonadoblastomas are considered benign, malignant transformation may occur if they are not excised. The most common malignant tumor to arise within a gonadoblastoma is a dysgerminoma.

Gorosito M, Pancera B, Sarancone S, et al: Gonadoblastoma: an unusual ovarian tumor. *Ann Diagn Pathol* 2010;14(4):247-250.

Talerman A, Roth LM: Recent advances in the pathology and classification of gonadal neoplasms composed of germ cells and sex cord derivatives. *Int J Gynecol Pathol* 2007;26(3):313-321.

8. c. Granular cell tumor, as depicted in the image, consists of numerous cells with small, dark, round nuclei within voluminous eosinophilic cytoplasm. The cytoplasm contains eosinophilic granules. Fibrous septa are often present. Granular cell tumor of the vulva is most often identified at a routine gynecologic examination, but it does not have a distinct clinical appearance, and the diagnosis must be made histologically. Granular cell tumors demonstrate strong, diffuse immunohistochemical staining for S100, leading many pathologists to believe that these neoplasms are of schwannian origin. The granules are also PAS positive and diastase resistant.

If a granular cell tumor arises in a subepithelial location, it may evoke a reaction of the overlying epithelium, known as *pseudoepitheliomatous hyperplasia*. In a biopsy specimen, especially if the underlying granular cell tumor is not sampled, pseudoepitheliomatous hyperplasia may be mistaken for squamous cell carcinoma. This is a well-known pitfall. Careful examination of the underlying tissue, if sampled, commonly reveals the granular cell tumor. Malignant granular cell tumors are suggested by several atypical histologic findings. Atypical features include prominent nucleoli, high nuclear-to-cytoplasmic ratios, pleomorphism, greater than 2 mitotic figures per 10 high-power fields, and spindling of the tumor cells. Malignant granular cell tumors recur rapidly after initial excision and have been reported to metastasize widely.

Horowitz JR, Copas P, Majmudar B: Granular cell tumors of the vulva. *Am J Obstet Gynecol* 1995;173(6):1710-1713; discussion 1713-1714.

Schmidt O, Fleckenstein GH, Gunawan B, et al: Recurrence and rapid metastasis formation of a granular cell tumor of the vulva. *Eur J Obstet Gynecol Reprod Biol* 2003;106(2):219-221.

9. d. The lesion in the image is an adult granulosa cell tumor. Adult granulosa cell tumors display various patterns, including diffuse, microfollicular, insular, and trabecular patterns. A mixture of patterns commonly may be demonstrated in a single patient, illustrating the importance of ample sampling of these neoplasms. This image depicts the microfollicular pattern; although this is not the most common pattern, it is the most easily recognizable. The spaces correspond to Call-Exner bodies, which contain eosinophilic cellular debris most commonly and are lined by haphazardly arranged grooved nuclei.

Adult granulosa cell tumors are well known to secrete estrogen; this is important clinically because increased unopposed estrogen can lead to endometrial hyperplasia or carcinoma. Grossly, adult granulosa cell tumors can have a tan-to-yellow appearance. Grossly yellow tumors are due to increased steroid production. Granulosa cell tumors are strongly and diffusely positive for inhibin, separating these tumors from many carcinomas, which are often inhibin negative. Stage remains the most important prognostic factor in granulosa cell tumors. Other prognostic factors include tumor size, age of the patient, presence or absence of tumor rupture, and mitotic activity.

Kommoss F, Oliva E, Bhan AK, et al: Inhibin expression in ovarian tumors and tumor-like lesions: an immunohistochemical study. *Mod Pathol* 1998;11(7):656-664.

Schumer ST, Cannistra SA: Granulosa cell tumor of the ovary. *J Clin Oncol* 2001;21(6):1180-1189.

10. b. The most diagnostic feature distinguishing serous neoplasms of low malignant potential from invasive serous carcinomas is lack of stromal invasion. Neoplasms of low malignant potential without evidence of stromal invasion have a much better prognosis than tumors with evidence of stromal invasion.

The micropapillary type of serous tumor of low malignant potential is a variant that is important to recognize because it is thought to have a poorer prognosis than the typical type. Micropapillae arise from either cyst walls or large fibrous or edematous papillae. The papillae are smoothly contoured. The micropapillae are lined by cuboidal cells with little to no cytoplasm with mildly to moderately atypical nuclei. The cells have high nuclear-to-cytoplasmic ratios. The micropapillary type tends to lack cilia, and the nuclei often contain small, prominent nucleoli. Micropapillary areas must measure at least 5 mm in one dimension on one slide to be diagnosed.

Bell DA, Longacre TA, Prat J, et al: Serous borderline (low malignant potential, atypical proliferative) ovarian tumors: workshop perspectives. *Hum Pathol* 2004;35(8):934-948.

11. a. Lichen sclerosus of the vulva can occur at any age but is seen primarily in two age groups: children and postmenopausal women, usually elderly white women. This condition manifests with severe pruritus. Examination of the lesion demonstrates a characteristic white "cigarette paper" appearance, with loss of the anatomy of the vulva with advanced disease, including loss of the labia minora, agglutination of the hood of the clitoris, and narrowing of the introitus, which leads to difficulty in sexual intercourse. The entire area from the clitoris to the anus may be involved.

A biopsy may be performed because lichen sclerosus can resemble other diseases of the genitalia. The edge is the best area from which to take a biopsy specimen of the lesion because sampling only eroded tissue may result in error of diagnosis. Adjacent normal tissue must be sampled. Direct immunofluorescence of skin adjacent to the lesion is needed to rule out other diseases, such as lichen planus, pemphigus, and pemphigoid, which may resemble lichen sclerosus.

HPV-negative invasive squamous cell carcinoma in elderly women is often associated with lichen sclerosus in the adjacent skin. The nature of this relationship is uncertain because lichen sclerosus is widely considered to be a benign condition.

Although most women with lichen sclerosus do not develop invasive squamous cell carcinoma, they are at a markedly increased risk. Some cases of lichen sclerosus have been shown to demonstrate monoclonality, increased p53 expression, allelic imbalance, and aneuploidy. These findings are independent of the presence or absence of atypia in the biopsy specimen.

Fox H, Wells M: Recent advances in pathology of the vulva. *Histopathology* 2003;42(3):209-216.
Smith YR, Haefner HK: Vulvar lichen sclerosus: pathophysiology and treatment. *Am J Clin Dermatol* 2004;5(2):105-125.

12. e. The image demonstrates a vaginal biopsy specimen containing subepithelial glands, some of which have undergone squamous metaplasia (left side of the image).

Mucus-secreting cervical-type glands are identified on the right side of the image. These findings are the hallmark of adenosis. Although squamous metaplasia is present in the left portion of the image, it is not present on the right side. The image demonstrates glands in tissue that is not normally glandular; this finding is the major feature of the image.

Condyloma acuminatum is an exophytic lesion that exhibits blunt papillae. Karyomegaly; nuclear enlargement, often with binucleation; nuclear membrane irregularity; and nuclear hyperchromasia are present. Vaginal intraepithelial neoplasia consists of low-grade lesions and high-grade lesions. In the low-grade lesions, which include exophytic condylomata and flat condylomata, surface atypia is present, and koilocytes are readily identifiable. High-grade vaginal intraepithelial lesions are similar to lesions seen in the cervix, where atypia is demonstrated in greater than half the thickness of the epithelium. Hyperchromasia and nuclear membrane irregularity are prominent. Mitotic activity is identified close to the surface of the epithelium. Loss of maturation from the basal cells to the surface is evident.

Bartholin duct cysts are associated with the Bartholin gland of the vulva. Bartholin duct cysts are thought to be due to obstruction of the Bartholin gland and may be accompanied by infection or abscess. The cyst is lined by transitional or squamous epithelium. The specimen also often contains the associated Bartholin gland and skeletal muscle, which are important in making the diagnosis.

Chattopadhyay I, Cruikshan DJ, Packer M: Non diethylstilbestrol induced vaginal adenosis—a case series and review of literature. *Eur J Gynaecol Oncol* 2001;22(4):260-262.
Kurita T, Mills AA, Cunha GR: Roles of p63 in the diethylstilbestrol-induced vaginal adenosis. *Development* 2004;131(7):1639-1649.
Robboy SJ, Hill EC, Sandberg EC, et al: Vaginal adenosis in women born prior to the diethylstilbestrol era. *Hum Pathol* 1986; 17(5):488-492.

13. d. The Arias-Stella reaction is composed of secretory endometrial glands with markedly enlarged cells that often fill the gland space or protrude into the lumen as tufts of cells. The cytoplasm is vacuolated or eosinophilic sometimes with eosinophilic inclusions. The nuclei contain optically clear, vacuolated, or smudged chromatin with rare to no mitotic figures. The Arias-Stella reaction is a clue that the patient either was very recently or is currently pregnant. However, the Arias-Stella reaction is not an indication as to whether the pregnancy is intrauterine versus ectopic.

The endometrial malignancy in the differential diagnosis for this condition is clear cell carcinoma of the endometrium. Clear cell carcinoma occurs in women who are not pregnant. It does not occur in secretory endometrium. It is much more likely to be seen in postmenopausal women. The nuclei have high-grade characteristics, including hyperchromasia and large prominent nucleoli. Endometrial hyperplasia is classified by the degree of glandular crowding (known as gland-to-stroma ratio) and by nuclear features. The process shown in the image contains intervening stroma between each of the distended glands. Hyperplastic glands tend to resemble proliferative endometrium in appearance.

Arias-Stella J: The Arias-Stella reaction: facts and fancies four decades after. *Adv Anat Pathol* 2002;9(1):12-23.

Arias-Stella J Jr, Arias-Velasquez A, Arias-Stella J: Normal and abnormal mitoses in the atypical endometrial change associated with chorionic tissue effect. *Am J Surg Pathol* 1994; 18(7):694-701.

14. c. The illustrated lesion is a Brenner tumor, characterized by nests of urothelial-type epithelium within a fibrous stroma. The cells in the nests have nuclear grooves. Glandular spaces are common, as is mucinous metaplasia. The urothelium of Brenner tumors shares the same immunohistochemical characteristics as the urothelium of the genitourinary tract—the lesions are positive for cytokeratin 7 and uroplakin III. However, transitional cell carcinomas of the ovary are negative for markers of urothelial differentiation.

Eichhorn JH, Young RH: Transitional cell carcinoma of the ovary: a morphologic study of 100 cases with emphasis on differential diagnosis. *Am J Surg Pathol* 2004;28(4):453-463.

Riedel I, Czernobilsky B, Lifschitz-Mercer B, et al: Brenner tumors but not transitional cell carcinomas of the ovary show urothelial differentiation: immunohistochemical staining of urothelial markers, including cytokeratins and uroplakins. *Virchows Arch* 2001;438(2):181-191.

15. b. The image demonstrates numerous cells in which mucin has pushed the nucleus to the edge of the cell. This finding is known as a signet ring cell. Carcinomas of the gastrointestinal tract, primarily carcinomas of the colon and stomach, can have the histologic appearance shown. According to most studies, these tumors are the most common primary malignancies with this appearance to metastasize to the ovary. They commonly occur bilaterally and are classically described as Krukenberg tumors.

Breast carcinoma also can metastasize to the ovary in this fashion. Lobular carcinoma of the breast in particular can have the histologic appearance demonstrated in the image. Lung carcinoma has been reported rarely to metastasize to the ovary. However, this carcinoma would be unlikely to have a signet ring appearance because this appearance is uncommon in the lung.

Melanoma is a great mimic of many malignant tumors and should always be considered in the work-up of a lesion that appears to be metastatic. Cervical carcinomas uncommonly metastasize to the ovary. However, this carcinoma is unlikely to have a signet ring appearance as shown in the image.

Moore RG, Chung M, Granai CO, et al: Incidence of metastasis to the ovaries from nongenital tract primary tumors. *Gynecol Oncol* 2004;93(1):87-91.

Seidman JD, Kurman RJ, Ronnett BM: Primary and metastatic mucinous adenocarcinomas in the ovaries: incidence in routine practice with a new approach to improve intraoperative diagnosis. *Am J Surg Pathol* 2003;27(7):985-993.

16. b. In contrast to the more common warty and basaloid patterns of VIN, differentiated VIN is *not* associated with HPV infection. Differentiated VIN accounts for 2% to 10% of all cases of VIN, making it the least common of the VIN subtypes. It occurs in postmenopausal women, with the mean age at presentation being 67 years in one study; this is 2 to 3 decades later than what is seen with the more common warty and basaloid

variants. One quarter of patients have a history of cigarette use.

Clinically, the lesions of differentiated VIN are small, ranging in size from 0.5 to 3.5 cm in greatest dimension. They often manifest as focal gray-white discolorations with a roughened surface or an ill-defined raised, thickened white plaque. Some lesions manifest as discrete elevated nodules. The lesions occasionally may be multifocal. Histologically, these lesions can be extremely difficult to identify because they demonstrate a high degree of cellular maturation with a lack of widespread architectural abnormality, nuclear pleomorphism, and cellular atypia. When atypia is present, it tends to be confined to the basal layer.

The differential diagnostic pitfall for differentiated VIN is the benign mimic squamous cell hyperplasia, especially in superficial biopsy specimens. However, close inspection of differentiated VIN reveals abnormal squamous cells in the epithelium. They are conspicuously enlarged with large vesicular nuclei, usually with macronucleoli. Rare cells may be binucleated. The cytoplasm is abundant and brightly eosinophilic, indicative of premature differentiation or keratinization. Intercellular bridges typically are very prominent. These findings are the hallmark of differentiated VIN.

Hart WR: Vulvar intraepithelial neoplasia: historical aspects and current status. *Int J Gynecol Pathol* 2001;20(1):16-30.

17. a. Sarcoma botryoides of the cervix is a rare tumor that occurs during adolescence and early adulthood. It typically appears as a polypoid, grapelike mass protruding from the vagina. It is an embryonal rhabdomyosarcoma and may be deceptively bland with low cellularity. A hallmark is the relatively denser accumulation of neoplastic cells under the surface described as the cambium layer. These findings are seen in the image and correlate with the clinical history.

Yolk sac tumor of the vagina occurs in children but does not have the features of the lesion shown in the image. Sarcoma botryoides of the vagina is a rare tumor that occurs in children younger than 5 years old. Similar to sarcoma botryoides of the cervix, it is an embryonal rhabdomyosarcoma. The histologic features are identical; however, sarcoma botryoides of the vagina is more aggressive than its cervical counterpart. Condyloma acuminatum and condyloma latum (syphilis) are completely different clinical and pathologic entities and are more likely to be seen in an older patient.

Daya DA, Scully RE: Sarcoma botryoides of the uterine cervix in young women: a clinicopathological study of 13 cases. *Gynecol Oncol* 1988;29(3):290-304.

18. d. This patient has chronic endometritis. Neutrophils and lymphocytes are normally seen in the endometrial stroma. The numbers of these cells are increased around the time of menstruation. However, plasma cells are not normally seen in the endometrium and are a sign of chronic endometritis.

Although a cause is occasionally identified, most cases are nonspecific. There is an increased association between chronic endometritis and the presence of an IUD, but chronic endometritis is not rare in the absence of an IUD.

The decidualized stromal cells of pregnancy should not be mistaken for plasma cells. Dating of the secretory endometrium can be unreliable in the presence of chronic endometritis.

Mount S, Mead P, Cooper K: *Chlamydia trachomatis* in the endometrium: can surgical pathologists identify plasma cells? *Adv Anat Pathol* 2001;8(6):327-329.

Rotterdam H: Chronic endometritis. A clinicopathologic study. *Pathol Annu* 1978;13(Pt 2):209-231.

Smith M, Hagerty KA, Skipper B, et al: Chronic endometritis: a combined histopathologic and clinical review of cases from 2002-2007. *Int J Gynecol Pathol* 2009;29(1):44-50.

19. a. The image corresponds to low-grade endometrial stromal sarcoma. Low-grade endometrial stromal sarcomas and endometrial stromal nodules have similar cytologic features. The features that distinguish low-grade endometrial stromal sarcomas from endometrial stromal nodules are deep myometrial invasion, usually seen histologically in the form of tongues of spindle cells infiltrating into the myometrium, and vascular invasion. Histologic variants are known to obscure the histologic findings of endometrial stromal tumors. Morphologic variants that have been reported include epithelioid change, rhabdoid and rhabdomyoblastic differentiation, fibromyxoid change, sex cord differentiation, smooth muscle differentiation, and glandular differentiation. Fat and highly atypical cells have also been reported in this family of tumors.

There can be considerable overlap when attempting to differentiate low-grade endometrial stromal sarcoma from endometrial stromal nodules. Because curettage is unreliable, hysterectomy is needed to make the definitive diagnosis. High-grade or undifferentiated stromal sarcomas do not present this diagnostic difficulty. When also considering the variant morphologic appearances previously discussed, the differential diagnosis of endometrial stromal tumors includes cellular leiomyoma, intravenous leiomyomatosis, leiomyosarcoma, adenosarcoma, malignant mixed müllerian tumor, and perivascular epithelioid cell tumor. The differential diagnosis can often be resolved with an immunohistochemical panel. CD10, desmin, and h-caldesmon are useful in separating endometrial stromal tumors (CD10 positive, desmin negative, h-caldesmon negative) from smooth muscle tumors (CD10 negative, desmin positive, h-caldesmon positive).

The most frequently reported translocation in endometrial stromal sarcomas is t(7;17)(p15;q21) resulting in a JAZF1/SUZ12 fusion product.

Chiang S, Ali R, Melnyk N, et al: Frequency of known gene rearrangements in endometrial stromal tumors. *Am J Surg Pathol* 2011;35(9):1364-1372.

Dionigi A, Oliva E, Clement PB, et al: Endometrial stromal nodules and endometrial stromal tumors with limited infiltration: a clinicopathologic study of 50 cases. *Am J Surg Pathol* 2002; 26(5):567-581.

20. d. Histologically, müllerian adenosarcoma contains benign glands cuffed by malignant stroma, as is seen in the image. Some lesions exhibit features similar to phyllodes tumors. Müllerian adenosarcomas are most commonly seen in patients in their sixth decade and older, although younger patients have been described. They are predominately polypoid growths that fill the entire uterine cavity. Some may be deeply invasive. Müllerian adenosarcomas can undergo sarcomatous overgrowth. In these cases, the overgrown areas are of higher histologic grade than is associated with the typical adenosarcoma. Adenosarcomas with sarcomatous overgrowth are aggressive tumors with metastatic potential.

In contrast to malignant mixed müllerian tumors, which are high-grade malignant neoplasms, müllerian adenosarcomas are thought to be less aggressive. Most women who present with adenosarcomas have better survival rates stage for stage than women with malignant mixed müllerian tumors.

Arend R, Bagaria M, Lewin SN, et al: Long term outcome and natural history of uterine adenosarcomas. *Gynecol Oncol* 2010;119(2):305-308.

Clement PB: Müllerian adenosarcomas of the uterus with sarcomatous overgrowth. A clinicopathological analysis of 10 cases. *Am J Surg Pathol* 1989;13(1):28-38.

Clement PB, Scully RE: Müllerian adenosarcoma of the uterus. A clinicopathologic analysis of ten cases of a distinctive type of Müllerian mixed tumor. *Cancer* 1974;34(4):1138-1149.

21. e. Adenomatoid tumors of the fallopian tube are benign mesothelial neoplasms. They are usually well circumscribed grossly and measure less than 2 cm in greatest dimension. The histologic features are as shown in the image—most commonly irregular slitlike spaces surrounded by stroma and vacuoles that may contain basophilic material. The slitlike spaces are lined by mesothelial cells. Adenomatoid tumors are not associated with tubal ectopic pregnancy.

Salpingitis isthmica nodosa is a lesion of unknown cause characterized by multiple blind outpouchings of mucosa in the muscularis of the fallopian tube. These lesions are seen histologically as additional lumina cuffed by muscle and are thought to increase the risk of entrapping an ovum, leading to increased risk of tubal ectopic pregnancy. Chlamydial infection can lead to often silent salpingitis, which can lead to tubal scarring, and IUDs can be a cause of chronic salpingitis—both increase the risk of a tubal ectopic pregnancy. Follicular salpingitis is a potential manifestation of chronic salpingitis. It is characterized by the fusion of the delicate epithelial folds of the tube with the formation of multiple cystic spaces, a risk factor for tubal ectopic pregnancy.

Green LK, Kott ML: Histopathologic findings in ectopic tubal pregnancy. *Int J Gynecol Pathol* 1989;8(3):255-262.

Sangoi AR, McKenney JK, Schwartz EJ, et al: Adenomatoid tumors of the male and female genital tracts: a clinicopathologic and immunohistochemical study of 44 cases. *Mod Pathol* 2009; 22(9):1228-1235.

22. c. Most ovarian neoplasms in adolescents are of germ cell origin. The tumor depicted is a yolk sac tumor. Ovarian neoplasms are unusual in adolescents. These tumors represent less than 1% to 2% of all neoplasms occurring in girls younger than 16 years old. However, these neoplasms represent 60% to 70% of all gynecologic neoplasms in childhood and adolescence. These lesions are malignant in 29% to 55% of cases.

In adults, epithelial neoplasms are the most common ovarian neoplasms, representing approximately 90% of ovarian malignancies. Sex cord–stromal tumors and germ cell tumors account for about 5% of ovarian malignancies. In adolescents, germ cell tumors outnumber the other types; they represent approximately 62% of ovarian malignancies, whereas epithelial tumors represent only 20%. Epithelial tumors are much more likely to be benign in adolescent patients than in adult patients.

Germ cell tumors are the most common malignant neoplasms in the first 2 decades of life. They often express hormonal markers, which can also be traced in the blood and can be followed to assess for recurrence. Dysgerminoma is the most common malignant germ cell neoplasm, whereas mature teratoma is the most common benign germ cell neoplasm. Immature teratomas are important to recognize because patients need to be appropriately staged. Immature neural elements are the most common immature elements identified in immature teratoma. Juvenile granulosa cell tumors are the most common sex cord–stromal tumors in pediatric patients. In three quarters of the cases, the tumors secrete estrogen, which results in sexual pseudoprecocity in prepubescent girls. The 5-year survival rate has been reported to be 92%, and patients often require unilateral salpingo-oophorectomy only.

Fotiou SK: Ovarian malignancies in adolescence. *Ann N Y Acad Sci* 1997;816:338-346.

23. **a.** The lesion is an immature teratoma. These neoplasms are graded based on the amount of immature neuroepithelium in the tumor as follows: grade 1, immature neuroepithelium occupying less than 1 low-power (4 × objective) field on the worst slide; grade 2, immature neuroepithelium occupying no more than 3 low-power fields on the worst slide; grade 3, immature neuroepithelium occupying more than 3 low-power fields on any slide.

Yolk sac tumor is often identified in association with immature teratoma, resulting in a mixed germ cell tumor. Yolk sac tumors are thought to be an important risk factor for recurrence in immature teratomas. Yolk sac elements can be overlooked if patterns such as the hepatoid pattern are present because they resemble normal fetal tissues.

The only immature neural tissues that should be considered in the grading of immature teratomas are neural tubules and immature rosettes. Gliomatosis peritonei is defined as mature glial implants along the peritoneal surfaces or in the omentum. These are associated with approximately one quarter of immature teratomas. Low-grade immature teratomas are more likely to have predominately immature neural tissue, whereas high-grade immature teratomas tend to have less neural tissue and to have an abundance of other immature tissues.

Heifetz SA, Cushing B, Giller R, et al: Immature teratomas in children: pathologic considerations: a report from the combined Pediatric Oncology Group/Children's Cancer Group. *Am J Surg Pathol* 1997;22(9):1115-1124.

24. **d.** Choices a through c fit the case scenario presented in the question. The lesion in the image is an endometrioid adenocarcinoma of the uterus. Granulosa cell tumors are sex cord–stromal tumors, which have a well-known association

with estrogen production and overstimulation of the endometrium leading to endometrial carcinomas. Fibrothecomas, similar to granulosa cell tumors, have a well-known association with estrogen production and overstimulation of the endometrium leading to endometrial carcinomas. Steroid cell tumors are uncommon, occur across a wide age range, and can be estrogenic and virilizing.

Luteomas are seen in pregnancy, and they are a lesion of younger women. They would not be included in the differential diagnosis.

Aboud E: A review of granulosa cell tumours and thecomas of the ovary. *Arch Gynecol Obstet* 1997;259(4):161-165.

25. **c.** The image represents a partial hydatidiform mole. Partial hydatidiform moles are usually diandric triploids and have a much higher risk of progression to gestational trophoblastic neoplasia than partial hydatidiform moles. Partial moles are most commonly present as missed abortions. The histologic appearance may be subtle. In this regard, both the clinician and the pathologist may be fooled. Complete moles tend to show more trophoblastic proliferation than partial hydatidiform moles. Choice c is therefore not true and is the correct answer choice.

Cheung AN: Pathology of gestational trophoblastic diseases. *Best Pract Res Clin Obstet Gynaecol* 2003;17(6):849-868.
Genest DR: Partial hydatidiform mole: clinicopathological features, differential diagnosis, ploidy and molecular studies, and gold standards for diagnosis. *Int J Gynecol Pathol* 2001; 20(4):315-322.

26. **b.** The image shows a clear cell adenocarcinoma of the vagina. This neoplasm includes positivity for cytokeratin 7, CEA, cytokeratin 34βE12, CA 125, and CAM 5.2. Roughly two thirds of cases of clear cell adenocarcinoma of the vagina are linked to DES exposure in utero. However, other cases have been associated with vaginal endometriosis. Most cases of vaginal clear cell adenocarcinoma related to DES occur in young women—older than 12 years but younger than 30 years. Ultrastructurally, these tumors resemble the endometrial and ovarian counterparts seen in older women. Histologic sections show tubules and cysts lined by clear cells. Solid and papillary areas may be identified. Where tubules are present, hobnail cells protrude into the glandular lumina.

Hajek RA, King DW, Hernandez-Valero MA, et al: Detection of chromosomal aberrations by fluorescence in situ hybridization in cervicovaginal biopsies from women exposed to diethylstilbestrol in utero. *Int J Gynecol Cancer* 2006;16(1): 318-324.
Shah C, Pizer E, Veljovich DS, et al: Clear cell adenocarcinoma of the vagina in a patient with vaginal endometriosis. *Gynecol Oncol* 2006;103(3):1130-1132.
Vang R, Whitaker BP, Farhood AI, et al: Immunohistochemical analysis of clear cell carcinoma of the gynecologic tract. *Int J Gynecol Pathol* 2001;20(3):252-259.

27. **d.** The lesion depicted is a Sertoli cell tumor of the ovary. It is a pure Sertoli cell tumor because no Leydig cell elements are seen. A subset of the patients has Peutz-Jeghers syndrome, and the tumors may have abundant eosinophilic cytoplasm (the oxyphilic variant). The lipid-rich variant of Sertoli cell tumor is also known as *folliculoma lipidique*. The Sertoli cells contain abundant vacuolated cytoplasm

filled with lipid, which can be demonstrated with oil red O staining. Most Sertoli cell tumors manifest unilaterally. Sertoli cell tumors can manifest clinically with patients demonstrating signs of excess estrogen stimulation, excess androgen, or rarely a combination of both. Although pancytokeratin AE1/AE3 is positive in many Sertoli cell tumors, EMA has been shown to be consistently negative.

Oliva E, Alvarez T, Young RH: Sertoli cell tumors of the ovary: a clinicopathologic and immunohistochemical study of 54 cases. *Am J Surg Pathol* 2005;29(2):143-156.

Tavassoli FA, Norris HJ: Sertoli cell tumors of the ovary. A clinicopathologic study of 28 cases with ultrastructural observations. *Cancer* 1980;46(10):2281-2297.

Verdorfer I, Horst D, Höllrigl A, et al: Sertoli-Leydig cell tumors of the ovary and testis: a CGH and FISH study. *Virchows Arch* 2007;450(3):267-271.

28. a. The image shows endometrioid adenocarcinoma of the ovary. This entity is histologically similar to its counterpart in the uterine corpus. It is composed of glands and tubular structures that are lined by stratified columnar epithelial cells and contains luminal mucin.

The microglandular pattern of ovarian endometrioid adenocarcinoma can mimic an adult granulosa cell tumor. However, adult granulosa cell tumors, particularly of the microfollicular pattern, contain nuclei with prominent central grooves and a "coffee bean" shape. Call-Exner bodies are commonly present. Krukenberg tumors demonstrate numerous cells in which mucin has pushed the nucleus to the edge of the cell. This finding is known as a signet ring cell and is most commonly seen in metastatic adenocarcinomas to the ovary. Krukenberg tumors are often bilateral.

The diagnosis of endometriosis requires the presence of benign endometrial glands and stroma in a site outside the uterine corpus. The lesion in the image is not benign, although it may arise out of a focus of endometriosis. An endometrioid borderline tumor is a tumor of low malignant potential that is composed of atypical or frankly malignant-appearing glands or cysts. These glands or cysts are most commonly identified in a dense fibrous stroma. However, there is no evidence of stromal invasion. The lesion in the image has invaded into the stroma, and no cystic component is present.

Keita M, AinMelk Y, Pelmus M, et al: Endometrioid ovarian cancer and endometriotic cells exhibit the same alteration in the expression of interleukin-1 receptor II: to a link between endometriosis and endometrioid ovarian cancer. *J Obstet Gynaecol Res* 2011;37(2):99-107.

Kurman RJ, Shih L: The origin and pathogenesis of epithelial ovarian cancer—a proposed unifying theory. *Am J Surg Pathol* 2010;34(3):433-443.

Prat J: Ovarian carcinomas, including secondary tumors: diagnostically challenging areas. *Mod Pathol* 2005;18(Suppl 2):S99-S111.

29. e. The tumor in the image is a dysgerminoma, which is a germ cell tumor of the ovary. Germ cell tumors are the most common ovarian tumors in children and adolescents. PLAP is strongly positive in all germ cell tumors, including dysgerminoma. Testicular seminoma is histologically identical to ovarian dysgerminoma. Epithelioid granulomas are commonly seen in dysgerminomas. Their presence is

completely unrelated to tuberculosis infection, another cause of granulomas. In intersex disorders, gonadoblastomas may develop. Gonadoblastoma is a known precursor lesion of dysgerminoma and is the reason why removal of gonadoblastomas is so important.

Baker PM, Oliva E: Immunohistochemistry as a tool in the differential diagnosis of ovarian tumors: an update. *Int J Gynecol Pathol* 2004;24(1):39-55.

Cheng L, Roth LM, Zhang S, et al: KIT gene mutation and amplification in dysgerminoma of the ovary. *Cancer* 2011;117(10):2096-2103.

Talerman A: Germ cell tumors of the ovary. *Curr Opin Obstet Gynecol* 1997;9(1):44-47.

30. a. The lesion in the image is a leiomyosarcoma of the uterus. Coagulative (tumor cell) necrosis is the most important factor in determining malignancy of a smooth muscle tumor, provided that there is no confounding history, such as leuprolide administration, which can create a similar histologic finding.

In the absence of coagulative necrosis, a mitotic index of greater than 10 mitotic figures per 10 high-power fields is needed with diffuse moderate to severe atypia. A high mitotic rate alone is insufficient for the diagnosis of leiomyosarcoma. At least moderate to severe atypia is needed in concert with a high mitotic rate. Pleomorphism alone is insufficient to make the diagnosis of leiomyosarcoma. Leiomyomas can be highly cellular, as can leiomyosarcoma. The presence of increased cellularity alone is insufficient to make a diagnosis of leiomyosarcoma. Although leiomyomas are often multiple, leiomyosarcomas are overwhelmingly single. Multiple lesions are not a criterion for the diagnosis of leiomyosarcoma.

Chen E, O'Connell F, Fletcher CD: Dedifferentiated leiomyosarcoma: clinicopathological analysis of 18 cases. *Histopathology* 2011;59(6):1135-1143.

D'Angelo E, Prat J: Uterine sarcomas: a review. *Gynecol Oncol* 2010;116(1):131-139.

D'Angelo E, Espinosa I, Ali R, et al: Uterine leiomyosarcomas: tumor size, mitotic index, and biomarkers Ki-67 and Bcl-2 identify two groups with different prognosis. *Gynecol Oncol* 2011;121(2):328-333.

31. c. HPV 18 is a high-risk HPV that has been detected at a much higher rate than the other high-risk HPV options in this question (HPV 33, HPV 45). HPV is considered high risk if it has ever been detected in either a squamous cell carcinoma or an adenocarcinoma of the cervix.

HPV 16 and HPV 18 were the first HPVs to be detected in human cervical cancer, although they were first identified in squamous cell carcinoma of the cervix. HPV 16 and HPV 18 were found to be implicated in endocervical adenocarcinoma several years later. Early studies noted that HPV 18 was isolated most commonly in endocervical adenocarcinoma in situ and endocervical adenocarcinoma. More recent studies have shown that HPV 16 is becoming slightly more common, possibly reflecting the increased prevalence of HPV 16 in the population. Endocervical adenocarcinoma in situ is a histologically recognizable precursor to invasive endocervical adenocarcinoma. It is commonly multifocal and involves multiple quadrants of the cervix when examined histologically. Endocervical adenocarcinoma in situ can be treated in most cases by simple hysterectomy or cervical cone biopsy with close subsequent monitoring in cases when preservation of fertility is desired.

Duggan MA, Benoit JL, McGregor SE, et al: Adenocarcinoma in situ of the endocervix: human papillomavirus determination by dot blot hybridization and polymerase chain reaction amplification. *Int J Gynecol Pathol* 1994;13(2):143-149.

Quint KD, de Koning MNC, van Doorn LJ, et al: HPV genotyping and HPV16 variant analysis in glandular and squamous neoplastic lesions of the uterine cervix. *Gynecol Oncol* 2010; 117(2):297-301.

Yokoyama M, Tsutsumi K, Pater A, et al: Human papillomavirus 18-immortalized endocervical cells with in vitro cytokeratin expression characteristics of adenocarcinoma. *Obstet Gynecol* 1994;83(2):197-204.

Zaino RJ: Symposium part I: adenocarcinoma in situ, glandular dysplasia, and early invasive adenocarcinoma of the uterine cervix. *Int J Gynecol Pathol* 2002;21(4):314-326.

32. b. The lesion depicted is an invasive squamous cell carcinoma of the cervix. It is well known that cervical intraepithelial neoplasia is a precursor lesion to squamous cell carcinoma. It is highly likely that this patient has had abnormal Pap smears and has experienced postcoital bleeding. Patients who have squamous intraepithelial lesions of any site of the female genital tract, especially women who are immunocompromised, are at increased risk of developing intraepithelial neoplasia of other sites.

HPV 16 is the most common high-risk HPV to be detected in squamous cell carcinoma. It is highly likely that the patient has been previously exposed to HPV 16. Squamous cell carcinomas are well known to display positive immunohistochemical staining for cytokeratin 5/6 and p63.

Crum CP: Contemporary theories of cervical carcinogenesis: the virus, the host, and the stem cell. *Mod Pathol* 2000;13(3): 243-251.

Lax S: Histopathology of cervical precursor lesions and cancer. *Acta Dermatovenereol Alp Panonica Adriat* 2011;20(3):125-133.

McCluggage WG: Immunohistochemistry as a diagnostic aid in cervical pathology. *Pathology* 2007;39(1):97-111.

33. b. The classic histologic appearance of molluscum contagiosum is demonstrated in the image. The surface consists of an acanthotic squamous mucosa. Directly underlying the squamous mucosa are numerous epidermal cells containing large intracytoplasmic inclusion bodies, termed *molluscum bodies*. As the infected cells move toward the surface, the molluscum bodies increase in size. The nucleus appears as no more than a thin crescent at the periphery of the cell.

The image does not show features of the other answer choices. In herpes infection, the nuclei have three specific characteristics: (1) the nuclei tend to mold to one another, (2) the chromatin is marginated to the periphery as viral particles fill the nucleus, and (3) many of the lesional cells are multinucleate. Histologically, syphilis demonstrates two basic findings: (1) swelling and proliferation of endothelial cells and (2) a predominately perivascular infiltrate that is composed of plasma cells and lymphocytes. This histologic appearance of condyloma acuminatum demonstrates a lesion with surface hyperkeratosis with acanthosis of the underlying epithelium. Orderly maturation and cell polarity are preserved. Vacuolization of the cytoplasm with nuclear atypia (koilocytosis) is present.

Histologically, granuloma inguinale demonstrates four important features: (1) a massive granulation tissue response containing numerous plasma cells; (2) diffuse infiltration of neutrophils forming local collections; (3) rare, if any, lymphocytic infiltration; and (4) large mononuclear cells containing Donovan bodies, which are large, intracytoplasmic, encapsulated bodies. They have two poles.

Smith KJ, Yeager J, Skelton H: Molluscum contagiosum: its clinical, histopathologic, and immunohistochemical spectrum. *Int J Dermatol* 1999;38(9):664-672.

34. c. The correct diagnosis is placental site trophoblastic tumor. The image demonstrates a monotonous lesion with mildly eosinophilic, dense cytoplasm. Pleomorphism is present in occasional cells, but all nuclei demonstrate a wrinkled membrane. Chorionic villi and syncytiotrophoblasts are absent. Placental site trophoblastic tumors are composed predominately of intermediate trophoblasts without other trophoblastic elements present. The patients are usually of reproductive age, and the lesions are most commonly found after a term pregnancy.

Placental site trophoblastic tumors are extremely rare, and chemotherapy is not terribly effective in treating them. Surgery continues to be the mainstay of treatment for these patients.

Histologically, placental site trophoblastic tumors demonstrate monotonous, eosinophilic to amphophilic lesions. The nuclei are hyperchromatic with wrinkled membranes. Lymphovascular invasion is extremely common within the tumor. Chorionic villi and syncytiotrophoblasts are absent. Compared with choriocarcinoma, much less hemorrhage and necrosis are seen. Deep myometrial invasion with splitting of muscle fibers is the rule.

Despite deep myometrial invasion, most placental site trophoblastic tumors are adequately managed by hysterectomy. However, a subset of the lesions is extremely malignant and demonstrates aggressive behavior. These patients may die despite aggressive treatment with surgery and chemotherapy. Placental site trophoblastic tumors demonstrate strong immunohistochemical staining for human placental lactogen, supporting an origin from the intermediate trophoblast.

Chen Y, Zhang X, Xie X: Clinical features of 17 cases of placental site trophoblastic tumor. *Int J Obstet Gynecol* 2011;115(2): 204-205.

Cheung AN: Pathology of gestational trophoblastic diseases. *Best Pract Res Clin Obstet Gynaecol* 2003;17(6):849-868.

Lurain JR: Gestational trophoblastic disease I: epidemiology, pathology, clinical presentation and diagnosis of gestational trophoblastic disease, and management of hydatidiform mole. *Am J Obstet Gynecol* 2011;204(6):11-18.

35. e. The lesion depicted is a tubal ectopic pregnancy. An association with chronic salpingitis is present in 35% to 45% of all cases of tubal ectopic pregnancy. Salpingitis is usually secondary to PID. A common cause of PID is *Chlamydia trachomatis* infection. The histologic examination demonstrates numerous immature chorionic villi and trophoblastic cells. Tubal epithelium is observed on the left side of the image. On gross examination of the specimen, an embryo may be present. Tubal ectopic pregnancies have been reported to occur in the ampulla, isthmus, and fimbriated end of the fallopian tube. The ampulla is the most common site of tubal ectopic pregnancy.

A missed abortion is an important differential diagnostic consideration. Patients are usually evaluated by ultrasound to demonstrate absence of an intrauterine gestational sac. Ultrasound can be followed by endometrial dilatation and curettage, which would show the absence of chorionic villi, trophoblasts, or embryonal tissue.

Endometriosis can cause scarring of the fallopian tube. Fallopian tube scarring, most commonly caused by chronic salpingitis often in the presence of PID, is a risk factor for tubal ectopic pregnancy.

Shaw JL, Dey SK, Critchley HO, et al: Current knowledge of the aetiology of human tubal ectopic pregnancy. *Hum Reprod Update* 2010;16(4):432-444.
Shaw JL, Willis GS, Lee KF, et al: *Chlamydia trachomatis* infection increases fallopian tube PROKR2 via TLR2 and NFκB activation resulting in a microenvironment predisposed to ectopic pregnancy. *Am J Pathol* 2011;178(1):253-260.

36. e. The lesion in the image is a choriocarcinoma. Choriocarcinomas demonstrate an admixture of cytotrophoblasts, intermediate trophoblasts, and syncytiotrophoblasts without the presence of chorionic villi. Cytotrophoblasts tend to have clear cytoplasm, whereas intermediate trophoblasts have more eosinophilic cytoplasm. The syncytiotrophoblast is strongly positive for β-hCG and weakly positive for hPL. All three cell types within choriocarcinoma are strongly and diffusely positive for cytokeratins. Choriocarcinomas do not possess their own vessels or stroma, and this creates a propensity for extensive tumor necrosis. Commonly, the only viable tumor identified in resection specimens is at the periphery of the lesion.

Extraordinarily, intraplacental choriocarcinoma has been diagnosed immediately following pregnancy. This is an extremely rare lesion.

Cheung AN: Pathology of gestational trophoblastic diseases. *Best Pract Res Clin Obstet Gynaecol* 2003;17(6):849-868.
Wagner BJ, Woodward PJ, Dickey GE: From the archives of the AFIP. Gestational trophoblastic disease: radiologic-pathologic correlation. *Radiographics* 1996;16(1):131-148.
Wong SC, Chan AT, Chan JK, et al: Nuclear β-catenin and Ki-67 expression in choriocarcinoma and in its pre-malignant form. *J Clin Pathol* 2006;59(4):387-392.

37. b. The correct diagnosis is pulmonary-type small cell carcinoma, which is a primary small cell carcinoma of the ovary that resembles pulmonary small cell neuroendocrine carcinoma. Pulmonary-type small cell carcinoma is an extremely rare lesion with approximately 20 cases in the literature. The lesion may manifest unilaterally or bilaterally. They are most often solid, although cystic lesions and foci of necrosis are common. Histologically, the lesions resemble their pulmonary counterpart. The cells are small to medium in size with finely stippled chromatin. Nucleoli are absent. Nuclear molding is present, as is pyknosis and tumor cell necrosis. In the largest series to date comprising 11 cases, a surface epithelial-stromal neoplasm was present. The most common associated lesion is endometrioid adenocarcinoma.

Although hypercalcemic-type small cell carcinoma has been shown to demonstrate WT-1 positivity with much greater frequency, pulmonary-type small cell carcinoma

does not show the same level of consistency in WT-1 staining. Clinical work-up is essential in determining whether pulmonary-type small cell carcinoma is a primary ovarian lesion versus a metastatic lesion from the lung.

Pulmonary-type small cell carcinoma is an aggressive lesion. The prognosis is poor. In the original series, 7 of 11 cases had spread beyond the confines of the ovary on initial diagnosis. Of the 11 patients, 5 were dead within 13 months of diagnosis. Because the volume of cases is so low, little is known about optimal therapy. What is known is that the usual therapeutic regimens for other ovarian malignancies are ineffective in treating pulmonary-type small cell carcinoma.

Carlson JW, Nucci MR, Brodsky J, et al: Biomarker-assisted diagnosis of ovarian, cervical, and pulmonary small cell carcinomas: the role of TTF-1, WT-1, and HPV analysis. *Histopathology* 2007;51(3):305-312.
McCluggage WG: Ovarian neoplasms composed of small round cells. A review. *Adv Anat Pathol* 2004;11(6):288-296.

38. b. The lesion shown in the image is herpes simplex virus (HSV) infection. Several nuclei demonstrate ground-glass features and contain numerous viral particles. One of the main features of HSV infection is molding of the nuclei to each other. When examining nuclei infected by HSV, a dark rim at the edge of the nuclei is noticed. This feature is the margination of nuclear chromatin to the edges of the nucleus, which is another important histologic feature of HSV infection. Cowdry type A inclusions are eosinophilic inclusions seen in the center of some, but not all, HSV-infected nuclei. These inclusions are composed of nucleic acid and protein. They are also seen in varicella-zoster virus and vaccinia virus infection. However, Cowdry type B inclusions are a part of cytomegalovirus infection, not a part of HSV infection.

Sauerbrei A, Wutzler P: Herpes simplex and varicella zoster infections during pregnancy: current concepts of prevention, diagnosis and therapy. Part 1: herpes simplex virus infections. *Med Microbiol Immunol* 2007;196(2):89-94.
Sugiyama H, Yoshikawa T, Ihira M, et al: Comparison of loop-mediated isothermal amplification, real-time PCR, and virus isolation for the detection of herpes simplex virus in genital lesions. *J Med Virol* 2005;75(4):583-587.

39. a. The lesion shown in the image is a mature teratoma. It is a cystic lesion that often contains hair, keratinous debris, and sometimes teeth. The structure containing the tooth is known as a Rokitansky protuberance. Rarely, malignant neoplasms may arise within mature teratomas. Of all malignancies that have been reported, squamous cell carcinoma is the most common.

Papillary thyroid carcinoma, rhabdomyosarcoma, osteosarcoma, and melanoma also have been reported in association with mature teratoma. However, these lesions are not as commonly associated with mature teratoma as squamous cell carcinoma.

Chiang AJ, La V, Peng J, et al: Squamous cell carcinoma arising from mature cystic teratoma of ovary. *Int J Gynecol Cancer* 2011;21(3):466-474.
Kikkawa F, Ishikawa H, Tamakoshi K, et al: Squamous cell carcinoma arising from mature cystic teratoma of the ovary: a clinicopathologic analysis. *Obstet Gynecol* 1997;89(6): 1017-1022.

Sakuma M, Otsuki T, Yoshinaga K, et al: Malignant transformation arising from mature cystic teratoma of the ovary: a retrospective analysis of 20 cases. *Int J Gynecol Cancer* 2010;20(5):766-771.

40. c. The gross image represents a carcinosarcoma, or malignant mixed müllerian tumor. Carcinosarcoma is most commonly a disease of elderly, postmenopausal women. The image is an excellent representation of what often occurs with the tumor. The image shows a large, bulky polypoid lesion with foci of hemorrhage. Foci of necrosis are present. The neoplasm fills the endometrial cavity. Patients with carcinosarcoma present with vaginal bleeding and abdominal mass or pelvic pain. The lesion may prolapse through the cervix to produce an upper vaginal mass.

Histologically, the lesion exhibits epithelial and mesenchymal components. There are two types: homologous and heterologous. The mesenchymal elements in homologous tumors are of tissue types that would normally arise in the uterine corpus, such as smooth muscle or endometrial stroma. The mesenchymal elements in heterologous tumors are of tissue types that would normally arise outside the uterine corpus, such as bone, cartilage, or adipose tissue. Deep myometrial invasion is frequent in carcinosarcomas. Some lesions invade through the full thickness of the uterine wall and involve other pelvic structures by direct extension. The malignant epithelial element of carcinosarcoma is most commonly of glandular origin. Rarely, the malignant epithelial element may be squamous or undifferentiated carcinoma.

Kempson RL, Hendrickson MR: Smooth muscle, endometrial stromal, and mixed Müllerian tumors of the uterus. *Mod Pathol* 2000;13(3):328-342.

Silverberg SG, Major FJ, Blessing JA, et al: Carcinosarcoma (malignant mixed mesodermal tumor) of the uterus. A Gynecologic Oncology Group pathologic study of 203 cases. *Int J Gynecol Pathol* 1990;9(1):1-19.

41. d. The lesion demonstrates the classic features of a papillary thyroid carcinoma. Papillary thyroid carcinomas have been reported to arise within struma ovarii; these tumors are sometimes designated as malignant struma ovarii. Struma ovarii is a specialized teratoma that is predominately composed of thyroid tissue. It is usually not a diagnostic difficulty. Patients may present with symptoms of a primary thyroid neoplasm, which must be excluded.

In serous carcinoma, glands are noted back to back without intervening stroma. Examination of the nuclei results in marked pleomorphism with prominent nucleoli. Mitotic figures are present and may be atypical. Giant tumor cells also may be seen. Serous cystadenomas are typically lined by cells resembling the lining cells of the fallopian tube, although they may also be lined by nonciliated cuboidal or columnar epithelium that resembles ovarian surface epithelium. Mucinous cystadenoma is a cystic lesion lined by a single layer of mucin-containing columnar cells. The cells resemble cells seen in the normal endocervix. Brenner tumor is characterized by nests of urothelial-type epithelium within a fibrous stroma. The cells in the nests have nuclear grooves. Glandular spaces are common, as in mucinous metaplasia. Papillary thyroid carcinoma has not been reported to arise in any of these conditions.

Hatami M, Breining D, Owers RL, et al: Malignant struma ovarii—a case report and review of the literature. *Gynecol Obstet Invest* 2008;65(2):104-107.

Marti JL, Clark VE, Harper H, et al: Optimal surgical management of well differentiated thyroid carcinoma arising in struma ovarii: a series of 4 patients and a review of 53 reported cases. *Thyroid* 2012;22(4):400-406.

Schmidt J, Derr V, Heinrich MC, et al: BRAF in papillary thyroid carcinoma of the ovary (malignant struma ovarii). *Am J Surg Pathol* 2007;31(9):1337-1343.

42. e. There are approximately 130 known genotypes of HPV. They are categorized into low-risk and high-risk types. Worldwide, HPV 16 is the most common HPV detected in both invasive cervical cancer and cervical precancers; it is detected in 50% to 70% of invasive cervical carcinomas. Other high-risk types include HPV 18, HPV 31, HPV 33, and HPV 45. At any point in time, approximately 10% of women with normal cervical cytologic appearance will test positive for HPV DNA by molecular methods.

Genital HPV infections are common worldwide. They are sexually transmitted and are most frequent in men and women 18 to 30 years old. Risk factors for HPV infection include early age of first intercourse, numerous sexual partners throughout life, and sexual contact with high-risk partners. In most patients, HPV infection clears spontaneously. However, in 10% to 20% of patients, HPV infection persists. In these patients, there is a significantly increased risk of progression to high-grade squamous intraepithelial lesions and invasive cervical carcinomas. HPVs are small, double-stranded DNA viruses that are specific only for humans. They are also exquisitely tissue-tropic because they can complete their infectious cycle only in fully differentiating squamous epithelium.

Castellsagué X: Natural history and epidemiology of HPV infection and cervical cancer. *Gynecol Oncol* 2008; 110(3 Suppl 2):S4-S7.

Stanley M: Pathology and epidemiology of HPV infection in females. *Gynecol Oncol* 2010;117(2 Suppl):S5-S10.

43. b. The image illustrates a *Schistosoma* species, which is usually identified as ova in biopsy specimens. Live specimens at the time of biopsy contain miracidia within the ova. Calcified ova are also commonly identified in histologic sections. These parasites are endemic in Malawi. Travel history is always important when attempting to identify microorganisms.

H. capsulatum is a fungal disease that is identified as multiple small encapsulated organisms within histiocytes. It is endemic in the Ohio and Mississippi River valleys. It is most commonly a pulmonary illness, although dissemination can occur in immunocompromised patients. Histologically, the organisms of *C. immitis* are seen within large, round, thick-walled spherules. Each spherule contains hundreds to thousands of highly infectious endospores. If this infection is suspected, it is important to warn the microbiology laboratory because special culture techniques must be employed. *C. neoformans* is a ubiquitous fungus with a worldwide distribution. It is most commonly seen in immunocompromised patients. Its natural habitat is soil. Round budding yeasts are seen histologically. They have a mucinous capsule, which stains readily with mucicarmine staining. Classically, *Blastomyces* undergoes broad-based budding, which can be seen on histologic sections. The organisms are better seen after applying Gomori-Grocott methenamine silver staining. Similar to *Histoplasma, Blastomyces* is endemic in the Mississippi and Ohio River valleys.

Helling-Giese G, Sjaastad A, Poggensee G, et al: Female genital schistosomiasis (FGS): relationship between gynecological and histopathological findings. *Acta Trop* 1996;62(4): 257-267.

Wright ED, Chiphangwi J, Hutt MSR: Schistosomiasis of the female genital tract. A histopathologic study of 176 cases from Malawi. *Trans R Soc Trop Med Hyg* 1982;76(6):822-829.

44. c. Merkel cell carcinoma, as seen in the image, is a neuroendocrine neoplasm of the skin. It demonstrates a solid or trabecular architectural pattern. The lesion has oval to polygonal nuclei with scant cytoplasm. The chromatin pattern is fine and evenly distributed, classically described as a "salt and pepper" pattern.

Poorly differentiated squamous cell carcinoma is in the differential diagnosis of this lesion. However, poorly differentiated squamous cell carcinoma does not have such fine, evenly distributed nuclear chromatin. It also does not display a solid and trabecular architectural pattern and tends to have more cytoplasm as well as prominent nucleoli. Diffuse large B-cell lymphoma does not display a nested or cohesive pattern; rather, patternless sheets of large, pleomorphic lymphocytes would be seen. Basal cell carcinoma, in contrast to what is seen in this image, demonstrates atypical basaloid cells often present in nests (although other growth patterns are well described) with peripheral palisading at the edges. Differentiated VIN demonstrates surface hyperkeratosis, with underlying acanthosis of the squamous epithelium. Intracellular bridges are prominent. Prominent keratin pearls are seen. When cytologic atypia is present, it is most commonly seen only in the basal layers. Nucleoli are prominent. These features are not seen in the image.

Chen KT: Merkel's cell (neuroendocrine) carcinoma of the vulva. *Cancer* 1994;73(8):2186-2191.

Iavazzo C, Terzi M, Arapantoni-Dadioti P, et al: Vulvar Merkel cell carcinoma: a case report. *Case Rep Med* 2011;2011:546972.

45. b. The lesion in the image is an aggressive angiomyxoma. This lesion is most commonly reported in patients in their reproductive years and is more common in the vulva than in the vagina where it has also been reported. Despite the locally aggressive behavior, metastasis is not a part of the clinical picture. It is a low to moderately cellular lesion set in a myxoid stroma with numerous medium-sized to large blood vessels with hyalinized walls. Because of its local aggressiveness and the risk of recurrence, negative margins are essential for a better outcome. HGMA2 immunohistochemistry is positive in approximately 50% of cases of aggressive angiomyxoma. In cases when immunohistochemistry is positive, the marker can be used to assess the surgical margins.

Dahiya K, Jain S, Duhan N, et al: Aggressive angiomyxoma of the vulva and vagina: a series of three cases and review of the literature. *Arch Gynecol Obstet* 2011;283(5):1145-1148.

McCluggage WG: Recent developments in vulvovaginal pathology. *Histopathology* 2009;54(2):156-173.

46. a. Ovarian tuberculosis is more common in areas where tuberculosis is endemic but has been reported worldwide. One difficulty encountered in managing this condition is that it is nearly impossible clinically to differentiate tuberculosis from ovarian neoplasia because the abdominoperitoneal presentation is similar. Several reports have shown that CA 125 levels may be elevated in patients with ovarian tuberculosis, further complicating preoperative diagnosis. Ovarian tuberculosis has been demonstrated in adolescent patients, and because germ cell tumors are of concern in this age group, the diagnosis is difficult to exclude preoperatively. Some studies have shown correlation between female genital organ tuberculosis and infertility. In areas where tuberculosis infection is endemic, it is reasonable to consider the diagnosis in young women presenting with fertility problems. The worldwide emergence of HIV has increased the incidence of tuberculosis, and unusual presentations of this illness are increasing.

Namavar Jahromi B, Parsanezhad ME, Ghane-Shirazi R: Female genital tuberculosis and infertility. *Int J Gynecol Obstet* 2001; 75(3):269-272.

Sharma JB, Jain SK, Pushparaj M, et al: Abdomino-peritoneal tuberculosis masquerading as ovarian cancer: a retrospective study of 26 cases. *Arch Gynecol Obstet* 2010;282(6):643-648.

47. b. The lesion shown in the image is an endometrioid endometrial adenocarcinoma. As in most lesions, increased Ki-67 is related to poor prognosis in these patients. Low p21 levels, especially when combined with microsatellite instability and high survivin expression, results in poor prognosis in endometrial carcinoma even in low-grade lesions. Microsatellite instability was shown to be involved in endometrial carcinomas in the late 1990s. It is distributed among all FIGO (International Federation of Gynecology and Obstetrics) stages. High survivin expression is a marker of poor prognosis in endometrioid endometrial adenocarcinoma, especially when combined with low p21 activity and microsatellite instability. Although increased p53 activity is much more common in serous carcinomas of the uterus, it can be demonstrated in endometrioid endometrial carcinomas as well, and if it is present, it is a marker of poor prognosis.

Lax SF, Kurman RJ: A dualistic model for endometrial carcinogenesis based on immunohistochemical and molecular genetic analyses. *Verh Dtsch Ges Pathol* 1997;81:228-232.

Markova I, Duskova M, Lubusky M, et al: Selected immunohistochemical prognostic factors in endometrial cancer. *Int J Gynecol Cancer* 2010;20(4):576-582.

Steinbakk A, Malpica A, Slewa A, et al: Biomarkers and microsatellite instability analysis of curettings can predict the behavior of FIGO stage I endometrial endometrioid adenocarcinoma. *Mod Pathol* 2011;24(9):1262-1271.

48. e. Mixed germ cell tumors of the ovary with teratomatous components have been shown to demonstrate isochromosome 12p; this is thought to be similar to the pathogenesis in the testis. In contrast, pure mature and immature teratomas do not demonstrate isochromosome 12p; this supports the possible dual pathogenesis of teratomas of the ovary. Fluorescence in situ hybridization can be used to isolate isochromosome 12p amplification in germ cell tumors of the ovary.

Dysgerminoma, similar to seminoma in the testis, shows both isochromosome 12p and polysomy of chromosome 12p; in contrast, gonadoblastomas do not demonstrate either isochromosome 12p or polysomy of chromosome 12p; this suggests a role for chromosome 12p in the malignant evolution of the dysgerminoma. Chromosome 12p may serve as a useful diagnostic tool in cases when the germ cell origin of an ovarian neoplasm is unclear.

Cossu-Rocca P, Zhang S, Roth LM, et al: Chromosome 12p abnormalities in dysgerminoma of the ovary: a FISH analysis. *Mod Pathol* 2006;19(4):611-615.

Poulos C, Cheng L, Zhang S, et al: Analysis of ovarian teratomas for isochromosome 12p: evidence supporting a dual histogenetic pathway for teratomatous elements. *Mod Pathol* 2006;19(6):766-771.

49. e. The image shows embryonal carcinoma. This entity is rarely seen in pure form and is much more commonly seen as a component of a mixed germ cell tumor. CD30 is a major marker used in the differential diagnosis of embryonal carcinoma with other neoplasms. AFP immunohistochemical staining is often identified in embryonal carcinomas. This is one of the reasons why it can be difficult to differentiate yolk sac tumor from embryonal carcinoma.

OCT4 immunohistochemical staining has been noted to be highly sensitive in the detection of embryonal carcinomas and dysgerminomas. D2-40 was originally thought to be a marker of seminoma/dysgerminoma. It has since been demonstrated to be positive in embryonal carcinomas as well. CD117 is the immunohistochemical marker of the *KIT* gene. This gene is known to be involved in dysgerminoma—hence the positive staining in that tumor. However, CD117 is negative in most embryonal carcinomas.

Baker PM, Oliva E: Immunohistochemistry as a tool in the differential diagnosis of ovarian tumors: an update. *Int J Gynecol Pathol* 2004;24(1):39-55.

Ulbright TM: Germ cell tumors of the gonads: a selective review emphasizing problems in differential diagnosis, newly appreciated, and controversial issues. *Mod Pathol* 2005; 18(Suppl 2):S61-S79.

50. c. The image shows microglandular hyperplasia. The glands are tightly packed and are of varying size. Cystic dilatation of some glands is present. The nuclei are bland. Mitoses are absent. Inflammatory cells are seen in the scant stroma and within the gland lumina.

Microglandular hyperplasia can be easily confused with endocervical adenocarcinoma in situ when the specimen is scant. Endocervical adenocarcinoma in situ demonstrates nuclear atypia and mitoses that are not seen in microglandular hyperplasia. Microglandular hyperplasia can also be difficult to differentiate from well-differentiated endometrioid endometrial adenocarcinoma. However, the lack of nuclear atypia and mitoses in most cases can aid in making the correct diagnosis. Microglandular hyperplasia is also a diagnosis most commonly seen in reproductive-age women, whereas endometrial adenocarcinoma is more common in postmenopausal women. The histologic features of tubal metaplasia are not seen in this image. No ciliated cells are present. The lesion in the image is glandular. No squamous differentiation is evident on the slide, so squamous metaplasia is not a consideration.

Medeiros F, Bell DA: Pseudoneoplastic lesions of the female genital tract. *Arch Pathol Lab Med* 2010;134(3):393-403.

Roh MH, Agostin E, Birch C, et al: P16 immunohistochemical patterns in microglandular hyperplasia of the cervix and their significance. *Int J Gynecol Pathol* 2009;28(2):107-113.

51. a. The image demonstrates a yolk sac tumor. Three Schiller-Duval bodies are identified in the image. There is no embryonal variant of yolk sac tumor.

The endodermal sinus variant is the variant of yolk sac tumor most easily recognized because it tends to have many Schiller-Duval bodies. The hepatoid variant, a more recently described variant of yolk sac tumor, can be pure or seen as a component of yolk sac tumor with mixed patterns. The reticular pattern is the most common pattern of yolk sac tumor. It is formed by a loose, basophilic stroma containing a network of microcystic spaces lined by primitive germ cells. Atypia is variable. The polyvesicular vitelline pattern of yolk sac tumor is a rare variant of the tumor. It appears as multiple large dilated spaces lined by flattened cells resembling mesothelium.

Young RH: New and unusual aspects of ovarian germ cell tumors. *Am J Surg Pathol* 1993;17(12):1210-1224.

CHAPTER 11

BREAST PATHOLOGY

Hanina Hibshoosh, Lorenzo Memeo, and Aqeel Ahmed

QUESTIONS

Questions 1-15 in this chapter refer to a photo or photomicrograph.

1. Which of the following statements regarding the relative risk of developing an invasive carcinoma is TRUE?
   a. The relative risk associated with the lesion shown in the image is 1.5 to 2.
   b. The relative risk associated with atypical ductal hyperplasia is 8 to 10.
   c. The relative risk associated with nonatypical proliferative disease is 4 to 5.
   d. The relative risk associated with usual ductal hyperplasia is 1.5 to 2.
   e. The relative risk of ductal carcinoma in situ is 4 to 5.

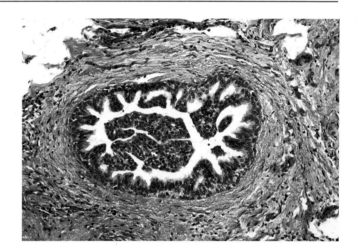

2. All of the following statements regarding the lesion shown in the image are true EXCEPT:
   a. The lesion is three to four times more common among Hispanic immigrants (particularly women from Central and South America) and Asian American women than whites.
   b. The stromal component of this lesion has been shown to be clonal in most examined cases.
   c. The high-grade malignant form of this tumor may show heterologous differentiation.
   d. Cellular fibroadenoma is not a part of the differential diagnosis.
   e. Tumors in this category can be divided into histologically benign (most tumors) and high-grade and low-grade malignant variants.

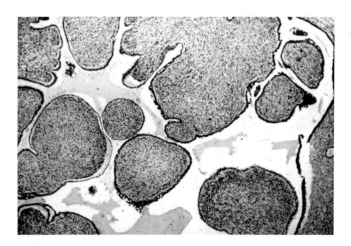

3. All of the following statements regarding vascular lesions that may occur in the breast and the associated region are true EXCEPT:

   a. Benign vascular lesions include perilobular hemangioma, papillary endothelial hyperplasia, and atypical vascular lesion (benign lymphangiomatous papule).

   b. Lymphangiosarcoma occurring in the arms of patients who have undergone modified radical mastectomy is also known as Stewart-Treves syndrome.

   c. The image shown could not have been taken from a high-grade angiosarcoma.

   d. Angiosarcoma in the skin of the breast after lumpectomy and radiation therapy is primarily high grade but may be low grade.

   e. The median age of primary mammary angiosarcoma is the 30s and 40s, and survival is related to the grade (i.e., presence of numerous mitoses, blood lakes, and necrosis).

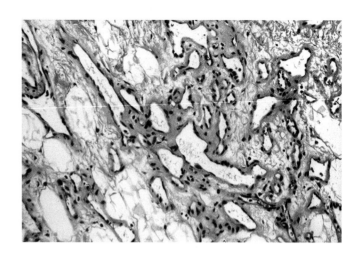

4. Medullary, tubular, and mucinous types of invasive breast cancer generally have a prognosis that is:

   a. Equivalent to the lesion depicted in the image

   b. Similar to carcinoma with central fibrotic focus

   c. Similar to invasive micropapillary carcinoma

   d. Similar to invasive ductal carcinoma of no special type (NST)

   e. Better than all of the above

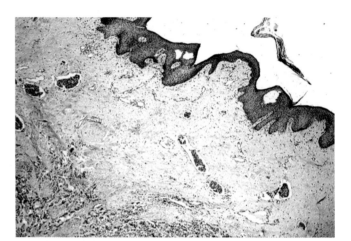

5. Invasive lobular carcinoma is characterized by:

   a. A classic pattern of growth characterized by an Indian file pattern and targetoid arrangement of cells as depicted in the image

   b. A higher rate of estrogen receptor and progesterone receptor positivity relative to ductal carcinoma not otherwise specified and less likely to be *ERBB2* (*HER2/neu*) positive

   c. Variants of lobular carcinoma, including a solid pattern of growth, alveolar pattern, pleomorphic and tubulolobular pattern, and skip pattern of distribution in invasive lobular cancer

   d. A prominent signet ring cell feature, apocrine differentiation, or a histiocytoid or pleomorphic variant

   e. All of the above, including commonly showing E-cadherin loss and a significant percentage showing E-cadherin mutations

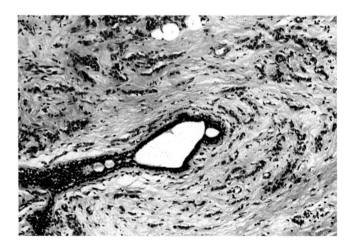

6. All of the following statements regarding the lesion depicted in the image (the panel on the right is a *p63* immunostain) are true EXCEPT:

a. Intraductal and invasive carcinomas do not arise from this lesion.

b. This lesion is microglandular adenosis.

c. The differential diagnosis includes sclerosing adenosis and tubular carcinoma.

d. This bland-appearing but infiltrating lesion lacks myoepithelial cells and reactivity with epithelial membrane antigen or gross cystic disease fluid protein (GCDFP-15).

e. Type IV collagen can be demonstrated around the tubular structures.

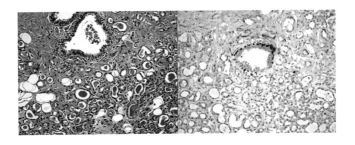

7. All of the following statements regarding breast development are true EXCEPT:

a. During the fifth week of gestation, thickening of the epidermis begins, forming the milk line, which extends from the axilla to the groin region.

b. The mammary ridge involutes except in the region of the chest, and subsequently downward growth of the epithelium into stroma is seen during the 15th week of gestation.

c. Supernumerary breast tissue or polythelia or both occur as a consequence of failure of the milk line to involute.

d. Breast tissue identified in the axilla may represent either ectopic breast tissue or the axillary tail of the breast.

e. Ectopic breast tissue cannot demonstrate the changes seen in the image.

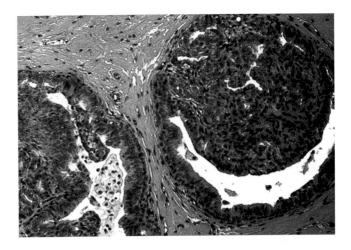

8. All of the following statements are true regarding the location of breast lesions EXCEPT:

a. The terminal duct lobular unit is the site of changes of the lesion depicted in the image and peripheral papillomas.

b. The nipple or areolar region may show Paget disease, solitary papilloma, florid papillomatosis of the nipple (nipple adenoma), duct ectasia in the subareolar region, squamous metaplasia of lactiferous ducts with subareolar abscess, and subareolar sclerosing duct hyperplasia.

c. Interlobular stroma is associated with fat necrosis, lipoma, mesenchymal tumors including fibromatosis and sarcoma, and pseudoangiomatous stromal hyperplasia.

d. Skin is the only site of angiosarcoma.

e. Intralobular stroma and periductal stroma are associated with fibroadenoma and phyllodes tumor, respectively.

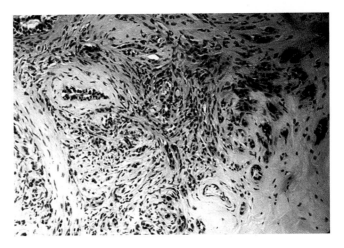

9. Infiltrative lesions of the breast include all of the following EXCEPT:

a. Sclerosing papilloma

b. Syringomatous adenoma of the nipple

c. Tubular carcinoma

d. Microglandular adenosis

e. Granular cell tumor

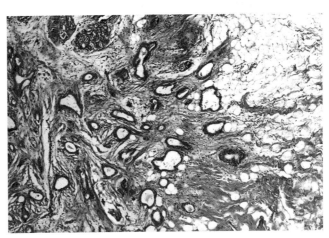

10. All of the following statements regarding the lesion depicted in the image are true EXCEPT:
    a. The differential diagnosis may include fibromatosis, fascicular pseudoangiomatous stromal hyperplasia, spindle cell carcinoma, postbiopsy scar, myofibroblastoma, and phyllodes tumor.
    b. The tumor primarily occurs in postmenopausal women.
    c. The lesion generally lacks mitoses or has only a rare mitotic figure and is typically seen in patients in their 20s to 40s.
    d. The lesion is infiltrative but not metastasizing.
    e. Lymphoid follicles may be seen at the edge of infiltrating lesional cells, and the lesion is associated with a significant recurrence rate, particularly if not excised with a wide margin.

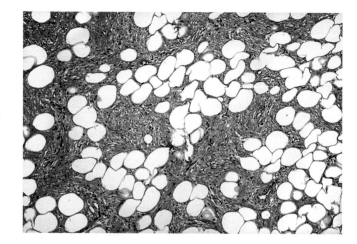

11. All of the following statements regarding the class of lesions of the breast seen in the image are true EXCEPT:
    a. Multiple intraductal papillomas arising from the terminal duct lobular unit are generally thought to be associated with a 1.5- to 2-fold increased risk of developing invasive cancer, and this risk is not observed in solitary intraductal papilloma.
    b. The presence of a myoepithelial and luminal cell layer excludes the possibility of intraductal papillary carcinoma and the presence of any carcinoma within the duct.
    c. Intraductal papilloma may additionally harbor atypical ductal hyperplasia or ductal carcinoma in situ within the duct.
    d. Papillary ductal carcinoma in situ comes in two varieties: intraductal micropapillary ductal carcinoma lacking fibrovascular cores and intraductal papillary ductal carcinoma containing fibrovascular cores but without myoepithelial cells.
    e. Atypical ductal hyperplasia noted in association with an intraductal papilloma is associated with a 4- to 5-fold relative risk of developing invasive cancer, which is primarily ipsilateral.

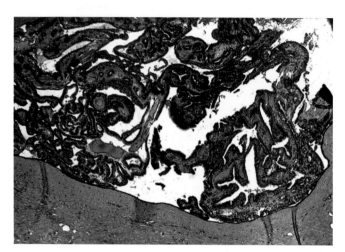

12. All of the following statements regarding lobular carcinoma in situ are true EXCEPT:
    a. Lobular carcinoma in situ is depicted in the image and shows a similar cell population to atypical lobular hyperplasia but shows a greater degree of distention of the acini and involvement of the terminal duct lobular unit.
    b. Lobular carcinoma in situ typically shows weak to no E-cadherin staining and is generally positive for high-molecular-weight cytokeratin (34βE12).
    c. Lobular carcinoma in situ is commonly multifocal and bilateral in distribution.
    d. Most carcinomas arising on a background of lobular carcinoma in situ are invasive ductal carcinomas and overwhelmingly have an ipsilateral distribution.
    e. The magnitude of the relative risk of development of an invasive cancer is similar in lobular carcinoma in situ and ductal carcinoma in situ.

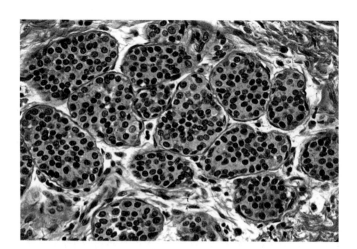

13. The classic yet rare tumor of the nipple that is depicted in the image is characterized by all of the following EXCEPT:
    a. The tumor is nonmetastasizing.
    b. The tumor may be confused with some forms of a florid papillomatosis of the nipple or tubular carcinoma.
    c. The tubules formed by the tumor never form comma-shaped glands.
    d. The tumor classically occurs in the nipple.
    e. The tumor may recur if incompletely excised.

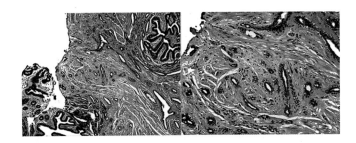

14. All of the following statements regarding the breast lesion shown in the image are true EXCEPT:
    a. This is the most common lesion identified in the male breast.
    b. A similar-appearing lesion is never seen in females.
    c. This lesion has a bimodal age distribution that includes puberty and old age.
    d. The early forms of this lesion show florid intraductal epithelial hyperplasia, which may be mistaken for carcinoma.
    e. Patients with this condition do not have an increased incidence of breast carcinoma.

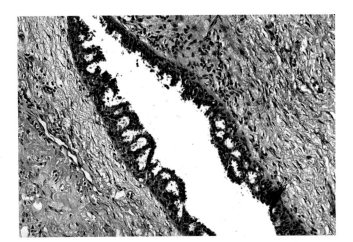

15. The tumor depicted in the image is associated with all of the following characteristics EXCEPT:
    a. The tumor has a prognosis equivalent to invasive ductal carcinoma not otherwise specified.
    b. A central fibrotic focus may vary with respect to its cellularity in the fibrotic focus from high to low. The acellular zone is this lesion's key feature.
    c. The tumor has a high risk of brain and lung metastasis.
    d. The fibrotic focus is associated with death by cancer independent of nodal status and tumor size, and the tumor has a worse prognosis compared with invasive ductal carcinoma of equivalent grade and size.
    e. The central fibrotic focus is a scarlike area that may be associated with necrosis and is related to intratumoral hypoxia.

16. Key features of male breast cancer include all of the following EXCEPT:
    a. Male breast cancer corrected for stage is associated with a worse prognosis than female breast cancer.
    b. Male breast cancer is more likely to be estrogen receptor positive than female breast cancer.
    c. Hereditary forms of male breast cancer are associated with *BRCA2* germline mutations.
    d. Risk factors include living in Western countries, increasing age, obesity, exposure to estrogens and ionizing radiation, and Klinefelter syndrome.
    e. Male breast cancer generally manifests at a more advanced stage than female breast cancer.

17. Which of the following is a well-confirmed factor that increases breast cancer risk?
    a. Geographic region of Asia and Africa, early age of first full-term pregnancy, and high parity
    b. High breast density on mammography
    c. Breastfeeding of long duration and obesity in premenopausal women
    d. Nonproliferative cystic disease
    e. Use of tamoxifen or other selective estrogen receptor modulators

18. All of the following statements regarding prognostic and predictive factors of breast carcinoma are true EXCEPT:

a. In the Elston-Ellis modification of the Bloom-Richardson grading scheme, the field diameter is not relevant in establishing the mitotic count as long as 10 high-power fields are examined.

b. The Elston-Ellis modification of the Bloom-Richardson grading scheme can be applied to invasive ductal and lobular carcinoma.

c. Estrogen receptor, progesterone receptor, and *HER2/neu* expression status are both predictive and prognostic factors in invasive breast cancer.

d. Prognostic factors for breast cancer include lymph node status, histologic grade, tumor size, and special histologic type.

e. *HER2/neu* gene amplification and overexpression are both prognostic and predictive factors in invasive breast cancer because the status of *HER2/neu* may be used in selecting patients for trastuzumab therapy.

19. Which of the following statements regarding patterns of genomic changes noted in breast cancer is TRUE?

a. Genomic changes suggest that low-grade carcinoma does not generally transition to high-grade breast carcinoma except in ~50% of luminal B tumors.

b. No concordance is seen between grade and genomic changes in in situ and associated invasive cancer.

c. Transitioning from low-grade to high-grade carcinoma is a common event in triple negative breast cancer.

d. In high-grade carcinoma, 16q loss is typical.

e. Pleomorphic lobular carcinoma does not arise in a background of classic lobular carcinoma.

20. Gene expression profiling in breast cancer has led to which realization?

a. Breast cancer is not a diverse set of diseases but rather a single disease.

b. Luminal breast cancers are defined by estrogen receptor expression and proliferation levels.

c. Proliferation levels are not important in prognostication of estrogen receptor–positive cancers, but they are important in prognostication of *HER2* and basal cancers.

d. Prognostic gene signatures can replace conventional prognostic factors such as size and stage.

e. Array-based gene expression profiling provides little information beyond classification and prognostication.

21. Which of the following statements regarding gene expression profiling–based classification of breast cancer is TRUE?

a. Discordance between classifications defined by gene expression profiling and immunohistochemistry-based classification raises questions regarding their definition.

b. *HER2* subtype is enriched for estrogen receptor–negative tumors expressing genes identified on the *HER2* amplicon. The luminal subtypes (A and B) correspond to estrogen receptor–positive tumors with low proliferation.

c. Basallike tumors are triple-negative tumors that do not express cytokeratin 5/6 or epidermal growth factor receptor.

d. Normallike breast cancer subtype likely represents an artifact seen in tumors of high purity.

e. Claudin-low breast cancers are characterized by estrogen receptor negativity, high proliferation, characteristics resembling mature cells, and expression of genes associated with epithelial mesenchymal transition.

22. Gene expression profiling of special histologic subtypes of breast cancer would reveal which of the following?

a. Tubular carcinoma of the breast is primarily luminal B type.

b. Neuroendocrine and cribriform subtypes of breast cancer are similar molecularly to adenoid cystic carcinoma of the breast.

c. Pleomorphic lobular carcinoma maps to the same molecular subtype as classic lobular carcinoma.

d. Invasive micropapillary carcinoma maps to claudin-low subtype.

e. Virtually all recognized histologic subtypes of breast cancer are more uniform than breast cancers of no special type.

23. Features of basallike breast cancer include which of the following?

a. By immunohistochemistry, basallike cancers are always triple negative and cytokeratin 5/6 positive or epidermal growth factor receptor positive.

b. Basallike cancers are unlikely to be interval cancers.

c. Of triple-negative cancers defined by immunohistochemistry, approximately 71% are basallike cancers by gene expression.

d. Basallike cancers are histologically uniform.

e. *BRCA1* germline mutated basallike cancers arise from myoepithelial cells.

24. Which of the following statements regarding Oncotype DX and MammaPrint is TRUE?

a. MammaPrint is a test approved by the U.S. Food and Drug Administration that is based on a 70-gene signature performed on node-negative invasive breast cancer, independent of estrogen receptor status, which classifies patients in low-risk and high-risk groups.

b. Oncotype DX is a prognostic test for invasive estrogen receptor–positive breast cancer, but it is not predictive.

c. Oncotype DX and MammaPrint provide information that has been shown to be dependent on clinicopathologic risk assessment.

d. Oncotype DX is based on a 21-gene signature that provides a dichotomous result of good and bad prognosis.

e. Oncotype DX is a prognostic signature for estrogen receptor–positive and estrogen receptor–negative invasive carcinoma.

25. All of the following statements describe features of encapsulated papillary carcinoma EXCEPT:

a. Encapsulated papillary carcinoma is a well-circumscribed papillary lesion lacking myoepithelial cells in papillae and at its periphery.

b. The lesion may have a solid papillary or cystic character.

c. Encapsulated papillary carcinoma is considered by some experts to be a low-grade invasive carcinoma with expansile growth.

d. Encapsulated papillary carcinoma is associated with an expression pattern of invasion-associated markers, which is typical of invasive cancer.

e. Intracystic papillary carcinoma is associated with conventional invasion at a rate of approximately 27%, whereas solid papillary carcinoma is associated with a conventional invasion rate of approximately 63%.

26. Which of the following features are typical of secretory breast cancer?

  a. Associated with a chromosomal translocation t(12;15)
  b. Occurs exclusively in young girls
  c. Regarded as an aggressive carcinoma
  d. Characterized as a hormone receptor–positive tumor
  e. Associated with high mitotic activity

27. All of the following statements regarding *ERBB2* (*HER2/neu*)-positive breast cancer are true EXCEPT:

  a. Amplification of *HER2/neu* gene or overexpression of its protein product or both have been found in 25% to 30% of human breast cancers.
  b. *HER2/neu* breast cancers are associated with poorer outcomes compared with *HER2*-normal breast cancer.
  c. The combination of trastuzumab with adjuvant chemotherapy has shown significant benefit in disease-free survival, overall survival, locoregional recurrence, and distant recurrence compared with chemotherapy alone.
  d. Nine weekly doses of adjuvant trastuzumab is the standard of care for *HER2/neu*-positive early breast cancer.
  e. Clinical evaluation before treatment with trastuzumab should include careful screening for cardiac risk factors.

28. All of the following statements regarding diabetic mastopathy are true EXCEPT:

  a. It is a fibroinflammatory breast disease characterized by dense fibrosis with perivascular, periductal, and perilobular lymphocytic infiltrates and associated ductitis and sclerosing lobulitis.
  b. It is always associated with type 1 diabetes mellitus.
  c. Patients with diabetic mastopathy are not at an increased risk for developing breast cancer.
  d. On physical examination, a hard, nontender, palpable breast mass clinically suspicious for carcinoma is frequently found.
  e. Diabetic mastopathy is prone to single or multiple recurrences in the same breast or the contralateral breast.

29. All of the following statements regarding mammographic density are true EXCEPT:

  a. Mammographic density refers to the radiopaque portion of the breast that appears white on a mammogram.
  b. Mammographic density is one of the most important indicators of breast cancer risk.
  c. Mammographic density can mask some radiologic features of the breast and increase the difficulty in detecting tumors.
  d. More extensive density was found to be associated with risk of estrogen receptor–positive tumors.
  e. Mammographic density has consistently been found to be less widespread in older women.

ANSWERS

1. d. The image shows atypical ductal hyperplasia with atypical micropapillary features. In view of the irregular lumen, relatively short papillae, and crowding and hyperchromasia of the cells at the tip of the micropapillae, this lesion is associated with a relative risk of 4 to 5. Proliferative cystic disease with atypia, both atypical ductal hyperplasia and atypical lobular hyperplasia, is associated with a relative risk of 4 to 5. The relative risk for developing invasive carcinoma given a biopsy specimen showing a particular histologic appearance represents the ratio of the incidence of cancer in the population that underwent biopsy over the general incidence of cancer. As identified by the pioneering work of Page, nonproliferative cystic disease is associated with a relative risk of 1 (i.e., no increased risk over the general population). Pathologic lesions included in this category are cysts (macroscopic and microscopic), apocrine change, mild hyperplasia, and fibroadenoma without complex features. Proliferative cystic disease without atypia is associated with a relative risk of developing invasive carcinoma of 1.5 to 2. This category includes moderate to florid intraductal epithelial hyperplasia; sclerosing adenosis; peripheral papillomas, but not central ones (i.e., identified in the nipple); radial scar; and complex fibroadenomas, which may have a higher (3) increased relative risk. Lobular carcinoma in situ and ductal carcinoma in situ have a relative risk of 8 to 10. The grade of ductal carcinoma in situ may influence the level of risk with higher grade ductal carcinoma in situ associated with a higher relative risk. For all of the described entities except ductal carcinoma in situ, the risk is bilateral. The risk is primarily ipsilateral (95%) for ductal carcinoma in situ. Traditionally it was thought that patients with a family history of breast cancer with proliferative cystic disease with atypia have a relative risk similar to that of ductal carcinoma in situ of 8 to 10. Also it was thought that the risk of developing cancer in proliferative disease with or without atypia was primarily in the first 10 years after the diagnosis. The risk subsequently was thought to decrease by two thirds, a reduction not seen in in situ cancer. Both of these observations are challenged by a study from Degnim et al. and supported by more recent data suggesting that family history does not impact ADH risk level, and the risk associated with ADH does not decline over many decades.

Dumitrescu RG, Cotarla I: Understanding breast cancer risk—where do we stand in 2005? *J Cell Mol Med* 2005;9(1):208-221.
Degnim AC: Startification of breast cancer risk in women with atypia: A Mayo cohort study. *J Clin Oncol* 2007;25:2671–2677.

2. d. The image shows cystosarcoma phyllodes. Cystosarcoma phyllodes may be classified as histologically benign (most common), borderline malignant (low-grade malignant), or high-grade malignant. In this fibroepithelial tumor, the epithelium for the most part has been shown to be polyclonal, whereas the stroma is clonal. This finding is in contrast to what has been observed in most, but not all, fibroadenomas, in which both the epithelial and the stromal components are polyclonal. Phyllodes tumor has been increasing in incidence, which may be due partly to increasing awareness of the diagnostic criteria of this lesion. Also, there is a high incidence of this tumor among immigrant Hispanic women, particularly women from

Central and South America, and Asian American women. The differential diagnosis of cystosarcoma phyllodes includes cellular fibroadenoma and juvenile fibroadenoma; in addition, the tumor may be confused with fibroadenoma with fascicular pseudoangiomatous stromal hyperplasia or sclerosing lobular hyperplasia. Features favoring phyllodes tumor include periductal stromal hypercellularity with zonation suggesting greater cellularity near the ducts rather than away from the ducts. Juvenile fibroadenoma typically has an even distribution of stromal hypercellularity with respect to ducts and a greater number of ductal structures (terminal duct lobular unit) per unit area. A prominent intracanalicular pattern is more commonly seen in phyllodes tumor. As cystosarcoma phyllodes becomes more malignant, the mitotic rate increases, although scattered mitoses may be seen in histologically benign cases; no mitoses are required for the diagnosis. Stromal overgrowth (absence of epithelium in a low-power field), stromal invasion, increasing mitotic activity, and cellularity are typical of the low-grade and high-grade malignant variants. High-grade malignant tumors typically have a sarcomatous appearance and may no longer show a prominent intracanalicular pattern. Histologically benign lesions may recur but generally do not metastasize, whereas high-grade malignant lesions may metastasize at a rate of 25% to the lung. Cystosarcoma phyllodes generally does not involve draining lymph nodes and does not require a node dissection unless the nodes are clinically positive. The peak age at diagnosis is 50, although in high-risk populations it is frequently seen in the 30s and 40s. Cystosarcoma phyllodes may also be seen in teenagers; it has a similar histologic appearance to tumors in adults but is associated with a lower rate of recurrence and a more benign course.

Bernstein L, Deapen D, Ross RK: The descriptive epidemiology of malignant cystosarcoma phyllodes tumors of the breast. *Cancer* 1993;71(10):3020-3024.

Lerwill MF: Biphasic lesions of the breast. *Semin Diagn Pathol* 2004;21(1):48-56.

3. c.   The image depicts a low-grade angiosarcoma. Most high-grade angiosarcomas also have areas of low-grade angiosarcoma, which is why sampling is important for appropriate grading. Numerous benign vascular lesions may be seen in the breast. Angiolipomas are delimited lesions characterized by increased vascularity toward the outer capsule without interanastomosing channels, with bland cells lining the vessels with scattered microthrombi. Perilobular hemangiomas, angiomatosis, and other forms of hemangioma may be seen in the breast and are relatively circumscribed without interanastomosing vessels. Malignant vascular tumors of the breast in this region include primary mammary angiosarcoma, postmastectomy lymphangiosarcoma of the arm (also known as Stewart-Treves syndrome), and postirradiation angiosarcoma of the skin and underlying breasts in patients treated by lumpectomy and radiation therapy. Primary angiosarcoma of the breast typically occurs in younger individuals and may be graded from 1 to 3. In one study, patients with grade 1 angiosarcoma had a median age of 43, whereas median age in grade 2 was 34 and in grade 3 was 29. Patients with grade 1 and grade 2 tumors have a disease-free survival of about 12 to 15 years and a 5-year survival rate of approximately 76% (grade 1) and 70% (grade 2). Patients with grade 3 tumors

have a disease-free survival of approximately 15 months and a 15% 5-year survival rate. Both high-grade and intermediate-grade angiosarcomas are typically easily identified by their abundant cellularity and mitotic activity. However, low-grade angiosarcoma may be extremely bland in appearance and can easily be missed. It typically shows interanastomosing channels with only mild endothelial atypia and ectatic vascular channels dissecting adipose tissue. In addition, both intermediate-grade and high-grade angiosarcomas may be largely composed of low-grade angiosarcomatous areas. Nascimento et al. challenged the view that grade affects outcome in angiosarcoma, but most authors seem to believe it does. Postradiation angiosarcoma may occur in the skin or subcutaneous tissue or underlying breast parenchyma. Angiosarcomas are primarily high-grade tumors, although low-grade tumors have been identified. In contrast to most postradiation sarcomas, postradiation angiosarcomas have been reported to occur with a short latency period characterized by several years. The incidence of this type of angiosarcoma has been estimated to range from 0.2% to about 1% in patients who have undergone irradiation. The differential diagnosis, in addition to the previously mentioned benign conditions, includes papillary endothelial hyperplasia. Papillary endothelial hyperplasia is also known as Masson vegetant intravascular hemangioendothelioma; distinction from angiosarcoma includes circumscription, intravascular location, thrombus, and papillary architecture with a bland cytologic appearance. Papillary endothelial hyperplasia is primarily an intravascular condition most likely representing abnormal thrombus organization. The circumscribed nature of the lesion and its intravascular location are important in arriving at the correct diagnosis. Not all vascular lesions after radiation are malignant. Atypical vascular lesion, also known as benign lymphangiomatous papules of the skin, has been described in irradiated skin. The lesion comprises dilated, occasionally interanastomosing, vascular channels, which are circumscribed but may contain endothelial cells that are prominent but not overtly malignant appearing. Atypical vascular lesion shows marked dilated lymphaticlike spaces that may be associated with lymphoid follicles. The vessels are capacious and show projection of stroma into lumina. These lesions may be confused with angiosarcoma but are benign. Atypical vascular lesion may recur. The lesions typically occur 2 to 5 years after radiotherapy and are smaller than 1 cm.

Brenn T, Fletcher CD: Radiation associated cutaneous atypical vascular lesions and angiosarcoma: clinicopathologic analysis of 42 cases. *Am J Surg Pathol* 2005;29(8):983-996.

Kaklamanos IG, Birbas K, Syrigos KN, et al: Breast angiosarcoma that is not related to radiation exposure: a comprehensive review of the literature. *Surg Today* 2011;41(2):163-168.

Nascimento AF, Raut CC, Fletcher CD: Primary angiosarcoma of the breast: clinicopathologic analysis of 49 cases suggesting that grade is not prognostic. *Am J Surg Pathol* 2008; 32(12):1896-1904.

4. e.   Subtypes of invasive breast carcinoma associated with a good prognosis include mucinous, tubular, cribriform, and medullary if strict definitions are used. Tumors associated with a bad prognosis include inflammatory carcinoma of the breast (shown in the image), which currently is defined primarily on clinical grounds—having an erythematous or peau d'orange skin appearance and carcinoma anywhere in the breast. Invasive micropapillary carcinoma is an aggressive tumor, which is associated with a high lymphatic and lymph node metastasis rate (75%) regardless of tumor size, even for T1a lesions. Tumors with a central fibrotic focus also have been associated with a poor prognosis and enrich for a basal phenotype. Tumors in the poor prognosis group including luminal B, *HER2* amplified, and most (but not all) basal-type cancers have a worse prognosis than invasive ductal carcinoma NST. Pure medullary carcinoma, secretory carcinoma, and adenoid cystic carcinoma are some of the basal-type cancers associated with a good prognosis. The subtypes (e.g., luminal A) associated with a good prognosis have a better prognosis than NST cancers.

Colleoni M, Russo L, Dellapasqua S: Adjuvant therapies for special types of breast cancer. *Breast* 2011;20(Suppl 3):S153-S157.

Rakha EA, Lee AH, Evans AJ, et al: Tubular carcinoma of the breast: further evidence to support its excellent prognosis. *J Clin Oncol* 2010;28(1):99-104.

Simpson JF, Page DL: Pathology of preinvasive and excellent prognosis breast cancer. *Curr Opin Oncol* 2001;13(6):426-430.

5. e. Invasive lobular carcinoma may occur in tumors with apparently mixed ductal and lobular differentiation. Given the relatively small size of the cells of most invasive lobular carcinomas, cytokeratin staining might be valuable in evaluating lymph nodes for metastasis to reduce the false-negative rate (approximately 30% to 40%). Invasive ductal carcinoma may show an Indian file pattern, and sometimes an E-cadherin stain might be useful in differentiating it from invasive lobular carcinoma. In these instances, the cells of ductal carcinoma frequently are larger, and the cords may be more than one cell thick. A typical immunophenotype of a lobular carcinoma is E-cadherin negative, high-molecular-weight cytokeratin positive, estrogen receptor and progesterone receptor positive, and *HER2* negative. By expression array, the classic variant of invasive lobular carcinoma is typically of the luminal A intrinsic subtype. Intracytoplasmic vacuolization is commonly seen, and these tumors are mucicarmine positive. The overall rate of invasive lobular carcinoma is approximately 10% of all invasive tumors. These tumors are associated with a higher rate of bilaterality (10% to 20%) compared with invasive ductal carcinoma (5%). Subdiaphragmatic involvement by breast cancer frequently shows a signet ring cell pattern of invasive lobular carcinoma that must be distinguished from gastric or other organs of origin. Invasive lobular carcinoma is less responsive to adjuvant and neoadjuvant therapy compared with invasive ductal carcinoma. E-cadherin germline mutation is associated with both lobular carcinoma and diffuse gastric carcinoma. Loss of expression of β-catenin is common in invasive lobular carcinoma. β-Catenin typically is expressed in invasive ductal carcinoma. In addition, p120 is reported to be present in most invasive lobular carcinomas in the cytoplasm as a result of E-cadherin loss, with which it normally forms a complex. In contrast, in invasive ductal carcinoma, p120 is present in the membrane/variable but shows limited cytoplasmic distribution. E-cadherin may be seen in normal or reduced amounts in classic invasive lobular carcinoma in 10% to 15% of cases. These cases show similar histopathologic and clinical features as seen in E-cadherin-negative invasive lobular carcinoma. Cases of classic invasive ductal carcinoma, particularly if poorly differentiated, may show a loss of E-cadherin expression complicating interpretation. Tubulolobular carcinoma is typically E-cadherin positive in both components (tubules and lobular-appearing areas). So-called mixed ductal and lobular carcinoma primarily expresses E-cadherin, but in one study, 24% were negative for E-cadherin, whereas 17% showed composite positive and negative areas for E-cadherin expression.

Cocquyt V, Van Belle S: Lobular carcinoma in situ and invasive lobular cancer of the breast. *Curr Opin Obstet Gynecol* 2005; 17(1):55-60.

de Deus Moura R, Wludarski SC, Carvalho FM, et al: Immunohistochemistry applied to the differential diagnosis between ductal and lobular carcinoma of the breast. *Appl Immunohistochem Mol Morphol* 2013;21(1):1-12.

6. a. The lesion depicted in the image is microglandular adenosis, which is a proliferative infiltrating lesion that may mimic carcinoma clinically and pathologically but is nonmetastasizing. The lesion comprises small microglandular structures with eosinophilic secretions within the lumen typically lined by bland cells. The lesions lack myoepithelial cells as demonstrated by the absence of *p63* and smooth muscle actin staining. They show strong positivity for S100 and pancytokeratin and are negative for estrogen receptor and progesterone receptor, *p53*, *HER2/neu*, GCDFP-15, and epithelial membrane antigen. Type IV collagen typically surrounds the microglandular structures. Microglandular adenosis may appear to be infiltrative or may have a more lobulated architecture. Varying degrees of atypia and both in situ and invasive carcinoma have been reported to arise from this lesion. Microglandular adenosis is considered a nonobligatory precursor of basal-type/triple-negative (estrogen receptor, progesterone receptor, and *HER2* negative) carcinoma and has been shown sometimes to be clonal. Sclerosing adenosis can be distinguished from microglandular adenosis by its lobulocentric distribution and its myoepithelial cells. Although tubular carcinoma shares with microglandular adenosis the absence of myoepithelial cells, type IV collagen is not present. Tubular carcinoma has tubules that tend to be larger and more angulated and are lined by more clearly neoplastic cells. Epithelial membrane antigen and estrogen receptor and progesterone receptor expression suggest a tubular carcinoma.

Acs G, Simpson JF, Bleiweiss IJ, et al: Microglandular adenosis with transition into adenoid cystic carcinoma of the breast. *Am J Surg Pathol* 2003;27(8):1052-1060.

Khalifeh IM, Albarracin C, Diaz LK, et al: Clinical, histopathologic, and immunohistochemical features of microglandular adenosis and transition into in-situ and invasive carcinoma. *Am J Surg Pathol* 2008;32(4):544-552.

7. e. In normal breast development, thickening of the epidermis with the formation of the milk line occurs during the fifth week of gestation. The milk line is also known as the mammary ridge; it forms bilaterally and extends from the axilla to the groin region. Subsequent involution of the mammary ridge except in the region of the chest results in normally located breast tissue in the chest wall. Failure to involute may result in ectopic breast tissue or polythelia (supernumerary nipple) or both. Supernumerary nipples were reported in one study in 2.4% of infants.

This abnormality apparently is more common in African Americans than whites. Ectopic breast parenchyma along the milk line can be seen in both males and females, although it is clinically more apparent in females. The incidence of ectopic breast tissue in women is variably reported to be less than 5%. Polythelia can be found anywhere along the anterior chest wall, most commonly above and below the normal breast tissue. In most patients, ectopic breast parenchyma is found in the axilla. Nevertheless it can be found anywhere along the milk line from the axilla to the groin and vulva region. The image depicts proliferative cystic disease. Any change that can be identified in the normal breast parenchyma, including cystic disease, proliferative changes with or without atypia, and carcinoma, can be seen in ectopic breast parenchyma. Occasionally, breast tissue identified in the axilla represents the axillary extension of the breast and not a separate or discrete focus of ectopic breast tissue. In addition, breast tissue may be identified outside the region of the mammary ridge and milk line that is histologically indistinguishable from both ectopic breast tissue (along the milk line) and normal breast tissue.

Howard BA, Gusterson BA: Human breast development. *J Mamm Gland Biol Neoplasia* 2000;5(2):119-137.

Rosen PP: Abnormalities of mammary growth and development. In Rosen PP (ed): *Rosen's Breast Pathology,* 2nd ed. Philadelphia: Lippincott Williams & Wilkins, 2001, pp 23-27.

8. d. The image shows confluent sclerosing adenosis—note the lobulated growth pattern. Lesions of the breast typically are associated with specific locations in the breast, although the distribution is not always strict. Angiosarcoma may be primary in the breast or may manifest in skin usually after irradiation in the setting of conservative therapy (i.e., lumpectomy). Additionally, angiosarcoma may be seen away from the breast primarily in the skin of the upper extremity after lymph node dissection and lymphatic obstruction. In all of these instances, angiosarcoma may secondarily involve compartments from which it does not arise. The terminal duct lobular unit is the site of origin of changes typically characterized by cystic disease, including usual ductal hyperplasia, adenosis and sclerosing adenosis, atypical ductal or lobular hyperplasia, and lobular and ductal carcinoma in situ. Stem cells in this location are thought to give rise to both ductal and lobular tumors. The intralobular stroma is thought to be associated with the formation of fibroadenoma, and primarily periductal stroma is thought to be associated with phyllodes tumor. Peripheral papilloma, characterized by a mildly increased risk (1.5 to 2 relative risk) of development of invasive carcinoma, arises in the terminal duct lobular unit.

The nipple and subareolar region are associated with numerous lesions, including Paget disease representing ductal carcinoma in situ arising in lactiferous ducts and extending into the epidermis. Also noted in the nipple is a potentially mass-forming lesion, florid papillomatosis of the nipple (also known as nipple adenoma); this lesion is characterized by ductular proliferation arising from lactiferous ducts and florid intraductal epithelial hyperplasia with varying degrees of atypia. Cancer may be associated with this lesion. Solitary intraductal papillomas, which are the most common cause of bloody nipple discharge, are seen in the subareolar region as well as in the nipple. Subareolar abscess formation may be seen in association with

lactiferous ducts with squamous metaplasia. Terminal duct obstruction leads to duct rupture proximally with abscess formation. This condition typically requires abscess and duct excision. Duct ectasia is characteristically found in the subareolar location along with a sclerosing lesion referred to as subareolar sclerosing duct hyperplasia. The latter lesion is characterized by a geographic area of duct sclerosis and stromal elastosis with florid epithelial proliferation; this lesion is in the family of radial sclerosing lesions but tends to show less cyst formation. Subareolar sclerosing duct hyperplasia may be associated with carcinoma; however, the lesion itself is not a carcinoma, and careful attention should be paid to the geographic nature of the lesion and the presence of myoepithelial cells surrounding the intraductal epithelial proliferation, which may be highlighted with a smooth muscle actin, smooth muscle myosin heavy chain, or *p63* immunostain. The smooth muscle actin immunostain should be interpreted carefully because sclerotic lesions may be strongly positive for smooth muscle actin. A rare lesion referred to as syringomatous adenoma of the nipple is a benign, locally infiltrating neoplasm histologically similar to the tumor of the skin. Syringomatous adenoma of the nipple does not appear to arise from skin, and it is not typically associated with intraductal epithelial proliferation. It should be distinguished from florid papillomatosis of the nipple (nipple adenoma). Syringomatous adenoma of the nipple comprises small tubular and ductular structures with elongated architecture in a teardrop shape. It has an infiltrative pattern that should not be confused with an invasive carcinoma, either well-differentiated or otherwise. The ducts are lined by one or more layers of small uniform cells.

Kumar V, Abbas AK, Fausto N, et al (eds): *Robbins and Cotran Pathologic Basis of Disease,* 8th ed. Philadelphia: Saunders, 2010.

9. a. Numerous lesions of the breast can be confused with invasive carcinoma by virtue of their infiltrating or pseudoinfiltrating growth pattern and epithelioid or epithelial morphologic appearance. Sclerosing intraductal papilloma is a noninfiltrative lesion and is characterized by a geographic distribution; given the sclerosis, a pseudoinfiltrating pattern is sometimes noted. Careful attention should be paid to the geographic distribution of the lesion and the presence of myoepithelial cells that on high power can be seen lining the sclerosed ductal structures. In doubtful cases or cases of attenuation of myoepithelial cells that, immunostains such as *p63*, smooth muscle myosin heavy chain, calponin, and smooth muscle actin (active sclerosis may hamper interpretation) can highlight the myoepithelial cells. A radial scar may be similarly confused with an invasive lesion. The image shows a tubular carcinoma with characteristic angulated but dilated infiltrating tubules radiating outward. Examples of benign but infiltrative epithelial lesions of the breast not representing carcinoma include syringomatous adenoma of the nipple and microglandular adenosis. The absence of myoepithelial cells in microglandular adenosis may confuse the issue of infiltrative carcinoma further. Granular cell tumor (positive for S100 protein, which is also true of many breast cancers, and negative for cytokeratin), a primarily benign mesenchymal tumor, comprises cells with granular cytoplasm. Because of its infiltrative pattern, granular cell tumor may be confused with invasive carcinoma with apocrine features. However, careful attention to the absence of glands in a granular cell tumor, the more granular versus acidophilic cytoplasm, and immunohistochemical stains can distinguish the two lesions.

Lerwill ML: Current practical applications of diagnostic immunohistochemistry in breast pathology. *Am J Surg Pathol* 2004;28(8):1076-1091.

10. b. The lesion depicted in the image is fibromatosis. It is a locally infiltrating, nonmetastasizing tumor of fibroblasts, similar in histologic appearance to classic abdominal desmoid, and may be seen in extraabdominal sites including the breast. These lesions typically are identified in the breasts of younger premenopausal women, although a wide age range is seen. The tumor comprises infiltrating fascicles of fibroblasts of moderate cellularity without significant or, for the most part, any mitotic activity. At the periphery of many of the lesions, lymphoid follicles are seen as the tumor cells infiltrate the stroma. Local recurrence rates are around 25%, particularly if a wide excision (>1 cm) has not been performed. The differential diagnosis includes a scar, and a previous history of trauma should always be considered. Generally, the moderate degree of stromal cellularity and the infiltrative pattern allow for the differentiation from a scar, although this is not always possible. Fascicular pseudoangiomatous stromal hyperplasia may be seen in the context of fibroepithelial lesions or elsewhere but is generally not seen with this infiltrative pattern. In addition, fibromatosis lacks the spaces typically identified adjacent to cells seen in pseudoangiomatous stromal hyperplasia. Spindle cell–type metaplastic carcinoma can be excluded by finding other areas of invasive carcinoma and by demonstrating cytokeratin-positive cells. Distinction from cystosarcoma phyllodes can be made if a ductal component and intracanalicular pattern are identified, but this occasionally may be difficult in needle biopsy material. A highly infiltrative nature is typically lacking in cystosarcoma phyllodes, unless the phyllodes tumor is of high grade (which would exclude fibromatosis). Myofibroblastoma of the breast is a benign spindle cell tumor that manifests as a well-circumscribed mass. It generally has a more epithelioid appearance and tends to be more cellular and usually lacks the intimate association with fibrosis.

Brogi E: Benign and malignant spindle cell lesions of the breast. *Semin Diagn Pathol* 2004;21(1):57-64.

Rosen PP, Ernsberger D: Mammary fibromatosis. A benign spindle cell tumor with significant risk for local recurrence. *Cancer* 1989;63(7):1363-1369.

11. b. Solitary intraductal papilloma arising from large ducts generally is not thought to be associated with increased risk of developing invasive carcinoma relative to the general population. These lesions may arise in lactiferous ducts or in the subareolar region. Trauma or infarction of such papillomas may result in bloody nipple discharge. The papillary structures tend to be broader than what is seen in intraductal papillary carcinoma, which also contains fibrovascular cores that are generally, but not always, quite thin. Multiple intraductal papillomas and peripheral papillomas arise in terminal duct lobular units and are associated with a 1.5- to 2-fold increased risk of developing invasive carcinoma. All papillomas, regardless of type, contain two cell types: myoepithelial and luminal. Variable epithelial proliferation and atypical ductal

hyperplasia may be seen in these papillomas. Atypical ductal hyperplasia is associated with a 4- to 5-fold increased risk of developing invasive cancer. In contrast to the bilateral risk of developing invasive cancer associated with atypical ductal hyperplasia that occurs in other settings, the risk for developing an invasive cancer in papillomas with atypical ductal hyperplasia is ipsilateral. In this respect, the risk is similar to that for ductal carcinoma in situ, not in magnitude but in its ipsilateral nature. Intraductal papillomas, particularly in the nipple, sometimes may be confused with a normal star-shaped structure of the lactiferous ducts. This normal ductal structure may undergo trauma, and an inflammatorylike lesion may form in its wall, which is not a true papilloma. In addition to atypical ductal hyperplasia associated with intraductal papilloma, ductal carcinoma in situ may arise or coexist in or with an intraductal papilloma. Although the presence of myoepithelial cells suggests that the underlying lesion is an intraductal papilloma and not an intraductal papillary carcinoma, this does not exclude the concurrent presence of ductal carcinoma in situ in the duct. The presence of myoepithelial cells along the papillae excludes an intraductal papillary carcinoma but does not exclude an incidental (rare) ductal carcinoma in situ arising in the background of a papilloma. Intracystic papillary cancer, so called when the ducts are large and cystlike and the papillae are negative for myoepithelial cells, are primarily a form of encapsulated papillary carcinoma, but their classification depends on the absence additionally of myoepithelial cells at the periphery of the lesion. If myoepithelial cells are present at the periphery, the lesion is a form of intraductal papillary carcinoma, a distinction aided by myoepithelial cell studies. Intraductal papillary carcinoma is an in situ carcinoma as long as the ducts are surrounded by myoepithelial cells, which may be associated with invasion at the periphery. The lesion is characterized by the absent to rare myoepithelial cells lining the papillae, although myoepithelial cells are present at the periphery of the duct from which they arise. At this location, the myoepithelial cells may be variably attenuated or quite prominent. Typically, but not always, the fibrovascular cores are quite thin. A stratified columnar epithelium is seen in most instances with large vesicular nuclei. Intracystic, encapsulated, or intraductal papillary carcinoma may have a solid variant in which the papillae are not as clearly visible. The diagnosis should be suspected in the presence of large ducts with abundant malignant epithelium because this tissue requires a blood supply, which is impossible given the size of the ducts without fibrovascular cores. If papillary lesions lack myoepithelial cells in both the papillae and the periphery of the ductal-appearing structures, the lesion represents an encapsulated papillary carcinoma; more recently, this is thought by most authors to represent a low-grade form of invasive cancer.

Gutman H, Schachter J, Wasserberg N, et al: Are solitary papillomas entirely benign? *Arch Surg* 2003;138(12):1330-1333.

MacGrogan G, Tavassoli FA: Central atypical papillomas of the breast: a clinicopathological study of 119 cases. *Virchows Arch* 2003;443(5):609-617.

12. d. Lobular carcinoma in situ is multifocal and bilateral in distribution and is generally considered to be a marker of an increased risk of developing invasive cancer that is bilateral in distribution. In this respect, lobular carcinoma in situ is similar to atypical ductal hyperplasia, not in magnitude but in its distribution of invasive cancer, and contrasts with ductal carcinoma in situ, which is associated primarily with an ipsilateral risk for development of invasive cancer. Atypical lobular hyperplasia demonstrates similar-appearing cells to lobular carcinoma in situ but quantitatively is less extensive. Features in favor of atypical lobular hyperplasia include a lesser degree of distention or involvement of the lobule, less than half of the terminal duct lobular unit involved by the lesional cells, and residual luminal formation with a greater degree of admixture of lesional cells to luminal cells than is seen in lobular carcinoma in situ. In contrast, lobular carcinoma in situ demonstrates complete distention by a uniform cell population that frequently shows intracytoplasmic vacuolization and variably discohesive cells. The latter two features should not be confused with residual lumina. Pagetoid spread of lobular carcinoma in situ may result in the appearance of a residual lumen but one not opposed by neoplastic cells, but rather by nonneoplastic luminal cells. Rarely, lobular carcinoma in situ may be associated with calcification and comedo-type necrosis. Some authors have applied the term *lobular neoplasia* to both atypical lobular hyperplasia and lobular carcinoma in situ in view of the difficulty of distinguishing between these two entities. In general, the cytokeratin 34βE12 is strongly positive in lobular carcinoma in situ, whereas it is variably positive in atypical ductal hyperplasia but generally strongly positive in usual ductal hyperplasia.

Bratthauer GL, Tavassoli FA: Lobular intraepithelial neoplasia: previously unexplored aspects assessed in 775 cases and their clinical implications. *Virchows Arch* 2002;440(2):134-138.

Oppong BA, King TA: Recommendations for women with lobular carcinoma in situ (LCIS). *Oncology (Williston Park)* 2011;25(11): 1051-1056,1058.

13. c.   The lesion depicted in the image is a syringomatous adenoma of the nipple. This infiltrating but benign neoplasm may be confused with the adenosis portion of florid papillomatosis of the nipple, tubular carcinoma or low-grade carcinoma not otherwise specified, and low-grade adenosquamous carcinoma. Syringomatous adenoma of the nipple classically shows tubular structures with a so-called comma-shaped appearance, as is typical for syringomatous tumors of the skin. Syringomatous adenoma lacks the intraductal epithelial proliferation that is seen in florid papillomatosis of the nipple. Tubular carcinoma lacks myoepithelial cells. However, syringomatous adenoma frequently shows strong *p63* immunopositivity both in its peripherally placed cells and occasionally in cells more centrally located. Low-grade adenosquamous carcinoma is a form of low-grade metaplastic carcinoma that typically occurs in the breast exclusive of the nipple. In contrast, nipple syringoma occurs in the nipple. Secondary involvement of adjacent regions by each of these lesions has been described. Syringomatous adenoma of the nipple is typically associated with collagenous stroma and lymphocytic infiltrate and shows a variable positive staining pattern with myoepithelial cell markers. Although benign, syringomatous adenoma of the nipple may recur if incompletely excised.

Carter E, Dyess DL: Infiltrating syringomatous adenoma of the nipple: a case report and a 20-year retrospective review. *Breast J* 2004;10(5):443-447.

Oo KZ, Xiao PQ: Infiltrating syringomatous adenoma of the nipple: clinical presentation and literature review. *Arch Pathol Lab Med* 2009;133(9):1487-1489.

14. b.   The lesion depicted in the image is florid gynecomastia, which is characterized by an intraductal epithelial hyperplasia and periductal increased cellularity and edema. Three stages are described: early florid, intermediate, and late inactive or fibrotic phase. Epithelial proliferation may be confused with carcinoma in the early florid phase. As the lesion progresses, epithelial proliferation subsides, and the surrounding stroma becomes fibrotic. Gynecomastialike hyperplasia is a proliferative lesion that may be seen in the female breast. Gynecomastia is the most common lesion of the male breast. It occurs in a bimodal distribution but may be seen in any age group including newborn male infants. Gynecomastia affects 30% to 60% of boys and approximately 30% of adults. Most gynecomastia lesions are estrogen receptor positive. Occasionally, breast lobules may be seen in gynecomastia. Gynecomastia has been linked pathophysiologically to a hormonal imbalance between growth-promoting estrogens and growth-suppressing androgens. Conditions that have been associated with gynecomastia include hyperthyroidism; cirrhosis of the liver; chronic renal failure; use of hormones; and use of numerous common drugs, including digitalis, cimetidine, and spironolactone. Patients with gynecomastia do not have an increased incidence of breast carcinoma. Pseudogynecomastia may be seen in obese males because of lipomastia (i.e., fat in the breast, lacking glandular proliferation).

Barros AC, Sampaio Mde C: Gynecomastia: physiopathology, evaluation and treatment. *Sao Paulo Med J* 2012;130(3): 187-197.

Harigopal M, Murray MP, Rosen P, et al: Prepubertal gynecomastia with lobular differentiation. *Breast J* 2005;11(1):48-51.

15. a.   The image depicts an invasive ductal carcinoma, which is an unusual tumor with a central fibrotic focus also known as a large central acellular zone. The central fibrotic focus is typically acellular (>3 mm), although it may show areas of necrosis and is surrounded by a thin rim of invasive ductal carcinoma. Carcinoma with a central fibrotic focus has been associated with a poor prognosis compared with tumors of equivalent stage and grade. Also, the fibrotic focus has been linked to central hypoxia (expresses hypoxia-inducible factor-1α, carbonic anhydrase 9, and vascular endothelial growth factor A), and the tumor cells may show myoepithelial differentiation. In addition, this tumor is more likely to metastasize to lung and brain. Although the precise incidence is unclear, invasive ductal carcinoma probably represents a small percentage of all invasive cancer. Metastasis may show similar morphologic appearance to the primary tumor. In at least one study, proliferative activity, as determined by MIB-1 labeling of the fibroblasts comprising the fibrotic focus, correlated positively with an increased risk of lymph node metastasis and distant organ metastasis. This phenotype enriches (60% of such tumors) for a basal type of carcinoma (triple negative) if the invasive growth pattern at the periphery is expansive/circumscribed and not highly infiltrative.

Colpaert CG, Vermeulen PB, Fox SB, et al: The presence of a fibrotic focus in invasive breast carcinoma correlates with the expression of carbonic anhydrase IX and is a marker of hypoxia and poor prognosis. *Breast Cancer Res Treat* 2003;81(2):137-147.

Tsuda H, Takarabe T, Hasegawa F, et al: Large, central acellular zones indicating myoepithelial tumor differentiation in high-grade invasive ductal carcinomas as markers of predisposition to lung and brain metastases. *Am J Surg Pathol* 2000;24(2):197-202.

Van den Eynden GG, Colpaert CG, Couvelard A, et al: A fibrotic focus is a prognostic factor and a surrogate marker for hypoxia and (lymph)angiogenesis in breast cancer: review of the literature and proposal on the criteria of evaluation. *Histopathology* 2007;51(4):440-451.

Van den Eynden GG, Smid M, Van Laere SJ, et al: Gene expression profiles associated with the presence of a fibrotic focus and the growth pattern in lymph node-negative breast cancer. *Clin Cancer Res* 2008;14(10):2944-2952.

16. a. Male breast cancer has an incidence of 1% of all breast cancers. It manifests at a more advanced stage (42% with stage III or IV) than female breast cancer and overall has a worse prognosis. However, when corrected for stage, it is associated with a prognosis equivalent to female breast cancer. Male breast cancer is overwhelmingly of the ductal type, although special subtypes of breast carcinoma have been identified rarely. Lobular carcinoma is exceedingly rare. Estrogen receptor and progesterone receptor expression rates are higher in male breast cancer compared with female breast cancer. *BRCA2* germline mutations are associated with male breast cancer (a 70-year-old male carrier has an approximately 6.8% risk of developing breast cancer). Male carriers of *BRCA1* have also been shown to have a 1.2% risk of breast cancer by age 70. Other infrequent germline mutations have been associated with male breast cancer, including androgen receptor mutations, *CHEK2* mutations (associated with Li-Fraumeni syndrome), *PTEN* (Cowden syndrome), *HNPCC* (Lynch syndrome), and *CYP17* polymorphism. Paget disease is statistically more common in males than in females. Many male patients with Paget disease have an associated mass that is frequently invasive breast cancer. Although randomized trials to guide therapy of male breast cancer are lacking, the therapeutic approach is similar to female breast cancer.

Giordano SH, Buzdar AU, Hortobagyi GN: Breast cancer in men. *Ann Intern Med* 2002;137(8):678-687.

Zygogianni AG, Kyrgias G, Gennatas C, et al: Male breast carcinoma: epidemiology, risk factors and current therapeutic approaches. *Asian Pac J Cancer Prev* 2012;13(1):15-19.

17. b. Established, well-confirmed factors that increase the incidence of breast cancer include increasing age, certain geographic locations including the United States and other Western countries, family history, and mutations in *BRCA1* and *BRCA2*. In addition, germline mutations in other high-penetrance genes, such as *PTEN*, *p53*, *CDH1*, *STK11*, *CHEK2*, and *ATM*, are associated with an increased risk. A history of nonproliferative cystic disease does not increase the risk above the general population. Early menarche (<12 years old), late menopause (>54 years old), nulliparity, and maternal age older than 30 years at first birth all increase the risk of breast cancer. High breast density on mammography is a risk factor for breast cancer in both premenopausal and postmenopausal women. A fivefold increased risk of developing breast cancer is seen in women with a greater than 75% increase in breast density compared with women with less than 5% increased breast density. Acting synergistically with this factor is nulliparity and low body weight. Combined hormone replacement therapy, oral contraceptive use, obesity in postmenopausal women, and alcohol consumption (dose related) are associated with a more modest increased risk. Factors that are associated with lower cancer risk are geographic location in Asia and Africa, hormonal factors such as early first pregnancy and high parity, and breastfeeding for a long duration. To a lesser extent, obesity in premenopausal women and physical activity decrease the risk. Chemotherapeutic agents, such as antiestrogens (tamoxifen) and selective estrogen receptor modulators, and nonsteroidal antiinflammatory drugs reduce the risk of breast cancer.

American Cancer Society: What are the risks of breast cancer?

Dumitrescu RG, Cotarla I: Understanding breast cancer risks—where do we stand in 2005? *J Cell Mol Med* 2005;9(1):208-221.

Turkoz FP, Solak M, Petekkaya I, et al: Association between common risk factors and molecular subtypes in breast cancer patients. *Breast* 2013;22(3):344-350.

18. a. In the Ellston-Ellis modification of the Bloom-Richardson histologic grading classification, the mitotic count per 10 high-power fields is dependent on the microscopic fields to establish the appropriate cutoffs for scores of 1, 2, and 3. Field diameter must be carefully determined to establish these cutoffs. In addition, a score of 1 to 3 is given for the extent of tubular formation (1, >75% tubules, and 3, <10% tubules). Nuclear grade is scored 1 to 3, with small/regular corresponding to a score of 1 and a nucleus with marked variation in shape and size corresponding to a score of 3. These scores are added, and a total score of 3, 4, or 5 corresponds to histologic grade 1, well-differentiated; a total score of 6 or 7 corresponds to histologic grade 2, moderately differentiated; and a total score of 8 or 9 corresponds to histologic grade 3, poorly differentiated. Prognostic factors are factors that predict the outcome of breast cancer and include lymph node status, histologic grade, tumor size, histologic type, and presence of vascular invasion. Predictive factors of breast carcinoma are factors that determine a population of patients likely to respond to therapy and include response to tamoxifen predicted by estrogen receptor, progesterone receptor, and *HER2/neu* positivity by immunohistochemistry and response to treatment with trastuzumab, a humanized monoclonal antibody against *HER2/neu*, by more predictive gene amplification. Estrogen receptor, progesterone receptor, and *HER2/neu* are also prognostic factors. In the past decade, Oncotype DX and MammaPrint prognostic and predictive tests for invasive breast carcinoma, which use an assortment of genes heavily relying on proliferation, were introduced. These tests provide assessment of risk of distant recurrence, which is independent of the classic clinicopathologic parameters used to evaluate breast cancer (size, lymph node status, and grade). However, these classic clinicopathologic parameters still contain prognostic information.

Espinosa E, Vara JÁ, Navarro IS, et al: Gene profiling in breast cancer: time to move forward. *Cancer Treat Rev* 2011;37(6):416-421.

Fitzgibbons PL, Page DL, Weaver D, et al: Prognostic factors in breast cancer. College of American Pathologists Consensus statement 1999. *Arch Pathol Lab Med* 2000;124(7):966-978.

Reis-Filho JS, Pusztai L: Gene expression profiling in breast cancer: classification, prognostication, and prediction. *Lancet* 2011;378(9805):1812-1823.

19. a. Genomic changes seen in low-grade tumors and lesions include deletions of 16q and gains in 1q and 16p. Few changes characterize a low-grade family of precursors (columnar cell change, columnar cell hyperplasia, columnar cell atypia, atypical ductal hyperplasia, atypical lobular hyperplasia) and cancers (lobular carcinoma in situ, low-grade ductal carcinoma in situ, low-grade invasive ductal and lobular carcinomas) that are estrogen receptor positive, *HER2* negative, and diploid. High-grade carcinomas exhibit more genomic changes than low-grade carcinomas, including amplification of 8q, 17q, and 20q and low rate of 16q deletions (approximately 10%). However, when 16q deletions are seen in high-grade tumors, they are a result of a different mechanism than low-grade tumors. At least two main nonoverlapping pathways or states of carcinoma are seen, low grade and high grade—shifting the multistep pathway paradigm to multiple multistep pathways. The exception to this appears to be in ~50% of the luminal B tumors that arise from luminal A tumors. Genomic changes correlate more closely with grade, not stage. Transitioning from low grade to high grade is uncommon except for ~50% of the luminal B tumors and in pleomorphic lobular carcinoma (16q loss is common in low-grade carcinoma and uncommon in high-grade carcinoma). When 16q loss is seen in high-grade cancer, it is due to a different mechanism (the mechanism is physical loss in low-grade cancer versus loss of heterozygosity and mitotic recombination in high-grade cancer). In usual ductal hyperplasia, there are no or rare genomic changes, and it is rarely clonal. Usual ductal hyperplasia is a nonobligate precursor of some low-grade cancers similar to atypical ductal hyperplasia and low-grade ductal carcinoma in situ. Among atypical ductal hyperplasia, 50% of cases show genetic changes linking atypical ductal hyperplasia to low-grade cancer genotype; atypical lobular hyperplasia and lobular carcinoma in situ are genomically closely linked, with losses more common than gains. Lobular carcinoma in situ is linked genomically to adjacent invasive lobular carcinoma; it is a nonobligatory precursor and shares features of low-grade ductal cancers, suggesting a family of low-grade tumors.

Cleton-Jansen AM, Buerger H, Haar Nt, et al: Different mechanism of chromosome 16 loss of heterozygosity in well- versus poorly differentiated ductal breast cancer. *Genes Chromosom Cancer* 2004;41(2):109-116.

Geyer FC, Marchio C, Reis-Filho JS: The role of molecular analysis in breast cancer. *Pathology* 2009;41(1):77-88.

20. b. Gene expression profiling has stressed the importance of viewing breast cancer not as a single entity, but rather as different disease entities with unique molecular correlates and corresponding prognostic and therapeutic implications. Gene expression profiling further provides additional information and parameters to characterize tumors molecularly and has substantiated that estrogen receptor, progesterone receptor, *HER2*, and proliferation are key components to be used for classification. Gene expression profiling supports the view that grade and

molecular profiling may represent unique intrinsic qualities that are not captured by and are distinct from size and lymph node status. A molecular profile may be related to prognosis as well as predict response to therapy. Response to therapy is not associated with stage. Prognosis depends on gene expression profiling in a manner independent from stage. The exact number, nature, and definition of molecular subtypes of cancer are still debated; however, broadly speaking, a category of luminal-type cancers exists dominated by expression of genes related to estrogen receptor and progesterone receptor. Although these cancers likely represent a continuum of tumor types, they are frequently categorized as the two ends of a spectrum—luminal A and luminal B. Other subtypes include *HER2* and basal. Also included as distinct subtypes are normallike breast cancer (many doubt its existence and relate it to tumors containing a large amount of stroma) and claudin-low breast cancer. An alternative classification identified a poor-prognosis, molecular apocrine type of cancer typically with an estrogen receptor–negative and androgen receptor–positive phenotype. Although numerous prognostic gene expression profiling–based signatures have been defined in breast cancer, they appear to be driven by expression of proliferation-related genes. Expression of the proliferation cassette plays a prognostic role primarily in estrogen receptor–positive (luminal) cancers because all estrogen receptor–negative cancers invariably are predicted to have a poor prognosis given their high proliferation status. Rare estrogen receptor–negative, low-proliferating tumors show only a limited prognostic difference. Although second-generation prognostic signatures use immune response signatures (correlates with level of inflammation associated with the tumor) to show better prognosis in association with high immune response, the number of relapses remains too high to avoid chemotherapy. Gene expression profiling–based signatures correlate well with response to chemotherapy because chemotherapy response is largely predicted by proliferation rate. Chemotherapy is most effective in highly proliferating tumors. Notwithstanding the more recent excitement regarding the emergence of prognostic and predictive gene expression profiling signatures in breast cancer, a growing body of evidence suggests that their contribution in prognosticating breast cancer may be limited when one integrates conventional pathologic parameters (stage and grade) and immunohistochemistry-based semiquantitation of estrogen receptor, progesterone receptor, *HER2* (immunohistochemistry and fluorescence in situ hybridization), and Ki-67. Venet et al. observed that 90% of all randomly generated signatures containing more than 100 genes correlate with outcome in breast cancer. These authors reasoned that the expression of the proliferation cassette has such an important prognostic value in breast cancer because given that the proliferation cassette is so large, capturing the essence of the cassette is virtually guaranteed in any signature that is simply large enough (invariably it would contain proliferation cassette members). This explanation should give pause to any conclusion that a particular gene is related to breast cancer simply because it is a member of a prognostic signature.

Cuzick J, Dowsett M, Pineda S, et al: Prognostic value of a combined estrogen receptor, progesterone receptor, Ki-67, and human epidermal growth factor receptor 2 immunohistochemical score and comparison with the Genomic Health recurrence score in early breast cancer. *J Clin Oncol* 2011;29(32):4273-4278.

Reis-Filho JS, Pusztai L: Gene expression profiling in breast cancer: classification, prognostication, and prediction. *Lancet* 2011;378(9805):1812-1823.

Venet D, Dumont JE, Detours V: Most random gene expression signatures are significantly associated with breast cancer outcome. *PloS Comput Biol* 2011;7(10):e1002240.

21. a. Lack of expression in some subtypes of cancers of their namesake (i.e., *HER2*) raises questions regarding the translatability of conventional College of American Pathologists (CAP)/American Society of Clinical Oncology (ASCO)–recommended determination methods of such parameters versus gene expression profiling. Gene expression profiling classification based on Perou and Sorlie "intrinsic genes"—genes whose expression varies more across different cancers than across different regions of the same breast cancer—are primarily based on the estrogen receptor cluster, the proliferation cluster, and, to a lesser extent, the *HER2*-related amplicon cluster. Gene expression profiling leads to a classification scheme that primarily, but not completely, overlaps or corresponds to immunohistochemistry-based classifications. For example, the *HER2* gene expression profiling–based cancers are only about 80% *HER2* overexpressed or amplified using ASCO/CAP guidelines. Luminal B gene expression profiling–defined cancers are associated with *HER2* positivity by immunohistochemistry and fluorescence in situ hybridization in 15% to 24% of cases. Given the large estrogen receptor–related cluster of genes, *HER2*-positive tumors expressing the estrogen receptor cluster are classified as luminal B, not *HER2*. Similarly, gene expression profiling–defined basal cancers are only 70% triple-negative by immunohistochemistry, and only 70% of triple-negative tumors by immunohistochemistry are basal by gene expression profiling. Luminal A tumors typically show high expression of estrogen receptor and progesterone receptor positivity, low proliferation, primarily low grade, good prognosis, and low benefit from chemotherapy (pathologic complete response of 0% to 5%). Luminal B tumors typically show a lower level of estrogen receptor expression, high proliferation, possible *HER2* positivity, intermediate to poor prognosis, and intermediate benefit from chemotherapy (pathologic complete response of 10% to 20%). Basallike breast cancers typically are triple-negative tumors (estrogen receptor–negative, progesterone receptor–negative, *HER2*-negative tumors), although by immunohistochemistry, 10% may be positive for estrogen receptor or progesterone receptor; may be highly proliferating, high-grade tumors; and represent 80% of *BRCA1* germline–associated tumors with poor outcome but with associated benefit from chemotherapy (pathologic complete response of 40%). *HER2*-positive tumors by gene expression profiling show 70% to 80% *HER2* positivity by immunohistochemistry and fluorescence in situ hybridization, high proliferation, high grade, and poor outcome; these tumors benefit from chemotherapy (pathologic complete response of 25% to 40%) but not as much as basal tumors. The tumor may

express estrogen receptor–related or progesterone receptor–related genes. Molecular apocrine–type cancers show some histologic apocrine features, are GCDFP-15 positive, are estrogen receptor negative and androgen receptor positive, and have high proliferation and grade. Androgen receptor is invariably positive in estrogen receptor–positive tumors but molecular apocrine cancers that are estrogen receptor negative and androgen receptor positive are associated with a poor prognosis. Based on estrogen receptor and androgen receptor, cancer can be divided into luminal (estrogen receptor positive, androgen receptor positive), basallike (estrogen receptor negative, androgen receptor negative), and molecular apocrine (estrogen receptor negative, androgen receptor negative). Claudin-low cancers are characterized by poorly differentiated tumors, are frequently metaplastic, show epithelial mesenchymal transition, and have a stem cell–like expression profile that appears less differentiated than basal cancers. Claudin-low cancers may show basal markers and low estrogen receptor expression. The prognosis is slightly better compared with basallike tumors, but claudin-low cancers show a slightly lower pathologic complete response (25% to 40%) than basal cancers.

Geyer FC, Marchio K, Reis-Filho JS: The role of molecular analysis in breast cancer. *Pathology* 2009;41(1):77-88.

Reis-Filho JS, Pusztai L: Gene expression profiling in breast cancer: classification, prognostication, and prediction. *Lancet* 2011;378(9805):1812-1823.

22. e. Approximately 25% of all breast cancers correspond to recognizable histologic subtypes. Molecular classification of these tumors suggests that they are less heterogeneous than breast cancers of no special subtype and that they represent molecularly distinct entities that are enriched for similarity. This idea is supported by unique translocations that are associated with some of these tumors, including secretory carcinoma t(12;15)(p13;q25) *ETV6-NTRK3* and adenoid cystic carcinoma t(6;9)(q22-23;p23-24) *MYB-NFIB*. Typical estrogen receptor–positive cancers that are low grade and have low mitotic activity are molecularly luminal in subtype. These cancers include tubular, classic lobular (most, but not all), neuroendocrine, mucinous, and low-grade invasive ductal carcinomas with osteoclastlike giant cells. Some cancer subtypes may map to more than one molecular subtype, such as invasive micropapillary cancer that maps to luminal or *HER2* subtypes. Classic lobular cancer primarily maps to luminal subtype but alternatively may map to *HER2* subtype. Adenoid cystic, secretory, and microglandular adenosis–associated carcinomas map to basallike subtype. Medullary and metaplastic carcinomas may map to basallike or claudin-low subtypes. Pleomorphic lobular carcinoma maps to luminal, *HER2*, or molecular apocrine subtypes. Apocrine carcinomas are heterogeneous and may map primarily to molecular apocrine or *HER2*. Despite mapping to a distinct or restricted set of molecular subtypes, the special histologic subtypes of breast cancer have been shown to be distinct transcriptomically from no special subtype invasive ductal carcinoma of the same molecular group. By analyzing these subtypes, it is possible that we may reduce the complexity and heterogeneity of the cohort studied, which potentially may aid in defining key drivers of breast cancer.

Weigelt B, Geyer FC, Reis-Filho JS: Histologic types of breast cancer: how special are they? *Mol Oncol* 2010;4(3):192-208.

Weigelt B, Horlings HM, Kreike B, et al: Refinement of breast cancer classification by molecular characterization of histological special subtypes. *J Pathol* 2008;216(2):141-150.

23. c. Basallike breast cancers, which account for approximately 15% of all breast cancers, as defined by gene expression correspond to a histologically heterogeneous group of high-grade tumors with high mitotic activity associated with a poor prognosis and early relapse rate. Notwithstanding these observations, these tumors are associated with the highest pathologic complete response rate (>40%) seen in breast cancer subtypes. Exceptions to the poor prognosis of basal tumors include adenoid cystic and secretory carcinomas of the breast. Correspondence between immunohistochemistry and gene expression profiling definitions of basallike tumors is only partially overlapping. Only 77% of basallike cancers are triple negative (negative for estrogen receptor, progesterone receptor, and *HER2*); higher levels of specificity (100%) and sensitivity (76%) for a basal phenotype are achieved if defined by immunohistochemistry as triple-negative and cytokeratin 5/6–positive and epidermal growth factor receptor–positive tumors. Triple-negative basallike tumors defined by immunohistochemistry (triple negative and cytokeratin 5/6 positive and epidermal growth factor receptor positive) have a worse prognosis than tumors that are triple negative only. Basallike cancers are associated with high rates of *p53* mutations and are seen at higher rates in premenopausal African American women (27%) versus postmenopausal women (15%). Basallike cancers, despite their name and initial suggestion of arising from the basal epithelium and myoepithelium in view of their partly shared phenotype, likely originate from luminal progenitor cells or have some stem cell characteristics. Basallike cancers lack classic myoepithelial cell phenotype (smooth muscle actin, calponin expression) and are positive for luminal cytokeratin 8/18 and frequently cytokeratin 5/6. *BRCA1*-associated basallike tumors have been targeted by poly adenosine diphosphate ribose polymerase (PARP)-1 inhibitors. PARP-1 inhibitors (targeting repair of single-strand breaks) in the context of mutation lead to accumulation of breaks in double-stranded DNA and cell death.

Eroles P, Bosch A, Pérez-Fidalgo JA, et al: Molecular biology in breast cancer: intrinsic subtypes and signalling pathways. *Cancer Treat Rev* 2012;38(6):698-707.

Irshad S, Ellis P, Tutt A: Molecular heterogeneity of triple-negative breast cancer and its clinical implications. *Curr Opin Oncol* 2011;23(6):566-577.

24. a. Oncotype DX and MammaPrint are prognostic and predictive tests for invasive breast carcinoma. These tests provide risk assessment of distant recurrence that is independent of the classic clinicopathologic parameters used to evaluate breast cancer (size, lymph node status, and grade); however, the classic clinicopathologic parameters still contain prognostic information. Oncotype DX is based on a 21-gene signature (16 cancer-related genes and 5 reference genes/controls). It is a quantitative reverse transcriptase polymerase chain reaction–based test performed on formalin-fixed paraffin-embedded tissue. It typically is performed on node-negative, estrogen receptor–positive invasive carcinoma. A recurrence score is generated that predicts the risk for distant relapse in 10 years for patients on tamoxifen therapy. The recurrence score may range from 0 to 100. A low recurrence score (<18) is associated with an estimated 7% risk of distant relapse in 10 years. An intermediate recurrence score (18 to 31) is associated with an average 14% risk of distant relapse in 10 years. A high recurrence score (≥31) is associated with a 30% risk of distant relapse rate in 10 years. MammaPrint is based on a 70-gene signature providing a dichotomous output: high risk and low risk. The high-risk category is associated with a 22% risk of distant metastasis in 5 years (30% in 10 years), and the low-risk category is associated with a 7% risk of distant metastasis in 5 years (10% in 10 years). MammaPrint was originally approved by the U.S. Food and Drug Administration as a test on frozen tissue only, but it has become available more recently on formalin-fixed paraffin-embedded tissue. MammaPrint is offered on node-negative invasive tumors of less than 5 cm that are either estrogen receptor positive or negative; however, it has limited discriminatory capacity in estrogen receptor–negative cancers because greater than 95% of estrogen receptor–negative cases are classified as high risk. Both Oncotype DX and MammaPrint are predictive tests. The test results suggest that the high-risk group benefits from chemotherapy and that the low-risk group does not (if they are both treated with adjuvant tamoxifen). This suggestion is in keeping with the observation that the high-risk group is highly proliferating, and it is this group that benefits from chemotherapy. In the case of Oncotype DX, an ongoing trial (TAILORx) is evaluating the role of chemotherapy in the intermediate-risk group. For MammaPrint, the MINDACT trial is comparing the outcome of patients treated with or without chemotherapy in cases of discordance of risk categorization between MammaPrint and traditional clinicopathologic criteria. Oncotype DX has been primarily applied to lymph node–negative cancers, but it is also prognostic in lymph node–positive disease. However, in disease with greater than three positive lymph nodes, the low-risk category absolute risk of distant recurrence is too high to avoid chemotherapy. Oncotype DX has limited utility in chemotherapy predictiveness in this setting (it has been suggested that Oncotype DX and MammaPrint have utility in predictive testing for chemotherapy in cancers with one to three positive lymph nodes). Some data suggest that the prognostic information offered by these tests may be limited if one integrates clinicopathologic parameters with immunohistochemistry-based determination of estrogen receptor, progesterone receptor, Ki-67, and *HER2*.

Paik S, Shak S, Tang G, et al: A multigene assay to predict recurrence of tamoxifen-treated, node-negative breast cancer. *N Engl J Med* 2004;351(27):2817-2826.

Reis-Filho JS, Pusztai L: Gene expression profiling in breast cancer: classification, prognostication, and prediction. *Lancet* 2011;378(9805):1812-1823.

van't Veer LJ, Dai H, van de Vijver MJ, et al: Gene expression profiling predicts clinical outcome of breast cancer. *Nature* 2002;415(6871):530-536.

25. d. Encapsulated papillary carcinoma is considered by some experts as a low-grade invasive carcinoma with an expansile growth pattern. It is defined as a form of well-circumscribed carcinoma (ductal carcinoma in situ–like in distribution) with papillary architecture lacking myoepithelial cells both in the papillae and at the periphery. Lymph node metastasis without associated conventional invasion (no special type [NST]) is rare. The differential diagnosis includes intraductal papilloma with or without secondary cancerization (ductal carcinoma in situ) and intraductal papillary carcinoma. Intraductal papilloma has myoepithelial cells in its papillae and at the periphery. Myoepithelial immunostains must be performed to resolve the differential diagnosis if myoepithelial cells are not clearly identified on hematoxylin-eosin stain or if their presence is in question. Ductal carcinoma in situ may cancerize an intraductal papilloma in part or in whole; this lesion has the same myoepithelial distribution as a papilloma but is lined by carcinoma cells. In intraductal papillary carcinoma (whether conventional, cystic, or rarely solid), myoepithelial cells are sparse to none in the papillae and are present at the periphery. Occasionally, the epithelial component may have usual ductal hyperplasia features, and the diagnosis depends on the demonstration of the absence of myoepithelial cells in the papillae only (while being present at the periphery). This form of ductal carcinoma in situ may be associated with conventional invasion. Encapsulated papillary carcinoma may be associated with a conventional invasive component (i.e., showing architectural complexity in that component). Rarely, a diffuse aggressive nonlocalized form of this tumor is present that is multifocally invasive; on biopsy, this may be impossible to distinguish from the localized form with a good prognosis. When conventional invasion is absent or limited in extent, lymph node metastasis is rare regardless of its association with either encapsulated papillary carcinoma or intraductal papillary carcinoma. Encapsulated papillary carcinoma is associated with an expression pattern of invasion-associated markers that is intermediate between ductal carcinoma in situ and invasive cancer. Higher expression levels of matrix metalloproteinases MMP-1 and MMP-9 are seen in encapsulated papillary carcinoma and in invasive carcinoma compared with ductal carcinoma in situ. Expression of matrix metalloproteinases MMP-2 and MMP-7 in encapsulated papillary carcinoma is similar to expression in ductal carcinoma in situ and lower than expression in invasive cancer. These findings support the view of an indolent cancer.

Collins LC, Schnitt SJ: Papillary lesions of the breast: selected diagnostic and management issues. *Histopathology* 2008; 52(1):20-29.
Rakha EA, Gandhi N, Climent F, et al: Encapsulated papillary carcinoma of the breast: an invasive tumor with excellent prognosis. *Am J Surg Pathol* 2011;35(8):1093-1103.
Rakha EA, Tun M, Junainah E, et al: Encapsulated papillary carcinoma of the breast: a study of invasion associated markers. *J Clin Pathol* 2012;65(8):710-714.

26. a. Secretory carcinoma is a rare special subtype of breast carcinoma. Initially described in children and young women, it subsequently was shown to occur over a wider age range with a median age of 25 years. It also was reported subsequently mostly in young men with a median age of 19 years. Secretory breast cancer is histologically characterized by eosinophilic secretions in intracellular and extracellular vacuoles, which are positive on PAS and diastase PAS stains. The cancer is typically immunoreactive for S100 protein and α-lactalbumin. Secretory breast cancer typically is a basallike tumor by gene expression profiling— triple negative and basal marker positive. It has a good prognosis highlighting the heterogeneity that may be seen in the basallike tumors despite their general poor prognosis. In this respect, it is similar to another good-prognosis basallike tumor, adenoid cystic carcinoma of the breast. Secretory breast cancer is characterized by a chromosomal translocation t(12;15) resulting in a fusion transcript *ETV6-NTRK3*. This chimeric tyrosine kinase transcript results in activation of both the Ras-Mek1 and pI3k-Akt pathways. Also, it is responsible for activation of mammary growth factor (also known as signal transducer and activator of transcription 5A), which is thought to be mechanistically linked to the observed secretory change. Prognosis is generally excellent, but if the tumor is large or metastatic, it demonstrates unfavorable behavior. The prognosis is better in children and adolescents and is noted to be slightly worse in adults.

Lambros MB, Tan DS, Jones RL, et al: Genomic profile of a secretory breast cancer with an ETV6-NTRK3 duplication. *J Clin Pathol* 2009;62(7):604-612.
Tognon C, Gamett M, Kenward E, et al: The chimeric protein tyrosine kinase ETV6-NTRK3 requires both Ras-Erk1/2 and PI3-kinase-Akt signaling for fibroblast transformation. *Cancer Res* 2001;61(24):8909-8916.
Vasudev P, Onuma K: Secretory breast carcinoma. *Arch Pathol Lab Med* 2011;135(12):1606-1610.

27. d. *HER2/neu* gene amplification identifies a biologically unique subset of aggressive breast tumors that are sensitive to growth inhibition and apoptosis induced by anti-*HER2/neu* targeted therapies. Because the only currently available predictor of responsiveness to trastuzumab is *HER2/neu* status, the ASCO recommends evaluation of all primary breast tumors for *HER2/neu* status. At the present time, two methods of measuring *HER2/neu* are approved by the U.S. Food and Drug Administration for selecting patients for trastuzumab-based therapy: immunohistochemistry and fluorescence in situ hybridization. *HER2/neu* staining by immunohistochemistry is expressed on a semiquantitative scale from 0 (no detectable HER2/neu protein) to 3+ (high HER2/neu protein expression). Tumors with a score of 3+ are most likely to respond to trastuzumab, and tumors with a score of 0 to 1+ are least likely to respond. Fluorescence in situ hybridization allows quantification of gene copy number to determine whether an invasive carcinoma is driven by *HER2/neu* gene amplification. This method is more specific and sensitive than immunohistochemistry. Fluorescence in situ hybridization should be routinely performed on tumors scored 2+ by immunohistochemistry because fluorescence in situ hybridization improves on the ability of immunohistochemistry to predict a response to trastuzumab in this subset of patients. Trastuzumab significantly improves disease-free survival and overall survival when used weekly or every 3 weeks for 1 year in patients with early *HER2/neu*-positive breast cancer. In four large multicenter randomized trials (NSABP B-31, NCCTG N9831, HERA, and BCTRG 006), addition of trastuzumab to the standard chemotherapy regimen (anthracycline-based regimens and a taxane-based regimen) in early *HER2/neu*-positive breast cancer showed a significant improvement in disease-free survival, increases in time to disease progression and overall survival, and reductions in the risk of recurrence rate and death in this group. The proposed mechanisms through which trastuzumab exerts its effects include (1) downregulation of the *HER2* receptor resulting in decreased amounts of available receptors; (2) inhibition of HER family dimerization, inhibiting activation of the signaling cascades; (3) reduction of the proteolytic cleavage of the extracellular domain, preventing the formation of a truncated, highly active receptor remnant; (4) inhibition of P13K/AKT and mitogen activated protein kinase pathways with resultant antiangiogenesis; (5) induction of *p27* with induction G_1 arrest; and (6) antibody-dependent cell-mediated cytotoxicity. Trastuzumab is not associated with typical side effects of chemotherapy, such as cytopenias, nausea, vomiting, or alopecia, and hypersensitivity reactions are rare. The most clinically significant side effect of trastuzumab is cardiotoxicity. Cardiotoxicity can be manifested as asymptomatic decreases in left ventricular ejection fraction or symptomatic congestive heart failure. Cardiotoxicity is reversible in most patients. Clinical evaluation before treatment with trastuzumab should include careful screening for cardiac risk factors. Lapatinib (a small molecule tyrosine kinase inhibitor that targets *HER1* and *HER2*), bevacizumab (which targets vascular endothelial growth factor), neratinib (a dual *HER1-HER2* inhibitor), and the peptide vaccines GP2 and AE37 all are in adjuvant trials for *HER2*-positive early-stage breast cancer.

Arteaga CL, Sliwkowski MX, Osborne CK, et al: Treatment of HER2-positive breast cancer: current status and future perspectives. *Clin Oncol* 2011;9(1):16-32.

Gonzalez-Angulo AM, Hortobágyi GN, Esteva FJ: Adjuvant therapy with trastuzumab for HER-2/neu-positive breast cancer. *Oncologist* 2006;11(8):857-867.

Murphy CG, Modi S: HER2 breast cancer therapies: a review. *Biologics* 2009;3:289-301.

28. b. Diabetic mastopathy is associated with type 1 or type 2 diabetes mellitus and has been reported in nondiabetic patients as well. Inflammatory infiltrates are composed of lymphocytes with variable numbers of plasma cells. In addition, dense keloidal fibrosis that contains embedded epithelioid fibroblasts has been described. Core biopsy can be used to monitor patients with recurrent lesions in a proven case of diabetic mastopathy because it can show ductal epithelial cells in clusters, lymphocytes, and epithelioid fibroblasts. Epithelioid fibroblasts appear uniquely in diabetic mastopathy and are diagnostic when found, although they are not present in all cases. The pathophysiology of this condition is unclear, although the most widely postulated theory relates to the production of nonenzymatically glycosylated proteins in diabetes. These proteins are often cross-linked and resistant to degradation and are deposited within the matrix of various tissues, including the breast, where they can stimulate an immunogenic response. Most cases are reported in women,

although a few cases have been reported in men, and an association with gynecomastia has been reported. It is widely reported that this condition occurs mainly in premenopausal women. Most mammograms of patients with diabetic mastopathy are reported with terms such as "dense breast parenchyma," "dense glandular tissue," "asymmetric densities," and "parenchymal deformity." A discrete mass lesion is typically not visualized.

Fong D, Lann MA, Finlayson C, et al: Diabetic (lymphocytic) mastopathy with exuberant lymphohistiocytic and granulomatous response. *Am J Surg Pathol* 2006;30(10):1330-1336.

Thorncroft K, Forsyth L, Desmond S, et al: The diagnosis and management of diabetic mastopathy. *Breast J* 2007;13(6):607-613.

29. d. The relative amounts of fat, connective tissue, and epithelial tissue determine the radiographic appearance of the breast on a mammogram. Fat appears as dark or radiologic lucent areas, whereas connective tissue and epithelial tissue appear as areas of high radiologic density; this is usually expressed as a percentage, when percent mammographic density is the percentage of the breast area observed on a mammogram that is radiodense or white. Percent mammographic density has been found to be one of the strongest independent predictors of breast cancer risk. Women with the most mammographically dense breasts have fourfold to sixfold increased risk of breast cancer compared with women with the least dense breasts. Breast density changes throughout a woman's lifetime; the proportion of the epithelial tissue tends to increase until the third or fourth decade of life and then declines progressively with increasing age. More pronounced reductions occur after each pregnancy and after menopause. Mammographic density also can be altered by endogenous and exogenous hormonal factors. Age, parity, and menopausal status account for only 20% to 30% of the percent mammographic density variation observed in the population. Genetic factors might explain a proportion of variation of percent mammographic density. Studies of twins suggest that percent mammographic density is a heritable quantitative trait. The American College of Radiology developed a four-category system, the BIRADS (Breast Imaging Reporting and Data System) classification of mammographic density: (1) breast is almost entirely fat (<25% glandular); (2) scattered fibroglandular densities (25% to 50%); (3) heterogeneously dense breast tissue (51% to 75%); and (4) extremely dense (>75% glandular).

Assi V, Warwick J, Cuzick J, et al: Clinical and epidemiological issues in mammographic density. *Nat Rev Clin Oncol* 2012;9(1):33-40.

Boyd NF, Martin LJ, Yaffe MJ: Mammographic density and breast cancer risk: current understanding and future prospects. *Breast Cancer Res* 2011;13(6):223-235.

Boyd NF, Rommens JM, Vogt K, et al: Mammographic breast density as an intermediate phenotype for breast cancer. *Lancet Oncol* 2005;6(10):798-808.

CHAPTER 12

BONE AND JOINT PATHOLOGY

May Parisien and Angela J. Yoon

Questions 1-40 refer to a photo or photomicrograph.

1. In a 28-year-old woman, a hard mass of the popliteal fossa was palpated. Radiographically, a large, mushroomlike lesion attached to the cortical surface of the distal femur was seen to protrude posteriorly. Which of the following statements does NOT apply to this lesion?
   a. A cartilaginous cap may be present.
   b. Surgical excision is the treatment of choice.
   c. This lesion is associated with a good prognosis.
   d. This lesion bears some histologic similarities to fibrous dysplasia.
   e. Dedifferentiation is not a feature of this lesion.

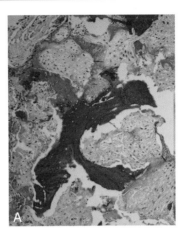

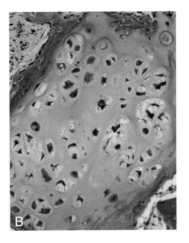

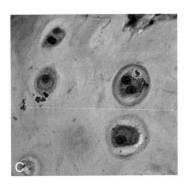

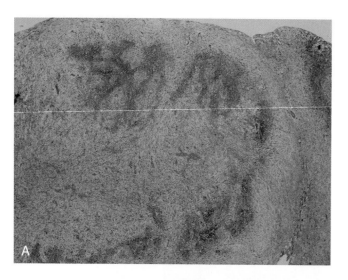

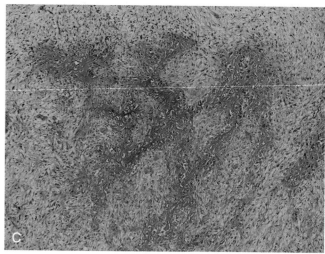

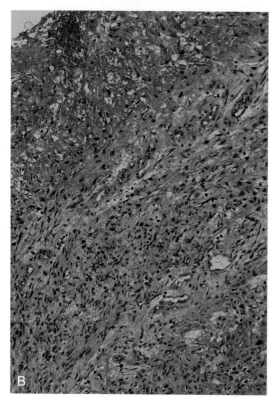

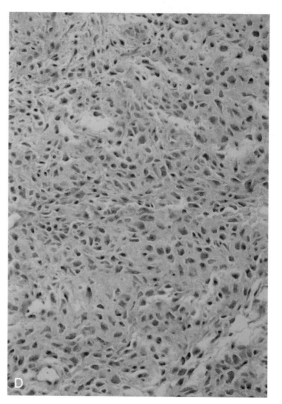

2. Which of the following entities corresponds BEST to the histologic changes observed in the photomicrographs in the image?

a. Juxtacortical osteosarcoma

b. Aggressive osteoblastoma invading soft tissue

c. Periosteal osteosarcoma

d. Exuberant fracture callus

e. Myositis ossificans circumscripta

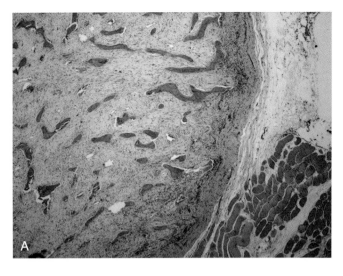

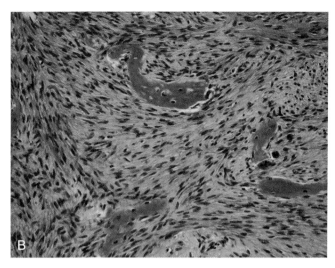

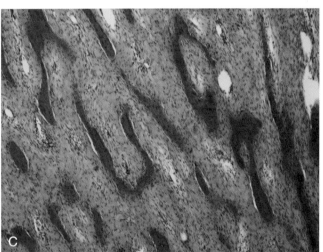

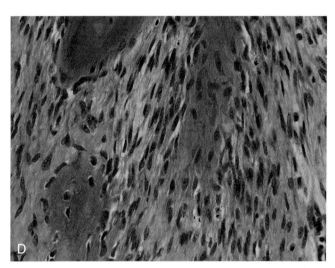

3. Which of the following statements is FALSE?
   a. This is the second most common malignant neoplasm of bone in adults.
   b. The lesion commonly arises from a preexisting benign cartilaginous tumor.
   c. The treatment of choice is surgical excision with wide margins.
   d. Common locations are the large bones of the axial skeleton, such as the pelvis.
   e. Radiographic signs are endosteal scalloping, cortical thickening, and the presence of a soft tissue mass.

4. The classic radiologic presentation of the lesion shown in the image is the "soap bubble" appearance. Which of the following statements is FALSE?
   a. This lesion is considered a reaction to injury.
   b. This lesion affects most frequently individuals in their second decade of life.
   c. This lesion may affect any bone with a slight predilection for the metaphyses of long bones and the vertebrae.
   d. Spontaneous regression is common.
   e. The cell population of the cyst lining includes numerous multinucleated giant cells.

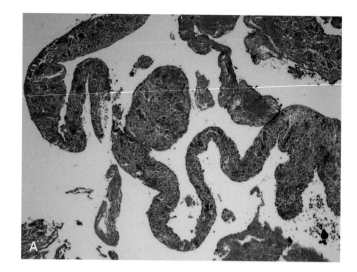

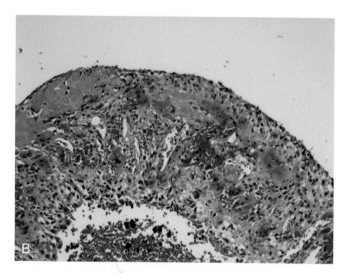

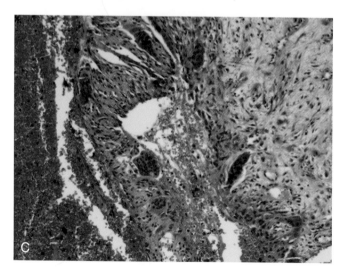

5. Which of the following is the LEAST likely diagnosis?
   a. Pigmented villonodular synovitis (PVNS)
   b. Lyme disease
   c. Systemic lupus erythematosus
   d. Rheumatoid synovitis
   e. Psoriasis

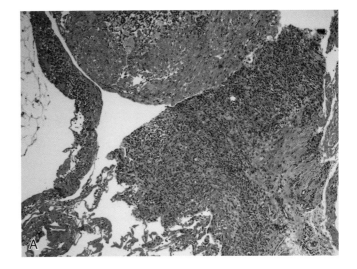

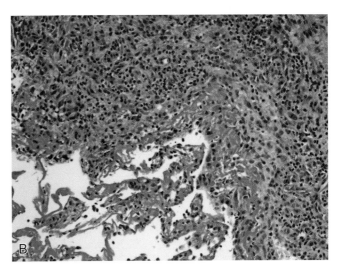

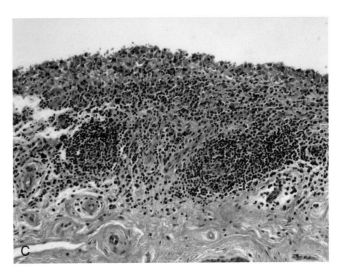

6. What is the probable diagnosis?
   a. Synovial chondromatosis
   b. Chondrosarcoma
   c. Chondroma (enchondroma)
   d. PVNS
   e. Chondromyxoid fibroma

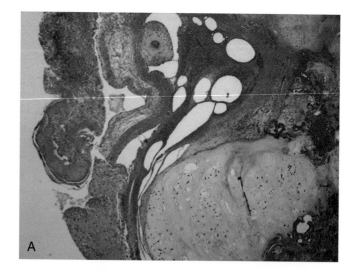

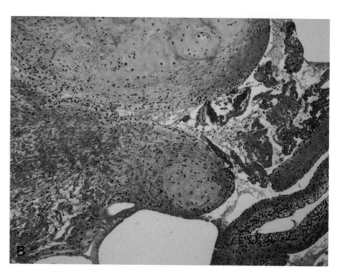

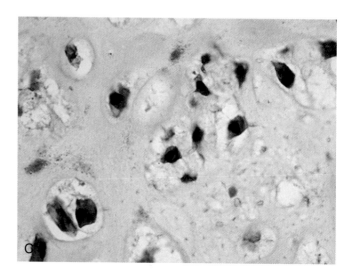

7. What is the MOST likely diagnosis?
   a. Central chondrosarcoma
   b. Chondromyxoid fibroma
   c. Intraosseous myxoid chondrosarcoma
   d. Fibromyxoma of bone
   e. Chondroblastoma

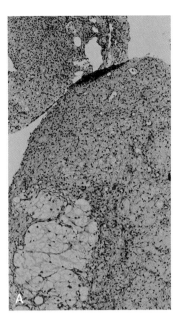

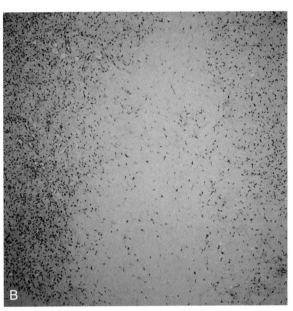

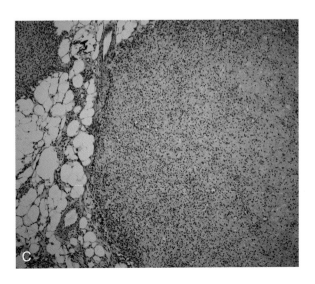

8. Which of the following is the CORRECT diagnosis?
   a. Gouty tophus
   b. Soft tissue calcinosis
   c. Pseudogout (calcium pyrophosphate dihydrate [CPPD] crystal deposition disease)
   d. Tumoral calcinosis
   e. Prosthetic or detritic synovitis

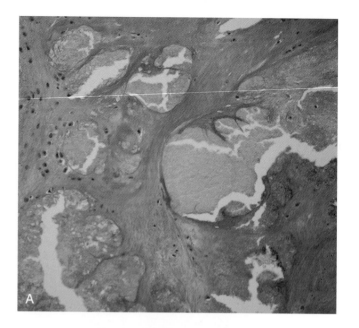

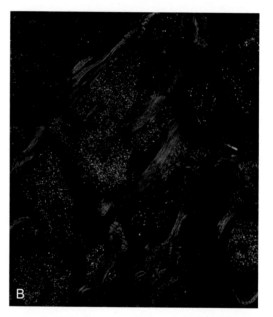

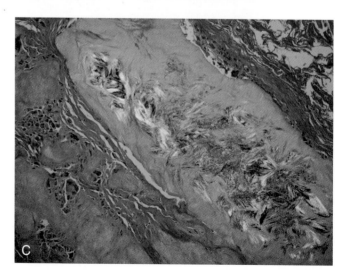

9. A 15-year-old high school athlete presented with pain in the right shoulder. Radiography showed an ill-defined radiolucent and radiopaque lesion of the proximal humerus associated with a soft tissue mass. Which of the following is the MOST likely diagnosis?

a. Osteoblastoma

b. Chondrosarcoma

c. Osteosarcoma

d. Chondroblastoma

e. Ewing sarcoma

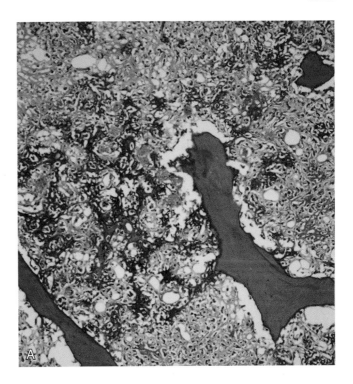

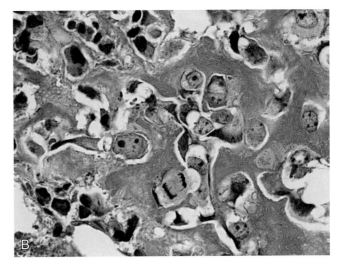

10. A 32-year-old man presented with a lesion in the proximal tibia that manifested as an ill-defined radiolucency. What is the MOST likely diagnosis?

    a. Ewing sarcoma/peripheral neuroectodermal tumor (PNET)

    b. Lymphoma

    c. Metastatic neuroblastoma

    d. Myxoid chondrosarcoma

    e. Small cell osteosarcoma

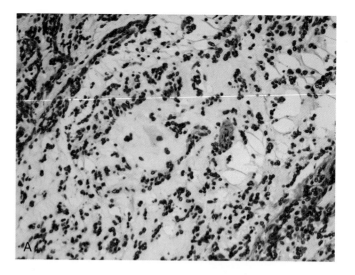

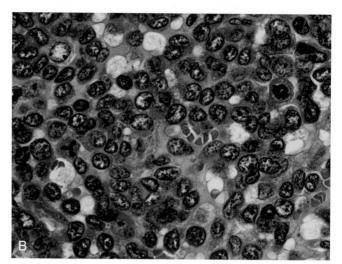

11. A 20-year-old woman complained of pain on mastication. A radiograph showed a destructive lesion of the left mandible extending to the temporomandibular joint. What is the MOST likely diagnosis?

a. Hemangiopericytoma

b. Monophasic, fibrous synovial sarcoma

c. Ewing sarcoma/PNET

d. Mesenchymal chondrosarcoma

e. Myxoid chondrosarcoma

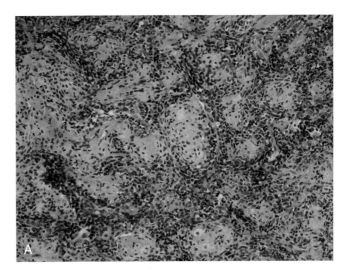

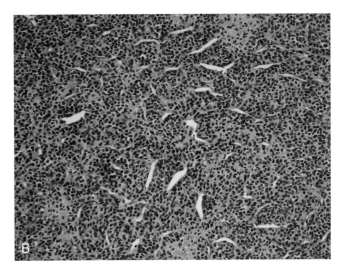

12. The lesion shown in the image is characterized by large multivacuolated cells. Which of the following statements is NOT correct?

   a. This tumor has a high metastatic rate.
   b. The lesion most commonly occurs after the sixth decade.
   c. The clinical presentation frequently includes severe constipation and a presacral mass.
   d. A lobulated architecture is a typical histologic finding.
   e. Radiologically, a solitary, large, central, expansile lucency is observed.

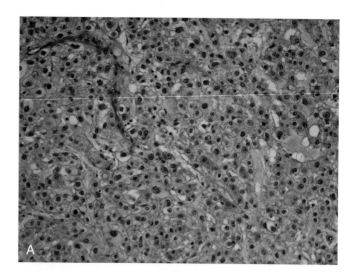

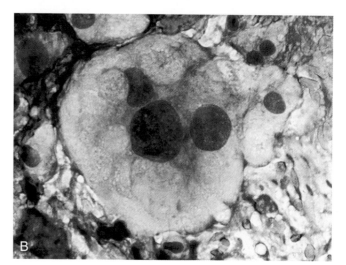

13. Which of the following statements is FALSE?
   a. The most common sites are the ribs, the facial bone, and the long bones.
   b. It is a benign fibroosseous lesion.
   c. The polyostotic form is less common than the monostotic form.
   d. Radiologic studies frequently show soft tissue extension with prominent periosteal reaction.
   e. G-protein mutations have been implicated in the cause of the polyostotic form and possibly of the monostotic form.

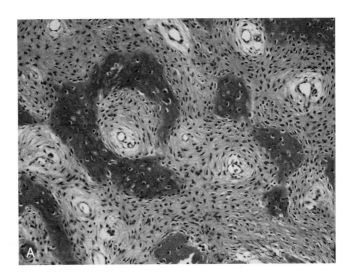

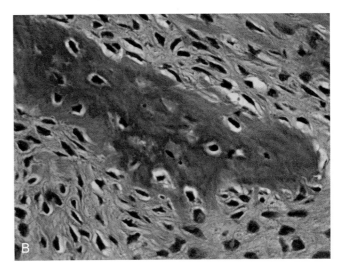

14. A 12-year-old child with normal serum calcium and
phosphorus presented with a large expansile radiolucency
involving the ascending ramus of the right mandible. What
is the CORRECT diagnosis?
   a. Giant cell tumor of bone
   b. Fracture callus
   c. Osteoblastoma
   d. Giant cell reparative granuloma
   e. Brown tumor of hyperparathyroidism

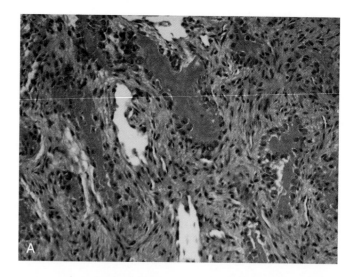

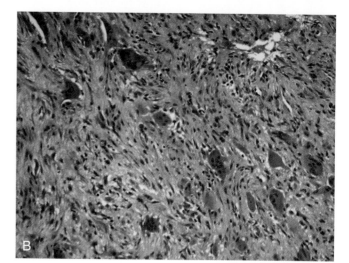

15. The lesion shown in the image is typically located in the epiphyses of long bones. Which of the following statements concerning this lesion is FALSE?

  a. The distal femur and proximal tibia are the most frequently involved sites.

  b. Malignant transformation occurs in 10% of cases.

  c. Histologically benign lesions can metastasize.

  d. Intravascular tumor observed at the periphery of the tumor indicates metastasis.

  e. Complete surgical excision is the treatment of choice.

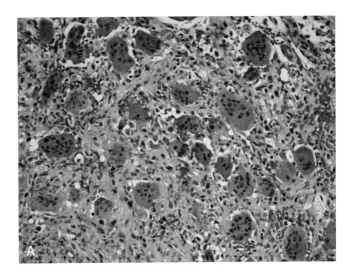

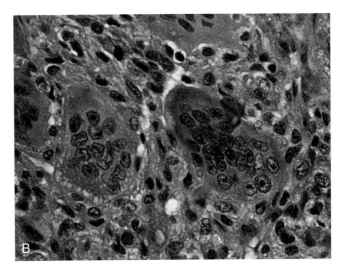

16. The tumor shown in the image is the second most common sarcoma of bone and soft tissue in children. Which of the following statements is NOT characteristic of this lesion?

   a. There is a predilection for the pelvis and long bones of the lower extremities.

   b. The characteristic radiologic appearance is moth-eaten bone destruction associated with "onion-layering" subperiosteal new bone.

   c. CD99 (gene product of *MIC2* gene), expressed in almost all cases, is the ultimate diagnostic marker.

   d. Bone involvement is frequently associated with soft tissue extension.

   e. The 5-year survival rate is 75% with proper therapy.

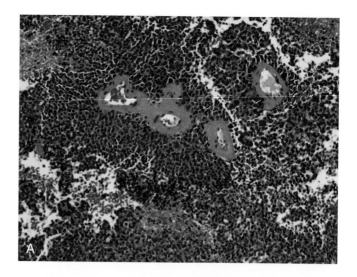

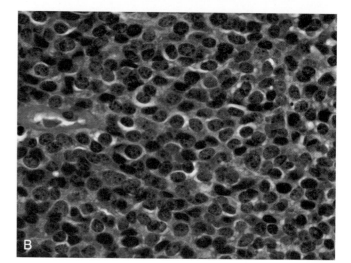

17. The tumor shown in the image typically involves the epiphyses of the long bones of young individuals and expresses S100 protein. Which of the following statements is FALSE?
   a. The local recurrence rate is approximately 15%.
   b. This tumor is associated with a grim prognosis.
   c. The most frequent sites are the distal femur and the proximal humerus.
   d. Most patients are 10 to 25 years old.
   e. Secondary aneurysmal bone cyst is a frequent development.

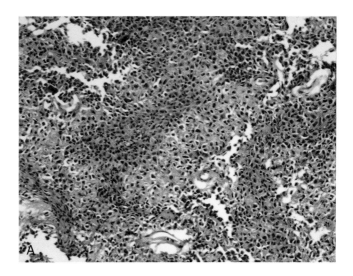

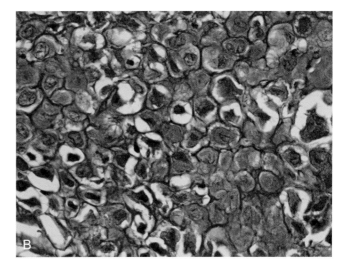

18. Which of the following statements is NOT correct for the intracortical lesion shown in the image?
   a. The lesion most often affects children and adolescents.
   b. The lesion has a predilection for long bones, particularly the proximal femur.
   c. A characteristic feature is pain, which is worse at night and is dramatically relieved by aspirin.
   d. The lesion has unlimited growth potential, reaching greater than 10 cm in some cases.
   e. A radiolucent center surrounded by a zone of cortical sclerosis is typical.

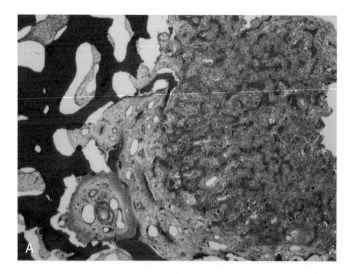

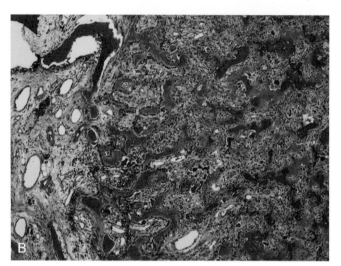

19. Which of the following is NOT a feature of the lesion shown in the image?
    a. Elevated levels of serum calcium and decreased alkaline phosphatase are observed.
    b. Transverse fracture of long bones (chalkstick fracture) is common.
    c. A single bone or multiple bones may be involved.
    d. The basic abnormality is disorderly, accelerated bone turnover.
    e. Sarcomas of bone are a possible complication.

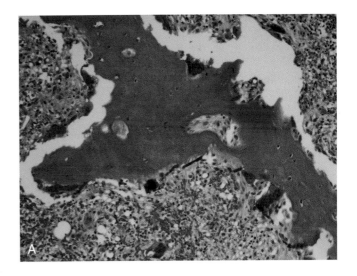

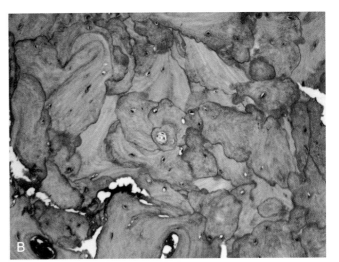

20. Which of the following statements concerning the lesion
shown in the image is NOT correct?

   a. The lesion involves the tibia and fibula almost exclusively.

   b. Histologic variants include spindle cell, basaloid, tubular,
   and squamous types.

   c. Vimentin, keratin, and endothelial monocyte antigen label
   the epithelial cells.

   d. Radiographically, a well-circumscribed, multiloculated,
   intracortical radiolucency with sclerotic margins is typical.

   e. The tumor is rapidly growing with a 70% metastatic rate.

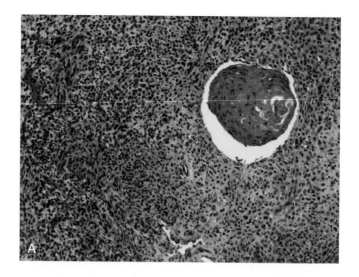

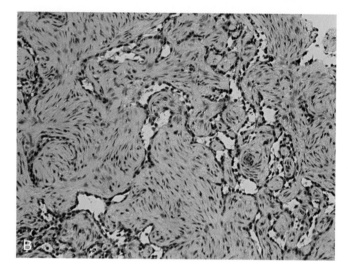

21. All of the following statements about this lesion are true EXCEPT:

   a. The recurrence rate is high.

   b. Erosion and destruction of bone is not a feature of this lesion.

   c. Systemic symptoms are not observed.

   d. The lesion most commonly involves the large joints.

   e. Patients commonly present with pain and swelling of a joint.

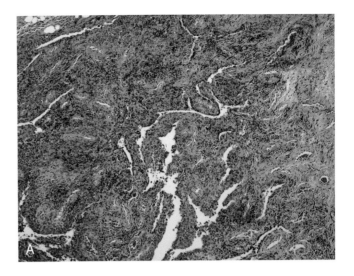

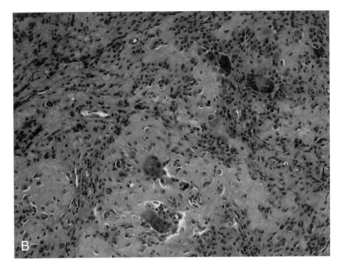

22. Which of the following conditions is MOST likely associated with the changes shown in the photomicrograph?

   a. Chondrosarcoma invading synovium

   b. Joint bodies secondary to osteochondritis dissecans

   c. Synovial chondromatosis/osteochondromatosis

   d. Reactive synovitis and joint bodies associated with osteoarthritis

   e. Villonodular synovitis

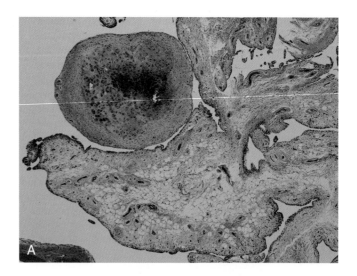

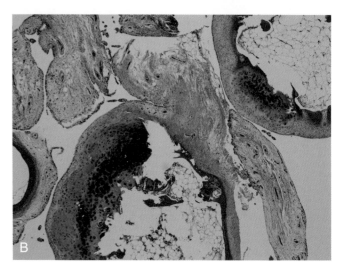

23. The histologic features demonstrated in the image are MOST compatible with what diagnosis?

   a. PVNS

   b. Hemosiderotic synovitis

   c. Nonspecific reactive synovitis

   d. Inflammatory synovitis and arthritis

   e. Synovial chondromatosis

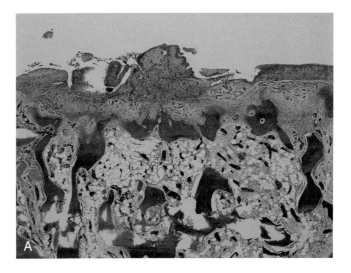

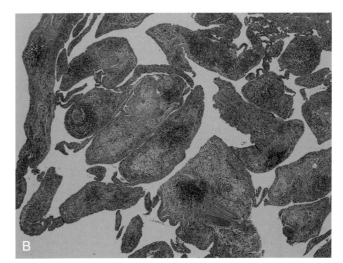

24. What is the MOST likely diagnosis?
  a. Rheumatoid arthritis
  b. Avascular necrosis
  c. Charcot joint (neurotrophic joint)
  d. Paget disease of bone
  e. Idiopathic osteoarthritis

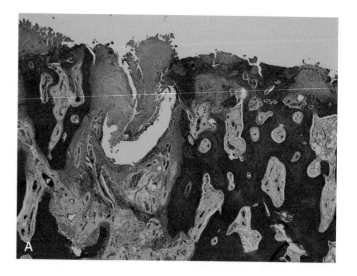

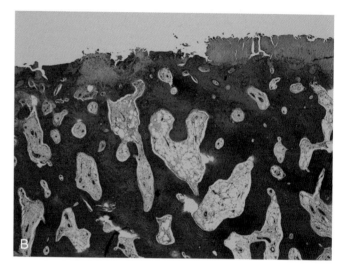

25. Which diagnosis is BEST suited to the histologic changes observed in the two panels shown in the image?

a. Paget sarcoma

b. Angiosarcoma with reactive bone

c. Poorly treated fracture with exuberant fracture callus

d. Fibrous dysplasia with complicating high-grade sarcoma

e. Well-differentiated osteosarcoma (intramedullary) with dedifferentiation

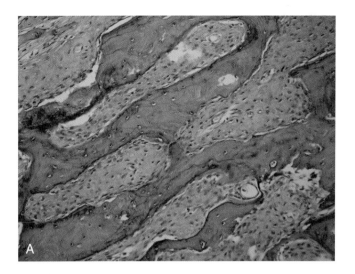

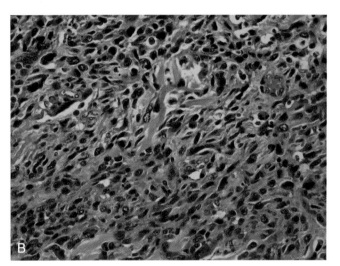

26. Which diagnostic entity would be MOST appropriate to the microscopic changes shown in the image?

a. Chondromyxoid fibroma
b. Osteochondroma
c. Bizarre parosteal osteocartilage proliferation (Nora lesion)
d. Periosteal chondroma
e. Grade 1 chondrosarcoma

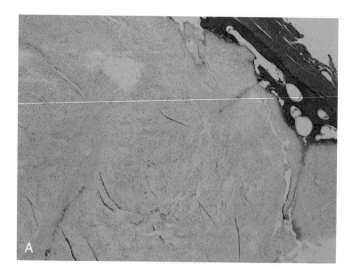

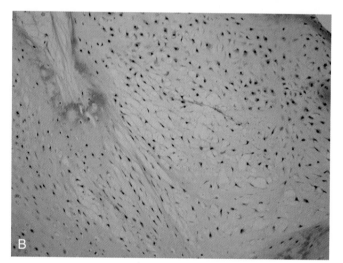

27. Judging from the photomicrographs shown in the image, which of the following entities is the CORRECT diagnosis?
    a. Niemann-Pick disease (sphingolipidosis)
    b. Lipogranulomatosis of bone (Chester-Erdheim disease)
    c. Gaucher disease (adult form; glucolipidosis)
    d. Hurler (mucopolysaccharidosis I) and Hunter (mucopolysaccharidosis II) syndromes
    e. Metastatic malignant granular cell tumor to bone

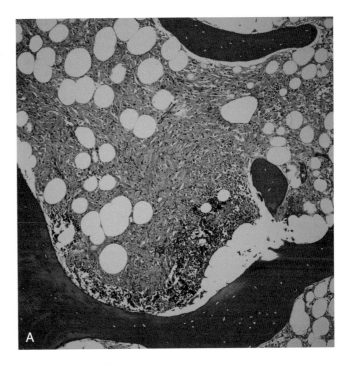

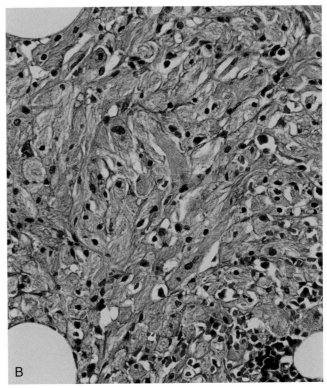

28. Based on the features shown in the image, what is the BEST
diagnosis?

   a. Chondroid chordoma
   b. Myxoid chondrosarcoma
   c. Conventional grade 1 chondrosarcoma
   d. Fibromyxoma of bone
   e. Conventional grade 2 chondrosarcoma

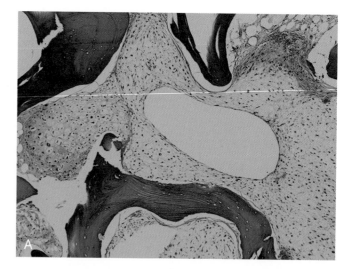

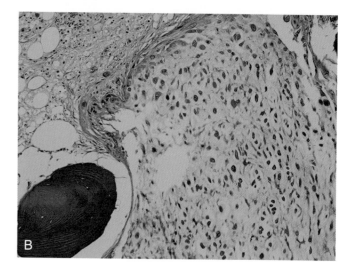

29. Which of the following entities is the CORRECT diagnosis?
   a. Metastatic adenocarcinoma with sarcomatoid reaction
   b. Metastatic mesothelioma
   c. Biphasic synovial sarcoma
   d. Metastatic malignant melanoma
   e. Epithelioid sarcoma

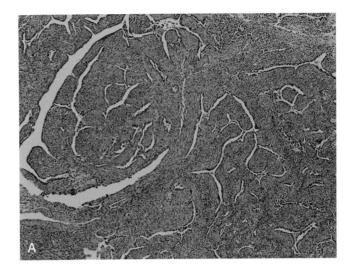

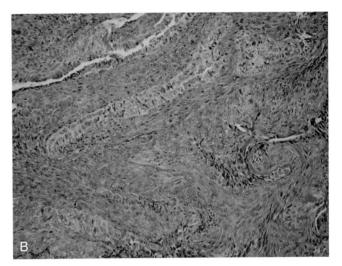

30. Which of the following entities is the CORRECT diagnosis?
   a. Dedifferentiated low-grade osteosarcoma (intramedullary)
   b. Metastatic sarcomatoid or spindle cell carcinoma
   c. High-grade fibrosarcoma
   d. Malignant fibrous histiocytoma of bone
   e. High-grade sarcoma complicating fibrous dysplasia

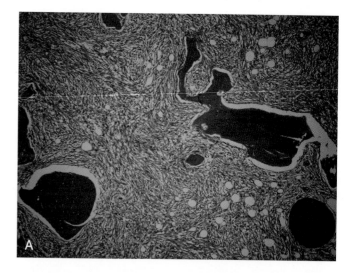

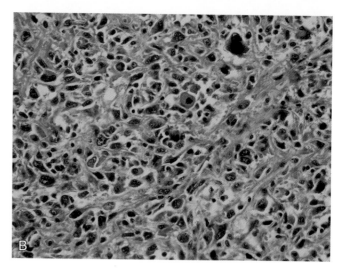

31. Which of the following entities is BEST described by the microscopic changes seen in the image?
   a. Central chondrosarcoma of bone
   b. Periosteal chondroma
   c. Periosteal osteosarcoma
   d. Osteochondroma
   e. Extraskeletal myxoid chondrosarcoma

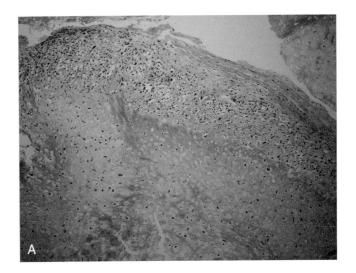

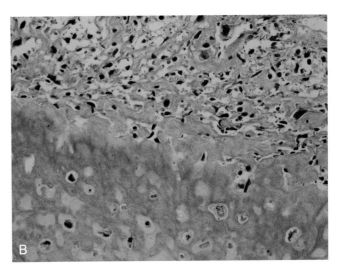

32. Based on the findings seen in the image, what is the MOST likely diagnosis?
   a. Paget disease
   b. Fracture healing
   c. Osteoblastoma
   d. Fibrous dysplasia
   e. Renal osteodystrophy

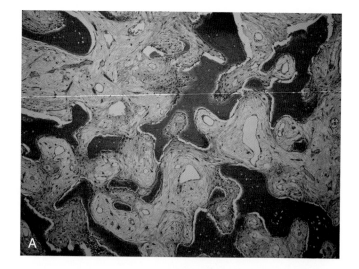

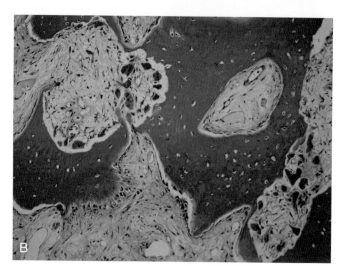

33. Based on the image, what is the CORRECT diagnosis?
    a. High-grade, monophasic synovial sarcoma
    b. Fibrosarcoma
    c. Hemangiopericytoma
    d. Ewing sarcoma/PNET
    e. Mesenchymal chondrosarcoma

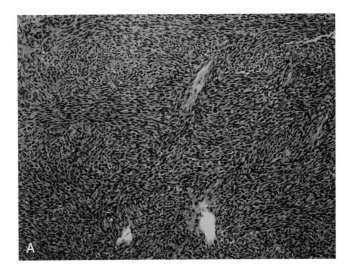

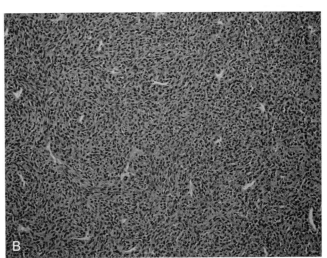

34. What is the CORRECT diagnosis?
    a. Low-grade, intramedullary osteosarcoma
    b. Conventional high-grade osteosarcoma
    c. Fibrous dysplasia
    d. Osteofibrous dysplasia (ossifying fibroma of long bones)
    e. Fibrosarcoma

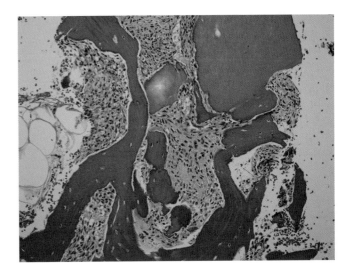

35. Which of the following lesions is the CORRECT diagnosis?
   a. Paget disease
   b. Renal osteodystrophy (osteitis fibrosa–type)
   c. Idiopathic osteoarthritis
   d. Camurati-Engelmann disease
   e. Melorheostosis

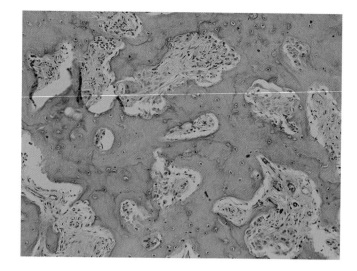

36. Which of the following neoplasms would be characterized BEST by the changes observed in the image?
   a. High-grade fibrosarcoma
   b. High-grade leiomyosarcoma
   c. High-grade osteosarcoma
   d. Dedifferentiated chondrosarcoma
   e. Mesenchymal chondrosarcoma

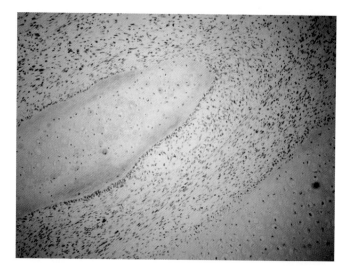

37. Which of the following entities would be described BEST by the changes observed in the image?
   a. Well-differentiated intramedullary osteosarcoma of bone
   b. Monostotic fibrous dysplasia
   c. Grade 2 chondrosarcoma
   d. Fibromyxoma of bone
   e. Xanthogranuloma of bone

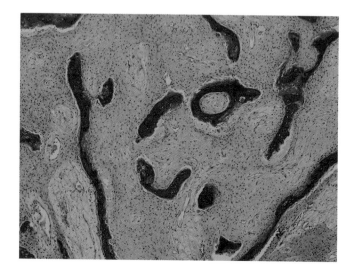

38. Which of the following is the MOST probable diagnosis?
   a. Metastatic clear cell carcinoma of breast
   b. Chondrosarcoma
   c. Metastatic renal cell carcinoma
   d. Chordoma
   e. Metastatic clear cell carcinoma of lung

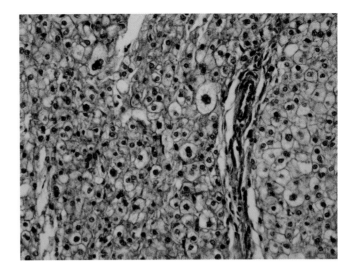

39. Based on interpretation of the histologic changes shown in the image, what is the MOST likely diagnosis?
   a. High-grade surface osteosarcoma
   b. Juxtacortical myositis ossificans
   c. Osteochondroma
   d. Periosteal osteosarcoma
   e. Juxtacortical (parosteal) osteosarcoma

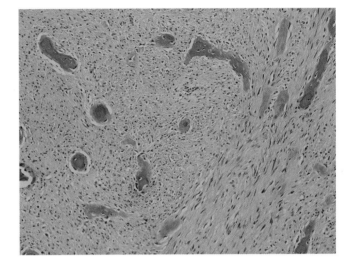

40. What is the MOST likely diagnosis?
   a. Metastatic renal cell carcinoma
   b. Chordoma
   c. Metastatic clear cell carcinoma of thyroid
   d. Metastatic clear cell carcinoma of lung
   e. Metastatic carcinoma of ovaries

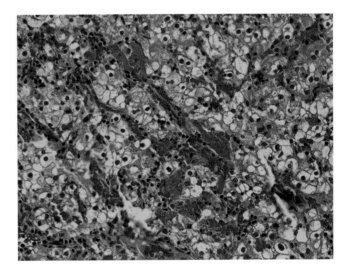

41. Osteosarcoma is associated with all of the following genetic abnormalities EXCEPT:
  a. Germline mutation at 13q14
  b. Single allelic mutation at 13q14 with "second hit" somatic mutation
  c. Amplification of *MDM2* with inactivation of *p53*
  d. t(11;22)(q24;q12)
  e. Loss of heterozygosity on chromosomes 3, 17, and 18

42. Which of the following is associated with a high risk of osteosarcoma?
  a. Germline mutation of *p53*
  b. Reciprocal X;18 translocation
  c. Nonreciprocal translocations and deletions in numerous chromosomes
  d. 1p rearrangements
  e. Nonrandom 9;22 translocation

43. Which of the following statements regarding multiple enchondromas (Ollier disease) is NOT true?
  a. The distribution of multiple enchondromas is bilateral and symmetric.
  b. Approximately one third of tumors undergo malignant transformation.
  c. The tumors are frequently on the cortical surface (juxtacortical or periosteal chondromas).
  d. The most common site is the short tubular bone of the hands.
  e. Histologically, chondromas show higher cellularity, atypia, and myxoid matrix.

44. All of the following should be included in the histologic differential diagnosis of osteosarcoma EXCEPT:
  a. Malignant fibrous histiocytoma
  b. Fibrosarcoma
  c. Chondrosarcoma
  d. Aneurysmal bone cyst
  e. Osteochondroma

45. All of the following statements regarding adamantinoma of long bones are true EXCEPT:
  a. The most common histologic variants are basaloid, spindle cell, squamoid, and tubular types.
  b. The epithelial component expresses cytokeratin 8 and cytokeratin 18.
  c. In patients with classic adamantinoma, younger age is associated with a worse prognosis.
  d. An osteofibrous dysplasia–like type is the least common histologic variant.
  e. Pain at presentation is associated with a less favorable prognosis.

46. All of the following statements regarding osteoblastoma, a bone-forming neoplasm, are true EXCEPT:
  a. Osteoblastoma may be histologically indistinguishable from osteoid osteoma.
  b. The tumor has a predilection for the spine and long bones.
  c. Osteoblastoma affects individuals in the first 2 decades.
  d. Osteoblastoma has unlimited growth potential and may reach a large size.
  e. Blood-filled spaces (aneurysmal change) are an ominous histologic sign.

ANSWERS

1. e. Parosteal osteosarcoma is a well-differentiated, bone-forming tumor, which manifests as a large bony mass affixed to the cortical surface of a long bone. The posterior aspect of the distal femur is the most common location. Histologically, this tumor comprises well-formed bony trabeculae immersed in a spindle cell stroma, which replaces the normal bone marrow. These spindle cells resemble fibroblasts and show minimal atypia and mitotic activity and have a deceptively benign appearance. The trabeculae are immature with a marbled basophilic appearance and lack the osteoblastic rimming expected in immature bone. The tumor can be mistaken for osteochondroma. However, in contrast to osteochondroma, the intraosseous compartment of the tumor is completely isolated from the medullary space of the parent bone. The prognosis is generally excellent, but incomplete surgical excision results in recurrence and possible dedifferentiation.

Cotran RS, Kumar V, Collins T (eds): *Robbins Pathologic Basis of Disease*, 6th ed. Philadelphia: Saunders, 1999.
Fletcher CDM, Unni KK, Mertens F (eds): *World Health Organization Classification of Tumours*. Lyon: IARC Press, 2002.

2. e. Myositis ossificans circumscripta is a soft tissue mass composed of a core of organizing blood, immature bone, and proliferating fibroblasts surrounded by a shell of mature trabecular bone. Also termed *posttraumatic myositis ossificans*, it occurs most often in reaction to trauma in athletic adolescents and young adults with a peak incidence in the second and third decades. The preferred location is the deep soft tissues (muscles) of the upper and lower extremities. The typical clinical history is mirrored in serial radiographs. The first sign is a radiolucent soft tissue mass, which appears shortly after trauma and evolves on a timetable similar to that of fracture callus. At 4 to 6 weeks, vague, fluffy radiopacities appear, forming a shell around the radiolucent center and becoming gradually more visible. This shell is separated from the cortical surface of the bone by a radiolucent zone indicating its extraosseous location. Initially worrisome, this mass is characteristic of myositis ossificans when fully mature. A biopsy performed too early before the correlating radiologic signs necessary for proper interpretation would reveal worrisome histologic changes. At this stage, proliferating spindle cells are seen in a myxoid stroma with ill-defined osteoid formation in a background of skeletal muscle, which may be misinterpreted as sarcomatous. It is believed that performance of an early biopsy interferes with the maturation process of the lesion and stimulates the formation of more immature, aggressive-looking tissues. At a later stage, an important "zoning" pattern is defined by a center of residual hemorrhage, granulation tissue, and proliferating fibroblasts surrounded by a zone of maturing trabeculae of new bone, crowned by a mantle of completely mature, calcified trabeculae wrapped in fibrous tissue. The presence of a lining of active osteoblasts on the trabecular surfaces is of great importance. Frequently, foci of cartilage may be present amid bone. To ensure the correct diagnosis, it is recommended that the clinician in close consultation with the radiologist perform the biopsy at the proper time. Resection can be performed successfully after maturity of the lesion is complete.

Dorfman HD, Czerniak B (eds): *Bone Tumors*. St. Louis: Mosby, 1998.

3. b. Chondrosarcoma is a malignant tumor of cartilage that most commonly affects the large, flat bones of the axial skeleton, such as the pelvis, scapula, and sternum, and less frequently affects the long bones. It is the second most common malignant neoplasm of bone in adults. Radiographic signs include endosteal scalloping, cortical thickening, and the presence of a soft tissue mass. Classic chondrosarcoma is divided into three grades, based on cellularity, nuclear pleomorphism, and degree of atypia. Most chondrosarcomas are grades 1 and 2. In the long bones, borderline malignancy (locally aggressive tumor) is suggested by a moderate increase in cellularity and relatively mild atypia. The natural history of chondrosarcoma is characterized by repeated local recurrences before metastases (grade 2 and 3 tumors). The treatment of choice is wide surgical excision. Adjunctive radiotherapy and chemotherapy is reserved for dedifferentiated tumors. Most chondrosarcomas arise de novo and are thought to originate from uncommitted precursor cells.

Bullough PG: *Orthopaedic Pathology,* 4th ed. St. Louis: Mosby, 2004.
Cotran RS, Kumar V, Collins T (eds): *Robbins Pathologic Basis of Disease,* 6th ed. Philadelphia: Saunders, 1999.
Dorfman HD, Czerniak B (eds): *Bone Tumors.* St. Louis: Mosby, 1998.

4. d. Aneurysmal bone cyst is a benign lesion of bone, which tends to occur in young individuals. The multiloculated radiolucent "soap bubble" appearance is typical on radiograph. This lesion may affect any bone but has a slight predilection for the metaphyses of long bones and the vertebrae. It most likely represents a local reaction to injury to the intraosseous capillary network or to intraosseous hemorrhage. Most lesions occur de novo, and some develop secondarily in a preexisting bone lesion. Aneurysmal bone cyst is a multiloculated hemorrhagic cyst comprising large blood-filled spaces separated by fibrous septa that are lined by mononucleated cells and multinucleated giant cells. The septa contain a mixed, reactive cell population in a fibroblastic stroma showing reactive new bone in strands. These strands impart rigidity to the cyst chambers. This feature, together with the absence of smooth muscle, explains the propensity for hemorrhage during surgery. Surgery alone or preceded by embolization is the treatment of choice. Simple curettage is followed by a high recurrence rate (20% to 70% within 2 years). The procedure of choice is a complete curettage, often assisted by cryotherapy and bone grafting.

Milgram JW, Gruhn JG (eds): *Radiologic and Histologic Pathology of Nontumorous Diseases of Bones and Joints,* Vols. 1 and 2. New Berlin: Northbrook Publishing, 1990.
Wold LE, Adler CP, Sim FH, et al (eds): *Atlas of Orthopaedic Pathology,* 2nd ed. Philadelphia: Saunders, 2004.

5. a. Rheumatoid arthritis, Lyme disease, systemic lupus erythematosus, and psoriasis are part of the group of inflammatory arthritides; PVNS is an exception. Rheumatoid arthritis, an autoimmune disorder and the prototypic member of this group, is a chronic, systemic inflammatory disorder affecting many tissues and organs, especially synovial joints. It has a predilection for women, occurs between the ages of 30 and 50 years, and is almost always polyarticular. The most commonly affected joints are the joints of the hands and feet and the large joints of the extremities. The exact mechanism of rheumatoid arthritis is uncertain. Tumor necrosis factor, interleukin 1, interleukin 6, chemokines, and proteases are possible mediators of the inflammatory reaction that induces synovitis and joint destruction. T and B lymphocytes, macrophages, and dendritic cells invade the synovial membrane, establishing a nidus that promotes inflammation and tissue destruction. It is believed that prostaglandin E stimulates the production of interleukin 6 in the chondrocytes of the joint surfaces, inducing self-destruction of the chondrocytes.

In rheumatoid synovitis (the lesion shown in the image), the synovial membrane characteristically demonstrates villous formation, hyperplasia and hypertrophy of lining cells, fibrinoid necrosis, and chronic inflammatory infiltration in a vascularized stroma. In the acute phase, the synovium demonstrates hyperemia and an inflammatory exudate, which includes an infiltration of neutrophils, lymphocytes, and plasma cells. In the more chronic phase, the infiltrate comprises nodules of lymphocytes surrounded by loose aggregates of plasma cells. Treatment depends on the severity of the disease and is generally aimed at reducing the inflammatory reaction. In severe cases, the treatment includes antiinflammatory agents and cytotoxic drugs such as methotrexate. Surgical treatment, supplemented by physiotherapy, is aimed at improving the functionality and correcting the deformities of the joints.

Milgram JW, Gruhn JG (eds): *Radiologic and Histologic Pathology of Nontumorous Diseases of Bones and Joints,* Vols. 1 and 2. New Berlin: Northbrook Publishing, 1990.
Sternberg SS, Antonioli, DA, Carter D, et al (eds): *Diagnostic Surgical Pathology,* Vol. 1, 3rd ed. Philadelphia: Lippincott Williams & Wilkins, 1999.

6. a. Synovial chondromatosis is an intraarticular lesion characterized by the presence of multiple nodules of hyaline cartilage in the synovial membrane. The cartilaginous nodules are formed by metaplasia and are typically located superficially underneath the synovial lining cells and may become separated to form joint bodies. When the nodules ossify by endochondral ossification, the entity is termed *synovial osteochondromatosis.* This lesion affects a wide range of individuals, from the second to the eighth decade. Most commonly affected are the large joints of the knee, shoulder, hip, and elbow. The radiographic signs of synovial chondromatosis are joint bodies recognized by multiple circumscribed calcific opacities often associated with erosion of the articular margins. Magnetic resonance imaging (MRI) and computed tomography (CT) show signal voids within the membrane. Within the cartilage nodules, chondrocytes are arranged in clusters along the periphery. Malignant change is suggested by loss of this peripheral, cluster arrangement and a more diffuse distribution of the cells associated with the presence of spindle cells. This lesion is benign, and mild to moderate nuclear atypia represented by nuclear hyperchromasia and binucleated cells is common and should not be overinterpreted. In the active, intrasynovial phase of the disease, the treatment is synovectomy because of the high recurrence rate. In the inactive phase, after separation of the nodules, excision of the joint bodies is sufficient.

Milgram JW, Gruhn JG (eds): *Radiologic and Histologic Pathology of Nontumorous Diseases of Bones and Joints,* Vols. 1 and 2. New Berlin: Northbrook Publishing, 1990.

Sternberg SS, Antonioli, DA, Carter D, et al (eds): *Diagnostic Surgical Pathology,* Vol. 1, 3rd ed. Philadelphia: Lippincott Williams & Wilkins, 1999.

7. b. Chondromyxoid fibroma is characterized by pseudolobules of cellular myxoid and chondroid tissue separated by stalks of connective tissue. These stalks contain blood vessels, mononuclear cells, and scattered giant cells. The periphery of the lobules comprises a dense population of small spindle, often stellate cells in a myxoid stroma containing microcysts. Toward the center of the lobules, differentiation to immature cartilage is represented by round chondrocytes in a focally chondroid stroma. Chondrocytes often show hyperchromasia and double nucleation but no mitoses. The immaturity of the cartilage and the presence of atypia may lead to misinterpretation of the lesion as chondrosarcoma. Chondromyxoid fibroma is a very rare tumor of bone representing 1% of all bone tumors. It affects young individuals, with a peak incidence in the second and third decades. It involves primarily the metaphyses of long bones, particularly distal femur and proximal tibia, and less often involves the bones of the foot and the ilium. Patients usually present with pain and local discomfort, which may be of some duration, sometimes associated with local swelling. The radiologic features are very helpful and should be correlated with the microscopic findings. Radiographic images show a sharply demarcated, purely lytic lesion located in the metaphysis of a long bone and with an orientation parallel to the long axis of the bone. Distinctly eccentric, its medullary margins are scalloped and sclerotic, suggesting a benign lesion. Its peripheral margin may be expanded by secondary aneurysmal transformation. The lesion may extend into the epiphysis or diaphysis of the bone but usually does not transgress an open growth plate. The treatment of choice is en bloc excision. Chondromyxoid fibroma has an overall recurrence rate of 20%.

Bullough PG: *Orthopaedic Pathology,* 4th ed. St. Louis: Mosby, 2004.

Dorfman HD, Czerniak B (eds): *Bone Tumors.* St. Louis: Mosby, 1998.

8. c. Pseudogout (CPPD disease) may be hereditary or sporadic and associated with numerous metabolic derangements, such as gout, hyperparathyroidism, hypothyroidism, and hemochromatosis, or may be triggered by trauma or surgery. The reported clinical incidence is much lower than recorded in pathology material. It occurs in individuals 20 to 40 years old and most frequently involves the knees, ankles, wrists, elbow, hips, and shoulders. Most patients are asymptomatic, and the disease is frequently discovered in surgical or autopsy materials. Symptomatic patients present with syndromes mimicking rheumatoid arthritis, osteoarthritis, or other arthritic conditions; the acute attacks often resemble attacks of gout. Symptoms may be monoarticular or involve a cluster of joints. Radiographs show punctate or linear radiopacities in articular cartilage (chondrocalcinosis) and various radiopaque deposits in periarticular structures and synovium. Chalky white

aggregates are observed grossly in poorly vascularized periarticular collagenous structures or in intraarticular structures such as articular cartilage, menisci, and synovium. Microscopically, deposits appear as finely fragmented basophilic aggregates surrounded in vascularized tissues by histiocytes and a foreign body giant cell reaction. In avascular tissues, deposits are lodged in tissue defects lacking the cellular reaction. In articular cartilage, deposits are seen in defects left by degenerated chondrocytes and are surrounded by mucoid pools. From there, the deposits are released into the joint, causing an inflammatory reaction. Under polarized light, tissue deposits show weak positive birefringence and are seen as rhomboid-shaped or as short rods with squared ends in synovial fluid; rarely, the deposits can be needle-shaped. They are light blue when oriented parallel to the line of the compensation filter and yellow when perpendicular to the latter. Treatment is symptomatic and aimed at controlling the inflammatory process.

Bullough PG: *Orthopaedic Pathology,* 4th ed. St. Louis: Mosby, 2004.

9. c. Osteosarcoma is a malignant bone-forming neoplasm. It most commonly affects individuals in the second decade and favors the distal femur and proximal tibia. Osteosarcoma appears on radiograph as an ill-defined lesion with mixed radiolucencies and radiopacities in the metaphyses of long bones. There is frequently evidence of cortical destruction and, in most cases, soft tissue extension. The histologic appearance of osteosarcoma is characterized by malignant bone matrix infiltrating the bone marrow spaces between the mature trabeculae. The malignant bone is typically deposited in a lacelike pattern, encircling the neoplastic mesenchymal cells. After the diagnosis is confirmed by biopsy, the patient receives a full course of multidrug chemotherapy aimed at reducing the size of the tumor, making it amenable to en bloc surgical resection with allograft replacement (limb salvage procedure). The resection specimen is examined microscopically to determine the extent of tumor necrosis; at least 95% of necrosis indicates a good response. The postoperative chemotherapy protocol is modified accordingly.

Cotran RS, Kumar V, Collins T (eds): *Robbins Pathologic Basis of Disease,* 6th ed. Philadelphia: Saunders, 1999.

Fletcher CDM, Unni KK, Mertens F (eds): *World Health Organization Classification of Tumours.* Lyon: IARC Press, 2002.

10. d. Myxoid chondrosarcoma is a rare variant of chondrosarcoma that may occur in soft tissue or bone. Histologically, the tumor is composed of a monotonous proliferation of uniform, relatively small cells demonstrating deeply acidophilic cytoplasm and vesicular nuclei. The cells are arranged in sheets and cords in a very myxoid stroma. None of the other listed pathologic entities is associated with a myxoid stroma on histologic examination. Median age at presentation is 40s to 50s, and men are affected twice as often as women. Wide surgical excision is the treatment of choice. Despite a slow, protracted course, late recurrences and metastases occur commonly.

Cotran RS, Kumar V, Collins T (eds): *Robbins Pathologic Basis of Disease,* 6th ed. Philadelphia: Saunders, 1999.

Dorfman HD, Czerniak B (eds): *Bone Tumors.* St. Louis: Mosby, 1998.

Rosai J (ed): *Rosai and Ackerman's Surgical Pathology,* 9th ed. St. Louis: Mosby, 2004.

11. d. Mesenchymal chondrosarcoma is a highly malignant, aggressive neoplasm that typically has a biphasic appearance. It most often occurs in the jaw bones and ribs of young adults. Histologic appearance is characterized by the presence of small immature mesenchymal cells associated with foci of relatively well-differentiated cartilage in a stroma frequently demonstrating hemangiopericytomalike vascularity. This tumor has an aggressive clinical course marked by frequent local recurrences and a high metastatic rate. Differentiation of this neoplasm from other small, round, blue cell tumors, such as Ewing sarcoma/PNET and hemangiopericytoma, depends on the recognition of the biphasic morphologic pattern, particularly of cartilage differentiation.

Cotran RS, Kumar V, Collins T (eds): *Robbins Pathologic Basis of Disease,* 6th ed. Philadelphia: Saunders, 1999.
Fletcher CDM, Unni KK, Mertens F (eds): *World Health Organization Classification of Tumours.* Lyon: IARC Press, 2002.

12. a. Chordoma is a low-grade to intermediate-grade malignancy showing notochordal differentiation. It accounts for 3% to 4% of primary bone tumors. The lesion commonly occurs in adults, most frequently in individuals in the fifth and sixth decades. It most frequently involves the sacrococcygeal region (50%), less frequently the base of the skull (the sphenooccipital region; 30%), and rarely the mobile spine. In the spine, the cervical vertebrae are most commonly involved, particularly in children and adolescents. Chordoma is speculated to originate from notochordal rests at the ends of the spine. Although no direct evidence is available, the lectin-binding pattern of chordoma strongly supports its origin in the notochord. In the mobile spine, the tumor arises from rests located in the body of the vertebrae rather than in the intervertebral disks. The tumor comprises cells with lightly acidophilic, vacuolated cytoplasm, arranged in solid sheets, cords, or single cells floating in an abundant myxoid stroma. Physaliferous cells, typical of chordoma, are large with pale, multivacuolated cytoplasm and prominent nucleoli. There may be moderate nuclear atypia, but mitoses are infrequent. The cells typically coexpress S100 and epithelial markers such as cytokeratin and endothelial monocyte antigen. The rate of local and regional recurrences is high, but true distant metastases, most commonly to the lungs, are rare and occur in less than 10% of patients. The 5-year survival rate is 65%. Survival after 10 years is extremely rare.

Dorfman HD, Czerniak B (eds): *Bone Tumors.* St. Louis: Mosby, 1998.
Fletcher CDM, Unni KK, Mertens F (eds): *World Health Organization Classification of Tumours.* Lyon: IARC Press, 2002.
Sternberg SS, Antonioli, DA, Carter D, et al (eds): *Diagnostic Surgical Pathology,* Vol. 1, 3rd ed. Philadelphia: Lippincott Williams & Wilkins, 1999.

13. d. Fibrous dysplasia is a dysplastic condition of the bone-forming mesenchyme. It is characterized by the inability to produce mature bone, either at a single skeletal site (monostotic form) or at multiple locations (polyostotic form). The ribs, facial bones, and long bones are most commonly involved. Radiologically, fibrous dysplasia manifests as an intramedullary lesion, showing various degrees of opacity depending on the amount of bone formed and having a typical ground-glass appearance. Fibrous dysplasia causes bone expansion, often thinning one cortex, without associated soft tissue mass or periosteal reaction. Histologically, the stroma is fibrocellular with bland oval spindle cells and contains maloriented, curvilinear trabeculae typically composed of woven bone, without a recognizable border of osteoblasts. Round, calcified, cementumlike spherules are commonly seen, especially in facial bone lesions.

Cotran RS, Kumar V, Collins T (eds): *Robbins Pathologic Basis of Disease,* 6th ed. Philadelphia: Saunders, 1999.
Neville BW, Damm DD, Allen CM, et al (eds): *Oral and Maxillofacial Pathology,* 3rd ed. Philadelphia: Saunders, 2009.

14. d. Reparative granuloma (formerly termed *giant cell reparative granuloma*) is a benign, reactive lesion of bone of unknown cause. It is composed of a fibroblastic and collagenous stroma containing small hemorrhagic cysts, scattered lymphocytes, and multinucleated giant cell clusters. The giant cells are irregularly distributed within the stroma and tend to aggregate around areas of hemorrhage and foci of reactive new bone. Reparative granuloma affects individuals 10 to 25 years old. There is a predilection for facial bones such as the mandible and maxilla. The second most common site is the bones of the hands and feet. The long bones and the vertebrae are rarely affected. The lesion usually manifests as a local swelling in the area of the mandible, maxilla, or hands and feet secondary to the expansion of the contour of the underlying bone. Radiographically, the lesion appears as a round or oval lucency with fine trabeculations and well-defined margins. The lesion may expand the contours of the bone and cause cortical thinning. There is usually no cortical destruction or periosteal new bone formation. Simple surgical curettage is the treatment of choice. However, the recurrence rate is high (33% to 50%) in the lesions of the hands and feet. In these locations, reparative granulomas that show destructive behavior are best treated by amputation or ray resection.

Dorfman HD, Czerniak B (eds): *Bone Tumors.* St. Louis: Mosby, 1998.
Neville BW, Damm DD, Allen CM, et al (eds): *Oral and Maxillofacial Pathology,* 3rd ed. Philadelphia: Saunders, 2009.
Wold LE, Adler CP, Sim FH, et al (eds): *Atlas of Orthopaedic Pathology,* 2nd ed. Philadelphia: Saunders, 2004.

15. d. Giant cell tumor of bone is a locally aggressive neoplasm that occurs in skeletally mature individuals (>20 years old) and is typically located in the epiphyses of long bones. The most common sites are distal femur, proximal tibia, distal radius, and sacrum. Histologically, the lesion comprises a crowded population of relatively small oval or spindle-shaped cells (stromal cells), intermixed with innumerable osteoclastlike giant cells showing uniform distribution. The giant cells have numerous centrally located nuclei. The neoplastic stromal cells are a mixture of macrophages and mesenchymal (spindle-shaped) cells. Mitoses are not unusual in the stromal cells. Although histologically benign-appearing, indolent metastases to the lungs may be observed in 1% to 2% of cases. These metastases are successfully treated by surgical excision. Most giant cell tumors, although locally aggressive, are benign. Approximately 10% undergo malignant transformation. The presence of intravascular tumor near the margins of the lesion does not indicate metastasis and has no prognostic significance.

Cotran RS, Kumar V, Collins T (eds): *Robbins Pathologic Basis of Disease,* 6th ed. Philadelphia: Saunders, 1999.

Fletcher CDM, Unni KK, Mertens F (eds): *World Health Organization Classification of Tumours.* Lyon: IARC Press, 2002.

16. c. Ewing sarcoma/PNET, a tumor of bone and soft tissue characterized by small round cells, is the second most common sarcoma of bone in children and the third most common bone sarcoma overall. It is rare in African Americans. Histologically, the tumor comprises sheets of uniform small round cells showing indistinct cytoplasmic margins. Areas of necrosis are frequently observed. Preferred skeletal sites are the pelvis and the long bones, where the tumor has a predilection for the diaphysis and metadiaphyseal junction. Most tumors (95%) express CD99 (gene product of *MIC2* gene), which, although helpful, is not specific because it is commonly expressed in other soft tissue tumors, such as rhabdomyosarcoma and synovial sarcoma. The most frequent genetic abnormality is a reciprocal translocation between chromosomes 11 and 22 [t(11;22) (q24;q11)] resulting in the fusion of the *Fli-1* and *EWS* genes. Isolation of the chimeric product by reverse transcriptase polymerase chain reaction or fluorescence in situ hybridization is diagnostic. With advances in treatment modalities, the previously dismal prognosis of Ewing/PNET has dramatically improved with a 5-year survival rate of 75%.

Fletcher CDM, Unni KK, Mertens F (eds): *World Health Organization Classification of Tumours.* Lyon: IARC Press, 2002.

Wold LE, Adler CP, Sim FH, et al (eds): *Atlas of Orthopaedic Pathology,* 2nd ed. Philadelphia: Saunders, 2004.

17. b. Chondroblastoma is an uncommon benign cartilage-forming neoplasm of bone. It occurs most frequently in young individuals—50% occur in skeletally immature individuals—and involves the epiphyses of long bones, typically the proximal humerus and the distal femur. The radiograph shows a round lytic lesion with well-defined, sclerotic borders (measuring between <3.0 cm and 5.0 cm). Fine opacities representing focal calcifications may be present. Chondroblastoma comprises sheets of immature cartilage-forming cells (chondroblasts) admixed with a variable number of irregularly distributed osteoclastlike giant cells. The cells are relatively uniform, round or oval, and densely arranged in a sheetlike architecture. The presence of foci of chondroid matrix and a pericellular network of fine calcifications ("chicken-wire" calcifications) is helpful diagnostically. Secondary aneurysmal change is common. Although rare cases have aggressive behavior, the prognosis is excellent in most cases. Simple curettage is the treatment of choice. The recurrence rate is approximately 14% to 18%. Malignant transformation is extremely rare. The large number and even distribution of the giant cells in giant cell tumor of bone distinguish this entity from chondroblastoma.

Bullough PG: *Orthopaedic Pathology,* 4th ed. St. Louis: Mosby, 2004.

Dorfman HD, Czerniak B (eds): *Bone Tumors.* St. Louis: Mosby, 1998.

Fletcher CDM, Unni KK, Mertens F (eds): *World Health Organization Classification of Tumours.* Lyon: IARC Press, 2002.

18. d. Osteoid osteoma is a benign bone-forming tumor best defined by its small size (<2.0 cm), characteristic radiologic appearance, typical pain pattern, and limited growth potential. It is usually seen in children and adolescents, although it is occasionally seen in older individuals. Any bone may be involved, but the long bones, especially the proximal femur, are most commonly involved. Osteoid osteoma commonly manifests as an intracortical lesion, radiographically appearing as a round or oval lucency measuring less than 1.5 cm (the nidus), surrounded by a thick zone of sclerotic bone. Its size distinguishes it from osteoblastoma, a larger, histologically similar lesion. Histologically, the nidus is composed of small trabeculae in a vascularized, cellular stroma containing osteoblasts and osteoclasts. The treatment of choice is simple surgical curettage. The prognosis is excellent, and recurrences are rare. Some lesions have been reported to regress on their own after incomplete removal.

Milgram JW, Gruhn JG (eds): *Radiologic and Histologic Pathology of Nontumorous Diseases of Bones and Joints,* Vols. 1 and 2. New Berlin: Northbrook Publishing, 1990.

Wold LE, Adler CP, Sim FH, et al (eds): *Atlas of Orthopaedic Pathology,* 2nd ed. Philadelphia: Saunders, 2004.

19. a. Paget disease is characterized by waves of increased osteoclastic resorption (seen as radiolucencies), rapidly followed by increased bone formation. A single bone (monostotic form) or multiple bones (polyostotic form) may be involved. The basic abnormality is disorderly acceleration of bone turnover. In the quiescent phase, there is an accumulation of architecturally abnormal sclerotic bone. This pattern appears as irregular patches of lamellar bone with scalloped margins separated by numerous cement lines ("mosaic" pattern). When the disease is widespread, the patient has skeletal deformities resulting from the widening and bowing of long bones, widening of the pelvis, and enlargement of the skull. Chalkstick or "snapped-carrot" fracture—pathologic fracture of long bones—is an important complication of widespread disease. In the polyostotic form, high levels of serum alkaline phosphatase and normal serum calcium and phosphate are observed. Sarcomas of bone, especially osteosarcoma, are a rare complication and include osteosarcoma, fibrosarcoma, chondrosarcoma, malignant fibrous histiocytoma, lymphomas, and myeloma. Giant cell tumor is a well-known occurrence in Paget disease.

Milgram JW, Gruhn JG (eds): *Radiologic and Histologic Pathology of Nontumorous Diseases of Bones and Joints,* Vols. 1 and 2. New Berlin: Northbrook Publishing, 1990.

Wold LE, Adler CP, Sim FH, et al (eds): *Atlas of Orthopaedic Pathology,* 2nd ed. Philadelphia: Saunders, 2004.

20. e. Adamantinoma is a rare, low-grade malignancy of bone, typically located intracortically in the diaphysis of the tibia and less frequently the fibula. It is a biphasic tumor resulting from the differentiation of the multipotential mesenchymal cell along various cell lines. The most common histologic types are spindle, basaloid, tubular, and squamous variants. Tubular spaces are lined by flattened or cuboidal cells. Basaloid nests are compact or may show central spaces resembling vascular channels. The tumor follows an indolent course, spanning many years. However, with inadequate treatment, the metastatic rate is 25% with localization primarily in lungs and lymph nodes.

Cotran RS, Kumar V, Collins T (eds): *Robbins Pathologic Basis of Disease,* 6th ed. Philadelphia: Saunders, 1999.
Fletcher CDM, Unni KK, Mertens F (eds): *World Health Organization Classification of Tumours.* Lyon: IARC Press, 2002.

21. b. PVNS is an aggressive, proliferative lesion that frequently affects the large joints and causes erosion of adjacent bones. A nodular form (diffuse nodular synovitis) may involve the large joints with the knees much more frequently affected than the hips and ankles. A single nodule may occur in a large joint such as the knee (localized nodular synovitis) but is very common in the tendon sheaths around the finger joints (localized nodular tenosynovitis). Clinically, the affected joint is usually swollen and not painful or only slightly painful, and there may be symptoms of internal derangement. Systemic symptoms are not observed in PNVS. Radiologically, swelling in and around the joint, joint narrowing, erosion of the articular margins, and lytic defects of the bone are often seen. MRI and CT often show punctate signal voids within the lesion. A typical intraoperative finding of PVNS is the rusty brown color of the joint fluid and synovial surfaces, which have both a fernlike villous and grossly nodular appearance. Histologically, PVNS is characterized by striking villous hypertrophy of the synovial surface lined by hyperplastic cells that are heavily laden with hemosiderin pigment. The villous component coexists with large nodules formed by coalescence of the villi. The membrane is hypervascular and is crowded with aggregates of lipid-laden macrophages, scattered giant cells, and occasional lymphocytes. The treatment of choice is surgical excision. However, recurrences are common because of the difficulty of complete surgical removal.

Rosai J (ed): *Rosai and Ackerman's Surgical Pathology,* 9th ed. St. Louis: Mosby, 2004.
Sternberg SS, Antonioli, DA, Carter D, et al (eds): *Diagnostic Surgical Pathology,* Vol. 1, 3rd ed. Philadelphia: Lippincott Williams & Wilkins, 1999.

22. c. Synovial chondromatosis/osteochondromatosis is a monarthric disease that affects predominantly the large joints such as hip, knee, and shoulder. It is characterized by metaplastic transformation of the sublining cells of synovium into hyaline cartilage and formation of multiple joint bodies. The age range of affected patients is large (second to eighth decade), and men are affected twice as often as women. Patients usually present with a history of gradual onset of pain and swelling of a joint, most frequently the knee, with "locking" of other large joints such as hip, shoulder, and elbow frequently associated. Clinical signs include joint effusion. The key to this diagnosis is the presence on radiographs of multiple small intraarticular radiopacities secondary to calcification or ossification of the cartilage. However, calcifications are not always present, and MRI may be necessary to detect joint bodies. Grossly, the synovial surface is hypertrophied and raised by a multitude of small nodules. Microscopically, numerous nodules of hyaline cartilage of various sizes occupy the synovial villi. In the early phase of the disease, the nodules are small and entirely cartilaginous and are intimately related to—and thought to arise from—the sublining cells of the membrane. The chondrocytes are typically arranged in clusters along the periphery of the

nodules. Loss of this pattern with diffuse distribution of the chondrocytes and the presence of spindle cells raises concern about the possibility of malignancy. The cartilage is usually hypercellular and frequently shows signs of mild atypia such as hyperchromasia and double nucleation; this feature may lead to an erroneous diagnosis of chondrosarcoma. As the disease progresses, large nodules occupy the enlarged villi and are covered by lining cells (synovial chondromatosis). Cartilage nodules eventually undergo endochondral ossification to become osteocartilaginous (synovial osteochondromatosis) and separate from the synovial surface, becoming loose bodies. Treatment depends on the phase of the disease. In the early phase (active intrasynovial disease without formation of joint bodies), arthroscopic synovectomy is recommended; in the late phase (inactive, "burned-out" phase with joint bodies but no intrasynovial disease), removal of the joint bodies is performed without synovectomy.

Bullough PG: *Orthopaedic Pathology,* 4th ed. St. Louis: Mosby, 2004.
Parisien S: *Techniques in Therapeutic Arthroscopy.* New York: Raven Press, 1993.

23. d. In inflammatory synovitis and arthritis, the synovial surface shows villous hypertrophy and inflammation. The inflammation is exudative and cellular and associated with fibrinoid necrosis. In the more chronic phase, nodules of lymphocytes and plasma cells showing germinal centers are featured. The articular surface becomes eroded by a pannus of inflamed connective tissue. The underlying bone is osteopenic, in contrast to subarticular sclerosis observed in osteoarthritis. Although both PVNS and rheumatoid synovitis demonstrate villous hypertrophy, the rust color of the membrane and the unique combination of a villous component associated with large nodules containing aggregates of hemosiderin-laden histiocytes are pathognomonic of PVNS. In contrast to rheumatoid synovitis, which is most often a polyarticular disease, hemosiderotic synovitis is monoarticular. Hemosiderotic synovitis is usually associated with a history of repeated hemarthroses secondary to a hemorrhagic diathesis such as hemophilia or a history of repetitive traumatic events. In addition, no significant inflammation is observed microscopically. Nonspecific reactive synovitis, often associated with osteoarthritis as well as with nonspecific circumstances, is characterized by synovium showing only hypertrophy and hyperplasia and is devoid of any significant inflammatory infiltration. Although villous hypertrophy is a shared feature between synovial chondromatosis and rheumatoid synovitis, nodules of hyaline cartilage occupying the substance of the villi and forming loose bodies are exclusive to this disease.

Rosai J (ed): *Rosai and Ackerman's Surgical Pathology,* 9th ed. St. Louis: Mosby, 2004.
Wang P, Zhu F, Konstantopoulos K: Interleukin-6 synthesis in human chondrocytes is regulated via the antagonistic actions of prostaglandin (PG)E2 and 15-deoxy-ΔPGJ(2). *PloS One* 2011;6(11):e27630.

24. e. Idiopathic osteoarthritis is a degenerative joint disease characterized by gradual degeneration, erosion, and eventually loss of articular cartilage. It occurs in individuals after the fourth decade or in younger individuals as a result of predisposing conditions, such as congenital hip dysplasia,

Legg-Calvé-Perthes disease, or fracture. As a result of loss of the cushioning effect of articular cartilage, the underlying bone is unprotected from the joint forces and is subject to microfractures. It affects most often the stress-bearing joints (hips, knees, shoulders, elbows, and ankles). Pain is the most common complaint associated with joint stiffness. In advanced stages, there is difficulty in ambulation and in the function of the joints involved. Plain radiographs reveal narrowing and eventually complete loss of the radiolucent zone ("joint space" representing the thickness of cartilage). In advanced stages, sclerosis and deformities of the joint surfaces are seen. Subchondral cysts, if large, may be seen in plain radiographs but are better visualized by MRI. Degenerative changes cause loss of integrity of articular cartilage. Microscopic changes include erosion of cartilage, which shows surface fibrillization, fissures, and gradually erosion and loss of the full thickness of cartilage. Complete exposure of the underlying bone eventually occurs. Because of direct friction of joint surfaces, microfractures caused by joint stresses heal with foci of fibrocartilage, which, in the absence of vascularity, degenerate and become subarticular cysts. As a result of constant, slow remodeling and osteoblastic response to mechanical stimulation, the exposed bone and underlying trabecular systems become consolidated (sclerotic), causing the polished (eburnated) appearance observed on gross examination of a resected femoral head. The sclerotic bone has a mature, lamellar architecture. As part of the remodeling process, osteocartilaginous growths (osteophytes) develop along the non–weight-bearing articular margins and are a constant finding. The treatment of idiopathic osteoarthritis is aimed at controlling the pain with analgesics, weight reduction in overweight individuals, and joint replacement surgery in severe stages.

Bullough PG: *Orthopaedic Pathology,* 4th ed. St. Louis: Mosby, 2004.

25. e.   Dedifferentiation of a low-grade neoplasm (in this case well-differentiated osteosarcoma), a phenomenon shared by many tumors, is defined by the uncontrolled growth of a subclone of the precursor cell in a low-grade neoplasm giving rise to a lethal tumor. Dedifferentiated osteosarcoma (intramedullary) occurs in the same age group and at the same skeletal locations as the low-grade tumor. The clinical symptoms are pain, discomfort, and possibly a palpable swelling of several months' duration, with a recent height in intensity of the symptoms and a rapid increase in the size of the mass. Radiographs show a significant radiolucent component superimposed on a tumor with features strongly suggestive of intramedullary low-grade osteosarcoma. This very aggressive component destroys cortical bone and forms a soft tissue mass. In the present case, the biopsy was performed because of the recent rapid growth of the tumor, and the specimen included only a pleomorphic, vascular component producing malignant osteoid matrix (*Panel A*). This case is a good example of sampling error. As shown in multiple samples through the resected fibula, this neoplasm began as a slow-growing tumor that later dedifferentiated. The predominantly well-differentiated component (*Panel B*) abruptly transitioned with the highly malignant component in patterns typical of dedifferentiation. The proper perspective could be obtained on exchange of material between two institutions. At the molecular level, patterns of alterations in *bcl-2*, *p53*, and *Rb* gene expressions

(owing to extensive loss of genetic material on 17p chromosome) are common to dedifferentiating tumors. It is important to diagnose and treat properly well-differentiated osteosarcoma (at an early stage) after ruling out fibrous dysplasia, the most important pitfall in the diagnosis. Dedifferentiated tumor has a poor prognosis with widespread metastases occurring rapidly despite surgery. The survival rate is very low. Chemotherapy is the only palliative option.

Dorfman HD, Czerniak B (eds): *Bone Tumors*. St. Louis: Mosby, 1998.

26. d.   Periosteal chondroma comprises a mass of lobulated hyaline cartilage nestled in a saucer of the outer cortex. Periosteal chondroma is a surface lesion, whereas chondromyxoid fibroma is intraosseous. Although there are histologic similarities (cellularity, atypia, myxoid stroma), periosteal chondroma is composed of moderately differentiated cartilage. Both periosteal osteosarcoma and osteochondroma manifest as a protruding mass on the surface of the bone, but osteochondroma is a developmental abnormality, not a neoplasm. In contrast to the lobular architecture of periosteal chondroma, the cartilaginous cap of osteochondroma has a structure identical to that of a growth plate. Nora lesion is located in the soft tissues adjacent to the bone and demonstrates a zonation and bizarre mixture of calcified cartilage, bone, and fibrous tissue. Periosteal chondroma is most frequently located in the small bones of the hands and feet; however, chondrosarcoma has a predilection for bones of the axial skeleton. Although the mild cellularity and atypia of periosteal chondroma have no bearing on the prognosis, such changes would be indicative of chondrosarcoma in an axially located cartilage lesion.

Bullough PG: *Orthopaedic Pathology,* 4th ed. St. Louis: Mosby, 2004.
Dorfman HD, Czerniak B (eds): *Bone Tumors*. St. Louis: Mosby, 1998.

27. c.   The lesion in Gaucher disease (adult form; glucolipidosis) comprises aggregates of large cells with acidophilic, striated cytoplasm replacing bone marrow. These cells are due to the accumulation of large amounts of glucocerebrosides in the phagocytes (Gaucher cells) of bone marrow. These accumulations are caused by a functional deficiency of the acid β-glucocerebrosidase. Gaucher disease is a rare inborn error of glycosphingolipid metabolism most often seen in patients of Ashkenazi Jewish ancestry and is caused by a functional deficiency of acid β-glucocerebrosidase. This deficiency is due to a mutation in the gene (*GBA1*) that encodes this enzyme, causing an inability for the enzyme to cleave the glucose residue from ceramide. Phagocytes are unable to digest complex glucosides and gangliosides. Glucocerebrosides, formed by the catabolism of glycolipids from the cell membranes of aging erythrocytes and leukocytes, accumulate in large amounts in the phagocytes of some organs (bone marrow, liver, spleen, lymph nodes). In patients with more severe type I disease, radiographic images show thinning of the cortices of long bone and vertebrae that have a trabeculated appearance, osteopenia, vertebral deformities, and collapse. Flaring of the diametaphysis of the distal femur, proximal tibia, and humerus secondary to a modeling failure causes the "Erlenmeyer flask" deformity. Avascular necrosis of the femoral head is frequently seen in type I disease. Three forms are recognized: type I (adult; nonneuronopathic), type II (infantile; acute neuronopathic with early death), and type III (juvenile; neuronopathic). In most patients, the chronic asymptomatic form of the disease is not discovered until adulthood. In other patients, complications include hepatomegaly and often dramatic splenomegaly causing thrombocytopenia and pancytopenia (hypersplenism). Erosion of bone by numerous phagocytic aggregates in the enlarged bone marrow space results in osteoporosis, fractures, and pain. The diagnostic tool of choice is measurement of glucocerebrosidase in peripheral leukocytes and skin fibroblasts; measurement of chitotriosidase (markedly elevated in Gaucher disease) also is a fairly specific marker. Histologically, the typical cell of Gaucher disease is a large phagocyte that can measure 100 μm, has a small dark nucleus, and has abundant acidophilic cytoplasm showing fine striations. These striations confer to the cytoplasm a wrinkled ("crumpled paper") appearance, which is typical of this disease. These striations correspond on electron microscopy to stacks of elongated lysosomes that store the accumulated glucocerebroside. Recombinant glucocerebrosidase has been used more recently for treatment with good results.

Cotran RS, Kumar V, Collins T (eds): *Robbins Pathologic Basis of Disease,* 6th ed. Philadelphia: Saunders, 1999.
Cox TM: Gaucher disease: clinical profile and therapeutic developments. *Biologics* 2010;4:299-313.
Rosai J (ed): *Rosai and Ackerman's Surgical Pathology,* 9th ed. St. Louis: Mosby, 2004.

28. e. Chondrosarcoma is the second most common primary sarcoma of bone (25%). It affects individuals older than 50 years. It most frequently affects the axial skeleton (particularly the pelvis and ribs); the ilium is the most commonly involved bone, followed by the femur and the humerus. The acral bones (hands and feet) are rarely involved. The most frequent mode of presentation is pain or dull aching usually of several months' duration. The pain may be associated with a mass secondary to expansion of the contour of the bone around the tumor or a soft tissue mass. Pain unrelated to trauma is an important clinical parameter in the evaluation of a cartilage neoplasm because benign cartilage tumors are asymptomatic. The radiographic changes almost always include calcifications characteristic of cartilaginous tumors. The images vary with the amount of calcifications and range from a completely lytic, often loculated lesion to a completely radiopaque mass. However, most lesions show fine or coarser calcifications on a radiolucent background. The contour of the bone is frequently expanded with scalloping erosions of the endosteal cortex. There can be thinning of the cortex or reactive thickening secondary to slow infiltration of the haversian canals. The outer surface of the cortex may show periosteal new bone occurring as parallel layers ("onion skinning"). In advanced cases, destruction of the cortex is associated with a soft tissue mass.

Most chondrosarcomas are grades 1 and 2; grade 3 tumors account for only 5% to 10% of chondrosarcomas. Chondrosarcomas arise de novo and not from preexisting chondromas. Grade 1 chondrosarcoma has a lobulated architecture; resembles chondroma; and comprises round, lacunar cells with large, vesicular nuclei and large nucleoli. Double-nucleated cells are present. Grade 2 chondrosarcoma shows a loss of lobulation and is composed of sheets of smaller, more uniform cells in a myxoid stroma. The cells are frequently spindle-shaped and admixed with groups of lacunar cells. Grade 3 chondrosarcoma comprises cells demonstrating hyperchromasia, marked nuclear atypia, and mitoses. Regardless the grade of a tumor, evidence of infiltration of intertrabecular spaces is proof of malignancy. Chondrosarcoma has an indolent course, with many patients having a history of an enlarging mass of many years' duration. The histologic grade of chondrosarcoma correlates well with the prognosis. Grade 1 tumors are indolent and prone to local recurrences but do not cause metastases. Grade 2 tumors have a high recurrence rate and a metastatic rate of approximately 15%. Grade 3 tumors have a high metastatic rate and are associated with a poor prognosis; metastases occur to lung, lymph nodes, and liver. Surgery is the primary treatment of chondrosarcoma and consists of wide excision with clear margins when possible. Chemotherapy and radiotherapy are reserved for high-grade and dedifferentiated tumors. Of chondrosarcomas, 10% may undergo dedifferentiation and have a lethal course.

Dorfman HD, Czerniak B (eds): *Bone Tumors*. St. Louis: Mosby, 1998.

29. c. Synovial sarcoma is a neoplasm of soft tissue that most often occurs in adolescents and young adults (age range, 15 to 40 years). The tumor occurs around large joints of the lower extremity, most often the knees and ankles, and rarely involves the joint itself. The second most common location is the head and neck, followed by the upper extremity; the chest wall and abdominal cavity are less frequent locations. Synovial sarcoma clinically manifests as a deep-seated, palpable mass associated with pain and tenderness. A history of slow growth over 2 to 4 years or longer is frequently reported. Tumors at other locations may have site-related symptoms. The radiographic findings are most often a round or oval mass of intermediate density located around large joints and showing spotty opacifications secondary to calcifications; ossification is a less frequent finding (15% to 20%). Erosion of adjacent bone is frequent (20%). This typically biphasic neoplasm comprises well-formed glandular and slitlike structures lined by cuboidal epithelium associated with dense fascicles of spindle cells. In addition, acinar structures and epithelioid clusters lie in a focally myxoid stroma. Epithelioid differentiation is emphasized by reticulin stain. Small amounts of mucin are present in both glands and stroma. Focally, deposits of hyalinized material in the stroma become foci of calcification and less often ossification. The tumor coexpresses vimentin; epithelial markers, especially cytokeratin 7 and cytokeratin 19; and endothelial monocyte antigen. CD34 is always negative, a point of distinction with other spindle cell sarcomas. Additionally, S100 may be positive in 60% to 70% of cases, and *bcl-2* is expressed in 75% to 100%. Most cases express CD99 (O13), a gene product of *MIC2* gene. At the molecular level (reverse transcriptase polymerase chain reaction or fluorescence in situ hybridization), most cases demonstrate a unique translocation t(x:18) (p11.2;q11.2) with fusion of the *SYT* gene (chromosome 18) and *SSX1* and *SSX2* (on the X chromosome). Synovial sarcoma is a slow-growing tumor that eventually metastasizes in 50% of cases to lung, lymph nodes, and bone marrow. The 5-year survival rate is 36% to 76% but may reach 82%. The 10-year survival rate of 20% to 63% reflects the occurrence of late metastases. Positive factors in regard to prognosis are young age, tumor size (<5.0 cm), distal extremity location, low tumor stage, and heavy calcifications microscopically. Negative histologic factors in regard to prognosis are tumor necrosis, rhabdoid features, high mitotic index, and nuclear grade. At the molecular level, *SYT/SSX2* is associated with a better prognosis than the *SYT/SSX1* fusion transcript. The treatment of choice is radical, local excision with adjunctive radiotherapy; this approach is preferred to amputation. Adjunctive chemotherapy is being evaluated.

Rosai J (ed): *Rosai and Ackerman's Surgical Pathology,* 9th ed. St. Louis: Mosby, 2004.
Weiss S, Goldblum JR: *Enzinger and Weiss's Soft Tissue Tumors,* 4th ed. St. Louis: Mosby, 2001.

30. d.   Malignant fibrous histiocytoma is a rare tumor of bone that accounts for less than 2% of primary malignant neoplasms of bone. The age distribution is wide; however, most tumors affect individuals older than 50 years. Malignant fibrous histiocytoma most frequently involves the bones of the lower extremity, particularly distal femur and proximal tibia, although any bone can be affected. In the trunk, the ilium is the most frequent site. The most frequent mode of presentation is pain associated with expansion of the bone and frequently a soft tissue mass. Clinical radiographs show an ill-defined, purely lytic, destructive lesion with permeative, moth-eaten margins. The lesion frequently destroys cortical bone with pathologic fracture and soft tissue invasion. Malignant fibrous histiocytoma is a biphasic neoplasm characterized by a fibrous component demonstrating fascicular growth and frequent storiform patterns associated with a high-grade pleomorphic component; the latter comprises a cellular population of large mesenchymal cells showing marked nuclear atypia and mitoses. Both components infiltrate bone marrow spaces around thickened trabeculae showing unusual shapes. These trabeculae are centered by cores of necrotic bone showing empty osteocytic lacunae surrounded by layers of reactive woven bone irregularly opposed to the surface of the dead bone. This appearance raises the possibility that this tumor may have occurred at the site of a previous bone infarct, a well-known association. The tumor evolves rapidly and has a poor prognosis—the 5-year survival rate with surgery alone is approximately 18%. The best treatment is a multimodality approach that includes aggressive surgery with adjunctive chemotherapy and radiotherapy. This approach is associated with improvement of prognosis. Tumors associated with predisposing conditions have a very poor prognosis. Metastases occur in lungs and rarely in lymph nodes.

Dorfman HD, Czerniak B (eds): *Bone Tumors.* St. Louis: Mosby, 1998.
Rosai J (ed): *Rosai and Ackerman's Surgical Pathology,* 9th ed. St. Louis: Mosby, 2004.

31. c.   Although periosteal osteosarcoma predominantly comprises lobules of hyaline cartilage, it is a grade 2 osteosarcoma. Grade 2 osteosarcoma arises subperiosteally

on the surface of the bone and represents 2% of osteosarcomas. This tumor occurs in young individuals, with a peak incidence in the second and third decades of life. It involves the long bones of the extremities, most frequently the tibia and less often the femur, and occupies the diaphysis of the bone. The tumor is most often discovered by swelling of the leg or thigh, which may be associated with pain and evolve over a relatively short time. The most frequent radiologic sign is a fusiform, broad-based radiolucency located on the surface of the bone. The tumor arises under the periosteum, which is lifted and causes a buttress of reactive new bone along the edges of the mass (Codman triangle); this is often associated with the "sunburst pattern" owing to reactive periosteal new bone represented by radiopaque streaks perpendicularly oriented toward the periphery of the lesion. The surface of the cortex may show irregular erosions. However, the medullary canal characteristically remains uninvolved. Microscopically, the tumor comprises lobules of moderately differentiated, atypical hyaline cartilage covered by a rim of small mesenchymal cells, which is covered by periosteum. The cartilaginous component is of high grade. The mesenchymal cells are immature and round, oval, or spindle-shaped and show central, small and dark or larger vesicular nuclei demonstrating frequent pleomorphism and hyperchromasia. These cells together with closely related thin strands of malignant osteoid are the hallmark of this tumor and indicate its true bone-forming nature. Well-differentiated, osteoblast-covered trabeculae of new bone document reactive new bone formation (radiologic Codman and "sunburst pattern"). The treatment of choice is en bloc resection of the tumor with clean margins of uninvolved bone supplemented in recent years by chemotherapy. The prognosis of this tumor is better than the prognosis of conventional high-grade osteosarcoma. If treatment is inadequate, recurrences occur. Metastases to lung and other skeletal sites may occur.

Dorfman HD, Czerniak B (eds): *Bone Tumors.* St. Louis: Mosby, 1998.

32. e.   Renal osteodystrophy is caused by an increase in parathyroid hormone (PTH) secretion secondary to parathyroid hyperplasia. The parathyroid hyperplasia occurs in response to a gradual deterioration of renal function (glomerular filtration rate <30%) caused by chronic disease, most frequently diabetes mellitus. It occurs in end-stage renal disease in patients on long-term hemodialysis. Pathophysiologically, the diseased renal parenchyma is no longer able to synthesize 1α-hydroxylase, which converts the inactive $25(OH)D_3$ form of vitamin D into the active $1,25(OH)_2D_3$ form. Decreased intestinal absorption of calcium and phosphate and decreased osteoclastic resorption of bone result, with a low level of ionized calcium. As a result of the feedback mechanism, PTH secretion increases with poor response from the renal parenchyma; this results in poor conservation of calcium and increased retention of phosphate by the distal renal tubules. Serum chemistry reveals elevated levels of serum phosphate, which signifies end-stage renal disease together with low levels of ionized calcium (despite elevated PTH). Histologically, trabeculae show severe osteoclastic erosion and, in alternating areas, are lined by rows of active osteoblasts, as shown in the image. Resorption is revealed by deep scalloping defects (Howship lacunae) containing numerous large osteoclasts, which cause deep furrows into the trabeculae ("dissecting resorption," "tunneling resorption") similar to severe primary hyperparathyroidism. Typically, bone marrow fibrosis showing a peritrabecular distribution is associated with increased erosion. Osteitis fibrosa, the most common form of renal osteodystrophy, reflects increased bone turnover, the typical response to increased PTH secretion. The treatment is high doses of $1,25(OH)_2D_3$ and renal transplantation.

Parisien M, Silverberg SJ, Shane E, et al: Bone disease in primary hyperparathyroidism. *Endocrinol Metab Clin North Am* 1990;19(1):19-34.

33. a. Synovial sarcoma affects predominantly adolescents and young adults (age range, 15 to 40 years). It occurs around large joints, most commonly situated in the lower extremity, affecting the ankle and hip joints and most frequently the knee joint. The head and neck is the next most common site followed by the upper extremity. It may also arise in the chest and abdominal walls as well as various other locations. The tumor occupies the deep soft tissues causing a palpable mass associated with pain and tenderness. Tumors in unusual locations are often clinically misinterpreted, causing delays in diagnosis. The radiographic findings are most often a round or oval, deep-seated, lobulated mass of intermediate density located around large joints and showing spotty radiopacities owing to calcifications and less often ossification (15% to 20% of cases). Erosion of adjacent bone occurs frequently (20% of cases). CT and MRI have become indispensable in evaluating the margins of the mass and its extent into the soft tissues. A high-grade, monophasic fibrous tumor is characterized by an extremely cellular population of densely packed, spindle-shaped mesenchymal cells. The cells are small and uniform and arranged in sheets showing a fascicular growth pattern and pseudorosettes focally. Vascularity is abundant and hemangiopericytoid. Mitoses are frequent (three to four per high-power field). Zones of necrosis attest to the high level of cellularity and paucity of supporting stroma. This histologic type overlaps with that of other small round cell neoplasms listed in the question. Immunohistochemically, vimentin is positive; endothelial monocyte antigen is focally positive; cytokeratin, CD45, S100, desmin, and smooth muscle actin are negative; and CD31 is positive in blood vessels. CD99, gene product of *MIC2* gene, is frequently positive. Although some soft tissue sarcomas express cytokeratins (cytokeratin 8 and cytokeratin 18 in epithelioid sarcoma), synovial sarcoma uniquely expresses cytokeratin 7 and cytokeratin 19. Reverse transcriptase polymerase chain reaction shows a diagnostic chromosomal translocation t(x:18) (p11.2; q11.2) that causes a fusion between the *SYT* gene on chromosome 18 and *SSX1* or *SSX2* on chromosome X with the fusion transcript *SYT/SSX1* (present in all biphasic tumors) or *SYT/SSX2* (present in some monophasic tumors). The prognosis of synovial sarcoma was traditionally thought to be dismal. In recent years, the 5-year survival rate has been stated to be 50%. With factors favorable to the prognosis (young age, distal location, small size, absence of necrosis, low mitotic rate), the 5-year survival rate approaches 80%. The tumor frequently recurs, and distant metastases occur in regional lymph nodes and lungs.

Rosai J (ed): *Rosai and Ackerman's Surgical Pathology*, 9th ed. St. Louis: Mosby, 2004.
Weiss S, Goldblum JR: *Enzinger and Weiss's Soft Tissue Tumors*, 4th ed. St. Louis: Mosby, 2001.

34. a. Low-grade, intramedullary osteosarcoma is a deceptively benign-appearing lesion of bone that is composed of immature trabeculae devoid of osteoblastic lining in a fibrous stroma. Well-differentiated intramedullary osteosarcoma is a very rare tumor of bone, accounting for 1% of all osteosarcomas. Compared with conventional osteosarcoma and fibrous dysplasia, it occurs in an older population with 50% of cases being discovered in the third decade. It has a predilection for the metaphyses of the long bones of the extremities, mostly the femur (50%) and tibia. Pain of a few months' duration is the most common presentation, in contrast to the much shorter duration of symptoms of conventional osteosarcoma. There may be an associated palpable mass. Occasionally, well-differentiated intramedullary osteosarcomas that are erroneously diagnosed as fibrous dysplasia may recur after treatment. On routine radiographs, the tumor usually appears as an ill-defined mixture of coarse radiodensities and lytic areas or as coarsely trabeculated radiopacities that may extend into the epiphysis. The tumor also may extend far into the diaphysis, causing cortical infiltration. Cortical infiltration is marked by expansion of the cortex, indicating the slow growth of the tumor, and may be associated with the formation of a soft tissue mass. A buttress of periosteal new bone (Codman triangle) is rarely present. Abnormal bone is formed in a fibrous, hypercellular stroma populated by fibroblastlike spindle cells. The bony trabeculae are generally well developed with an alignment reproducing the alignment of parosteal osteosarcoma in the medullary cavity. The trabeculae sometimes may be delicate, curvilinear trabeculae similar to trabeculae of fibrous dysplasia, making fibrous dysplasia the most difficult differential diagnosis. In many cases, there is a tendency for the malignant bone to be deposited in a peritrabecular fashion either in continuous layers ("mantlelike" pattern) or in redundant, acellular patches apposed to the surfaces of preexisting trabeculae ("stuccolike" pattern). The infiltrative spindle cell stroma of low-grade osteosarcoma is more cellular than the stroma of fibrous dysplasia and shows a degree of atypia that is frequently subtle. Hyperchromasia and mitoses are consistently present. Low-grade osteosarcoma is an indolent tumor that evolves over a long period, causing delays in diagnosis. Dedifferentiation can occur if the tumor is inadequately treated. En bloc resection with wide margins if possible is the ideal treatment and is preferred to amputation. Adjunctive chemotherapy is recommended for cases showing areas of dedifferentiation. The overall metastatic rate is 15%.

Bullough PG: *Orthopaedic Pathology*, 4th ed. St. Louis: Mosby, 2004.
Dorfman HD, Czerniak B (eds): *Bone Tumors*. St. Louis: Mosby, 1998.

35. a. Paget disease is characterized by high bone turnover represented by extensive resorption—Howship lacunae containing large osteoclasts and increased osteoblastic activity. The bone trabeculae are sclerotic and show an abnormal architecture ("mosaic" pattern). Renal osteodystrophy shares with Paget disease the general characteristics of increased bone turnover. However, high bone turnover is focal or multifocal in Paget disease, and it is systemic in osteitis fibrosa (secondary hyperparathyroidism). The "mosaic" pattern typical of Paget disease is inconsistent with osteitis fibrosa. Although sclerosis of bony trabeculae is often seen in idiopathic osteoarthritis, the latter process shows neither the high level of bone remodeling nor the "mosaic" architecture seen in Paget disease. These changes are seen only in osteoarthritis secondary to Paget disease. Camurati-Engelmann disease (diaphyseal dysplasia) causes sclerosis of long bones (femur, tibia). It occurs in individuals in the first decade, whereas Paget disease affects middle-aged individuals. Camurati-Engelmann disease affects predominantly the long bones and rarely the skull and axial bones, whereas Paget disease has a predilection for the axial skeleton. Paget disease typically shows signs of increased bone remodeling, whereas Camurati-Engelmann disease shows bone formation unchecked by resorption and lacks the "mosaic" pattern characteristic of Paget disease. Although Paget disease and melorheostosis share common features of bone pain and skeletal sclerosis, Paget disease affects middle-aged individuals, and melorheostosis occurs in children. Melorheostosis most often affects the long bones and shows unique features such as fibrosis of periarticular soft tissues, joint contractures and deformities, and vascular malformations of skin and subcutaneous tissues. Most importantly, melorheostosis shows the unique radiologic sign of new bone formation with the "candle dripping" appearance pathognomonic of this disease and lacks the microscopic "mosaic" pattern typical of Paget disease.

Bullough PG: *Orthopaedic Pathology,* 4th ed. St. Louis: Mosby, 2004.

36. d. Dedifferentiation occurs in approximately 10% of all chondrosarcomas. This phenomenon is due to the uncontrolled growth of a population of undifferentiated mesenchymal cells in a previously well-differentiated chondrosarcoma, both components of this tumor having been shown to arise from a common precursor cell. It affects individuals in the sixth decade and older and has a skeletal distribution similar to conventional chondrosarcoma. However, the femur is the most frequently involved bone followed by the pelvis, humerus, scapula, and ribs. The clinical presentation is typically a longstanding mass, present from 1 to 10 years, with multiple recurrences after surgeries, showing recent rapid enlargement. The recent event is associated with pain. The radiographic images reflect the coexistence of a low-grade component showing stippled or ringlike opacities and a radiolucent, destructive, high-grade component disrupting cortical bone and forming a soft tissue mass. Microscopically, well-differentiated hyaline cartilage coexists side by side and abruptly transitions with a poorly differentiated, heterologous component (in this case a cellular spindle cell component forming fascicles resembling "herringbone" patterns). The heterologous component most frequently resembles fibrosarcoma or malignant fibrous histiocytoma, other components being osteosarcomatous, angiomatous, pleomorphic with giant cells, and rhabdomyosarcomatous. Well-differentiated chondrosarcoma has a protracted course marked by local recurrence with a low probability of metastases, whereas dedifferentiated chondrosarcoma is a rapidly growing, highly lethal tumor with a 1-year survival rate of 10%. Despite surgery, widespread hematogenous metastases occur. The tumor is resistant to both adjunctive radiotherapy and chemotherapy.

Bullough PG: *Orthopaedic Pathology,* 4th ed. St. Louis: Mosby, 2004.
Dorfman HD, Czerniak B (eds): *Bone Tumors.* St. Louis: Mosby, 1998.

37. b. Monostotic fibrous dysplasia is represented by multiple abnormally structured trabeculae of woven bone lacking a lining of osteoblasts in a fibrocellular, bland stroma. Well-differentiated intramedullary osteosarcoma of bone occurs in an older population compared with fibrous dysplasia. Although both lesions show abnormal bone lacking a border of osteoblasts, fibrous dysplasia shows curvilinear profiles, whereas well-differentiated intramedullary osteosarcoma of bone typically shows a "stucco" effect of neoplastic bone in the normal trabeculae. In contrast to fibrous dysplasia, the stroma of well-differentiated intramedullary osteosarcoma of bone shows consistent, albeit subtle, atypia. Although sheets of uniform small cells in a light-staining, seemingly myxoid stroma may suggest grade 2 chondrosarcoma, the bland nature of the stroma and absence of nuclear atypia argue in favor of fibrous dysplasia. The trabeculae of fibrous dysplasia are an intrinsic part of the lesion and do not represent preexisting bone. Although the sheets of small, uniform, light-staining stromal cells of fibrous dysplasia may show a vague resemblance to fibromyxoma of bone, the presence of dysplastic trabeculae strongly argues against this diagnosis. The presence of degenerative clusters of lipid-laden cells seen in many foci superficially raises the possibility of a xanthogranuloma of bone. However, the lack of focal hemorrhage, hemosiderin, and cholesterol clefts does not support this diagnosis.

Bullough PG: *Orthopaedic Pathology,* 4th ed. St. Louis: Mosby, 2004.
Chapurlat RD, Orcel P: Fibrous dysplasia of bone and McCune-Albright syndrome. *Best Pract Res Clin Rheumatol* 2008;22(1):55-69.
Dorfman HD, Czerniak B (eds): *Bone Tumors.* St. Louis: Mosby, 1998.

38. d. The diagnosis of chordoma is established by the presence of sheets and cords of large cells with clear, vacuolated cytoplasm rich in glycogen, particularly multivacuolated and multinucleated cells (physaliferous cells). Breast carcinoma can show a clear cell variant with large cells rich in glycogen; can demonstrate positivity for low-molecular-weight cytokeratin, endothelial monocyte antigen, and in some cases S100; and can mimic chordoma. However, it lacks the typical physaliferous cells characteristic of chordoma. Also, breast carcinoma shows positivity for lactalbumin and in some cases carcinoembryonic antigen, B72.3, gross cystic disease fluid protein 15, and chromogranin, which chordoma does not. Chordoma and chondrosarcoma may contain foci of cartilage (mostly sphenooccipital lesions) and be positive for S100. However, only chordomas express epithelial markers. Metastatic renal cell carcinoma, which frequently causes a solitary metastasis to bone, shares with chordoma its rich glycogen content and vimentin, CD10, and endothelial monocyte antigen positivity. However, renal cell carcinoma shows a distinct pattern of hypervascularity not present in chordoma and lacks the large multivacuolated and multinucleated cells (physaliferous cells), positivity for S100, and lectin-binding pattern typical of notochordal tissue. Although metastatic clear cell carcinoma of lung may include a dominant glycogen-rich and mucin-rich clear cell population and may share with chordoma the immunoreactivity for low-molecular-weight cytokeratin, endothelial monocyte antigen, and S100, it does not show the physaliferous cells typical of chordoma. Instead, positivity for cytokeratin 7, cytokeratin 20, and thyroid transcription factor-1 strongly supports the diagnosis of lung metastasis.

Dorfman HD, Czerniak B (eds): *Bone Tumors*. St. Louis: Mosby, 1998.
Rosai J (ed): *Rosai and Ackerman's Surgical Pathology,* 9th ed. St. Louis: Mosby, 2004.

39. e. Juxtacortical (parosteal) osteosarcoma is a grade 1 osteosarcoma composed of irregular trabeculae of immature bone typically lacking a lining of osteoblast in a neoplastic spindle cell stroma. Low-grade or juxtacortical osteosarcoma is a surface fibroosseous malignancy of bone accounting for 3% of osteosarcoma. It affects older individuals (20 to 30 years old) compared with conventional osteosarcoma. It has a predilection for the long bones of the lower extremities; 80% affect the posterior surface of the distal femoral metaphysis. The most common clinical feature is the presence of a conspicuous, palpable hard mass protruding in the popliteal space and causing pain and discomfort. The duration of symptoms is several months as opposed to several weeks with conventional osteosarcoma. The clinical radiographic images are diagnostic, revealing a mushroom-shaped, lobulated mass of bone protruding from the posterior aspect of the distal metaphysis of the femur and attached to the cortical surface by a broad base. The center is densely radiopaque, whereas the periphery is more lucent, which is an important differential diagnostic point with myositis ossificans. The mass reflects over the surface of the adjacent cortex from which it is separated by a radiolucent line. There is no Codman triangle. In contrast to osteochondroma, the mass does not communicate with the medullary cavity of the femur. The lesion comprises a mass of well-differentiated, seemingly benign trabeculae of woven bone lacking a border of active osteoblasts in a fibrous stroma and appears deceptively benign. The trabeculae often show a directionality, streaming in parallel arrangement and frequently admixed with round, dotlike profiles. It may contain foci of cartilage. It may be difficult to distinguish between this lesion and fibrous dysplasia because both lesions share trabeculae lacking a lining of osteoblasts as well as a fibrous stroma. The trabeculae are most often delicate and curvilinear (resembling letters of the alphabet) in fibrous dysplasia, a feature seen less often in parosteal osteosarcoma. This tumor has a cellular spindle cell stroma with fascicular patterns compared with the hypocellular, bland stroma of fibrous dysplasia. In this neoplasm, a subtle blending between the spindle cells and the trabecular margins is best seen in the fibrous periphery of the tumor. Although the degree of atypia is often subtle, hyperchromasia and mitoses are consistently present. This tumor is slow-growing, and the prognosis is better than conventional osteosarcoma. If treated early and appropriately, a cure can be achieved.

The recommended treatment is en bloc resection with wide margins of uninvolved tissue. This lesion can dedifferentiate if treatment is inadequate.

Bullough PG: *Orthopaedic Pathology,* 4th ed. St. Louis: Mosby, 2004.
Dorfman HD, Czerniak B (eds): *Bone Tumors*. St. Louis: Mosby, 1998.

40. a. Renal cell carcinoma frequently presents as a solitary skeletal metastasis while the primary initially remains clinically silent (30%). Renal cell carcinoma is also known for its ability to metastasize to unusual sites. Although tumor metastases characteristically do not occur below the elbow or knee, renal cell carcinoma may be localized in distal parts of the skeleton (bones of hands and feet). The lesions are frequently discovered because of pain at the involved site associated with pathologic fracture. Radiography shows a solitary, lytic lesion with ill-defined, infiltrative margins and evidence of cortical destruction frequently leading to pathologic fracture and extension into the soft tissues. Metastatic renal cell carcinoma is represented by sheets and cords of epithelial cells with optically clear cytoplasm separated by fine connective tissue stalks containing small blood vessels. This optical clarity is due to the abundance of glycogen and fat in the tumor cells in the absence of intracellular mucin. The coexpression of vimentin and cytokeratins (cytokeratin 8 and cytokeratin 18) and positivity for CD10 are of diagnostic importance. Renal cell carcinoma frequently overexpresses *p53* and produces various proteins, including endothelial monocyte antigen, carcinoembryonic antigen, CD68, the α-subunit of S100 protein, Lewis blood group isoantigens, erythropoietin, angiotensin-converting enzyme, epidermal growth factor, and transthyretin. Because regression of metastases (partial or complete) sometimes occurs spontaneously or after surgery, resection of a solitary metastasis significantly prolongs life. Metastatectomy along with nephrectomy reduces the tumor burden with the hope of stabilization and regression of the neoplastic process. Because of the marked vascularity of the tumor, preoperative embolization is recommended. Dissemination occurs eventually in 50% of patients originally treated for solitary disease. Dedifferentiation into a spindle cell or pleomorphic sarcoma occurs in 10% and is associated with a worse prognosis.

Dorfman HD, Czerniak B (eds): *Bone Tumors*. St. Louis: Mosby, 1998.
Rosai J (ed): *Rosai and Ackerman's Surgical Pathology,* 9th ed. St. Louis: Mosby, 2004.

41. d. In contrast to the basic genetic abnormalities associated with osteosarcoma, a reciprocal translocation, t(11;22) (q24;q12), with fusion of *FLI-1* and *ESW* genes is characteristic of Ewing sarcoma and occurs in most cases. Most osteosarcomas contain clonal chromosomal aberrations. The most frequently altered chromosomal regions include 1p11-13, 1q11-12, 1q21-22, 11p14-15, 14q11-13, 15p11-13, 17p, and 19q13. Gene amplification in 8q23 is evident in 50% of osteosarcomas, and amplification in 8q24 (*MYC* gene) is evident in 44%. Loss of heterozygosity is evident in osteosarcomas involving chromosome arms 3q, 13q, 17p, and 18q. Amplication and overexpression of *MDM2*, *PRIM1*, and *CDK4* has been implicated in the genetic abnormalities of osteosarcoma.

A germline mutation of 13q14 (RB locus) is associated with hereditary retinoblastoma and a 500 times greater risk of osteosarcoma. A single mutation of the *RB* gene followed by an acquired somatic mutation ("second hit") causes an increased risk of osteosarcoma with or without retinoblastoma.

Fletcher CDM, Unni KK, Mertens F (eds): *World Health Organization Classification of Tumours.* Lyon: IARC Press, 2002.
Wold LE, Adler CP, Sim FH, et al (eds): *Atlas of Orthopaedic Pathology,* 2nd ed. Philadelphia: Saunders, 2004.

42. a. Li-Fraumeni syndrome (caused by an inherited mutant *p53* allele) is associated with a greater risk of sarcomas (and other malignancies), in particular, a 500 times greater risk of osteosarcoma. In sporadic osteosarcoma, loss of heterozygosity at 17p and *TP53* mutation are evident in 30% of osteosarcomas. A reciprocal X;18 translocation is characteristic of synovial sarcoma. Multiple nonreciprocal translocations and deletions involving various chromosomes and 1p rearrangements were reported in conventional chondrosarcoma. A nonrandom translocation 9;22 has been implicated in extraskeletal myxoid chondrosarcoma.

Fletcher CDM, Unni KK, Mertens F (eds): *World Health Organization Classification of Tumours.* Lyon: IARC Press, 2002.
Wold LE, Adler CP, Sim FH, et al (eds): *Atlas of Orthopaedic Pathology,* 2nd ed. Philadelphia: Saunders, 2004.

43. a. Ollier disease is a nonhereditary disease characterized by multiple enchondromas most frequently affecting the appendicular skeleton and the long bones (forearm and femur). Ollier disease usually manifests in early childhood, with patients frequently presenting with swelling of the fingers. Enchondromas in the metaphyseal regions of long bones may result in deformity and limb asymmetry and pathologic fracture. Enchondromas seen in association with Ollier disease are typically unilateral and asymmetric, with all or most lesions localized to one side of the body. Histologically, chondroma associated with Ollier disease tends to be hypercellular, and the chondrocyte nuclei are enlarged and irregular. Patients with Ollier disease have a 15% to 30% increased risk of developing malignant bone tumors, in particular, chondrosarcomas.

Fletcher CDM, Unni KK, Mertens F (eds): *World Health Organization Classification of Tumours.* Lyon: IARC Press, 2002.
Wold LE, Adler CP, Sim FH, et al (eds): *Atlas of Orthopaedic Pathology,* 2nd ed. Philadelphia: Saunders, 2004.

44. e. There is great diversity in the morphologic patterns of osteosarcoma sharing similar histologic features with many other disease entities. The fibroblastic subtype of osteosarcoma may mimic malignant fibrous histiocytoma and fibrosarcoma, the chondroblastic subtype may be misdiagnosed as chondrosarcoma, and the telangiectatic subtype often resembles a benign aneurysmal bone cyst in its general architecture. Making the correct diagnosis depends on the recognition of malignant osteoid generally deposited in anarchic, fine lacy patterns around malignant mesenchymal cells. Clinical and radiologic correlations are also important in making the diagnosis of osteosarcoma. Osteochondroma is a benign bone-forming and cartilage-forming lesion that is easily recognized by its bulk of cancellous bone. This bone is

formed by endochondral ossification from a cap of hyaline cartilage that has a structure identical to a growth plate. In contrast to osteosarcoma, there is no malignant bone in this lesion.

Bullough PG: *Orthopaedic Pathology,* 4th ed. St. Louis: Mosby, 2004.
Cotran RS, Kumar V, Collins T (eds): *Robbins Pathologic Basis of Disease,* 6th ed. Philadelphia: Saunders, 1999.
Dorfman HD, Czerniak B (eds): *Bone Tumors.* St. Louis: Mosby, 1998.

45. b. Adamantinoma is a rare, low-grade malignancy of bone. It is typically located intracortically in the diaphysis of the tibia and less frequently in the fibula. Synchronous involvement of both tibia and fibula is reported in 50% of cases. Classic adamantinoma occurs after age 20 years, whereas the differentiated variant typically occurs in the first 2 decades of life. Adamantinoma is a biphasic tumor resulting from the differentiation of the multipotential mesenchymal cell along various cell lines. The most common histologic types are spindle, basaloid, tubular, and squamous variants. Tubular spaces are lined by flattened or cuboidal cells. Basaloid nests either are compact or may show central spaces resembling vascular channels. The fibrous tissue is vimentin positive, and the epithelial cells are positive for cytokeratins (cytokeratin 5, cytokeratin 14, and cytokeratin 19), endothelial monocyte antigen, and vimentin. Adamantinoma follows an indolent course, spanning many years. However, the tumor metastasizes primarily in lungs and lymph nodes at a rate of 25% within 2 to 5 years. Metastases seem to occur exclusively in classic adamantinoma. Young age, pain at presentation, and short duration of symptoms are associated with increased rates of recurrence or metastasis. Differentiated adamantinoma (osteofibrous dysplasia type) has a different prognosis and does not tend to metastasize.

Cotran RS, Kumar V, Collins T (eds): *Robbins Pathologic Basis of Disease,* 6th ed. Philadelphia: Saunders, 1999.
Fletcher CDM, Unni KK, Mertens F (eds): *World Health Organization Classification of Tumours.* Lyon: IARC Press, 2002.

46. e. Osteoblastoma is a rare benign bone-forming lesion that produces woven bone spicules bordered by prominent osteoblasts. It is seen in young individuals 10 to 40 years old; however, the peak incidence is in the second and third decades. Men are affected more often than women. Pain is a common symptom; it may be dull or more significant and is relieved by antiinflammatory medication. However, it lacks the typical pattern of pain relief with aspirin that is characteristic of osteoid osteoma. Osteoblastoma has a predilection for the medullary (cancellous) compartment of the bone, whereas osteoid osteoma has an intracortical location. The skeletal distribution also differs from osteoid osteoma. Osteoblastoma has a predilection for the spine (40% of cases), affecting less frequently the long bones, whereas osteoid osteoma predominantly involves the long bones of the extremities, particularly the neck of the femur (22% of cases); osteoid osteoma affects the spine in only 5% of cases. Osteoblastoma is larger (>2.0 cm) than osteoid osteoma, and size is an important feature in distinguishing between the two tumors. Osteoblastoma has a greater potential for unlimited growth, and it may grow to 10.0 cm or more. Osteoblastoma comprises a nidus containing numerous small trabeculae of bone in a cellular, vascular stroma populated by osteoclasts and osteoblasts. Large osteoblasts proliferate in clusters in the stroma of osteoblastoma; this is not found in osteoid osteoma. Osteoid matrix may be deposited as very small, immature trabeculae. However, the bone is always covered by active osteoblasts and is not deposited in "lacy" patterns or "streamers" characteristic of osteosarcoma. In contrast to osteosarcoma, cellular atypia and mitoses are not present. Osteoblastoma never shows infiltration of preexisting trabecular bone.

Bullough PG: *Orthopaedic Pathology,* 4th ed. St. Louis: Mosby, 2004.

Dorfman HD, Czerniak B (eds): *Bone Tumors*. St. Louis: Mosby, 1998.

Fletcher CDM, Unni KK, Mertens F (eds): *World Health Organization Classification of Tumours*. Lyon: IARC Press, 2002.

CHAPTER 13

SKIN PATHOLOGY

Jennifer V. Nguyen, Suthinee Rutnin, and Adam I. Rubin

QUESTIONS

Questions 1-47 refer to a photo or photomicrograph.

1. Which one of the following infections does NOT demonstrate the histologic findings in the image?
   a. Cytomegalovirus
   b. Herpes simplex
   c. Herpes zoster
   d. Varicella

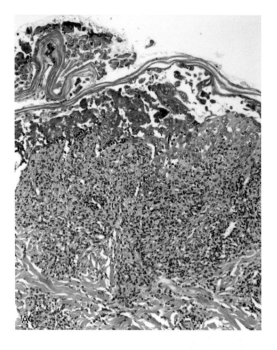

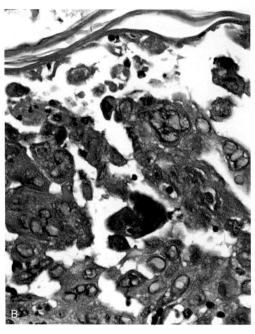

2. A 60-year-old man complained of a very pruritic papular eruption predominantly involving the chest and back. A biopsy specimen of the lesion is shown. The BEST histologic diagnosis is:

   a. Scabies

   b. Grover disease (transient acantholytic dermatosis)

   c. Varicella

   d. Pemphigus vulgaris

   e. Hailey-Hailey disease

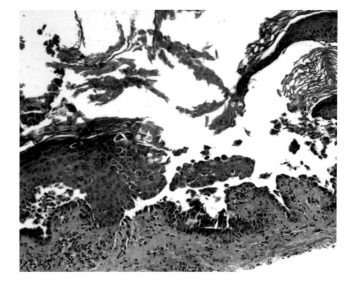

3. A skin biopsy specimen is shown that demonstrates papillary dermal edema and a dense, diffuse interstitial infiltrate of neutrophils involving the upper half of the reticular dermis. The BEST diagnosis is:

   a. Leukocytoclastic vasculitis

   b. Sweet syndrome

   c. Dermatophytosis

   d. Dermatitis herpetiformis

   e. Lepromatous leprosy

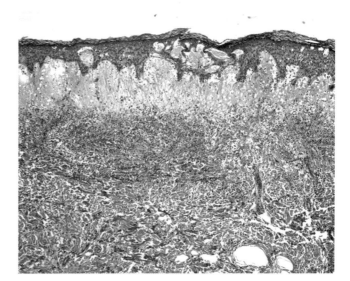

4. A shave biopsy specimen is shown that is characterized by alternating orthokeratosis and parakeratosis and unaffected epithelium surrounding the intraepidermal component of adnexal structures. These histologic findings are characteristic of:

   a. Extramammary Paget disease

   b. Psoriasis vulgaris

   c. Seborrheic dermatitis

   d. Seborrheic keratosis

   e. Actinic keratosis (solar keratosis)

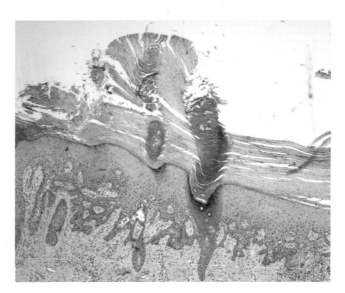

5. A 45-year-old woman complained of exquisitely painful subcutaneous nodules on both legs of 4 weeks' duration. The lesions have not ulcerated. The biopsy specimen shows inflammation primarily within the septa between fat lobules. The BEST diagnosis is:

   a. Subcutaneous T-cell lymphoma
   b. Tumid lupus erythematosus
   c. Panniculitis secondary to pancreatic carcinoma
   d. Erythema nodosum
   e. Nodular vasculitis

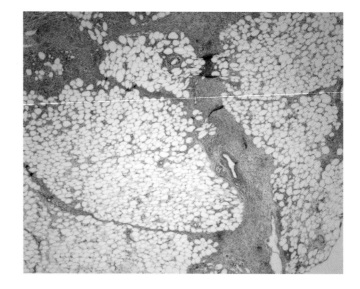

6. An 83-year-old man complained of a generalized rash characterized by oval erythematous asymptomatic patches over the entire torso. The eruption had waxed and waned for more than 10 years and previous biopsy specimens had been "nondiagnostic." The BEST diagnosis based on the biopsy specimen shown is:

   a. Spongiotic dermatitis
   b. Psoriasis vulgaris
   c. Cutaneous T-cell lymphoma (mycosis fungoides)
   d. Lichen planus

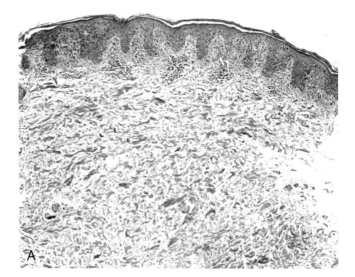

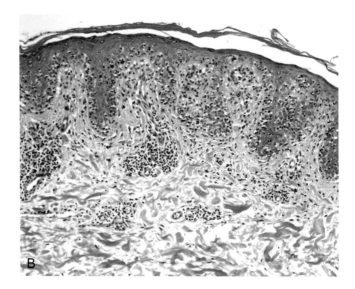

7. A 6-year-old boy presented with a 0.5-cm red nodule on the forearm that first appeared 4 months ago. A biopsy specimen is shown. The BEST histologic diagnosis is:
   a. Nodular melanoma
   b. Juvenile xanthogranuloma
   c. Spitz nevus
   d. Dysplastic nevus
   e. Molluscum contagiosum

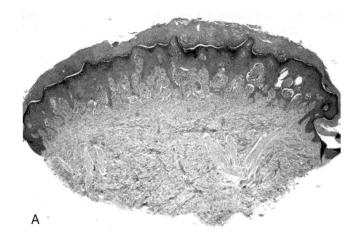

A

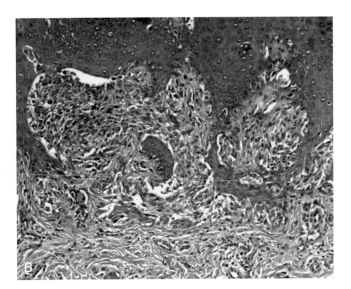

B

8. Which one of the following diagnoses is correct based on the biopsy specimen shown?
  a. Lentigo maligna melanoma in situ
  b. Simple lentigo
  c. Pigmented actinic keratosis
  d. Macular seborrheic keratosis
  e. Bowen disease

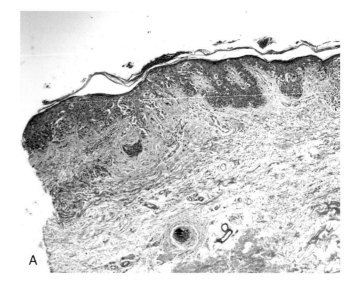

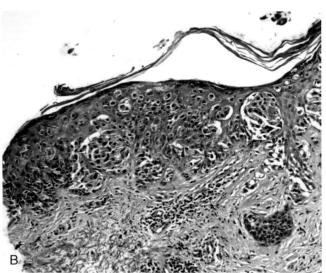

9. Which one of the following entities is NOT in the differential diagnosis of the biopsy specimen shown?
  a. Contact dermatitis
  b. Nummular dermatitis
  c. Photoallergic dermatitis
  d. Atopic dermatitis
  e. Lupus erythematosus

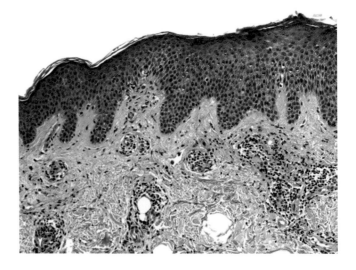

10. A 15-year-old boy presented with asymptomatic papulonodules on the dorsum of the hands, histologically characterized by foci of mucin deposition surrounded by a palisade arrangement of histiocytes. The BEST diagnosis is:

a. Reticulohistiocytosis

b. Multiple granular cell tumors

c. Granuloma annulare

d. Arthropod bite reaction

e. Sarcoidosis

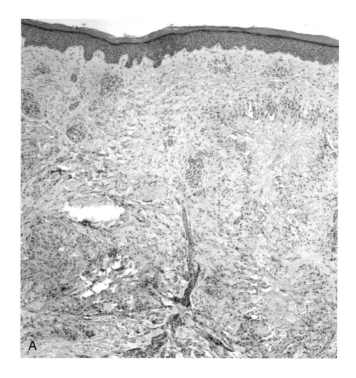

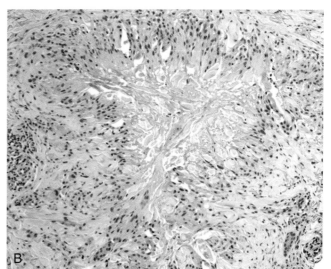

11. A 25-year-old man presented with a generalized eruption, clinically resembling a drug eruption of 1 week's duration. He was otherwise asymptomatic. A biopsy specimen of the lesion is shown. Based on the histologic findings, the BEST diagnosis is:

   a. Erythema multiforme
   b. Secondary syphilis
   c. Discoid lupus erythematosus
   d. Psoriasis
   e. Viral exanthem

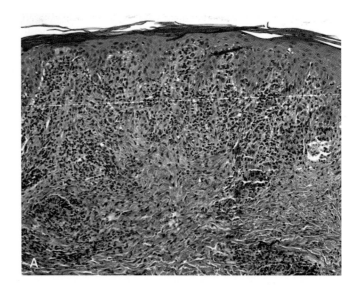

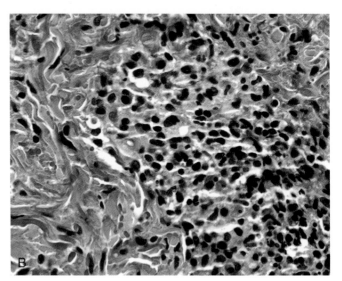

12. A 70-year-old man complained of a rough, slightly tender lesion on the forehead that had been present for months. A specimen from a shave biopsy is shown. The diagnosis is:

   a. Squamous cell carcinoma
   b. Basal cell carcinoma
   c. Eccrine poroma
   d. Inflamed seborrheic keratosis
   e. Clear cell acanthoma

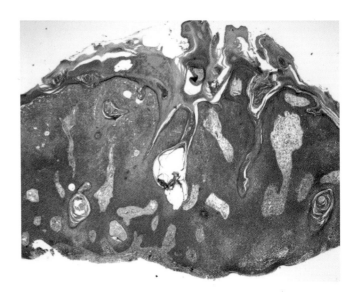

13. A 46-year-old woman presented with a 1.5-cm, flesh-colored, deeply indurated nodule on the upper lip that had been slowly enlarging for at least 5 years. A biopsy specimen is shown. The diagnosis is:

   a. Morpheaform basal cell carcinoma

   b. Syringoma

   c. Pseudoglandular squamous cell carcinoma

   d. Adenocarcinoma metastatic to skin

   e. Microcystic adnexal carcinoma

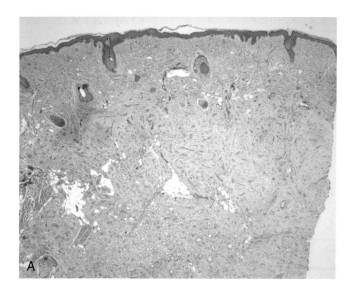

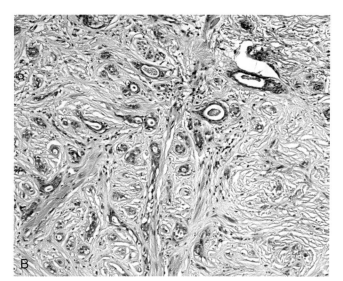

14. A 70-year-old man was noted to have a 2-cm, white, "scarlike" plaque on the left side of the nose extending onto the cheek. There was no history of prior injury or a previous surgical procedure at the site. The BEST interpretation of the biopsy specimen shown is:

a. Morpheaform basal cell carcinoma
b. Desmoplastic trichoepithelioma
c. Microcystic adnexal carcinoma
d. Adenocarcinoma metastatic to skin
e. Cutaneous lymphadenoma

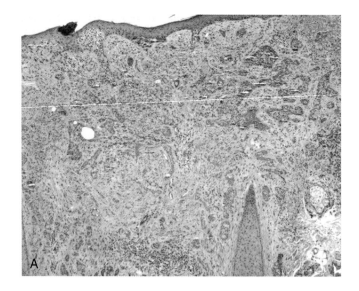

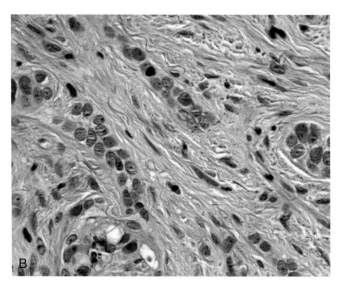

15. A 72-year-old woman presented with a 2.3 cm × 1.7 cm brown macule on the sole of the left foot. The asymptomatic lesion had been present for approximately 4 years and was enlarging slowly. A biopsy specimen is shown. It is correctly interpreted as:

a. Tinea nigra
b. In situ acral lentiginous melanoma
c. Lentiginous junctional nevus
d. Lentigo simplex
e. Macular seborrheic keratosis

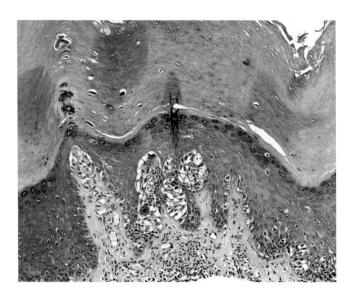

16. A 60-year-old man reported the sudden appearance of a 1-cm red nodule on the back of the neck that was friable and bled easily. Past history included a melanoma 2.3 cm in thickness, which had been excised 3 years ago from the lower back and was followed by a course of interferon-α, and renal cell carcinoma 10 years ago, which was treated by total nephrectomy. The lesion was removed for biopsy, and a specimen is shown. The diagnosis is:

a. Metastatic melanoma (amelanotic)
b. Metastatic renal cell carcinoma
c. Kaposi sarcoma
d. Pyogenic granuloma
e. Bacillary angiomatosis

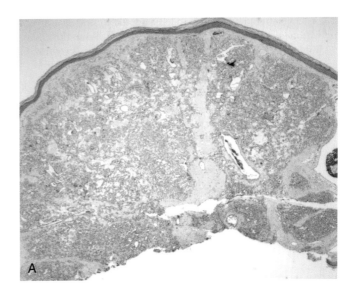

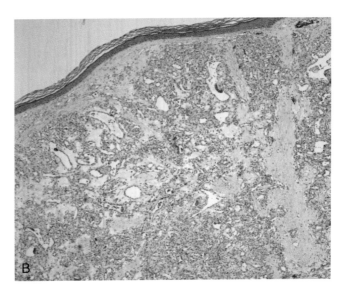

17. A 35-year-old, HIV-positive man presented to the dermatologist with a 1-cm, nontender, asymptomatic brown nodule on the calf. A biopsy specimen is shown. The correct diagnosis is:

 a. Dermatofibroma
 b. AIDS-related Kaposi sarcoma
 c. Granuloma annulare
 d. Dermatofibrosarcoma protuberans
 e. Desmoplastic melanoma

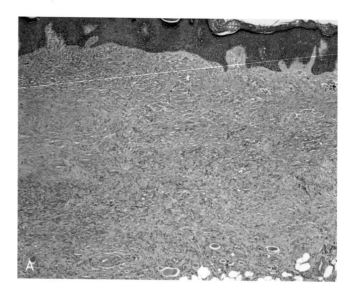

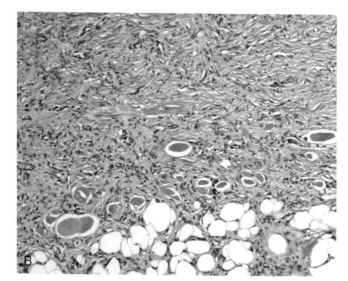

18. A 55-year-old woman had a "mole" removed from her chest. The lesion was said to have been "benign" on histologic evaluation. Within 6 months, she had developed a slightly tender, 8-mm, raised nodule at the surgical site. A biopsy of the nodule was performed, and the biopsy specimen is shown. The BEST histologic diagnosis is:
   a. Desmoplastic melanoma
   b. Recurrent leiomyoma
   c. Keloid
   d. Dermatofibroma
   e. Neurofibroma

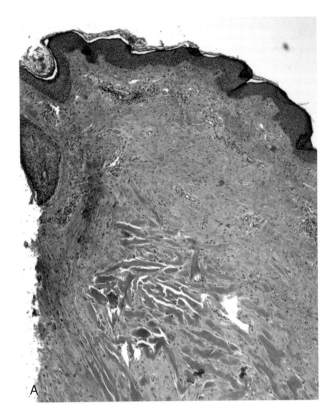

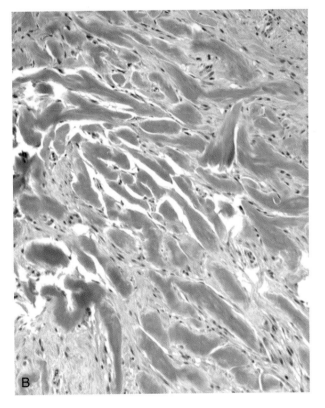

19. A 30-year-old woman had a "mole" removed from her chest. The surgical site healed, and later a blue-black macule developed in the central area of the scar. Excision of the site was performed, and the biopsy specimen is shown. The correct diagnosis is:

a. Junctional nevus
b. Recurrent (persistent) nevus phenomenon
c. Halo nevus phenomenon
d. Blue nevus
e. Metastatic adenocarcinoma of the breast

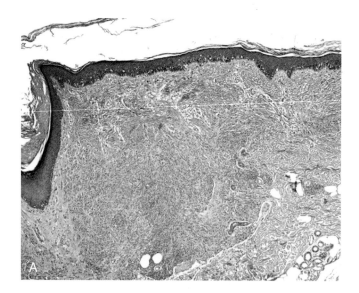

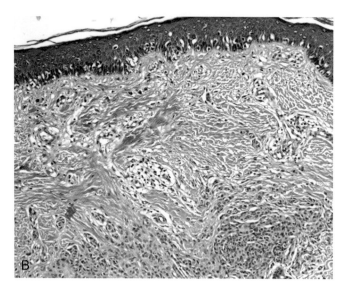

20. A 45-year-old man noticed a slowly enlarging, indurated nodule of the skin of the right thigh. The lesion was raised above the surface and measured approximately 3 cm in diameter. A biopsy was performed. Which of the following statements is correct regarding the histologic finding shown?

a. Immunostain for CD34 would be positive.
b. Immunostain for factor XIIIa would be positive.
c. Immunostain for S100 protein would be positive.
d. Immunostain for cytokeratin would be positive.
e. Immunostain for smooth muscle actin (SMA) would be positive.

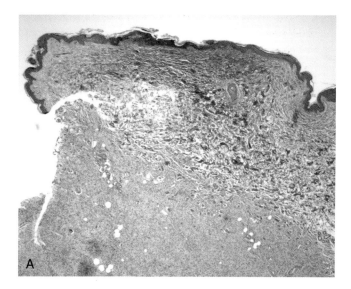

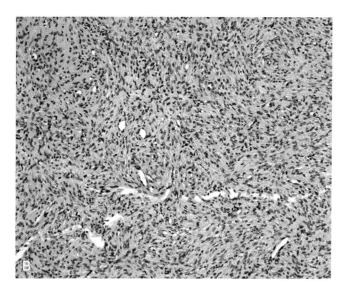

21. A 60-year-old woman presented with a painful ulcerated lesion of the pinna of the right ear. A biopsy specimen of the lesion is shown. This biopsy specimen confirms a diagnosis of:

a. Squamous cell carcinoma
b. Actinic keratosis
c. Basal cell carcinoma
d. Angiosarcoma
e. Chondrodermatitis nodularis chronica helicis

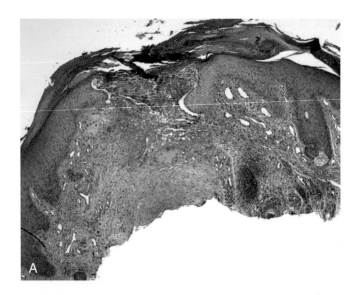

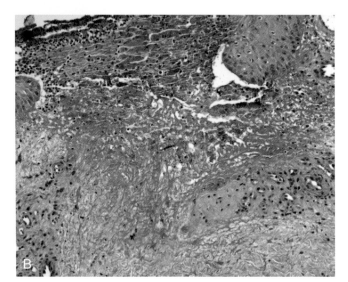

22. A 30-year-old man developed a raised firm nodule on the buttock. The lesion measured approximately 1.5 cm in diameter. The biopsy specimen shown demonstrates:
   a. Squamous cell carcinoma
   b. Tuberous xanthoma
   c. Granular cell tumor
   d. Condyloma accuminatum
   e. Dermatofibroma

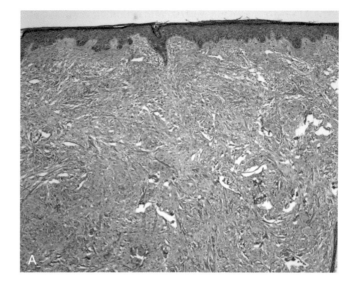

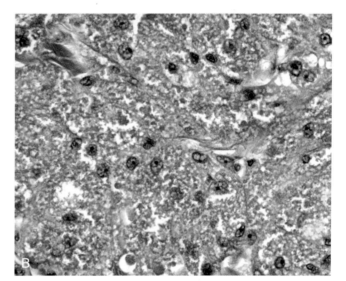

23. A 45-year-old man has multiple nodules on the forehead and scalp that appeared at puberty and have been asymptomatic. His mother and sister have similar lesions. The biopsy specimen shown confirms a diagnosis of:

  a. Trichoepithelioma

  b. Basal cell carcinoma

  c. Cylindroma

  d. Spiradenoma

  e. Pilomatricoma

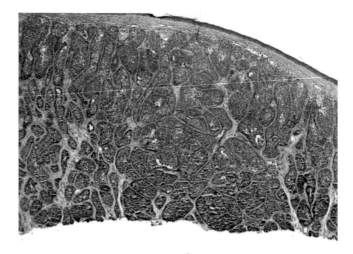

A

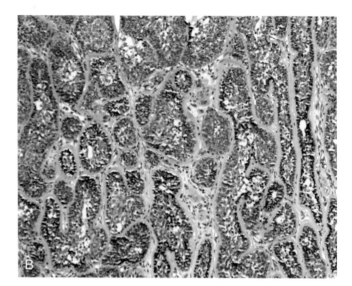

B

24. A 2-year-old boy presented with a slightly yellow nodule of the scalp that was "itchy" but otherwise asymptomatic. The correct diagnosis, based on the biopsy specimen shown, is:

a. Intradermal nevus
b. Glomus tumor
c. Juvenile xanthogranuloma
d. Mastocytoma
e. Arthropod bite reaction

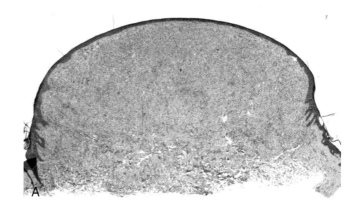

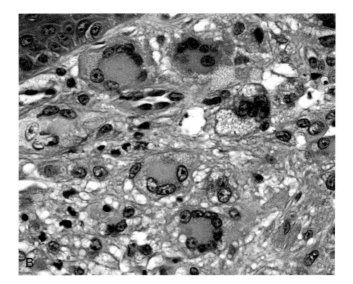

25. A 6-year-old boy was referred to a dermatologist for evaluation of a nodular lesion of the left cheek. The biopsy specimen shows aggregates of basaloid cells in association with granulomatous inflammation. The BEST diagnosis is:

   a. Basal cell carcinoma

   b. Trichoepithelioma

   c. Pilar cyst

   d. Pilomatricoma

   e. Acute folliculitis

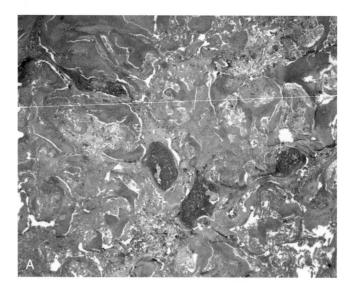

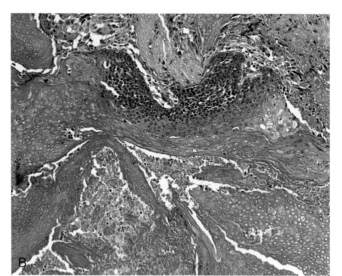

26. A 40-year-old woman presented with a 5-mm, flesh-colored papule of the right nasolabial fold. The biopsy specimen shows a:

a. Basal cell carcinoma
b. Trichoepithelioma
c. Trichilemmoma
d. Cylindroma
e. Merkel cell carcinoma

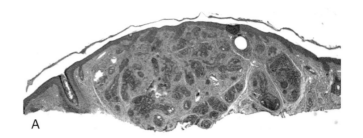

A

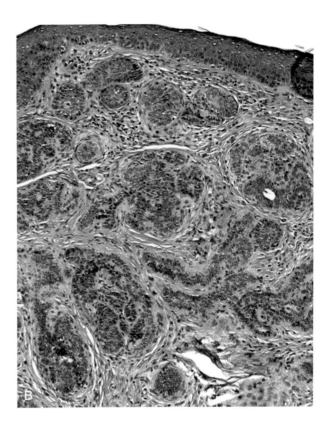

B

27. A 54-year-old-man presents with a translucent cystic nodule with a bluish hue on his upper eyelid. A biopsy specimen of the lesion is shown. The BEST histologic diagnosis is:

a. Apocrine hidrocystoma
b. Pilar cyst
c. Venous lake
d. Epidermal inclusion cyst
e. Superficial lymphangioma

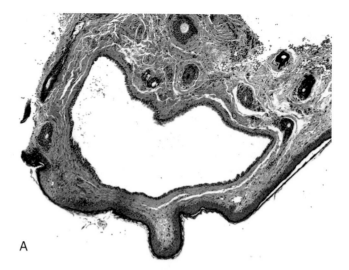

A

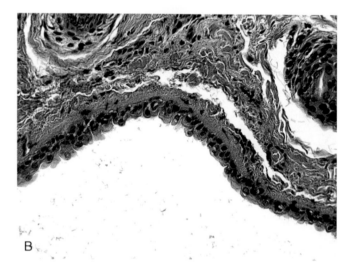

B

28. A 48-year-old man presents with a soft, dome-shaped, tan, 8-mm papule on his upper back. A biopsy specimen of the lesion is shown. The lesion is asymptomatic and has been present for an unknown duration. The BEST histologic diagnosis is:

a. Nodular melanoma

b. Piloleiomyoma

c. Neurofibroma

d. Dermal nevus

e. Dermatofibroma

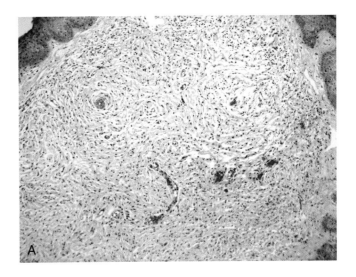

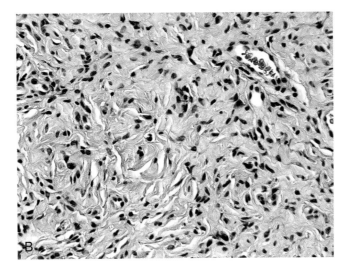

29. A 25-year-old African American woman presents with multiple red-brown papules on her face. A chest x-ray study demonstrates bilateral hilar adenopathy. A skin biopsy specimen is shown. The BEST diagnosis is:

   a. Multicentric reticulohistiocytosis
   b. Sarcoidosis
   c. Juvenile xanthogranuloma
   d. Foreign body granuloma
   e. Tuberculoid leprosy

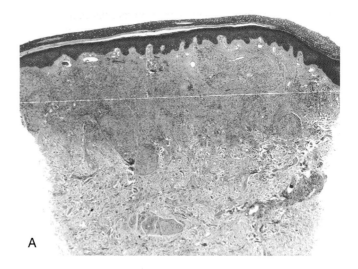

A

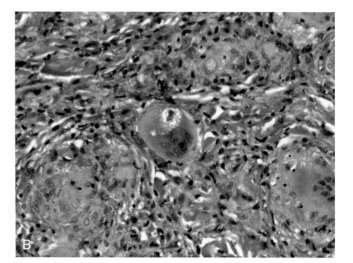

B

30. An 8-year-old boy presents with numerous flat-topped, skin-colored papules on the back of his hands. A biopsy specimen of the lesion is shown. The BEST histologic diagnosis is:

a. Tinea versicolor
b. Epidermodysplasia verruciformis
c. Lichen planus
d. Verrucae plana
e. Verrucae vulgaris

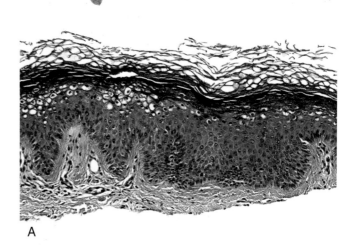
A

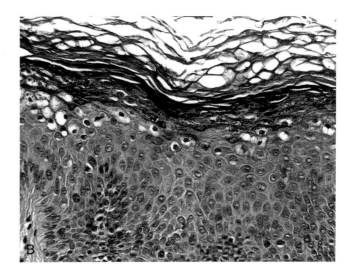
B

31. A 53-year-old man has multiple annular, pink patches, each
with a thin, threadlike border, scattered on his dorsal arms and
lower legs. The lesions are less than 1 cm in diameter. He has a
history of extensive sun exposure. A biopsy specimen of the
lesion is shown. The BEST histologic diagnosis is:
   a. Verruca plana
   b. Granuloma annulare
   c. Porokeratosis (disseminated superficial actinic type)
   d. Subacute cutaneous lupus erythematosus
   e. Tinea corporis

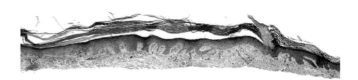

A

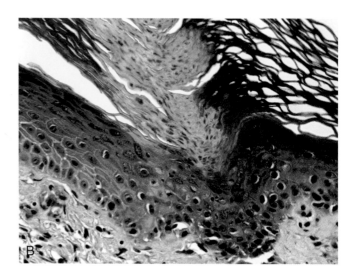

B

32. A 67-year-old man complains of multiple nodules on his elbows, which sometimes discharge a white, chalky material. A biopsy specimen of the lesion is shown. The BEST diagnosis is:

a. Calcinosis cutis
b. Tuberous xanthoma
c. Granuloma annulare
d. Gout
e. Rheumatoid nodule

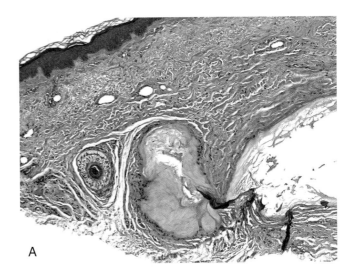

A

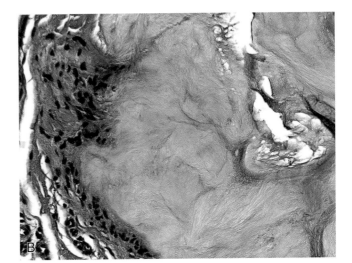

B

33. A 44-year-old woman presents with severe pruritus of the vulvar region. Physical examination demonstrates smooth, porcelain-white plaques of the labia minora and perianal region. A biopsy specimen of the lesion is shown. The BEST histologic diagnosis is:

   a. Condyloma latum
   b. Lichen sclerosus et atrophicus
   c. Morphea
   d. Lichen planus
   e. Cicatricial pemphigoid

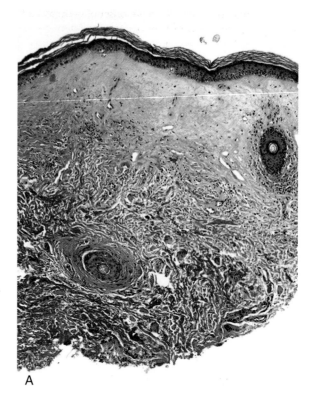

A

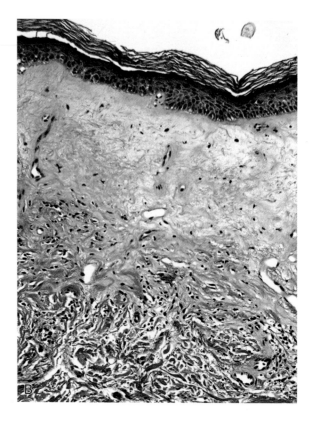

B

34. A 36-year-old man presents with acute onset of widespread erythematous macules and papules on his extremities bilaterally. The lesions have a targetoid appearance. He reports developing a "cold sore" on his upper lip 2 weeks ago. A skin biopsy specimen is shown. The BEST histologic diagnosis is:

   a. Acute generalized exanthematous pustulosis

   b. Erythema multiforme

   c. Fixed drug eruption

   d. Subacute cutaneous lupus erythematosus

   e. Viral exanthem

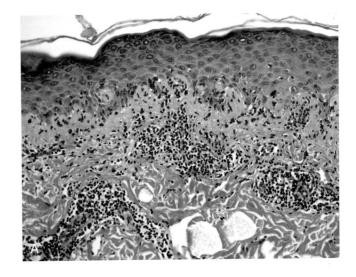

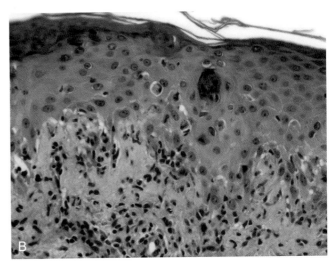

35. A 46-year-old man presents with a 2-year history of severely itchy lesions all over his body, particularly over his elbows, knees, trunk, and buttocks. He was treated for scabies without improvement. Physical examination reveals multiple excoriated papules, erosions, and a few vesicles. Direct immunofluorescence was performed on perilesional skin, and the specimen is shown. The BEST diagnosis is:

   a. Bullous pemphigoid

   b. Dermatitis herpetiformis

   c. Linear IgA disease

   d. Pemphigus vulgaris

   e. Lichen planus

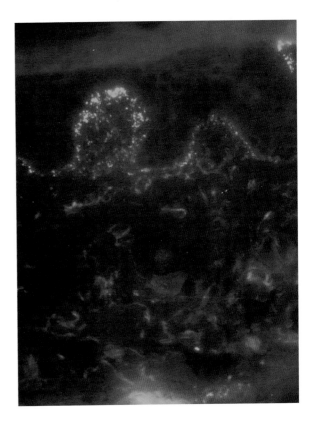

36. A 2-year-old boy presents with multiple widespread tan-brown
macules and papules scattered over his body. On examination,
a lesion exhibits a wheal-and-flare reaction in response to
rubbing. A biopsy specimen of one of the papules is shown.
The BEST histologic stain to confirm the diagnosis is:

   a. Alcian blue stain
   b. Verhoeff–Van Gieson stain
   c. Giemsa stain
   d. Warthin-Starry stain
   e. Von Kossa stain

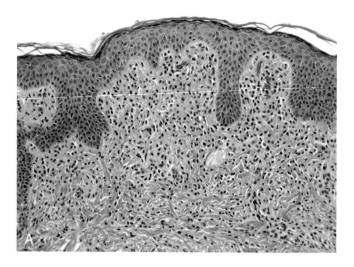

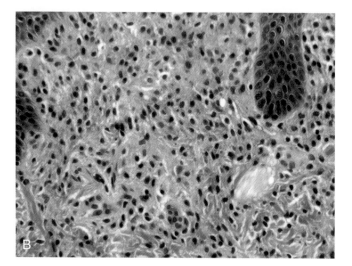

37. A 5-year-old boy presented with a 1-month history of multiple discrete, skin-colored, dome-shaped umbilicated papules on the face, trunk, and extremities, ranging from 2 to 5 mm in diameter. A biopsy specimen of the lesion is shown. Which of the following is a key histologic feature on this biopsy specimen?

   a. Henderson-Patterson bodies
   b. Koilocytotic (raisin) nuclei
   c. Mikulicz cells
   d. Multinucleated giant cells with intranuclear inclusions
   e. Donovan bodies

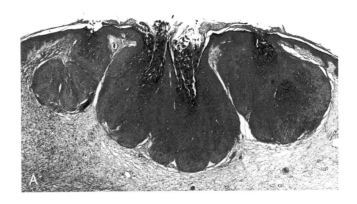

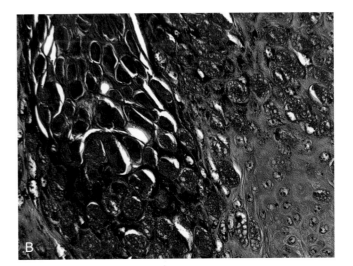

38. A 20-year-old man presents with an abrupt onset of multiple areas of palpable purpura on both lower extremities. Approximately 3 to 4 weeks before his presentation, he had been given a diagnosis of streptococcal pharyngitis, for which he received an oral antibiotic. He has no systemic symptoms. The biopsy specimen is shown. The BEST diagnosis is:

a. Sweet syndrome
b. Leukocytoclastic vasculitis
c. Pigmented purpuric dermatosis
d. Erythema nodosum
e. Polyarteritis nodosa

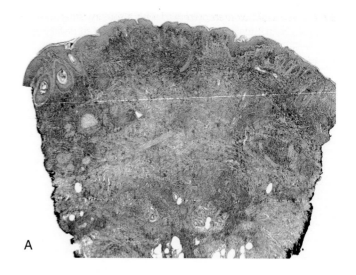

A

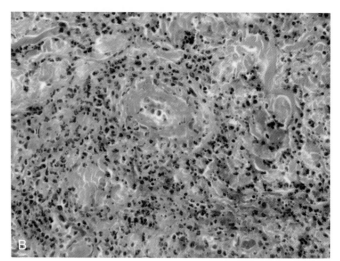

B

39. A 35-year-old woman presented with a solitary, small, erythematous tender nodule on the left dorsal third finger. A biopsy was performed, and the histologic finding is shown. Which of the following immunohistochemical stains is the MOST useful to confirm the diagnosis?

a. S100 protein
b. Epithelial membrane antigen (EMA)
c. Smooth muscle actin (SMA)
d. Desmin
e. CD34

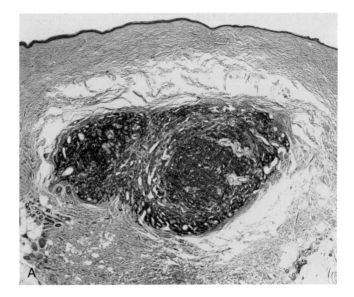

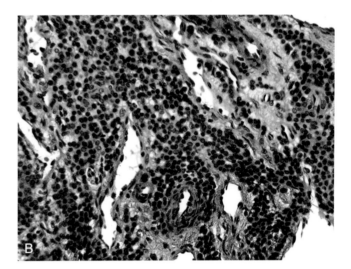

40. A 60-year-old man presented with multiple small, pruritic, tan-brown papules coalescing into large plaques on the anterior surface of the lower extremities. A biopsy was performed, and the specimen is shown. Which of the following stains is useful to confirm the diagnosis?

a. Congo red
b. Verhoeff–Van Gieson
c. Masson trichrome
d. Alcian blue
e. Colloidal iron

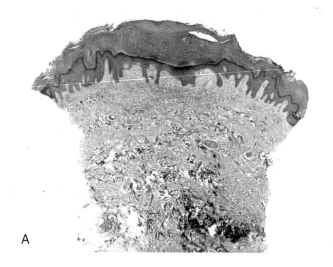

A

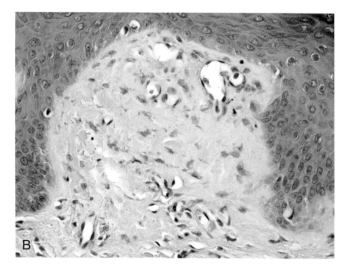

B

41. A 40-year-old HIV-seropositive man presented with a 6-month history of asymptomatic progressive purplish patches and plaques over his arms and trunk. A biopsy was performed, and the specimen is shown. Which of the following immunohistochemical stains is the most useful tool to confirm the diagnosis?

  a. Human herpesvirus (HHV)-8 antibody

  b. CD31

  c. CD34

  d. D2-40

  e. *Ulex europaeus* agglutinin I

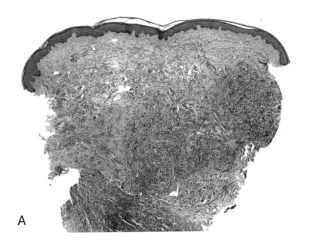

A

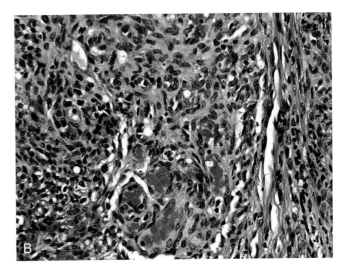

B

42. A 45-year-old man with HIV infection was noncompliant with his antiretroviral medications and developed multiple umbilicated papules on the face. A biopsy specimen of one of the lesions is shown and identifies the diagnosis as:

   a. Coccidioidomycosis

   b. Cryptococcosis

   c. Molluscum contagiosum

   d. Keratoacanthoma

   e. Reactive perforating collagenosis

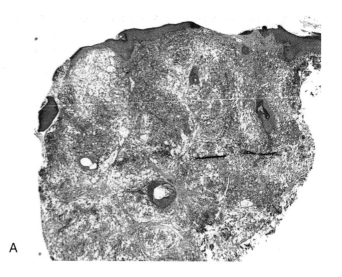

A

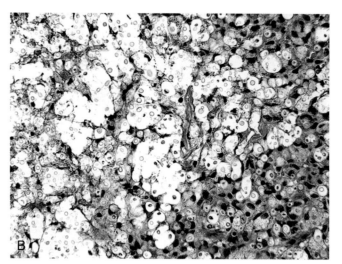

B

43. A 75-year-old man developed a single pink nodule on his scalp. A biopsy was performed, and the specimen is shown. The cells in Panel B show positive immunostaining with cytokeratin 20 in a perinuclear dot pattern. The tumor is negative for S100 protein, melan-A (MART-1), CD99, CD3, CD20, CD79a, and CD45 (leukocyte common antigen). The combined features are features of:

a. Metastatic melanoma
b. Merkel cell carcinoma
c. B-cell lymphoma
d. Leukemia cutis
e. Dermatofibrosarcoma protuberans

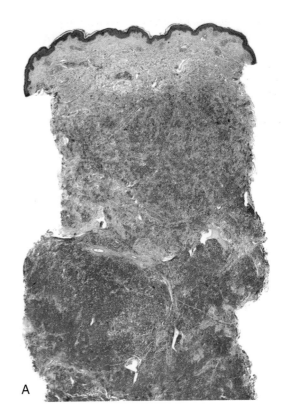

A

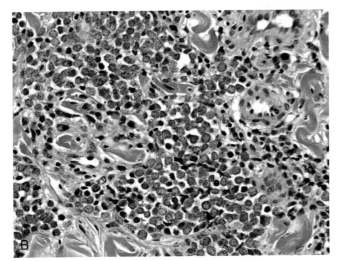

B

44. A 35-year-old woman developed widespread blisters on the trunk and extremities. A biopsy specimen of one of the blisters is shown. Panel B shows a direct immunofluorescence stain for IgG on perilesional skin. Based on the specimen, the diagnosis is:

a. Bullous pemphigoid
b. Contact dermatitis
c. Linear IgA bullous dermatosis
d. Porphyria cutanea tarda
e. Pemphigus vulgaris

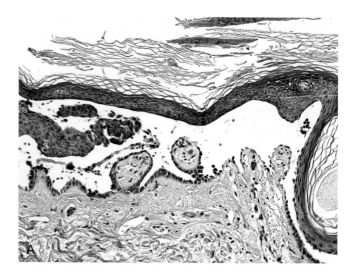

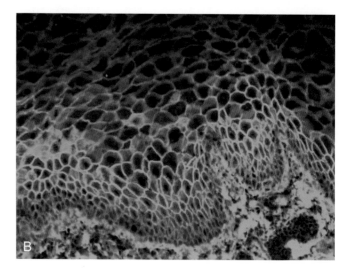

45. A 20-year-old woman has a history of developing pruritic violaceous papules and macules on the dorsum of multiple fingers and toes around the same time each year. The biopsy specimen shown identifies the process as:

a. Lichen planus
b. Erythema multiforme
c. Contact dermatitis
d. Necrolytic acral erythema
e. Pernio

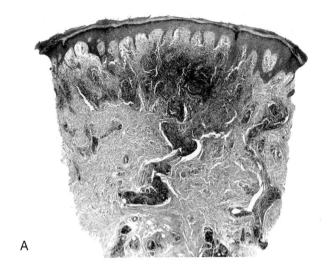

A

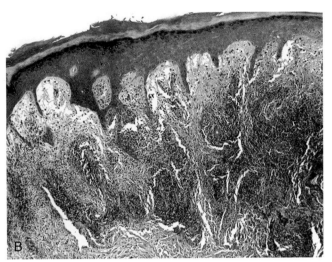

B

46. A 65-year-old woman developed a persistent scaly plaque on the vulva. A biopsy specimen of the lesion shows the cells in the epidermis to be positive for cytokeratin (CK) 7 and negative for CK20. The diagnosis is:

a. Kaposi sarcoma

b. Extramammary Paget disease

c. Basal cell carcinoma

d. Psoriasis

e. Melanoma in situ

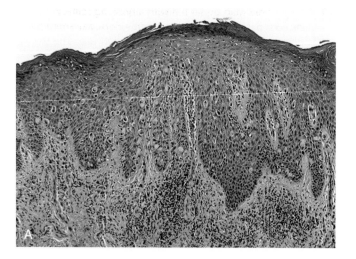

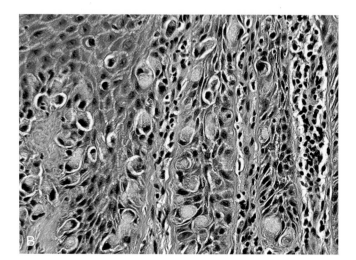

47. A 45-year-old man presented with a growing solitary skin-colored nodule on the left chest. The biopsy specimen is shown. The diagnosis is:
   a. Dermatofibroma
   b. Sclerotic fibroma
   c. Keloid
   d. Myofibroma
   e. Traumatic neuroma

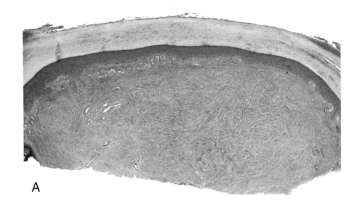

A

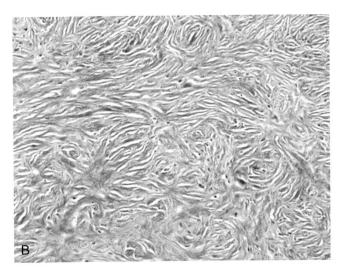

B

48. Which of the following histopathologic findings is the LEAST important prognostic parameter in a biopsy specimen of melanoma?
   a. Tumor thickness (Breslow measurement)
   b. Presence or absence of ulceration
   c. Presence or absence of inflammation
   d. Dermal mitotic rate (mitoses/mm^2)

49. Which of the following histopathologic findings is NOT associated with psoriasis vulgaris?
   a. Confluent parakeratosis
   b. Neutrophils in the parakeratotic horn
   c. Bandlike mononuclear infiltrate in the dermis
   d. Loss of the granular layer
   e. Spongiform pustules of Kogoj

50. Which of the following histologic features is NOT typically associated with lichen planus?
   a. Prominent granular layer
   b. Compact orthokeratosis
   c. Necrotic keratinocytes in the basal layer
   d. Regular acanthosis of the epidermis
   e. A bandlike dermal lymphocytic infiltrate approximating the epidermis

51. Which of the following entities is NOT characterized by subepidermal bulla formation?
   a. Bullous pemphigoid
   b. Pemphigus vulgaris

   c. Porphyria cutanea tarda
   d. Dermatitis herpetiformis
   e. Linear IgA bullous dermatosis

52. Which of the following conditions is NOT characterized by a grenz zone of normal collagen separating the epidermis and dermal infiltrate?
   a. Lepromatous leprosy
   b. Patch stage cutaneous T-cell lymphoma (mycosis fungoides)
   c. Acute myelomonocytic leukemia
   d. Granuloma faciale
   e. Cutaneous marginal zone lymphoma

53. Which of the following histologic features is NOT characteristic of lupus erythematosus?
   a. Hydropic alteration of the basal layer
   b. Thickened basement membrane
   c. Mucin deposition in the dermis
   d. Periadnexal lymphocytic infiltrate
   e. Eosinophils at the dermal-epidermal junction

54. All of the following entities would be in the differential diagnosis of a subcorneal vesicle EXCEPT:
   a. Impetigo
   b. Bullous pemphigoid
   c. Pemphigus foliaceus
   d. Staphylococcal scalded skin syndrome

55. All of the following conditions are associated with mucin deposition in the dermis EXCEPT:
   a. Lupus erythematosus
   b. Papular mucinosis (lichen myxedematosus)
   c. Granuloma annulare
   d. Necrobiosis lipoidica
   e. Basal cell carcinoma

56. A section of skin at "scanning power" looks normal. Which one of the following diagnoses would NOT appear "normal" (i.e., invisible dermatosis) on low magnification?
   a. Macular amyloidosis
   b. Psoriasis vulgaris
   c. Tinea versicolor
   d. Urticaria
   e. Viral exanthem

57. A 50-year-old man developed a rapidly enlarging nodule on the dorsum of the hand. The histologic findings included a craterlike architecture, neutrophilic microabscesses in the proliferating epithelium, and severe dysplasia at the base of the epithelial proliferation. The BEST histologic diagnosis is:
   a. Prurigo nodularis
   b. Keratoacanthoma
   c. Inflamed wart
   d. Deep fungal infection
   e. Reactive perforating collagenosis

58. A 75-year-old man with recently diagnosed lung cancer developed widespread bullae on the extremities. There were no oral lesions. A perilesional skin biopsy specimen was sent for direct immunofluorescence and showed linear deposition of IgG and C3 along the epidermal basement membrane zone. The BEST diagnosis is:
   a. Pemphigus vulgaris

   b. Paraneoplastic pemphigus
   c. Bullous pemphigoid
   d. Dermatitis herpetiformis
   e. Pemphigus foliaceus

59. A 50-year-old woman developed bullae on the extremities and intertriginous areas. She was hospitalized for elective surgical excision of colon carcinoma. In the postoperative period, she developed a wound infection caused by methicillin-resistant *Staphylococcus aureus* and was treated with intravenous vancomycin. A skin biopsy was performed, and a perilesional skin specimen was obtained. Direct immunofluorescence showed linear deposition of IgA at the epidermal basement membrane zone. The BEST diagnosis is:
   a. Paraneoplastic pemphigus
   b. Linear IgA disease
   c. Pemphigus vulgaris
   d. Bullous pemphigoid
   e. Pemphigus foliaceus

60. Which one of the following immunostains is MOST likely to show diffuse positivity in desmoplastic melanoma?
   a. S100 protein
   b. HMB-45
   c. MART-1
   d. MITF

61. Electron microscopy reveals Birbeck granules in:
   a. Langerhans cells
   b. Merkel cells
   c. Melanocytes
   d. Keratinocytes
   e. Mast cells

A NSWERS

1. a. The histologic features of herpes zoster, herpes simplex, and varicella are identical. Early changes in herpes simplex virus (HSV) and varicella-zoster virus (VZV) lesions include nuclear swelling of keratinocytes and individual cell necrosis, and later changes include acantholysis and vesicle formation. Multinucleated giant cells, margination of nuclear chromatin, and molding of nuclei may be present. Clinically, HSV manifests as painful vesicles or punched-out erosions commonly in the orofacial region (HSV-1) or genital region (HSV-2).

Cutaneous cytomegalovirus infection demonstrates enlarged endothelial cells in the dermal vessels. Large nuclear eosinophilic inclusions in endothelial cells, macrophages, or fibrocytes may be seen. Epidermal acantholysis and vesiculation are not characteristic.

Choi YL, Kim JA, Jang KT, et al: Characteristics of cutaneous cytomegalovirus infection in non-acquired immune deficiency syndrome, immunocompromised patients. *Br J Dermatol* 2006;155(5):977-982.

Fatahzadeh M, Schwartz RA: Human herpes simplex virus infections: epidemiology, pathogenesis, symptomatology, diagnosis, and management. *J Am Acad Dermatol* 2007;57(5): 737-763; quiz 764-766.

Weinberg JM: Herpes zoster: epidemiology, natural history, and common complications. *J Am Acad Dermatol* 2007;57(6 Suppl): S130-S135.

2. b. Grover disease, which is shown in the image, is characterized by acantholysis with suprabasilar clefting and keratinocyte dyskeratosis. The pathologic changes may be focal in the biopsy specimen. Clinically, Grover disease resembles an arthropod bite reaction or drug eruption.

Scabies may manifest as an intensely pruritic eruption but on histologic examination characteristically shows a mite, larvae, or excreta in the stratum corneum. Curved, pink "pigtails" in the stratum corneum represent egg fragments or casings left behind by a mite. An eosinophilic infiltrate in the dermis may be present. Varicella demonstrates keratinocyte acantholysis and vesicle formation. Multinucleated giant cells, margination of nuclear chromatin, and molding of nuclei may be present. Clinically, varicella manifests as a vesicular eruption. Pemphigus vulgaris demonstrates a suprabasilar blister and acantholysis, resulting in a "tombstone" appearance of basal keratinocytes that remain attached to the dermis. Acantholysis may extend down adnexal structures. Patients present with mucocutaneous erosions and flaccid blisters rather than pruritic papules. Hailey-Hailey disease is characterized by epidermal intercellular edema and full-thickness acantholysis, resulting in a "dilapidated brick wall" appearance of the epidermis. Dyskeratotic cells are rare. Hailey-Hailey disease is an uncommon genodermatosis that manifests clinically with erythematous plaques, vesicles, and erosions, often in the neck and intertriginous areas.

Fernández-Figueras MT, Puig L, Cannata P, et al: Grover disease: a reappraisal of histopathological diagnostic criteria in 120 cases. Am J Dermatopathol 2010;32(6):541-549.
Leinonen PT, Myllylä RM, Hägg PM, et al. Keratinocytes cultured from patients with Hailey-Hailey disease and Darier disease display distinct patterns of calcium regulation. Br J Dermatol 2005;153(1):113-117.

3. b. The best diagnosis is Sweet syndrome (acute febrile neutrophilic dermatosis), which is characterized by papillary dermal edema and a dense, bandlike infiltrate of neutrophils and leukocytoclasis throughout the papillary dermis and in the upper two thirds of the reticular dermis.

Leukocytoclastic vasculitis is characterized by a neutrophilic infiltrate similar to Sweet syndrome. However, in leukocytoclastic vasculitis, the neutrophils surround or infiltrate the walls of blood vessels in the dermis. It is frequently associated with "nuclear debris" and fibrinoid necrosis of vessel walls. Such vascular damage is not typically seen in Sweet syndrome. Dermatophytosis (tinea infections) most often shows histologic features of an eczematous dermatitis, unless the infection also involves hair follicles, in which case there is typically a suppurative folliculitis. PAS stain shows fungal organisms in the stratum corneum or in hair follicles. Dermatitis herpetiformis is characterized by small collections of neutrophils localized to the dermal papillae, rather than diffusely distributed throughout the dermis as in Sweet syndrome. A subepidermal blister may be seen. Lepromatous leprosy is characterized by a grenz zone of normal collagen separating the epidermis from an infiltrate of foamy histiocytes containing the lepra bacillus. A diffuse neutrophilic infiltrate is not seen.

Dabade TS, Davis MD: Diagnosis and treatment of the neutrophilic dermatoses (pyoderma gangrenosum, Sweet's syndrome). Dermatol Ther 2011;24(2):273-284.
Von den Driesch P: Sweet's syndrome (acute febrile neutrophilic dermatosis). J Am Acad Dermatol 1994;31(4):535-556; quiz 557-560.
Wallach D, Vignon-Pennamen MD: From acute febrile neutrophilic dermatosis to neutrophilic disease: forty years of clinical research. J Am Acad Dermatol 2006;55(6):1066-1071.

4. e. Actinic keratoses, as seen here, are caused by ultraviolet light exposure, resulting in keratinocyte dysplasia. The lesions demonstrate parakeratosis, keratinocyte atypia, and solar elastosis in the dermis.

Extramammary Paget disease demonstrates a pagetoid proliferation of atypical cells in the epidermis with abundant pale cytoplasm containing mucin and large pleomorphic nuclei. The mucin in the cells may be highlighted with mucicarmine, alcian blue at pH 2.5, colloidal iron, and PAS stain. Clinically, extramammary Paget disease manifests as erythematous scaly patches in the genital area. Psoriasis vulgaris is characterized by regular epidermal hyperplasia, loss of the granular layer, and parakeratosis with neutrophils in the stratum corneum. There is a sparse perivascular lymphocytic infiltrate. Atypia of keratinocytes is not seen. Seborrheic dermatitis may demonstrate an acute, subacute, or chronic spongiotic dermatitis. Lesions often have overlying scale crust containing a few neutrophils and may be centered on a hair follicle. Psoriasiform hyperplasia of the epidermis and focal parakeratosis may be seen. Atypia of keratinocytes is not seen. A seborrheic keratosis demonstrates epidermal papillomatosis, acanthosis, and a variable number of horn cysts. No significant cytologic atypia is present.

Sober AJ, Burstein JM: Precursors to skin cancer. Cancer 1995; 75(2 Suppl):645-650.
Uhlenhake EE, Sangueza OP, Lee AD: Spreading pigmented actinic keratosis: a review. J Am Acad Dermatol 2010;63(3):499-506.

5. d. Erythema nodosum is a septal panniculitis. Edema and fibrosis of the septa in the subcutaneous fat are demonstrated. The septal infiltrate is predominantly lymphocytic, with varying numbers of giant cells.

Subcutaneous T-cell lymphoma characteristically demonstrates rimming of neoplastic lymphocytes around individual adipocytes. The atypical lymphocytes have hyperchromatic, irregular nuclei. Erythrophagocytosis ("beanbag cells") by histiocytes may be seen. In contrast to erythema nodosum, there is a prominent lobular inflammatory infiltrate of the fat. Tumid lupus erythematosus demonstrates a superficial and deep lymphoplasmacytic inflammatory infiltrate in the dermis, associated with increased dermal mucin. The subcutaneous fat is not involved. Erythematous plaques often appear on sun-exposed areas on the face and upper trunk. Pancreatic panniculitis is a form of lobular panniculitis, most commonly associated with acute pancreatitis and rarely with pancreatic carcinoma. On histologic examination, pancreatic panniculitis characteristically shows fat necrosis, forming the outlines of dead adipocytes (ghost cells). Nodular vasculitis is a form of lobular panniculitis with granulomatous inflammation and vasculitis. Caseation necrosis may be seen, particularly in cases associated with tuberculosis. Patients often present with painful nodules on the calves.

Gilchrist H, Patterson JW: Erythema nodosum and erythema induratum (nodular vasculitis): diagnosis and management. Dermatol Ther 2010;23(4):320-327.
Requena L, Yus ES: Panniculitis. Part I. Mostly septal panniculitis. J Am Acad Dermatol 2001;45(2):163-183; quiz 184-186.
Requena L, Sánchez Yus E: Erythema nodosum. Semin Cutan Med Surg 2007;26(2):114-125.

6. c. The best diagnosis is cutaneous T-cell lymphoma (mycosis fungoides), which demonstrates exocytosis of atypical mononuclear cells into the epidermis. The lymphocytes in the epidermis are hyperchromatic, have irregular nuclear contours, and typically have a white halo surrounding each one or surrounding small collections, which are referred to as Pautrier microabscesses.

Spongiotic dermatitis is characterized by intercellular edema between keratinocytes, with varying degrees of hyperkeratosis, epidermal acanthosis, and perivascular inflammation. Allergic contact dermatitis, nummular dermatitis, and atopic dermatitis are examples of spongiotic dermatitides. Although lymphocytic exocytosis may be seen in cutaneous T-cell lymphoma, the lymphocytes in a spongiotic dermatitis do not demonstrate hyperchromasia or nuclear irregularity. Psoriasis vulgaris shows epidermal hyperplasia, loss of the granular layer, and parakeratosis with neutrophils in the stratum corneum. There is a sparse perivascular lymphocytic infiltrate. Exocytosis of atypical lymphocytes is not seen. Lichen planus demonstrates a bandlike lymphocytic inflammatory infiltrate at the dermal-epidermal junction, associated with epidermal hyperkeratosis, wedge-shaped hypergranulosis, and peg-shaped rete ridges. There is basal layer vacuolar alteration and colloid body formation, owing to degenerated keratinocytes. Lymphocyte atypia and exocytosis are not prominent features.

Diamandidou E, Colome-Grimmer M, Fayad L: Transformation of mycosis fungoides/Sezary syndrome: clinical characteristics and prognosis. *Blood* 1998;92(4):1150-1159.
Vergier B, de Muret A, Beylot-Barry M, et al: Transformation of mycosis fungoides: clinicopathological and prognostic features of 45 cases. French Study Group of Cutaneous Lymphomas. *Blood* 2000;95(7):2212-2218.
Wilcox RA: Cutaneous T-cell lymphoma: 2011 update on diagnosis, risk-stratification, and management. *Am J Hematol* 2011;86(11):928-948.

7. c. The best histologic diagnosis is Spitz nevus. Spitz nevi are symmetric, well-circumscribed melanocytic proliferations that can be junctional, compound, or dermal. The epidermis is acanthotic, and the melanocytes may be spindled, epithelioid, or both. Ovoid nests of cells often hang vertically in the epidermis and exhibit artifactual clefting from the adjacent epidermal cells.

A nodular melanoma demonstrates atypical collections of melanocytes in the dermis, forming a nodular proliferation. Epidermal involvement is usually not prominent and may be restricted to the area above the dermal nodule. Juvenile xanthogranuloma often manifests as an isolated papule on a child, similar to Spitz nevi. However, on histologic examination, juvenile xanthogranuloma demonstrates a dense, dermal proliferation of histiocytes with characteristic Touton giant cells, which are enlarged histiocytes with foamy cytoplasm surrounded by a wreath of nuclei. A dysplastic nevus demonstrates irregular junctional nests and single melanocytes. The melanocytes show varying degrees of cytologic atypia with enlarged, hyperchromatic nuclei. The papillary dermis shows lamellar fibrosis. A dermal component of nested melanocytes may be present. Spindled and epithelioid melanocytes of Spitz nevi are not a feature of dysplastic nevi. Molluscum contagiosum is due to poxvirus infection and demonstrates endophytic squamous lobules with large eosinophilic inclusions within keratinocytes. These characteristic inclusions are termed Henderson-Patterson bodies. A melanocytic proliferation is not seen.

Sulit DJ, Guardiano RA, Krivda S: Classic and atypical Spitz nevi: review of the literature. *Cutis* 2007;79(2):141-146.
Weedon D, Little JH: Spindle and epithelioid cell nevi in children and adults. A review of 211 cases of the Spitz nevus. *Cancer* 1977;40(1):217-225.

8. a. Melanoma in situ of the lentigo maligna type is the correct diagnosis. Lentigo maligna melanoma in situ demonstrates an increased number of single melanocytes

and confluent nests of melanocytes in the lower epidermis. Solar elastosis is often present in the dermis. Pagetoid melanocytes in the upper portion of the epidermis may be seen but are less common than in the superficial spreading type of melanoma.

A simple lentigo may show an increased number of single melanocytes in the basal layer; however, the melanocytes are neither confluent nor atypical as in lentigo maligna melanoma in situ. There is usually regular elongation of the rete ridges with basal layer hyperpigmentation. A pigmented actinic keratosis demonstrates enlarged and crowded keratinocytes in the epidermis, often associated with parakeratosis and solar elastosis. Increased pigmentation of the basal keratinocytes is present. Melanocytes are neither significantly increased in number nor atypical. Seborrheic keratoses exhibit epidermal acanthosis, hyperkeratosis, and papillomatosis, often with the formation of horn pseudocysts. Melanocytes are neither atypical nor confluent in the epidermis. Bowen disease is a form of squamous cell carcinoma in situ in which there is a "windblown" appearance of the epidermis owing to full-thickness keratinocyte disorganization and atypia. Mitoses and dyskeratotic keratinocytes may be seen, but melanocyte atypia or confluence in the epidermis is not seen.

Cohen LM: Lentigo maligna and lentigo maligna melanoma. *J Am Acad Dermatol* 1995;33(6):923-936; quiz 937-940.
Helm K, Findeis-Hosey J: Immunohistochemistry of pigmented actinic keratoses, actinic keratoses, melanomas in situ and solar lentigines with Melan-A. *J Cutan Pathol* 2008;35(10):931-934.

9. e. Lupus erythematosus would not be part of the differential diagnosis. It typically demonstrates hydropic alteration of the basal layer of the epidermis, thickening of the basement membrane zone, and a periadnexal lymphocytic infiltrate. Spongiosis is not a significant feature of lupus.

Contact dermatitis, nummular dermatitis, photoallergic dermatitis, and atopic dermatitis all are "eczematous dermatoses," the histologic hallmark of which is spongiosis (intercellular edema). The distinction is usually made clinically. Intraepidermal vesicles and eosinophils may be present in acute contact dermatitis. Nummular dermatitis often demonstrates a subacute spongiotic dermatitis, with spongiosis, moderate irregular epidermal acanthosis, and parakeratosis. Photoallergic dermatitis demonstrates variable spongiosis and a lymphohistiocytic inflammatory infiltrate. Eosinophils may be seen in photoallergic reactions from systemic medications. Atopic dermatitis demonstrates variable spongiosis. Chronic lesions may show less spongiosis and inflammation and demonstrate epidermal hyperplasia.

Kamsteeg M, Bergers M, de Boer R: Type 2 helper T-cell cytokines induce morphologic and molecular characteristics of atopic dermatitis in human skin equivalent. *Am J Pathol* 2011; 178(5):2091-2099.
Phelps RG, Miller MK, Singh F: The varieties of "eczema": clinicopathologic correlation. *Clin Dermatol* 2003;21(2): 95-100.

10. c. The best diagnosis is granuloma annulare. Granuloma annulare is a dermal process characterized by foci of altered connective tissue (necrobiosis) often containing mucin and surrounded by a palisade arrangement of histiocytes. The overlying epidermis is normal.

Multicentric reticulohistiocytosis can manifest with papulonodules on the dorsum of the hands. However, it is typically associated with arthritis and is histologically characterized by a diffuse dermal infiltrate of large cells (histiocytes) showing a ground-glass appearance of the cytoplasm. Altered collagen, mucin, and palisading granulomas are not a feature. Granular cell tumors are characterized by large, polygonal cells with small nuclei and granular-appearing cytoplasm. When the infiltrate involves the superficial dermis, there is pseudoepitheliomatous hyperplasia of the epidermis, which can be mistaken for squamous cell carcinoma. Altered collagen, mucin, and palisading granulomas are not a feature. Arthropod bite reactions are characterized by a superficial and deep perivascular and interstitial infiltrate of mononuclear cells and numerous eosinophils. Altered collagen, mucin, and palisading granulomas are not a feature. Cutaneous lesions of sarcoidosis are characteristically a dermal infiltrate of histiocytes and multinucleated giant cells forming a nodular, tuberclelike pattern. Surrounding lymphocytic inflammation is minimal. Altered collagen, mucin, and palisading granulomas are not characteristic.

Boulton AJ, Cutfield RG, Abouganem D, et al: Necrobiosis lipoidica diabeticorum: a clinicopathologic study. *J Am Acad Dermatol* 1988;18(3):530-537.

Dabski K, Winkelmann RK: Generalized granuloma annulare: clinical and laboratory findings in 100 patients. *J Am Acad Dermatol* 1989;20(1):39-47.

11. b. Secondary syphilis is the best diagnosis. The histologic features of secondary syphilis are variable. Typically, biopsy specimens demonstrate psoriasiform hyperplasia; a lichenoid dermatitis; basal layer vacuolization; and a superficial and deep perivascular or periadnexal infiltrate composed of lymphocytes, histiocytes, and granulomas. Numerous plasma cells are characteristic.

Erythema multiforme may show an interface dermatitis at the dermal-epidermal junction associated with basal layer vacuolization, similar to secondary syphilis. However, erythema multiforme is characterized by necrotic keratinocytes in the epidermis, which can result in confluent areas of epithelial necrosis, and a sparse superficial perivascular infiltrate. Discoid lupus erythematosus typically demonstrates hydropic alteration of the basal layer of the epidermis and a periadnexal lymphoplasmacytic infiltrate. Increased dermal mucin, thickening of the basement membrane zone, and follicular plugging also may be seen; these features are not associated with secondary syphilis. Clinically, discoid lupus erythematosus manifests as atrophic, scarred areas with dyspigmentation on sun-exposed skin. Psoriasis demonstrates epidermal hyperplasia, loss of the granular layer, and parakeratosis with neutrophils in the stratum corneum. There is a sparse perivascular lymphocytic infiltrate. In contrast to syphilis, basal layer vacuolization and prominent plasma cells are not typical. Viral exanthems may manifest as a generalized eruption; however, on histologic examination, they typically show a very sparse superficial, perivascular lymphocytic infiltrate and are often close to resembling normal skin.

Abell E, Marks R, Jones EW: Secondary syphilis: a clinico-pathological review. *Br J Dermatol* 1975;93(1):53-61.

Müller H, Eisendle K, Bräuninger W, et al: Comparative analysis of immunohistochemistry, polymerase chain reaction and focus-floating microscopy for the detection of Treponema pallidum in mucocutaneous lesions of primary, secondary and tertiary syphilis. *Br J Dermatol* 2011;165(1):50-60.

12. d. The diagnosis is inflamed seborrheic keratosis. Seborrheic keratoses exhibit epidermal acanthosis, hyperkeratosis, and papillomatosis, often with the formation of horn pseudocysts. Inflamed seborrheic keratoses are associated with a brisk lymphocytic dermal infiltrate, which may be in a lichenoid or eczematous pattern. Squamous cell carcinomas exhibit irregular lobules of atypical, enlarged keratinocytes that extend from the epidermis into the dermis. Keratin pearl formation can be seen. In contrast to squamous cell carcinomas, seborrheic keratoses usually demonstrate a flat, uniform base, without significant cytologic atypia of keratinocytes. Basal cell carcinoma, as distinguished from a seborrheic keratosis, is a predominantly dermal lesion composed of basaloid islands with a peripheral palisade arrangement of nuclei, which exhibit stromal retraction and cell necrosis. They often have a connection with the overlying epidermis. Eccrine poromas demonstrate epidermal acanthosis and a monotonous proliferation of small cuboidal cells. On low magnification, eccrine poromas resemble seborrheic keratoses; however, they often exhibit ductal formation and do not have horn pseudocysts. They most often occur on the palms and soles. Clear cell acanthomas have glycogen-filled cytoplasm, which imparts a clear cell appearance to a very well circumscribed lesion in the epidermis. Some authors believe these lesions are a variant of seborrheic keratosis. They manifest as red papules, most commonly located on the legs.

Noiles K, Vender R: Are all seborrheic keratoses benign? Review of the typical lesion and its variants. *J Cutan Med Surg* 2008; 12(5):203-210.

Sim-Davis D, Marks R, Wilson-Jones E: The inverted follicular keratosis. A surprising variant of seborrheic wart. *Acta Derm Venereol* 1976;56(5):337-344.

13. e. The diagnosis is microcystic adnexal carcinoma. Microcystic adnexal carcinomas are poorly circumscribed eccrine tumors that demonstrate infiltrative epithelial cords associated with a sclerotic stroma. Horn cysts, ducts, and glandlike structures may be seen. Tumor cells may extend into the subcutis and skeletal muscle, and perineural invasion is common.

Morpheaform basal cell carcinoma clinically manifests as a white, scarlike patch or plaque with ill-defined borders. Histologically, the tumor forms cords and strands of basaloid cells that infiltrate a dense collagen stroma. Although the histologic appearance is similar to microcystic adnexal carcinoma, basal cell carcinomas usually do not have ductal structures or horn cysts, and they may exhibit features of typical basal cell carcinomas, such as stromal retraction and mucin deposition. Syringomas are benign eccrine neoplasms that exhibit small ducts embedded in a sclerotic stroma. The ducts may have elongated tails of epithelial cells, forming tadpolelike structures. Deep infiltration of epithelial cells is not seen as in microcystic adnexal carcinoma. Pseudoglandular squamous cell carcinoma demonstrates a proliferation of atypical keratinocytes that form invasive, glandular structures. Ductal structures are not seen. Metastatic adenocarcinoma shows atypical, pleomorphic cells forming glandular structures in the dermis. Mucin deposition may be present. These lesions do not demonstrate the horn cysts or ductal structures that are characteristic of microcystic adnexal carcinoma.

Antley CA, Carney M, Smoller BR: Microcystic adnexal carcinoma arising in the setting of previous radiation therapy. *J Cutan Pathol* 1999;26(1):48-50.

Krahl D, Sellheyer K: Monoclonal antibody Ber-EP4 reliably discriminates between microcystic adnexal carcinoma and basal cell carcinoma. *J Cutan Pathol* 2007;34(10):782-787.

14. a. The best interpretation of the biopsy specimen shown in Panels A and B of the image is morpheaform basal cell carcinoma. Desmoplastic trichoepithelioma histologically resembles morpheaform basal cell carcinoma, but the lesion is differentiated by the presence of multiple horn cysts and calcification. Mitoses and apoptotic bodies are rare compared with basal cell carcinomas. Clinically, desmoplastic trichoepithelioma, similar to morpheaform basal cell carcinoma, typically appears on the face as a small plaque with a raised border or a slightly umbilicated nodule. Microcystic adnexal carcinoma demonstrates infiltrative epithelial cords associated with a sclerotic stroma. Horn cysts and ductal structures may be seen. Tumor cells may extend into the subcutis and skeletal muscle, and perineural invasion is common. Metastatic adenocarcinoma shows atypical, pleomorphic cells forming glandular structures in the dermis. Basaloid cords and islands are not typically seen. Cutaneous lymphadenoma shows basaloid islands of cells with characteristic central, intraepithelial lymphocytes. Cutaneous lymphadenoma is believed to be a variant of trichoblastoma.

Kirchmann TT, Prieto VG, Smoller BR: CD34 staining pattern distinguishes basal cell carcinoma from trichoepithelioma. *Arch Dermatol* 1994;130(5):589-592.

Mamelak AJ, Goldberg LH, Katz TM: Desmoplastic trichoepithelioma. *J Am Acad Dermatol* 2010;62(1):102-106.

Merritt BG, Snow SN, Longley BJ: Desmoplastic trichoepithelioma, infiltrative/morpheaform BCC, and microcystic adnexal carcinoma: differentiation by immunohistochemistry and determining the need for Mohs micrographic surgery. *Cutis* 2010;85(5):254-258.

15. b. This biopsy specimen can be correctly interpreted as in situ acral lentiginous melanoma, which demonstrates increased density of single and nested melanocytes in the basal layer of the epidermis. As the lesion progresses, singly displaced melanocytes can be seen in the upper epidermis as well.

Tinea nigra may manifest similarly to acral lentiginous melanoma as a brown patch on the palm or sole. A biopsy specimen demonstrates brown hyphal elements in the stratum corneum of acral surfaces. No melanocyte atypia is seen. A lentiginous junctional nevus shows single cells and orderly nests of banal melanocytes located in the basal epidermis. The melanocytes are localized to the tips and sides of elongated rete ridges. There is not a contiguous proliferation of melanocytes or cytologic atypia. Lentigo simplex is a 3- to 4-mm lesion characterized by elongated rete ridges and basal layer hyperpigmentation. An increase in the concentration of melanocytes in the basal layer

may be seen, particularly in the rete ridges, but they do not demonstrate contiguous growth or cytologic atypia. Seborrheic keratoses exhibit acanthosis, hyperkeratosis, and papillomatosis. They can show increased pigmentation of the keratinocytes, but they do not exhibit melanocyte atypia or a significant increase in the number of melanocytes.

Bravo Puccio F, Chian C: Acral junctional nevus versus acral lentiginous melanoma in situ: a differential diagnosis that should be based on clinicopathologic correlation. *Arch Pathol Lab Med* 2011;135(7):847-852.

Hutcheson AC, McGowan JW 4th, Maize JC Jr: Multiple primary acral melanomas in African-Americans: a case series and review of the literature. *Dermatol Surg* 2007;33(1):1-10.

16. d. The lesion shown in Panels A and B of the image was diagnosed as pyogenic granuloma, which demonstrates a lobular proliferation of capillaries, an epidermal "collarette," and an edematous stroma. Epidermal atrophy and ulceration are commonly seen.

Amelanotic melanoma may appear as a friable, red papule, similar to a pyogenic granuloma. However, on histologic examination, it is composed of poorly differentiated, pleomorphic melanocytes in the dermis that demonstrate confluent growth and can show pagetoid spread in the epidermis. A lobular proliferation of vessels is not seen. Metastatic renal cell carcinoma usually manifests as a firm, subcutaneous nodule with a predilection for the scalp. On histologic examination, it has a highly vascular stroma. However, it demonstrates poorly circumscribed sheets of "clear cells" that exhibit pleomorphism and mitoses. Nodular Kaposi sarcoma is characterized by a proliferation of hyperchromatic spindle cells that form a vascular slit pattern with extravasated erythrocytes. Nuclear pleomorphism may be seen, and the nuclei stain positively with HHV-8. The lobular architecture of pyogenic granulomas is not characteristic. Bacillary angiomatosis is due to bacterial infection by *Bartonella* species most commonly in HIV-infected patients and may manifest as red, vascular papules similarly to pyogenic granulomas. Bacillary angiomatosis shows a vascular proliferation on histologic examination, but it may be distinguished from pyogenic granuloma by more prominent neutrophilic inflammation throughout the lesion and clumps of bacilli that stain positively with Warthin-Starry or Giemsa stains.

Fortna RR, Junkins-Hopkins JM: A case of lobular capillary hemangioma (pyogenic granuloma), localized to the subcutaneous tissue, and a review of the literature. *Am J Dermatopathol* 2007;29(4):408-411.

Requena L, Sangueza OP: Cutaneous vascular proliferation. Part II. Hyperplasias and benign neoplasms. *J Am Acad Dermatol* 1997;37(6):887-919; quiz 920-922.

17. a. The correct diagnosis is dermatofibroma. Dermatofibroma is characterized by acanthosis of the overlying epidermis with hyperpigmentation of the basal layer. Within the dermis, there is a proliferation of spindle cells that course between and wrap around collagen bundles, producing so-called collagen balls at the periphery of the lesion.

AIDS-related Kaposi sarcoma may show a similar histologic appearance to dermatofibroma, with a proliferation of spindle cells in the dermis. However,

Kaposi sarcoma shows slender spindle cells with focal formation of cleftlike spaces containing red blood cells. These irregular, often jagged, vascular channels tend to separate collagen bundles and surround normal adnexal structures and preexisting blood vessels. Granuloma annulare manifests as annular papules on the extremities of young adults. The histologic finding shows foci of degenerative collagen with mucin surrounded by a palisade arrangement of histiocytes and multinucleated giant cells. Collagen trapping by spindle cells is not typically seen. Dermatofibrosarcoma protuberans is a spindle cell proliferation that may histologically mimic dermatofibroma. However, dermatofibrosarcoma protuberans usually has a normal-appearing epidermis. The spindle cell proliferation forms a storiform pattern in the deep dermis that infiltrates the subcutaneous adipose tissue, yielding a honeycomb pattern. Immunohistochemistry is often used to differentiate dermatofibroma from dermatofibrosarcoma protuberans because dermatofibroma is usually factor XIIIa positive and CD34 negative, whereas dermatofibrosarcoma protuberans is factor XIIIa negative and CD34 positive. Desmoplastic melanoma resembles a scar on histopathology, but the spindle cells are usually oriented perpendicular to the epidermis, and there may be an atypical melanocytic proliferation in the overlying epidermis. Nodular lymphoid aggregates may also be present. The spindle cells label with S100 protein staining. Collagen trapping by spindle cells is not typically seen.

Abenoza P, Lillemoe T: CD34 and factor XIIIa in the differential diagnosis of dermatofibroma and dermatofibrosarcoma protuberans. *Am J Dermatopathol* 1993;15(5):429-434.

Gershtenson PC, Krunic AL, Chen HM: Multiple clustered dermatofibroma: case report and review of the literature. *J Cutan Pathol* 2010;37(9):e42-e45.

Kahn HJ, Fekete E, From L: Tenascin differentiates dermatofibroma from dermatofibrosarcoma protuberans: comparison with CD34 and factor XIIIa. *Hum Pathol* 2001;32(1):50-56.

Kim HJ, Lee JY, Kim SH, et al: Stromelysin-3 expression in the differential diagnosis of dermatofibroma and dermatofibrosarcoma protuberans: comparison with factor XIIIa and CD34. *Br J Dermatol* 2007;157(2):319-324.

18. c.   The best histologic diagnosis is keloids. Keloids are characterized by spindle cells that are associated with thickened, ribbonlike bands of hyalinized eosinophilic connective tissue.

Desmoplastic melanoma demonstrates a spindle cell proliferation that may resemble a scar. However, the thickened ribbons of hyalinized collagen, typical of a keloid, are absent. Leiomyomas are characterized by a poorly circumscribed, fascicular arrangement of spindled smooth muscle cells. The smooth muscle cells have blunt-ended, cigar-shaped nuclei that appear to have a clear halo around them on cross section. Thickened, hyalinized collagen bundles are not seen. Although focal keloidal changes have been reported in dermatofibromas, other characteristic features of dermatofibromas are typically present, such as epidermal acanthosis and spindle cells that course between and wrap around collagen bundles producing collagen balls at the periphery of the lesion. Neurofibromas contain delicate spindle cells with comma-shaped, tapered nuclei

and abundant cytoplasm. There is a pale or myxoid stroma. Thickened, hyalinized collagen bundles are not typically seen.

Busam KJ: Desmoplastic melanoma. *Clin Lab Med* 2011;31(2):321-330.

Seifert O, Mrowietz U: Keloid scarring: bench and bedside. *Arch Dermatol Res* 2009;301(4):259-272.

19. b.   Recurrent (persistent) nevus phenomenon, as seen here, is histologically characterized by a flattened epidermis and scar in the dermis. An asymmetric epidermal melanocytic proliferation is demonstrated with confluent nests of melanocytes and singly displaced melanocytes, confined to the area above the scar.

A junctional nevus is a symmetric, intraepidermal melanocytic proliferation characterized by discrete nests of melanocytes localized to the base of rete ridges. Scar tissue should not be present unless a prior procedure was performed. A halo nevus manifests clinically with a white, depigmented ring surrounding a flesh-colored or pigmented papule, which may appear similar to a recurrent nevus. On histologic examination, a halo nevus demonstrates nested melanocytic cells in association with a dense bandlike lymphocytic infiltrate in the superficial dermis that partially obscures the nests of melanocytes. A blue nevus is characterized by pigmented spindle and dendritic melanocytes localized to the reticular dermis in association with thickened collagen bundles. Scar tissue should not be present unless a prior procedure was performed. Metastatic adenocarcinoma of the breast rarely has an intraepidermal component and is characterized by atypical cells in the dermis, forming glandular structures or infiltrative cords of cells. A junctional melanocytic proliferation and scar tissue are not seen in the epidermis.

Hoang MP, Prieto VG, Burchette JL, et al: Recurrent melanocytic nevus: a histologic and immunohistochemical evaluation. *J Cutan Pathol* 2001;28(8):400-406.

Sommer LL, Barcia SM, Clarke LE, et al: Persistent melanocytic nevi: a review and analysis of 205 cases. *J Cutan Pathol* 2011;38(6):503-507.

20. a.   The history of a slowly enlarging, indurated nodule on the proximal extremity, as shown, is highly suggestive of dermatofibrosarcoma protuberans. CD34 positivity in dermatofibrosarcoma protuberans is useful in differentiating the lesions from dermatofibromas, which are CD34 negative and factor XIIIa positive.

Traditionally, a dermatofibroma is factor XIIIa positive and CD34 negative. In addition to dermatofibromas, factor XIIIa is positive in angiosarcomas, Kaposi sarcomas, fibrous papules, atypical fibroxanthomas, xanthogranulomas, and atypical cells in radiation dermatitis. S100 protein can be detected in a large variety of cells, including melanocytes, Langerhans cells, eccrine and apocrine gland cells, nerve cells, muscle cells, Schwann cells, myoepithelial cells, chondrocytes, and adipocytes. Dermatofibrosarcoma protuberans is usually negative for S100 protein staining. Cytokeratin stains the epidermis, its appendages, and their tumors. Squamous cell carcinomas and adenocarcinomas are positive, whereas lymphomas, sarcomas, and melanomas are negative. Dermatofibrosarcoma protuberans is cytokeratin negative. SMA stains myofibroblastic cells, smooth muscle cells, and their tumors.

Dermatofibrosarcoma protuberans is negative for SMA staining.

Harvell JD, Kilpatrick SE, White WL: Histogenetic relations between giant cell fibroblastoma and dermatofibrosarcoma protuberans: CD34 staining showing the spectrum and a simulator. *Am J Dermatopathol* 1998;20(4):339-345.

Llombart B, Monteagudo C, Sanmartín O, et al: Dermatofibrosarcoma protuberans: a clinicopathological, immunohistochemical, genetic (COL1A1-PDGFB), and therapeutic study of low-grade versus high-grade (fibrosarcomatous) tumors. *J Am Acad Dermatol* 2011; 65(3):564-567.

21. e. The biopsy specimen confirmed a diagnosis of chondrodermatitis nodularis chronica helicis, a lesion on the ear helix and antihelix for which biopsy is commonly indicated. The clinical differential diagnosis often includes basal cell carcinoma and squamous cell carcinoma. The lesion is often ulcerated. Histologically, the epidermis is ulcerated, and beneath the epidermis there is altered hypocellular eosinophilic staining material. There is an increased number of ectatic blood vessels lateral to this area.

Chondrodermatitis nodularis chronica helicis clinically may mimic a squamous cell carcinoma; however, on histologic examination, squamous cell carcinomas consist of irregular masses of epidermal cells that proliferate downward into the dermis. The cells have abundant eosinophilic cytoplasm and large atypical, often vesicular, nuclei. There is variable keratinization and keratin pearl formation, depending on the degree of differentiation of the tumor. An actinic keratosis is characterized by atypical basilar keratinocytes in the epidermis and can be associated with the presence of parakeratosis. Solar elastosis is prominent. These keratoses usually manifest as rough, erythematous papules on sun-exposed skin. Chondrodermatitis nodularis chronica helicis also may mimic a basal cell carcinoma clinically; however, on histologic examination, basal cell carcinomas are composed of islands or nests of basaloid cells, with palisade arrangement of the cells at the periphery and haphazard arrangement of cells in the centers of the islands. The tumor cells have hyperchromatic nuclei with relatively little, poorly defined cytoplasm. Clefting at the stromal-tumor interface with mucin is common. Cutaneous angiosarcomas usually manifest on the head and neck as an enlarging macular area or nodule, which may be ulcerated. However, on histologic examination, angiosarcomas demonstrate irregular anastomosing vascular channels lined by enlarged atypical endothelial cells that dissect between collagen bundles.

Moncrieff M, Sassoon EM: Effective treatment of chondrodermatitis nodularis chronic helicis using a conservative approach. *Br J Dermatol* 2004;150(5):892-894.

Oelzner S, Elsner P: Bilateral chondrodermatitis nodularis chronica helicis on the free border of the helix in a woman. *J Am Acad Dermatol* 2003;49(4):720-722.

22. c. The biopsy specimen showed a granular cell tumor. These tumors are histologically characterized by a monomorphous dermal infiltrate of polygonal cells that have small round nuclei and granular-appearing cytoplasm.

Squamous cell carcinomas consist of irregular masses of epidermal cells that proliferate downward into the dermis.

The cells have abundant eosinophilic cytoplasm and large atypical, often vesicular, nuclei. There is variable central keratinization and keratin pearl formation, depending on the differentiation of the tumor. Intracytoplasmic granules are not seen. Tuberous xanthomas consist of aggregates of foamy cells throughout the dermis, which represent lipid-laden histiocytes. Fibroblasts are increased in number in older lesions, leading to the progressive deposition of collagen. Cholesterol clefts may be found. Polygonal cells with intracytoplasmic granules are not seen. Clinically, tuberous xanthomas are yellowish nodules usually overlying joints. Condyloma accuminatum are caused by human papillomavirus infection and may manifest as papules in the genital region. The histologic finding shows marked acanthosis, with papillomatosis and hyperkeratosis. Although vacuolization of granular cells and koilocytic changes are not as prominent as in classic verrucae vulgaris, the presence of these characteristic features aids in the diagnosis. Lesions may resemble seborrheic keratosis clinically and histologically. Dermatofibromas are characterized by acanthosis of the overlying epidermis with hyperpigmentation of the basal layer. Within the dermis, there is an infiltrate of spindle cells that course between collagen bundles, producing so-called "collagen balls" at the periphery of the lesion. Dermatofibromas usually manifest on the extremities as firm, hyperpigmented nodules.

Gokaslan ST, Terzakis JA, Santagada EA: Malignant granular cell tumor. *J Cutan Pathol* 1994;21(3):263-270.

Janousková G, Campr V, Konkol'ová R, et al: Multiple granular cell tumour. *J Eur Acad Dermatol Venereol* 2004;18(3):347-349.

23. c. The biopsy specimen confirmed a diagnosis of cylindroma. Cylindromas are characterized by aggregates of basaloid cells surrounded by a distinctive eosinophilic cuticle or basement membrane. The configuration of the tumor aggregates resembles the pieces of a jigsaw puzzle. Tubular lumina are sometimes present.

Trichoepitheliomas may be familial; they usually manifest as skin-colored papules or nodules on the face. On histologic examination, trichoepitheliomas are characterized by a lacelike arrangement of basaloid cells. Tumor aggregates are surrounded by an onion-skin pattern of spindle cells, which are probably fibrocytes. Horn cysts and papillary mesenchymal bodies, which consist of basaloid cells that cup around fibroblastic cells, are usually present. Basal cell carcinoma may appear clinically similar to a cylindroma; however, on histologic examination, basal cell carcinoma demonstrates islands or nests of basaloid cells, with a palisade arrangement of the cells at the periphery and a haphazard arrangement of cells in the centers of the islands. The tumor cells have a hyperchromatic nucleus with little, poorly defined cytoplasm. Clefting at the stromal-tumor interface with mucin is common. Papillary mesenchymal bodies are not a feature. Eccrine spiradenomas may appear as nodules on the face and scalp, similar to cylindromas. On histologic examination, spiradenomas are well-circumscribed lobules that appear as "blue balls" in the dermis. They are composed of two cell types: cells with small dark nuclei located at the periphery and large pale nuclei located in the center of the aggregates. Eosinophilic PAS-positive basement membrane material may be seen in the lobules. Histologic features of spiradenoma and cylindroma may occur in the same lesion. Pilomatricomas often manifest as solitary nodules on the head and neck. Histopathologically, they are characterized by aggregates of basaloid cells that transition to enucleated shadow or ghost cells. Granulomatous inflammation, calcification, and occasionally cartilage or bone are often present.

Schirren CG, Wörle B, Kind P, et al: A nevoid plaque with histological changes of trichoepithelioma and cylindroma in Brooke-Spiegler syndrome. An immunohistochemical study with cytokeratins. *J Cutan Pathol* 1995;22(6):563-569.

Szepietowski JC, Wasik F, Szybejko-Machaj G, et al: Brooke-Spiegler syndrome. *J Eur Acad Dermatol Venereol* 2001; 15(4):346-349.

24. c. The correct diagnosis is juvenile xanthogranuloma. Juvenile xanthogranuloma is characterized by a dense diffuse arrangement of histiocytes and multinucleated giant cells of the Touton type in the dermis. The overlying epidermis is flattened, and the infiltrate abuts the epidermis. Eosinophils are common.

Intradermal nevus may appear clinically similar to juvenile xanthogranuloma but on histopathologic examination would show nests and cords of banal nevus cells in the upper dermis without a junctional component. Glomus tumor displays a well-circumscribed solid mass composed of uniform round cells with pale cytoplasm and central punched-out nuclei. Small blood vessels are distributed in the tumor. In contrast to juvenile xanthogranuloma, glomus tumor usually manifests as blue-red papules or nodules on the extremities, particularly the subungual area, and may be painful. Mastocytoma most commonly manifests in young children as a red or yellow plaque that may urticate when stroked. Histologically, mast cells lie closely packed in tumorlike aggregates within dermal papillae and the dermis. Their nuclei are cuboidal and show ample granular cytoplasm. Eosinophils may be present in the lesion. Arthropod bites usually manifest as erythematous, pruritic papules. The classic histopathology of an arthropod bite is a superficial and deep, perivascular and interstitial inflammatory dermal infiltrate composed of lymphocytes and eosinophils, often in association with an overlying focus of epidermal spongiosis.

Asarch A, Thiele JJ, Ashby-Richardson H, et al: Cutaneous disseminated xanthogranuloma in an adult: case report and review of the literature. *Cutis* 2009;83(5):243-249.

Hernandez-Martin A, Baselga E, Drolet BA, et al: Juvenile xanthogranuloma. *J Am Acad Dermatol* 1997;36(Pt 1):355-367; quiz 368-369.

Zvulunov A, Barak Y, Metzker A: Juvenile xanthogranuloma, neurofibromatosis, and juvenile chronic myelogenous leukemia: world statistical analysis. *Arch Dermatol* 1995;131(8):904-908.

25. d. The best diagnosis is pilomatricoma, which is characterized by aggregates of basaloid cells that transition to enucleated shadow or ghost cells. Granulomatous inflammation, calcification, and occasionally cartilage or bone are present. Pilomatricoma usually manifests as a solitary lesion on the head, neck, or upper extremities of young children.

Basal cell carcinoma may appear as a solitary skin-colored lesion, similar to a pilomatricoma. However, basal cell

carcinomas are composed of islands or nests of basaloid cells, with a palisade arrangement of the cells at the periphery and a haphazard arrangement of the cells in the centers of the islands. The tumor cells have a hyperchromatic nucleus with little, poorly defined cytoplasm. Clefting at the stromal-tumor interface with mucin is common. Basal cell carcinoma would be highly unlikely in a young child. Trichoepitheliomas often manifest as skin-colored papules or nodules on the face. However, on histologic examination, trichoepitheliomas are characterized by islands of basaloid cells in the dermis. Tumor aggregates are surrounded by an onion-skin pattern of fibrocytes. Horn cysts are usually present as well as papillary mesenchymal bodies, which consist of basaloid cells that cup around fibroblastic cells, recapitulating the follicular papillary mesenchyme. Pilar or trichilemmal cysts may manifest as solitary nodules on the head and neck area. Histologically, these cysts are lined by stratified squamous epithelium showing trichilemmal keratinization without formation of a granular layer. The cells in the lining increase in bulk and vertical diameter toward the lumen. The cyst contains compact, homogeneous eosinophilic material. Acute folliculitis shows an area of perifollicular inflammation with numerous neutrophils. Although granulomatous inflammation may be present, basaloid cells transitioning to shadow cells are not seen.

Hardisson D, Linares MD, Cuevas-Santos J, et al: Pilomatrix carcinoma: a clinicopathologic study of six cases and review of the literature. *Am J Dermatopathol* 2001;23(5):394-401.

Julian CG, Bowers PW: A clinical review of 209 pilomatricomas. *J Am Acad Dermatol* 1998;39(2 Pt 1):191-195.

Marrogi AJ, Wick MR, Dehner LP: Pilomatrical neoplasms in children and young adults. *Am J Dermatopathol* 1992;14(2): 87-94.

26. b. The image depicts trichoepithelioma, which is characterized by islands of basaloid cells surrounded by an onion-skin pattern of fibrocytes. Occasional horn cysts and abortive hair follicles may be present. The lesions often contain papillary mesenchymal bodies, which consist of basaloid cells that cup around fibroblastic cells, recapitulating the follicular papillary mesenchyme. Stromal retraction of tumor islands is not seen.

Similar to trichoepithelioma, basal cell carcinoma comprises islands or nests of basaloid cells. A palisade arrangement of the cells at the periphery of the islands may be seen in both basal cell carcinoma and trichoepithelioma. However, basal cell carcinoma demonstrates a haphazard arrangement of cells in the centers of the islands, often with necrotic cells. The tumor cells have a hyperchromatic nucleus with little, poorly defined cytoplasm. Clefting at the stromal-tumor interface with mucin deposition is common. Horn cysts and papillary mesenchymal bodies are not typically seen. A trichilemmoma usually manifests as a flesh-colored papule on the face or neck, sometimes with a verrucous surface. Histologically, it is characterized by an endophytic, lobular proliferation of pale-staining keratinocytes, which contain glycogen. An eosinophilic hyaline cuticle lines the periphery of the lobules. Multiple trichilemmomas may be a marker for Cowden disease. Cylindroma may manifest as a flesh-colored papule or nodule on the scalp or face. Histologically, it is characterized by aggregates of basaloid cells surrounded by a distinctive eosinophilic cuticle composed of basement membrane material. The configuration of the tumor aggregates resembles the pieces of a jigsaw puzzle. Merkel cell carcinoma may appear as a flesh-colored nodule often on the face, head, or neck of an older individual. On histologic examination, it is composed of small, round-to-oval blue cells of uniform size with a vesicular nucleus and multiple small nucleoli. Mitoses and apoptotic bodies are usually numerous.The cytoplasm is scanty and amphophilic, and the cell borders are vaguely defined. Merkel cell carcinoma demonstrates positive cytokeratin 20 staining in a perinuclear dot pattern. Horn cysts and papillary mesenchymal bodies are not seen.

Abdelsayed RA, Guijarro-Rojas M, Ibrahim NA, et al: Immunohistochemical evaluation of basal cell carcinoma and trichepithelioma using Bcl-2, Ki67, PCNA and P53. *J Cutan Pathol* 2000;27(4):169-175.

Bettencourt MS, Prieto VG, Shea CR: Trichoepithelioma: a 19-year clinicopathologic re-evaluation. *J Cutan Pathol* 1999;26(8): 398-404.

Kirchmann TT, Prieto VG, Smoller BR: CD34 staining pattern distinguishes basal cell carcinoma from trichoepithelioma. *Arch Dermatol* 1994;130(5):589-592.

Pham TT, Selim MA, Burchette JL Jr, et al: CD10 expression in trichoepithelioma and basal cell carcinoma. *J Cutan Pathol* 2006;33(2):123-128.

27. a. The best diagnosis is apocrine hidrocystoma, which demonstrates a large cystic space in the dermis, lined by a row of columnar cells exhibiting decapitation secretion. Decapitation secretion is characteristic of apocrine glands. The lesions usually manifest as translucent cystic nodules on the face.

Pilar cysts typically manifest as subcutaneous nodules on the scalp. On histologic examination, a well-circumscribed cyst is filled with homogeneous eosinophilic keratin, and the lining exhibits abrupt keratinization without a granular layer. Venous lakes manifest as soft, compressible, blue papules on sun-exposed skin, most often on the face, lips, and ears. Histologic appearance demonstrates a dilated vascular space with erythrocytes, lined by a single layer of flattened endothelial cells. Decapitation secretion is not seen. Epidermal inclusion cyst often manifests as a subcutaneous nodule, usually with a central punctum. Histologic appearance demonstrates a keratin-filled cyst lined by stratified squamous epithelium with a granular layer present. Superficial lymphangioma (lymphangioma circumscriptum) often occurs in infancy and manifests as clear, cystic, vesiclelike lesions. Histologic examination shows one or more dilated, thin-walled lymphatic vessels in the dermis that closely abut the epidermis. The vessels may contain eosinophilic lymph fluid or red blood cells. Decapitation secretion is not seen.

de Viragh PA, Szeimies RM, Eckert F: Apocrine cystadenoma, apocrine hidrocystoma, and eccrine hidrocystoma: three distinct tumors defined by expression of keratins and human milk fat globulin 1. *J Cutan Pathol* 1997;24(4):249-255.

Sarabi K, Khachemoune A: Hidrocystomas—a brief review. *MedGenMed* 2006;8(3):57.

28. c. The best histologic diagnosis is neurofibroma, which demonstrates a well-circumscribed, nonencapsulated proliferation of spindle cells with wavy nuclei and scant cytoplasm. The lesion is embedded in a pale, loose collagen stroma. Mast cells are often present.

Nodular melanoma demonstrates a confluent proliferation of atypical single and nested melanocytes in the dermis. The lesion is poorly circumscribed and asymmetric, and the dermal cells often show mitoses and nuclear pleomorphism. Although melanomas may comprise spindle cells, the cells typically do not have the wavy nuclei characteristic of a neurofibroma. Piloleiomyoma is a benign smooth muscle tumor derived from the arrector pili muscle. Histologic appearance demonstrates poorly circumscribed fascicles of spindle cells in the dermis. As opposed to the wavy nuclei of neural cells, smooth muscle cells can be identified by their blunt-ended, cigar-shaped nuclei with a perinuclear vacuole. Dermal nevi can appear clinically similar to neurofibromas. However, on histologic examination, a dermal nevus demonstrates uniform nests of banal, cuboidal melanocytes within the dermis. Spindle cell proliferation is not seen. Dermatofibromas manifest as hyperpigmented, firm nodules. On histologic examination, there is proliferation of spindle cells in the dermis that often wrap around collagen bundles at the periphery of the lesion, forming collagen balls. Epidermal hyperplasia and basal layer pigmentation are usually present.

Boyd KP, Korf BR, Theos A: Neurofibromatosis type 1. *J Am Acad Dermatol* 2009;61(1):1-14.

Jouhilahti EM, Peltonen S, Callens T, et al: The development of cutaneous neurofibromas. *Am J Pathol* 2011;178(2):500-505.

29. b. The best diagnosis is sarcoidosis, which is a granulomatous disorder. On histologic examination, sarcoidosis demonstrates nodular collections in the dermis composed of epithelioid histiocytes and multinucleated giant cells, with minimal surrounding inflammation. Caseation necrosis is absent or minimal.

Multicentric reticulohistiocytosis manifests with nodules on the dorsal hands and is typically associated with a mutilating arthritis. In contrast to the nodular collections of histiocytes seen in sarcoidosis, multicentric reticulohistiocytosis is characterized by a diffuse dermal proliferation of large cells with a ground-glass appearance of the cytoplasm. The cells may be multinucleated. Juvenile xanthogranuloma often manifests in children as an isolated, yellowish papule. On histologic examination, juvenile xanthogranuloma demonstrates a dense, dermal proliferation of histiocytes with characteristic Touton giant cells, which are enlarged histiocytes containing foamy cytoplasm surrounded by a wreath of nuclei. A foreign body granuloma may demonstrate noncaseating granulomas composed of histiocytes and giant cells, similar to sarcoidosis. However, polariscopic examination shows doubly refractile material, such as silica. Knife marks in the tissue are also suggestive of foreign material. The presence of polarizable material on histopathologic examination should not exclude a concurrent diagnosis of sarcoidosis, which may occur in sites of trauma or scars. Tuberculoid leprosy can be difficult to distinguish histologically from sarcoidosis. However, the granulomas in tuberculoid leprosy often appear elongated because they follow nerves and are more likely to demonstrate central necrosis. The inflammatory infiltrate is usually more pronounced in tuberculoid leprosy granulomas compared with sarcoid granulomas.

Cardoso JC, Cravo M, Reis JP, et al: Cutaneous sarcoidosis: a histopathological study. *J Eur Acad Dermatol Venereol* 2009; 23(6):678-682.

Marchell RM, Judson MA: Cutaneous sarcoidosis. *Semin Respir Crit Care Med* 2010;31(4):442-451.

Miida H, Ito M: Tuberculoid granulomas in cutaneous sarcoidosis: a study of 49 cases. *J Cutan Pathol* 2010;37(4):504-506.

30. d. Verrucae plana (flat warts) are caused by HPV infection, usually HPV-3 and HPV-10. They demonstrate basket-weave hyperkeratosis and acanthosis, with diffuse vacuolization of the cells of the granular and upper spinous layers and pyknotic nuclei, creating a "bird's eye" appearance of the cells. Hypergranulosis is common.

Tinea versicolor often manifests with tan, slightly scaly patches on the trunk and extremities that may appear similar to flat warts. On histologic examination, tinea versicolor demonstrates multiple hyphae and spores in the stratum corneum, which can be highlighted with PAS staining. Epidermodysplasia verruciformis is a genetic disorder that predisposes to HPV infection by multiple strains, including HPV-3, HPV-5, and HPV-8. The flat warts seen in epidermodysplasia verruciformis infection are usually more persistent and widespread than verrucae plana. Although the histologic appearance may resemble verrucae plana, epidermodysplasia verruciformis usually demonstrates large cells in the granular and spinous layers. The cells have a blue-gray cytoplasm, a clear nucleoplasm, and a perinuclear halo. Although lichen planus can manifest with multiple flat-topped papules, they are usually violaceous in color and pruritic. On biopsy, lichen planus demonstrates a bandlike lymphocytic inflammatory infiltrate in the superficial dermis, associated with epidermal hyperkeratosis, wedge-shaped hypergranulosis, and peg-shaped rete ridges. There is basal layer vacuolar alteration and colloid body formation owing to degenerated keratinocytes. Verrucae vulgaris are also caused by HPV infection. However, in contrast to verrucae plana, verrucae vulgaris classically demonstrate marked epidermal acanthosis and hyperkeratosis, with columns of parakeratosis overlying papillomatous projections. The valleys of the projections show vacuolated, koilocytic cells with pyknotic nuclei and clumping of keratohyaline granules.

Nuovo GJ, Ishag M: The histologic spectrum of epidermodysplasia verruciformis. *Am J Surg Pathol* 2000;24(10):1400-1406.

Stierman S, Chen S, Nuovo G, et al: Detection of human papillomavirus infection in trichilemmomas and verrucae using in situ hybridization. *J Cutan Pathol* 2010;37(1):75-80.

31. c. The best histologic diagnosis is porokeratosis (disseminated superficial actinic type). On histologic examination, all forms of porokeratosis demonstrate a cornoid lamella, which is a column of parakeratotic cells beneath which there is absence or diminution of the granular layer as well as dyskeratotic or vacuolated keratinocytes. The cornoid lamella corresponds clinically to the raised, keratotic or threadlike rim that is seen in lesions of porokeratosis. Solar elastosis is often found in the dermis in lesions of disseminated superficial actinic porokeratosis.

Verrucae plana are caused by HPV infection, usually HPV-3 and HPV-10. They appear as multiple pink or tan papules on the extremities. On histologic examination, verrucae plana demonstrate hyperkeratosis, hypergranulosis, and acanthosis, with diffuse vacuolization of the cells of the granular and upper spinous layers. Granuloma annulare may manifest with multiple annular lesions. On histologic examination, granuloma annulare is a dermal process characterized by foci of altered connective tissue containing mucin and surrounded by a palisade arrangement of histiocytes. The overlying epidermis is normal. Subacute cutaneous lupus erythematosus may manifest with multiple annular, scaly papules and plaques on sun-exposed areas. On histologic examination, subacute cutaneous lupus erythematosus demonstrates a lymphocytic interface dermatitis at the dermal-epidermal junction, associated with vacuolar degeneration of the basal layer and increased mucin in the dermis. Cornoid lamellae are not seen. Tinea corporis also may manifest with annular, scaly papules and plaques. On histologic examination, multiple hyphae are present in the stratum corneum that can be highlighted by PAS staining. Cornoid lamellae are not seen.

Murase J, Gilliam AC: Disseminated superficial actinic porokeratosis co-existing with linear and verrucous porokeratosis in an elderly woman: update on the genetics and clinical expression of porokeratosis. *J Am Acad Dermatol* 2010;63(5):886-891.

Sertznig P, von Felbert V, Megahed M: Porokeratosis: present concepts. *J Eur Acad Dermatol Venereol* 2012;26(4):404-412.

32. d. The best diagnosis is gout. On formalin-fixed biopsy specimens, gouty tophi demonstrate aggregates of amorphous white material, which are often walled off by a rim of macrophages and multinucleated giant cells. On high-power views, the amorphous material displays needle-shaped, radial clefts, where the urate crystals have dissolved.

Calcinosis cutis may manifest with subcutaneous nodules over joints that discharge white material. The condition may be idiopathic, metastatic secondary to hypercalcemia, or associated with diseases such as dermatomyositis and systemic scleroderma. On histologic examination, calcinosis cutis demonstrates deposits of deeply basophilic material in the dermis or subcutaneous tissue. The deposits stain black with Von Kossa staining. Tuberous xanthomas may manifest with large nodules on the elbows, most commonly in patients with hyperlipidemia. On histologic examination, the lesions demonstrate diffuse dermal aggregates of foam cells, which represent lipid-laden macrophages. Inflammation is minimal. The lipid within the foam cells can be highlighted with oil red O staining of frozen sections. Granuloma annulare manifests with papular lesions on the extremities, and deep granuloma annulare may form nodular lesions. On histologic examination, granuloma annulare is characterized by foci of altered connective tissue in the dermis, which often contain mucin and are surrounded by a palisade arrangement of histiocytes. The mucin in the center of the palisade areas forms so-called "blue granulomas." Rheumatoid nodules may occur over joints, similar to gout. However, on histologic examination, rheumatoid nodules demonstrate areas of histiocytes in a palisade arrangement that surround areas of necrobiosis and fibrin within the deep dermis and subcutis. The central necrobiotic areas are usually homogeneous and eosinophilic, forming "red granulomas."

Falasca GF: Metabolic diseases: gout. *Clin Dermatol* 2006;24(6): 498-508.
Nielsen GP, Rosenberg AE, O'Connell JX, et al: Tumors and diseases of the joint. *Semin Diagn Pathol* 2011;28(1):37-52.
Thissen CA, Frank J, Lucker GP: Tophi as first clinical sign of gout. *Int J Dermatol* 2008;47(Suppl 1):49-51.

33. b. The best histologic diagnosis is lichen sclerosus et atrophicus, which most commonly involves the genital region, although extragenital lesions may occur. Histologic appearance demonstrates epidermal atrophy, hyperkeratosis, and follicular plugging. A vacuolar interface dermatitis is present, and subepidermal collagen demonstrates a zone of edematous or pink, homogenized collagen. There is a perivascular, bandlike lymphocytic infiltrate beneath this zone. This infiltrate is pushed downward as the zone of homogenized collagen expands.

Condyloma latum is a manifestation of secondary syphilis and manifests as moist, white papules in the genital region. Histologic appearance demonstrates epidermal hyperplasia and a lichenoid inflammatory infiltrate with numerous plasma cells. Staining with Warthin-Starry stain or immunoperoxidase techniques may reveal the *Treponema pallidum* causative organism. The homogenization of collagen seen in lichen sclerosus et atrophicus is not present. Histologically, morphea and lichen sclerosus et atrophicus may appear similar because they share many overlapping features, such as thickening and eosinophilia of collagen bundles. However, morphea is distinguished by sclerotic collagen in the lower dermis and subcutaneous fat, and it lacks basal layer vacuolar alteration, follicular plugging, or bandlike edema of the superficial dermis. Clinically, morphea occurs as indurated plaques on the trunk and extremities. Lichen planus may manifest with white, sometimes reticulated, patches on mucosal surfaces, including the anogenital region. It may also show a lichenoid infiltrate as is seen in lichen sclerosus. However, the edema and homogenization of superficial collagen of lichen sclerosus is not seen in lichen planus. Cicatricial pemphigoid is an autoimmune blistering disorder that may cause blisters, erosions, and scarring of mucosal surfaces. Histologic appearance demonstrates subepidermal blister formation and mixed inflammatory infiltrate, usually with eosinophils. Although dermal fibrosis may be present, bandlike homogenization of collagen and basal layer vacuolar alteration are not features of cicatricial pemphigoid.

Murphy R: Lichen sclerosus. *Dermatol Clin* 2010;28(4):707-715.
Ross SA, Sànchez JL, Taboas JO: Spirochetal forms in the dermal lesions of morphea and lichen sclerosus et atrophicus. *Am J Dermatopathol* 1990;12(4):357-362.
Zollinger T, Mertz KD, Schmid M, et al: Borrelia in granuloma annulare, morphea and lichen sclerosus: a PCR-based study and review of the literature. *J Cutan Pathol* 2010;37(5):571-577.

34. b. The best histologic diagnosis is erythema multiforme. Erythema multiforme demonstrates a sparse, lymphocytic interface dermatitis associated with basal layer vacuolization. Dyskeratotic keratinocytes are present at all levels of the epidermis, which may result in confluent epidermal necrosis. The stratum corneum shows basket-weave orthokeratosis. Eosinophils are rare in erythema multiforme except in cases that are medication-induced. The most common cause of erythema multiforme is orolabial HSV infection.

Acute generalized exanthematous pustulosis is a widespread eruption that is often secondary to medications. Multiple pinpoint pustules are seen on physical examination, and a biopsy specimen shows subcorneal neutrophils. The histologic appearance of a fixed drug eruption may appear identical to erythema multiforme, with a vacuolar interface dermatitis and epidermal dyskeratosis. However, compared with erythema multiforme, fixed drug eruptions tend to show a greater amount of pigment incontinence, a polymorphous inflammatory infiltrate with eosinophils and neutrophils, and a deeper infiltrate. Fixed drug eruptions usually manifest as a solitary, dusky plaque, which can be bullous. Subacute cutaneous lupus erythematosus may manifest as a lymphocytic vacuolar interface dermatitis, as seen in erythema multiforme; however, it typically does not exhibit full-thickness epidermal dyskeratosis and more likely shows compact hyperkeratosis and edema of the dermis with increased mucin. Subacute cutaneous lupus erythematosus clinically manifests as annular, scaly patches in sun-exposed areas. Viral exanthems typically show a very sparse superficial, perivascular lymphocytic infiltrate and are often close to resembling "normal skin." Significant dyskeratosis is not seen. Clinically, a viral exanthem manifests as a morbilliform, erythematous eruption.

Brice SL, Krzemien D, Weston WL, et al: Detection of herpes simplex virus DNA in cutaneous lesions of erythema multiforme. *J Invest Dermatol* 1989;93(1):183-187.
Wetter DA, Davis MD: Recurrent erythema multiforme: clinical characteristics, etiologic associations, and treatment in a series of 48 patients at Mayo Clinic, 2000 to 2007. *J Am Acad Dermatol* 2010;62(1):45-53.

35. b. The best diagnosis is dermatitis herpetiformis. On histologic examination, dermatitis herpetiformis demonstrates neutrophilic microabscesses localized to the dermal papillae, associated with subepidermal blister formation. Direct immunofluorescence of noninvolved perilesional skin reveals IgA deposition at the dermal-epidermal junction and in the dermal papillae in a granular pattern.

Hematoxylin-eosin staining of bullous pemphigoid demonstrates a subepidermal blister with eosinophils. Direct immunofluorescence demonstrates deposition of IgG and C3 at the basement membrane zone in a linear pattern. Hematoxylin-eosin staining of linear IgA disease shows a subepidermal blister with neutrophils. Direct immunofluorescence testing is diagnostic, revealing linear deposition of IgA at the basement membrane zone, in contrast to the granular pattern of IgA seen in dermatitis herpetiformis. Hematoxylin-eosin staining of pemphigus vulgaris demonstrates a suprabasilar blister and acantholysis. Direct immunofluorescence of pemphigus vulgaris is characterized by deposition of IgG between the cells of the epidermis, forming a "fishnet" pattern. Direct immunofluorescence of lichen planus shows colloid bodies containing IgM, linear and shaggy deposition of fibrinogen at the dermal-epidermal junction, and occasionally granular deposits of IgM or linear deposits of C3 with or without IgG at the basement membrane zone.

Rose C, Armbruster FP, Ruppert J, et al: Autoantibodies against epidermal transglutaminase are a sensitive diagnostic marker in patients with dermatitis herpetiformis on a normal or gluten-free diet. *J Am Acad Dermatol* 2009;61(1):39-43.

Templet JT, Welsh JP, Cusack CA: Childhood dermatitis herpetiformis: a case report and review of the literature. *Cutis* 2007;80(6):473-476.

36. c. The patient's history and biopsy specimen suggest a diagnosis of cutaneous mastocytosis (i.e., urticaria pigmentosa, which is the most common childhood form). Giemsa stain is a metachromatic stain that is used to identify the granules in mast cells. Mast cell granules stain purple, eosinophils stain bright pink, and lymphocytes stain blue. Giemsa stain can also be used to identify infectious organisms, such as spirochetes, protozoa, and cutaneous *Leishmania*.

Alcian blue stains acid mucopolysaccharides blue. Sulfated mucopolysaccharides, such as chondroitin sulfate and heparan sulfate, stain at a pH of 2.5 and 0.5, whereas nonsulfated mucopolysaccharides (e.g., hyaluronic acid) stain at a pH of 2.5 only. Alcian blue is useful for detecting acidic mucin in neoplasms; inflammatory conditions; and dermatoses, including granuloma annulare, lupus erythematosus, and pretibial myxedema. Verhoeff–Van Gieson stain is a silver stain that stains elastic fibers blue-black to black. This stain is useful for detecting elastic fiber abnormalities as well as for identifying the elastic lamina of vessels. Warthin-Starry stain is a silver stain that is used to highlight bacterial organisms, such as spirochetes, including *Treponema pallidum*, and *Bartonella* bacilli. The organisms stain black, and the background stains golden yellow. Von Kossa stain is a silver stain that stains calcium deposits black.

Briley L, Phillips C: Cutaneous mastocytosis: a review focusing on the pediatric population. *Clin Pediatr* 2008;47(8):757-761.

Valent P, Akin C, Sperr WR, et al: Mastocytosis: pathology, genetics, and current options for therapy. *Leuk Lymphoma* 2005;46(1):35-48.

37. a. Eosinophilic inclusion bodies that form in the cytoplasm of keratinocytes in molluscum contagiosum are called Henderson-Patterson bodies or molluscum bodies. Henderson-Patterson bodies are a key histologic feature on the biopsy specimen shown.

Epithelial cells infected by human papillomavirus classically demonstrate koilocytotic nuclei, which are pyknotic and shriveled ("raisinoid") in appearance and demonstrate distinct perinuclear vacuolization. Koilocytic nuclei can be seen in verrucae vulgaris and condylomata acuminata. Mikulicz cells are large mononuclear cells with vacuolated cytoplasm found in lesions of rhinoscleroma. Within the cytoplasm of these cells, many bacilli (gram-negative rod *Klebsiella pneumoniae* subsp. *rhinoscleromatis*) can be seen. Rhinoscleroma manifests as nodules of the upper respiratory tract that may lead to extensive disfigurement. Multinucleated giant cells with intranuclear inclusions are found in herpesvirus infections, including herpes simplex, varicella, and herpes zoster. Other histologic features of herpesvirus infections include epidermal acantholysis, margination of nuclear chromatin, and molding of nuclei. Donovan bodies are vacuolated macrophages that contain multiple bacilli (the gram-negative rod *K. granulomatis*) in their cytoplasm. Donovan bodies are characteristically seen in biopsy specimens of granuloma inguinale, a sexually transmitted disease that clinically manifests as chronic beefy red, ulcerating nodules in the genital region.

Cribier B, Scrivener Y, Grosshans E: Molluscum contagiosum: histologic patterns and associated lesions. A study of 578 cases. *Am J Dermatopathol* 2001;23(2):99-103.

Dohil MA, Lin P, Lee J, et al: Epidemiology of molluscum contagiosum in children. *J Am Acad Dermatol* 2006;54(1):47-54.

38. b. Leukocytoclastic vasculitis is the best diagnosis. Leukocytoclastic vasculitis is characterized by neutrophils surrounding or infiltrating the walls of blood vessels in the dermis. It is frequently associated with "nuclear debris" (leukocytoclasis) and fibrinoid necrosis of the vessel wall. Streptococcal infection and medications are common causes of leukocytoclastic vasculitis.

Sweet syndrome (acute febrile neutrophilic dermatosis) is characterized by papillary dermal edema and a dense bandlike infiltrate of neutrophils throughout the papillary dermis and in the upper two thirds of the reticular dermis. Although endothelial cell swelling and mild vascular injury may be seen, frank leukocytoclastic vasculitis is not a feature of Sweet syndrome. Pigmented purpuric dermatosis may manifest with purpura on the lower extremities, but lesions are typically not palpable. On histologic examination, it is characterized by a lymphocytic perivascular infiltrate limited to the papillary dermis associated with extravasated red blood cells and hemosiderin-laden macrophages. Although mild vascular damage may be present, frank vessel wall necrosis and neutrophilic inflammation are not features. Erythema nodosum is the prototype of a septal panniculitis. Although streptococcal infection and medications may trigger erythema nodosum, the histopathologic picture differs from leukocytoclastic vasculitis. Early lesions of erythema nodosum show edema of the septa with a predominantly lymphohistiocytic infiltrate. Later lesions show widening and fibrosis of the septa, with chronic inflammation at the septal edges. Granulomas and multinucleated giant cells are commonly seen. Vascular injury with fibrinoid necrosis is not a characteristic feature. Polyarteritis nodosa is characterized by a panarteritis involving medium and small arteries and usually manifests with subcutaneous nodules or livedo reticularis. As in leukocytoclastic vasculitis, the histopathologic examination shows a necrotizing leukocytoclastic vasculitis, but polyarteritis nodosa affects medium-sized arteries, which are usually located in the lower dermis or the subcutis. Intimal proliferation and thrombosis may lead to occlusion of the lumen and subsequent ulceration. The small vessels of the upper dermis often remain intact.

Fiorentino DF: Cutaneous vasculitis. *J Am Acad Dermatol* 2003; 48(3):311-340.

Grzeszkiewicz TM, Fiorentino DF: Update on cutaneous vasculitis. *Semin Cutan Med Surg* 2006;25(4):221-225.

39. c. SMA stains myofibroblastic cells, smooth muscle cells, and their tumors. Glomus cells are thought to be of smooth muscle origin and often stain positively with SMA. Glomus cells typically do not stain positively with S100 protein, EMA, or CD34. S100 protein can be detected in a

of staining with S100 protein and MART-1 excludes this diagnosis. Many types of B-cell lymphoma can involve the skin, either as a primary or as a secondary process. The histologic features vary with the type of lymphoma present. In the scenario presented, the lack of staining with the B-cell markers CD20 and CD79a exclude this diagnosis. Leukemia cutis is seen on histologic examination as atypical cells infiltrating between collagen bundles in the dermis; the atypical cells can form sheetlike areas in the dermis. The lack of staining with CD45, or leukocyte common antigen, excludes this diagnosis. Dermatofibrosarcoma protuberans is characterized histologically by a spindle cell proliferation in the dermis that overtakes the adipose tissue and stains positively for CD34. These histologic features are not seen in the image.

Chang Y, Moore PS: Merkel cell carcinoma: a virus-induced human cancer. *Annu Rev Pathol* 2012;7:123-144.

Wang TS, Byrne PJ, Jacobs LK, et al: Merkel cell carcinoma: update and review. *Semin Cutan Med Surg* 2011;30(1):48-56.

Wong HH, Wang J: Merkel cell carcinoma. *Arch Pathol Lab Med* 2010;134(11):1711-1716.

44. e. On histologic examination, pemphigus vulgaris has the features of an intraepidermal blister that demonstrates acantholysis. A characteristic feature is the presence of "tombstones," which refer to basal layer keratinocytes that remain attached to the basement membrane zone.

A biopsy specimen taken from a blister of a patient with bullous pemphigoid would show a subepidermal blister, which usually demonstrates a prominent eosinophilic infiltrate, although a paucicellular variant is also recognized. Contact dermatitis histologically demonstrates epidermal spongiosis. If the reaction is prominent, spongiotic vesicles can be seen in the epidermis. Eosinophils can be seen in spongiotic areas of the epidermis (eosinophilic spongiosis) or in the dermis. Linear IgA bullous dermatosis demonstrates a subepidermal blister associated with a neutrophilic inflammatory infiltrate on routinely stained sections. Porphyria cutanea tarda demonstrates a paucicellular subepidermal blister with "festooning" of the dermal papillae. Clinically, lesions are generally localized to sun-exposed areas.

Guillen S, Khachemoune A: Pemphigus vulgaris: a short review for the practitioner. *Dermatol Nurs* 2007;19(3):269-272.

Mihai S, Sitaru C: Immunopathology and molecular diagnosis of autoimmune bullous diseases. *J Cell Mol Med* 2007;11(3):462-481.

Parker SR, MacKelfresh J: Autoimmune blistering diseases in the elderly. *Clin Dermatol* 2011;29(1):69-79.

Schmidt E, Zillikens D: Modern diagnosis of autoimmune blistering skin diseases. *Autoimmun Rev* 2010;10(2):84-89.

45. e. The image shows pernio, or chilblains. Pernio is characterized by a superficial and deep perivascular and perieccrine inflammatory infiltrate that usually is seen in skin biopsy specimens of acral skin.

Although lichen planus manifests with pruritic violaceous lesions and can affect acral skin sites, the histopathologic picture is that of a lichenoid dermatitis, with a bandlike inflammatory infiltrate that abuts the epidermis and is associated with epidermal hyperplasia. Erythema multiforme usually affects acral sites, but the histologic appearance is characterized by an interface dermatitis

without involvement of the deep dermal adnexal structures or perivascular areas. Clinically, one could consider contact dermatitis in a case in which a rash cyclically appears. However, the histologic features of contact dermatitis typically show a spongiotic dermatitis, and the deep perivascular and periadnexal areas are unaffected. Although necrolytic acral erythema occurs on acral sites, the lesions are characterized histologically by the presence of pallor of the epidermis, focal necrosis, spongiosis, and parakeratosis.

Almahameed A, Pinto DS: Pernio (chilblains). *Curr Treat Options Cardiovasc Med* 2008;10(2):128-135.

Boada A, Bielsa I, Fernández-Figueras MT, et al: Perniosis: clinical and histopathological analysis. *Am J Dermatopathol* 2010;32(1):19-23.

Simon TD, Soep JB, Hollister JR: Pernio in pediatrics. *Pediatrics* 2005;116(3):e472-e475.

46. b. The diagnosis is extramammary Paget disease, which is characterized histologically by atypical cells present at all levels of the epidermis. Kaposi sarcoma is characterized histologically by spindle cell proliferation in the dermis that forms slitlike vascular spaces and is positive for HHV-8. Basal cell carcinoma can manifest as a scaly patch but is characterized by a proliferation of basaloid cells that show a peripheral palisade arrangement of nuclei, necrosis, and retraction artifact. Psoriasis is commonly located on the genitals, but the histologic appearance demonstrates psoriasiform epidermal hyperplasia and dilated capillaries in the papillary dermis. Although melanoma in situ typically shows atypical cells in a pagetoid pattern, the melanocytes are usually pigmented and are not positive for CK7.

Hegarty PK, Suh J, Fisher MB, et al: Penoscrotal extramammary Paget's disease: the University of Texas M. D. Anderson Cancer Center contemporary experience. *J Urol* 2011;186(1):97-102.

Lam C, Funaro D: Extramammary Paget's disease: summary of current knowledge. *Dermatol Clin* 2010;28(4):807-826.

Mendivil AA, Abaid L, Epstein HD, et al: Paget's disease of the vulva: a clinicopathologic institutional review. *Int J Clin Oncol* 2012;17(6):569-574.

Stranahan D, Cherpelis BS, Glass LF, et al: Immunohistochemical stains in Mohs surgery: a review. *Dermatol Surg* 2009;35(7):1023-1034.

47. b. The diagnosis is sclerotic fibroma. Sclerotic fibroma is characterized histologically by the presence of thickened, hyalinized collagen bundles that are hypocellular and form a distinctive "plywood" or storiform pattern. Dermatofibroma demonstrates a fibrohistiocytic proliferation in the dermis with collagen wrapping at the periphery and associated epidermal hyperplasia. Keloid is a form of a hypertrophic scar that is characterized by the presence of thickened, eosinophilic collagen bundles, associated with scar tissue. Myofibroma is characterized by nodular collections of myofibroblasts that are surrounded at the periphery by vascular channels. Traumatic neuroma is characterized by collections of nerve fascicles that are embedded in scar tissue. The fascicles of nerves are surrounded by fibrous tissue.

González-Vela MC, Val-Bernal JF, González-López MA, et al: Pure sclerotic neurofibroma: a neurofibroma mimicking sclerotic fibroma. *J Cutan Pathol* 2006;33(1):47-50.

González-Vela MC, Val-Bernal JF, Martino M, et al: Sclerotic fibroma-like dermatofibroma: an uncommon distinctive variant of dermatofibroma. *Histol Histopathol* 2005;20(3): 801-806.

High WA, Stewart D, Essary LR, et al: Sclerotic fibroma-like change in various neoplastic and inflammatory skin lesions: is sclerotic fibroma a distinct entity? *J Cutan Pathol* 2004;31(5): 373-378.

48. c. The least important prognostic parameter in a biopsy specimen of melanoma is the presence or absence of inflammation. The significance of inflammation in melanomas has been controversial, partly because the assessment of the host lymphocytic infiltrate has a significant subjective component. Although the presence of tumor-infiltrating lymphocytes influences the prognosis in some studies, inflammation is not a significant factor that influences therapeutic decision making.

Maximum tumor (Breslow) thickness is measured from the granular layer of the overlying epidermis or base of a superficial ulceration to the deepest malignant cells invading the dermis. In most prognostic studies, the measured depth of a melanoma is considered to be the most powerful independent factor for prediction of lymph node metastasis and survival. Ulceration is defined as tumor-induced full-thickness loss of the epidermis with subjacent dermal tumor and reactive dermal changes. The presence of ulceration has been found to be an adverse independent prognostic factor in melanomas. Mitotic rate is measured as the number of dermal mitoses per square millimeter. The mitotic rate should be reported in any melanoma showing a vertical growth phase component. Several large studies have emphasized the prognostic importance of the mitotic rate in melanomas.

Bichakjian CK, Halpern AC, Johnson TM, et al: Guidelines of care for the management of primary cutaneous melanoma. *J Am Acad Dermatol* 2011;65(5):1032-1047.

Piris A, Mihm MC Jr, Duncan LM: AJCC melanoma staging update: impact on dermatopathology practice and patient management. *J Cutan Pathol* 2011;38(5):394-400.

49. c. A bandlike mononuclear infiltrate in the dermis that hugs the overlying epidermis is characteristic of lichen planus and is not typical of psoriasis. Confluent parakeratosis (retention of nuclei in the keratinocytes of the stratum corneum) is best seen in fully developed plaque lesions of psoriasis. It is often associated with underlying hypogranulosis in the epidermis. Mounds of parakeratosis with neutrophils in the stratum corneum, also known as Munro microabscesses, represent an early key diagnostic feature of psoriatic lesions. Other key diagnostic features are a diminished to absent granular layer and the presence of spongiform pustules of Kogoj, formed by collections of neutrophils in the spinous and granular layers.

Griffiths CE, Barker JN: Pathogenesis and clinical features of psoriasis. *Lancet* 2007;370(9583):263-271.

Nestle FO, Kaplan DH, Barker J: Psoriasis. *N Engl J Med* 2009; 361(5):496-509.

50. d. The epidermal acanthosis in lichen planus is irregular, giving a saw-toothed appearance to the rete ridges. Regular acanthosis of the epidermis is characteristic of a psoriasiform dermatitis. Lichen planus demonstrates wedge-shaped,

nonconfluent areas of a thickened granular layer, termed *wedge-shaped hypergranulosis.* The cornified layer of lichen planus often shows compact orthokeratosis. The presence of parakeratosis suggests a lichenoid drug eruption. Necrotic keratinocytes are present in the basal layer of lichen planus and may appear as dull, pink globules, which are referred to as colloid, hyaline, cytoid, or Civatte bodies. The infiltrate in the upper dermis in lichen planus is bandlike and composed almost entirely of lymphocyte intermingled with macrophages.

Boyd AS, Neldner KH: Lichen planus. *J Am Acad Dermatol* 1991; 25(4):593-619.

Scully C, Carrozzo M: Oral mucosal disease: lichen planus. Br J Oral Maxillofac Surg 2008;46(1):15-21.

51. b. Pemphigus vulgaris is characterized by suprabasal separation with intraepidermal acantholysis. Although the basal cells lose their intercellular bridges, they remain attached to the dermis, resulting in a "tombstone" appearance.

Bullous pemphigoid is characterized by a subepidermal bulla with a prominent infiltrate of eosinophils in the dermis and blister cavity. Porphyria cutanea tarda results in a cell-poor, subepidermal blister with preservation of the dermal papillae in the floor, called "festooning." PAS-positive material is often found around the vessel walls in the dermal papillae and upper dermis. Dermatitis herpetiformis shows a subepidermal blister with an intense inflammatory infiltrate of neutrophils and some eosinophils. In early lesions, the presence of dermal papillary neutrophilic microabscesses is a characteristic feature. Linear IgA bullous dermatosis is a subepidermal blistering disease in which neutrophils are the predominant cell type in the blister cavity or along the dermal-epidermal junction. In contrast to dermatitis herpetiformis, the lesions have a lower tendency to form papillary microabscesses.

Korman N: Bullous pemphigoid. *J Am Acad Dermatol* 1987; 16(5 Pt 1):907-924.

Kolanko E, Bickle K, Keehn C, et al: Subepidermal blistering disorders: a clinical and histopathologic review. *Semin Cutan Med Surg* 2004;23(1):10-18.

Mutasim DF, Adams BB: Immunofluorescence in dermatology. *J Am Acad Dermatol* 2001;45(6):803-822.

52. b. Patch stage mycosis fungoides shows a patchy bandlike infiltrate of lymphocytes that approximates the dermal-epidermal junction within a fibrotic papillary dermis. The epidermis is characterized by tagging of atypical lymphocytes along the basement membrane and exocytosis of atypical lymphocytes within the epidermis. The lymphocytes have hyperchromatic nuclei and are surrounded by a clear "halo." Pautrier microabscesses, defined as clustered epidermotropic atypical lymphocytes within the epidermis, are highly characteristic of mycosis fungoides. A grenz zone is not typically seen in patch stage cutaneous T-cell lymphoma.

Lepromatous leprosy is characterized by a grenz zone of normal collagen separating the epidermis from a dermal infiltrate of foamy histiocytes containing the lepra bacillus. In cutaneous infiltrates of acute myelomonocytic leukemia, there is a monomorphous infiltrate of atypical leukemic cells through the dermis with the presence of a grenz zone in the superficial dermis. In granuloma faciale, beneath the grenz zone of normal collagen, there is a diffuse mixed inflammatory infiltrate, often including neutrophils, eosinophils, and mononuclear cells. Vasculitic changes, including perivascular inflammation with nuclear dust and vessel wall damage, may be seen. In cutaneous marginal zone lymphoma, there is a dermal cellular infiltrate that may extend into the subcutis with preservation of a grenz zone in the superficial dermis and sparing of the epidermis. The infiltrate has a nodular or diffuse pattern characterized by neoplastic cells that infiltrate around reactive lymphoid follicles. The cells of marginal zone lymphoma are composed of centrocytelike cells with cleaved nuclei, monocytoid cells with round nuclei and more prominent pale cytoplasm, or lymphoplasmacytoid cells.

Baldassano MF, Bailey EM, Ferry JA, et al: Cutaneous lymphoid hyperplasia and cutaneous marginal zone lymphoma: comparison of morphologic and immunophenotypic features. *Am J Surg Pathol* 1999;23(1):88-96.

Ortonne N, Wechsler J, Bagot M, et al: Granuloma faciale: a clinicopathologic study of 66 patients. *J Am Acad Dermatol* 2005;53(6):1002-1009.

Wong TY, Suster S, Bouffard D, et al: Histologic spectrum of cutaneous involvement in patients with myelogenous leukemia including the neutrophilic dermatoses. *Int J Dermatol* 1995;34(5):323-329.

53. e.   Eosinophils are rarely seen in connective tissue disorders such as lupus erythematosus. Their presence should suggest an alternative diagnosis. Eosinophils lining the dermal-epidermal junction is a histologic feature characteristic of bullous pemphigoid.

Hydropic alteration of the basal layer manifests as vacuolization and swelling of basal cells in the epidermis. Hydropic alteration is a feature of all vacuolar interface dermatitides, including lupus erythematosus, and is usually associated with an inflammatory infiltrate at the dermal-epidermal junction. Lupus erythematosus is usually associated with a thickened basement membrane, particularly in established lesions. A PAS stain highlights basement membrane thickening. Increased dermal mucin, both superficially and deep, is seen in lupus erythematosus but can also be seen in other connective tissue disorders, such as dermatomyositis. The mucin can be highlighted with alcian blue or colloidal iron stain. Lesions of lupus erythematosus, particularly the discoid and tumid variants, often show periadnexal lymphocytic inflammation around hair follicles and eccrine glands. Plasma cells may also be found.

Cozzani E, Christana K, Rongioletti F, et al: Lupus erythematosus tumidus: clinical, histopathological and serological aspects and therapy response of 21 patients. *Eur J Dermatol* 2010; 20(6):797-801.

Fabbri P, Amato L, Chiarini C, et al: Scarring alopecia in discoid lupus erythematosus: a clinical, histopathologic and immunopathologic study. *Lupus* 2004;13(6):455-462.

França AF, de Souza EM: Histopathology and immunohistochemistry of depigmented lesions in lupus erythematosus. *J Cutan Pathol* 2010;37(5):559-564.

54. b.   Bullous pemphigoid demonstrates a subepidermal blister, often with numerous eosinophils in the inflammatory infiltrate. Early lesions may demonstrate eosinophilic spongiosis. Subcorneal vesicles are not a characteristic feature, so it would not be included in the differential diagnosis.

Impetigo contagiosa typically demonstrates a vesicopustule in the subcorneal layer, with numerous neutrophils. Many gram-positive cocci are present within the pustule. Pemphigus foliaceus is an autoimmune blistering disorder that demonstrates a blister in the subcorneal or upper epidermal layers with acantholytic keratinocytes and dyskeratotic granular cells. Neutrophils may be present in the blister cavity. Pemphigus foliaceus demonstrates intercellular IgG antibody deposition in the epidermis using direct immunofluorescence. Staphylococcal scalded skin syndrome may demonstrate subcorneal splitting of the epidermis as well as a few acantholytic cells and sparse neutrophils in the blister cavity. There is a sparse, mixed inflammatory infiltrate in the underlying dermis.

Hanakawa Y, Stanley JR: Mechanisms of blister formation by staphylococcal toxins. *J Biochem* 2004;136(6):747-750.

Stanley JR, Amagai M: Pemphigus, bullous impetigo, and the staphylococcal scalded-skin syndrome. *N Engl J Med* 2006; 355(17):1800-1810.

55. d.   Necrobiosis lipoidica is not characterized by mucin deposition. It typically shows thickened, hyalinized collagen bundles arranged parallel to the epidermis in a tiered pattern, associated with a patchy lymphoplasmacytic infiltrate.

Characteristic histopathologic findings of cutaneous lupus erythematosus are vacuolar (hydropic) alteration of the basal layer of the epidermis, a thickened basement membrane, interstitial mucin deposition in the superficial and deep dermis, and a lymphocytic inflammatory infiltrate. Papular mucinosis (lichen myxedematosus) demonstrates diffuse mucin deposition, increased collagen, and fibroblast proliferation that replaces the dermal connective tissue. Granuloma annulare is characterized by a dermal process with foci of altered connective tissue containing mucin, which are surrounded by a palisade arrangement of histiocytes, forming so-called blue granulomas. Basal cell carcinoma is characterized by mucin deposition within and surrounding the tumor aggregates. The mucin at the periphery of the tumor results in retraction of the tumor nodules from the surrounding stroma.

Güneş P, Göktay F, Mansur AT, et al: Collagen-elastic tissue changes and vascular involvement in granuloma annulare: a review of 35 cases. *J Cutan Pathol* 2009;36(8):838-844.

Lloyd J, Flanagan AM: Mammary and extramammary Paget's disease. *J Clin Pathol* 2000;53(10):742-749.

Rongioletti F, Rebora A: Updated classification of papular mucinosis, lichen myxedematosus, and scleromyxedema. *J Am Acad Dermatol* 2001;44(2):273-281.

56. b.   Psoriasis vulgaris is not on the differential diagnosis for a "normal" skin biopsy specimen. It is characterized by regular epidermal hyperplasia, loss of the granular layer, and parakeratosis with neutrophils in the stratum corneum. Neutrophilic microabscesses may be seen in the upper spinous and granular layers. There is also usually a sparse perivascular lymphocytic infiltrate.

Macular amyloidosis may appear unremarkable on a low-power view. Hematoxylin-eosin staining reveals subtle, amorphous, pink deposits of amyloid in the papillary dermis. Melanophages are often seen within the dermal deposits. The amyloid can be highlighted with Congo red staining, crystal violet and methyl violet, and cotton pagoda red dye. On a low-power view, tinea versicolor may appear normal, with a mild, superficial perivascular inflammatory infiltrate and mild epidermal hyperkeratosis and acanthosis. In the stratum corneum, there are numerous round budding yeasts and septate hyphae, giving a "spaghetti and meatballs" appearance. The causative *Pityrosporum* organisms are clearly seen on hematoxylin-eosin stain but may be highlighted with PAS stain. Urticaria may look normal on a low-power view. A higher power examination reveals a perivascular and interstitial distribution of lymphocytes, eosinophils, and neutrophils in the dermis. A variable amount of dermal edema is present. Small blood vessels may be dilated with swollen endothelial cells. Viral exanthems typically show a very sparse superficial, perivascular lymphocytic infiltrate and are often close to resembling normal skin.

Mendez-Tovar LJ: Pathogenesis of dermatophytosis and tinea versicolor. *Clin Dermatol* 2010;28(2):185-189.

Schreml S, Szeimies RM, Vogt T, et al: Cutaneous amyloidoses and systemic amyloidoses with cutaneous involvement. *Eur J Dermatol* 2010;20(2):152-160.

Toppe E, Haas N, Henz BM: Neutrophilic urticaria: clinical features, histological changes and possible mechanisms. *Br J Dermatol* 1998;138(2):248-253.

57. b. The best histologic diagnosis is keratoacanthoma, which demonstrates an exoendophytic squamous proliferation of well-differentiated, eosinophilic, large keratinocytes. It has a keratin-filled crater and is circumscribed by an epidermal buttress. There is often a dense dermal inflammatory infiltrate containing neutrophils and eosinophils. Clinically, keratoacanthoma manifests as a rapidly growing lesion that may exhibit spontaneous involution.

Prurigo nodularis demonstrates a dome-shaped lesion exhibiting irregular epidermal hyperplasia, hyperkeratosis, and hypergranulosis. The papillary dermis shows fibroplasia and an increased number of small vessels. It is caused by chronic scratching. An inflamed wart (verruca vulgaris) may manifest as an enlarging, crateriform or verrucous nodule. On histologic examination, warts characteristically demonstrate marked epidermal acanthosis and hyperkeratosis, with columns of parakeratosis overlying the papillomatous projections. The valleys of the projections show vacuolated, koilocytic cells with pyknotic nuclei and clumping of keratohyaline granules. Keratinocyte dysplasia is not seen. Pseudoepitheliomatous hyperplasia, which is characteristic of a deep fungal infection, can mimic the epidermal features of both keratoacanthoma and well-differentiated squamous cell carcinoma. However, deep fungal infections typically are associated with granulomatous inflammation, often together with small neutrophilic abscesses in the dermis (in contrast to neutrophilic abscesses in the epithelium in keratoacanthoma). PAS or Gomori methenamine silver staining highlights fungal organisms. Reactive perforating collagenosis demonstrates a saucer-shaped invagination containing neutrophilic debris and vertically oriented strands of collagen that have perforated through the epidermis.

Ko CJ: Keratoacanthoma: facts and controversies. *Clin Dermatol* 2010;28(3):254-261.

Mandrell JC, Santa Cruz D: Keratoacanthoma: hyperplasia, benign neoplasm, or a type of squamous cell carcinoma? *Semin Diagn Pathol* 2009;26(3):150-163.

Petrie M, Eliezri Y, Campanelli C: Keratoacanthoma of the head and neck with perineural invasion: incidental finding or cause for concern? *Dermatol Surg* 2010;36(7):1209-1213.

58. c. The best diagnosis is bullous pemphigoid. The classic direct immunofluorescence pattern of bullous pemphigoid includes deposition of IgG or C3 or both at the epidermal basement membrane zone.

Pemphigus vulgaris shows a direct immunofluorescence pattern of intercellular IgG deposition in the epidermis. Paraneoplastic pemphigus shows a direct immunofluorescence pattern of IgG or C3 deposition in the intercellular and basement membrane zones of the epidermis. Dermatitis herpetiformis shows a direct immunofluorescence pattern of granular deposits of IgA in the dermal papillae and the basement membrane zone in perilesional skin. The direct immunofluorescence pattern of pemphigus foliaceus is intercellular deposition of IgG and C3. This intercellular staining is sometimes localized solely to the upper epidermal cell layers.

Charneux J, Lorin J, Vitry F, et al: Usefulness of BP230 and BP180-NC16a enzyme-linked immunosorbent assays in the initial diagnosis of bullous pemphigoid: a retrospective study of 138 patients. *Arch Dermatol* 2011;147(3):286-291.

Di Zenzo G, Della Torre R, Zambruno G, et al: Bullous pemphigoid: from the clinic to the bench. *Clin Dermatol* 2012;30(1):3-16.

Schmidt E, Della Torre R, Borradori L: Clinical features and practical diagnosis of bullous pemphigoid. *Dermatol Clin* 2011;29(3):427-438; viii-ix.

59. b. Findings of direct immunofluorescence are classic for linear IgA disease. Direct immunofluorescence shows deposition of IgA in a linear pattern at the epidermal basement membrane zone. Vancomycin is a well-known trigger of linear IgA disease.

Direct immunofluorescence of paraneoplastic pemphigus shows IgG or C3 deposition in the intercellular and basement membrane zones of the epidermis. Clinically, paraneoplastic pemphigus usually manifests with prominent oropharyngeal erosions and ulcerations, in addition to skin lesions. Pemphigus vulgaris shows a direct immunofluorescence pattern of intercellular IgG deposition in the epidermis. It manifests with erosions and flaccid blisters of mucocutaneous areas. The direct immunofluorescence pattern of bullous pemphigoid shows linear deposition of IgG or C3 or both at the epidermal basement membrane zone. The direct immunofluorescence pattern of pemphigus foliaceus shows intercellular deposition of IgG and C3. The intercellular staining is sometimes localized solely to the upper epidermal cell layers.

Fortuna G, Marinkovich MP: Linear immunoglobulin A bullous dermatosis. *Clin Dermatol* 2012;30(1):38-50.

Mintz EM, Morel KD: Clinical features, diagnosis, and pathogenesis of chronic bullous disease of childhood. *Dermatol Clin* 2011;29(3):459-462; ix.

Palmer RA, Ogg G, Allen J, et al: Vancomycin-induced linear IgA disease with autoantibodies to BP180 and LAD285. *Br J Dermatol* 2001;145(5):816-820.

60. a. Although tumor cells in desmoplastic melanoma usually do not produce melanin, they stain positively for S100 protein in approximately 95% of cases. Generally, other melanocytic markers, such as HMB-45, MART-1, and MITF, are negative in desmoplastic melanoma and are not useful in confirming the diagnosis. HMB-45 is a monoclonal antibody that targets a melanocyte-specific melanosome membrane protein. Although it is routinely used in the diagnosis of cutaneous malignant melanomas and other melanocytic tumors, it is generally negative in desmoplastic melanomas. MART-1 is a melanocyte differentiation antigen located on melanosomes and endoplasmic reticulum. MART-1 is a specific melanocyte marker that is routinely used in the diagnosis of cutaneous malignant melanomas and other melanocytic tumors, but it is generally negative in desmoplastic melanomas. MITF is a melanocytic nuclear protein that is critical for the development and survival of melanocytes. Although MITF staining may be positive in some melanomas, it is usually negative in desmoplastic melanomas. In addition, it is nonspecific and may stain macrophages, smooth muscle cells, and Schwann cells.

Baer SC, Schultz D, Synnestvedt M, et al: Desmoplasia and neurotropism. Prognostic variables in patients with stage I melanoma. *Cancer* 1995;76(11):2242-2247.

Ramos-Herberth FI, Karamchandani J, Kim J, et al: SOX10 immunostaining distinguishes desmoplastic melanoma from excision scar. *J Cutan Pathol* 2010;37(9):944-952.

Yeh I, McCalmont TH: Distinguishing neurofibroma from desmoplastic melanoma: the value of the CD34 fingerprint. *J Cutan Pathol* 2011;38(8):625-630.

61. a. The Birbeck granule or Langerhans granule is characteristically found in the cytoplasm of Langerhans cells. This organelle, when cut in cross section, is often recognizable because of its resemblance in shape to a tennis racquet.

Merkel cells are normally present in the basal layer of the epidermis. They function in mechanoreception and are found in touch-sensitive areas in glabrous and hairy skin. Electron microscopy shows neurosecretory granules in the cytoplasm. Electron microscopy of a melanocyte shows cytoplasmic melanosomes in different stages of development. Electron microscopy of a keratinocyte shows bundles of tonofibrils in the cytoplasm. Melanosomes may also be seen. Electron microscopy of a mast cell shows densely packed, cytoplasmic granules, which appear similar to cylindrical membrane scrolls.

Hussein MR: Skin-limited Langerhans' cell histiocytosis in children. *Cancer Invest* 2009;27(5):504-511.

Koch S, Kohl K, Klein E, et al: Skin homing of Langerhans cell precursors: adhesion, chemotaxis, and migration. *Allergy Clin Immunol* 2006;117(1):163-168.

CHAPTER 14

MUSCLE AND PERIPHERAL NERVE PATHOLOGY

Kurenai Tanji

QUESTIONS

Questions 1-17 refer to a photograph or photomicrograph.

1. Which one of the following statements is CORRECT for normal skeletal muscle?
   a. Type II muscle fibers (the darkly stained fibers by adenosine triphosphatase [ATPase] in panel B) are slow-twitch, and the lightly stained type I are fast-twitch.
   b. Energy for type II fiber contraction is derived mainly from anaerobic glycolysis.
   c. Type II fibers are rich in mitochondria.
   d. Type II fibers are slow to fatigue.
   e. Type II fibers become hypertrophic in steroid myopathy.

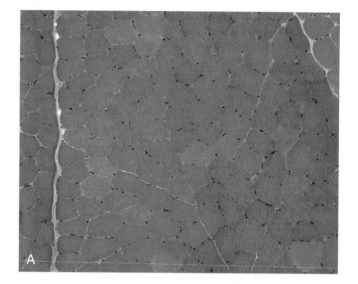

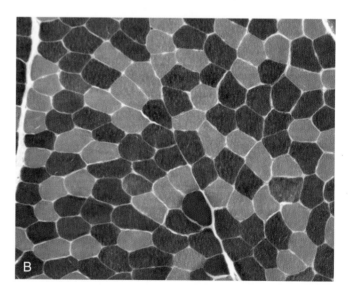

2. Which one of the following diseases MOST likely causes the change depicted in Panel A by ATPase staining and in Panel B by nicotine adenine dehydrogenase (NADH)?
   a. Cushing syndrome
   b. Muscular dystrophy
   c. Fibromyalgia
   d. Charcot-Marie-Tooth disease
   e. Dermatomyositis

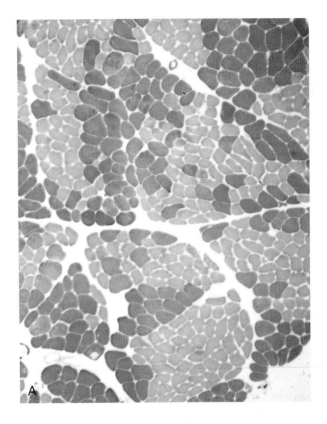

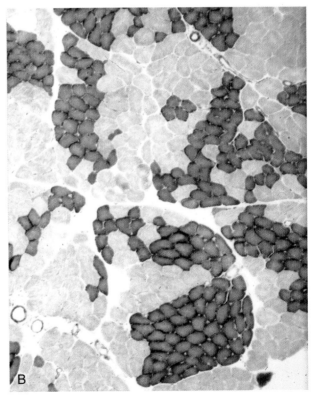

3. Which one of the following statements is INCORRECT for the condition represented in this hematoxylin-eosin–stained frozen section?

   a. Large groups of atrophic muscle fibers are seen.

   b. Individual fibers may show target structures.

   c. Fiber type grouping (fibers of same histochemical type occur in groups) may be demonstrated by ATPase histoenzymatic staining.

   d. Extensive muscle necrosis/regeneration is associated with severe endomysial fibrosis.

   e. Compensatory hypertrophy may be seen in nonatrophic fibers.

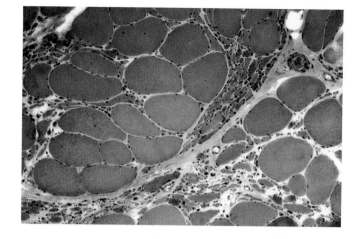

4. Which one of the following conditions is the MOST likely cause of the change seen in the myofibers shown in the figure?

   a. Nemaline myopathy

   b. Inclusion body myositis (IBM)

   c. Myotonic dystrophy

   d. Limb-girdle muscular dystrophy

   e. Peripheral neuropathy

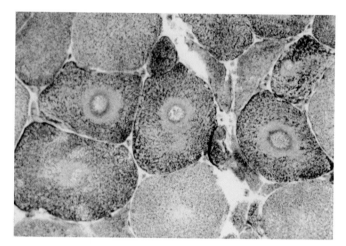

5. Which one of the following is the CORRECT diagnosis for the disease shown in this muscle biopsy from a 5-year-old boy?
   a. Familial amyloidosis
   b. Inclusion body myositis (IBM)
   c. Pompe disease
   d. Spinal muscular atrophy (SMA)
   e. Duchenne muscular dystrophy (DMD)

6. Which one of the following statements is CORRECT regarding the molecular basis of the disease described in Question 5?
   a. The causative gene is among the smallest identified in humans.
   b. The gene is located on chromosome 5q.
   c. The gene product is a nuclear envelope protein.
   d. The protein links actin to the extracellular matrix.
   e. The protein is thought to functionally control beta-oxidation in mitochondria.

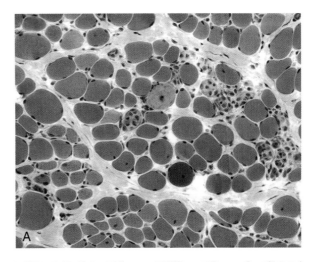

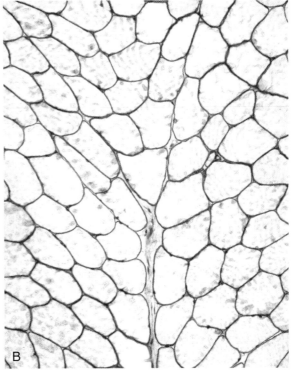

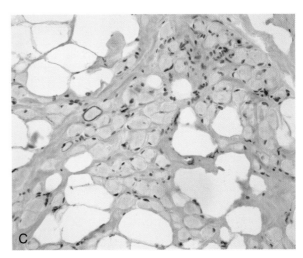

7. A 37-year-old woman presented with seizures and right temporal headache. She subsequently developed visual hallucinations, and had five more generalized tonic-clonic seizures. She also showed aphasia, left hemiplegia, and left hemineglect. A brain magnetic resonance imaging (MRI) scan showed restricted diffusion and T2 FLAIR hyperintensity in the right thalamus and temporal, parietal, and occipital lobes, with contrast enhancement of the adjacent meninges. Her muscle biopsy showed changes depicted in the picture. What is the diagnosis?

   a. Amyotrophic lateral sclerosis
   b. Multiple sclerosis
   c. Polymyositis
   d. Duchenne muscular dystrophy
   e. Mitochondrial encephalomyopathy

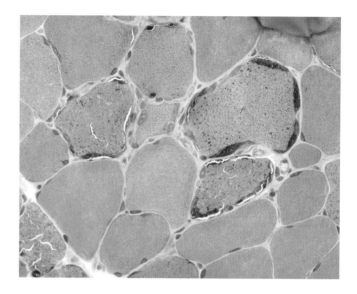

8. A 73-year-old woman complains of a proximal muscle weakness and pain for approximately 2 months. Her past medical history includes hypertension, hypercholesterolemia, and a colon cancer surgically removed 2 months ago followed by chemotherapy. She recalled skin rash in her chest and face during the course of chemotherapy. A muscle biopsy from the quadriceps shows features depicted in the figures. What is the diagnosis?

   a. Chemotherapy-induced toxic myopathy
   b. Dermatomyositis
   c. Steroid-induced myopathy
   d. Inclusion body myositis
   e. Lambert-Eaton syndrome

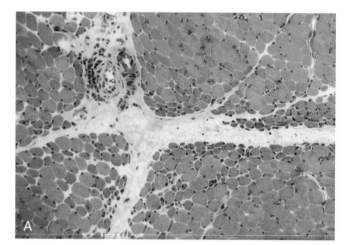

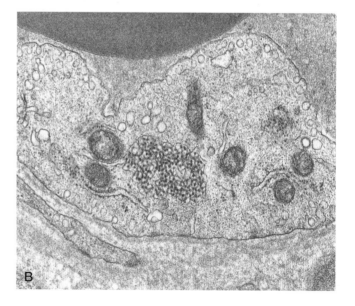

9. Which one of the following conditions is the MOST likely cause of the muscle disease shown at the arrow in panels A (hematoxylin-eosin) and B (CD3 immunohistochemical staining)?

   a. Polymyositis
   b. Dermatomyositis
   c. Sarcoidosis
   d. Inclusion body myositis
   e. Lyme disease

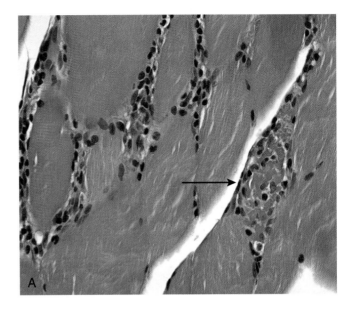

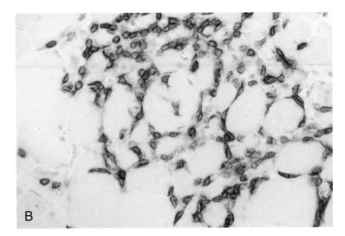

10. A 72-year-old man developed slowly progressive, proximal-dominant muscle weakness. He has had difficulty in climbing stairs and arising from a seated position for approximately 6 months. A neurologist noticed that he also has a mild weakness in the neck and in the finger flexors. He does not have abnormality in sensation. Deep tendon reflexes were hypoactive and plantar responses were flexor. Laboratory tests were normal except for an elevated creatine kinase of 1015 (normal range: 51 to 294) IU/L. A muscle biopsy disclosed focal, chronic inflammation mainly in the endomysium, and abnormalities depicted in the panels A, B, and C. Which is the CORRECT statement about this disease?

a. This disease may show on biopsy amyloid deposition in vacuolated muscle fibers, and is known to be often associated with Alzheimer disease.

b. This disease shows a bimodal pattern of age distribution. The one peak is in the 20s, and the other is in the 60s.

c. This disease is typically resistant for steroid or other immunosuppressive therapy.

d. This disease is seen equally in men and women.

e. This disease is considered to be an autoimmune response after unknown toxic exposure.

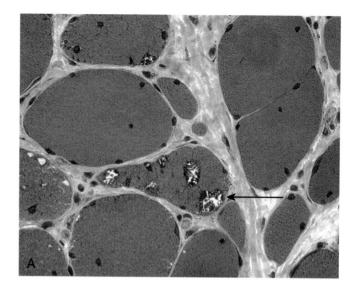

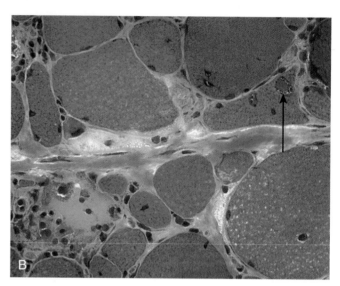

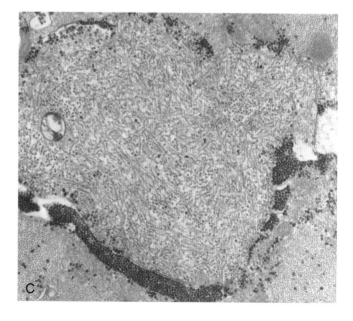

11. This image illustrates the microscopic findings in muscle of a
5-month-old girl with profound hypotonia. The MOST
likely diagnosis is:
   a. Central core disease
   b. Duchenne muscular dystrophy
   c. Werdnig-Hoffmann disease
   d. Amyotrophic lateral sclerosis
   e. Infantile dermatomyositis

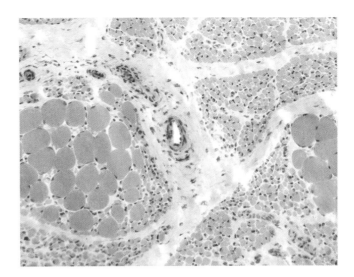

12. Which one of the following statements is CORRECT to describe
the disease depicted in the biopsy?
   a. This biopsy represents nemaline myopathy, one of the most
   common congenital myopathies.
   b. This biopsy represents central core disease, one of the most
   common congenital myopathies.
   c. This biopsy represents lipid storage myopathy.
   d. This biopsy represents mitochondrial myopathy.
   e. This biopsy represents Werdnig-Hoffmann disease.

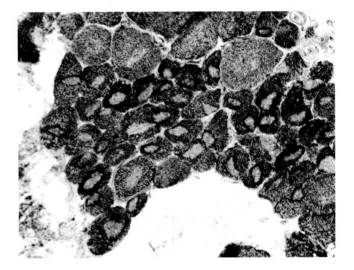

13. A 38-year-old man with no significant past medical history presented with bilateral weakness of the legs along with pins-and-needles sensation. He had had an episode of diarrhea 10 days prior to the onset. The weakness of the legs progressed to paraplegia within 20 hours, and further spread to the arms, trunk, and face. A cerebrospinal fluid (CSF) analysis shows a mild elevation of protein without any cells. Which one of the following statements is CORRECT for the disease described in this clinical history and demonstrated in the figures?

a. Acute, idiopathic wallerian degeneration of peripheral nerve axons is the cause of the disease.

b. CD8+ cyotoxic T cells attack the peripheral axons, resulting in axonal degeneration.

c. This is a self-limited complication of gastrointestinal viral infection, as antiviral therapy is effective for most patients.

d. This disease is considered to be an autoimmune demyelinating disease, but no association with specific HLA (human leukocyte antigen) haplotype has been reported.

e. This disease is known to be closely associated with cerebrovascular disease.

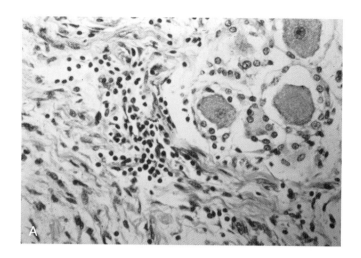

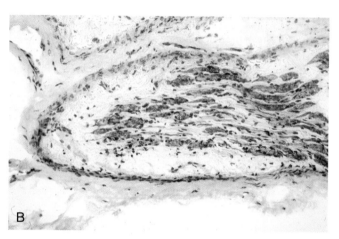

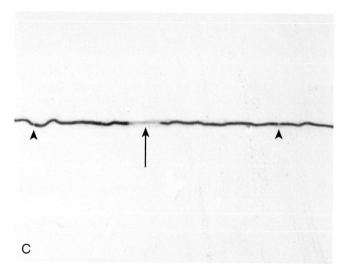

14. Which one of the following conditions is the MOST likely cause of the abnormality of myelinated fiber shown in the epoxy resin section of sural nerve stained by toluidine blue?
  a. This phenomenon is called "onion bulb" and reflects axonal regeneration (sprouting).
  b. This phenomenon is called "onion bulb" and is typically seen in traumatic neuroma.
  c. This lesion is produced by repeated cycles of segmental remyelination and demyelination, and takes weeks to months to develop.
  d. This lesion is a characteristic finding of acute inflammatory polyneuropathy (Guillain-Barré syndrome [GBS]).
  e. This lesion is a characteristic finding of vasculitic neuropathy.

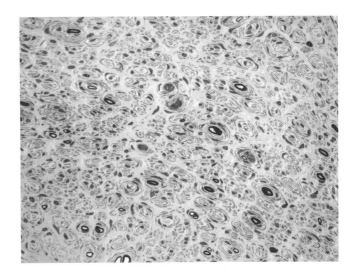

15. Which one of the following statements is CORRECT to describe the lesion shown in the figure?
  a. The main neurologic consequence of this disease is usually an acute demyelinating neuropathy.
  b. This is a common cause of infantile axonopathy.
  c. Unmyelinated fibers are more susceptible in this pathologic process as compared to myelinated fibers.
  d. CSF examination shows significant elevation of protein in about 80% of patients.
  e. This lesion can be seen in the peripheral nervous system either as part of systemic disease or as nonsystemic neuropathy.

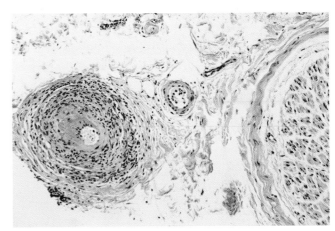

16. Which one of the following statements regarding the disease depicted here is INCORRECT?
  a. Familial or inherited forms of this condition show accumulation of β-amyloid in the central nervous system.
  b. On biopsy, affected nerve exhibits nodular amyloid deposits in the endoneurium accompanied by nerve fiber loss.
  c. Unmyelinated fibers and small-diameter myelianted fibers are more severely affected than large fibers.
  d. Primary amyloidosis associated with multiple myeloma or plasma cell dyscrasia is the most common type of amyloidotic neuropathy in the United States.
  e. Neuropathy is not a significant complication of secondary (reactive) amyloidosis.

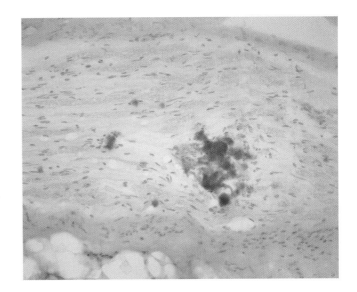

17. Which one of the following conditions is the MOST likely cause of the skeletal muscle lesions seen on the biopsy from a 14-month-old boy with profound muscle weakness and heart enlargement?

   a. Mitochondrial myopathy

   b. Inclusion body myositis

   c. Freezing artifact of unfixed muscle tissue

   d. Pompe disease (Glyocogen storage disease type II)

   e. X-linked vacuolar myopathy with excessive autophagy (XMEA)

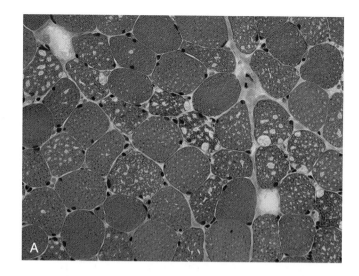

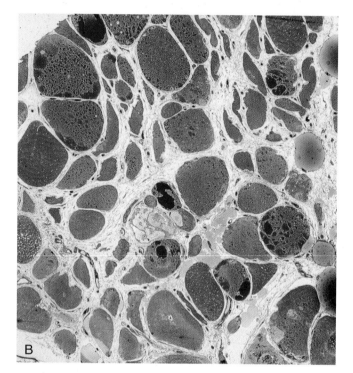

18. Certain inherited muscle disorders, known as congenital myopathies, can cause profound hypotonia in infancy. Which one of the following disorders is not considered to be in this group?
    a. Nemaline myopathy
    b. Myotubular (cetronuclear) myopathy
    c. Central core myopathy
    d. Congenital fiber type disproportion
    e. Werdnig-Hoffmann disease

19. Which one of the following statements is CORRECT regarding mitochondrial disease?
    a. Mitochondrial diseases are caused by gene abnormalities either in the mitochondrial DNA (mtDNA) or the nuclear DNA (nDNA).
    b. Ragged red fibers (RRFs) are specific findings in muscle biopsy from the patients with mitochondrial myopathy.
    c. Functional activities of the respiratory chain (RC) are relatively well preserved, as compared to those of β-oxidation.
    d. Cardiac muscle and extraocular muscles are spared in virtually all cases.
    e. In RRFs, mitochondria are significantly reduced in number.

20. Which organism is LEAST likely a cause of acquired peripheral neuropathy?
    a. *Borrelia burgdorferi*
    b. Human immunodeficiency virus (HIV)
    c. Herpes zoster virus (HZV)
    d. *Trichinella spiralis*
    e. *Mycobacterium leprae*

21. Which one of the following statements is CORRECT with regard to muscle fiber necrosis and regeneration?
    a. Myofibers are postmitotic cells, and there is no restorative mechanism for the necrotized cytostructure.
    b. Satellite cells are usually dormant until activated by myonecrosis. Their main function is phagocytosis of the muscle necrotic debris.
    c. Satellite cells are postmitotic cells and do not replicate.
    d. Activated satellite cells form elongated syncytium, and replace the entire length (tendon to tendon) of muscle fibers.
    e. Activated satellite cells form myoblasts, which eventually fuse to each other and to both ends of intact parts of the fiber to form a regenerating segment.

22. Which one of the following statements is CORRECT for diabetic neuropathy?
    a. Diabetes mellitus (DM) is a rare cause of peripheral neuropathy.
    b. Diabetic neuropathy can be presented as focal and multifocal neuropathies or polyneuropathies.
    c. The cause of diabetic polyneuropathy remains unknown, and the onset of neuropathy does not seem to correlate to the duration of hyperglycemia.
    d. Autonomic dysfunctions are rarely associated with diabetic polyneuropathy.
    e. The diagnostic feature in nerve biopsy from the patients with diabetic polyneuropathy is necrotizing vasculitis.

ANSWERS

1. **b.** Human skeletal muscle fibers can be divided into two histochemical types based on the standard histoenzymatic ATPase reaction (pH 9.4). By this histochemical method, type I fibers are lightly stained, and type II fibers show dark reactions. Normally, type I and II fibers are randomly distributed to show on section a "checkerboard pattern," using the ATPase reaction. In denervation followed by reinnervation of the muscle, the distribution patterns of type I and II fibers are altered (see Question 2). Type I fibers are slow-twitch, resistant to fatigue, and dependent upon oxidative metabolism, but type II fibers are fast-twitch, dependent largely on glycolytic metabolism, and fatigue quickly. Mitochondria that produce adenosine triphosphate (ATP) through oxidative phosphorylation are abundant in type I, and are less abundant in type II. Selective type II myofiber atrophy occurs in various conditions, including disuse atrophy of muscle, steroid myopathy, Cushing syndrome, collagen vascular disease, endocrine myopathy, cancer, starvation, and others. Distinction of type I fibers from type II can also be done using immunohistochemical method, using antibodies against specific types of myosin heavy chains.

   Dubowitz V, Sewry CA: *Muscle Biopsy,* 3rd ed. Philadelphia: Saunders Elsevier, 2007, pp 3-247.

2. **d.** Panels A and B show the phenomenon called "fiber type grouping" consisting of groups of myofibers of the same histochemical properties (compare with normal muscle in Question 1). The ATPase histoenzymatic staining is considered the gold standard for fiber typing. Other stains, such as the NADH in panel B, may also distinguish fiber types, but are less reliable. By NADH, type I fibers are stained dark blue. Fiber type grouping is thought to be a consequence of collateral reinnervation of muscle fibers occurring over a period of months or longer. In human disease, this change is diagnostic of chronic conditions causing denervation/reinnervation, namely neurogenic disorders including peripheral neuropathy, such as Charcot-Marie-Tooth disease, plexopathy, radiculopathy, and motor neuron disease. Myopathies do not exhibit neurogenic abnormalities. Cushing syndrome is known to be associated with selective atrophy of type II myofibers (see Question 1).

   Dubowitz V, Sewry CA: *Muscle Biopsy,* 3rd ed. Philadelphia: Saunders Elsevier, 2007, pp 3-247.

3. **d.** This hematoxylin-eosin–stained frozen section shows grouped atrophy of muscle fibers. Group atrophy is one of the characteristic features of neurogenic disorders. The other two are fiber type grouping (see Question 2) and target fibers (see Question 4). The three "neurogenic features" help to distinguish this group of disorders from primary muscle diseases (myopathies). In myopathy, the muscle often exhibits atrophic fibers, but those fibers do not form large groups: they may be singly present surrounded by

nonatrophic fibers or may form small clusters. Many myopathies are chronic and show increased variation of fiber size, necrosis/regeneration of myofibers, frequent presence of internally nucleated fibers, and prominent endomysial fibrosis. "Neurogenic features" are seen on biopsy in peripheral neuropathy, plexopathy, radiculopathy, and motor neuron disease. In denervation atrophy, atrophic muscle fibers are usually either type I or type II.

Dubowitz V, Sewry CA: *Muscle Biopsy,* 3rd ed. Philadelphia: Saunders Elsevier, 2007, pp 3-247.

4. e. This phenomenon is called "target fibers." In muscle biopsy, there are three major features that are nearly diagnostic of neurogenic disorders: large groups of atrophic fibers; fiber type grouping (see Question 2); and target fibers. Target fibers are well demonstrated by the NADH-tetrazolium histoenzymatic stain as seen in the figure, which shows a clear central zone devoid of oxidative enzymatic activity surrounded by a densely stained area. Target fibers are usually seen in denervating disease, most commonly in chronic peripheral neuropathies or more acute recovering neuropathies. Experimental studies suggest that they may occur during reinnervation. Ultrastructurally, the target area consists of Z-line irregularities and no mitochondria. Distinction of target structures from central cores can sometimes be difficult.

Dubowitz V, Sewry CA: *Muscle Biopsy,* 3rd ed. Philadelphia: Saunders Elsevier, 2007, p 105.
Karpati G (ed): *Structural and Molecular Basis of Skeletal Muscle Disease.* Oxford, UK: International Society of Neuropathology, 2002, pp 5-45.

5. e. DMD and Becker muscular dystrophy (BMD) are X-linked recessive disorders, and are the most common form of childhood muscular dystrophy. The incidence of DMD is approximately 1 in 3500 male births. Clinical symptoms of DMD and BMD do not become evident until the child is 3 to 5 years old, but motor development may be delayed. Affected children cannot raise their knees properly, and soon toe walking and waddling gait become evident. Patients have difficulty rising from the ground, and use a characteristic maneuver called Gower sign (climbing sign). DMD and BMD are caused by mutations in the dystrophin gene at Xp21, and genetically are called dystrophinopathies. Mutations associated with DMD cause frame-shift to create a stop codon in the gene, although those with BMD are in-frame mutations. Accordingly, DMD immunohistochemically shows on biopsy a near or complete absence of dystrophin in muscle fibers. By Western blot, the protein is undetectable. In BMD, weak staining or discontinuities of dystrophin may be detectable at the fiber surface. Western blot typically reveals the protein of a smaller molecular weight in a reduced quantity. Histologically, muscle biopsy shows so-called dystrophic changes: myonecrosis; regeneration; significantly increased variation in fiber size; and interstitial fibrosis. In advanced stage, the muscle tissue is replaced by adipose tissue, which may be clinically observed as pseudohypertrophy of muscle. These dystrophic changes on biopsy are not specific to DMD or BMD, and are shared with other muscular dystrophies, including limb-girdle muscular dystrophies (LGMD). Mutations in a variety of genes are increasingly

linked to LGMD, including those that encode sarcoglycans (α-, β-, γ-, and δ-sarcoglycan), merosin (α2 chain laminin), dysferlin, emerin, caveolin 3, calpain 3, dystroglycans, myotilin, telethonin, and others. Some of these gene products can be immunohistochemically tested in muscle biopsies using commercially available antibodies.

Karpati G (ed): *Structural and Molecular Basis of Skeletal Muscle Disease.* Oxford, UK: International Society of Neuropathology, 2002, pp 6-23.

6. d. The amino-terminal domain of dystrophin binds to actin, and the carboxy-terminus is linked to the extracellular matrix via a sarcolemmal protein, dystroglycan, and other dystrophin-associated glycoproteins. DMD and BMD are X-linked recessive disorders (see Question 5). Dystrophin gene is among the largest genes identified in humans so far. The gene spans about 2.4 megabases and is located on chromosome Xp21. The gene product is a large-molecular-weight protein of 427 kD, and is located along the inner surface of the plasma membrane. The amino-terminal domain of dystrophin binds to actin, and the carboxy-terminus is linked to the extracellular matrix via a sarcolemmal protein, dystroglycan, and other dystrophin-associated glycoproteins. The main function of the protein is thought to stabilize the sarcolemma during cycles of contraction and relaxation of muscle fibers.

Karpati G (ed): *Structural and Molecular Basis of Skeletal Muscle Disease.* Oxford, UK: International Society of Neuropathology, 2002, pp 6-23.

7. e. Strokelike episodes and seizures involving a relatively young individual are suggestive of an inherited type of encephalopathy. RRFs, depicted in the image, are a histologic hallmark of mitochondrial encephalomyopathy associated with mtDNA abnormalities. Amyotrophic lateral sclerosis is a motor neuron disease in which upper and lower motor neurons undergo degeneration. As a result, it shows on biopsy neurogenic changes, such as grouped atrophic fibers, fiber type grouping, and target fibers. Multiple sclerosis is a demyelinating disease that mainly involves the central nervous system. Usually, muscle biopsies do not reveal diagnostic abnormalities. PM is an immune-mediated inflammatory myopathy. Patients do not clinically present encephalopathic features. Muscle biopsy usually reveals T-cell dominant inflammation. In muscular dystrophies in general, muscle biopsy usually reveals myofiber necrosis and regeneration, along with endomysial/perimysial fibrosis. When myofiber necrosis is actively ongoing, chronic inflammation including phagocytizing macrophages and lymphocytes may be associated.

DiMauro S, Hirano M, Schon EA: *Mitochondrial Medicine.* London: Informa Healthcare, 2006, pp 7-26.
Karpati G (ed): *Structural and Molecular Basis of Skeletal Muscle Disease.* Oxford, UK: International Society of Neuropathology, 2002, pp 202-213.

8. b. The image of hematoxylin-eosin stain shows a frozen muscle section of a patient suffering from dermatomyositis. Note that the atrophic fibers are more frequent at the periphery of muscle fascicles, a phenomenon known as "perifascicular atrophy." This pattern is nearly specific for the disorder and is thought to be caused by ischemic injury secondary to an angiopathy. Dermatomyositis is characterized by a subacute clinical course that evolves over a period of weeks or a few months. Patients present with progressive proximal muscle weakness, often associated with pain (myalgia), and characteristic skin rash. Dermatomyositis exhibits a bimodal pattern of age distribution. One peak occurs in children between 5 and 14 years of age, and the other peak occurs in those between 45 and 64 years old. Roughly 25% (in some studies 40% of patients over age 39) of adult dermatomyositis patients have malignancy. The presentation of myopathy may precede that of malignancy. Myositis-specific autoantibodies including anti-Jo-1 and anti-Mi-2 are detected in approximately 20% of dermatomyositis and PM patients. Jo-1 antibody positive dermatomyositis is frequently associated with interstitial lung disease. The electron micrograph depicts a reticulotubular aggregate in the endothelial cell of an endomysial capillary. This ultrastructure is not specific to dermatomyositis, as it can be observed in systemic lupus erythematosus, mixed connective tissue disease, HIV infection, and other diseases.

Dubowitz V, Sewry CA: *Muscle Biopsy,* 3rd ed. Philadelphia: Saunders Elsevier, 2007, pp 519-540.

9. a. Polymyositis (PM) is the most likely cause of the disease shown. PM is a disorder of skeletal muscle of diverse causes, and is one of the three major categories of inflammatory myopathy. The other two are dermatomyositis and inclusion body myositis (IBM). PM and dermatomyositis affect women more commonly than men, whereas IBM is more common in men than in women. PM and dermatomyositis are characterized by progressive weakness of proximal limb muscles of acute or subacute onset and possible intervals of improvement of symptoms. Progression from onset to peak weakness is measured in weeks or in months, not years as in IBM. PM is considered an autoimmune disease of disordered cellular immunity; however, the nature of the antigen and of the immunologic aberration is not known. It can be associated with collagen-vascular disease, Crohn disease, biliary cirrhosis, graft-versus-host disease, and HIV and HTLV-1 infection. It may be associated with interstitial pulmonary disease. Anti-Jo-1 antibodies are found in about a half of patients with both PM and pulmonary fibrosis. Typically, muscle biopsy shows infiltration of lymphocytes in the endomysium. When T-cell markers are immunohistochemically applied, sections may capture CD8+ cytotoxic T cells infiltrating into nonnecrotic muscle fibers. Unlike dermatomyositis, no perifascicular pattern of disease is observed in PM. PM is treated with steroids and immunosuppressive drugs. Although PM or IBM can be seen in the patients with malignancy, it is much less frequent than the association of malignancy with dermatomyositis.

Dubowitz V, Sewry CA: *Muscle Biopsy,* 3rd ed. Philadelphia: Saunders Elsevier, 2007, pp 519-540.
Rowland LP: Polymyosiyis, inclusion body myositis, and related myopathies. In Rowland LP (ed): *Merritt's Neurology.* Philadelphia: Lippincott Williams & Wilkins, 2010, pp 897-901.

10. c. The clinical history and the muscle biopsy indicate that this patient has inclusion body myositis (IBM). IBM is the most common inflammatory myopathy in patients over the age of 50, and affects men more than women. As a rule, the disease is resistant to steroid or immunosuppressive agents. The muscle biopsies of IBM are similar to those of polymyositis, but there are important differences. First, the muscle typically reveals vacuoles within muscle fibers as seen in the question. The vacuoles are rimmed by basophilic, granular material, and are called "rimmed vacuoles." The muscle fibers often contain sparse eosinophilic inclusions, usually within or near the vacuoles, a finding that gave rise to the name inclusion body myositis. The inclusions are weakly congophilic. The recent recognition of insoluble protein aggregates associated with rimmed vacuoles prompted the usage of antibodies, including phosphorylated tau, β-amyloid, TAR DNA binding protein-43 (TDP43), and others, but no single protein appears pathogenic for vacuole formation in IBM. The morphologic distinction of IBM from other inflammatory myopathy is important, because IBM does not respond to steroid treatment or other immunosuppressive agents, despite lymphocytic infiltration of the muscle.

Dubowitz V, Sewry CA: *Muscle Biopsy,* 3rd ed. Philadelphia: Saunders Elsevier, 2007, pp 519-540.
Rowland LP: Polymyositis, inclusion body myositis, and related myopathies. In Rowland LP (ed): *Merritt's Neurology.* Philadelphia: Lippincott Williams & Wilkins, 2010, pp 897-901.

11. c. The muscle section shows neurogenic abnormalities (large-group atrophy of muscle fibers) of a patient with Werdnig-Hoffmann disease (infantile SMA type I). More than 95% of SMA patients carry a homozygous deletion in the survival motor neuron (SMN) gene on chromosome 5q11-q13. Based on age at onset and severity of symptoms, SMA has been historically classified into three types: infantile SMA type I (Werdnig-Hoffmann syndrome); SMA type II; and SMA type III (Kugelberg-Welander syndrome). The three are all allelic and clinically are a continuous spectrum with phenotypic overlap. All are autosomal recessive. SMA type I is clinically the most severe phenotype, and hypotonia is evident at birth or soon thereafter. This is one of the most common causes of floppy infant syndrome. Proximal muscles are affected before distal muscles, but ultimately flaccid quadriplegia results. Without proactive care, most patients die before age 2. The SMN gene has two almost identical forms (*SMN1* and *SMN2*) on chromosome 5q. The clinical severity of the disease is correlated with the copy numbers of *SMN2* genes. *SMA1* gene mutation is embryonically lethal in the absence of *SMA2*. A study has shown that 80% of SMA type I patients had one or two *SMN2* copies, 82% of SMA type II patients three *SMN2* copies, and 96% of SMA type III patients three or four *SMN2* copies.

Kaufmann P, De Vivo DC: Spinal muscular atrophies of childhood. In Rowland LP (ed): *Merritt's Neurology.* Philadelphia: Lippincott Williams & Wilkins, 2010, pp 810-811.
Rowland LP, Mitsumoto H, Predborski S: Amyotrophic lateral sclerosis, progressive muscular atrophy, and primary lateral sclerosis. In Rowland LP (ed): *Merritt's Neurology.* Philadelphia: Lippincott Williams & Wilkins, 2010, pp 802-808.

12. b. This biopsy represents central core disease (CCD), one of the most common congenital myopathies. The characteristic cores are single, circular, centrally placed, sharply demarcated, and detectable in the majority of type I myofibers. They are devoid of mitochondria and sarcoplasmic reticulum, and are, thus, deficient in oxidative enzymatic activities, including NADH, succinate dehydrogenase, and cytochrome c oxidase. Congenital myopathies are named after the characteristic morphologic features in muscle biopsies. Most common forms are nemaline (rods) myopathy, core (central or multi/mini core) myopathies, myotubular/centronuclear myopathy, and fiber type disproportion. Several causative genes have been identified in each morphologic group, and the gene abnormalities associated with congenital myopathy are rapidly expanding. CCD is inherited in an autosomal dominant fashion in the vast majority of the cases with variable expression and incomplete penetrance in terms of the clinical phenotypes. The most common gene mutations causing CCD are in the *RYR1* (ryanodine receptor-1 gene). Identification of disease-causing mutations in the *RYR1* in patients with CCD and malignant hyperthermia (MH) disclosed the link between myopathy and MH susceptibility. Although CCD is associated with an increased risk of MH, the association between MH and CCD is complex: most patients with MH have histologically normal muscle, and approximately 28% of patients with CCD have MH susceptibility. CCD and MH are both genetically heterogeneous, and it has not been clearly understood why the same *RYR1* mutations can present with clinical different phenotypes.

Dubowitz V, Sewry CA: *Muscle Biopsy,* 3rd ed. Philadelphia: Saunders Elsevier, 2007, pp 407-442.
North K: Congenital myopathy. In Engel AG, Franzini-Armstrong C (eds): *Myology,* 3rd ed. New York: McGraw-Hill, 2004, pp 1473-1533.

13. d.   The clinical signs and symptoms, and the pathologic changes demonstrated in the figures, are features of acute inflammatory polyneuropathy, Guillain-Barre syndrome (GBS). GBS is the most frequent acquired demyelinating neuropathy, with an incidence of 0.6 to 1.9 cases per 100,000 population. Viral respiratory or gastrointestinal infection, immunization, or surgery often precedes neurologic symptoms by 5 days to 4 weeks. The CSF protein content is elevated in most patients with GBS. The CSF cell count is usually normal, exhibiting cell-protein dissociation. Antecedent *Campylobacter jejuni* infection, infectious mononucleosis, cytomegalovirus (CMV) infection, viral hepatitis, HIV infection, or other viral diseases may be documented by serologic studies. The cause of GBS is incompletely understood. There is evidence that it is immune-mediated: there is inflammation involving peripheral nerve and dorsal root ganglions as demonstrated in the figures A and B; patients usually improve with immunomodulatory therapy. Although a similar disease can be introduced in experimental animals immunized with certain antigens, including peripheral myelin, myelin basic protein, or galactocerebroside, the target antigen has not been clearly identified. Histologically, GBS is characterized by focal segmental demyelination (figure C) with perivascular and endoneurial infiltration of lymphocytes and monocytes. The earliest pathologic change is migration of lymphocytes across the walls of venules into the endoneurium, and blood-borne monocytes enter the endoneurium shortly after. These monocytes, rather than lymphocytes, attack and strip away the myelin sheath,

based on electron microscopic observation. The debris of myelin fragments is phagocytized by monocytes, which acquire the morphologic features of macrophages. Lesions are scattered throughout the nerves, nerve roots, and cranial nerves. In severe cases, there is both demyelination and axonal degeneration. After roughly 1 week, the Schwann cells begin to form new myelin sheaths along the denuded segments. The rate of clinical recovery varies. In some cases with rapid recovery, patients restore normal functions within a few weeks. In most, however, recovery is slow and not complete for many months. In untreated cases, about 35% of patients have permanent residual hyporeflexia, atrophy, and weakness of distal or facial muscles.

Brannagan TH, Weimer LH: Acquired neuropathies. In Rowland LP (ed): *Merritt's Neurology.* Philadelphia: Lippincott Williams & Wilkins, 2010, pp 822-837.
Mandell JR, Kissel JT, Cornbath DR (eds): *Diagnosis and Management of Peripheral Nerve Disorders.* New York: Oxford University Press, 2001, pp 145-172.

14. c.   The lesion called "onion-bulb" is produced through repetitive cycles that build up the concentric array of flattened Schwann cell processes and their basement membranes. Animal models have demonstrated that a single demyelinating/remyelinating event is insufficient to create onion bulbs, whereas recurrent and continuing demyelinating insults can produce onion bulbs in great numbers. Human diseases in which demyelination is occurring constantly with remyelination for prolonged periods often show onion bulbs on biopsy. These diseases include inherited hypertrophic neuropathies (Charcot-Marie-Tooth disease type I) and chronic inflammatory demyelinating polyradiculoneuropathy. By observations in human disease and experimental models, the presence of onion bulbs suggests that a demyelinating process has been active for at least several months. The longer the duration of the demyelinating process, the more onion bulbs are seen. Although onion bulbs are far more likely seen in diseases of primary demyelination, demyelination secondary to axonal disease may also cause onion bulb formation. This occurrence depends on the chronicity of the process and on how many times the axon sheds its myelin sheath before dying.

Kissel JT, Mendell JR: Chronic inflammatory demyelinating polyradiculopathy. In Mendell JR, Kissel JT, Cornblath DR (eds): *Diagnosis and Management of Peripheral Nerve Disorders.* New York: Oxford University Press, 2001, pp 173-191.
Midroni G, Bilbao JM: Schwann cells and myelin in the peripheral nervous system. In Midroni G, Bilbao JM: *Biopsy Diagnosis of Peripheral Neuropathy.* Boston: Butterworth-Heinemann, 1995, pp 75-103.

15. e.   This figure depicts vasculitic neuropathy. The most commonly involved nerves include peroneal, posterior tibial, and ulnar nerves. Involved vessels show characteristic pathologic features in common: inflammation and structural damage to blood vessels walls, leading to ischemic, hemorrhagic, and thrombotic damage to the nerves supplied by those vessels. Vasculitis/vasculitides can be classified into two groups: one group results from direct bacterial, fungal, rickettsial, or viral infection, and the other results from immunologic mechanism. For the most immune-mediated vasculitic syndromes, the inciting events that trigger the vasculitis and the precise pathogenic mechanism of vascular damage are not well understood.

Immune-mediated vasculitic neuropathy can be the primary disease process as in polyarteritis nodosa or Wegener granulomatosis, or can be associated with some other connective tissue disorder, such as rheumatoid arthritis or systemic lupus erythematosus. A tissue diagnosis is absolutely essential for the management of patients with suspected vasculitis. Active lesions are characterized by transmural inflammation with concurrent necrosis. Endothelial cell necrosis with hemorrhage may also occur. Mononuclear cells infiltrating the vessels are predominantly T cells and macrophages. Vasculitic neuropathy is predominantly axonopathy, and nerve biopsy usually demonstrates varying degrees of nerve fiber loss, with undergoing wallerian degeneration depending on the age of the lesion. Unmyelinated fibers are more resistant to ischemic insults than larger myelinated fibers.

Kissel JT, Collins MP, Mendell JR: Vasculitic neuropathy. In Mendell JR, Kissel JT, Cornblath DR (eds): *Diagnosis and Management of Peripheral Nerve Disorders*. New York: Oxford University Press, 2001, pp 202-255.

16. a. Amyloid is deposited in tissue in the form of nonbranching fibrils with an underlying three-dimensional structure of β-pleated sheet. Many different proteins can be deposited in the nerve as amyloid, including immunoglobulin light chains, serum amyloid A, transthyretin, apolipoprotein A-I, gelsolin, and others. Primary amyloidosis is the most common form of amyloidotic neuropathy. Monoclonal light chain deposits in tissue, and the immunoglobulin protein is more often λ than κ. Most of the patients have a detectable level of monoclonal paraprotein in the serum and/or urine. Neuropathy is not a significant complication in secondary (reactive) amyloidosis. Familial amyloid polyneuropathy (FAP) shows the accumulation of one of three plasma proteins: transthyretin, apolipoprotein A-1, or gelsolin. Most FAPs are associated with transthyretin, a normal protein that transports thyroxine and retinol. Amyloid neuropathy often affects unmyelinated fibers and small myelinated fibers more severely than large fibers. Symptoms include numbness and pain. Orthostatic hypotension and other autonomic dysfunction often appear at onset, and most patients show some degree of cardiac or renal involvement. Weakness due to involvement of the large motor fibers develops later in the clinical course.

Nerve biopsy and simultaneous muscle biopsies are often diagnostic of amyloidosis. Because the amyloid deposits are focal and scanty, sections from deeper levels of the blocks may be required in a suspected case. If the biopsies are negative, a rectal biopsy (positive in roughly 80% of patients), abdominal fat aspirate (70%), or bone marrow aspirate (50%) may be helpful to establish the diagnosis.

Kissel JT, Mendell JR: Neuropathies associated with monoclonal gammopathies. In Mendell JR, Kissel JT, Cornblath DR (eds): *Diagnosis and Management of Peripheral Nerve Disorders*. New York: Oxford University Press, 2001, pp 272-296.
Rowland LP, Pedley TA: *Merrit's Neurology*. Philadelphia: Lippincott Williams & Wilkins, 2009.

17. d. This biopsy reveals a vacuolar myopathy. Vacuoles may contain stainable material, or may appear optically empty either because their contents have been dissolved from vacuoles or because they do not stain. They could also be created as an artifact from inadequately freezing unfixed muscle tissue. Glycogen and neutral lipid are particularly liable to be dissolved from vacuoles so that they often appear empty. Methods of tissue preparation can thus influence the appearance of vacuoles. In this particular biopsy, a significant accumulation of glycogen (PAS-stained) is demonstrated by toluidine blue–PAS double stain on epoxy resin plastic sections generated from the glutaraldehyde-fixed tissue (panel B). Acid maltase is a lysosomal glycosidase that hydrolyzes both α-1,4- and β-1,6-glycosidic linkage, and can degrade glycogen completely. In the absence of acid maltase, glycogen is accumulated in skeletal muscle, heart, and liver. There is a clinical spectrum associated with acid maltase deficiency (AMD) including infantile, childhood, and adult forms. All types of AMD are transmitted by autosomal recessive inheritance. Infantile AMD presents within the first few months of life with rapidly progressive weakness and hypotonia and enlargement of heart, tongue, and liver. Respiratory and feeding problems are common, and death is usually caused by cardiorespiratory failure before the age of 2. The childhood type of AMD presents clinically in infancy or early childhood as a myopathy. The disease progresses relatively slowly, and the usual cause of death is respiratory failure. Few patients survive beyond the second decade. Liver, heart, and tongue enlargement infrequently occurs. The adult form of AMD presents after age 20 either as slowly progressive myopathy that clinically mimics polymyositis, or limb-girdle dystrophy, with symptoms of respiratory failure. Biochemical deficiency of acid maltase has been documented in muscle, liver, heart, leukocytes, and cultured fibroblasts, but not in kidney.

DiMauro S, Hays AP, Tsujino S: Metabolic disorders affecting muscle. In Engel AG, Franzini-Armstrong C (eds): *Myology*, 3rd ed. New York: McGraw-Hill, 2004, pp 1535-1558.
Engel AG, Hirschhorn R, Huie M: Acid maltase deficiency. In Engel AG, Franzini-Armstrong C (eds): *Myology*, 3rd ed. New York: McGraw-Hill, 2004, pp 1559-1586.

18. e. Werdnig-Hoffmann disease is not in the same group as the other answer choices. It is infantile SMA type I. More than 95% of SMA patients carry a homozygous deletion in the *SMN* gene on chromosome 5q11-q13 (see Question 11). Congenital myopathies are named after the characteristic morphologic features in muscle biopsies. Most common forms are nemaline (rods) myopathy, core (central or multi/mini core) myopathies, myotubular/centronuclear myopathy, and fiber type disproportion. Several causative genes have been identified in each morphologic group, and the gene abnormalities associated with congenital myopathy are rapidly expanding. Myotubular (centronuclear) myopathy is defined pathologically by the presence of centrally located nuclei in the majority of extrafusal muscle fibers. X-linked myotubular myopathy is clinically associated with severe phenotypes with severe floppiness and weakness, feeding difficulties, and respiratory distress that often requires assisted ventilation. Nemaline bodies and cores are forms of disorganized myofilamentous structure. Nemaline bodies, also known as rods, appear with the Gomori trichrome (not clearly visible by hematoxylin-eosin) as dark red granules or tiny rods. They generally measure about 3 to 6 μm in length and 1 to 3 μm in width, and are originated from the Z-disk. Central cores are sharply demarcated areas within fibers where myofibrillar organization is different from that in the rest of the fiber (see Question 12). They longitudinally run from end to end of the fiber and are not invariably central. Within cores, myofibrils are not demarcated from one another, and the Z-disk is not straight (Z-line streaming). Recognition of CCD is important because of its association with MH. The diagnostic abnormality of CFTD is a discrepancy in size: type I (slow-twitch) fibers are smaller than type II (fast-twitch) fibers by at least 12%. Electron microscopically, fibers show normal cytoarchitecture, regardless of size. Because there are many secondary causes of relative type I fiber hypotrophy or atrophy, CFTD is a diagnosis of exclusion.

North K: Congenital myopathy. In Engel AG, Franzini-Armstrong C (eds): *Myology,* 3rd ed. New York: McGraw-Hill, 2004, pp 1473-1533.

19. a. We refer to mitochondrial disease as a group of disorders, often multisystemic, associated with primary dysfunction of the mitochondrial RC. The RC consists of five complexes (I to V), four of which, except for complex II, are encoded by mtDNA and nDNA. Complex II is entirely encoded by nDNA; therefore, either mtDNA or nDNA gene mutations can result in a profoundly dysfunctional state of the RC, namely mitochondrial disease. RRF is a histologic hallmark of mitochondrial myopathy, especially diseases caused by mtDNA mutations; however, it is not completely specific to mitochondrial myopathy, and can be seen in other chronic myopathies, including inflammatory myopathy. Muscle biopsy from elderly people may show it at a low frequency. RRF represents focal and segmental increase of mitochondria. The precise mechanism of mitochondrial proliferation is not well understood, but is believed to be a compensation mechanism for faulty mitochondrial RC function. Hyperplasia of mitochondria is often accompanied with ultrastructural abnormality of the organelle, such as bizarre, convoluted arrangements of cristae with or without abnormal, intramitochondrial inclusions. Many mitochondrial diseases are multisystemic, as mitochondrial RC defects tend to significantly affect tissues that are highly dependent on oxidative phosphorylation as an energy source including brain, skeletal muscle, cardiac muscle, kidney, and liver.

DiMauro S, Bonilla E: Mitochondrial encephalomyopathies. In Engel AG, Franzini-Armstrong C (eds): *Myology,* 3rd ed. New York: McGraw-Hill, 2004, pp 1623-1662.
DiMauro S, Hirano M, Schon EA (eds): *Mitochondrial Medicine.* London: Informa Healthcare, 2006, pp 7-26.

20. d. Of the answer choices, *Trichinella spiralis* is least likely a cause of acquired peripheral neuropathy. Trichinellosis manifests as a systemic infection stemming from larval migration. Muscle pain and tenderness (muscle invasion by the organism) is not uncommon, and the organism can be detectable in a biopsy of the affected muscle, together with features of myositis.

Many infectious diseases can be associated with acquired peripheral neuropathy, including various viral infections (e.g., HCV, CMV, HIV, HZV, EBV, etc.), leprosy, diphtheria, Lyme disease, and others. *Campylobacter jejuni* infections

may precede Guillain-Barre syndrome (GBS), probably by the mechanism of molecular mimicry (see Question 13). Infection can affect the peripheral nervous system either directly in the form of axonopathy or demyelinating disease, or in the form of vasculitic neuropathy. HIV-related neuropathies are complex. Several forms of neuropathy affect patients, depending on the stage of the illness and the immunocompetence of the patient: acute demyelinating disease indistinguishable from GBS, early in the course of infection; subacute demyelinating disease clinically indistinguishable from idiopathic CIDP (chronic inflammatory demyelinating polyneuropathy), usually found in HIV-positive patients before there is any evidence of AIDS; or distal sensorimotor polyneuropathy, usually seen in patients who fulfill diagnostic criteria of AIDS. Other forms of neuropathy involving HIV-infected patients include diffuse lymphocytosis syndrome (DILS), mononeuropathy multiplex that can be associated with opportunistic infections such as CMV, and iatrogenic neuropathy secondary to antiretroviral medications. Lyme neuropathy (neuroborreliosis) can also cause various forms of neuropathy. The most common features of neuroborreliosis are a painful sensory radiculitis, appearing about 3 weeks after the erythema migrans. Cranial nerve involvement, especially facial nerve, is relatively frequently seen (61%). In general, treatments for neuropathies associated with infection are designated to eradicate the causative organism and to prevent secondary immune reactions; however, some antiorganism medications are neurotoxic (e.g., dapsone for leprosy, dideoxynucleotide antiretroviral agents for HIV).

Brannagan TH, Weimer LH: Acquired neuropathies. In Rowland LP (ed): *Merritt's Neurology.* Philadelphia: Lippincott Williams & Wilkins, 2010, pp 828-833.

21. e. Segmental necrosis of muscle fibers is found in many different inherited and acquired myopathies. Populations of reserve cells called satellite cells are normally dormant, and are activated by muscle injury. Satellite cells are considered to be committed stem cells, and play a major role in muscle maintenance and regeneration. Skeletal muscle fibers are of mesenchymal origin. Embriologically, the limb and trunk muscles develop from the mesoderm of the somites. During the first week of gestation, certain mesenchymal cells become premyoblast. When those cells begin to synthesize cytoskeletal proteins or receptors, they become recognized as myoblasts. Myoblasts undergo intense proliferation, and by 7 weeks of gestation, they are ready to fuse to each other to form multinucleated, primary myotubes. Subsequently, secondary myotubes form until the total number of primary and secondary myotubes eventually corresponds to the ultimate number of muscle fibers in a given muscle. As myotubes mature, their myofibrils increase in number and in size, the nuclei become peripherally located, and the cells become surrounded by their own basal lamina. Under the basal lamina of these immature muscle fibers, each bears for a time adherent undifferentiated cells. They probably continue to divide and fuse with the muscle cells until about the 30th week of development. Some of them, however, withdraw from the cell cycle and become quiescent, and constitute the satellite cell population. A satellite cell cannot be, therefore, distinguished from a muscle fiber by routine histologic examination, but it can be identified by electron microscopy as a separate small cell in which it is enclosed by the same basal lamina that surrounds each myofiber. Immunohistochemically, a certain type of neural cell adhesion molecule (N-CAM) binds to quiescent satellite cells. Muscle fiber injury triggers activation of the satellite cells to become myoblasts. They subsequently undergo mitosis and cell division. Within 2 days of the onset of fiber injury, the myoblasts begin to fuse to each other and to the ends of the intact residual fiber segments. Activated nuclei with prominent nucleoli move to the center of the regenerating fibers where they produce abundant RNA for synthesis of new proteins. By hematoxylin-eosin, the cytoplasm of these regenerating fibers is basophilic due to the high content of RNA. Under optimal conditions, regeneration can eventually restore the function of the muscle to a normal state as quickly as 2 to 3 weeks in humans following an episode of muscle fiber necrosis (often referred to as rhabdomyolysis).

Bischoff R, Franzini-Armstrong C: Satellite cells and stem cells in muscle regeneration. In Engel AG, Franzini-Armstrong C (eds): *Myology,* 3rd ed. New York: McGraw-Hill, 2004, pp 66-86.

Carpenter S, Karpati G: General aspects of skeletal muscle biology. In Carpenter S, Karpati G: *Pathology of Skeletal Muscle.* New York: Oxford University Press, 2001, pp 28-62.

Carpenter S, Karpati G: Major pathological reactions and their consequences for skeletal muscle cells. In Carpenter S, Karpati G: *Pathology of Skeletal Muscle.* New York: Oxford University Press, 2001, pp 63-130.

22. b.   DM is the most common cause of peripheral neuropathy in the Western world. In a population-based cohort, 66% of type 1 and 59% of type 2 diabetics had objective evidence of neuropathy. The advent of better methods of glucose control may improve these statistics in the future. Various forms of neuropathy are associated with DM. In the form of focal and multifocal neuropathies, patients may present cranial neuropathies, mononeuropathies, diabetic thoracolumbar radiculopathy, or diabetic lumbosacral radiculoplexus neuropathy. The other form of neuropathy associated with DM is polyneuropathies, which include diabetic polyneuropathy, acute painful diabetic neuropathy, and treatment-induced neuropathy (insulin neuritis). Among various neuropathies associated with DM, a distal symmetric sensorimotor polyneuropathy is the most common form. It occurs either in type 1 or type 2 DM. In type 1 DM, it develops after chronic and prolonged hyperglycemia for many years. In type 2, the onset of polyneuropathy is more variable, but it is possibly because the patients might have unrecognized periods of hyperglycemia, prior to the diagnosis. Autonomic manifestations accompany distal symmetric sensory polyneuropathy and correlate with the severity of the somatic nerve abnormality. Those manifestations include cardiovascular symptoms such as severe postural hypotension, genitourinary symptoms such as erectile dysfunction and bladder atony, and gastrointestinal dysfunctions such as gastroparesis secondary to vagal denervation. In diabetic polyneuropathy, nerve biopsy shows loss of myelinated and unmyelinated nerve fibers. Axonal degeneration and regeneration is the predominant feature, and secondary myelin changes may be seen. The microvasculature reveals markedly thickened basement membrane and loss of pericytes; however, those features are not specific to DM, and nerve biopsy per se is not diagnostic. The clinical and electrodiagnostic results, and assay of blood glucose according to the established criteria, preclude the need for nerve biopsy; however, preexisting nerve disease in diabetics is so extensive that few other conditions can be diagnosed. In patients with asymmetric neuropathies, a possibility of necrotizing vasculitis may provide the indication for nerve biopsy, but other vascular changes in the nerves of diabetics may confound the diagnosis. Pathogenesis of diabetic neuropathy remains to be clarified, and the heterogeneity of clinical forms of diabetic neuropathy makes it difficult to identify a singular cause. The major theories for nerve damage include altered polyol metabolism and myoinositol depletion, formation of advanced glycosylation end products, altered neurotrophic factors, oxidative stress, altered essential fatty acid metabolism, and vascular hypothesis. Those theories are by no means mutually exclusive. The most important factor in the treatment of diabetic neuropathy is tight control of hyperglycemia.

Mendell JR: Diabetic neuropathies. In Mendell JR, Kissel JT, Cornblath DR (eds): *Diagnosis and Management of Peripheral Nerve Disorders.* New York: Oxford University Press, 2001, pp 373-399.

CHAPTER 15

NEUROPATHOLOGY

Julio A. Valentín and James E. Goldman

QUESTIONS

Questions 1-23 refer to a photo or photomicrograph.

1. This squamous cell lesion located in the suprasellar space represents:
   a. Epidermoid cyst
   b. Craniopharyngioma
   c. Teratoma
   d. Dermoid cyst
   e. Metastatic squamous cell carcinoma

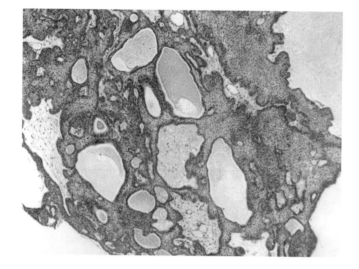

2. The neuronal disease illustrated in this section of hippocampus reflects:
   a. Alzheimer disease (AD)
   b. Hexosaminidase A deficiency
   c. Acute ischemic change
   d. Frontotemporal dementia
   e. Acute Wernicke disease

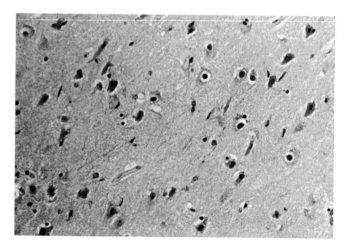

3. This neocortical biopsy from a patient with a rapidly progressive dementia is characteristic of:

a. AD

b. Transmissible spongiform encephalopathies

c. Multiinfarct dementia associated with CADASIL (cerebral autosomal dominant arteriopathy with subcortical infarcts and leukoencephalopathy)

d. Neocortical lesions associated with amyotrophic lateral sclerosis (ALS) dementia

e. Neocortical lesions associated with Lewy body disease

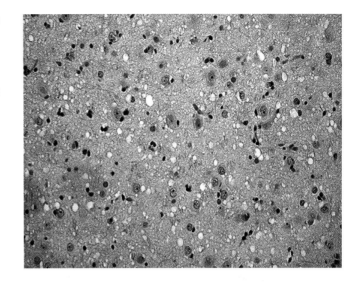

4. The disease in this section of neocortex, visualized with a silver stain, represents:

a. Neurofibrillary tangles and neuritic plaques in AD

b. Astrocyte disease in corticobasal degeneration

c. Pick bodies

d. Oligodendrocyte disease in multiple system atrophy

e. Fungal cerebritis

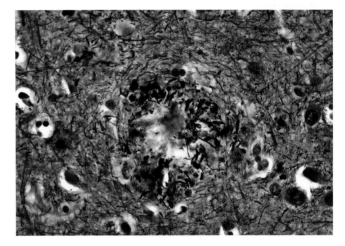

5. A 40-year-old man suffered an intracerebral hemorrhage. This image illustrates what was removed. The diagnosis is:

a. Arteriovenous malformation (AVM)

b. Berry aneurysm

c. Hypertensive arteriopathy

d. Cavernous hemangioma

e. Angiomatous meningioma

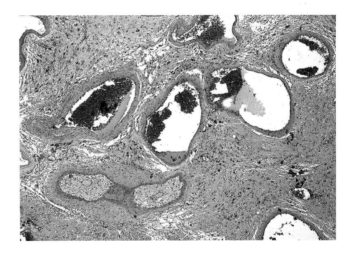

6. A 25-year-old woman who was born and raised in Central America presented with focal seizures. Magnetic resonance imaging (MRI) showed a ringlike enhancing mass in the right cerebral hemisphere. The surgical specimen contained the illustrated image, which represents:

  a. Central nervous system (CNS) schistosomiasis
  b. Toxoplasmosis
  c. Encysted *Taenia solium* larvae
  d. Fungal abscess
  e. Tuberculoma

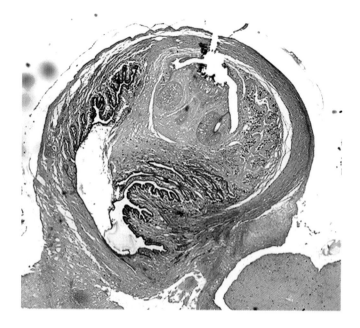

7. This spindle cell neoplasm was removed from the spinal subdural space. Its immune profile included the following: epithelial membrane antigen (EMA) positive, S100 beta negative, HMB-45 negative, desmin negative. The MIB-1 labeling index was less than 1%. The MOST likely diagnosis is:

  a. Schwannoma
  b. Meningioma
  c. Spindle cell melanoma
  d. Leiomyoma
  e. Astrocytoma

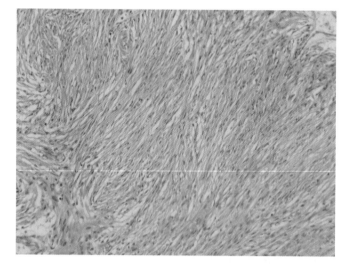

8. The pathology represents:

  a. Diffuse axonal injury
  b. Acute atherothrombotic occlusion of proximal middle cerebral artery (MCA)
  c. Acute atherothrombotic occlusion of anterior cerebral artery (ACA)
  d. Diffuse astrocytoma
  e. Gliomatosis cerebri

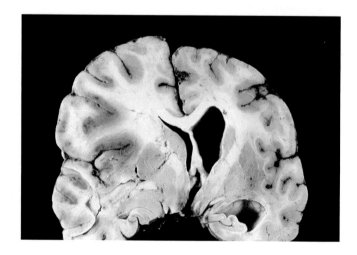

9. All of the following are true of this lesion, the pathology of which is shown in this elastic stain, EXCEPT:
   a. It is thought to be congenital.
   b. It will increase in size over time.
   c. It will rupture into the subarachnoid space.
   d. It will occur at branch points in the circle of Willis.
   e. The risk of rupture is not associated with hypertension.

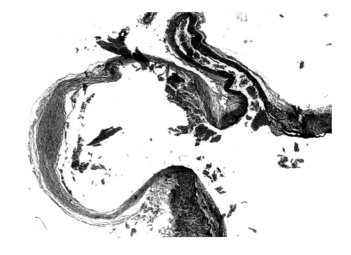

10. This horizontal section of spinal cord, visualized with a silver stain, shows a lesion associated with:
   a. Syphilis
   b. Multiple sclerosis (MS)
   c. Vitamin B_{12} deficiency (subacute combined degeneration)
   d. HIV myelopathy
   e. ALS

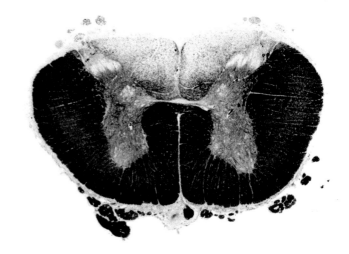

11. These argyrophilic structures in the AD brain are composed of abnormal polymers of:
   a. α-Synuclein
   b. Tau
   c. β-Amyloid
   d. Glucose
   e. Tubulin

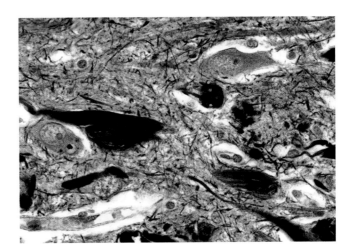

12. The patient whose brain is illustrated here suffered from:
    a. Mutations in the tau gene
    b. Mutations in the β-amyloid precursor protein (APP) gene
    c. Mutations in the α-synuclein gene
    d. Expanded triplet repeats in the huntingtin gene
    e. Expanded triplet repeats in the androgen receptor gene

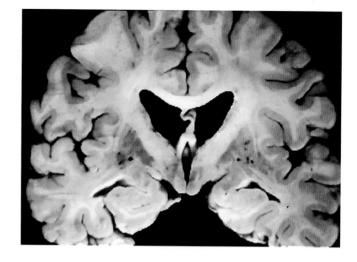

13. The pathology in the substantia nigra is associated with:
    a. Involuntary movement disorder
    b. Myoclonic seizures
    c. Bradykinesia, resting tremor
    d. Rapidly progressive dementia
    e. Loss of recent memory

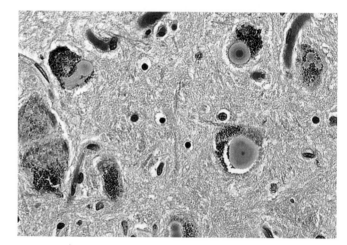

14. The pathology in this brain is characteristic of:
    a. Glioblastoma (World Health Organization [WHO] grade IV)
    b. Diffuse astrocytoma (WHO grade II)
    c. Metastatic lung adenocarcinoma
    d. Acute MCA occlusion
    e. Intraventricular meningioma

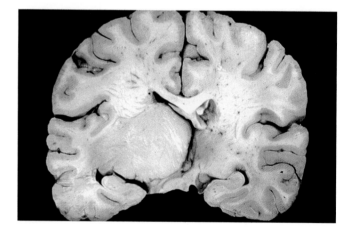

15. The pathology illustrated in this micrograph is characteristic of:
   a. Diffuse astrocytoma (WHO grade II)
   b. Medulloblastoma (WHO grade IV)
   c. Ependymoma (WHO grade II)
   d. Schwannoma (WHO grade I)
   e. Meningioma

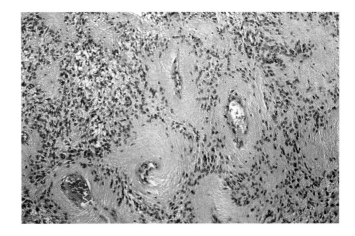

16. Which of the following is TRUE of this neoplasm?
   a. It is more frequently found in adults than in children.
   b. Its most common location is the spinal cord.
   c. It is associated with neurofibromatosis type 2 (NF2).
   d. It is potentially curable with resection.
   e. It is commonly associated with mutations in the *TP53* gene.

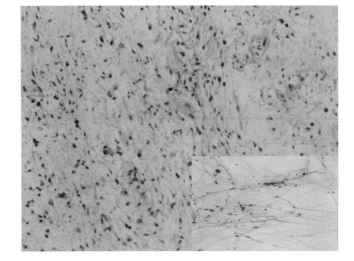

17. The glial disease illustrated here is MOST likely to be a consequence of:
   a. Severe hypoxia or hypoglycemia
   b. Posthepatic cirrhosis
   c. Parkinson disease (PD)
   d. AD
   e. Multiple system atrophy

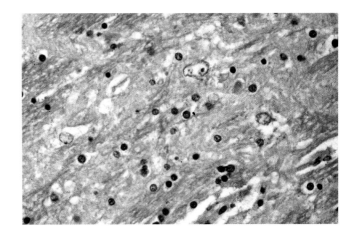

18. The consequences of meningeal infection caused by the organisms shown in this mucicarmine stain include:
    a. Granulomatous meningitis
    b. Acute neutrophilic exudates
    c. Subarachnoid hemorrhage
    d. Lymphocytic meningitis
    e. Little inflammatory reaction in the meninges

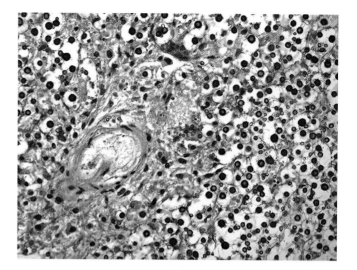

19. The lesion in this picture is the result of:
    a. Uncal herniation
    b. MS
    c. Rapid correction of hypernatremia or hyponatremia
    d. Intrathecal methotrexate treatment
    e. Descending tract degeneration in ALS

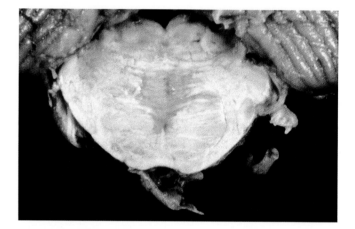

20. In addition to macroscopically complete removal of the lesion shown, these other features are also associated with a favorable outcome EXCEPT:
    a. Absence of microvascular proliferation
    b. Deletion of 1p and 19q
    c. Increased p53 positivity
    d. Low mitotic activity
    e. Lack of contrast enhancement on neuroimaging

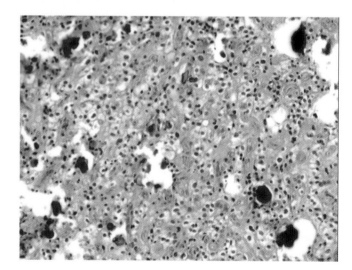

21. The cerebellar lesion shown has the following immunophenotype: inhibin positive, EMA negative, and CD10 negative. It is associated with which of the following syndromes?
    a. Von Hippel-Lindau
    b. Neurofibromatosis type 1 (NF1)
    c. Tuberous sclerosis
    d. Nevoid basal cell carcinoma syndrome
    e. Li-Fraumeni syndrome

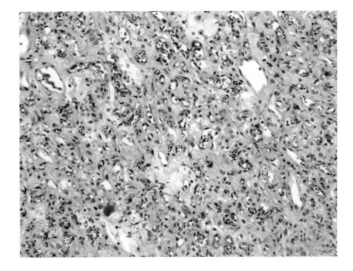

22. Resection of an enhancing lesion in the basal ganglia from a 58-year-old HIV positive man showed predominantly necrotic tissue and the microscopic findings shown in the picture. These findings are compatible with a diagnosis of:
    a. Coccidiodomycosis
    b. Toxoplasmosis
    c. Progressive multifocal leukoencephalopathy
    d. Cryptococcal meningitis
    e. Herpes simplex encephalitis

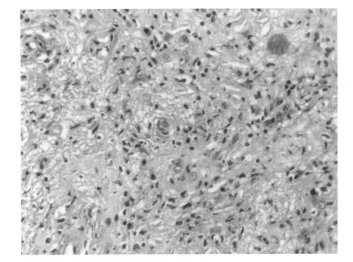

23. Which of the following immunoprofiles corresponds to the biopsy shown from a multicentric lesion in a 62-year-old woman?
    a. CD20 positive, synaptophysin negative, INI1 positive
    b. EMA positive, INI1 positive, glial fibrillary acidic protein (GFAP) negative
    c. CD20 negative, synaptophysin negative, GFAP positive
    d. EMA positive, INI1 negative, CD20 negative
    e. Synaptophysin positive, GFAP positive, cytokeratin negative

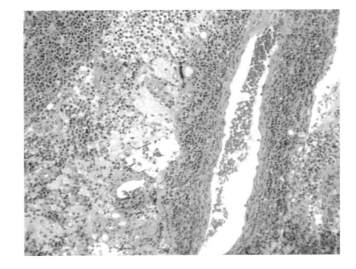

24. A 32-week premature infant suffered a severe hypotensive episode and was successfully resuscitated. A cranial ultrasound examination revealed bilateral areas of congestion in the subcortical white matter that evolved to small cystic areas over the following several weeks. After resuscitation, the infant remained lethargic. The MOST likely diagnosis is:
    a. Germinal matrix hemorrhage
    b. Porencephaly
    c. Status marmoratus
    d. Periventricular leukomalacia (PVL)
    e. Multicystic encephalopathy

25. Which of the following associations between an organism and the cell type(s) it infects is INCORRECT?
    a. Rabies virus—astrocyte
    b. Cytomegalovirus—ependymal cells
    c. HIV-1—cerebral microglia/monocyte/macrophage cells
    d. JC virus—oligodendrocytes, astrocytes
    e. Herpes simplex virus type 1—cortical neurons

26. Lesions of NF1 include all of the following EXCEPT:
    a. Multiple subcutaneous neurofibromas
    b. CNS meningiomas
    c. Café-au-lait spots
    d. Bilateral schwannomas of the seventh cranial nerve
    e. Gene mutations on chromosome 17

27. All of the following are true statements about carcinomas metastatic to the brain EXCEPT:
    a. MRI often shows one or more ring-enhancing lesions.
    b. The tumor cells usually show the histologic features of the primary tumor.
    c. Tumor cells typically express high levels of GFAP.
    d. Carcinoma of the lung is the most common tumor to metastasize to the brain.
    e. Metastatic tumors typically show a noninfiltrative growth pattern.

28. An infant develops hydrocephalus after resolution of *Escherichia coli* meningitis. The cause of this hydrocephalus is MOST likely due to:
    a. Communicating hydrocephalus due to block in cerebrospinal fluid (CSF) resorption
    b. Proliferation of the choroid plexus, overproducing CSF
    c. Obstructive hydrocephalus due to occlusion of the aqueduct of Sylvius
    d. a, b, and c
    e. a and c

29. All of the following histologic features are used to grade diffuse astrocytomas EXCEPT:
    a. Nuclear atypia
    b. Mitoses
    c. Endothelial proliferation
    d. Necrosis
    e. Degree of infiltration

30. An acute MS plaque is distinguishable from a chronic plaque by which of the following criteria?
    a. A well-circumscribed border
    b. The presence of large numbers of macrophages and enlarged astrocytes
    c. Lymphocytes in the lesion and in perivascular accumulations
    d. Complete loss of axons
    e. A periventricular location

31. Herpes simplex encephalitis MOST commonly involves which regions of the CNS:
    a. Midbrain and pons
    b. Basal ganglia and thalamus
    c. Frontal and temporal lobes
    d. Posterior columns of the spinal cord
    e. Ependymal lining of the ventricles

32. Which of the following genetic abnormalities are MOST commonly seen in meningiomas?
    a. p53 mutations
    b. PTEN (phosphatase and tensin homolog) mutations
    c. Deletions of chromosome 22
    d. Estrogen receptor mutations
    e. Deletions of chromosome 17

33. A motor vehicle accident in which an individual experiences severe, linear, and rotational accelerative-decelerative forces, but does not strike the head, can result in all of the following EXCEPT:
    a. Tearing of axons in subcortical white matter and corpus callosum
    b. Epidural hematoma, due to tearing of the middle meningeal artery
    c. Subdural hematoma
    d. Hemorrhages in subcortical white matter
    e. Atlanto-occipital dislocation

34. Multiple brain abscesses, often with hemorrhage, are characteristic of:
    a. MS
    b. Progressive multifocal leukoencephalopathy
    c. CNS borreliosis
    d. Acute demyelinating encephalomyelitis
    e. Aspergillosis cerebritis

35. A better response to temozolomide has been demonstrated in patients with glioblastomas showing:
    a. Hypermethylation of O(6)-methylguanine-DNA methyltransferase (MGMT)
    b. Loss of 1p and 19q
    c. P53 mutations
    d. IDH mutations
    e. PTEN mutations

ANSWERS

1. b. Craniopharyngiomas are slowly growing epithelial neoplasms in the suprasellar region. Patients can present with increased intracranial pressure due to compression of CSF flow, visual disturbances due to compression of the optic pathways, and endocrine deficiencies due to compression of the hypothalamus or pituitary. Grossly, craniopharyngiomas can have a mixture of solid and cystic components. The solid component can contain foci of calcifications and the cystic component may contain a dark brown thick liquid ("machine oil"-like). There are two variants of craniopharyngiomas: adamantinomatous and papillary. Adamantinomatous craniopharyngiomas are characterized by cords or lobules of squamous epithelium, often surrounded by a peripheral palisade of columnar cells. Loosely cohesive clusters of squamous cells (stellate reticulum), nodules of wet keratin, calcifications, and cholesterol clefts are typical of this type of craniopharyngioma. Papillary craniopharyngiomas are adult neoplasms and are characterized by a papillary architecture and well-differentiated squamous epithelium lacking surface maturation; calcifications are rare. Other suprasellar lesions include epidermoid cysts, characterized by a squamous epithelium with orderly maturation and dermoid cysts, which contain adnexal structures. Rathke cleft cysts occur in the suprasellar region or pituitary and consist of cyst(s) spaces lined by cuboidal epithelium. Pituitary adenomas, although most common in the sellar region, can extend to the suprasellar region and consist of monotonous sheets of small oval or polyhedral cells.

Louis DN, Ohgaki H, Wiestler OD, Cevenee WK (eds): *WHO Classification of Tumours of the Central Nervous System*, 4th ed. Lyon: IARC Press, 2007.
Perry A, Brat DJ (eds): *Practical Surgical Neuropathology: A Diagnostic Approach*. Philadelphia: Elsevier, 2010.

2. c. Neurons are especially vulnerable to damage by hypoxia, more so than astrocytes. Histologic features of hypoxic/ischemic cell change include shrinkage of the cell body and increased cytoplasmic acidophilia (red neuron), condensation of nuclear chromatin, and nuclear pyknosis. Acidophilic neurons can remain hours to days after injury. These acidophilic or red neurons are important to distinguish from dark neurons. Dark neurons are the result of biopsy artifact due to perturbed neurons at the time of fixation. Dark neurons are not eosinophilic, but have pyknotic nuclei; condensed, darkly staining cell bodies; and irregular dendrites. Certain types of neurons are more vulnerable than others to hypoxic/ischemic damage. These neurons include the pyramidal neurons in the CA1 region of the hippocampus, thalamus, and layers three and five of the neocortex, and Purkinje cells in the cerebellum. Ischemic changes can present as a result of either local or global ischemia. Local brain ischemia usually results from arterial stenosis or thrombosis, or from atheroemboli or thromboembolic arterial occlusion, and involves the area supplied by the affected vessel. An ischemic infarction would then occur if the ischemia is more profound or prolonged. Global brain ischemia occurs when there is a pronounced decrease in cerebral perfusion pressure, such as a consequence of severe hypotension or cardiac failure. The damage is more pronounced in watershed, or border zone, regions (regions at the borders of major arterial territories), especially in the depths of sulci. Global ischemia can be transient or permanent depending on when circulation returns.

Ellison D, Love S, Chimelli L, et al (eds): *Neuropathology: A Reference Text of CNS Pathology*, 3rd ed. Edinburgh: Mosby Elsevier, 2013.
Love S, Louis DN, Ellison DW (eds): *Greenfield's Neuropathology*, 8th ed. London: Hodder Arnold, 2008.

3. b. Prion diseases or transmissible spongiform encephalopathies are caused by the accumulation of an abnormal form of a normal cellular protein (prion). In the brain, neuronal death, gliosis, synaptic loss, and microvacuolation, or spongiform change, are present. Prion diseases display transmissibility to humans and other mammalian species. The molecular pathologic process of prion diseases involves the conversion of a normal cellular protein, called prion protein (PrP), into an abnormal configuration. The gene *PRNP* for PrP is located on chromosome 20. Four different human prion diseases have been identified: Creutzfeldt-Jakob disease (CJD) and variant Creutzfeldt-Jakob diseases (vCJD), Gerstmann-Sträussler-Scheinker disease (GSS), fatal familial insomnia (FFI), and kuru. GSS and FFI are inherited forms of the disease caused by mutations in the *PRNP* gene. vCJD and kuru are contracted by eating prion-containing tissues (bovine in the former, and human brain tissue in the latter). The annual incidence of sporadic CJD is one to two cases per 1 million population. Clinical presentation includes rapidly progressive dementia with ataxia and myoclonus. Pseudoperiodic synchronous discharges (PSDs) can be seen on the electroencephalogram (EEG). Computed tomography (CT) and MRI studies may show variable cerebral and cerebellar atrophy. Histologically, neuronal loss (especially in cortical layers III to V), gliosis, and vacuolation of the neuropil are seen in affected areas. The vacuoles are diffuse or focally clustered and are typically round and small. The vacuoles are intracellular and mainly occur in gray matter. The most common affected areas are the cerebral and cerebellar cortices, but basal ganglia and the thalamus can also be involved. Decontamination procedures should take place after conduction of autopsies of suspected prion disease. Instruments and surfaces can be decontaminated by immersion in or application of 2 *N* sodium hydroxide for 1 hour. Tissue for histologic examination should be treated with formic acid before processing.

Dickson DW, Weller RO (eds): *Neurodegeneration: The Molecular Pathology of Dementia and Movement Disorders*, 2nd ed. Oxford, UK: Wiley-Blackwell: International Society of Neuropathology, 2011.
Ellison D, Love S, Chimelli L, et al (eds): *Neuropathology: A Reference Text of CNS Pathology*, 3rd ed. Edinburgh: Mosby Elsevier, 2013.

4. a. AD is the most common cause of dementia and presents with early memory dysfunction and progresses to disorders of frontal and parietal lobe function, such as difficulties with executive function, spatial orientation, and aphasias. The brain in AD shows atrophy most prominently in the medial temporal regions (hippocampus), but also in the frontal, inferior temporal, and parietal regions. Significant ventricular enlargement can be present, as well as reduced brain weight. The major pathologic changes include extracellular deposits of a specific amyloid in the brain (amyloid plaques), intraneuronal filamentous inclusions (neurofibrillary tangles), and distortion of neuronal processes to form dystrophic neurites and neuropil threads, and loss of neurons in later stages. The amyloid plaques are composed of extracellular aggregates of Aβ peptide, which is derived from the normal neuronal membrane called APP. The gene of APP is located on chromosome 21 (association with Down syndrome). Silver stain and immunostaining for tau can demonstrate neuronal accumulation of fibrillary, hyperphosphorylated tau. In AD, tau may accumulate in the cell body (neurofibrillary tangles) or it may accumulate in neuronal processes (neuropil threads). Amyloid deposition can also occur in the arteries and arterioles in the cerebral and cerebellar cortex and leptomeninges leading to cerebral amyloid angiopathy. Amyloid angiopathy increases the risk of cerebral hemorrhage.

Dickson DW, Weller RO (eds): *Neurodegeneration: The Molecular Pathology of Dementia and Movement Disorders*, 2nd ed. Oxford, UK: Wiley-Blackwell: International Society of Neuropathology, 2011.
Ellison D, Love S, Chimelli L, et al (eds): *Neuropathology: A Reference Text of CNS Pathology*, 3rd ed. Edinburgh: Mosby Elsevier, 2013.

5. a. AVMs are the most common malformation producing brain hemorrhages and the second most common cause of subarachnoid hemorrhage. Although congenital, AVMs can become symptomatic at any age and can present with brain hemorrhage, subarachnoid hemorrhage, ischemia, seizure, or severe headaches. By angiography, a nidus is identified composed of a "feeding" artery/arteries and draining veins. AVMs are commonly supratentorial, occurring on the surface of the cerebral hemispheres. AVMs contain arteries, with muscular and elastic laminae, and dilated veins due to the pressure generated by the shunting of blood. The veins can have thin to thick walls and no elastic laminae. Arterialized veins are those with a thick collagenous wall but no elastic laminae. The vessels of the AVMs are usually embedded within brain parenchyma, which can show neuronal loss and gliosis. AVMs have been associated with hereditary hemorrhagic telangiectasia (Osler-Weber-Rendu syndrome). The second most common type of vascular malformation is the cavernous hemangioma. Cavernous hemangiomas have a tightly packed collection of dilated vessels without an intervening brain parenchyma.

Ellison D, Love S, Chimelli L, et al (eds): *Neuropathology: A Reference Text of CNS Pathology*, 3rd ed. Edinburgh: Mosby Elsevier, 2013.
Love S, Louis DN, Ellison DW (eds): *Greenfield's Neuropathology*, 8th ed. London: Hodder Arnold, 2008.

6. c. Cysticercosis is the most common parasitic infection. The clinical presentation varies but it can include seizures, papilledema, headache, vomiting and ataxia, focal motor and sensory deficits, dementia, and acute hydrocephalus. It is most common in the developing world and is caused by infection with the larval form of the pork tapeworm, *Taenia solium*. The disease can present 2 months to 30 years after infection. One or multiple cysts can occur in the parenchyma, meninges, or ventricles. A viable intraparenchymal cysticercus contains a single invaginated scolex. After degeneration, they become fibrotic and present as a firm white nodule (a calcified lesion on imaging). Histologically, the cyst wall is sparsely cellular and consists of three distinct layers: an outer, eosinophilic layer with microvilli; a middle cellular layer; and an inner reticular layer. Encysted larvae can be visible with minimal surrounding parenchymal reaction. During degeneration of the cyst, an inflammatory response is initiated, predominantly composed of neutrophils with variable amounts of granulation tissue, eosinophils, and fibrosis. When the cysticercus dies, it calcifies and the inflammation diminishes.

Ellison D, Love S, Chimelli L, et al (eds): *Neuropathology: A Reference Text of CNS Pathology*, 3rd ed. Edinburgh: Mosby Elsevier, 2013.
Love S, Louis DN, Ellison DW (eds): *Greenfield's Neuropathology*, 8th ed. London: Hodder Arnold, 2008.

7. b. Meningiomas arise from meningothelial (arachnoid) cells and occur throughout the CNS, where they are typically attached to the dura mater. They occur most commonly in woman and in middle-aged and elderly patients. Meningiomas consist of sheets or lobules of oval cells with intervening dense collagenous tissue. A syncytial growth pattern is present where cytologic borders are indistinct. Whorls and psammoma bodies are characteristic features, as well as nuclear clearing and nuclear pseudoinclusions. Meningiomas are immunoreactive to vimentin and EMA; meningiomas have a wide range of histologic patterns including fibrous, psammomatous, secretory, chordoid, clear cell, rhabdoid, and papillary. Of these, clear cell and chordoid meningiomas are graded as WHO grade II tumors, and papillary and rhabdoid meningiomas are graded as WHO grade III tumors. A meningioma is graded as "atypical," WHO grade II, if brain invasion or more than four mitotic figures in 10 high-power fields are identified. For "anaplastic" meningiomas, WHO grade III, more than 20 mitoses in 10 high-power fields are required. The differential diagnosis of a neoplasm in the subdural spaces in the spinal cord should include schwannomas. Antoni A and B patterns and Verocay bodies are histologic features of schwannomas. Immunohistochemistry is also helpful in differentiating meningiomas versus schwannomas, because the latter is S100 positive and EMA negative.

Louis DN, Ohgaki H, Wiestler OD, Cevenee WK (eds): *WHO Classification of Tumours of the Central Nervous System*, 4th ed. Lyon: IARC Press, 2007.
Perry A, Brat DJ (eds): *Practical Surgical Neuropathology: A Diagnostic Approach*. Philadelphia: Elsevier, 2010.

8. b. Inadequate perfusion of a brain territory due to arterial occlusion (e.g., thrombosis or embolism) leads to an ischemic infarction. Different gross and microscopic findings can be seen in an infarct at different times. Changes seen in acute infarction (8 to 36 hours) include blurring of the gray/white matter junction, a dusky discoloration of the gray matter, and slight softening. Microscopically, vacuolation of the neuropil and shrunken hypereosinophilic neurons are seen. Neutrophilic infiltration begins around 24 hours. In subacute infarction (5 to 30 days), cerebral edema is the most prominent abnormality; dusky gray discoloration and blurring of the gray/white matter junction are also present. Microscopic pathologic examination includes necrotic tissue, anecrotic and reactive microvessels, reactive astrocytes, and microglial activation with the presence of macrophages. Chronic infarction (months to years) is characterized by cavitation. The cystic cavity is surrounded by reactive astrocytes and may contain residual macrophages. The ACA supplies the most medial parts of the frontal lobes and superomedial parietal lobes. The MCA supplies the lateral surface of the hemispheres as well as the basal ganglia and the internal capsule. The posterior cerebral artery (PCA) supplies the occipital lobe.

Ellison D, Love S, Chimelli L, et al (eds.): *Neuropathology: A Reference Text of CNS Pathology*, 3rd ed. Edinburgh: Mosby Elsevier, 2013.
Love S, Louis DN, Ellison DW (eds): *Greenfield's Neuropathology*, 8th ed. London: Hodder Arnold, 2008.

9. e. Berry aneurysms occur at major branch points in the circle of Willis and at the basilar artery bifurcation. The aneurysm can be uni- or multilobular. The aneurysmal pouch consists of a thin wall of an endothelial layer and fibrous connective tissue. There is neither muscular tunica media nor internal elastic lamina in the aneurysm wall. Atherosclerotic changes can also be seen. Although thought to be congenital, the risk of developing aneurysms is increased by hypertension, AVM, systemic vascular disease, polycystic kidney disease, and defective vascular collagen, smooth muscle or elastic tissue. Rupture of a berry aneurysm produces a subarachnoid hemorrhage, although occasionally one can rupture into the brain if the aneurysm is embedded within the brain parenchyma. Hypertension increases the likelihood of rupture. Cigarette smoking, alcohol consumption, and cocaine abuse can also precipitate rupture of an aneurysm.

Ellison D, Love S, Chimelli L, et al (eds): *Neuropathology: A Reference Text of CNS Pathology*, 3rd ed. Edinburgh: Mosby Elsevier, 2013.
Love S, Louis DN, Ellison DW (eds): *Greenfield's Neuropathology*, 8th ed. London: Hodder Arnold, 2008.

10. a. Tabes dorsalis involves selective degeneration of the dorsal spinal nerve roots and ganglia with associated degeneration of the posterior columns of the spinal cord. Tabes dorsalis can present 15 to 20 years after the initial syphilis infection as pain or paresthesias in the distribution of the involved nerve roots. With time, loss of pain and proprioceptive sensation can occur. The histologic findings include marked loss of neurons from the dorsal root ganglia, with associated proliferation of satellite cells and inflammatory cells (lymphocytes and plasma cells). As a result, secondary wallerian degeneration of the posterior column occurs. Tabes dorsalis can be seen in tertiary syphilis. Syphilis infection is caused by the spirochete *Treponema pallidum* and can be divided into three stages: primary (development of a chancre), secondary (maculopapular rash, condylomata lata), and tertiary syphilis (cardiovascular, ocular, and gummatus forms). Involvement of the CNS by syphilis can also include syphilitic meningitis (1 to 2 years after infection with perivascular inflammation composed of plasma cells and lymphocytes) and gummatous neurosyphilis (solitary space-occupying lesions with central necrosis-gummas).

Ellison D, Love S, Chimelli L, et al (eds): *Neuropathology: A Reference Text of CNS Pathology*, 3rd ed. Edinburgh: Mosby Elsevier, 2013.
Love S, Louis DN, Ellison DW (eds): *Greenfield's Neuropathology*, 8th ed. London: Hodder Arnold, 2008.

11. b. Protein aggregation is a common finding in neurodegenerative diseases and can help classified diseases according to the protein that accumulates in different groups, such as AD, prion disease, tauopathies, and α-synucleinopathies. Aggregation of proteins can be the result of protein misfolding, in the case of tau accompanied by hyperphosphorylation. In AD, β-amyloid deposits form extracellular aggregates called amyloid plaques. Tauopathies, such as progressive supranuclear palsy, corticobasal degeneration, and frontotemporal lobe dementia, share with AD the presence of cytoplasmic, fibrillar aggregates of tau protein termed neurofibrillary tangles. In Pick disease, a tauopathy, basophilic, round, and well-demarcated cytoplasmic inclusions are seen and are called Pick bodies. These inclusions also stain with the antitau antibodies that react with neurofibrillary tangles. PD and dementia with Lewy bodies reveal cytoplasmic accumulations of α-synuclein called Lewy bodies. In multiple system atrophy, cytoplasmic inclusions positive for α-synuclein are seen predominantly in oligodendrocytes and are called glial cytoplasmic inclusions. In prion diseases, misfolded and aggregated versions of the normal cellular PrP are identified.

Dickson DW, Weller RO (eds): *Neurodegeneration: The Molecular Pathology of Dementia and Movement Disorders*, 2nd ed. Oxford, UK: Wiley-Blackwell: International Society of Neuropathology, 2011.
Ellison D, Love S, Chimelli L, et al (eds): *Neuropathology: A Reference Text of CNS Pathology*, 3rd ed. Edinburgh: Mosby Elsevier, 2013.

12. d. A large number of neurodegenerative diseases can be caused by genetic mutations or abnormalities. Genetic abnormalities can include single gene mutations and microsatellite repeat instability leading to expansion of tandem triplet repeats. Mutations in the gene for α-synuclein, *SNCA*, cause some familial cases of PD. α-Synuclein is a protein that forms the pathologic inclusions (Lewy body) in PD, diffuse Lewy bodies, and multiple system atrophy. In Huntington disease, an increase in the number of repeats of the CAG sequence is seen in the *HTT* gene localized in the short arm of chromosome 4 and coding for the protein huntingtin. Mutations in the *APP* gene have been associated with autosomal dominant forms of AD. The *APP* gene is located on chromosome 21 (thus, the association of AD and Down syndrome) and codes for the APP. The tau gene, *MAPT*, is located on chromosome 17 and codes for the microtubule-associated protein, tau. Mutations in this gene are associated with chromosome 17-linked frontotemporal lobar dementia. In X-linked bulbospinal neuronopathy (like Kennedy disease), a CAG repeat region in the first exon of the androgen receptor gene on the X chromosome causes slowly progressive lower motor neuron weakness of facial, bulbar, and proximal limb muscles.

Dickson DW, Weller RO (eds): *Neurodegeneration: The Molecular Pathology of Dementia and Movement Disorders*, 2nd ed. Oxford, UK: Wiley-Blackwell: International Society of Neuropathology, 2011.
Ellison D, Love S, Chimelli L, et al (eds): *Neuropathology: A Reference Text of CNS Pathology*, 3rd ed. Edinburgh: Mosby Elsevier, 2013.

13. c. PD is a neurodegenerative disorder with a clinical picture that includes bradykinesia or akinesia, resting tremors, rigidity, and postural instability. Also associated are autonomic dysfunction, cognitive disturbances, and dysphagia. It has a mean age of onset of 61 years. Pallor of the substantia nigra and locus coeruleus is seen in brains of patients with PD, due to the loss of pigmented neurons. Cerebral atrophy and ventricular enlargement can also be present. The histopathologic features of PD include widespread α-synuclein accumulations in neurons and dystrophic neurites throughout the CNS. Lewy body accumulation in isocortical neurons is a hallmark of diffuse Lewy body disease. In addition, variable neuronal loss occurs in many nuclei, in particular the substantia nigra, locus coeruleus, nucleus basalis of Meynert, and dorsal motor nucleus of the vagus nerve. The prominent lesions of PD are α-synuclein-positive Lewy bodies. Lewy bodies are spherical, cytoplasmic, intraneuronal inclusions with a hyaline eosinophilic core, concentric lamellar bands, and a narrow pale-stained halo. Mutations in the gene for α-synuclein, *SNCA*, have been associated with some familial cases of PD. There are patients with dementia whose brains contain both PD (Lewy bodies) and AD (amyloid plaques and neurofibrillary tangles).

Dickson DW, Weller RO (eds): *Neurodegeneration: The Molecular Pathology of Dementia and Movement Disorders*, 2nd ed. Oxford, UK: Wiley-Blackwell: International Society of Neuropathology, 2011.
Ellison D, Love S, Chimelli L, et al (eds): *Neuropathology: A Reference Text of CNS Pathology*, 3rd ed. Edinburgh: Mosby Elsevier, 2013.

14. b. Diffuse fibrillary astrocytomas occur throughout the CNS, generally in adults, and are most frequently located within the cerebral hemispheres. The lesions are composed of individual tumor cells that infiltrate widely throughout the brain parenchyma, and can be graded according to cellular density, degree of anaplasia, and other findings. Due to the diffuse infiltration, the neoplasms are poorly demarcated. In diffuse astrocytomas (grade II), the neoplastic cells show mild atypia, such as nuclear pleomorphism and hyperchromasia, and fibrillar processes, which are highlighted by GFAP immunostain. A low rate of mitotic activity is characteristic of diffuse astrocytomas, which are diagnosed as grade II astrocytomas. An increase in mitotic activity and atypia, but without necrosis and microvascular proliferation, would be diagnostic of a grade III astrocytoma or anaplastic astrocytoma. The presence of endothelial proliferation and necrosis, especially pseudopalisading necrosis, in a diffuse astrocytoma corresponds to a diagnosis of glioblastoma or grade IV astrocytoma. *IDH1* gene mutations are common in low-grade gliomas, both diffuse astrocytomas and oligodendrogliomas, and in secondary glioblastomas, but very rarely seen in primary glioblastomas. The presence of mutant IDH1 protein in tumor cells can be detected by immunohistochemistry. Mutations in TP53 are much more characteristic of diffuse astrocytomas than oligodendrogliomas. Accumulation of the mutant p53 in tumor cell nuclei can be detected by immunocytochemistry. PTEN and EGFR (epidermal growth factor receptor) are mutated more commonly in primary glioblastomas than in secondary glioblastomas, which arise from lower grade gliomas.

Louis DN, Ohgaki H, Wiestler OD, Cevenee WK (eds): *WHO Classification of Tumours of the Central Nervous System*, 4th ed. Lyon: IARC Press, 2007.
Perry A, Brat DJ (eds): *Practical Surgical Neuropathology: A Diagnostic Approach*. Philadelphia: Elsevier, 2010.

15. c. Ependymomas are generally slow-growing tumors originating from the wall of the ventricles or spinal canal. Ependymomas can be either infratentorial or supratentorial and are more frequent in children and young adults. Ependymomas grow as circumscribed masses generally related to the ventricular system. They occur most commonly in the posterior fossa, where they can fill the fourth ventricle. Histologically the tumor is composed of sheets of uniform cells with indistinct borders and "salt and pepper" chromatin. Perivascular pseudorosettes are a feature of ependymomas and appear as a perivascular anuclear zone of fibrillary processes surrounded by the cell bodies of the neoplastic cells. Also seen are ependymal (true) rosettes with a central lumen surrounded by columnar cells. Ependymomas can be grade II or grade III. Increased pleomorphism, mitotic activity, necrosis, and capillary endothelial proliferation would classify an ependymoma as a grade III or anaplastic ependymoma. Other types of ependymomas include subependymomas (grade I) and myxopapillary ependymomas (grade I). GFAP immunoreactivity is seen in ependymomas, especially in the perivascular pseudorosettes. EMA positivity can be seen along the borders of ependymal rosettes and as dotlike cytoplasmic positivity in scattered cells.

Louis DN, Ohgaki H, Wiestler OD, Cevenee WK (eds): *WHO Classification of Tumours of the Central Nervous System*, 4th ed. Lyon: IARC Press, 2007.
Perry A, Brat DJ (eds): *Practical Surgical Neuropathology: A Diagnostic Approach*. Philadelphia: Elsevier, 2010.

16. d. Pilocytic astrocytomas are relatively well circumscribed, slow-growing tumors that can appear radiologically as cysts with an enhancing mural nodule. Pilocytic astrocytomas are more common in children and young adults. The preferred sites include cerebellum, optic nerve and chiasm, brain stem, hypothalamus, and temporal lobe. The tumor has a biphasic appearance: compact areas with fascicles consisting of elongated cells with long thick processes and microcystic areas within a network of long processes. Rosenthal fibers and eosinophilic granular bodies are common findings. Nuclear pleomorphism can be increased and is not of prognostic significance, most likely representing degenerative change. Tandem duplications of the *BRAF* gene are present in a large number of pilocytic astrocytomas. In comparison to diffuse astrocytomas, IDH1/2 and TP53 mutations are absent in pilocytic astrocytomas. Pilocytic astrocytomas are classified as a grade I neoplasm. They very rarely progress to an anaplastic form. Similar histologic findings can be seen in the gliomatous part of gangliogliomas, but these also contain dysmorphic ganglion cells.

Louis DN, Ohgaki H, Wiestler OD, Cevenee WK (eds): *WHO Classification of Tumours of the Central Nervous System*, 4th ed. Lyon: IARC Press, 2007.
Perry A, Brat DJ (eds): *Practical Surgical Neuropathology: A Diagnostic Approach*. Philadelphia: Elsevier, 2010.

17. b. Hepatic encephalopathy is a neurologic complication of liver disease. Patients can present with short-term memory problems, confusion, and drowsiness. The characteristic histologic finding in hepatic encephalopathy is the presence of Alzheimer type II astrocytes. These cells have enlarged, irregular, lucent nuclei with marginated chromatin and scanty cytoplasm. Alzheimer type II astrocytes are commonly found in the caudate nucleus, putamen, thalamus, dentate nucleus of the cerebellum, and deep layers of the cerebral cortex.

Ellison D, Love S, Chimelli L, et al (eds): *Neuropathology: A Reference Text of CNS Pathology*, 3rd ed. Edinburgh: Mosby Elsevier, 2013.
Love S, Louis DN, Ellison DW (eds): *Greenfield's Neuropathology*, 8th ed. London: Hodder Arnold, 2008.

18. e. Cryptococcal infection of the CNS can present as meningoencephalitis or cryptococcal abscesses due to hematogenous spread to the CNS, more commonly in immunosuppressed patients. The fungus *Cryptococcus neoformans* is a spherical/oval budding yeast with a thick polysaccharide capsule, which stains with mucin. The yeasts can also be visualized by PAS or methenamine silver impregnation. The leptomeningeal inflammation associated with infection is usually scant and can include lymphocytes, plasma cells, eosinophils, and multinucleated giant cells. The fungal organisms can be seen within the giant cells. The fungus can move along the Virchow-Robin spaces to spread into the brain parenchyma. Another yeast infection involving the CNS is candidiasis, which usually presents as a late manifestation of systemic candidiasis. The findings include scattered hemorrhagic infarcts due to thrombosed vessels. Budding yeasts and pseudohyphae can be seen in hematoxylin-eosin, PAS, and Gomori methenamine silver (GMS) preparations. Other yeast forms—*Histoplasma*, *Blastomyces*, and *Coccidioides*—can also infect the CNS when systemic infection occurs, but these cases are rare.

Ellison D, Love S, Chimelli L, et al (eds): *Neuropathology: A Reference Text of CNS Pathology*, 3rd ed. Edinburgh: Mosby Elsevier, 2013.
Love S, Louis DN, Ellison DW (eds): *Greenfield's Neuropathology*, 8th ed. London: Hodder Arnold, 2008.

19. c. Central pontine myelinolysis occurs as a complication of rapid correction of hypo- or hypernatremia. Clinically, the patient can present with rapid onset of confusion, seizures, limb weakness, conjugate gaze palsies, dysarthria, dysphagia, and hypotension. Gray discoloration and softness in the basis pontis is present. The lesions can also extend to the upper parts of the pons and can have a symmetrical, triangular shape. Other parts of the CNS can also be involved, including the basal ganglia and lateral geniculate bodies. Active demyelination is seen microscopically characterized by large numbers of foamy, lipid-laden macrophages; most axons are preserved. Methotrexate toxicity, associated with high dosage or intrathecal administration, reveals multiple discrete or confluent foci of coagulative necrosis with myelin loss in the cerebral and spinal white matter.

Ellison D, Love S, Chimelli L, et al (eds): *Neuropathology: A Reference Text of CNS Pathology*, 3rd ed. Edinburgh: Mosby Elsevier, 2013.
Love S, Louis DN, Ellison DW (eds): *Greenfield's Neuropathology*, 8th ed. London: Hodder Arnold, 2008.

20. c. Oligodendrogliomas are diffusely infiltrating gliomas usually present in adulthood and most often in the cerebral hemispheres (predominantly in the frontal lobes). Oligodendrogliomas are composed of uniform cells with round nuclei and perinuclear halos ("fried egg" appearance) on paraffin sections. Microcystic degeneration and dystrophic calcifications can be present. A delicate vasculature consisting of branching capillaries runs through the neoplasm ("chicken-wire"). Increase in mitotic activity and presence of microvascular proliferation indicate a more aggressive behavior consistent with an anaplastic oligodendroglioma, WHO grade III. Absence of these features, as well as necrosis, is compatible with a WHO grade II oligodendroglioma. Concurrent deletion of chromosomal arms 1p and 19q is a hallmark alteration in oligodendrogliomas. This genetic signature is associated with both prolonged survival time and a favorable response to various chemotherapy agents or radiation therapy. Favorable prognostic indicators for oligodendrogliomas include young age, WHO grade 2, less than 5% ki-67 labeling index, and 1p/19q loss.

Louis DN, Ohgaki H, Wiestler OD, Cevenee WK (eds): *WHO Classification of Tumours of the Central Nervous System*, 4th ed. Lyon: IARC Press, 2007.
Perry A, Brat DJ (eds): *Practical Surgical Neuropathology: A Diagnostic Approach*. Philadelphia: Elsevier, 2010.

21. a. Von Hippel-Lindau syndrome (VHL) is an autosomal dominant familial cancer syndrome. The VHL tumor suppressor gene is present on chromosome 3p25. CNS hemangioblastoma, retinal angiomas, renal cysts, renal cell carcinoma (RCC), pancreatic cysts, or epididymal papillary cystadenoma can occur in affected patients. Hemangioblastomas are slow-growing tumors that usually present in the cerebellar hemispheres, but can occur in the brain stem, spinal cord, and, rarely, in the cerebrum and can be multiple. Cerebellar hemangioblastomas frequently present as cysts with a mural nodule. Hemangioblastomas are composed of vascular and stromal cells. Endothelial cells and pericytes form a dense network of small vascular channels. Interstitial cells often contain lipid and variable amounts of glycogen (foamy stromal cells) and often show nuclear pleomorphism and hyperchromasia. In VHL patients, distinction between metastatic RCC and hemangioblastomas is warranted. Immunohistochemistry can help distinguish these two entities because hemangioblastomas show positivity for inhibin-alpha and are negative for CD10; in contrast, RCCs are negative for inhibin-alpha and usually positive for CD10.

Louis DN, Ohgaki H, Wiestler OD, Cevenee WK (eds): *WHO Classification of Tumours of the Central Nervous System*, 4th ed. Lyon: IARC Press, 2007.
Perry A, Brat DJ (eds): *Practical Surgical Neuropathology: A Diagnostic Approach*. Philadelphia: Elsevier, 2010.

22. b. Toxoplasmosis is usually acquired by consumption of undercooked meat containing the parasitic cysts of *Toxoplama gondii*. Infection most commonly produces neurologic disease in patients with immunosuppression (e.g., HIV). The clinical picture is usually one of a mass lesion causing seizures or focal neurologic signs. Clinical suspicion should be increased in patients with HIV infection or other reasons for immunosuppression. Imaging studies demonstrate single or multiple ring-enhancing lesions, which are most commonly seen in the basal ganglia, thalamus, and gray-white matter junction. Microscopically, necrotizing abscesses or foci of coagulative necrosis surrounded by reactive astrocytes, microglial nodules, and inflammation characterize the initial lesions. Fibrous encapsulation, fibrinoid necrosis, and perivascular hemorrhage can also be present. Intracellular and extracellular *Toxoplasma* tachyzoites are oval or crescent-shaped organisms. Bradyzoites, the more slowly proliferating stage, accumulate within small cysts.

Ellison D, Love S, Chimelli L, et al (eds): *Neuropathology: A Reference Text of CNS Pathology*, 3rd ed. Edinburgh: Mosby Elsevier, 2013.
Love S, Louis DN, Ellison DW (eds): *Greenfield's Neuropathology*, 8th ed. London: Hodder Arnold, 2008.

23. a. CNS lymphomas may be primary or secondary. Primary CNS lymphomas are confined to the brain or spinal cord, most commonly involving the hemispheres. The majority of primary CNS lymphomas are diffuse, large B-cell lymphomas. Secondary CNS lymphomas spread to the brain or spinal cord from a primary site outside the CNS. Lymphomas present as space-occupying lesions causing raised intracranial pressure, focal neurologic deficit, or seizures. Imaging reveals irregular, sometimes multifocal, contrast-enhancing masses. Lymphomas are characterized by sheets of tumor cells separated by areas of necrosis. The cells tend to invade the walls of small cerebral blood vessels and accumulate in perivascular spaces. Like a glioma, lymphomas can diffusely invade CNS tissue and can also spread to the subarachnoid space. The differential diagnosis of lymphoma in the CNS include: oligodendroglioma, primitive neuroectodermal tumor, small cell carcinoma, and gliomas (infiltrative pattern). CNS lymphomas respond rapidly to steroid therapy.

Ellison D, Love S, Chimelli L, et al (eds): *Neuropathology: A Reference Text of CNS Pathology*, 3rd ed. Edinburgh: Mosby Elsevier, 2013.
Louis DN, Ohgaki H, Wiestler OD, Cevenee WK (eds): *WHO Classification of Tumours of the Central Nervous System*, 4th ed. Lyon: IARC Press, 2007.
Perry A, Brat DJ (eds): *Practical Surgical Neuropathology: A Diagnostic Approach*. Philadelphia: Elsevier, 2010.

24. d. PVL or white matter necrosis is a developmental lesion consisting of focal or more extensive regions of softening in the white matter. Premature infants (24 to 32 weeks) are at greatest risk for PVL. Microscopically, PVL shows foci of necrosis in the periventricular regions and a surrounding, diffuse, reactive gliosis and microglial activation. In older lesions, cavitation, a microcystic parenchyma, and calcifications can be present. A glial scar can be found in the previously necrotic component. Germinal matrix hemorrhages are mainly seen in low-birth-weight premature infants. They can occur anywhere in the periventricular tissue and can extend into the ventricles and adjacent brain parenchyma. Porencephaly and multicystic encephalopathy are fetal lesions due to hypoxic-ischemic injury. Porencephaly consists of smooth-walled defects in the cerebral mantle, and multicystic encephalopathy produces multiple cysts from third trimester injury.

Ellison D, Love S, Chimelli L, et al (eds): *Neuropathology: A Reference Text of CNS Pathology*, 3rd ed. Edinburgh: Mosby Elsevier, 2013.
Love S, Louis DN, Ellison DW (eds): *Greenfield's Neuropathology*, 8th ed. London: Hodder Arnold, 2008.

25. a. The classic histologic feature of rabies includes the presence of Negri bodies, which are delineated, round to oval eosinophilic inclusions in the cytoplasm of neurons. Perivascular lymphocytic infiltrates, neuronophagia, and clusters of microglia (Babes nodules) can be present in a limited degree. Cytomegalovirus infection can present as a necrotizing encephalitis or ventriculoencephalitis with infiltration by lymphocytes and macrophages and the presence of microglial nodules and typical cytomegalic inclusion cells. Neurons, glia, and endothelial cells can be infected, especially in the subependymal region. HIV infects mainly microglial cells or macrophages, which can produce a leukoencephalopathy or leukoencephalitis. In HIV encephalitis, the presence of multinucleated giant cells is characteristic. Progressive multifocal leukoencephalopathy is caused by the JC papovavirus, which produces a demyelinating disease. Viral inclusions can be detected in infected oligodendrocytes. Astrocytes are also infected. Specific diagnosis is made using antibodies to SV40 T antigen. Herpes simplex virus produces a necrotizing encephalitis; affected nuclei of neurons, glia, and endothelial cells can contain homogenous eosinophilic inclusions and a rim of condensed marginated chromatin. Cowdry type A inclusions, seen as an eosinophilic material separated of the marginated chromatin by a clear zone, can be found in infected cells.

Ellison D, Love S, Chimelli L, et al (eds): *Neuropathology: A Reference Text of CNS Pathology*, 3rd ed. Edinburgh: Mosby Elsevier, 2013.
Love S, Louis DN, Ellison DW (eds): *Greenfield's Neuropathology*, 8th ed. London: Hodder Arnold, 2008.

26. d. NF1 is an autosomal dominant disease associated with the NF1 gene on chromosome 17q11, which codes for neurofibromin. Neoplasms associated with NF1 include: neurofibromas, malignant nerve sheath tumors, optic nerve gliomas, rhabdomyosarcomas, pheochromocytomas, and carcinoid tumors. Other findings in NF1 patients include café-au-lait spots, Lisch nodules, and axillary freckling. NF2 is an autosomal dominant disease associated with the NF2 gene on chromosome 22q12, which codes for merlin. Neoplasms associated with NF2 include schwannomas, neurofibromas, ependymomas, and meningiomas. Patients with NF2 can present with bilateral eighth cranial nerve schwannomas.

Louis DN, Ohgaki H, Wiestler OD, Cevenee WK (eds): *WHO Classification of Tumours of the Central Nervous System*, 4th ed. Lyon: IARC Press, 2007.
Perry A, Brat DJ (eds): *Practical Surgical Neuropathology: A Diagnostic Approach*. Philadelphia: Elsevier, 2010.

27. c. Metastatic neoplasms can present as either single or multiple lesions causing raised intracranial pressure, focal neurologic deficits, or epilepsy. Metastatic carcinomas are the most common CNS neoplasms. The most common metastatic neoplasms are lung cancer, breast cancer, and melanoma. Sometimes metastases to the CNS present clinically before any signs or symptoms of the primary carcinoma. Immunohistochemistry can help determine the organ of origin. The majority of brain metastases are located in the cerebral hemispheres, especially in arterial border zones and at the junction of cerebral cortex and white matter. Usually more than one lesion is present. Hemorrhage into the neoplasm is characteristic of malignant melanoma, choriocarcinomas, and metastatic RCC. Histologically, the neoplasm is usually well demarcated from adjacent brain parenchyma and usually shows features identical or similar to those of the primary carcinoma.

Louis DN, Ohgaki H, Wiestler OD, Cevenee WK (eds): *WHO Classification of Tumours of the Central Nervous System*, 4th ed. Lyon: IARC Press, 2007.
Perry A, Brat DJ (eds): *Practical Surgical Neuropathology: A Diagnostic Approach*. Philadelphia: Elsevier, 2010.

28. a. Bacterial meningitis presents with fever, headache, vomiting, nuchal rigidity, and photophobia, some of which are symptoms associated with increased intracranial pressure. The principal etiologic agent causing meningitis varies by age group. In neonates, it is usually caused by gram-negative bacilli (mostly *E. coli*). In children, *Haemophilus influenzae* type b and *Neisseria meningitidis* are the most common. In adults, *Streptococcus pneumoniae* accounts for more than 50% of cases. Histologically, an exudate containing large numbers of neutrophils and necrotic debris extending along perivascular spaces into the brain parenchyma is seen. Bacteria (intra- and extracellular) can usually be demonstrated by Gram stain. Complications of acute meningitis include obstructive or communicating hydrocephalus (thick meninges block the arachnoid granulations) and cavitation of cerebral gray and white matter. Other complications include cerebral edema, infarctions, and subdural effusions. Bacterial infections can also lead to the formation of brain abscesses. An encapsulated brain abscess is composed of a necrotic center, a surrounding rim of granulation tissue, and a capsule composed of fibroblasts, collagen, and inflammatory cells.

Ellison D, Love S, Chimelli L, et al (eds): *Neuropathology: A Reference Text of CNS Pathology*, 3rd ed. Edinburgh: Mosby Elsevier, 2013.
Love S, Louis DN, Ellison DW (eds): *Greenfield's Neuropathology*, 8th ed. London: Hodder Arnold, 2008.

29. e. Diffuse astrocytomas can be graded according to histologic features into three different grades: diffuse astrocytomas (grade II), anaplastic astrocytomas (grade III), and glioblastomas (grade IV). Diffuse astrocytomas present more commonly in the third and fourth decades. By radiology, low-grade astrocytomas are generally ill-defined and nonenhancing and diffusely expand the white matter. They are reflections of the infiltration of CNS tissue by diffuse astrocytomas. They are most commonly located in the cerebral hemispheres. Cortical invasion and edema can produce expansion of the gyri. The neoplastic cells show mild atypia, such as nuclear pleomorphism and hyperchromasia, and fibrillar processes, which are highlighted by GFAP immunostain. Low-grade diffuse astrocytomas can contain IDH1 and TP53 mutations. Increased mitotic activity and atypia, but without necrosis and microvascular proliferation, would be diagnostic of a

grade III astrocytoma or anaplastic astrocytoma. The presence of endothelial proliferation and necrosis, especially pseudopalisading necrosis, in a diffuse astrocytoma corresponds to a diagnosis of glioblastoma, or grade IV astrocytoma. The low-grade tumors have a tendency to progress to a higher grade. When they become glioblastomas, they are referred to as secondary glioblastomas, in contrast to glioblastomas that arise de novo.

Louis DN, Ohgaki H, Wiestler OD, Cevenee WK (eds): *WHO Classification of Tumours of the Central Nervous System*, 4th ed. Lyon: IARC Press, 2007.
Perry A, Brat DJ (eds): *Practical Surgical Neuropathology: A Diagnostic Approach*. Philadelphia: Elsevier, 2010.

30. b. MS is the most common demyelinating disease of the CNS. MS is typically multifocal and the lesions can be of different ages. Clinically, the disease can have a relapsing and remitting course or a progressive course over many years. It is most common in women and its symptoms vary according to the location of the lesions and can include optic neuritis, diplopia, weakness, paresthesia, and sensory loss of one or more limbs. Areas of demyelination (plaques) appear as well-demarcated regions varying in size and shape at the junction between the cerebral gray and white matter and within the cortical gray matter and deep gray nuclei. Plaques can also be present in the cerebellar white matter, brain stem, and spinal cord. Active plaques contain a dense perivascular and parenchymal infiltrate of lymphocytes and macrophages, greatest at the edge of the lesion. Complete or almost complete demyelination is seen in the plaques. Axons are usually relatively preserved, although axonal swellings are common. Chronic inactive plaques are densely gliotic lesions with loss of oligodendrocytes and myelin and usually axonal loss. Inflammatory component is minimal to none.

Ellison D, Love S, Chimelli L, et al (eds): *Neuropathology: A Reference Text of CNS Pathology*, 3rd ed. Edinburgh: Mosby Elsevier, 2013.
Love S, Louis DN, Ellison DW (eds): *Greenfield's Neuropathology*, 8th ed. London: Hodder Arnold, 2008.

31. c. The clinical picture of herpes simplex encephalitis involves nonspecific features of encephalitis (headache, neck stiffness) and focal neurologic signs (e.g., dysphagia, hemiparesis, and focal seizures). CSF examination may reveal a moderate leukocytosis and elevated protein levels. Acute presentation is characterized by bilateral, usually asymmetrical, congestion and hemorrhagic necrosis involving the temporal lobes. The lesions can extend from the pial surface through the cerebral cortex and into the white matter. A mild to moderate lymphocytic infiltrate is present in the leptomeninges and some is seen within the parenchyma. Affected cells (neurons, glia, and endothelial cells) have a slightly hypereosinophilic cytoplasm and the nuclei are pyknotic and can contain homogeneous eosinophilic inclusions. An irregular rim of condensed marginated chromatin can be seen. Cowdry type A inclusions, eosinophilic inclusions surrounded by a clear halo, and marginated chromation can be present in infected cells, especially along the periphery of the lesion. Immunocytochemistry provides a sensitive assay for herpes. In long-term survivors, affected parts of the brain are shrunken and cavitated. A glial scar replaces the normal gray and white matter and some inflammatory component may remain.

Ellison D, Love S, Chimelli L, et al (eds): *Neuropathology: A Reference Text of CNS Pathology*, 3rd ed. Edinburgh: Mosby Elsevier, 2013.

Love S, Louis DN, Ellison DW (eds): *Greenfield's Neuropathology*, 8th ed. London: Hodder Arnold, 2008.

32. c. Monosomy of chromosome 22 is the most common cytogenetic abnormality in meningiomas. Loss of heterozygosity for chromosome 22q markers is also seen. NF2 (22q12) mutation frequently accompanies allelic loss on chromosome 22q. Patients with NF2 can therefore develop meningiomas. TP53 gene mutations are considered to be early events in neoplastic progression of astrocytomas and are common in diffuse astrocytomas and secondary glioblastomas. Accumulation of nuclear p53 in tumor cells can be detected by immunohistochemistry. IDH mutations have been found to be common in low-grade gliomas, including oligodendrogliomas, but are very rarely seen in primary glioblastomas. PTEN is mutated more commonly in primary glioblastomas than in secondary glioblastomas.

Louis DN, Ohgaki H, Wiestler OD, Cevenee WK (eds): *WHO Classification of Tumours of the Central Nervous System*, 4th ed. Lyon: IARC Press, 2007.

Perry A, Brat DJ (eds): *Practical Surgical Neuropathology: A Diagnostic Approach*. Philadelphia: Elsevier, 2010.

33. b. Traumatic axonal injury can result from acceleration and deceleration forces to the head, the most severe being diffuse axonal injury (DAI). The main regions affected are the superior, parasagittal cerebral white matter, corpus callosum, subcortical fiber tracts, superior cerebellar peduncles, and brain stem. Histologic changes in DAI include axonal swellings in the white matter and accumulations of APP, due to an interruption of fast axonal transport. Weeks and months after the insult, one sees loss of axons and myelin and clusters of microglia. DAI leads to cognitive, motor, and sensory abnormalities, and in severe form a persistent vegetative state. Rapid accelerative-decelerative forces can produce stretching, deformation, and tearing of small blood vessels causing diffuse vascular damage. This can show as petechial hemorrhages, mostly in the frontal and temporal white matter, diencephalon, and brain stem. Acute subdural hematomas can be the result of the head being subjected to rapid acceleration or deceleration. This movement causes traction on, and tearing of, bridging veins between brain and dura. Gliding contusions are usually associated with diffuse axonal injury and are seen as hemorrhages involving the deep layers of the cortex and white matter.

Ellison D, Love S, Chimelli L, et al (eds): *Neuropathology: A Reference Text of CNS Pathology*, 3rd ed. Edinburgh: Mosby Elsevier, 2013.

Love S, Louis DN, Ellison DW (eds): *Greenfield's Neuropathology*, 8th ed. London: Hodder Arnold, 2008.

34. e. CNS infection by the fungus *Aspergillus* (aspergillosis) can occur from hematogenous spread from the lungs or by direct extension from paranasal sinuses, middle ears, or orbit. The clinical presentation can include headaches, hemiparesis, focal neurologic deficits, seizures, cranial nerve palsies, and increased intracranial pressure. Patients with immunosuppression are at major risk of infection. Hematogenous spread can lead to single or multiple lesions involving more commonly the cerebral cortex, white matter, and basal ganglia. Early lesions resemble necrotic and hemorrhagic infarcts with surrounding edema. Abscess formation can be present. Infiltration by fungal hyphae of blood vessels causes thrombosis, hemorrhage, and infarction, accompanied by a variable inflammatory infiltrate. Fungal hyphae are demonstrated by methenamine silver impregnation. In chronic cases, a granulomatous inflammation with giant cells and fibrosis can be present.

Ellison D, Love S, Chimelli L, et al (eds): *Neuropathology: A Reference Text of CNS Pathology*, 3rd ed. Edinburgh: Mosby Elsevier, 2013.

Love S, Louis DN, Ellison DW (eds): *Greenfield's Neuropathology*, 8th ed. London: Hodder Arnold, 2008.

35. a. Glioblastoma is the most frequent primary brain tumor and the most malignant. Histologically, glioblastomas show nuclear atypia of astrocytic cells, increased mitotic activity, microvascular proliferation, and necrosis. Glioblastomas are highly resistant to therapy, which can include aggressive surgical resection, radiation therapy, and maximum tolerated doses for chemotherapy. Many of the chemotherapeutic agents used to treat glioblastoma, including temozolomide, are agents that cross-link DNA by alkylating at the O(6) position of guanine. DNA cross-linking is reversed by the DNA repair enzyme MGMT. Tumors with low levels of MGMT expression would, therefore, be expected to demonstrate a better response to alkylating agents, because there is reduced repair. The expression level of MGMT is determined in large part by the methylation status of the gene's promoter. Increased methylation leads to decreased MGMT levels. Promoter methylation status can be assessed on polymerase chain reaction (PCR)-based tests of genomic DNA. Epigenetic silencing of MGMT in glioblastoma is associated with a longer survival period among patients treated with temozolomide and radiotherapy. In addition, promoter methylation also seems to have a positive prognostic effect independent of therapy.

Louis DN, Ohgaki H, Wiestler OD, Cevenee WK (eds): *WHO Classification of Tumours of the Central Nervous System*, 4th ed. Lyon: IARC Press, 2007.

Perry A, Brat DJ (eds): *Practical Surgical Neuropathology: A Diagnostic Approach*. Philadelphia: Elsevier, 2010.

CHAPTER 16

SOFT TISSUE PATHOLOGY
Fabrizio Remotti

*Q*UESTIONS

Questions 1-20 refer to a photograph or photomicrograph.

1. The microscopic fields correspond to a recent onset spindle cell proliferation involving the subcutaneous tissue of a 35-year-old man. Which one of the following is the MOST likely diagnosis?
   a. Superficial angiomyxoma
   b. Benign fibrous histiocytoma (BFH)
   c. Desmoid fibromatosis
   d. Myxofibrosarcoma
   e. Nodular fasciitis

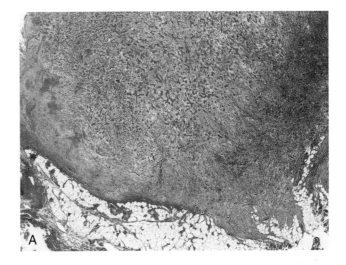

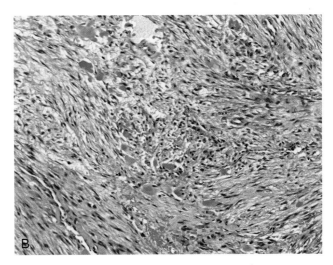

2. The pictures are from a deep-seated soft tissue mass from the popliteal region of a middle-aged man. The lesion had been present for several months and had been growing slowly.

Which one of the following is the MOST likely diagnosis?

a. Chordoma
b. Intramuscular myxoma (IM)
c. Extraskeletal myxoid chondrosarcoma (ESMC)
d. Myxoid liposarcoma
e. Ossifying fibromyxoid tumor (OFT)

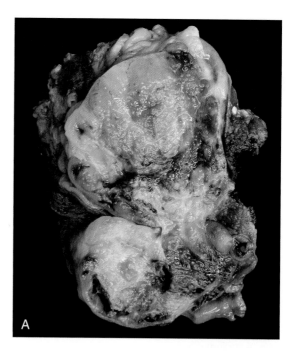

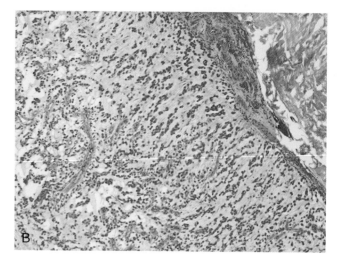

3. The gross and microscopic pictures are of a lesion from the deep soft tissue of the back of a middle-aged man. Which one of the following is the MOST likely diagnosis?
   a. Extrapleural solitary fibrous tumor (SFT)
   b. Leiomyosarcoma
   c. Desmoid fibromatosis
   d. Myofibroma
   e. Dermatofibrosarcoma protuberans (DFSPs)

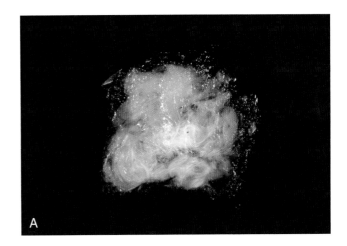

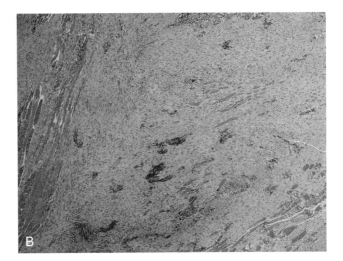

4. The gross and microscopic pictures are of a lesion in the skin of the lower back of a middle-aged man. The lesion has been present for several years and has been enlarging slowly. Which one of the following is the MOST likely diagnosis?

   a. DFSPs

   b. Neurofibroma

   c. BFH

   d. Plexiform fibrohistiocytic tumor (PFHT)

   e. Atypical fibroxanthoma

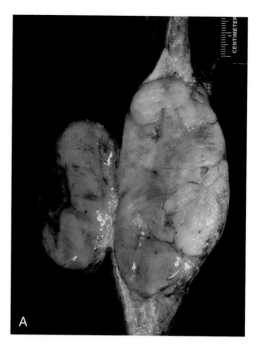

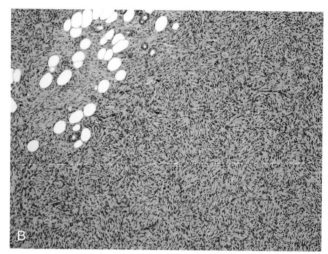

5. The microscopic images are from a fatty lesion involving the subcutaneous tissue of the volar aspect of the forearm of a 25-year-old man. What is the MOST likely diagnosis?
   a. Lipoma
   b. Spindle cell lipoma
   c. Angiolipoma
   d. Hemangioma
   e. Fat atrophy

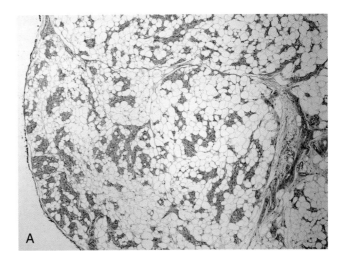

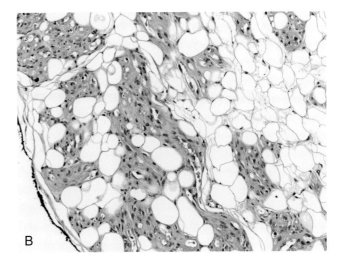

6. The low-magnification picture represents a painful nodule in the subcutis of the ankle of a 55-year-old woman. Which one of the following is the MOST likely diagnosis?

a. Cutaneous leiomyoma
b. Cutaneous leiomyosarcoma
c. Myofibroma
d. Glomangiomyoma
e. Angioleiomyoma (vascular leiomyoma)

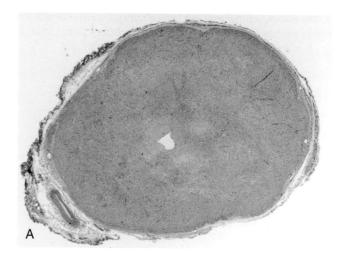

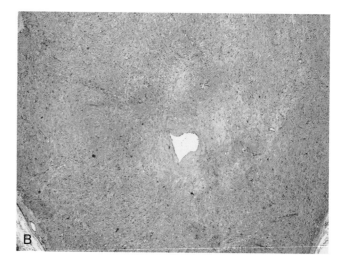

7. The low-power microscopic image shows a superficial soft
   tissue lesion from the chest wall of a young man. Which one of
   the following is the MOST likely diagnosis?
   a. Rhabdomyoma, adult type
   b. Hibernoma
   c. Granular cell tumor
   d. Leiomyoma
   e. Granular cell dermatofibroma

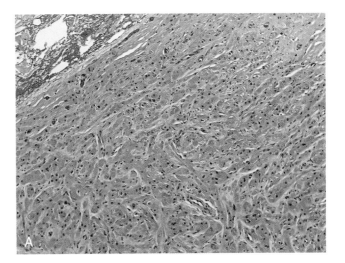

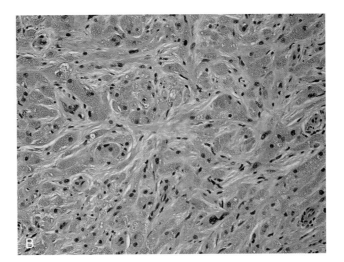

8. The image shows a rapidly growing, violaceous plaque lesion from the forehead of a 75-year-old man. Which one of the following is the MOST likely diagnosis?

   a. Kaposi sarcoma
   b. Spindle squamous cell carcinoma
   c. Desmoplastic melanoma
   d. Cutaneous angiosarcoma
   e. Atypical fibroxanthoma

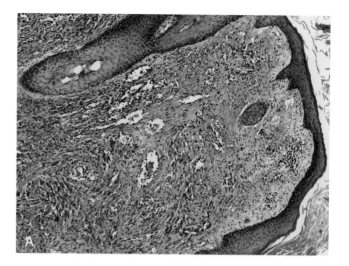

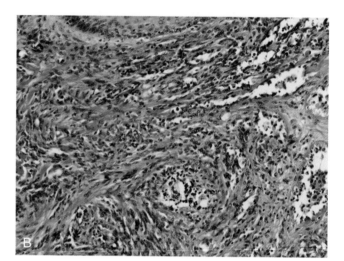

9. The microscopic image represents a slowly growing 7-cm soft tissue mass in the thigh of a 65-year-old woman. Which one of the following is the MOST likely diagnosis?
   a. Synovial sarcoma
   b. Hemangiopericytoma (HPC)
   c. Cellular schwannoma
   d. Low-grade fibromyxoid sarcoma
   e. Leiomyosarcoma

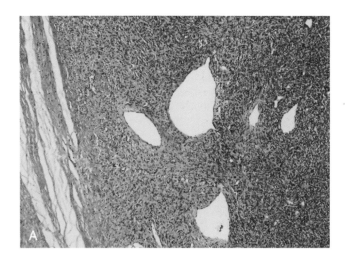

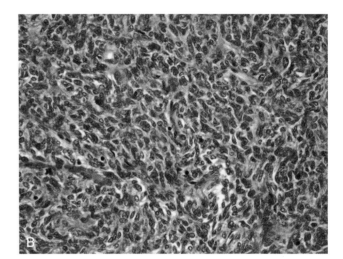

10. The image represents an intramuscular myxoid neoplasm in the thigh of a 75-year-old man. Which one of the following is the MOST likely diagnosis?
    a. Low-grade fibromyxoid sarcoma
    b. Myxoid liposarcoma
    c. IM
    d. Nodular fasciitis
    e. ESMC

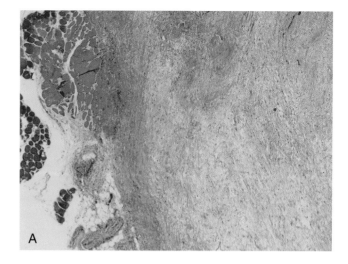

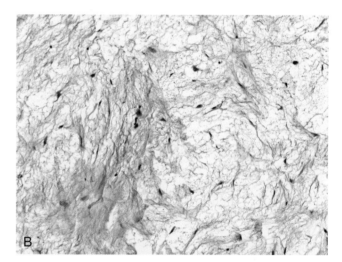

11. The image is representative of a lesion from a 28-year-old previously healthy woman with a slow-growing deep soft tissue mass in the ankle. Which one of the following is the MOST likely diagnosis?
    a. Malignant melanoma
    b. Cellular blue nevus
    c. Malignant peripheral nerve sheath tumor (MPNST)
    d. Synovial sarcoma
    e. Clear cell sarcoma (CCS) of tendons and aponeuroses

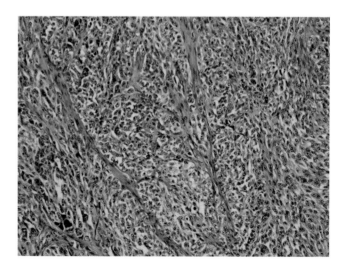

12. Which one of the following is the MOST likely diagnosis?
   a. Synovial sarcoma
   b. Schwannoma
   c. Intraneural neurofibroma
   d. Extrapleural SFT
   e. MPNST

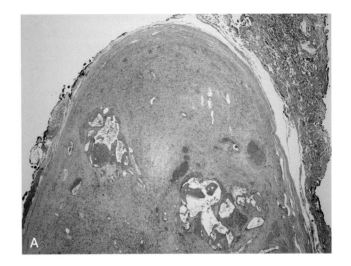

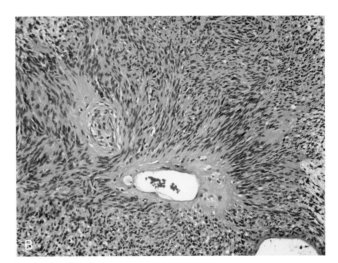

13. Which one of the following is the MOST likely diagnosis?
- **a.** Metastatic malignant melanoma
- **b.** Dendritic reticulum cell tumor
- **c.** Angiomatoid fibrous histiocytoma (AFH)
- **d.** Atypical fibroxanthoma
- **e.** Cavernous hemangioma

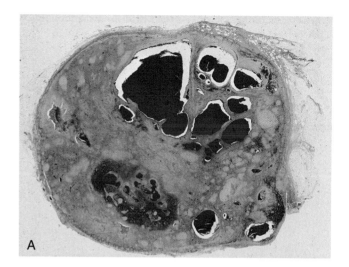

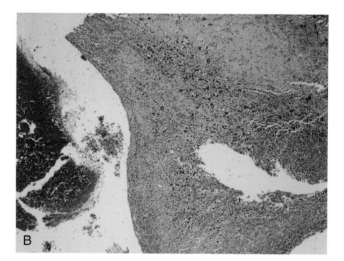

14. Which one of the following is the MOST likely diagnosis?

   a. Squamous cell carcinoma
   b. Malignant melanoma
   c. Epithelioid sarcoma (ES)
   d. Deep granuloma annulare (necrobiotic granuloma)
   e. Rheumatoid nodule

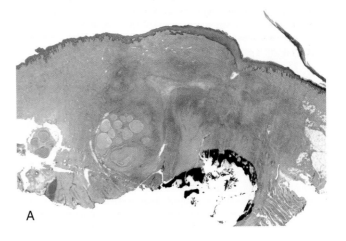

A

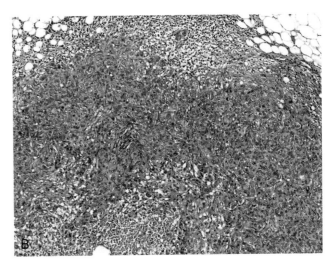

B

15. Which one of the following is the MOST likely diagnosis?
   a. Metastatic renal cell carcinoma (RCC)
   b. Alveolar soft part sarcoma (ASPS)
   c. Metastatic malignant melanoma
   d. Paraganglioma
   e. Granular cell tumor

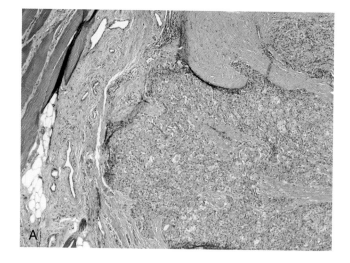

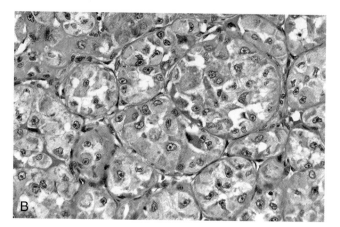

16. Which one of the following is the MOST likely diagnosis?

    a. DFSP

    b. Myofibroma

    c. Leiomyosarcoma

    d. Cellular BFH

    e. Spindle cell carcinoma

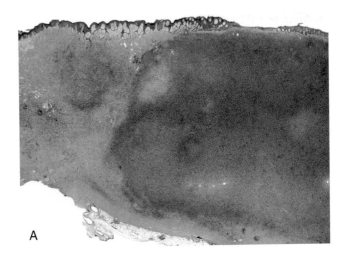

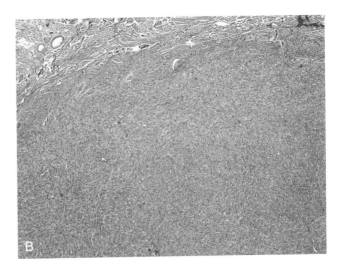

17. Which one of the following is the MOST likely diagnosis?
   a. Nodular fasciitis
   b. Giant cell fibroblastoma
   c. Fibrous hamartoma of infancy
   d. PFHT
   e. Deep granuloma annulare

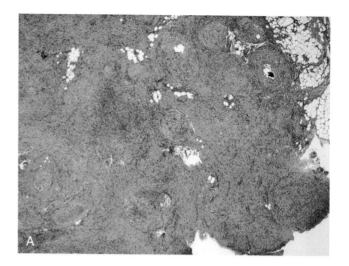

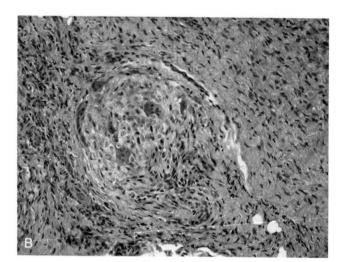

18. Which one of the following is the MOST likely diagnosis?
   a. HPC
   b. Phosphaturic mesenchymal tumor (PMT)
   c. Extraskeletal mesenchymal chondrosarcoma
   d. Soft tissue chondroma
   e. Spindle cell hemangioma (SCH)

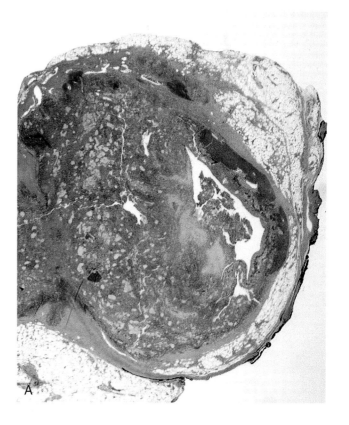

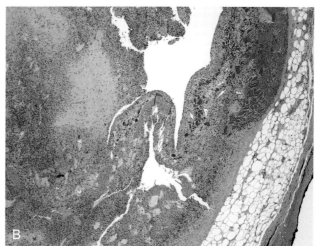

19. Which one of the following is the MOST likely diagnosis?
   a. Cellular angiofibroma (CA)
   b. Myxoid liposarcoma
   c. IM
   d. Low-grade fibromyxoid sarcoma
   e. Spindle cell lipoma

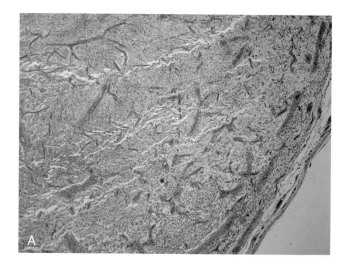

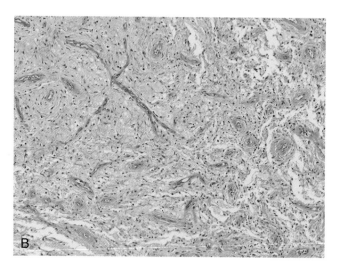

20. Which one of the following is the MOST likely diagnosis?

   a. Classic Kaposi sarcoma

   b. SCH

   c. Angiosarcoma

   d. Cavernous hemangioma

   e. Kaposiform hemangioendothelioma

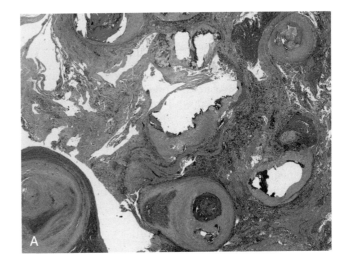

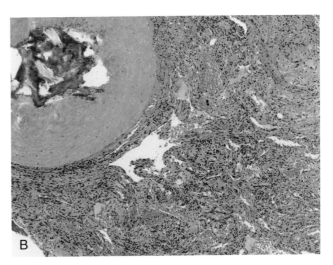

*A*NSWERS

1. e. Nodular fasciitis is a rapidly growing lesion that comes to surgery within 1 to 2 months of clinical onset. Although it may affect almost any district, it has a predilection for the upper extremity. Nodular fasciitis, including special types (intravascular and cranial), is a small and superficial lesion that is centered in the subcutis. Skeletal muscle involvement may be seen in certain anatomic sites, such as the head and neck. Involvement of bone is common in cranial fasciitis, a process involving the scalp of infants and children less than 2 years old. Nodular fasciitis has a limited growth potential. If untreated, it spontaneously regresses within a few months after onset, leaving behind scar tissue. Even with limited local excision, local recurrence is very rare (less than 2% of cases). If well sampled and relatively intact, nodular fasciitis is a straightforward diagnosis. Other entities may enter the differential diagnosis in limited biopsies, when clinical history, size, and depth of the lesion are not known. The differential diagnosis includes desmoid fibromatosis extending to the subcutis; however, desmoids have a more uniform fascicular architecture, have a more uniform vascular pattern, and lack the distinct "zonation" of fasciitis, with myxoid center and fibroblastic periphery. In cranial

fasciitis, myofibroma should be considered in the differential diagnosis, especially in larger lesions. In older individuals, cytologic atypia and larger size should alert one to a low-grade sarcoma, such as a myxofibrosarcoma.

Bernstein KE, Lattes R: Nodular (pseudosarcomatous) fasciitis, a nonrecurrent lesion: clinicopathologic study of 134 cases. *Cancer* 1982;49(8):1668-1678.

Montgomery EA, Meis JM: Nodular fasciitis. Its morphological spectrum and immunohistochemical profile. *Am J Surg Pathol* 1991;15(10):942-948.

Rosenberg AE: Pseudosarcomas of soft tissue. *Arch Pathol Lab Med* 2008;132(4):579-586.

2. c. ESMC is a painless mass in middle-aged adults, with slight male predilection, involving the deep soft tissues of the lower and upper extremities, trunk, paraspinal region, retroperitoneum, and head and neck region. The thigh is the most commonly affected site. Originally ESMC was considered a low-grade sarcoma; however, late metastases are common, and the survival rate of patients significantly drops with extended clinical follow-up. The survival rate at 5, 10, and 15 years is 90%, 70%, and 60%, respectively. Most

ESMCs are intramuscular, but in 25% of the cases there can be subcutaneous tissue involvement. ESMC is circumscribed and nodular, with a fibrous pseudocapsule, and fibrous septa transecting the mass. The cut surface is myxoid. The tumor cells are arranged in cords and nests with a cribriform architecture. The tumor cells are uniform and round to spindle shaped, with small, uniform hyperchromatic nuclei. The cytoplasm is moderately abundant and eosinophilic. Higher-grade lesions exist with cytologic atypia, rhabdoid features, mitotic activity, and solid growth. Immunohistochemically, ESMCs are positive for vimentin and variably positive for S100 protein, Leu-7, and epithelial membrane antigen (EMA). They are generally negative for cytokeratin and may be positive for glial-fibrillary acidic protein (GFAP). Some cases with rhabdoid phenotype have been reported negative for INI-1. Specific recurrent translocations have been reported, the most common being t(9; 22) (q22; q12), identified in 70% to more than 90% of cases, which generates an EWS/NR4A3 gene fusion. Other translocations include t(9; 17) (q22; q11), generating a gene fusion between TAF15 (an EWS-related gene) with NR4A3. Proximal location, large size, high cellularity and pleomorphism, recurrence, and metastases are adverse prognostic factors.

Kohashi K, Oda Y, Yamamoto H, et al: SMARCB1/INI1 protein expression in round cell soft tissue sarcomas associated with chromosomal translocations involving EWS: a special reference to SMARCB1/INI1 negative variant extraskeletal myxoid chondrosarcoma. *Am J Surg Pathol* 2008;32:1168-1174.

Meis-Kindblom JM, Bergh P, Gunterberg B, Kindblom LG: Extraskeletal myxoid chondrosarcoma: a reappraisal of its morphologic spectrum and prognostic factors based on 117 cases. *Am J Surg Pathol* 1999;23(6):636-650.

Wang W-L, Mayordomo E, Czerniak BA, et al: Fluorescence in situ hybridization is a useful ancillary diagnostic tool for extraskeletal myxoid chondrosarcoma. *Mod Pathol* 2008; 21(11):1303-1310.

3. c. More than 50% of desmoids are extraabdominal and most commonly affect adults between 20 and 40 years of age with a marked female predominance (3:1). The most common sites are the shoulder (approximately 25% of the cases), followed by the chest wall, thigh, and neck. The remaining cases involve the back, upper and lower extremities, and head. Desmoids vary in size, with most tumors between 3 cm and 15 cm in the largest dimension. They are usually intramuscular and have irregular borders owing to the infiltrative nature of the process. They are arranged in large fascicles composed of uniform spindle cells embedded in abundant fibrous matrix that may contain keloidlike collagen fibers. The fascicles are lined by elongated vessels with open lumina. Individual tumor cells have indistinct cell boundaries, eosinophilic cytoplasm, and ovoid nuclei with small nucleoli. Mitotic activity is generally low, not exceeding 2 to 3 mitoses per 10 high-power fields (HPFs), and atypical forms are absent. Nuclear staining for β-catenin is present in the majority of cases. They also stain for vimentin and have variable focal positivity for smooth muscle actin (SMA) and desmin. They are uniformly negative for CD34, S100 protein, and bcl-2. The treatment of choice is surgical excision, possibly with negative surgical margins; however, preservation of function should be pursued, considering that the rate of recurrence between

cases excised with negative and focally positive surgical margins is essentially the same (approximately 25% of cases). The majority of recurrences occur within 2 years of surgery. When complete surgical excision is not an option, radiation therapy may be considered; however, the use of adjuvant radiation therapy does not influence the rate of local recurrence regardless of the margin status.

Bhattacharya B, Dilworth HP, Iacobuzio-Donahue C, et al: Nuclear β-catenin expression distinguishes deep fibromatosis from other benign and malignant fibroblastic and myofibroblastic lesions. *Am J Surg Pathol* 2005;29(5):653-659.

Merchant NB, Lewis JJ, Woodruff JM, et al: Extremity and trunk desmoid tumors: a multifactorial analysis of outcome. *Cancer* 1999;86(10):2045-2052.

Pignatti G, Barbanti-Brodano G, Ferrari G, et al: Extraabdominal desmoid tumor. A study of 83 cases. *Clin Orthop Related Res* 2000;375:205-213.

4. a. DFSP is a slow-growing neoplasm that mainly affects young adults and shows a male predominance. It favors the trunk and the proximal extremities where early lesions have a plaquelike appearance and late lesions are multinodular with skin ulceration. DFSP is a low-grade sarcoma with a high propensity for local recurrence if incompletely excised. Complete excision, however, requires wide margins because of the capacity of DFSP to infiltrate beyond the grossly visible margins. Recurrence rates of 20% within 2 years of surgery are common. Mohs surgery significantly reduces the rate of recurrence (less than 2%). Grossly the lesion is firm and fibrous and varies from a small dermis-based plaquelike area or nodule to a large multinodular lesion that ulcerates the overlying skin and deeply involves the underlying adipose tissue. Occasionally DFSP may be purely subcutaneous. Microscopically DFSP consists of a proliferation of uniform, mildly atypical spindle cells, arranged in a tight, repetitive storiform pattern. It infiltrates the dermis surrounding the epidermal appendages and infiltrates the fat in a checkerboard or beaded pattern. The lesional cells are uniformly CD34 positive. DFSP may contain fascicular areas that are indistinguishable from fibrosarcoma. These areas are composed of intersecting fascicles of spindle cells with increased atypia and mitotic activity (>10 mitoses per 10 HPFs); however, to be considered fibrosarcomatous, these areas have to represent at least 5% of the entire lesion. DFSP with fibrosarcomatous transformation has a small but definite metastatic potential that varies between 5% and 10%. The lung is the most common site of dissemination.

Abbott JJ, Oliveira AM, Nascimento AG: The prognostic significance of fibrosarcomatous transformation in dermatofibrosarcoma protuberans. *Am J Surg Pathol* 2006;30 (4):436-443.

Sandberg AA, Bridge JA: Updates on the cytogenetics and molecular genetics of bone and soft tissue tumors: dermatofibrosarcoma protuberans and giant cell fibroblastoma. *Cancer Genet Cytogenet* 2003;140(1):1-12.

Taylor HB, Helwig EB: Dermatofibrosarcoma protuberans: a study of 115 cases. *Cancer* 1962;15(4):717-725.

5. c. Angiolipoma is a relatively common subcutaneous neoplasm composed of adipose tissue and clustered capillaries with fibrin thrombi. It is generally small and circumscribed and may be tender. It affects young individuals in the second and third decades of life and shows a male predominance. The single most affected site is the volar aspect of the forearm, followed by the upper chest, including the breast, upper arm, abdominal wall, and thigh. The majority of lesions are solitary, but 10% of the cases may be multiple. Up to 5% of the cases may be familial. The typical lesion is predominantly composed of adipose tissue with peripheral clusters of capillaries containing fibrin thrombi. Rare cases are predominantly vascular and may be confused with hemangioma subtypes, such as SCHs and juvenile capillary hemangiomas. Occasionally borderline and malignant neoplasms may enter the differential diagnosis. No cytogenetic abnormalities have been found. Simple excision is curative.

Howard WR, Helwig EB: Angiolipoma. *Arch Dermatol* 1960; 82(6):924-931.

Hunt SJ, Santa Cruz DJ, Barr RJ: Cellular angiolipoma. *Am J Surg Pathol* 1990;14(1):75-81.

Sciot R, Akerman M, Dal Cin P, et al: Cytogenetic analysis of subcutaneous angiolipoma: further evidence supporting its difference from ordinary pure lipomas: a report of the CHAMP study group. *Am J Surg Pathol* 1997;21(4):441-444.

6. e. Angioleiomyomas (ALs) are very common, generally solitary benign smooth muscle tumors that involve the subcutis and dermis of the extremities of patients between the fourth and sixth decades. ALs are usually rounded, sharply circumscribed white to brown lesions that on average measure 1 to 2 cm. Three subtypes are recognized: solid, cavernous, and venous. Microscopically, the solid variant consists of thickened criss-crossing bundles of smooth muscle that compress numerous slitlike vascular spaces. The cavernous subtype is mainly composed of dilated vascular channels in which the smooth muscle of the vessels subtly blends with the smooth muscle of the neoplasm. In the venous subtype there is a proliferation of vascular channels with compressed lumina and thickened muscular walls that blend with the lesional smooth muscle bundles. AL stains for SMA and desmin. AL is biologically benign and local excision is curative.

Hachisuga T, Hashimoto H, Enjoji M: Angioleiomyoma. A clinicopathologic reappraisal of 562 cases. *Cancer* 1984;54 (1):126-130.

Hasegawa T, Seki K, Yang P, et al: Mechanism of pain and cytoskeletal properties in angioleiomyomas: an immunohistochemical study. *Pathol Int* 1994;44(1):66-72.

Nilbert M, Mandahl N, Heim S, et al: Cytogenetic abnormalities in an angioleiomyoma. *Cancer Genet Cytogenet* 1989;37(1):61-64.

7. c. Granular cell tumor is a neoplasm of schwannian origin. Granular cell tumor may affect all age groups, but the majority of cases are seen between the third and sixth decades. Women are predominantly affected. It is most commonly seen in the superficial soft tissue of the upper extremity, trunk, and thigh, but the muscle may be affected. Many cases involve the mucosa of deep organs, most commonly of the aerodigestive tract. The lesions are usually small and circumscribed but unencapsulated, with yellowish cut surfaces. The tumors are arranged in sheets or clusters limited by fibrous bands. The individual tumor cells are large and polygonal to spindly, with abundant finely granular cytoplasm with scattered large granules. The nuclei may be small and uniform, but larger nuclei with prominent nucleoli may be seen as well as random cytologic atypia. Mitoses are

rare and typical. The tumor cells are consistently positive for S100 protein. The majority of lesions are benign, but 1% to 2% of the cases may be biologically aggressive to malignant. Features that have been associated with a malignant behavior are large size, high mitotic activity (more than 2 mitoses per 10 HPFs), significant cytologic atypia with prominent nucleoli, spindling and necrosis of the tumor cells, and Ki67 index more than 10%. Complete local excision is curative.

Fanburg-Smith JC, Meis-Kindblom JM, Fante R, Kindblom LG: Malignant granular cell tumor of soft tissue: diagnostic criteria and clinicopathologic. *Am J Surg Pathol* 1998;142:221-229.

Miettinen M, Lehtonen E, Lehtola H, et al: Histogenesis of granular cell tumor—an immunohistochemical and ultrastructural study. *J Pathol* 1984;6:186-203.

Ordonez NG: Granular cell tumor: a review and update. *Adv Anat Pathol* 1999;6:186-203.

8. d. Cutaneous AS is the most common variant of angiosarcoma (approximately 40% of the cases) and affects the sun-exposed skin of the head and neck of fair-skinned elderly patients. Less common variants of AS are secondary to radiation therapy or arise in lymphedematous limbs (10% of the cases), followed by AS arising in breast parenchyma of young women (less than 10% of the cases), bone (10% of the cases), and deep soft tissues, including large vessels (approximately 25% of the cases) and deep organs, such as liver and spleen. The morphologic spectrum of AS is quite wide, varying from well-differentiated and clearly vasoformative cases to primitive neoplasms with no clear endothelial differentiation. AS stains variably for the markers of vascular differentiation CD31, CD34, and factor VIII, with CD31 being the most reliable. It is important to remember that AS, especially the higher-grade epithelioid subtypes, regularly stain for cytokeratin, mainly CK18, CK7, and CK8. AS is a highly aggressive sarcoma with high potential for local recurrence and metastasis. Metastases are more common to the lung and bone. The overall 5-year survival rate is around 40%, with longer survival rates seen in lower-grade and superficial sites.

Abraham JA, Hornicek FJ, Kaufman AM, et al: Treatment and outcome of 82 patients with angiosarcoma. *Ann Surg Oncol* 2007;14(6):1953-1967.

Maddox JC, Evans HL: Angiosarcomas of skin and soft tissue: a study of forty-four cases. *Cancer* 1981;48(8):1907-1921.

Mendenhall WM, Mendenhall CM, Werning JW, et al: Cutaneous angiosarcoma. *Am J Clin Oncol* 2006;29(5):524-528.

9. b. HPC/extrapleural solitary fibrous tumor is a slow-growing tumor of deep soft tissue, mainly localized to retroperitoneum and proximal extremities, with a small subset affecting the meninges. It mainly affects adults, with a peak in the fourth and fifth decades of life. HPC has a female predominance. HPCs are solid, circumscribed, stroma-poor lesions composed of uniform cells associated with delicate compressed to gaping, irregularly shaped vascular channels. The tumor cells are consistently CD34 positive. A wide immunohistochemical panel should be performed to exclude mimics, both benign and malignant. HPC of deep soft tissue is generally benign. Features that may be associated with malignancy are large size, cytologic atypia and tumor necrosis, and more than 4 mitoses per 10 HPF. Although a few cases have been associated with cytogenetic abnormalities, no consistent translocations are associated with HPC.

Enzinger FM, Smith BH: Hemangiopericytoma. An analysis of 106 cases. *Hum Pathol* 1976;7(1):61-82.

Espat NJ, Lewis JJ, Leung D, et al: Conventional hemangiopericytoma: modern analysis of outcome. *Cancer* 2002;95(8):1746-1751.

Sreekantaiah C, Bridge JA, Rao UN, et al: Clonal chromosomal abnormalities in hemangiopericytoma. *Cancer Genet Cytogenet* 1991;54(2):173-181.

10. c. IM is a slow-growing benign neoplasm characterized by bland spindle cells embedded in abundant mucin with sparse vessels. It affects adults between the fourth and seventh decade of life and predilects females. It involves the musculature of the proximal extremities, and the thigh is the most commonly affected site. The majority of cases are solitary, but multiple lesions are seen in 5% to 10% of the cases. The association of multiple myxomas with fibrous dysplasia is known as Mazabraud syndrome. McCune-Albright syndrome is the association of multiple myxomas with cutaneous hyperpigmentation and endocrine abnormalities. Individual lesions are circumscribed but unencapsulated with some degree of muscle infiltration. They are composed of myxoid matrix with sparse vascularity in the form of delicate capillaries. The tumor cells are widely spaced and are spindle to stellate in shape. The cytoplasm is scant and the nuclei small, ovoid, and hyperchromatic. Mitoses are generally absent. IM is positive for vimentin and may be focally positive for SMA and CD34. Desmin and S100 protein are negative. A small subset of IM shows increased cellularity and vascularity (cellular IM). IM, solitary or multiple, is associated with a point mutation of the *GNAS1* gene, the same point mutation seen in fibrous dysplasia of bone. Complete conservative excision is curative.

Miettinen M, Hockerstedt K, Reitamo J, Totterman S: Intramuscular myxoma: a clinicopathological study of 23 cases. *Am J Clin Pathol* 1985;84(3):265-272.

Nielsen GP, O'Connell JX, Rosenberg AE: Intramuscular myxoma: a clinicopathologic study of 51 cases with emphasis on hypercellular and hypervascular variants. *Am J Surg Pathol* 1998;22:1222-1227.

Szendroi M, Rahoty P, Antal I, Kiss J: Fibrous dysplasia associated with intramuscular myxoma (Mazabraud's syndrome): a long term follow-up of three cases. *J Cancer Res Clin Oncol* 1998;124:401-406.

11. e. CCS affects the deep soft tissue of distal extremities of individuals in the second and third decades of life. The majority of cases affect the foot and ankle (50% of cases), followed by the leg and upper extremity. The lesion is in relationship with tendons and aponeuroses with larger tumors extending to the subcutaneous fat. The overlying epidermis is unremarkable. CCS is composed of uniform spindle cells arranged in small clusters, nests, and short fascicles surrounded by delicate fibrous septa. The tumor cells have clear to eosinophilic cytoplasm, and uniform round to oval nuclei with vesicular chromatin and large nucleoli. Mitoses are generally rare, and nuclear pseudoinclusions are sometimes seen as well as scattered multinucleated tumor giant cells. Melanin is present in approximately 50% of the cases, and melanosomes may be identified on electron microscopy. CCS is reactive for S100 protein, and HMB-45, tyrosinase, melan A, and microphthalmia transcription factor. CCS has a specific

t(12; 22) (12q13; 22q12) translocation. It is a very aggressive and chemoresistant tumor with high potential for local recurrence. Metastases to lymph nodes, liver, bone, and lung occur in 50% or more of cases. The 5-year survival rate is slightly above 50%.

Bridge JA, Sreekantaiah C, Neff JR, Sandberg AA: Cytogenetic findings in clear cell sarcoma of tendons and aponeuroses. Malignant melanoma of soft parts. *Cancer Genet Cytogenet* 1991;52(1):101-106.

Enzinger FM: Clear-cell sarcoma of tendons and aponeuroses. An analysis of 21 cases. *Cancer* 1965;18(9):1163-1174.

Lucas DR, Nascimento AG, Sim FH: Clear cell sarcoma of soft tissue. Mayo Clinic experience with 35 cases. *Am J Surg Pathol* 1992;16(12):1197-1204.

12. b. Schwannomas are benign nerve sheath tumors that may occur superficially or deep within the soft tissues. The extremities and the head and neck region are most commonly involved, followed by the spine at the emergence of the spinal roots, the posterior mediastinum, and the retroperitoneum. The majority of schwannomas are sporadic and solitary or they may be multiple, as in schwannomatosis. A small subset is associated with the NF2 syndrome, manifesting as bilateral vestibular lesions. There are special variants of schwannoma that include cellular, epithelioid, plexiform, and psammomatous melanotic schwannoma, the last commonly associated with the Carney complex. Schwannoma is characterized by alternating cellular and hypocellular regions. The cellular regions are composed of tightly packed Schwann cells with frequent nuclear palisading (Verocay bodies), often referred to as Antoni A areas. The hypocellular regions, referred to as Antoni B areas, are more rarefied, with myxoid matrix containing histiocytes. Schwannomas are diffusely positive for S100 protein. EMA highlights perineurial cells in the capsule and CD34 stains sparse fibroblastic cells. Cytokeratin and GFAP may be positive.

Das Gupta TK, Brasfield RD, Strong EW, Hajdu SI: Benign solitary schwannomas (neurilemomas). *Cancer* 1969;24(2):355-366.

Woodruff JM, Godwin TA, Erlandson RA, et al: Cellular schwannoma: a variety of schwannoma sometimes mistaken for a malignant tumor. *Am J Surg Pathol* 1981;5(8):733-744.

Woodruff JM, Selig AM, Crowley K, Allen PW: Schwannoma (neurilemoma) with malignant transformation. A rare, distinctive peripheral nerve tumor. *Am J Surg Pathol* 1994; 18(9):882-895.

13. c. AFH is a soft tissue neoplasm that involves the deep dermis and subcutaneous tissue. Neoplasms are generally small, measuring on average between 1 cm and 3 cm. AFH mainly affects children and young adults (mean age 20 years) and has a predilection for the extremities, followed by the trunk and the head and neck region. It is characterized by a thick fibrous pseudocapsule with a prominent lymphoplasmacytic infiltrate with germinal centers surrounding a center containing epithelioid and spindle fibrohistiocytic cells, and large blood-filled spaces. AFH is variably positive for desmin in 50% to 80% of the cases, and it has been suggested that it originates from myoid cells of lymphoid tissue. AFH is characterized by several specific translocations. The most common is a t(2; 22) (q34; q12) translocation affecting the *EWSR1* and *CREB1* genes. The tumor has an indolent clinical course with local recurrences in less than 10% of the cases. Rare metastases have been reported.

Antonescu CR, Dal Cin P, Nafa K, et al: EWSR1-CREB1 is the predominant gene fusion in angiomatoid fibrous histiocytoma. *Genes Chromosom Cancer* 2007;46(12):1051-1060.

Enzinger FM: Angiomatoid malignant fibrous histiocytoma: a distinct fibrohistiocytic tumor of children and young adults simulating a vascular neoplasm. *Cancer* 1979;44(6):2147-2157.

Fanburg-Smith JM, Miettinen M: Angiomatoid "malignant" fibrous histiocytoma: a clinicopathologic study of 158 cases and further exploration of the myoid phenotype. *Hum Pathol* 1999;30(11):1336-1343.

14. c. ES mainly occurs in the distal extremities of young adults and shows a male predominance. The most commonly affected sites are the fingers, hands, and forearms. The neoplasm tends to spread along the aponeuroses in a centripetal pattern and may involve ulcerating the skin. ES appears as a single or multiple well-circumscribed nodules, which occasionally may ulcerate. The tumor nodules are composed of a mixture of epithelioid and spindle cells with nuclei that have complex outlines and generally inconspicuous nucleoli. The center of the nodules may undergo necrosis, giving it a pseudogranulomatous appearance.

ES is positive for vimentin, cytokeratin, and EMA, and for CD34 in over 50% of the cases. HHF-35, desmin, and S100 may be focally positive. ES may recur locally in 30% to 80% of the cases, and it metastasizes in up to 40% of cases, mainly to lung, lymph nodes, soft tissues, and central nervous system. Metastases may occur late, with a survival rate of less than 70% at 5 years and 50% at 10 years.

Enzinger FM: Epithelioid sarcoma. A sarcoma simulating a granuloma or a carcinoma. *Cancer* 1970;26(5):1029-1041.

Miettinen M, Fanburg-Smith JC, Virolainen M, et al: Epithelioid sarcoma: an immunohistochemical analysis of 112 classical and variant cases and a discussion on the differential diagnosis. *Hum Pathol* 1999;30(8):934-942.

Spillane AJ, Thomas JM, Fisher C: Epithelioid sarcoma: the clinicopathological complexities of this rare soft tissue sarcoma. *Ann Surg Oncol* 2000;7(3):218-225.

15. b. ASPS is a rare sarcoma that constitutes less than 1% of all soft tissue sarcomas. The majority of the patients are children and young adults. Pediatric cases show a female predilection, whereas cases affecting patients older than 30 years old are more commonly seen in men. Pediatric ASPS is mainly localized to the tongue, head and neck, and orbit and measures 2.5 cm on average. Tumors in young adults mainly affect the lower extremity, with thigh and buttock being the most common locations. Tumors of the extremities and deep soft tissue usually are larger than 5 cm. The histologic appearance shows a tumor composed of tightly packed tumor nodules lined by a delicate vascular meshwork. Many of the tumor nodules have an alveolar pattern due to loss of cohesion or degeneration of the tumor cells. The tumor cells have abundant pale to eosinophilic cytoplasm and contain distinctive rhomboidal crystals that are PAS positive and diastase resistant. The tumor cells show variable positivity for desmin in more than 50% of the cases, but myogenin and MyoD1 are consistently negative. Vimentin is negative in a high percentage of cases. Cytokeratin, chromogranin, synaptophysin, and S100 protein are negative. ASPS has a characteristic

unbalanced translocation t(X; 17) (p11.2; q25) that fuses the TFE3 transcription factor gene at Xp11 to a novel gene at 17q25, designated ASPL (alveolar soft part locus). An identical but balanced translocation has been identified in a subset of pediatric RCCs. ASPS follows a relatively indolent and prolonged clinical course if metastases are not present at diagnosis. Unfortunately, more than 50% of the patients will already have metastasis at the time of diagnosis, usually to the lung. Factors that favorably influence the prognosis are small size of the tumor (<5 cm) and young age.

Ladanyi M, Lui MY, Antonescu CR, et al: The der (17) t(X; 17) (p11; q25) of human alveolar soft part sarcoma fuses the TFE3 transcription factor gene to ASPL, a novel gene at 17q25. *Oncogene* 2001;20(1):48-57.

Lieberman PH, Brennan MF, Kimmel M, et al: Alveolar soft-part sarcoma. A clinico-pathologic study of half a century. *Cancer* 1989;63(1):1-13.

Portera CA, Ho V, Patel SR, et al: Alveolar soft part sarcoma: clinical course and patterns of metastasis in 70 patients treated at a single institution. *Cancer* 2001;91(3):585-591.

16. d. BFH is one of the most common benign cutaneous neoplasms. It is most commonly diagnosed in young adults between the second and fourth decades of life, and it shows a slight predilection for the female sex. It is more common in the extremities, followed by the trunk and the head and neck region. Several variants of BFH exist that may be confused with malignant neoplasms, such as leiomyosarcoma and DFSPs. One of these subtypes is the cellular variant of fibrous histiocytoma (CBFH). CBFH occurs mainly in young adults and favors the extremities, is more common in male patients, and recurs in 25% of the cases. The majority of CBFHs consist of slightly elevated lesions with ill-defined margins that frequently involve the subcutis. CBFH lacks the distinct cellular polymorphism of common fibrous histiocytoma. Its central portion is very cellular and composed of short fascicles with numerous but typical mitoses (up to 10 mitoses per 10 HPFs). Only at the periphery, CBFH may show areas typical of common BFH. CBFH stains like BFH but is more consistently and diffusely positive for SMA, calponin, and heavy-caldesmon, markers of myofibroblastic differentiation. Owing to this potential for local recurrence, wider excision may be considered in cases excised with close surgical margins.

Calonje E, Mentzel T, Fletcher CDM: Cellular benign fibrous histiocytoma. Clinicopathologic analysis of 74 cases of a distinctive variant of cutaneous fibrous histiocytoma with frequent recurrence. *Am J Surg Pathol* 1994;18(7):668-676.

Han TY, Chang HS, Lee JH, et al: A clinical and histopathological study of 122 cases of dermatofibroma (benign fibrous histiocytoma). *Ann Dermatol* 2011;49(8):185-192.

Luzar B, Calonje E: Cutaneous fibrohistiocytic tumours—an update. *Histopathology* 2010;56(1):148-165.

17. d. PFHT affects children and young adults, with one third of the patients younger than 10 years old. The majority of the cases (60%) affect the dermis and subcutis of the upper extremity and shoulder girdle, with the remaining cases equally divided between the lower extremity, trunk, and head and neck region. PFHT is generally solitary and affects the deep dermis and subcutis with occasional extension to the upper dermis or skeletal muscle. The majority of cases are small with average size around 2 cm. The typical lesion is composed of discrete nodules made of histiocytes and scattered osteoclastlike multinucleated giant cells that are surrounded and connected to each other by a plexus of fibroblastlike spindle cells arranged in fascicles. Immunohistochemical stains are positive for histiocytic markers in the nodules (CD68 and CD163) and myofibroblastic markers in the spindle cells (SMA and HHF35). No recurrent cytogenetic abnormalities have been described. PFHT is a locally aggressive tumor that may recur locally if incompletely excised. Rare cases may metastasize to regional lymph nodes and lung.

Billings SD, Folpe AL: Cutaneous and subcutaneous fibrohistiocytic tumors of intermediate malignancy. *Am J Dermatopathol* 2004;26(2):141-155.

Enzinger FM, Zhang R: Plexiform fibrohistiocytic tumor presenting in children and young adults. An analysis of 65 cases. *Am J Surg Pathol* 1988;12(11):818-826.

Remstein ED, Arndt CAS, Nascimento AG: Plexiform fibrohistiocytic tumor: clinicopathologic analysis of 22 cases. *Am J Surg Pathol* 1997;23(6):662-670.

18. b. PMT is a very rare mesenchymal tumor that is associated with oncogenic osteomalacia. The symptoms are secondary to the production of fibroblast growth protein-23 by the tumor cells. This protein regulates renal tubular phosphate resorption. The majority of cases of PMT affect the soft tissue, where they have been described as PMTs of mixed connective tissue variant, but rare cases may occur in bone, where they resemble osteoblastoma or nonossifying fibroma. Microscopically the tumor is reminiscent of HPC, but additionally it may contain areas of cartilaginous metaplasia with "grungy" calcification, adipose and fibrous tissue, and osteoclastlike multinucleated giant cells. PMT is positive for FGF-23 and negative for CD34. The majority of cases are biologically benign and complete excision is curative, followed by complete resolution of the symptoms.

Folpe AL, Fanburg-Smith JC, Billings SD, et al: Most osteomalacia-associated mesenchymal tumors are a single histopathologic entity: an analysis of 32 cases and a comprehensive review of the literature. *Am J Surg Pathol* 2004;28(1):1-30.

Shimada T, Mizutani S, Muto T, et al: Cloning and characterization of FGF23 as a causative factor of tumor-induced osteomalacia. *Proc Natl Acad Sci U S A* 2001;98(11):6500-6505.

Weidner N, Santa Cruz D: Phosphaturic mesenchymal tumors. A polymorphous group causing osteomalacia or rickets. *Cancer* 1987;59(8):1442-1454.

19. a. CA is a slow-growing soft tissue neoplasm that affects the sexes equally and involves predominantly the vulvovaginal, inguinal, and paratesticular regions. It affects adults in a wide age range (third to eighth decades) but has a peak in the fifth decade in women and in the sixth decade in men. It is generally small, with most tumors between 3 and 5 cm in the largest dimension, but larger tumors may occur, especially in men. CA tends to be circumscribed and is frequently surrounded by a fibrous pseudocapsule, but some may have indistinct boundaries. CA is variably cellular and composed of uniform short spindle cells with bland ovoid nuclei and scant pale eosinophilic cytoplasm. Mitotic activity may be prominent, especially in cases affecting women, but there are no atypical mitoses. The tumor matrix varies from edematous to fibrotic with delicate to thickened

collagen fibers. The vascular component is prominent and composed of regularly spaced vessels with conspicuous perivascular fibrosis. CA may contain adipocytes, but these are a minor component of the tumor (<5%) and are generally concentrated at the periphery of the lesion. The tumors are variably reactive for CD34, SMA, and desmin. Estrogen and progesterone receptors are also frequently positive, both in men and women, raising speculation regarding the role of hormonal stimulation in the pathogenesis of this lesion. CA is characterized by recurrent rearrangements involving chromosome 13. CA is benign; complete local excision is curative, and recurrences are very rare.

Flucke U, van Krieken HJM, Mentzel T: Cellular angiofibroma: analysis of 25 cases emphasizing its relationship to spindle cell lipoma and mammary-type myofibroblastoma. *Mod Pathol* 2011;24(1):82-89.

Iwasa Y, Fletcher CDM: Cellular angiofibroma. Clinicopathologic and immunohistochemical analysis of 51 cases. *Am J Surg Pathol* 2004;28(11):1426-1435.

Laskin WB, Fetsch JF, Mostofi FK: Angiomyofibroblastoma-like tumor of the male genital tract. *Am J Surg Pathol* 1998; 22(1):6-16.

20. b. SCH preferentially affects the distal extremities of young adults, with the majority of cases involving the hand and foot. There is no sex predilection. A small percentage of patients are affected by Maffucci syndrome, a nonhereditary and congenital form of mesodermal dysplasia that manifests with multiple encondromas and hemangiomas. Rare cases may be seen in Klippel-Trenaunay syndrome and Milroy disease. SCH is usually located in the dermis and subcutis, but it may occasionally involve the deep soft tissue or be purely intravascular. SCH appears as a red to bluish nodule that elevates the skin and measures from a few millimeters to several centimeters in diameter. The majority of the lesions are single, but many patients have multiple lesions in the same area at presentation. The histologic appearance shows cavernous spaces that are frequently thrombosed or contain phleboliths that are separated by a cellular proliferation of bland spindle cells and collapsed vascular spaces. Some of the spindle cells have vacuolated cytoplasm. No cytologic atypia or significant mitotic activity is present. Generally, all the lesions are in relationship with large-diameter vessels. SCH is treated with complete local excision, but 50% of the patients will experience additional lesions in the same area, which are probably the result of multifocal growth of the lesions along the vessels of the area rather than a true recurrence of the neoplasm.

Ding J, Hashimoto H, Imayama S, et al: Spindle cell haemangioendothelioma: probably a benign vascular lesion not a low-grade angiosarcoma. A clinicopathological, ultrastructural and immunohistochemical study. *Virchow Arch A Pathol Anat Histopathol* 1992;420(1):77-85.

Perkins P, Weiss SW: Spindle cell hemangioendothelioma. An analysis of 78 cases with reassessment of its pathogenesis and biologic behavior. *Am J Surg Pathol* 1996;20(10):1196-1204.

Weiss SW, Enzinger SW: Spindle cell hemangioendothelioma. A low-grade angiosarcoma resembling a cavernous hemangioma and Kaposi's sarcoma. *Am J Surg Pathol* 1986; 10(8):521-530.

CHAPTER 17

THYROID AND PARATHYROID GLAND PATHOLOGY

Andrew Turk and Karl H. Perzin

QUESTIONS

Questions 1-36 refer to a photograph or photomicrograph.

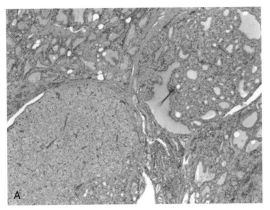

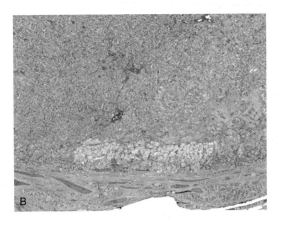

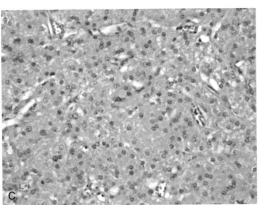

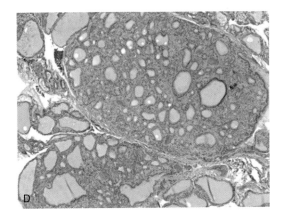

1. A 30-year-old man with a familial *PTEN* mutation underwent total thyroidectomy, in order to relieve symptoms caused by massive enlargement of his thyroid. The surgical specimen weighed 133 g. Representative histologic images are shown. No evidence of malignancy was detected, either clinically or histologically. Mutation of *PTEN* is most strongly associated with which of the following thyroid cancers?
   a. Papillary carcinoma, solid variant
   b. Papillary carcinoma, cribriform-morular variant
   c. Follicular carcinoma
   d. Medullary carcinoma
   e. Anaplastic (undifferentiated) carcinoma

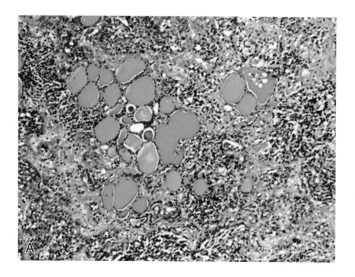
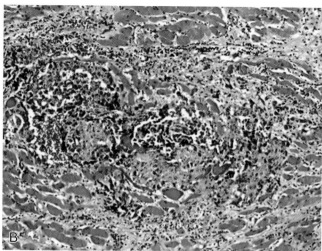
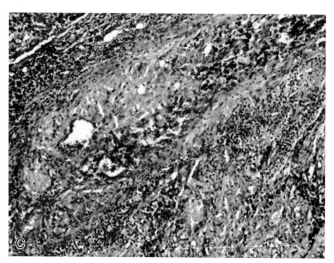
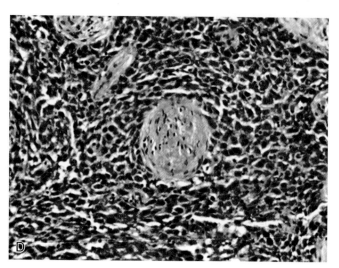

2. An 84-year-old woman underwent thyroid lobectomy. Histologic examination of the tumor led to a diagnosis of undifferentiated (anaplastic) thyroid carcinoma (UTC). Which one of the following statements regarding this case is INCORRECT?

   a. This patient's age is consistent with the typical clinical scenario of UTC.

   b. This lesion possibly arose from a better differentiated carcinoma, or possibly de novo.

   c. The mortality rate of UTC is more than 90%.

   d. Based on the involvement of skeletal muscle (as shown), this is a T3 tumor.

   e. Positive immunohistochemical staining for thyroglobulin would be unexpected in this lesion.

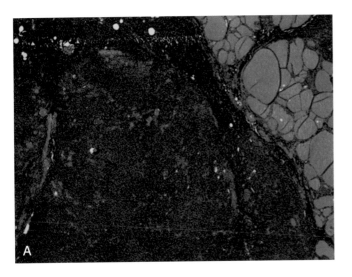

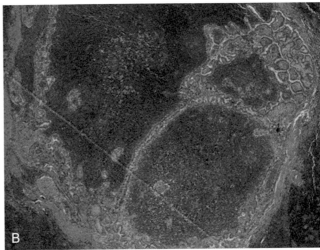

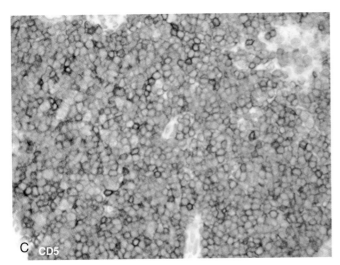

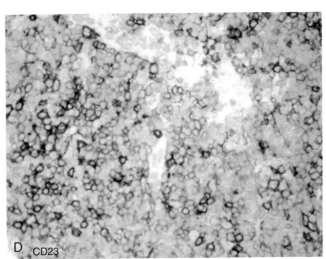

3. The illustration shows the histologic appearance and (selected) immunohistochemical staining properties of a thyroidectomy specimen removed from a 73-year-old woman. Which one of the following options represents the CORRECT diagnosis?

   a. Extranodal marginal zone B-cell lymphoma (EMZBCL)/ mucosa-associated lymphoid tissue (MALT) lymphoma

   b. Diffuse large B-cell lymphoma (DLBCL)

   c. Follicular lymphoma (FL)

   d. Small lymphocytic lymphoma (SLL)

   e. Hodgkin lymphoma

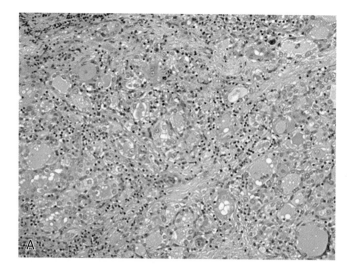

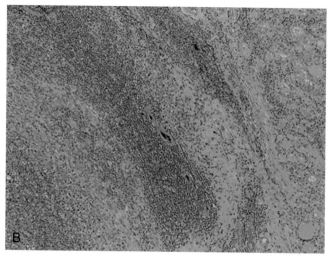

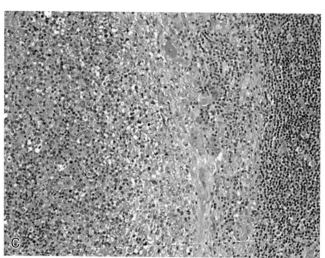

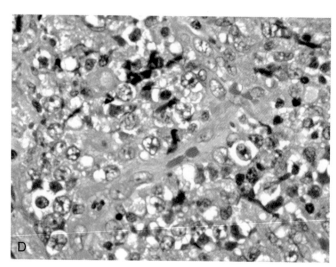

4. A 70-year-old man brought himself to an emergency department for urgent management of airway obstruction and decreasing ability to speak. Physical examination revealed a large neck mass. Fine needle aspiration (FNA) of the mass showed scattered lymphocytes and benign-appearing thyroid follicular cells. The patient underwent surgery. Histologic examination of the surgical specimen revealed the histologic features shown in the illustration. The lesional cells stained negatively for thyroid transcription factor-1 (TTF-1) and thyroglobulin, and positively for CD20 and Bcl-6. Cytogenetic analysis revealed the translocation t(3;14)(q27;q32). Which one of the following options represents the CORRECT diagnosis?
   a. EMZBCL/MALT lymphoma
   b. DLBCL
   c. FL
   d. SLL
   e. Hodgkin lymphoma

5. Which one of the following options represents the most common type of primary thyroid lymphoma?
   a. EMZBCL/MALT lymphoma
   b. DLBCL
   c. FL
   d. SLL
   e. Hodgkin lymphoma

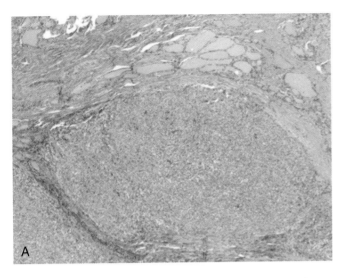
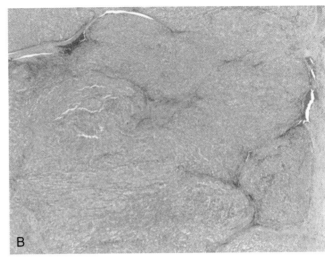
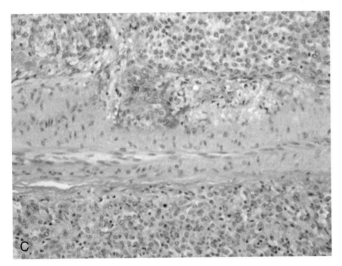
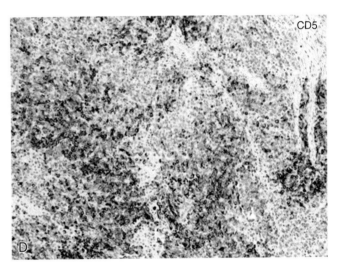

6. The illustration displays four foci of a 3.2-cm mass resected from a 77-year-old man. Based on the histologic and immunohistochemical features shown, which one of the following options represents the MOST likely diagnosis?
   a. UTC
   b. Primary squamous cell carcinoma of the thyroid
   c. Carcinoma showing thymuslike differentiation (CASTLE)
   d. Papillary thyroid carcinoma, solid variant
   e. Follicular thyroid carcinoma, microfollicular variant

7. A 52-year-old woman had clinical hyperthyroidism and a nodule in the right thyroid lobe. A thyroid scan showed an autonomous/hyperfunctioning ("hot") nodule, with suppression of the remaining thyroid. The patient did not respond to antithyroid medications. A right thyroid lobectomy was performed. The cut surface showed a well-circumscribed nodule measuring 4 cm in greatest dimension; the remaining thyroid tissue appeared grossly normal. The illustration shows a representative section of the nodule. Which one of the following statements regarding this case is INCORRECT?

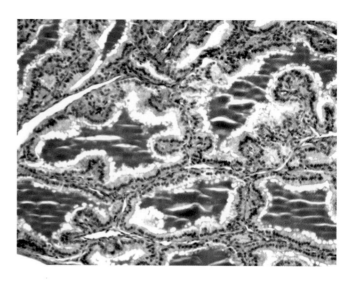

- **a.** In most autonomous thyroid nodules, variable areas of hyperplasia are found (as shown in this illustration), similar to the diffuse hyperplasia that characterizes Graves disease.
- **b.** These nodules are generally well circumscribed lesions composed of variably sized follicles, frequently having the low-power appearance of nonfunctional nodules (i.e., nontoxic nodular goiter).
- **c.** As in Graves disease, clinical and laboratory evidence indicates that autonomous nodules result from an autoimmune process.
- **d.** Clinical hyperthyroidism usually occurs in association with autonomous nodules measuring more than 3 cm in greatest dimension.
- **e.** Hyperfunctional nodules associated with clinical hyperthyroidism are frequently described in the literature as "toxic adenomas."

8. A 56-year-old woman with clinical hyperthyroidism underwent bilateral subtotal thyroidectomy. The illustration shows a representative section of the thyroid. The histologic changes are most consistent with which one of the following entities?

- **a.** Graves disease
- **b.** Nodular goiter
- **c.** Palpation thyroiditis
- **d.** Amiodarone treatment
- **e.** Diffuse colloid goiter

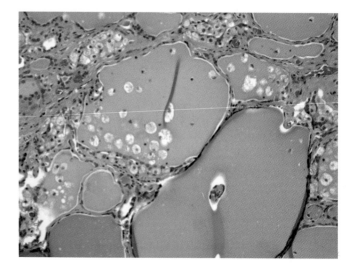

9. A 42-year-old woman presented with a 3-cm nodule in the right lobe of her thyroid. A thyroid scan showed a "cold" nodule. FNA of the nodule showed benign-appearing follicular cells, consistent with a follicular neoplasm. A right thyroid lobectomy was performed. The cut surface showed a well-circumscribed tan nodule. Histologic examination showed a lesion composed of small follicles. Which one of the following statements regarding this case is INCORRECT?

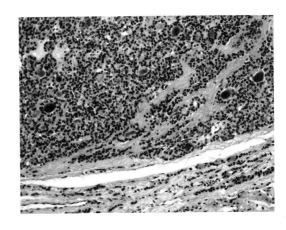

   a. The entire edge of the lesion should be examined histologically.
   b. Foci of fibrosis that extend into the lesion should not be interpreted as invasive carcinoma.
   c. Invasion of neoplastic tissue through the capsule into adjacent thyroid tissue justifies the diagnosis of follicular carcinoma.
   d. Most follicular neoplasia of the thyroid (adenoma and carcinoma) presents clinically as a solitary nodule.
   e. In most follicular carcinomas, the cells show obviously malignant cytologic features, with large pleomorphic nuclei and numerous mitotic figures.

10. A 60-year-old man presented with a nodule in the left lobe of his thyroid. FNA showed follicular cells, consistent with a diagnosis of follicular neoplasm. A lobectomy was performed. The cut surface showed a well-circumscribed tan nodule measuring 5 cm in greatest dimension. The entire edge of the tumor was submitted for histologic analysis. Which one of the following statements regarding this case is INCORRECT?

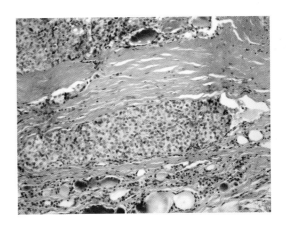

   a. The mass in the capsule shows the "arm-in-sleeve" appearance of large tumor nests plugging capsular veins.
   b. The small finger of tumor pushing into the capsule (upper left) may represent invasion into the fibrous capsule, or invasion into a small vein.
   c. Controversy exists concerning the significance of invasion by follicular neoplasia into only the fibrous capsule (i.e., without invasion into vessels).
   d. Identification of capsular invasion may suggest that additional, potentially more extensive, invasive foci are present elsewhere.
   e. When metastasis of follicular carcinoma occurs, regional lymph nodes are usually involved.

11. A 60-year-old man underwent right thyroid lobectomy for removal of a mass lesion. The cut surface of the resected specimen showed a firm tan/gray mass that measured 5 cm in greatest dimension. The entire edge of the lesion was submitted for histologic analysis. A representative image of the lesion is shown. Which one of the following statements is FALSE?

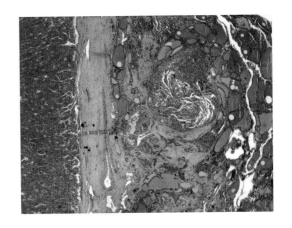

   a. The diagnosis is follicular thyroid carcinoma.
   b. For many cases in which follicular carcinoma invades the adjacent thyroid, direct extension through the capsule is identified.
   c. In some cases, foci of capsular penetration are unapparent, potentially due to the plane of the section.
   d. When follicular carcinoma extends through its capsule into veins within the adjacent thyroid, there is a substantial chance that the tumor will metastasize.
   e. Follicular thyroid carcinoma frequently involves both lobes of the gland.

12. The nuclear clearing that characterizes papillary thyroid carcinoma represents an artifact of formalin fixation. Which of the following findings also represents an artifact of tissue processing?
    a. The "fried egg" appearance of oligodendroglioma
    b. Stromal retraction in basal cell carcinoma
    c. Clefting in salivary gland adenoid cystic carcinoma
    d. Retraction in micropapillary carcinoma of the breast
    e. All of the above

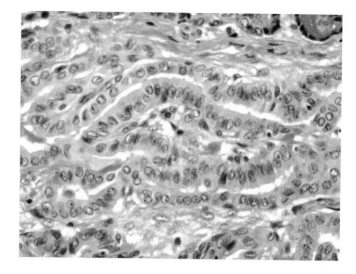

13. This photograph shows a Fontana-stained section of a thyroidectomy specimen. This patient's medication history likely included which one of the following drugs?
    a. Interferon-α
    b. Interleukin 2
    c. Amiodarone
    d. Minocycline
    e. Radioactive iodine

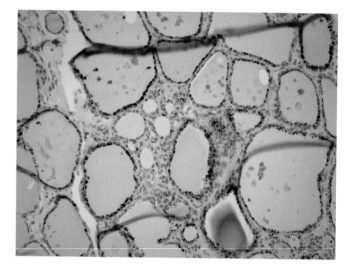

14. A 56-year-old woman underwent thyroid lobectomy for removal of a follicular adenoma. A portion of the lesion's capsule is evident in the lower left corner of the illustration. The central portion of the photograph displays the histologic features of the surrounding parenchyma. This patient's medication history likely includes which one of the following drugs?
    a. Interferon-α
    b. Interleukin 2
    c. Amiodarone
    d. Minocycline
    e. Radioactive iodine

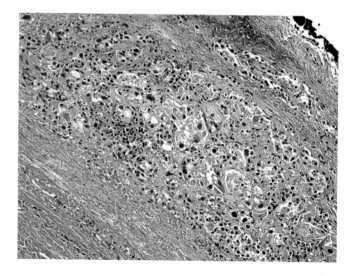

15. A 28-year-old woman had thyroid surgery. The illustration shows a section taken from the resected thyroid tissue. This patient has which of the following conditions?
   a. Graves disease (diffuse toxic goiter)
   b. Toxic nodular goiter
   c. Nodular goiter (nontoxic)
   d. Papillary carcinoma, classical type
   e. Papillary carcinoma, tall cell variant

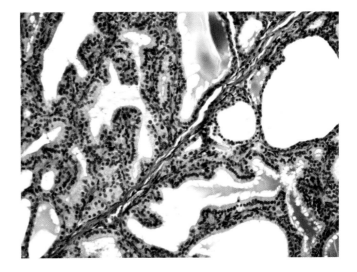

16. A 38-year-old woman underwent thyroidectomy for hyperthyroidism that was refractory to medical therapy. Prior to surgery, her treatment course had included propylthiouracil, propranolol (initially), radioactive iodine (subsequently), and potassium iodide (in preparation for surgery). The illustration shows a representative section of her thyroid. Which one of the following statements IS INCORRECT?
   a. The diagnosis is Hashimoto thyroiditis.
   b. Scattered cells containing large, atypical, hyperchromatic nuclei are characteristic of patients who have undergone radioactive iodine treatment.
   c. Treatment with β-blockers or potassium iodide does not usually produce nuclear abnormalities in follicular epithelial cells.
   d. The cells in this image are not diagnostic of papillary carcinoma.
   e. Cases of UTC developing subsequent to radioactive iodine treatment have been reported.

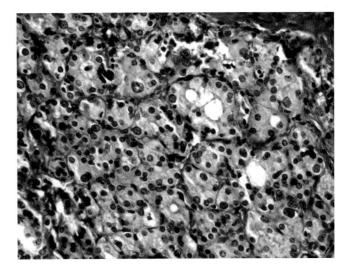

17. This illustration shows a thyroid lobectomy specimen containing a well-circumscribed 2-cm nodule. The specimen was submitted for intraoperative analysis by frozen section. Which one of the following options corresponds to the MOST likely frozen section diagnosis?
   a. Nodular goiter
   b. Follicular neoplasm
   c. Follicular carcinoma
   d. Papillary carcinoma
   e. Medullary carcinoma

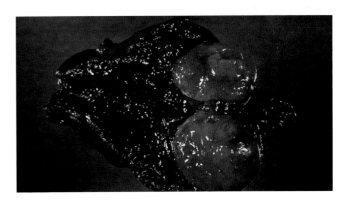

18. Which one of the following cellular features is LEAST frequently associated with a diagnosis of papillary thyroid carcinoma?
    a. "Optically clear" nuclei
    b. Nuclear grooves
    c. Numerous mitotic figures
    d. Intranuclear inclusions
    e. Nuclear crowding and stratification

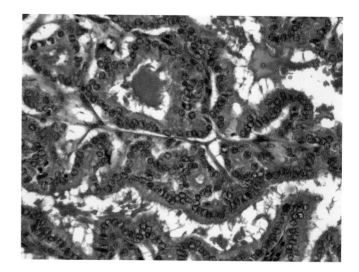

19. A 42-year-old woman underwent thyroid lobectomy for removal of a 4-cm nodule in the right lobe of her gland. Gross inspection of the resected specimen showed a firm gray/tan mass with irregular borders. Based on the results of a frozen section, the patient underwent total thyroidectomy. The illustration shows a representative image of the lesion. Which one of the following statements is FALSE?
    a. This tumor shows features of medullary carcinoma.
    b. The amorphous material between nests of tumor cells is amyloid, which stains positively with congo red and crystal violet.
    c. Like papillary carcinoma, these lesions generally metastasize via lymphatic vessels rather than veins.
    d. These tumors generally stain positively for calcitonin and negatively for thyroglobulin.
    e. Medullary carcinoma generally portends a worse prognosis than papillary or follicular thyroid carcinoma.

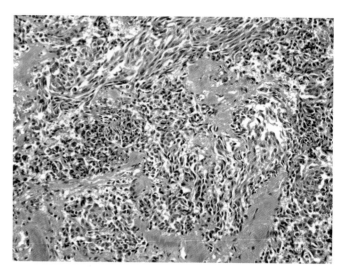

20. A 52-year-old woman sought medical attention for right flank pain, and was diagnosed with nephrolithiasis. Additional work-up showed hypercalcemia and high serum levels of parathyroid hormone (PTH). Neck exploration revealed an enlarged (1.5 cm) parathyroid gland, which was resected. The histologic appearance of the gland was consistent with adenoma, surrounded by a rim of compressed nonneoplastic parathyroid. Which one of the following statements regarding this case is INCORRECT?
    a. Follicular structures may be found either focally or extensively within parathyroid adenomas.
    b. Basally situated nuclei and densely stained nuclei may be diagnostically useful findings, in terms of distinguishing follicles of parathyroid adenoma from thyroid follicles.
    c. Parathyroid adenomas generally consist of chief cells, but oxyphil cells and "water-clear" cells may be present in various proportions.
    d. The upper limit of normal parathyroid gland size is approximately 0.6 to 0.7 cm in greatest dimension.
    e. Large pleomorphic nuclei within parathyroid neoplasia provide a strong indication of malignancy.

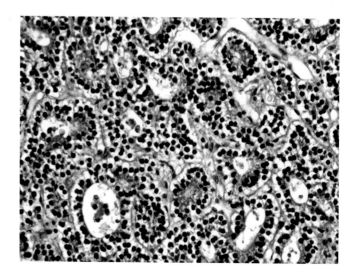

21. A 35-year-old man was found to have hypercalcemia when routine studies were performed during his annual physical examination. Subsequent work-up showed elevated serum PTH concentration. His renal function was normal. Neck exploration revealed an enlarged (2 cm) parathyroid gland, which was resected. Three other parathyroid glands, all of apparently normal size, were identified. Which one of the following statements is INCORRECT?
   a. The histologic features illustrated here are those of parathyroid hyperplasia.
   b. Parathyroid adenomas generally consist of a single nodule devoid of fat.
   c. Lipoadenoma is considered a variant of parathyroid adenoma.
   d. Biopsy sampling of this patient's three remaining (normal-sized) glands may be warranted.
   e. Parathyroidectomy is curative in cases such as this, and further parathyroid-related problems would be unusual and unexpected.

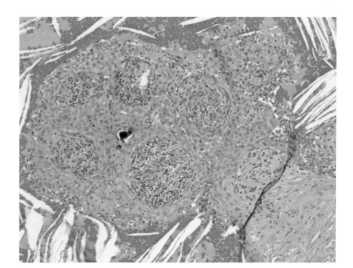

22. A 68-year-old woman underwent FNA of a thyroid nodule, which led to a diagnosis of papillary carcinoma. She subsequently underwent total thyroidectomy. Histologic examination of the resection specimen confirmed the diagnosis of papillary carcinoma, and also revealed reactive and degenerative changes at the FNA site, including squamous metaplasia. Which of the following nonneoplastic thyroid conditions may be associated with squamous metaplasia?
   a. Follicular adenomatous hyperplasia
   b. Lymphocytic thyroiditis
   c. Ultimobranchial body remnants/solid cell nests
   d. Thymic rests
   e. All of the above

23. An association has been recognized between Hashimoto thyroiditis and which of the following entities and/or phenomena?
   a. Immune complex deposition
   b. Human leukocyte antigen (HLA) alleles HLA-DR3, HLA-DR4, and HLA-DR5
   c. Turner syndrome
   d. Down syndrome
   e. All of the above

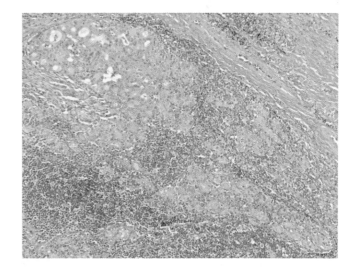

24. The illustration shows a representative image of a total
thyroidectomy specimen from a 33-year-old woman. Which of
the following options MOST likely describes this patient's
laboratory values at the time of surgery?
  a. Elevated serum thyroxine (T_4), elevated serum
    triiodothyronine (T_3), elevated serum thyroid-stimulating
    hormone (TSH)
  b. Elevated serum T_4, elevated serum T_3, low serum TSH
  c. Normal serum T_4, normal serum T_3, elevated
    serum TSH
  d. Normal serum T_4, normal serum T_3, low serum TSH
  e. Low serum T_4, low serum T_3, elevated serum TSH

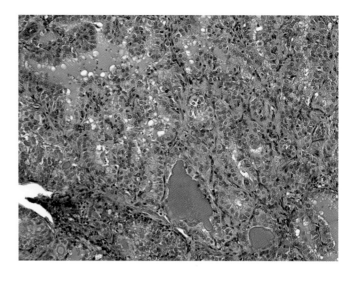

25. This patient is MOST likely to have elevated titers of which of
the following antibodies?
  a. Anti-Coxsackievirus antibodies
  b. Antithyroglobulin antibodies
  c. Antithyroid-stimulating hormone receptor (anti-TSHR)
    antibodies
  d. Antithyroid peroxidase antibodies
  e. Antimicrosomal antibodies

26. Which one of the following HLAs has been associated with an
increased risk for development of this condition?
  a. HLA-DR3
  b. HLA-DR4
  c. HLA-DR5
  d. HLA-Bw35
  e. HLA-B8

27. A 65-year-old woman underwent total thyroidectomy,
following a diagnosis of papillary carcinoma established by
FNA. Histologic examination of the tumor revealed prominent
nuclear pseudoinclusions, as shown in the photograph. Which
of the following tumors also display(s) nuclear inclusions or
pseudoinclusions?
  a. Hepatocellular carcinoma
  b. Melanoma
  c. Pulmonary adenocarcinoma
  d. Parathyroid carcinoma
  e. All of the above

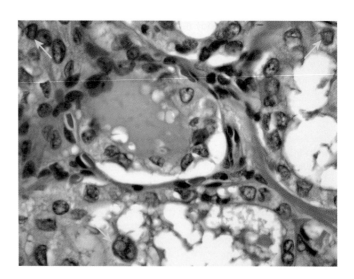

28. A 70-year-old woman with primary hyperparathyroidism underwent parathyroidectomy. Histologic examination revealed vascular invasion by the tumor; the pathologist consequently rendered a diagnosis of parathyroid carcinoma. Laboratory work-up of this patient would LEAST likely reveal which one of the following findings?

a. Elevated serum PTH level
b. Elevated serum alkaline phosphatase activity
c. Hypercalcemia
d. Hyperphosphatemia
e. Hypercalciuria

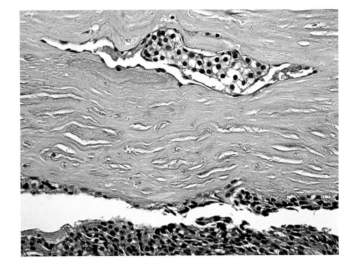

29. A 67-year-old man on amiodarone sought medical attention for difficulty sleeping. Laboratory work-up showed low TSH and high free T_4. Nuclear medicine studies showed low radionuclide uptake. He underwent total thyroidectomy, a representative image of which is shown. Which of the following options BEST describes/most closely pertains to this clinical scenario?

a. Primary hyperthyroidism
b. Secondary hyperthyroidism
c. Thyrotoxicosis
d. Acute thyroiditis
e. Subacute thyroiditis

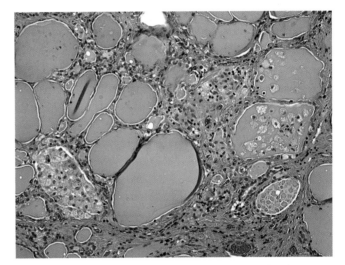

30. A 73-year-old woman underwent total thyroidectomy. Histologic examination of the gland revealed an incidental papillary carcinoma that showed prominent nuclear grooves, as shown in the photograph. Which of the following tumors also display(s) nuclear grooves?

a. Granulosa cell tumor, adult type
b. Solid pseudopapillary tumor of the pancreas
c. Chondroblastoma
d. Pulmonary adenocarcinoma in situ (bronchioloalveolar carcinoma)
e. All of the above

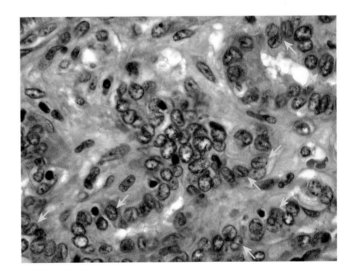

31. A 40-year-old woman underwent FNA of a 2.4-cm nodule in the right lobe of her thyroid. The findings were consistent with papillary carcinoma, and she underwent total thyroidectomy. Histologic examination of the surgical specimen resulted in a diagnosis of hyalinizing trabecular tumor (HTT). Among thyroid tumors, this lesion exhibits a unique staining pattern with which of the following immunohistochemical markers?
    a. TTF-1
    b. Thyroglobulin
    c. Ki-67
    d. Calcitonin
    e. Galectin-3

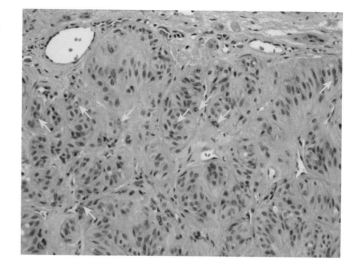

32. The illustration displays a calcitonin-stained section of thyroid. With which one of the following syndromes is this condition MOST characteristically associated?
    a. Familial adenomatous polyposis (FAP)
    b. Cowden syndrome
    c. Multiple endocrine neoplasia type 1 (MEN 1)
    d. MEN 2A and MEN 2B
    e. Werner syndrome

33. Assuming this finding results from a genetic syndrome, which one of the following findings would be LEAST likely in the same patient?
    a. Primary hyperparathyroidism
    b. Pheochromocytoma
    c. Pituitary adenoma
    d. Mucosal neuroma of the tongue
    e. Ganglioneuromatosis of the intestine

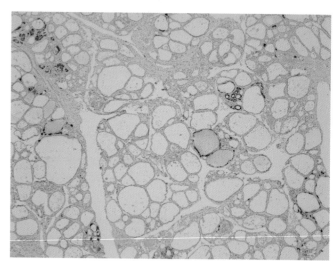

34. A 49-year-old man with primary hyperparathyroidism underwent surgery for a suspected parathyroid adenoma. Histologic examination revealed neural invasion by the tumor; the pathologist consequently rendered a diagnosis of parathyroid carcinoma. No other features of malignancy were evident, but this finding was considered sufficient evidence of malignancy. Which one of the following features, as a solitary finding, is LEAST likely to independently result in a diagnosis of parathyroid carcinoma?
    a. Abnormal mitotic figures
    b. Nuclear pleomorphism
    c. Coagulative tumor necrosis
    d. Invasion beyond the capsule into another structure (thyroid, skeletal muscle, etc.)
    e. Vascular invasion

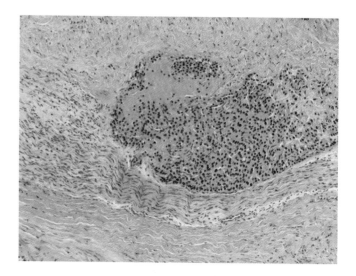

35. A 55-year-old woman underwent FNA of a thyroid nodule, which revealed no definitive evidence of neoplasia. The nodule continued to grow over several months following the procedure, and the patient subsequently underwent thyroidectomy. Histologic examination revealed a nodule comprising normal-appearing follicles, surrounded by a fibrous rim. The follicular architecture within the nodule did not differ significantly from that of the remaining uninvolved gland. Careful examination of the lesion's edge revealed the finding shown in the photograph. Which one of the following options BEST describes this lesion?

   a. Follicular adenoma, showing a fibrous capsule without invasion
   b. Follicular carcinoma, showing capsular invasion
   c. Hyperplastic nodule, showing post-FNA changes
   d. Palpation thyroiditis, showing multinucleated giant cells
   e. Subacute thyroiditis, showing multinucleated giant cells

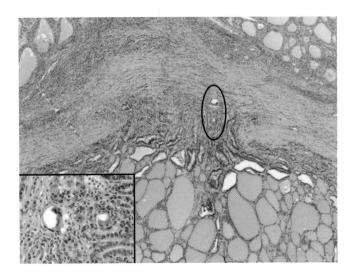

36. A 56-year-old woman underwent surgery for removal of a nodule in her right thyroid lobe. Careful histologic examination revealed the nuclear features of papillary carcinoma. Multiple foci within the tumor also displayed prominent interfollicular fibrosis, as shown in the illustration. This finding is suggestive of which of the following lesions?

   a. Papillary thyroid carcinoma, classical type
   b. Papillary thyroid carcinoma, columnar cell variant
   c. Papillary thyroid carcinoma, tall cell variant
   d. Papillary thyroid carcinoma, follicular variant
   e. Papillary thyroid carcinoma, solid variant

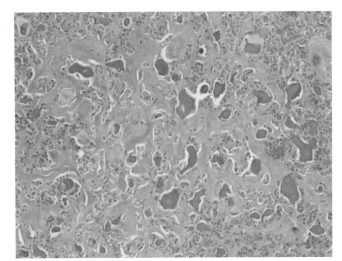

37. Which one of the following statements concerning poorly differentiated carcinoma of the thyroid is INCORRECT?

   a. Poorly differentiated carcinoma is an uncommon neoplasm derived from thyroid follicular cells.
   b. Poorly differentiated carcinoma confers a prognosis worse than that of follicular carcinoma, but better than that of UTC.
   c. Poorly differentiated carcinoma comprises solid nests of cells ("insulae") that show moderate atypia and mitotic activity.
   d. Morphologic overlap may complicate the distinction between poorly differentiated carcinoma and medullary carcinoma.
   e. Unlike undifferentiated carcinoma, poorly differentiated carcinoma is not generally associated with other types of carcinoma.

38. Which one of the following statements concerning UTC is INCORRECT?

   a. The typical clinical scenario of anaplastic carcinoma is an elderly patient with a rapidly growing neck mass.
   b. In many cases, anaplastic carcinoma causes death by growing into the larynx or trachea and obstructing the airway.
   c. Histologic examination of anaplastic carcinoma may show areas of better differentiated (papillary, follicular, or medullary) carcinoma within the tumor.

   d. Anaplastic carcinoma generally shows diffuse immunohistochemical staining for thyroglobulin, and for calcitonin in a few cases.
   e. Sheets of large, bizarre cells constitute the characteristic histologic appearance of anaplastic carcinoma.

39. Which one of the following statements concerning medullary carcinoma of the thyroid is INCORRECT?

   a. Medullary carcinoma arises from C cells (or their precursors), which migrate from the region of the fourth/fifth branchial pouch to the lateral upper two thirds of each thyroid lobe.
   b. Approximately 10% to 20% of medullary carcinoma cases occur as part of a familial syndrome.
   c. Elevation of serum calcitonin concentration in a patient without a clinically evident thyroid mass may nonetheless warrant additional work-up.
   d. Immunohistochemistry may be necessary to distinguish between medullary carcinoma and HTT, which share morphologic similarities.
   e. Medullary thyroid carcinoma is less common than papillary carcinoma, but more common than follicular carcinoma.

40. Which one of the following statements concerning Graves disease (diffuse toxic goiter) is INCORRECT?
    a. Graves disease is an autoimmune disease.
    b. Scattered collections of lymphocytes are normally found throughout the thyroid in cases of Graves disease.
    c. Exophthalmos in Graves disease is caused by high serum levels of T_4 or T_3.
    d. In Graves disease, hyperplastic thyroid tissue may be found in skeletal muscle adjacent to the thyroid.
    e. Some follicular cells in cases of Graves disease may show nuclear clearing, similar to the changes that characterize papillary thyroid carcinoma.

41. Which one of the following statements concerning thyroglossal duct cysts is INCORRECT?
    a. Partial resection of the hyoid bone is sometimes warranted during resection of a thyroglossal duct cyst.
    b. Thyroglossal duct cysts are lined by squamous epithelium, ciliated respiratory epithelium, or both.
    c. Medullary carcinoma is the most common neoplasm found in association with thyroglossal duct cysts.
    d. Ectopic salivary gland tissue is not unexpected in the connective tissue adjacent to thyroglossal duct cysts.
    e. Inflammatory complications of persistent thyroglossal duct structures are not unexpected.

ANSWERS

1. c. Germline mutations of the tumor suppressor *PTEN* are associated with various tumor syndromes, including Cowden syndrome, Bannayan-Riley-Ruvalcaba syndrome, and *Proteus* syndrome. Cowden syndrome confers increased risk for development of follicular thyroid carcinoma. Accordingly, this histologic type is the most common thyroid malignancy in patients with Cowden syndrome. An entity currently classified as the cribriform-morular variant of papillary carcinoma is associated with the FAP syndrome. This syndrome results from mutation of *APC*. Medullary carcinoma is associated with MEN 2A and MEN 2B. An association has been reported between anaplastic carcinoma and Werner syndrome, which results from mutation of the gene *WRN*.

Foulkes WD, Kloos RT, Harach HR, LiVolsi V: Familial non-medullary thyroid cancer. In DeLellis RA, Lloyd RV, Heitz PU, Eng C (eds): *Pathology and Genetics of Tumours of Endocrine Organs. World Health Organization Classification of Tumours.* Lyon: IARC Press, 2004, pp 257-261.
Harach HR, Williams GT, Williams ED: Familial adenomatous polyposis associated thyroid carcinoma: a distinct type of follicular cell neoplasm. *Histopathology* 1994; 25:549-561.
Marsh DJ, Coulon V, Lunetta KL, et al: Mutation spectrum and genotype-phenotype analyses in Cowden disease and Bannayan-Zonana syndrome, two hamartoma syndromes with germ line *PTEN* mutation. *Hum Mol Genet* 1998; 7:507-515.

2. d. All of the statements are true except d. UTC typically manifests as a rapidly expanding neck mass, usually in an elderly patient. Adequate sampling of UTC frequently reveals an association with a coexisting or preexisting better differentiated thyroid carcinoma. Alternatively, some cases are considered to arise de novo. The mortality rate of UTC is more than 90%. The average survival after diagnosis is approximately 6 months. All cases of UTC are staged as T4 tumors, by definition. UTC virtually always shows negative immunohistochemical staining for thyroglobulin. Staining for TTF-1 is usually negative as well.

Ordonez N, Baloch Z, Matias-Guiu, et al: Undifferentiated (anaplastic) carcinoma. In DeLellis RA, Lloyd RV, Heitz PU, Eng C (eds): *Pathology and Genetics of Tumours of Endocrine Organs. World Health Organization Classification of Tumours.* Lyon: IARC Press, 2004, pp 77-80.

3. d. The correct diagnosis is SLL. Lymphoma involving the thyroid can manifest as several different types or entities. In one series, 50% of patients had DLBCL, 23% had MALT lymphoma, 12% had FL, 7% had Hodgkin lymphoma, 4% had SLL, and 4% had Burkitt lymphoma. Among the small B-cell lymphoproliferative disorders (chronic lymphocytic leukemia [CLL]/SLL, prolymphocytic leukemia, hairy cell leukemia, lymphoplasmacytic lymphoma, marginal zone lymphoma, FL, and mantle cell lymphoma [MCL]), only CLL/SLL should show positive immunohistochemical staining with both CD5 and CD23. FL should show positive immunohistochemical staining with CD23, but this lesion should not stain with CD5. MCL should show positive immunohistochemical staining with CD5, but this lesion should not stain with CD23. Among thyroid tumors, CASTLE also shows positive immunohistochemical staining with CD5.

Abbondazo S, Aozasa K, Boerner S, Thompson LDR: Primary lymphoma and plasmacytoma. In DeLellis RA, Lloyd RV, Heitz PU, Eng C (eds): *Pathology and Genetics of Tumours of Endocrine Organs. World Health Organization Classification of Tumours.* Lyon: IARC Press, 2004, pp 109-111.
Thieblemont C, Mayer A, Dumontet C, et al: Primary thyroid lymphoma is a heterogeneous disease. *J Clin Endocrinol Metab* 2002;87:105-111.

4. b. and 5. b. DLBCL is the correct diagnosis in this case. The centroblastlike histologic appearance, immunohistochemical staining for Bcl-6, and t(3;14) (q27;q32) translocation are characteristic of DLBCL. Lymphoma involving the thyroid can manifest as several different types or entities. In one series, 50% of patients had DLBCL, 23% had MALT lymphoma, 12% had FL, 7% had Hodgkin lymphoma, 4% had SLL, and 4% had Burkitt lymphoma. The same series reported a 5-year survival rate of 44% among patients with DLBCL of the thyroid. Chromosomal translocations involving *BCL6*, located at band q27 of chromosome 3, are among the most common rearrangements in B-cell non-Hodgkin lymphoma. These translocations include t(3;14)(q27;q32), which places *BCL6* expression under transcriptional regulation by the IgH promoter. DLBCL likely arises from peripheral B cells of germinal center or postgerminal center origin. Primary thyroid lymphoma has a significantly higher incidence among patients with Hashimoto thyroiditis.

Abbondazo S, Aozasa K, Boerner S, Thompson LDR: Primary lymphoma and plasmacytoma. In DeLellis RA, Lloyd RV, Heitz PU, Eng C (eds): *Pathology and Genetics of Tumours of Endocrine Organs. World Health Organization Classification of Tumours.* Lyon: IARC Press, 2004, pp 109-111.

Baron BW, Nucifora G, McCabe N, et al: Identification of the gene associated with the recurring chromosomal translocations t(3;14)(q27;q32) and t(3;22)(q27;q11) in B-cell lymphomas. *Proc Natl Acad Sci U S A* 1993;90:5262-5266.

Thieblemont C, Mayer A, Dumontet C, et al: Primary thyroid lymphoma is a heterogeneous disease. *J Clin Endocrinol Metab* 200;87:105-111.

6. c. As shown in this case, a broadly invasive tumor front and architecture comprising variably sized solid nests are characteristic of CASTLE. In accordance with these histologic features, CASTLE tends to behave in a locally invasive manner, and frequently demonstrates early metastasis to regional lymph nodes. Based on its invasive growth pattern, and the squamoid and/or syncytial features of the lesional cells, CASTLE shares morphologic overlap with various lesions, such as UTC and squamous cell carcinoma. Positive immunohistochemical staining for CD5 facilitates distinction between CASTLE and potential mimics, such as those previously listed. CASTLE occurs slightly more frequently in women than in men.

Cheuk W, Chan JKC, Dorfman DM, Giordano T: Carcinoma showing thymus-like differentiation. In DeLellis RA, Lloyd RV, Heitz PU, Eng C (eds): *Pathology and Genetics of Tumours of Endocrine Organs. World Health Organization Classification of Tumours.* Lyon: IARC Press, 2004, pp 96-97.

7. c. All of the statements are correct except c. In contrast to Graves disease, there is no evidence that autonomous hyperfunctioning nodules result from an autoimmune process. In this illustration, extensive hyperplasia is apparent. Papillary foci are present. Follicles are lined by tall columnar cells with uniform, small, round, basally placed nuclei. Scalloping of colloid is seen. These histologic findings can be found in "hot" nodules, as well as in untreated Graves disease. Most patients with "hot" nodules smaller than 3 cm are clinically euthyroid. "Hot" nodules, sometimes described as "toxic adenomas," may cause clinical hyperthyroidism, as in this case.

Mills SE: *Sternberg's Diagnostic Surgical Pathology,* 5th ed. Vol. 1, Chap. 13. Philadelphia: Lippincott Williams & Wilkins, 2009.

Rosai J (ed): *Rosai and Ackerman's Surgical Pathology,* 10th ed. Vol. 1, Chap. 9. St. Louis: Mosby, 2004.

8. d. This section shows large and small colloid-filled follicles, some of which are markedly distended. Foamy macrophages are found in scattered follicles. Distended, disrupted follicles associated with foamy macrophages are not characteristic of Graves disease or nodular goiter. At least some areas of papillary hyperplasia should be seen in these conditions. In palpation thyroiditis, small disrupted follicles are found scattered throughout the gland. This condition is associated with histiocytic infiltration, but in palpation thyroiditis, most histiocytes should not have foamy cytoplasm. Colloid goiter is associated with diffuse

enlargement of the thyroid, but histologic examination would not show disrupted follicles. Furthermore, patients with diffuse colloid goiter are usually euthyroid. In patients with clinical hyperthyroidism secondary to amiodarone treatment, histologic examination of the thyroid shows distended and ruptured follicles. Thyrotoxicity in this context presumably results from follicular rupture, which leads to excessive release of thyroid hormones.

Martino E, Bartalena L, Bogazzi F, Braverman LE: The effects of amiodarone on the thyroid. *Endocr Rev* 2001;22(2):240-254.

Smyrk TC, Goellner JR, Brennan MD, Carney JA: Pathology of the thyroid in amiodarone-associated thyrotoxicosis. *Am J Surg Pathol* 1987;11(3):197-204.

9. e. All of the statements are correct except e. Follicular adenomas generally consist of cytologically benign follicular epithelial cells, with small, mildly pleomorphic nuclei. Most well-differentiated follicular carcinomas comprise follicular and trabecular structures containing cells with relatively bland nuclei, similar to those of follicular adenomas. Only a few (or no) mitotic figures are apparent. Invasion (capsular and/or vascular) constitutes the only finding that differentiates follicular carcinoma (invasive) from follicular adenoma (noninvasive). The entire edge of the lesion should be examined histologically, because invasion may occur only focally. Adenomas usually exhibit a sharp edge upon low-power examination. Most authors agree that invasion of neoplastic tissue through the tumor capsule into adjacent thyroid tissue justifies the diagnosis of follicular carcinoma. The significance of invasion into (but not through) the fibrous tissue of the tumor capsule, however, is controversial. In the majority of cases, differentiation between follicular adenoma and carcinoma cannot be done intraoperatively (by frozen section) because of sampling issues and difficulty of interpreting the frozen section material.

Mills SE: *Sternberg's Diagnostic Surgical Pathology,* 5th ed. Vol. 1, Chap. 13. Philadelphia: Lippincott Williams & Wilkins, 2009.

Rosai J (ed): *Rosai and Ackerman's Surgical Pathology,* 10th ed. Vol. 1, Chap. 9. St. Louis: Mosby, 2004.

Rosai J, Carcangiu ML, DeLellis RA: *Atlas of Tumor Pathology: Tumors of the Thyroid Gland,* Fascicle 5, 3rd series. Washington, DC: Armed Forces Institute of Pathology, 1993.

10. e. All of the statements are correct except e. Follicular thyroid carcinoma usually metastasizes hematogenously, and generally does not metastasize to cervical lymph nodes.

In foci of vascular invasion, endothelial cells may be found at the advancing tumor edge, as in this case. Immunohistochemical staining for endothelial cells (e.g., for CD34) may be helpful in identification of vascular invasion. In the absence of vascular invasion, many authors will diagnose a lesion as follicular carcinoma only when the tumor has invaded through the fibrous capsule into adjacent thyroid tissue. Only in rare cases is invasion of the fibrous capsule, in the absence of vascular invasion, associated with metastatic tumor. In all cases of follicular neoplasia, the entire capsule should be examined histologically. In difficult cases, deeper levels corresponding to foci suspicious for capsular/vascular invasion should be examined.

Mills SE: *Sternberg's Diagnostic Surgical Pathology,* 5th ed. Vol. 1, Chap. 13. Philadelphia: Lippincott Williams & Wilkins, 2009.
Rosai J (ed): *Rosai and Ackerman's Surgical Pathology,* 10th ed. Vol. 1, Chap. 9. St. Louis: Mosby, 2004.
Rosai J, Carcangiu ML, DeLellis RA: *Atlas of Tumor Pathology: Tumors of the Thyroid Gland,* Fascicle 5, 3rd series. Washington, DC: Armed Forces Institute of Pathology, 1993.

11. e. All of the statements are correct except e. Follicular thyroid carcinoma usually involves only one lobe. Follicular neoplasms (adenoma and carcinoma) are generally encapsulated and well circumscribed. These lesions frequently comprise variable percentages of follicles, trabecular structures, and solid nests. In follicular carcinoma, invasion occurs into adjacent thyroid tissue or into blood vessels. In some cases, distinction between follicular carcinoma and medullary carcinoma may be difficult, although medullary carcinoma is not usually encapsulated. Immunohistochemical studies may be helpful in this context.

Mills SE: *Sternberg's Diagnostic Surgical Pathology,* 5th ed. Vol. 1, Chap. 13. Philadelphia: Lippincott Williams & Wilkins, 2009.
Rosai J (ed): *Rosai and Ackerman's Surgical Pathology,* 10th ed. Vol. 1, Chap. 9. St. Louis: Mosby, 2004.
Rosai J, Carcangiu ML, DeLellis RA: *Atlas of Tumor Pathology: Tumors of the Thyroid Gland,* Fascicle 5, 3rd series. Washington, DC: Armed Forces Institute of Pathology, 1993.

12. e. All of the answer choices are correct. The nuclear features of papillary thyroid carcinoma include enlargement, irregular contours, chromatin dispersion/nuclear clearing, grooves, and pseudoinclusions containing cytoplasmic material. The nuclear clearing of papillary carcinoma represents an artifact of formalin fixation. Other artifacts that result from tissue processing include the "fried egg" appearance of oligodendroglioma, stromal retraction in basal cell carcinoma, clefting in salivary gland adenoid cystic carcinoma, and retraction in micropapillary carcinoma of the breast. The image depicts the tall cell variant of papillary carcinoma. This variant represents one of the biologically aggressive forms of papillary carcinoma. Other variants with stereotypically aggressive behavior include the diffuse sclerosing variant, the columnar cell variant, the solid variant, and papillary carcinoma with prominent hobnail features.

LiVolsi VA: Papillary thyroid carcinoma: an update. *Mod Pathol* 2011;24:S1-S9.
LiVolsi VA, Albores-Saavedra J, Asa SL, et al: Papillary carcinoma. In DeLellis RA, Lloyd RV, Heitz PU, Eng C (eds): *Pathology and Genetics of Tumours of Endocrine Organs. World Health Organization Classification of Tumours.* Lyon: IARC Press, 2004, pp 57-66.

13. d. and 14. e. This patient's medication history likely included minocycline, which is associated with deposition of granular black pigment in thyroid follicular epithelial cells, colloid, and macrophages. The mechanism of this process likely involves thyroid peroxidase. Investigators have demonstrated inhibition of thyroid peroxidase activity by minocycline. Patients receiving interferon-α or interleukin 2 may develop painless/"silent" thyroiditis. Interferon-α can also cause hyper- or hypothyroidism. These drugs are not associated with deposition of granular black pigment. Radioactive iodine can cause follicular epithelial changes, such as development of large, irregular, hyperchromatic nuclei (see Questions 14 and 16). The pathologic hallmark of amiodarone-induced thyrotoxicosis is accumulation of foamy macrophages within thyroid follicles, with or without disruption of follicular architecture (see Questions 8 and 29).

Jameson JL, Weetman AP: Disorders of the thyroid gland. In Longo DL, Fauci AS, Kasper DL, et al (eds): *Harrison's Principles of Internal Medicine,* 18th ed. New York: McGraw-Hill, 2012, pp 2911-2939.
Taurog A, Dorris ML, Doerge DR: Minocycline and the thyroid: antithyroid effects of the drug, and the role of thyroid peroxidase in minocycline-induced black pigmentation of the gland. *Thyroid* 1996;6:211-219.

15. a. The thyroid normally has a lobulated architecture, which may be somewhat difficult to detect histologically. The illustration shows two adjacent lobules, separated by a thin fibrous septum that runs diagonally across the picture. Normal follicles are lined by cuboidal cells. Follicular epithelial cells usually have round, somewhat dense nuclei as in this illustration. In Graves disease, these cells tend to become columnar and may produce papillary infoldings into follicles. In severe Graves disease, little or no colloid is stored in follicles. This patient received potassium iodide treatment, which manifests histologically as variable colloid storage and decreased cellularity relative to untreated Graves disease. Papillary hyperplasia may be found in nodules of nodular goiter, usually within large, dilated follicles. The cells found in papillary carcinoma have a different appearance than those found in Graves disease. This appearance includes nuclear features such as elongation, crowding, clearing, grooves, and cytoplasmic pseudoinclusions.

Mills SE: *Sternberg's Diagnostic Surgical Pathology,* 5th ed. Vol. 1, Chap. 13. Philadelphia: Lippincott Williams & Wilkins, 2009.
Rosai J (ed): *Rosai and Ackerman's Surgical Pathology,* 10th ed. Vol. 1, Chap. 9. St. Louis: Mosby, 2004.

16. a. All of the statements are correct except a. Nuclear changes occur in thyroid follicular epithelial cells following administration of radioactive iodine. Propylthiouracil, potassium iodide, and β-blockers do not usually produce nuclear abnormalities. Nuclear abnormalities may be found in Hashimoto thyroiditis, but the image does not show the histologic features of Hashimoto thyroiditis (oxyphil metaplasia, chronic inflammation, and fibrosis).

Mills SE: *Sternberg's Diagnostic Surgical Pathology,* 5th ed. Vol. 1, Chap. 13. Philadelphia: Lippincott Williams & Wilkins, 2009.
Rosai J (ed): *Rosai and Ackerman's Surgical Pathology,* 10th ed. Vol. 1, Chap. 9. St. Louis: Mosby, 2004.

17. b. The nodule in this illustration has a uniform, solid cut surface, most consistent with a follicular neoplasm (follicular adenoma or follicular carcinoma). The lesion grossly appears well circumscribed, but histologic examination is necessary to rule out capsular and vascular invasion. Nodules of nodular goiter usually have a glassy, somewhat glistening, variegated cut surface with light and dark areas. Fibrotic and cystic foci are often found. Medullary carcinoma may have a tan or tan/gray appearance, but is not usually as well circumscribed as this lesion. The diagnosis of follicular carcinoma frequently cannot be made intraoperatively, because the diagnostic foci of capsular and/or vascular invasion are not identified in the representative frozen piece.

Mills SE: *Sternberg's Diagnostic Surgical Pathology,* 5th ed. Vol. 1, Chap. 13. Philadelphia: Lippincott Williams & Wilkins, 2009.

Rosai J (ed): *Rosai and Ackerman's Surgical Pathology,* 10th ed. Vol. 1, Chap. 9. St. Louis: Mosby, 2004.

Rosai J, Carcangiu ML, DeLellis RA: *Atlas of Tumor Pathology: Tumors of the Thyroid Gland,* Fascicle 5, 3rd series. Washington, DC: Armed Forces Institute of Pathology, 1993.

18. c. This illustration shows a focus papillary carcinoma. "Optically clear" nuclei, nuclear grooves, and nuclear stratification, which constitute features of papillary carcinoma, are evident. Very few mitotic figures are generally evident in well-differentiated papillary carcinomas, which tend to grow slowly.

Mills SE: *Sternberg's Diagnostic Surgical Pathology,* 5th ed. Vol. 1, Chap. 13. Philadelphia: Lippincott Williams & Wilkins, 2009.

Rosai J (ed): *Rosai and Ackerman's Surgical Pathology,* 10th ed. Vol. 1, Chap. 9. St. Louis: Mosby, 2004.

Rosai J, Carcangiu ML, DeLellis RA: *Atlas of Tumor Pathology: Tumors of the Thyroid Gland,* Fascicle 5, 3rd series. Washington, DC: Armed Forces Institute of Pathology, 1993.

19. c. All of the statements are correct except c. Medullary carcinomas of the thyroid are composed of irregular solid nests of ovoid to spindle-shaped cells. Medullary carcinoma frequently metastasizes via both veins and lymphatic vessels. In various series, the 5-year survival rate for medullary carcinoma ranges from 20% to 40%. In contrast, the 5-year survival rate for follicular carcinoma ranges from 50% to 70%, and the 5-year survival rate for papillary carcinoma is more than 90%. Medullary carcinoma generally stains positively for calcitonin, synaptophysin, chromogranin, and carcinoembryonic antigen, and sometimes for other neuroendocrine markers, such as serotonin and adrenocorticotropic hormone. These tumors do not stain positively for thyroglobulin. Immunohistochemical findings may be misleading at the tumor edge, where it invades into (and may line follicles within) the adjacent thyroid parenchyma. In these areas, neoplastic cells that stain positively for calcitonin may be intermixed with nonneoplastic cells that stain positively for thyroglobulin.

Mills SE: *Sternberg's Diagnostic Surgical Pathology,* 5th ed. Vol. 1, Chap. 13. Philadelphia: Lippincott Williams & Wilkins, 2009.

Rosai J (ed): *Rosai and Ackerman's Surgical Pathology,* 10th ed. Vol. 1, Chap. 9. St. Louis: Mosby, 2004.

Rosai J, Carcangiu ML, DeLellis RA: *Atlas of Tumor Pathology: Tumors of the Thyroid Gland,* Fascicle 5, 3rd series. Washington, DC: Armed Forces Institute of Pathology, 1993.

20. e. All of the statements are correct except e. Follicular structures may be found either focally or extensively within parathyroid adenomas. Colloidlike material may be present within these follicles. Features of cells lining follicles in parathyroid adenomas include basally situated nuclei and densely stained nuclei. These features may be useful in distinguishing follicles of parathyroid adenoma from thyroid follicles. In some cases, immunohistochemical stains for PTH and thyroglobulin may be necessary to differentiate parathyroid adenoma from thyroid adenoma. Large, pleomorphic, and hyperchromatic nuclei are frequently found in parathyroid adenomas. These cells are most often identified focally, but may occur extensively. Mitotic figures are rarely abundant in cases of parathyroid adenoma. If mitotic figures are numerous, the lesion should be examined carefully for invasion and other findings that would establish a diagnosis of parathyroid carcinoma.

Mills SE: *Sternberg's Diagnostic Surgical Pathology,* 5th ed. Vol. 1, Chap. 13. Philadelphia: Lippincott Williams & Wilkins, 2009.

Rosai J (ed): *Rosai and Ackerman's Surgical Pathology,* 10th ed. Vol. 1, Chap. 9. St. Louis: Mosby, 2004.

21. e. All of the statements are correct except e. In the image, the parathyroid gland shows a lobular architecture, with enlarged hypercellular lobules containing scattered adipocytes. This is the stereotypical histologic appearance of parathyroid hyperplasia. Parathyroid adenomas generally consist of a single nodule devoid of fat, with or without a surrounding rim of compressed nonneoplastic parathyroid tissue. Patients with parathyroid hyperplasia may have a single enlarged gland, or multiple enlarged glands. In cases such as the one described previously, the surgeon may biopsy normal-appearing or slightly enlarged parathyroid glands, in order to rule out parathyroid proliferative disease that is grossly unapparent. Recurrent hypercalcemia may occur following surgery for either parathyroid hyperplasia or parathyroid adenoma. In such cases of parathyroid hyperplasia, patients may have hyperplasia of one or multiple remaining gland(s) at reoperation. Parathyroid adenomas sometimes occur doubly, either as synchronous or metachronous lesions. In cases of metachronous double adenomas, patients may develop recurrent hypercalcemia following resection of the first adenoma. In cases of synchronous double adenomas, both lesions may be identified during the first operation. Some patients with parathyroid hyperplasia and/or multiple parathyroid adenomas have MEN 1. This condition also includes hyperplasia and/or neoplasia involving pancreatic endocrine cells and the pituitary gland. Lipoadenoma is an uncommon type of parathyroid adenoma. These lesions are generally solitary, nonlobulated lesions that contain variable numbers of adipocytes, but otherwise show the histologic features of parathyroid adenoma.

Mills SE: *Sternberg's Diagnostic Surgical Pathology,* 5th ed. Vol. 1, Chap. 13. Philadelphia: Lippincott Williams & Wilkins, 2009.

Rosai J (ed): *Rosai and Ackerman's Surgical Pathology,* 10th ed. Vol. 1, Chap. 9. St. Louis: Mosby, 2004.

22. e. All of the conditions listed in the question can be associated with squamous metaplasia. Squamous metaplasia can occur as a reactive process within the thyroid following trauma, e.g., due to FNA, or within follicular adenomatous hyperplasia, ultimobranchial body remnants/solid cell nests, or thymic rests. Various reports have described squamous metaplasia within Hashimoto thyroiditis. Several thyroid tumors show squamous differentiation or metaplasia. These include the diffuse sclerosing variant of papillary carcinoma (which demonstrates extensive squamous metaplasia), primary squamous cell carcinoma, the cribriform-morular variant of papillary carcinoma, CASTLE, mucoepidermoid carcinoma, and UTC.

Dube VE, Joyce GT: Extreme squamous metaplasia in Hashimoto's thyroiditis. *Cancer* 1971;27:434-437.

Harcourt-Webster JN: Squamous epithelium in the human thyroid gland. *J Clin Pathol* 1966;19:384-388.

23. e.   An association has been recognized between Hashimoto thyroiditis and all of the answer choices. Several studies have demonstrated immune complex deposition within the context of Hashimoto thyroiditis. Laboratory work-up of patients with Hashimoto thyroiditis may reveal antithyroglobulin, antithyroid peroxidase, and antimicrosomal antibodies. These autoantibodies likely mediate thyrocyte dysfunction via deposition of immune complexes on the basement membranes of follicular epithelial cells, which leads to complement activation and thyrocyte necrosis. Hashimoto thyroiditis is associated with several HLA alleles including HLA-DR3, HLA-DR4, and HLA-DR5. The incidence of Hashimoto thyroiditis is increased among individuals with Turner syndrome and Down syndrome.

Kalderon AE, Bogaars HA: Immune complex deposits in Graves' disease and Hashimoto's thyroiditis. *Am J Med* 1977; 63:729-734.

Stassi G, De Maria R: Autoimmune thyroid disease: new models of cell death in autoimmunity. *Nat Rev Immunol* 2002;2:195-204.

24. b., 25. c., and 26. e.   Hyperthyroidism refers to excessive thyroid function. Causes of primary hyperthyroidism include Graves disease, "toxic" goiter, and "toxic" adenoma. Causes of secondary hyperthyroidism include pituitary adenoma and gestational thyrotoxicosis. Graves disease results from production of stimulatory anti-TSHR antibodies, which cause constitutive activation of follicular epithelial cells, and overproduction of T_3 and T_4. Laboratory work-up of patients with Hashimoto thyroiditis may reveal antithyroglobulin, antithyroid peroxidase, or antimicrosomal antibodies. Histologic features of Graves disease include papillary hyperplasia, follicles that show "scalloping" of colloid, follicles containing little or no colloid, and follicular epithelial cells with columnar morphologic appearance. Various HLAs have been associated with different autoimmune and inflammatory thyroid conditions. HLA-B8 has been associated with an increased risk for development of Graves disease. HLA-DR3, HLA-DR4, and HLA-DR5 have been associated with an increased risk for development of Hashimoto thyroiditis. HLA-Bw35 has been associated with an increased risk for development of subacute thyroiditis.

Jameson JL, Weetman AP: Disorders of the thyroid gland. In Longo DL, Fauci AS, Kasper DL, et al (eds): *Harrison's Principles of Internal Medicine,* 18th ed. New York: McGraw-Hill, 2012, pp 2911-2939.

Nyulassy S, Hnilica P, Buc M, et al: Subacute (de Quervain's) thyroiditis: association with HLA-BW35 antigen and abnormalities of the complement system, immunoglobulins and other serum proteins. *J Clin Endocrinol Metab* 1977; 45:270-274.

Thompson LD: Diffuse hyperplasia of the thyroid gland (Graves' disease). *Ear Nose Throat J* 2007;86:666-667.

27. e.   All of the lesions listed in the answer choices may display nuclear inclusions or pseudoinclusions. The nuclear features of papillary thyroid carcinoma include enlargement, irregular contours, chromatin dispersion/nuclear clearing, grooves, and pseudoinclusions containing cytoplasmic material. Some authors posit that the follicular variant is less likely to show robust nuclear inclusions, compared to other variants of papillary carcinoma. Hepatocellular carcinoma and melanoma also show prominent nuclear inclusions. Occasionally, nuclear inclusions are present in cases of parathyroid carcinoma. Invasive pulmonary adenocarcinoma and pulmonary adenocarcinoma in situ (bronchioloalveolar carcinoma) sometimes show nuclear pseudoinclusions or grooves. These features may be useful in terms of distinguishing adenocarcinoma in situ from benign reactive atypia.

Atkins KA: The diagnosis of bronchioloalveolar carcinoma by cytologic means. *Am J Clin Pathol* 2004;122:14-16.

LiVolsi VA: Papillary thyroid carcinoma: an update. *Mod Pathol* 2011;24:S1-S9.

LiVolsi VA, Albores-Saavedra J, Asa SL, et al: Papillary carcinoma. In DeLellis RA, Lloyd RV, Heitz PU, Eng C (eds): *Pathology and Genetics of Tumours of Endocrine Organs. World Health Organization Classification of Tumours.* Lyon: IARC Press, 2004, pp 57-66.

28. d.   Primary hyperparathyroidism results from oversecretion of the PTH. The direct effects of PTH include increased reabsorption of calcium from renal tubules, increased reabsorption of calcium from bone, and increased conversion of 25-OH-vitamin D to $1,25\text{-}(OH)_2$-vitamin D. This more active metabolite of vitamin D increases intestinal absorption of calcium, and further increases calcium reabsorption from renal tubules and bone. Laboratory work-up of patients with primary hyperparathyroidism reveals hypercalcemia and hypophospatemia (because PTH decreases reabsorption of phosphate by renal tubules). Severe hypercalcemia and extremely high PTH levels are generally more common in cases of parathyroid carcinoma, compared to cases of parathyroid adenoma.

Some authors posit that diagnosis of parathyroid carcinoma requires one of the following findings: abnormal mitotic figures, coagulative/geographic tumor necrosis, tumoral invasion into adjacent structures, vascular invasion, or (peri)neural invasion. Nuclear pleomorphism is common in both parathyroid carcinoma and adenoma. According to most series, 80% to 85% of primary hyperparathyroidism cases result from parathyroid adenoma, 15% to 20% result from primary chief cell hyperplasia, and less than 1% result from parathyroid carcinoma.

Bondeson L, Grimelius L, DeLellis RA, et al: Parathyroid carcinoma. In DeLellis RA, Lloyd RV, Heitz PU, Eng C (eds): *Pathology and Genetics of Tumours of Endocrine Organs. World Health Organization Classification of Tumours.* Lyon: IARC Press, 2004, pp 125-127.

DeLellis RA, Williams ED: Thyroid and parathyroid tumours: introduction. In DeLellis RA, Lloyd RV, Heitz PU, Eng C (eds): *Pathology and Genetics of Tumours of Endocrine Organs. World Health Organization Classification of Tumours.* Lyon: IARC Press, 2004, pp 51-56.

Thompson LDR: Parathyroid carcinoma. *Ear Nose Throat J* 2008;87:502-504.

29. c. Thyrotoxicosis refers to elevated levels of thyroid hormone. Hyperthyroidism refers to excessive thyroid function. Thyrotoxicosis can (but does not necessarily) result from hyperthyroidism. Thyrotoxicosis without hyperthyroidism (destructive thyroiditis) results from thyroid destruction (e.g., due to amiodarone, subacute thyroiditis, infarction of an adenoma, etc.). Amiodarone exerts various effects on thyroid function, and causes thyrotoxicosis via multiple different mechanisms. In individuals without underlying thyroid abnormalities, amiodarone-induced thyrotoxicosis manifests as destructive thyroiditis resulting from lysosomal activation. The pathologic hallmark of this condition is accumulation of foamy macrophages within thyroid follicles. The histologic appearance of subacute thyroiditis (also known as de Quervain thyroiditis, granulomatous thyroiditis, or viral thyroiditis) differs from the present case.

Acute thyroiditis is rare, and results from suppurative infection of the thyroid. Causes of primary hyperthyroidism include Graves disease, "toxic" goiter, and "toxic" adenoma. Causes of secondary hyperthyroidism include pituitary adenoma and gestational thyrotoxicosis.

Jameson JL, Weetman AP: Disorders of the thyroid gland. In Longo DL, Fauci AS, Kasper DL, et al (eds): *Harrison's Principles of Internal Medicine*, 18th ed. New York: McGraw-Hill, 2012, pp 2911-2939.

Martino E, Bartalena L, Bogazzi F, Braverman LE: The effects of amiodarone on the thyroid. *Endocr Rev* 2001;22(2):240-254.

Smyrk TC, Goellner JR, Brennan MD, Carney JA: Pathology of the thyroid in amiodarone-associated thyrotoxicosis. *Am J Surg Pathol* 1987;11(3):197-204.

30. e. All of the answer choices are correct. The nuclear features of papillary thyroid carcinoma include enlargement, irregular contours, chromatin dispersion/ nuclear clearing, grooves, and pseudoinclusions containing cytoplasmic material. Nuclear grooves sometimes occur in nonneoplastic contexts. In the thyroid, the nuclei of oncocytes can show grooves. Many other tumors characteristically demonstrate nuclear grooves. Grooved nuclei are typical of solid pseudopapillary tumor of the pancreas, and they represent a diagnostic feature of chondroblastoma. Among ovarian tumors, Brenner tumor and the adult type of granulosa cell tumor display nuclear grooves. Bronchioloalveolar carcinoma/pulmonary adenocarcinoma in situ sometimes shows nuclear pseudoinclusions and grooves. These features may be useful in terms of distinguishing this lesion from benign reactive atypia.

Atkins KA: The diagnosis of bronchioloalveolar carcinoma by cytologic means. *Am J Clin Pathol* 2004;122:14-16.

LiVolsi VA: Papillary thyroid carcinoma: an update. *Mod Pathol* 2011;24:S1-S9.

LiVolsi VA, Albores-Saavedra J, Asa SL, et al: Papillary carcinoma. In DeLellis RA, Lloyd RV, Heitz PU, Eng C (eds): *Pathology and Genetics of Tumours of Endocrine Organs. World Health Organization Classification of Tumours*. Lyon: IARC Press, 2004, pp 57-66.

31. c. HTT consists of trabeculae and nests within a delicate fibrovascular stroma. This tumor features nuclei with prominent grooves and cytoplasmic pseudoinclusions, and consequently mimics papillary carcinoma in FNA specimens. HTT characteristically demonstrates circumscription and is sometimes encapsulated. These features may facilitate distinction between HTT and medullary carcinoma in some cases. HTT displays a distinctive membranous immunohistochemical staining pattern with Ki-67. Like many other thyroid tumors, HTT generally shows positive staining with thyroglobulin and TTF-1, and negative staining with calcitonin.

Carney JA, Volante M, Papotti M, Asa S: Hyalinizing trabecular tumour. In DeLellis RA, Lloyd RV, Heitz PU, Eng C (eds): *Pathology and Genetics of Tumours of Endocrine Organs. World Health Organization Classification of Tumours*. Lyon: IARC Press, 2004, pp 104-105.

32. d. and 33. c. MEN 2A and MEN 2B are autosomal dominant syndromes that result from mutation of *RET*. Definitive diagnosis of MEN 2 relies almost exclusively upon *RET* mutational analysis. Features of MEN 2A include medullary thyroid carcinoma, pheochromocytoma, and primary hyperparathyroidism. Manifestations of MEN 2B also include neuroma of the tongue, but do not include primary hyperparathyroidism. Medullary thyroid carcinoma occurring within the context of MEN 2 is frequently associated with C-cell hyperplasia. This finding does not generally characterize sporadic cases of medullary carcinoma.

MEN 1, alternatively known as Wermer syndrome, is an autosomal dominant syndrome that results from mutation of the MEN 1 gene on chromosome 11. Diagnosis of MEN 1 requires at least two of the following findings: (1) parathyroid hyperplasia and/or adenoma, or recurrent primary hyperparathyroidism; (2) duodenal and/or pancreatic endocrine neoplasia; (3) anterior pituitary adenoma; (4) adrenal cortical neoplasia; (5) foregut (i.e., bronchial or thymic) carcinoid tumor; and (6) a first-degree relative with MEN 1.

Calender A, Morrison CD, Komminoth P, et al: Multiple endocrine neoplasia type 1. In DeLellis RA, Lloyd RV, Heitz PU, Eng C (eds): *Pathology and Genetics of Tumours of Endocrine Organs. World Health Organization Classification of Tumours*. Lyon: IARC Press, 2004, pp 218-227.

Foulkes WD, Kloos RT, Harach HR, LiVolsi V: Familial non-medullary thyroid cancer. In DeLellis RA, Lloyd RV, Heitz PU, Eng C (eds): *Pathology and Genetics of Tumours of Endocrine Organs. World Health Organization Classification of Tumours*. Lyon: IARC Press, 2004, pp 257-261.

Gimm O, Morrison CD, Suster S, et al: Multiple endocrine neoplasia type 2. In DeLellis RA, Lloyd RV, Heitz PU, Eng C (eds): *Pathology and Genetics of Tumours of Endocrine Organs. World Health Organization Classification of Tumours*. Lyon: IARC Press, 2004, pp 257-261.

34. b. Perineural invasion is almost always diagnostic of parathyroid carcinoma. Other than perineural invasion, some authors posit that diagnosis of parathyroid carcinoma requires one of the following findings: abnormal mitotic figures, coagulative/geographic tumor necrosis, tumoral invasion into adjacent structures, and vascular invasion. Nuclear pleomorphism is common in both parathyroid carcinoma and adenoma. According to most series, 80% to 85% of primary hyperparathyroidism cases result from parathyroid adenoma, 15% to 20% result from primary chief cell hyperplasia, and less than 1% result from parathyroid carcinoma. Primary hyperparathyroidism results from oversecretion of PTH. The direct effects of PTH include increased reabsorption of calcium from renal tubules, increased reabsorption of calcium from bones, and increased conversion of 25-OH-vitamin D to 1,25-(OH)$_2$-vitamin D. This more active metabolite of vitamin D increases intestinal absorption of calcium, and further increases calcium reabsorption from renal tubules and bones. Laboratory work-up of patients with primary hyperparathyroidism reveals hypercalcemia and hypophospatemia (because PTH decreases reabsorption of phosphate by renal tubules). Severe hypercalcemia and extremely high PTH levels are generally more common in cases of parathyroid carcinoma, compared to cases of parathyroid adenoma.

Bondeson L, Grimelius L, DeLellis RA, et al: Parathyroid carcinoma. In DeLellis RA, Lloyd RV, Heitz PU, Eng C (eds): *Pathology and Genetics of Tumours of Endocrine Organs. World Health Organization Classification of Tumours.* Lyon: IARC Press, 2004, pp 125-127.

DeLellis RA, Williams ED: Thyroid and parathyroid tumours: introduction. In DeLellis RA, Lloyd RV, Heitz PU, Eng C (eds): *Pathology and Genetics of Tumours of Endocrine Organs. World Health Organization Classification of Tumours.* Lyon: IARC Press, 2004, pp 51-56.

Thompson LDR: Parathyroid carcinoma. *Ear Nose Throat J* 2008;87:502-504.

35. c. The lesion shown is a hyperplastic nodule, showing post-FNA changes. Classification of follicular thyroid lesions is associated with/subject to significant interobserver variability. Diagnosis of these lesions represents a potentially difficult and controversial aspect of surgical pathology. According to some experts, follicular adenoma should show three features: (1) a distinct microfollicular, macrofollicular, or trabecular growth pattern; (2) distinct architecture that differs from the surrounding thyroid parenchyma; and (3) confinement within a capsule. Hyperplastic nodules sometimes undergo degenerative changes (fibrosis and calcification), which may result in formation of a fibrous pseudocapsule. Irregularities in the fibrous pseudocapsule of a hyperplastic nodule can simulate capsular invasion, and potentially result in misdiagnosis of follicular carcinoma. In this case, the architectural similarity between the lesion and the uninvolved parenchyma supports a diagnosis of hyperplastic nodule, rather than adenoma or carcinoma. The foreign body-type giant cells shown in the inset suggest a reactive/reparative process, such as the aftermath of FNA.

Baloch ZW, LiVolsi VA: Follicular-patterned lesions of the thyroid. The bane of the pathologist. *Am J Clin Pathol* 2002;117: 143-150.

36. d. Among the different variants of papillary carcinoma, interfollicular fibrosis is suggestive of the follicular variant, especially in circumscribed/encapsulated lesions. Some authors posit that the follicular variant is less likely to show robust nuclear inclusions, compared to other variants of papillary carcinoma. The columnar variant consists of cells that resemble adenomatous colonic epithelium. The tall cell variant shows 50% or more of cells with height more than or equal to twice their width. The solid variant shows a solid growth pattern in 50% or more of the tumor.

LiVolsi VA: Papillary thyroid carcinoma: an update. *Mod Pathol* 2011;24:S1-S9.

LiVolsi VA, Albores-Saavedra J, Asa SL, et al: Papillary carcinoma. In DeLellis RA, Lloyd RV, Heitz PU, Eng C (eds): *Pathology and Genetics of Tumours of Endocrine Organs. World Health Organization Classification of Tumours.* Lyon: IARC Press, 2004, pp 57-66.

37. e. All of the answers are correct except e. Poorly differentiated carcinoma confers a prognosis worse than that of follicular carcinoma, but better than that of UTC. In many cases of poorly differentiated carcinoma, areas of papillary or follicular carcinoma are evident. This association suggests a cause involving "dedifferentiation" of well-differentiated carcinoma. If areas of poorly differentiated carcinoma are found in what is otherwise a well-differentiated (papillary or follicular) carcinoma, the tumor often shows more aggressive clinical behavior, compared to "pure" papillary or follicular carcinoma. Morphologic overlap may complicate the distinction between poorly differentiated carcinoma and medullary carcinoma, as both lesions may grow with a "carcinoidlike" pattern. In contrast to medullary carcinoma, poorly differentiated carcinoma shows positive immunohistochemical staining for thyroglobulin, and negative staining for calcitonin.

Mills SE: *Sternberg's Diagnostic Surgical Pathology,* 5th ed. Vol. 1, Chap. 13. Philadelphia: Lippincott Williams & Wilkins, 2009.

Rosai J (ed): *Rosai and Ackerman's Surgical Pathology,* 10th ed. Vol. 1, Chap. 9. St. Louis: Mosby, 2004.

38. d. All of the answers are correct except d. Histologic examination of anaplastic thyroid carcinomas usually shows sheets of large bizarre cells. Tumoral giant cells may be seen. Numerous mitotic figures are typically evident, as well as necrosis and vascular invasion. "Squamoid" or "sarcomatoid" features are frequently identified. The immunohistochemical properties of anaplastic carcinoma are variable. These tumors are usually cytokeratin positive and thyroglobulin negative. "Positive" thyroglobulin staining, if present, generally occurs in only a few scattered cells. Calcitonin staining may be found in tumors that have apparently arisen within medullary carcinoma.

Mills SE: *Sternberg's Diagnostic Surgical Pathology,* 5th ed. Vol. 1, Chap. 13. Philadelphia: Lippincott Williams & Wilkins, 2009.

Rosai J (ed): *Rosai and Ackerman's Surgical Pathology,* 10th ed. Vol. 1, Chap. 9. St. Louis: Mosby, 2004.

Rosai J, Carcangiu ML, DeLellis RA: *Atlas of Tumor Pathology: Tumors of the Thyroid Gland,* Fascicle 5, 3rd series. Washington, DC: Armed Forces Institute of Pathology, 1993.

39. e. In most series in the United States, papillary and follicular carcinomas occur more frequently than medullary carcinoma, with the following distribution: papillary carcinoma approximately 80% to 90%, follicular carcinoma approximately 10% to 15%, and medullary carcinoma approximately 5%. Medullary carcinoma is generally more aggressive than papillary or follicular carcinoma, and portends a worse prognosis. Medullary thyroid carcinoma shares histologic overlap with HTT, which generally consists of cords and trabeculae surrounded by hyalinized stroma. Unlike medullary carcinoma, HTTs are characteristically well circumscribed. Immunohistochemical studies of HTTs show positive staining for thyroglobulin, whereas medullary carcinoma stains positively for calcitonin and carcinoembryonic antigen. Approximately 10% to 20% of medullary carcinoma cases occur as part of MEN 2A or MEN 2B. These syndromes include medullary thyroid carcinoma, C-cell hyperplasia, pheochromocytoma, adrenal medullary hyperplasia, and parathyroid hyperplasia. MEN 2B also includes mucosal neuromas and gastrointestinal ganglioneuromas. In families affected by MEN 2A or MEN 2B, elevated serum calcitonin levels in individuals without detectable thyroid tumors may indicate C-cell hyperplasia or incipient medullary carcinoma.

Mills SE: *Sternberg's Diagnostic Surgical Pathology,* 5th ed. Vol. 1, Chap. 13. Philadelphia: Lippincott Williams & Wilkins, 2009.
Rosai J (ed): *Rosai and Ackerman's Surgical Pathology,* 10th ed. Vol. 1, Chap. 9. St. Louis: Mosby, 2004.
Rosai J, Carcangiu ML, DeLellis RA: *Atlas of Tumor Pathology: Tumors of the Thyroid Gland,* Fascicle 5, 3rd series. Washington, DC: Armed Forces Institute of Pathology, 1993.

40. c. All of the answers are correct except c. In Graves disease, some follicular cells may show nuclear clearing, similar to the changes that characterize papillary thyroid carcinoma. Nuclear clearing is not exclusively diagnostic of papillary thyroid carcinoma. Graves disease is an autoimmune disease in which antibodies attach to the TSH receptor on thyroid follicular cells, stimulating these cells and leading to hyperplasia. Periorbital edema and exophthalmos in Graves disease are believed to result from deposition of antigen-antibody complexes in periorbital tissues, especially muscle. Exophthalmos frequently persists in Graves disease even after pharmacologic treatment results in normalization of T_3 and T_4 and control of other stigmata of hyperthyroidism. Surgeons sometimes resort to resection of periorbital adipose tissue (in order to decompress the orbit) in Graves disease patients with persistent exophthalmos.

Mills SE: *Sternberg's Diagnostic Surgical Pathology,* 5th ed. Vol. 1, Chap. 13. Philadelphia: Lippincott Williams & Wilkins, 2009.
Rosai J (ed): *Rosai and Ackerman's Surgical Pathology,* 10th ed. Vol. 1, Chap. 9. St. Louis: Mosby, 2004.

41. c. All of the answers are correct except c. The thyroglossal duct originates in the foramen caecum of the posterior oral cavity, and extends along the midline to the ultimate position of the thyroid. Thyroid-type neoplasms may arise in thyroglossal duct cysts, or in ectopic thyroid tissue, which frequently exists adjacent to thyroglossal duct cysts. Papillary carcinoma is the most common thyroid-type neoplasm in this context. Medullary carcinoma arises from "C" cells (or their precursors), which migrate into the thyroid from the fourth/fifth branchial pouch. The thyroglossal duct does not contain "C" cells, and medullary carcinoma would, therefore, be highly unusual in thyroglossal duct remnants.

Mills SE: *Sternberg's Diagnostic Surgical Pathology,* 5th ed. Vol. 1, Chap. 13. Philadelphia: Lippincott Williams & Wilkins, 2009.
Rosai J (ed): *Rosai and Ackerman's Surgical Pathology,* 10th ed. Vol. 1, Chap. 9. St. Louis: Mosby, 2004.

CHAPTER 18

HEMATOPATHOLOGY

Bachir Alobeid and John C. Lee

QUESTIONS

Questions 1-30 in this chapter refer to a photograph or photomicrograph.

1. Which of the following is used to grade this lymphoma?
   a. Degree of cellular atypia
   b. Number of apoptotic bodies
   c. Number of mitoses
   d. Number of centroblastic cells
   e. Number of centrocytic cells

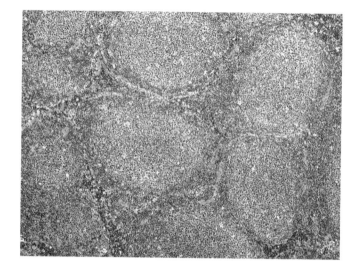

2. Which lymphoma/leukemia is characterized by these lymphoid infiltrates?
   a. Follicular lymphoma (FL)
   b. Chronic lymphocytic leukemia
   c. Marginal zone lymphoma
   d. Hairy cell leukemia (HCL)
   e. Splenic marginal zone lymphoma

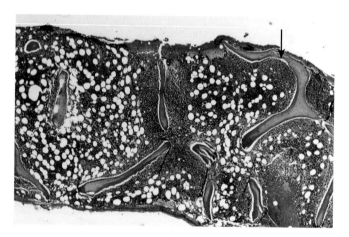

3. Which of the following statements regarding this leukemia is FALSE?

   a. The majority of cases that transform to acute leukemia are of myeloid lineage.

   b. This leukemia is characterized by t(8;21).

   c. The natural progression is transformation to an acute leukemia.

   d. The bone marrow is hypercellular with myeloid and megakaryocytic hyperplasia.

   e. Pseudo-Gaucher cells are commonly seen.

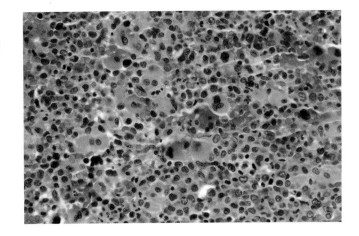

4. Which lymphoma is characterized by these cells?

   a. Nodular lymphocyte predominant Hodgkin lymphoma (NLPHL)

   b. Anaplastic large cell lymphoma (ALCL)

   c. Classical Hodgkin lymphoma, nodular sclerosis subtype

   d. Richter transformation

   e. Mantle cell lymphoma (MCL), blastoid variant

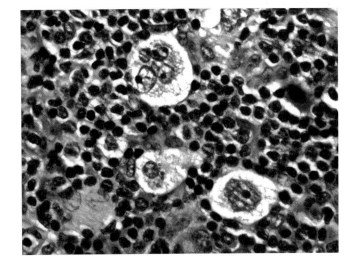

5. Which statement is FALSE regarding this lymphoma characterized by the cells indicated by arrows?

   a. It is a monoclonal B-cell neoplasm.

   b. Mediastinal and bone marrow involvement is common.

   c. Progressive transformation of germinal centers (PTGC) may be seen simultaneously in the same lymph node.

   d. The large cells show a CD20 positive, CD10 positive, Bcl-6 positive, and CD45 positive phenotype.

   e. Early stage lesions have a good prognosis.

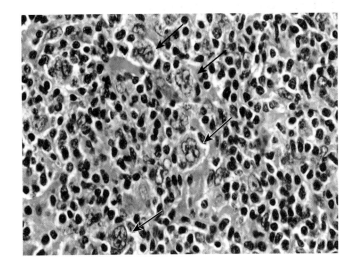

6. Which of the following statements is TRUE regarding this lymphoma?
   a. It is defined as a lymphoma expressing CD30.
   b. Most cases are Epstein-Barr virus (EBV) positive.
   c. Most cases are human herpesvirus (HHV)-8 positive.
   d. A t(2;5) with anaplastic lymphoma kinase (ALK) protein overexpression predicts a poor prognosis.
   e. Most cases express cytotoxic granule-associated proteins.

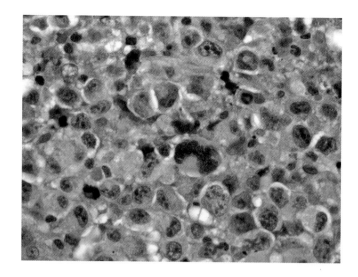

7. Which statement is FALSE regarding this leukemia/lymphoma?
   a. Splenomegaly is a characteristic finding.
   b. Interstitial infiltration of the marrow is typical.
   c. CD20 positive, CD5 negative, CD25 positive, CD103 positive, Annexin A1 positive, tartrate resistant acid phosphatase positive, and CD11c positive immunophenotype is typical.
   d. Nodular paratrabecular infiltration of the marrow is typical.
   e. Monocytopenia is typical.

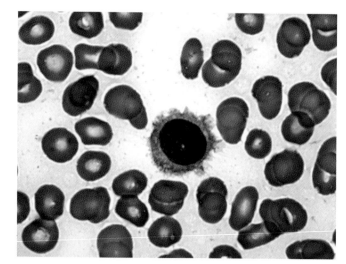

8. Which of the following statements is FALSE regarding this lymphoma?
   a. Diffuse marrow involvement has a worse prognosis.
   b. Cases with mutated immunoglobulin variable gene regions have a better prognosis.
   c. Cases with isolated 13q deletion usually have a more favorable clinical course.
   d. CD19 positive, CD20 dim, CD5 positive, CD23 positive, and cyclin D1 negative phenotype is characteristic.
   e. Cases with ZAP-70 or CD38 expression have a favorable prognosis.

9. Which of the following is characteristic of this lymphoma?

   a. Proliferation centers/pseudofollicles

   b. t(8;14)

   c. Aggressive clinical course

   d. A mixture of centrocytic and centroblastic cells

   e. t(11;14)

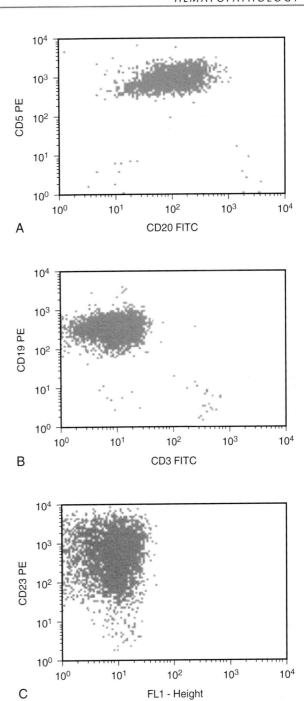

10. Which of the following are the postulated normal counterpart cells or cells of origin for the lymphoma seen in the figure?

a. Precursor thymic T cells
b. CD4⁺ follicular helper T cells
c. TCR γ/δ T cells
d. CD4⁺ T cells with cytotoxic features
e. NK (natural killer) cells or cytotoxic T cells

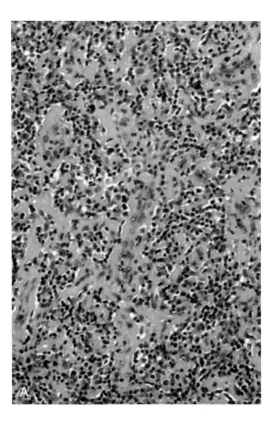

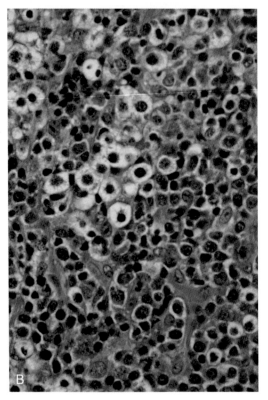

11. This hematolymphoid malignancy is associated with which cytogenetic/molecular abnormality?

a. Ras mutation

b. IgH-Bcl2 translocation

c. *BRAF* mutation

d. IgH-cyclin D1 translocation

e. IgH-myc translocation

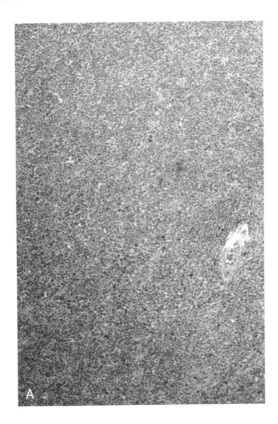

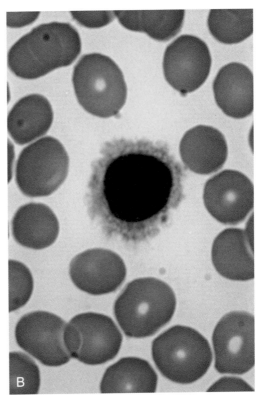

12. In the posttransplant setting, which of the following T/NK-cell lymphomas are the MOST common posttransplant lymphoproliferative disorders (PTLDs)?
   a. Extranodal NK/T-cell lymphoma
   b. Adult T-cell leukemia/lymphoma (ATLL)
   c. Hepatosplenic T-cell lymphoma
   d. Angioimmunoblastic T-cell lymphoma (AITL)
   e. ALCL

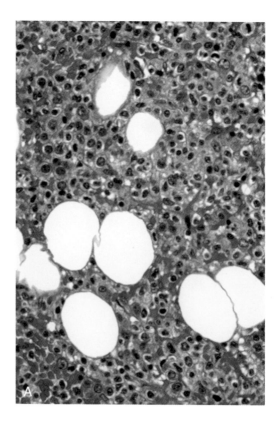

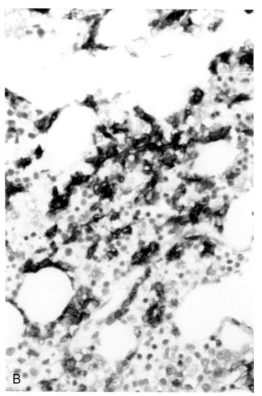

13. Which of the following is NOT a criterion in the diagnosis for systemic mastocytosis?

a. Multifocal compact clusters of 15 or more mast cells per aggregate

b. Spindled morphologic appearance in 25% or more of mast cells

c. Aberrant CD2 and/or CD25 expression in mast cells

d. Jak2 mutation

e. Serum tryptase level 20 ng/mL or higher

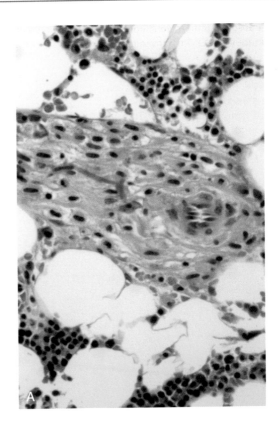

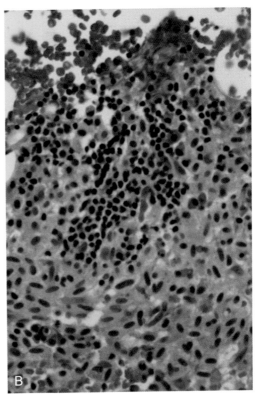

14. This cavity-based lymphoproliferative disorder is associated
with and attributable to which infectious agent?
   a. EBV
   b. Kaposi sarcoma herpesvirus (KSHV)
   c. Hepatitis C
   d. Human immunodeficiency virus
   e. Human T-lymphotropic virus (HTLV)

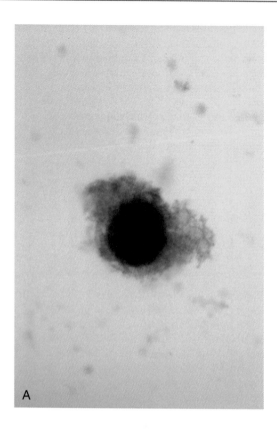

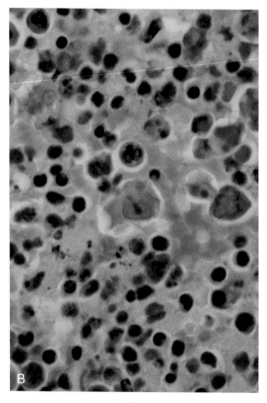

15. Which of the following translocations is characteristic of this leukemia?
    a. t(8;21)
    b. inv(16) or t(16;16)
    c. t(9;22)
    d. 11q23 translocations
    e. t(15;17)

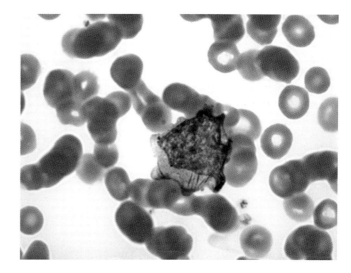

16. Which statement is FALSE regarding this lymphoma/leukemia?
    a. There are three types recognized: endemic, sporadic, and immunodeficiency-associated.
    b. This is the most common malignancy of childhood in equatorial Africa.
    c. EBV is identified to a varying extent in this malignancy.
    d. A predominant nodal involvement by this malignancy is characteristic.
    e. Genetic abnormalities involving the *MYC* gene on 8q24 play an essential role in pathogenesis.

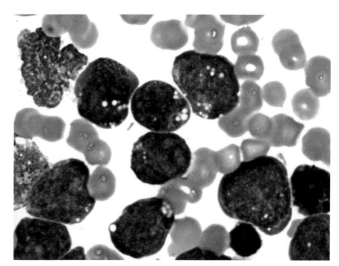

17. Which immunophenotype is MOST characteristic of these leukemic cells?
    a. CD19 positive, CD10 positive, CD34 positive, and cytoplasmic IgM positive
    b. CD34 negative, HLA-DR negative, CD117 positive, CD33 positive, and MPO positive
    c. CD11c positive, CD64 positive, CD33 positive, and CD13 positive
    d. CD19 positive, CD20 positive, CD11c positive, CD25 positive, and CD103 positive
    e. CD19 positive, CD20 positive, CD10 positive, and Bcl-2 positive

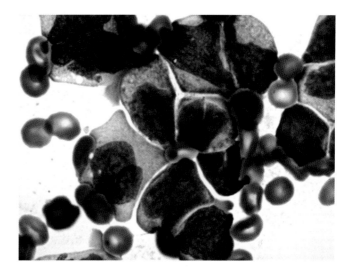

18. Which of the following statements is FALSE regarding the lymphoma?
  a. It is the most common lymphoma in developed countries.
  b. *MYC* gene rearrangements are seen in the vast majority of cases.
  c. It comprises a heterogeneous group of lymphomas.
  d. *BCL2* gene rearrangements are seen in 20% to 30% of cases.
  e. *BCL6* gene rearrangements can be seen in 30% of the cases.

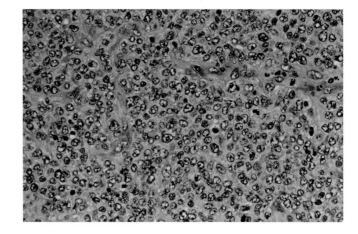

19. The lymphoid infiltrate shown in this gastric biopsy has the following immunophenotype: CD20 positive, CD43 positive, Bcl-2 positive, CD5 negative, and lambda positive. Which of the following microorganisms has been implicated in the pathogenesis of this lymphoma?
  a. *Mycobacterium avium* complex
  b. *Streptococcus suis*
  c. *Helicobacter pylori*
  d. *Borrelia burgdorferi*
  e. *Corynebacterium amycolatum*

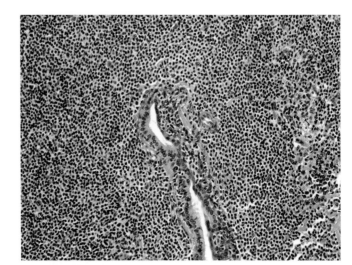

20. This intraabdominal lymphoma in a 12-year-old child shows the following immunophenotype: CD20 positive, CD19 positive, CD43 positive, CD10 positive, Bcl-6 positive, Bcl-2 negative, and surface Ig positive. Which of the following translocations is characteristically seen in this lymphoma?
  a. t(8:14)
  b. t(11;18)
  c. t(2;5)
  d. t(14;18)
  e. t(11;14)

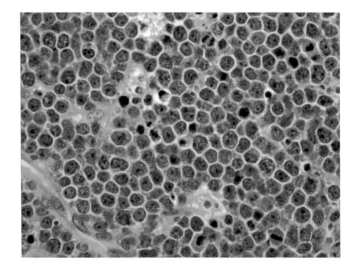

21. The leukemic cells in this testicular biopsy from an infant have the following immunophenotype: CD20 negative, CD19 positive, CD10 negative, CD34 positive, TdT positive, and sIg negative. Which of the following genes is MOST likely rearranged in this leukemia?
    a. *MLL*
    b. *RUNX1T1*
    c. *PML*
    d. *MYH11*
    e. *RUNX1*

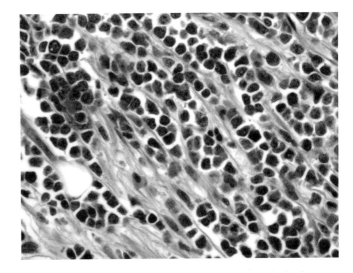

22. Which statement is FALSE regarding this lymphoma?
    a. Prognosis is dependent on the stage of the disease.
    b. The phenotype of the large cell shown is CD45 negative, CD30 positive, CD15 positive, MUM1 positive, and Pax5 positive.
    c. The large cell depicted in the picture is of histiocytic origin.
    d. Cervical and mediastinal lymph nodes are common sites of involvement.
    e. EBV can be detected in some cases.

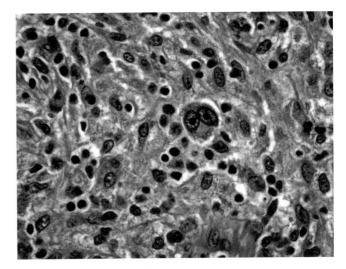

23. The cell depicted in the figure was seen on the peripheral blood smear from a patient with hypercalcemia. The atypical cells have the following immunophenotype: CD3 positive, CD7 negative, CD4 positive, CD8 negative, and CD25 positive. Which of the following T-cell lymphoproliferative disorders is MOST characterized by this morphologic appearance and immunophenotype?
    a. T-cell acute lymphoblastic leukemia (T-ALL)
    b. T-cell large granular lymphocytic (T-LGL) leukemia
    c. T-cell prolymphocytic leukemia (T-PLL)
    d. Adult T cell leukemia/lymphoma (ATLL)
    e. Sézary syndrome

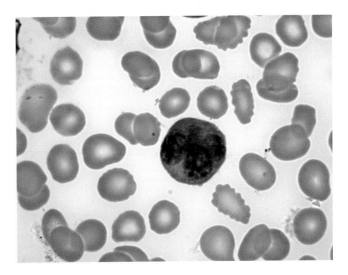

24. Which of the following mutations are associated with a worse prognosis in de novo acute myeloid leukemia (AML) with a normal karyotype?

   a. FLT3 mutations
   b. KIT mutations
   c. NPM1 mutations
   d. CEBPA mutations
   e. Jak2 mutations

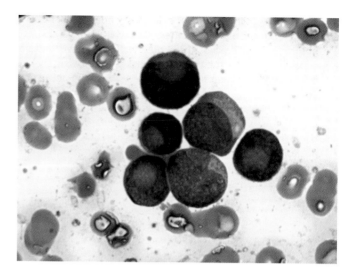

25. The leukemic cells depicted in the figure have the following immunophenotype: CD19 positive, CD10 positive, CD34 positive, and TdT positive. They also have a *bcr-abl* rearrangement. Which of the following protein isoforms encoded by the *bcr-abl* rearrangement is MOST often associated with this leukemia?

   a. p16
   b. p190
   c. p210
   d. p230
   e. p53

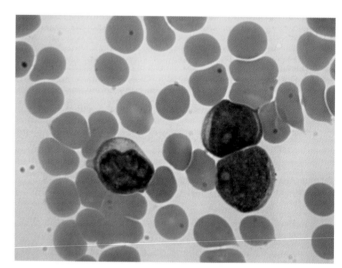

26. Which hematopoietic malignancy has the following immunophenotype: CD4 positive, CD56 positive, CD123 positive, TCL1 positive, CD2 positive/negative, TdT positive/negative, CD3 negative, CD5 negative, CD8 negative, CD34 negative, and EBV negative?

   a. Blastic plasmacytoid dendritic cell leukemia
   b. Aggressive NK-cell leukemia
   c. Hepatosplenic T-cell lymphoma
   d. Plasma cell leukemia
   e. Extranodal NK/T-cell lymphoma

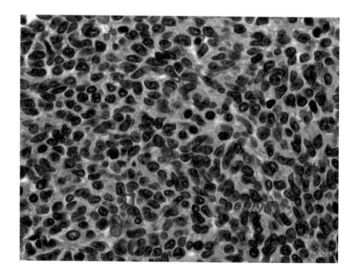

27. Which of the following is NOT a diagnostic criterion for chronic myelomonocyic leukemia (CMML)?
    a. Persistent peripheral blood monocytosis more than 1000 monocytes/mL or 1,000,000 monocytes/L
    b. Dysplasia present in one or more lineage (myeloid, erythroid, megakaryocytic)
    c. Fewer than 20% blasts or promonocytes
    d. Presence of a PDGFRA or PDGRB abnormality
    e. No Philadelphia chromosome or *bcr-abl* rearrangement

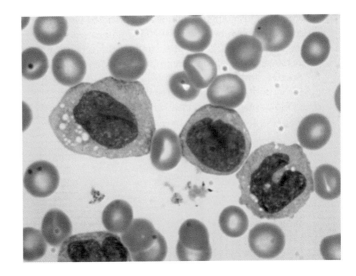

28. Extranodal marginal zone lymphoma involving the lacrimal gland or orbit is associated with which bacteria?
    a. *H. pylori*
    b. *Campylobacter jejuni*
    c. *Chlamydia psittaci*
    d. *Borrelia burgdorferi*
    e. *Mycobacterium tuberculosis*

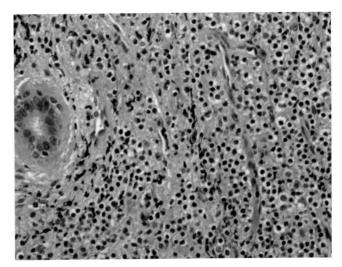

29. Which of the following is NOT a diagnostic criterion for juvenile myelomonocytic leukemia (JMML)?
    a. Peripheral blood monocytosis more than 1000 cells/mL or 1,000,000 cells/L
    b. Hemoglobin F increased for age
    c. NF1 mutation
    d. Clonal cytogenetic abnormality
    e. Granulocyte colony-stimulating factor (GCSF) hypersensitivity of myeloid cells in vitro

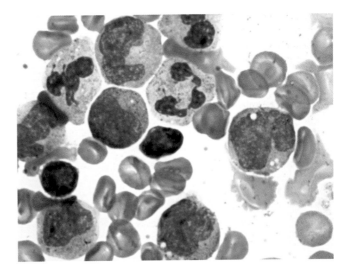

30. This process has neoplastic cells characterized by which of the following immunophenotypes?
    a. CD30 positive, CD15 positive, and pax5 positive (weak)
    b. CD30 positive, epithelial membrane antigen (EMA) positive, and ALK-1 positive
    c. CD34 positive, TdT positive, and CD10 positive
    d. CD68 positive, CD163 positive, and lysozyme positive
    e. S100 positive, CD1a positive, and langerin positive

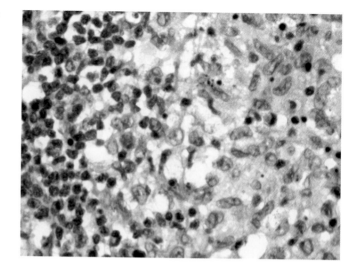

31. Which of the following statements is FALSE for lymphomatoid granulomatosis (LYG)?
    a. It is a lymphoproliferative disease with angiocentric and angiodestructive features.
    b. It represents an EBV-driven T-cell lymphoproliferative disease.
    c. It represents an EBV-driven B-cell lymphoproliferative disease.
    d. It most commonly presents as multiple pulmonary nodules.
    e. Histologic grading is clinically significant.

32. Which of the following cytogenetic abnormalities is associated with a favorable prognosis in B-cell acute lymphoblastic leukemia/lymphoma (B-ALL)?
    a. t(9;22)
    b. t(4;11)
    c. t(1;19)
    d. Hypodiploidy
    e. t(12;21)

33. Which of the following statements is FALSE regarding myelodysplastic syndrome (MDS) with isolated del(5q)?
    a. del(5q) or 5q deletion is the sole cytogenetic abnormality.
    b. It affects predominantly older men.
    c. The symptoms are most commonly related to anemia.
    d. Some patients have thrombocytosis.
    e. The megakaryocytes are small and show hypolobated nuclei.

34. Which of the following is FALSE regarding PTLDs?
    a. Most are EBV-driven B-cell lymphoproliferations.
    b. Early lesions may respond to reduction in immunosuppressive therapy.
    c. Presentation at extranodal sites is common.
    d. EBV-negative lesions tend to present early after transplantation.
    e. Risk is related to EBV status prior to transplantation.

35. Which of the following is FALSE regarding hepatosplenic T-cell lymphoma?
    a. Lymphoma cells show marked intrasinusoidal infiltration in the spleen, liver, and bone marrow.
    b. Lymphoma cells are usually of gamma/delta (γδ) T-cell receptor type.
    c. The lymphoma cells are cytotoxic T cells.

    d. The phenotype is usually CD3 positive, CD5 negative, CD4 negative, and CD8 negative/positive.
    e. It is EBV positive.

36. Which of the following is a FALSE statement regarding subcutaneous panniculitislike T-cell lymphoma?
    a. It is a cytotoxic T-cell lymphoma.
    b. It commonly involves lymph nodes.
    c. It is primarily associated with skin lesions.
    d. It is CD4 negative and CD8 positive.
    e. It can be complicated by a hemophagocytic syndrome.

37. Which of the following statements is FALSE regarding extranodal NK/T-cell lymphoma, nasal-type?
    a. Angiocentric/angiodestructive features and necrosis are typical.
    b. Most cases are true NK cell neoplasms.
    c. Isochromosome 7q is typical.
    d. It is EBV positive.
    e. Some cases are derived from CD56 negative cytotoxic T cells.

38. Which of the following statements is FALSE regarding ATLL?
    a. Most cases are CD4 negative and CD8 positive.
    b. The disease is caused by the human T-cell leukemia virus type 1 (HTLV-1).
    c. In addition to an acute/leukemic or lymphomatous presentation, patients can present with a chronic or smoldering presentation.
    d. Hypercalcemia is common.
    e. The "flower cell" morphologic appearance is characteristic for ATLL.

39. Which of the following statements is FALSE regarding mycosis fungoides (MF)?
    a. The disease is limited to the skin for a protracted period of time.
    b. It represents the most common type of T-cell lymphoma that arises primarily in the skin.
    c. Lymph node involvement can be seen in the later stages of disease.
    d. Inversion of chromosome 14 is seen in 80% of cases.
    e. A CD3 positive, CD5 positive, CD4 positive, CD7 negative, and CD8 negative phenotype is typical.

40. Which of the following is NOT a recurrent cytogenetic abnormality in AML?
    a. t(8;21)
    b. inv(16)
    c. t(1:19)
    d. 11q23 abnormalities
    e. t(15;17)

41. Which of the following is NOT characteristic of lymphoplasmacytic lymphoma (LPL)?
    a. A mixture of small lymphocytes, plasmacytoid lymphocytes, and plasma cells
    b. CD5 negative, CD10 negative, and cytoplasmic IgM positive phenotype
    c. Hyperviscosity
    d. CD19 positive, CD20 positive/negative, CD5 positive, CD23 positive, and IgM and IgD positive phenotype
    e. Increased mast cells in the bone marrow

42. Which of the following is NOT considered one of the diagnostic criteria of plasma cell myeloma?
    a. Bone marrow clonal plasma cells
    b. Cytologic atypia of plasma cells
    c. Plasmacytoma
    d. Monoclonal (M) protein in serum or urine
    e. Related organ or tissue impairment

43. Which site is MOST common for extraosseous (extramedullary) plasmacytoma?
    a. Gastrointestinal (GI) tract
    b. Urinary bladder
    c. Central nervous system
    d. Skin
    e. Upper respiratory tract

44. Which lymphoma is MOST commonly seen in patients with HIV infection?
    a. Primary effusion lymphoma (PEL)
    b. Peripheral T-cell lymphoma, not otherwise specified (NOS)
    c. Classical Hodgkin lymphoma
    d. Diffuse large B-cell lymphoma (DLBCL)
    e. Polymorphic lymphoproliferative disorder

45. Which of the following lymphomas MOST commonly present as lymphomatous polyposis?
    a. Extranodal marginal zone lymphoma of mucosa-associated lymphoid tissue (MALT)
    b. MCL
    c. FL
    d. LPL
    e. Chronic lymphocytic leukemia/small lymphocytic lymphoma (CLL/SLL)

46. Which of the following is MOST characteristic of MCL?
    a. Plasmacytic differentiation
    b. A mixture of centroblastic and centrocytic cells
    c. Presence of paraimmunoblastic cells
    d. Intrasinusoidal pattern of infiltration
    e. Diffuse or nodular proliferation of centrocytelike cells

47. Which of the following features is NOT characteristic of myeloproliferative neoplasms (MPN)?
    a. Myelofibrosis
    b. Organomegaly
    c. Leukocytosis
    d. Myelodysplasia
    e. Thrombocytosis

48. Which of the following is NOT characteristic of alkylating agent therapy-related myeloid neoplasms?
    a. 11q23 or *MLL* gene abnormalities
    b. Common initial presentation as MDS
    c. Occurs 5 to 10 years after exposure to therapy
    d. Cytogenetic abnormalities similar to those seen in MDS
    e. Short survival

49. Which of the following is the MOST common site of extranodal marginal zone lymphoma of MALT?
    a. Parotid gland
    b. Lung
    c. Ocular adnexae
    d. Skin
    e. GI tract

50. Which of the following features defines FL?
    a. t(14;18)
    b. Bcl-6 expression
    c. Bcl-2 expression
    d. A mixture of germinal center B cells, centrocytic and centroblastic, and at least a partial follicular growth pattern
    e. CD10 expression

51. Which of the following genes is rearranged in FL?
    a. *BCL1*
    b. *BCL2*
    c. *BCL6*
    d. *BCL10*
    e. *ALK*

52. Which of the following cytogenetic abnormalities is MOST common in gastric marginal zone lymphoma?
    a. t(14;18) translocation involving the *IgH* and *MALT1* genes
    b. Trisomy 3
    c. t(3;14) translocation
    d. Trisomy 18
    e. t(11;18) translocation

ANSWERS

1. d. The lymphoma in the photomicrograph shows a distinct nodular growth pattern with expansion of follicle centers. The follicle centers show loss of polarization and tingible body macrophages. These findings are consistent with FL. Degree of cellular atypia (a), number of apoptotic bodies (b), and number of mitoses (c) play no role in grading of FL. Centroblastic cells, not cetrocytic cells (e), are counted in multiple high-power fields (HPFs) and the grade is determined based on the average count (grades 1 to 2 have ≤15 centroblasts per HPF; grade 3 has >15 centroblasts per HPF).

Swerdlow SH, Campo E, Harris NL, et al: *WHO Classification of Tumours of Haematopoietic and Lymphoid Tissues.* Lyon, France: IARC, 2008.

2. a. The bone marrow trephine section shown in the photomicrograph shows dense and tight paratrabecular lymphoid infiltrates most characteristic of FL involving the bone marrow. MCL can occasionally show a similar pattern. Chronic lymphocytic leukemia in the marrow can show nonparatrabecular, random lymphoid aggregates and an interstitial/diffuse pattern of infiltration. Paratrabecular infiltrates are not typical (b) of this disease or of marginal zone lymphoma (c). HCL shows interstitial infiltration (d). Splenic marginal zone lymphoma shows nodular interstitial infiltrates with intrasinusoidal infiltrates being typical (e).

Swerdlow SH, Campo E, Harris NL, et al: *WHO Classification of Tumours of Haematopoietic and Lymphoid Tissues.* Lyon, France: IARC, 2008.

3. b. Chronic myelocytic leukemia (CML, also termed chronic granulocytic leukemia) has the characteristic t(9;22) or Philadelphia chromosome in 90% to 95% of cases (b). This translocation fuses the *BCR* gene on 22q11.2 with the *ABL* gene on 9q34. In the remainder of cases, the *BCR/ABL* fusion gene is present but not detectable by karyotype. In these cases the *BCR/ABL* fusion gene may be cryptic and may be detectable by alternate methods, such as fluorescence in situ hybridization, polymerase chain reaction, or Southern blot. t(8;21) translocation is a recurrent cytogenetic abnormality seen in de novo AML with myeloblasts showing neutophilic maturation (FAB-M2). The majority of transformations in CML are AML, which is seen in 70% of blast crises (a). Transformation to B-ALL is seen in 30%. Rarely transformation to T-ALL may be seen. The natural progression of CML is eventual transformation to acute leukemia (blast crisis). The presence of more than 20% blasts in the bone marrow or peripheral blood qualifies for transformation to acute leukemia (c). Marked hypercellularity and marked myeloid hyperplasia with maturation are characteristic findings in CML (d). Megakaryocytic hyperplasia with a predominance of small hypolobated megakaryocytes or "dwarf megakaryocytes" is also characteristic of CML. Pseudo-Gaucher cells, best seen on the bone marrow aspirate smear, are also typically seen in CML (e). Pseudo-Gaucher cells are not specific for CML and can be seen in other leukemias.

Swerdlow SH, Campo E, Harris NL, et al: *WHO Classification of Tumours of Haematopoietic and Lymphoid Tissues.* Lyon, France: IARC, 2008.

4. c. The Hodgkin-Reed-Sternberg (HRS) cells depicted in the photomicrograph have two or more large nuclei, each with a single prominent eosinophilic nucleolus and chromatin clearing around the nucleoli. These particular HRS cells have retraction of the cytoplasm characteristic of lacunar cells. The presence of lacunar cells is one of the diagnostic features of classical Hodgkin lymphoma, nodular sclerosis subtype. NLPHL (a) is characterized by the lymphocytic histiocytic (L&H) cells, or "popcorn cells." These cells have a single nucleus that is folded and multilobated, imparting a "popcorn" appearance. These cells also have multiple small basophilic nucleoli. ALCL (b) is characterized by "hallmark cells." These cells have eccentric kidney- or wreath-shaped nuclei with multiple small basophilic nucleoli and abundant eosinophilic cytoplasm. Richter transformation (d) is a DLBCL transformation in a patient with CLL/SLL. Just like de novo DLBCL, Richter transformation is characterized by sheets of large lymphoma cells. The blastoid variant of MCL (e) is characterized by a monomorphous population of medium-sized cells with blastoid morphologic appearance.

Swerdlow SH, Campo E, Harris NL, et al: *WHO Classification of Tumours of Haematopoietic and Lymphoid Tissues.* Lyon, France: IARC, 2008.

5. b. The cells indicated by the arrows are L&H cells or the so-called "popcorn" cells characteristic of NLPHL. NLPHL is a monoclonal B-cell lymphoma with a nodular, or a nodular and diffuse, pattern of growth (a). The nodules are rich in small reactive B lymphocytes and are associated with meshworks of CD21 positive follicular dendritic cells. In this background, scattered large L&H cells or "popcorn cells" (which are the neoplastic cells) are typically admixed. Cervical, axillary, and inguinal lymph nodes are the most common sites of involvement. Mediastinal (which is commonly seen in classical Hodgkin lymphoma) and bone marrow involvement are rare. The neoplastic popcorn cells are B cells of germinal center cell origin and have the characteristic phenotype of CD20 positive, CD10 positive, Bcl-6 positive, and CD45 positive (d). Stage I and II lesions have a very good prognosis (e). PTGC may be seen simultaneously in the same lymph node affected, or in previous or subsequent lymph node biopsies (c).

Swerdlow SH, Campo E, Harris NL, et al: *WHO Classification of Tumours of Haematopoietic and Lymphoid Tissues.* Lyon, France: IARC, 2008.

6. e. The photomicrograph shows a large cell lymphoma with pleomorphic/anaplastic cells with bizarre nuclear contours, including the so-called "hallmark cells" with horseshoe-shaped nuclei, consistent with ALCL. ALCL expresses cytotoxic granule-associated proteins, such as granzyme, perforin, and TIA-1. In addition, ALCL tends to be CD2 positive, CD3 negative/positive, CD5 positive, CD4 positive, CD8 negative, CD30 positive, CD15 negative, and EMA positive. ALCL is CD30 positive, but ALCL is not defined by CD30 expression. Other lymphomas can express CD30, such as classical Hodgkin lymphoma, primary cutaneous CD30 positive T-cell lymphoproliferative disorders, some DLBCLs, and other T-cell lymphomas. EBV (b) and HHV-8 (c) have not been detected in ALCL. Cases associated with t(2;5) translocation and subsequent ALK protein overexpression (ALCL, ALK positive) are generally associated with a more favorable prognosis compared to ALK-negative ALCL (d). In addition to prognosis, the ALK-positive subtype tends to be seen in pediatric and young adults, whereas the ALK-negative subtype tends to be seen in the middle aged to the elderly.

Swerdlow SH, Campo E, Harris NL, et al: *WHO Classification of Tumours of Haematopoietic and Lymphoid Tissues*. Lyon, France: IARC, 2008.

7. d. The hairy cell depicted in the picture is characteristic of HCL, which is a low-grade B-cell lymphoproliferative disorder characterized clinically by splenomegaly (a) and monocytopenia (e). In HCL, the marrow usually shows interstitial infiltration by leukemic cells (b), which are characterized by the phenotype of CD20 positive, CD5 negative, CD25 positive, CD103 positive, Annexin A1 positive, tartrate resistant acid phosphatase positive, and CD11c positive (c). Nodular paratrabecular pattern of infiltration of the marrow is not seen in HCL and is seen in FL (d).

Swerdlow SH, Campo E, Harris NL, et al: *WHO Classification of Tumours of Haematopoietic and Lymphoid Tissues*. Lyon, France: IARC, 2008.

8. e. The lymphoma depicted in the photomicrograph shows a proliferation of small, mature lymphoid cells with multiple proliferation centers/pseudofollicles. These vaguely defined and pale-looking areas are rich in paraimmunoblastic/prolymphocytic cells and are most characteristic of CLL/SLL. CD19 positive, CD20 dim, CD5 positive, CD23 positive, and cyclin D1 negative phenotype is characteristic (d). Diffuse marrow involvement may have a worse prognosis (a). Cases with mutated immunoglobulin variable gene regions have a better prognosis, as does CLL/SLL with 13q deletion (b). Trisomy 12 and a normal karyotype are associated with an intermediate prognosis. In contrast del 11q, del 17p, and del 6q are associated with a poorer prognosis. CLL/SLL with ZAP-70 or CD38 expression is associated with an unmutated status and, therefore, has a more aggressive course and adverse prognosis. ZAP-70 and CD38 have been used as surrogate markers for immunoglobulin gene mutational status (e).

Swerdlow SH, Campo E, Harris NL, et al: *WHO Classification of Tumours of Haematopoietic and Lymphoid Tissues*. Lyon, France: IARC, 2008.

9. a. The flow cytometric dot plots show a population of cells coexpressing dim CD20, CD19, CD5, and CD23. CLL/SLL is characterized by the following immunophenotype: CD19 positive, CD20 positive (dim), CD5 positive, CD23 positive, CD43 positive/negative, FMC7 negative to dim, and dim surface light chain immunoglobulin expression. CLL/SLL typically follows an indolent clinical course (c). t(8;14) is typical of Burkitt lymphoma (BL) and can be seen in other aggressive B-cell lymphomas (b). BL is CD20 bright, CD10 positive, Bcl-6 positive, CD43 positive, CD5 negative, and Bcl-2 negative, and t(11;14) is seen in MCL, which is CD20 bright, CD5 positive, and CD23 negative. Histologic examination, CLL/SLL will show vaguely defined, pale-looking areas rich

in paraimmunoblastic/prolymphocytic cells known as proliferation centers/pseudofollicles.

Swerdlow SH, Campo E, Harris NL, et al: *WHO Classification of Tumours of Haematopoietic and Lymphoid Tissues*. Lyon, France: IARC, 2008.

10. b. The lymphoma depicted in the figure is an example of AITL, which is derived from CD4[+] follicular helper T cells. AITL is characterized by diffuse or paracortical involvement showing increased arborizing high endothelial venules that are surrounded by polymorphous populations of cells; the neoplastic cells are typically medium-sized with abundant clear cytoplasm and distinct cell membrane staining. There are also admixed small reactive lymphocytes, plasma cells, and eosinophils. AITL recapitulates the phenotype of normal CD4[+] follicular helper T cells, which are normally found in the germinal centers of follicles and are thought to help mediate B-cell education in the germinal centers. AITL expresses CD10, Bcl-6, CXCL13, and PD-1. Also, CD21, CD23, or CD35 would highlight abnormal proliferations of extrafollicular follicular dendritic cell meshworks around the arborizing high endothelial venules.

Swerdlow SH, Campo E, Harris NL, et al: *WHO Classification of Tumours of Haematopoietic and Lymphoid Tissues*. Lyon, France: IARC, 2008.

11. c. In hematolymphoid malignancies, *BRAF* mutation is specific and sensitive for HCL. No other B-cell lymphomas or leukemias have the *BRAF* mutation. Ras mutations (a) in hematolymphoid malignancies are seen in myelodysplastic neoplasms, AML, and myelodysplastic/MPNs. IgH-Bcl-2 translocation (b) is seen in FL and a subset of DLBCL. IgH-cyclin D1 translocation (d) is seen in MCL. IgH-myc translocation (e) is seen in BL, B-cell lymphoma unclassifiable with features intermediate between DLBCL and BL, and a subset of DLBCL.

Swerdlow SH, Campo E, Harris NL, et al: *WHO Classification of Tumours of Haematopoietic and Lymphoid Tissues*. Lyon, France: IARC, 2008.
Tiacci E, Trifonov V, Schiavoni G, et al: BRAF mutations in hairy cell leukemia. *N Engl J Med* 2011;364:2305-2315.

12. c. Hepatosplenic T-cell lymphoma and peripheral T-cell lymphoma NOS are the most common T/NK-cell PTLD. T/NK-cell PTLD makes up only 15% of all PTLDs. Diagnosis of a T/NK-cell PTLD is based on diagnostic criteria for T/NK-cell lymphomas/leukemias seen in immunocompetent patients. Unlike B-cell PTLDs, only a minority (about a third) of T/NK-cell PTLDs are associated with EBV. The pathophysiology of T/NK-cell PTLD for most cases is unknown. In addition, T/NK-cell PTLDs arise typically at longer intervals after the start of immunosuppression and have a worse prognosis compared to B-cell PTLDs. Extranodal NK/T-cell lymphoma (a), ATLL (b), and ALCL (e) have all been reported in the transplant setting; however, they are not the most common T/NK-cell PTLD. AITL (d) has not been reported in the transplant setting.

Swerdlow SH, Campo E, Harris NL, et al: *WHO Classification of Tumours of Haematopoietic and Lymphoid Tissues*. Lyon, France: IARC, 2008.

13. d. Jak2 mutations are not associated with systemic mastocytosis. Jak2 mutations can be seen in polycythemia vera (PV), essential thrombocythemia (ET), and primary myelofibrosis (PMF). A diagnosis of systemic mastocytosis requires the presence of multifocal compact mast cell clusters that exceed 15 cells in either bone marrow or any extracutaneous organs (a). This criterion is a major one that must be fulfilled. Reactive mast cells may be increased; however, they are scattered interstitially and do not form clusters. There are a total of four minor criteria, of which three must be fulfilled for a diagnosis of systemic mastocytosis:

1. Spindled morphologic appearance in 25% or more of mast cells (b). Reactive mast cells are round. Neoplastic mast cells can show a spindled morphologic appearance.
2. Aberrant CD2 and/or CD25 expression in mast cells (c). Mast cells are normally CD117 positive and tryptase positive. Neoplastic mast cells can show aberrant CD2 and/or CD25 expression, which are not expressed by normal mast cells.
3. A persistently elevated serum tryptase level of 20 ng/mL or higher (e).
4. The presence of a *KIT* mutation involving codon 816.

Swerdlow SH, Campo E, Harris NL, et al: *WHO Classification of Tumours of Haematopoietic and Lymphoid Tissues.* Lyon, France: IARC, 2008.

14. b. PEL is associated with and attributable to KSHV, also known as HHV-8. PEL is the most common lymphoma primarily involving body cavity fluids and is typically seen in HIV positive patients. Large B-cell lymphoma arising in HHV-8-associated multicentric Castleman disease is another lymphoma associated with and attributable to KSHV. Classical Hodgkin lymphoma, BL, PTLDs, EBV positive DLBCL of the elderly, and LYG are associated with and attributable to EBV (a). None of these lymphomas are cavity based. PEL can be associated with EBV; however, it is thought that EBV is a coinfection and is not required in the pathogenesis of this lymphoma. Some cases of LPL and splenic marginal zone lymphoma have been associated with hepatitis C (c). Patients infected with HIV (d) are at a much higher risk to develop lymphoma, especially primary central nervous system lymphoma, BL, and DLBCL. Several pathogenetic mechanisms are involved in the development of lymphoma in the setting of HIV infection. Patients with PEL are typically HIV infected; however, PEL can be seen in elderly patients without HIV infection from areas with high prevalence for HHV-8 infection. ATLL (e) is associated with and attributable to HTLV. ATLL is not a cavity-based lymphoproliferative disorder.

Swerdlow SH, Campo E, Harris NL, et al: *WHO Classification of Tumours of Haematopoietic and Lymphoid Tissues.* Lyon, France: IARC, 2008.

15. e. The leukemic cell shown in the picture is an atypical promyelocytic cell with multiple Auer rods, known as "faggot cell," characteristic of acute promyelocytic leukemia (APL) or FAB-M3. APL is characterized by the t(15;17). The t(8;21) translocation (a), inv(16) (b), and 11q23 abnormalities (d) are the recurrent cytogenetic abnormalities in AML. The t(9;22) translocation (c) is typical of CML and is also retained in the blast crisis phase of CML.

Swerdlow SH, Campo E, Harris NL, et al: *WHO Classification of Tumours of Haematopoietic and Lymphoid Tissues.* Lyon, France: IARC, 2008.

16. d. The photomicrograph shows medium-sized lymphoid cells with round to oval nuclei and condensed chromatin pattern with deep blue vacuolated cytoplasm. These cytologic findings are consistent with BL/leukemia cells. There are three types of BL/leukemia: endemic, sporadic, and immunodeficiency-associated (in the setting of HIV infection) (a). BL, specifically the endemic subtype, is the most common malignancy of childhood in equatorial Africa (b), largely because of the endemic nature of EBV and malaria in equatorial Africa, as well as specific climatic factors. It is thought that both EBV and malaria may have a synergistic role in lymphomagenesis. In contrast, the sporadic subtype is typically seen in developed countries. EBV is identified in almost all cases of endemic BL, but only in 30% of sporadic BL, and 25% to 40% of immunodeficiency-associated BL (c). Extranodal sites in general are more often involved in BL. In the endemic subtype, the majority of cases present with a jaw or other facial bone mass. In the sporadic subtype, the majority of cases present with an ileocecal mass. In both the endemic and sporadic subtypes, involvement of the gonads, breasts, or kidneys can also be seen. The immunodeficiency-associated subtype is more frequently associated with node-based disease (d). Genetic abnormalities involving the *MYC* gene on 8q24 play an essential role in pathogenesis and are seen in up to 90% of BL. The most common translocations include t(8;14), t(8;22), and t(2;8). Translocations involving the *MYC* gene are not specific to BL. A subset of DLBCLs, as well as a "gray zone lymphoma" or B-cell lymphomas, unclassifiable with features intermediate between DLBCL and BL can also have a *MYC* translocation (e).

Swerdlow SH, Campo E, Harris NL, et al: *WHO Classification of Tumours of Haematopoietic and Lymphoid Tissues.* Lyon, France: IARC, 2008.

17. c. The leukemic cells shown in the picture are monoblasts and promonocytes characterized by the irregular, prominent, and delicate nuclear foldings, as well as abundant gray-blue cytoplasm. These cells express monocytic markers, such as CD11c and CD64, as well as myelomonocytic markers such as CD33 and CD13. A CD19 positive, CD10 positive, CD34 positive, and cytoplasmic IgM positive immunophenotype is characteristic of B-ALL (a). A CD34 negative, HLA-DR negative, CD117 positive, CD33 positive, and MPO positive immunophenotype is characteristic of APL (b). A CD19 positive, CD20 positive, CD11c positive, CD25 positive, and CD103 positive immunophenotype is seen in HCL. In addition, HCL is also positive for tartrate acid phosphatase (TRAP) and Annexin A1 (d). A CD19 positive, CD20 positive, CD10 positive, and Bcl-2 positive immunophenotype is typical of a lymphoma of follicle center origin, such as FL (e).

Swerdlow SH, Campo E, Harris NL, et al: *WHO Classification of Tumours of Haematopoietic and Lymphoid Tissues.* Lyon, France: IARC, 2008.

18. b. The photomicrograph shows a diffuse proliferation of large, monomorphic cells with frequent mitoses and apoptotic debris consistent with a DLBCL. DLBCL is the most common type of lymphoma seen in developed countries (a), and represents a heterogenous group of lymphoproliferations arising de novo or from preexisting low-grade lymphoproliferations (c). The t(14;18) or *BCL2* gene rearrangement common in FL is seen in 20% to 30% of DLBCLs (d). Abnormalities of the *BCL6* gene at 3q27 are seen in up to 30% of the cases and are the most common aberrations in DLBCL (e). Rearrangements of the *MYC* gene can be seen in a minority of DLBCLs (in up to 10%) and are usually associated with a complex pattern of cytogenetic aberrations. In contrast, BL is associated with a *MYC* gene rearrangement with no or few other cytogenetic aberrations (b).

Swerdlow SH, Campo E, Harris NL, et al: *WHO Classification of Tumours of Haematopoietic and Lymphoid Tissues*. Lyon, France: IARC, 2008.

19. c. The photomicrograph shows a gastric gland infiltrated by lymphoid cells forming a "lymphoepithelial lesion." Lymphoepithelial lesions with lymphoid infiltrates showing a CD20 positive, CD43 positive, CD5 negative, and Bcl-2 positive phenotype and light chain restriction are characteristic of extranodal marginal zone lymphoma of MALT type. *H. pylori* infection is implicated in the cause of MALT lymphomas of the stomach. An etiologic role has been proposed for *B. burgdorferi* infection in cutaneous marginal zone lymphoma (d). *M. avium* complex (a), *S. suis* (b), and *C. amycolatum* microorganisms (e) are not known to play an etiologic role in extranodal marginal zone lymphomas. Regression of MALT lymphoma of the stomach is sometimes seen with antibiotic treatment for *H. pylori*.

Swerdlow SH, Campo E, Harris NL, et al: *WHO Classification of Tumours of Haematopoietic and Lymphoid Tissues*. Lyon, France: IARC, 2008.

20. a. The photomicrograph shows an infiltrate of monomorphic, medium-sized lymphoid cells with round to oval nuclei. Mitoses, apoptotic bodies, and tingible body macrophages are seen. The frequent tingible body macrophages impart a "starry sky" appearance. The histologic appearance, clinical history, and immunophenotype are consistent with BL. The t(8;14) translocation between the immunoglobulin heavy chain and *MYC* genes is characteristically seen in BL. The *MYC* gene can also be rearranged in variant translocations, though less commonly, including t(2;8) and t(8;22) translocations with the kappa and lambda immunoglobulin light chain genes, respectively. The resultant deregulation of the *MYC* gene plays a major role in lymphomagenesis. Although *MYC* translocations are characteristic for BL, they are not entirely specific for BL. The t(11;18) (b) translocation is seen in extranodal marginal zone lymphomas of MALT, particularly in those involving the stomach, small intestine, or lung. The t(2;5) (c) translocation is seen in ALCL. The t(14;18) (d) translocation is seen in FL and a subset of DLBCL, and the t(11;14) (e) translocation is seen in MCL.

Swerdlow SH, Campo E, Harris NL, et al: *WHO Classification of Tumours of Haematopoietic and Lymphoid Tissues*. Lyon, France: IARC, 2008.

21. a. The age, histologic appearance, and immunophenotype (CD10 negative) are characteristic of infantile precursor B-cell lymphoblastic leukemia. The *MLL* gene on 11q23 is most commonly rearranged in infantile precursor B lymphoblastic leukemia/lymphoma, usually as a result of t(4;11). The *RUNX1T1* gene on 21q22 and *RUNX1* gene on 8q22 are rearranged in t(8;21), which is a recurrent cytogenetic abnormality in AML showing myeloblasts with neutrophilic maturation (b). The *PML* gene on 15q22 and *RARA* gene on 17q12 are rearranged in t(15;17), which is a recurrent cytogenetic abnormality in APL (c). The *CBFB* gene on 16q22 and *MYH11* gene on 16p13.1 are rearranged in inv(16) and t(16;16), which are recurrent cytogenetic abnormalities seen in AML showing myelomonocytic blasts with abnormal eosinophils (FAB-M4e) (d). The *RUNX1* gene on 8q22 and *RUNX1T1* gene on 21q22 are rearranged in t(8;21), which is a recurrent cytogenetic abnormality seen in up to 12% of AML (e).

Swerdlow SH, Campo E, Harris NL, et al: *WHO Classification of Tumours of Haematopoietic and Lymphoid Tissues*. Lyon, France: IARC, 2008.

22. c. The large cell depicted in the photomicrograph is a classical HRS cell typical of classical Hodgkin lymphoma. HRS cells are derived from follicle center B cells. The cells have the characteristic phenotype of CD45 negative, CD30 positive, CD15 positive, MUM1 positive, and Pax5 positive (b). Cervical and mediastinal lymph nodes are the most common sites of involvement, followed by axillary and paraaortic regions (d). Prognosis is heavily dependent on stage of disease. Histologic subtype is less important as a predictive factor (a). EBV is detected in a significant proportion of cases, but varies depending on histologic subtype (more frequent in mixed cellularity subtype). Most HIV-associated cases are EBV positive. In tropical regions, up to 100% of classical Hodgkin lymphoma cases are EBV positive. EBV is postulated to play a role in the pathogenesis of Hodgkin lymphoma (e).

Swerdlow SH, Campo E, Harris NL, et al: *WHO Classification of Tumours of Haematopoietic and Lymphoid Tissues*. Lyon, France: IARC, 2008.

23. d. The cell depicted in the figure is typical of ATLL. The cells are characterized by radiating flower- or clover-shaped nuclei with deeply invaginated nuclear indentations. The typical immunophenotype of ATLL is CD3 positive, CD7 negative, CD4 positive, CD8 negative, and CD25 positive. T-ALL (a) cells are characterized by blastic morphologic appearance. Typically, T-ALL cells are CD7 positive and express one or more of the following immaturity markers: TdT, CD34, CD10, and CD1a. T-LGL (b) is characterized by large granular lymphocytic cells with moderate to abundant cytoplasm with azurophilic granules. The immunophenotype of T-LGL is typically CD3 positive, CD4 negative, and CD8 positive.

T-PLL (c) is characterized by small to medium-sized cells with round/ovoid or irregular nuclear contours, prominent nucleoli, and cytoplasmic protrusions. T-PLL cells usually express CD7. Sézary syndrome (e) is characterized by cells with cerebriform nuclei that have highly convoluted nuclear membranes. The immunophenotype of Sézary cells can be similar: CD3 positive, CD7 negative, CD4 positive, CD8 negative, and CD25 positive.

Swerdlow SH, Campo E, Harris NL, et al: *WHO Classification of Tumours of Haematopoietic and Lymphoid Tissues.* Lyon, France: IARC, 2008.

24. a. FLT3 mutations are associated with a worse prognosis in AML with a normal karyotype. FLT3 mutations have also been reported in APL and AML with t(6;9)(p23;q24). KIT mutations (b) are seen in AML with t(8;21)(q22;q22) and AML with inv(16)(p13.1;q22) or t(16;16)(p13.1;q22). In both entities, KIT mutations are associated with a worse prognosis. The significance of KIT mutations in a normal karyotype AML is currently unknown. NPM1 mutations (c) are typically associated with a normal karyotype and are associated with a good prognosis. CEBPA mutations (d) are also typically associated with a normal karyotype and are associated with a good prognosis. Jak2 mutations (e) are typically not associated with de novo AML.

Swerdlow SH, Campo E, Harris NL, et al: *WHO Classification of Tumours of Haematopoietic and Lymphoid Tissues.* Lyon, France: IARC, 2008.

25. b. p190 is the most common protein isoform seen in acute B-ALL patients with *bcr-abl* rearrangement. p190 is the most common isoform seen in pediatric B-ALL patients. In contrast, in adult B-ALL patients (much less common than in pediatric B-ALL), about half of patients have the p190 isoform and the other half have the p210 isoform. p16 (a) is a tumor suppressor gene and is not a protein encoded by the *bcr-abl* rearrangement. In acute lymphoblastic leukemia p16 can show homozygous deletion and is associated with a poor prognosis. p210 (c) is the most common protein isoform seen in CML. p230 (d) is the second most common protein isoform seen in CML. The p230 isoform is associated with a prominent neutrophil maturation in CML. p53 (e) is a tumor suppressor gene and is not a protein encoded by the *bcr-abl* rearrangement. p53 mutation is associated with a poor prognosis in many malignancies, including hematolymphoid malignancies.

Swerdlow SH, Campo E, Harris NL, et al: *WHO Classification of Tumours of Haematopoietic and Lymphoid Tissues.* Lyon, France: IARC, 2008.

26. a. Blastic plasmacytoid dendritic cell leukemia essentially has the same immunophenotype as normal plasmacytoid dendritic cells (CD4 positive, CD123 positive), but with the additional aberrant expression of CD56 and TdT. Aggressive NK-cell leukemia (b) has the following immunophenotype: CD2 positive, surface CD3 negative, CD4 negative, CD5 negative, CD8 positive/negative, CD34 negative, CD56 positive, TdT negative, and EBV positive. Hepatosplenic T-cell lymphoma (c) has the following immunophenotype: CD2 positive, CD3 positive, CD4 negative, CD5 negative, CD8 negative/positive, CD19 negative, CD34 negative, CD56 positive/negative, TdT negative, and EBV negative. Plasma cell leukemia (d) has the following immunophenotype: CD2 negative, CD3 negative, CD4 negative, CD5 negative, CD8 negative, CD19 negative, CD34 negative, CD56 positive/negative, TdT negative, and EBV negative. In addition, the cells are CD138 positive, CD38 positive (bright), CD79a positive, and CD20

negative/positive. Extranodal NK/T-cell lymphoma (e) has the following immunophenotype: CD2 positive, surface CD3 negative, CD4 negative, CD5 negative, CD8 positive/negative, CD19 negative, CD34 negative, CD56 positive, TdT negative, and EBV positive.

Bain BJ, Clark DM, Wilkins BS: *Bone Marrow Pathology,* 4th ed. West Sussex, UK: Wiley-Blackwell, 2010.
Swerdlow SH, Campo E, Harris NL, et al: *WHO Classification of Tumours of Haematopoietic and Lymphoid Tissues.* Lyon, France: IARC, 2008.

27. d. Presence of a PDGFRA or PDGFRB abnormality is an *exclusion* criterion for CMML. CMML with eosinophilia commonly has a PDGFRB abnormality. PDGFRB abnormalities constitute translocations involving the 5q31~33 locus, the most common of which is t(5;12) (q31~q33;p12). Myeloid and lymphoid neoplasms with eosinophilia associated with a PDGFRA or PDGFRB abnormality were separately designated because these patients were responsive to imatinib (Gleevac). Persistent peripheral blood monocytosis is required for the diagnosis of CMML (a). Reactive causes of monocytosis must be ruled out. Persistent monocytosis is typically seen for at least 3 months. CMML is one of the overlapping myelodysplastic/MPNs and is characterized by increased blood counts and variable degrees of dysplasia (b). Dysplasia is seen in one or more lineages in CMML. If dysplasia is not present and a clonal cytogenetic or molecular abnormality is present, a diagnosis of CMML can still be made. The most common cytogenetic abnormalities in CMML are trisomy 8 and monosomy 7. *Ras* gene mutations are also common in CMML. If 20% or more are blasts or promonocytes (promonocytes are blast equivalents) (c), then a diagnosis of an acute myeloid or acute myelomonocytic leukemia should be made. The presence of a Philadelphia chromosome or *bcr-abl* rearrangement (e) is indicative of CML in the appropriate morphologic and immunophenotypic setting.

Swerdlow SH, Campo E, Harris NL, et al: *WHO Classification of Tumours of Haematopoietic and Lymphoid Tissues.* Lyon, France: IARC, 2008.

28. c. Lacrimal gland or orbital marginal zone lymphomas are associated with *C. psittaci.* In many different organ sites, it is thought that the acquisition of MALT secondary to chronic inflammatory disorders either due to an infection or autoimmune disease predisposes patients to extranodal marginal zone lymphoma. In addition to the infectious causes, patients with autoimmune conditions, such as Hashimoto thyroiditis and Sjögren disease, have a propensity for developing thyroid and salivary gland marginal zone lymphomas, respectively. Gastric marginal zone lymphomas are associated with *H. pylori* (a). Small intestinal marginal zone lymphoma or immunoproliferative small intestinal disease (IPSID) is associated with *C. jejuni* (b). Skin marginal zone lymphomas are associated with *B. burgdorferi* (d). No extranodal marginal zone lymphomas are associated with *M. tuberculosis* (e). Pyothorax-associated lymphoma (the most common form of DLBCL associated with chronic inflammation) is associated with tuberculous pleuritis or therapeutic artificial pneumothorax performed for pulmonary tuberculosis.

Swerdlow SH, Campo E, Harris NL, et al: *WHO Classification of Tumours of Haematopoietic and Lymphoid Tissues*. Lyon, France: IARC, 2008.

29. c. NF1 mutation is seen in 20% of JMML, and pediatric patients with NF1 mutation have an increased risk for developing JMML; however, NF1 mutation is not a criterion for JMML diagnosis. Other mutations seen in JMML include ras and PTPN11 (germ-line mutation seen in Noonan syndrome). Diagnostic criteria for JMML include the following: peripheral blood monocytosis more than 1000 cells/mL (a) and blasts and promonocytes less than 20% with absence of *bcr-abl* translocation; increased hemoglobin F (b); clonal cytogenetic abnormality (d). Monosomy 7 is the most common cytogenetic abnormality; however, most patients have a normal karyotype. GCSF hypersensitivity of myeloid cells in vitro is another criterion that can be used for JMML diagnosis (e). This assay, based on cell culture, is not often performed in a routine diagnostic setting. Other criteria that could be used for JMML include the presence of immature granulocytes in peripheral blood and white blood cell count more than 10,000 cells/mL or 10,000,000 cells/L.

Swerdlow SH, Campo E, Harris NL, et al: *WHO Classification of Tumours of Haematopoietic and Lymphoid Tissues*. Lyon, France: IARC, 2008.

30. e. The image shows Langerhans cells, which have elongated oval nuclei with longitudinal nuclear grooves, twisted or contorted nuclear contours, delicate nuclear membrane, clear chromatin, small to absent nucleoli, and abundant eosinophilic cytoplasm. There are also admixed small round lymphocytes as well as eosinophils. Langerhans cells are S100 positive, CD1a positive, and langerin positive. Birbeck granules can be identified by electron microscopy and are specific for Langerhans cells. Langerhans cell histiocytosis is a neoplastic proliferation of Langerhans cells with accompanying admixed histiocytes, eosinophils, and small lymphocytes. Langerhans cell histiocytosis can present with different clinical manifestations. It can present as a single solitary lesion, in which case it usually involves bone in older children and adults. It can also present as multifocal single system disease, in which case it usually involves bone in children. Lastly, it can present as multisystemic disease, in which case it can involve bone, bone marrow, skin, lymph nodes, liver, or spleen in infants. The prognosis is good when presenting as a single solitary lesion; however, the prognosis is poor when presenting as multisystemic disease. The HRS cells in classical Hodgkin lymphoma are CD30 positive, CD15 positive, and pax5 positive (weak) (a). HRS cells are markedly large cells that are mononucleated, binucleated, or multinucleated. They have round to oval nuclei with smooth but thick nuclear membranes, clear chromatin, and large inclusionlike prominent eosinophilic nucleoli. The background inflammatory component can comprise eosinophils, plasma cells, histiocytes, and small lymphocytes. The hallmark cells of ALCL are CD30 positive, EMA positive, and ALK-1 positive (b), and in addition they could be CD3 positive/negative, CD4 positive, granzyme positive, perforin positive, and TIA1 positive. The hallmark cells are large cells with horseshoe- or kidney-shaped nuclei, vesicular chromatin, and multiple small basophilic nucleoli.

Acute lymphoblastic leukemia (both B-ALL and T-ALL) is CD34 positive, TdT positive, and CD10 positive (c). Lymphoblasts are small to medium-sized cells with round nuclei, smooth nuclear contours, blastoid chromatin, small to absent nucleoli, and scant cytoplasm. Histiocytic sarcoma cells are CD68 positive, CD163 positive, and lysozyme positive (d). Histiocytic sarcoma cells are large with abundant granular eosinophilic or vacuolated cytoplasm, round to oval nuclei, and vesicular chromatin, and may show significant nuclear atypia. Multinucleation can sometimes be seen.

Swerdlow SH, Campo E, Harris NL, et al: *WHO Classification of Tumours of Haematopoietic and Lymphoid Tissues*. Lyon, France: IARC, 2008.

31. b. LYG is an angiocentric and angiodestructive lymphoproliferative disease (a). It represents an EBV-driven B-cell lymphoproliferative disease in which the neoplastic B cells comprise a minority of cells admixed with many reactive T cells (c). It is not a T-cell lymphoproliferative disease (b). LYG is a B-cell lymphoproliferative disease with many reactive T cells present in the background. LYG most commonly presents as multiple pulmonary nodules. Other common sites of involvement include the brain, kidney, and skin (d). Histologic grading is clinically significant. Grading is based on the presence of large cells with in situ hybridization for EBV (*EBER* gene) often being used to highlight the EBV-infected large cells. Grade I has less than 5 EBV positive cells per HPF, grade II has 5 to 20 EBV positive cells per HPF, and grade III has more than 50 EBV positive cells per HPF. Patients with grade III LYG are treated like DLBCL patients (e).

Swerdlow SH, Campo E, Harris NL, et al: *WHO Classification of Tumours of Haematopoietic and Lymphoid Tissues*. Lyon, France: IARC, 2008.

32. e. The t(12;21) confers a good prognosis. The t(12;21) juxtaposes the *ETV6* gene on 12p13 to the *RUNX1* gene on 21q22. In addition to t(12;21), hyperdiploidy defined by more than 50 chromosomes also confers a good prognosis. Both t(12;21) and hyperdiploidy are commonly seen in young children. Both are not seen in infants, are seen at a decreasing frequency in older children, and are rare in adults. The t(9;22) translocation (a), t(4;11) translocation (b), and hypodiploidy (d) are all associated with a poor prognosis. In both children and adults with B-ALL, the t(9;22) confers the worst prognosis. The t(9;22) juxtaposes the *BCR* gene on 22q11.2 to the *ABL1* gene on 9q34. The t(9;22) is more commonly seen in adults than in children and partially accounts for the worse prognosis seen overall in adults. The t(4;11) juxtaposes the *MLL* gene on 11q23 to the *AF4* gene on 4q21. The t(4;11) is most commonly seen in infants and is associated with a high leukocyte count often more than 100,000 cells/μL, central nervous system involvement, and CD10 negativity. The t(1;19) previously was associated with a poor prognosis; however, with modern chemotherapy it is associated with an intermediate prognosis. The t(1;19) juxtaposes the *E2A* gene on 19p13.3 to the *PBX* gene on 1q23. The t(1;19) is associated with CD34 negativity (c). Hypodiploid B-ALL is defined by having less than 46 chromosomes. Within hypodiploid B-ALL, prognosis worsens with decreasing number of chromosomes.

Swerdlow SH, Campo E, Harris NL, et al: *WHO Classification of Tumours of Haematopoietic and Lymphoid Tissues.* Lyon, France: IARC, 2008.

33. b. By definition, del(5q) is the sole cytogenetic abnormality in this syndrome (a). The presence of additional cytogenetic abnormalities does not allow such a classification. It affects predominantly middle-aged to older women, not men. Symptoms are most commonly related to anemia (c). One third to one half of patients have thrombocytosis. Thrombocytopenia is uncommon (d). Megakaryocytes in the marrow are usually small and show hypolobated nuclei known as micromegakaryocytes (e). Survival is usually long and cytogenetic evolution is uncommon.

Swerdlow SH, Campo E, Harris NL, et al: *WHO Classification of Tumours of Haematopoietic and Lymphoid Tissues.* Lyon, France: IARC, 2008.

34. d. The majority of PTLDs are EBV-driven B-cell proliferations, which tend to develop earlier (early onset) after transplantation (a). The early lesions (plasmacytic hyperplasia and infectious mononucleosislike lesions) are more likely to respond to reduction of immunosuppression therapy. Similarly polymorphic PTLD may also respond to reduction of immunosuppression therapy, unlike monomorphic PTLDs, which often require chemotherapy (b). Extranodal involvement is common, including the GI tract, lungs, and liver (c). Risk of developing a PTLD is related to the degree of immunosuppression (which in turn depends on the type of organ transplanted) and on EBV status prior to transplantation. A negative EBV status prior to transplantation carries a higher risk for developing PTLD (e).

Swerdlow SH, Campo E, Harris NL, et al: *WHO Classification of Tumours of Haematopoietic and Lymphoid Tissues.* Lyon, France: IARC, 2008.

35. e. Hepatosplenic T-cell lymphoma involves the spleen, liver, and bone marrow with lymph node involvement being uncommon (a). The lymphoma cells are cytotoxic T cells (c), usually of the γδ type; however, a minority of cases appear to be of α/β type (b). CD3 positive, CD5 negative, CD4 negative, and CD8 negative/positive is the characteristic immunophenotype of hepatosplenic T-cell lymphoma (d). Hepatosplenic T-cell lymphoma is not associated with EBV (e).

Swerdlow SH, Campo E, Harris NL, et al: *WHO Classification of Tumours of Haematopoietic and Lymphoid Tissues.* Lyon, France: IARC, 2008.

36. b. Subcutaneous panniculitislike T-cell lymphoma is a cytotoxic T-cell lymphoma (a), primarily involving the skin (c). Lymphadenopathy is usually absent. Subcutaneous panniculitislike T-cell lymphoma is CD4 negative and CD8 positive (d). It can be complicated by a hemophagocytic syndrome and can be fatal (e).

Swerdlow SH, Campo E, Harris NL, et al: *WHO Classification of Tumours of Haematopoietic and Lymphoid Tissues.* Lyon, France: IARC, 2008.

37. c. Prominent angiocentric/angiodestructive features and necrosis are seen in extranodal NK/T-cell lymphomas (a).

The majority of cases are of true NK-cell type (b); however, some cases are derived from CD56 negative cytotoxic T cells (e). Isochromosome 7q is seen in hepatosplenic T-cell lymphoma, but so far no specific cytogenetic abnormalities have been identified in extranodal NK/T-cell lymphoma. Extranodal NK/T-cell lymphoma is EBV positive (d).

Swerdlow SH, Campo E, Harris NL, et al: *WHO Classification of Tumours of Haematopoietic and Lymphoid Tissues.* Lyon, France: IARC, 2008.

38. a. A CD3 positive, CD5 positive, CD7 negative, CD4 positive, CD8 negative, and CD25 positive phenotype is characteristic of ATLL. It is caused by the HTLV-1 (b). It is common in areas such as southwestern Japan and the Caribbean basin where HTLV-1 is endemic. The latency period between HTLV-1 exposure and leukemia/lymphoma development is usually long with most patients being exposed early in life with a median age of presentation of 58 years old. In addition, only a subset of HTLV-1 carriers (for instance, 2.5% of Japanese carriers) actually develop the disease. Most patients have widespread disease and either present with an acute/leukemic or lymphomatous presentation. The acute/leukemic presentation is characterized by leukocytosis composed predominantly by leukemia cells, lymphadenopathy, hepatosplenomegaly, bone marrow involvement, skin involvement, increased lactate dehydrogenase (LD), and hypercalcemia. The lymphomatous presentation shows systemic involvement just like the acute/leukemic presentation; however, peripheral blood involvement is not seen. Occasionally patients can present with a chronic or smoldering presentation (c). The chronic phase, just like the acute/leukemic phase, has lymphocytosis; however, the chronic phase lacks the extensive systemic nature seen in the acute/leukemic phase, such as lymphadenopathy, hepatosplenomegaly, bone marrow involvement, increased lactate dehydrogenase, or hypercalcemia. The smoldering phase similarly lacks the extensive systemic nature seen in the chronic phase, but is also characterized by the lack of lymphocytosis. Both the chronic and smoldering phases can have skin involvement. Patients presenting in the chronic or smoldering phase have a better prognosis than the acute/leukemic or lymphomatous phase (with smoldering phase having a better prognosis than the chronic phase); however, patients in the chronic or smoldering phase can transform into the acute/leukemic phase. Hypercalcemia is common due to increased osteoclastic activity (d). As a result of increased osteoclastic activity, lytic bone lesions are also common. The "flower cell" is commonly seen in ATLL (e). The "flower cell" morphologic appearance is due to multiple deep invaginations of the nuclear membrane imparting a polylobated appearance.

Swerdlow SH, Campo E, Harris NL, et al: *WHO Classification of Tumours of Haematopoietic and Lymphoid Tissues.* Lyon, France: IARC, 2008.

39. d. Although inversion of chromosome 14 is seen in 80% of T-PLL cases, no specific cytogenetic abnormalities have been identified in MF. MF is the most common type of T-cell lymphoma that arises primarily in the skin, accounting approximately for 50% of all primary cutaneous lymphomas (b). The disease is, as a rule, confined to the skin for a protracted period of time (a). Extracutaneous dissemination may occur in advanced stages, mainly to lymph nodes, liver, spleen, lungs, and blood (c). A CD3 positive, CD5 positive, CD4 positive, CD7 negative, and CD8 negative phenotype is typical (e).

Swerdlow SH, Campo E, Harris NL, et al: *WHO Classification of Tumours of Haematopoietic and Lymphoid Tissues.* Lyon, France: IARC, 2008.

40. c. The t(8;21) translocation (a) is a recurrent cytogenetic abnormality in AML, which typically has a FAB-M2 morphologic appearance showing myeloblasts with neutrophil maturation. The t(8;21) juxtaposes the *RUNX1* gene on 21q22 to the *RUNX1T1* gene on 8q22. AML with t(8;21) often coexpresses B-cell markers, such as CD19 and pax5. The t(8;21) confers a good prognosis. The inv(16) or t(16;16) (b) is a recurrent cytogenetic abnormality in AML, which has a FAB-M4e morphologic appearance showing myelomonocytic blasts with abnormal eosinophils. The abnormal eosinophils are increased and show abnormal basophilic granules. The inv(16) or t(16;16) juxtaposes the *CBFB* gene on 16q22 to the *MYH1* gene on 16p13.1. The inv(16) or t(16;16) confers a good prognosis. Translocations involving 11q23 (d) or the *MLL* gene, particularly t(9;11), is a recurrent cytogenetic abnormality in AML, which has a FAB-M4 or M5 morphologic appearance showing myelomonocytic or monocytic blasts. Translocations involving 11q23 are also seen in therapy-related AML, specifically due to past treatment with the topoisomerase II inhibitors. Lastly, translocations involving 11q23 are seen in the infantile subset of B-lymphoblastic leukemia. Translocations involving 11q23 generally confer a worse prognosis. The t(15;17) translocation is a recurrent cytogenetic abnormality in AML and is also known as APL/FAB-M3 because of predominant abnormal promyelocytes that have reniform or bilobed nuclei, abundant azurophilic primary granules, and abundant Auer rods. The t(15;17) juxtaposes the *PML* gene on 15q22 to the *RARA* gene on 17q12. The t(15;17) confers a good prognosis; however, patients with AML with t(15;17) often present with disseminated intravascular coagulation, which can be fatal if the patient is not treated immediately with all-trans retinoic acid (ATRA). The t(1;19) translocation is seen in a subset of B-ALL. This subtype is associated with an intermediate to good prognosis.

Swerdlow SH, Campo E, Harris NL, et al: *WHO Classification of Tumours of Haematopoietic and Lymphoid Tissues.* Lyon, France: IARC, 2008.

41. d. The immunophenotype of CD19 positive, CD20 positive/negative, CD5 positive, CD23 positive, IgM positive, and IgD positive is characteristic for CLL/SLL, not LPL (d). All other features are characteristic or can be seen in LPL. A mixture of small lymphocytes, plasmacytoid lymphocytes, and plasma cells is characteristic (a), but not specific, because other low-grade B-cell lymphomas can present with plasma cell differentiation, especially marginal zone lymphoma. The CD5 negative, CD10 negative, and cytoplasmic IgM positive phenotype is typical for LPL (b). The most common heavy chain isotype expressed and secreted by LPL is IgM. Hyperviscosity occurs in up to 30% of LPL patients (c) and the syndrome defined by hyperviscosity

is known as Waldenström macroglobulinemia. Admixture of increased mast cells is often seen in the bone marrow of LPL patients (e).

Swerdlow SH, Campo E, Harris NL, et al: *WHO Classification of Tumours of Haematopoietic and Lymphoid Tissues.* Lyon, France: IARC, 2008.

42. b. Plasmacytoma (c) or bone marrow clonal plasma (a) cells are considered among the diagnostic criteria. No level of serum or urine M protein (d) is included as one of the diagnostic criteria of plasma cell myeloma. In fact, in nonsecretory plasma cell myelomas, an M protein can be absent. Manifestations of related end organ or tissue impairment (e) are the most important diagnostic criteria for symptomatic plasma cell myeloma (CRAB: hypercalcemia, renal insufficiency, anemia, lytic bone lesions). Other manifestations include hyperviscosity, amyloidosis, and recurrent infections. Cytologic atypia of plasma cells is not considered one of the diagnostic criteria of plasma cell myeloma because the cells can be cytologically indistinguishable from normal plasma cells.

Swerdlow SH, Campo E, Harris NL, et al: *WHO Classification of Tumours of Haematopoietic and Lymphoid Tissues.* Lyon, France: IARC, 2008.

43. e. Extraosseous (extramedullary) plasmacytoma is a localized plasma cell neoplasm forming a tumor mass at an extraosseous site. The upper respiratory tract is the most common site (80% of cases). Other less common locations include the GI (a), urinary bladder (b), central nervous system (c), and skin (d).

Swerdlow SH, Campo E, Harris NL, et al: *WHO Classification of Tumours of Haematopoietic and Lymphoid Tissues.* Lyon, France: IARC, 2008.

44. d. Aggressive B-cell lymphomas, such as DLBCL and BL, are the most common lymphomas encountered in HIV positive patients. Classic Hodgkin lymphoma (c) is common in HIV positive patients, but not as common as DLBCL. PEL (a) is most commonly seen in HIV positive patients; however, overall it is relatively uncommon. Rare cases of peripheral T-cell lymphoma, NOS (b), also occur in HIV positive patients. A polymorphic lymphoproliferative disorder (e) similar to the one described in the posttransplantation setting may be seen in HIV positive patients, but is overall relatively uncommon.

Swerdlow SH, Campo E, Harris NL, et al: *WHO Classification of Tumours of Haematopoietic and Lymphoid Tissues.* Lyon, France: IARC, 2008.

45. b. Most cases of multiple lymphomatous polyposis (multiple variably sized polyps due to involvement by lymphoma) represent MCL involving the GI tract. Waldeyer ring is the second most common extranodal site of involvement in MCL. Extranodal marginal zone lymphoma of MALT (a) and FL (c) can present in the GI tract as multiple lymphomatous polyposis, particularly primary intestinal FL in the latter case, but less commonly. LPL (d) commonly involves the bone marrow. Although some patients may have nodal involvement, LPL does not commonly involve extranodal sites, such as the GI tract. CLL/SLL (e) commonly involves the peripheral blood, bone marrow, and nodal sites.

CLL/SLL can involve extranodal sites, but usually presents as small perivascular infiltrates and rarely forms masslike lesions as would be seen in multiple lymphomatous polyposis.

Kodama T, Ohshima K, Nomura K, et al: Lymphomatous polyposis of the gastrointestinal tract, including mantle cell lymphoma, follicular lymphoma and mucosa-associated lymphoid tissue lymphoma. *Histopathology* 2005;47(5):467-478.

Swerdlow SH, Campo E, Harris NL, et al: *WHO Classification of Tumours of Haematopoietic and Lymphoid Tissues.* Lyon, France: IARC, 2008.

46. e. Classical MCL is most characterized by a diffuse or nodular proliferation of small to medium-sized centrocytelike cells. Plasmacytic differentiation (a) in MCL is exceptional. A mixture of centrocytic and centroblastic cells is seen in FL (b). Paraimmunoblastic cells are seen in the proliferation centers of CLL/SLL (c). Intrasinusoidal pattern of infiltration is most typical of ALCL and metastatic tumors (d).

Swerdlow SH, Campo E, Harris NL, et al: *WHO Classification of Tumours of Haematopoietic and Lymphoid Tissues.* Lyon, France: IARC, 2008.

47. d. MPNs are characterized by increased blood counts, with organomegaly (due to tissue infiltration by leukemic cells) (b) or myelofibrosis (a) being common. PMF, a subtype of MPN, is characterized by marked myelofibrosis. As for the other subtypes, CML and PV can also have myelofibrosis. ET rarely can have myelofibrosis. Varying degrees of leukocytosis (c) and thrombocytosis (e) can be seen in MPN, depending on the subtype and phase of disease. Leukocytosis is present in CML, PMF (especially the prefibrotic phase), and chronic neutrophilic leukemia. Myelodysplasia is not seen in MPN (d). Myelodysplasia is seen in MDSs and in the overlapping myelodysplastic/MPNs. MDS is characterized by cytopenia(s), myelodysplasia, and increased blast counts that are less than 20% of the peripheral blood and bone marrow aspirate differential. The myelodysplastic/MPNs have features of both MPN and MDS.

Swerdlow SH, Campo E, Harris NL, et al: *WHO Classification of Tumours of Haematopoietic and Lymphoid Tissues.* Lyon, France: IARC, 2008.

48. a. 11q23 or *MLL* gene abnormalities are not characteristic of alkylating agent therapy-related myeloid neoplasms. These gene abnormalities are characteristically seen in topoisomerase II inhibitor therapy-related myeloid neoplasms. Alkylating agent therapy-related myeloid neoplasms commonly present initially as MDS (b). Patients with prior history of treatment with an alkylating agent often present as therapy-related MDS (t-MDS). A minority of patients present as overt therapy-related AML (t-AML). The reverse is true for patients with prior treatment with topoisomerase II inhibitor, with most patients presenting with overt t-AML. Patients with an alkylating agent therapy-related myeloid neoplasm have a latency period of 5 to 10 years after therapy (c). In contrast, topoisomerase II inhibitor therapy-related myeloid neoplasms have a shorter

latency period of 1 to 5 years. Patients with an alkylating agent therapy-related myeloid neoplasm often present with cytogenetic abnormalties commonly seen in de novo MDS, such as monosomy 5 or monosomy 7, with or without a complex karyotype (d). Patients with this type of neoplasm have short survival; the 5-year overall survival rate is less than 10% (e). Prognosis is strongly influenced by the associated cytogenetic abnormalities and the comorbid condition of the underlying disease for which the alkylating agent chemotherapy was administered.

Swerdlow SH, Campo E, Harris NL, et al: *WHO Classification of Tumours of Haematopoietic and Lymphoid Tissues.* Lyon, France: IARC, 2008.

49. e. The GI tract is the most common site of extranodal marginal zone lymphoma of MALT (50% of cases). Within the GI tract, the stomach is the most common site (85%). The parotid gland (a), the lung (b), the ocular adnexae (c), and the skin (d) are other common sites.

Swerdlow SH, Campo E, Harris NL, et al: *WHO Classification of Tumours of Haematopoietic and Lymphoid Tissues.* Lyon, France: IARC, 2008.

50. d. FL is defined as a neoplastic proliferation of germinal center B cells, a mixture of centrocytic and centroblastic cells, and at least partial follicular growth (nodular) pattern. Although the t(14;18) translocation (a), Bcl-6 expression (b), Bcl-2 expression (c), and CD10 expression (e) are all typically seen in FL, they are not specific to it.

Swerdlow SH, Campo E, Harris NL, et al: *WHO Classification of Tumours of Haematopoietic and Lymphoid Tissues.* Lyon, France: IARC, 2008.

51. b. The *BCL2* gene is rearranged in up to 95% of FL cases due to t(14;18). The *BCL1* or cyclin *D1* gene (a) is rearranged due to t(11;14) in MCL and in some plasma cell neoplasms. The *BCL6* gene at 3q27 (c) is rearranged in up to 30% of DLBCL. The *BCL10* gene at 1p22 (d) is rearranged in a minority of extranodal marginal zone lymphomas of MALT. *ALK* (e) is rearranged in ALCL, most commonly due to t(2;5).

Swerdlow SH, Campo E, Harris NL, et al: *WHO Classification of Tumours of Haematopoietic and Lymphoid Tissues.* Lyon, France: IARC, 2008.

52. e. The t(11;18) translocation involves the *API2* and *MALT1* genes and is mainly detected in gastric and pulmonary MALT lymphomas. The t(14;18) translocation involving the *IgH* and *MALT1* genes (a) is mainly detected in MALT lymphoma arising in ocular adnexa/orbit and salivary gland lesions. Trisomy 3 (b) is a nonspecific abnormality frequently detected in MALT lymphomas. The t(3;14) translocation (c) involves the *IgH* and *FOXP1* genes and is mainly detected in MALT lymphomas of the thyroid, ocular adnexa/orbit, and skin. Trisomy 18 (d) is a nonspecific abnormality frequently detected in MALT lymphomas.

Swerdlow SH, Campo E, Harris NL, et al: *WHO Classification of Tumours of Haematopoietic and Lymphoid Tissues.* Lyon, France: IARC, 2008.

CHAPTER 19

INFECTIOUS DISEASE PATHOLOGY

Marcela Salomao and Heidrun Rotterdam

QUESTIONS

Questions 1-32 refer to a photo or photomicrograph.

1. A 60-year-old immigrant from East Africa presented with a 16-cm diameter splenic cyst. The cyst was resected, and contents included yellow-green fluid and cystic structures varying from 0.4 to 4 cm in diameter. Histologic sections showed a degenerated cyst wall with characteristic laminations. The diagnosis is:
   a. Cysticercosis
   b. *Diphyllobothrium* infection
   c. Echinococcosis
   d. Phaeomycotic cyst
   e. Sparganosis

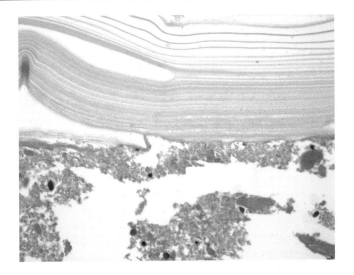

2. A 40-year-old man with dyspepsia underwent gastroscopy and gastric biopsy. The biopsy diagnosis resulted in triple antibiotic therapy, and his symptoms resolved. Which of the following statements about this infection is FALSE?
   a. Peptic ulcers, lymphoma, and gastric carcinoma have been described as complications.
   b. Infection is more common in cat owners and pig farmers.
   c. The biopsy specimen shows *Helicobacter pylori* gastritis, and response to treatment occurs in about 75% of cases.
   d. This infection is usually mild, and organisms are few in number.
   e. This type of gastritis accounts for 2% of gastritides in the Western world.

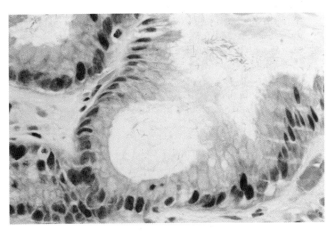

3. A 30-year-old, previously healthy man complained of right lower abdominal pain and intermittent diarrhea. The clinical impression was acute appendicitis. An appendectomy was performed. Grossly, the appendix appeared normal. Histologically, there was patchy chronic and focal acute inflammation. Which of the following statements about this infection is CORRECT?

   a. The patient is likely to have a colitis and should be treated appropriately.

   b. This infection is irrelevant and needs no further attention.

   c. This infection may be disseminated, and tests to discover additional foci are mandatory.

   d. This infection indicates that the patient has AIDS.

   e. A patient with this infection is likely to die within 6 months.

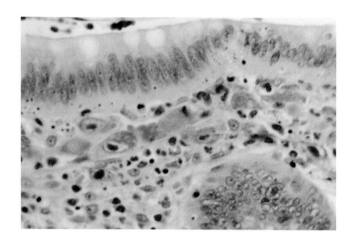

4. A Vietnam veteran who was recently diagnosed with lymphoma developed severe diarrhea, nausea, and vomiting. Upper gastrointestinal endoscopy revealed swollen duodenal mucosa covered with a thick layer of mucus. The biopsy diagnosis is infection with:

   a. *Enterobius vermicularis*

   b. *Necator americanus*

   c. *Ancylostoma duodenale*

   d. *Strongyloides stercoralis*

   e. *Ascaris lumbricoides*

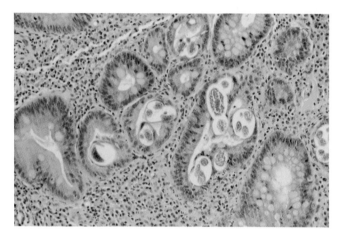

5. The image shows a Gram-stained section of lung from an 85-year-old man with multiple medical problems, who had been on a ventilator before he died from respiratory insufficiency. At autopsy, the lung demonstrated diffuse hemorrhagic pneumonitis. Which of the following statements about this bacterial infection is TRUE?

   a. It is seen only in elderly patients.

   b. It is an infection that causes bronchocentric pneumonitis.

   c. Bacteria have a special tendency to invade blood vessels.

   d. Lymphopenia predisposes to the infection.

   e. These bacteria colonize the nose of healthy individuals.

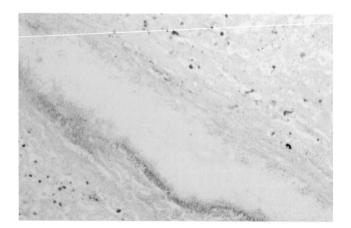

6. This segment of colon was taken from an autopsy case. All of the following statements about this condition are correct EXCEPT:

   a. Tissue damage is due to a toxin.

   b. Tissue damage is due to bacterial invasion of the mucosa.

   c. The white plaques consist of necrotic cell debris, fibrin, mucus, and neutrophils.

   d. The most common cause is infection with *Clostridium difficile*.

   e. It is usually associated with antibiotic treatment.

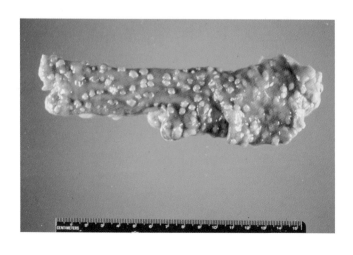

7. A 19-year-old hiker returned from a trip to the Grand Canyon. He developed a low-grade fever, nausea, anorexia, and mild diarrhea 10 days later. Stool examination for ova and parasites was negative. Symptoms persisted for another 2 weeks, and endoscopy was performed. The duodenal and proximal jejunal mucosa appeared slightly edematous. The biopsy diagnosis is:

   a. Cryptosporidiosis

   b. Microsporidiosis

   c. Blastocystosis

   d. Giardiasis

   e. Fascioliasis

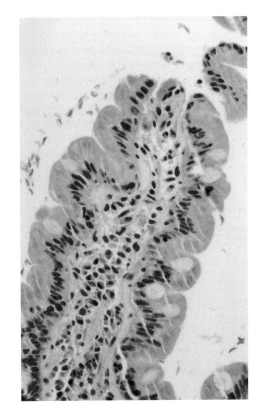

8. A 30-year-old intravenous drug user developed pneumonia. Antibiotic therapy was ineffectual. Bronchoscopy and biopsy were performed, and a Diff-Quik-stained touch preparation was done in the operating room. The pathologist can tell the clinician immediately that the diagnosis is:

   a. Bacterial infection, probably *Staphylococcus*

   b. Parasitic infection, probably toxoplasmosis

   c. Fungal infection, probably histoplasmosis

   d. Infectious organisms, not further classifiable

   e. *Pneumocystis jirovecii* pneumonia (PCP)

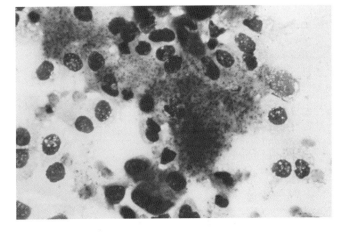

9. This gastric biopsy specimen shows an immunohistochemical stain positive for *H. pylori*. All of the following observations about this biopsy specimen are correct EXCEPT:

   a. The bacteria appear as clusters and singly scattered organisms in foveolar lumina.

   b. The bacterium is a curved rod.

   c. Some bacteria are attached to the luminal side of the foveolar epithelium.

   d. Rare bacteria can be seen in the lamina propria.

   e. The discrepancy between the large number of bacteria and the relatively mild inflammatory reaction suggests a low virulence strain.

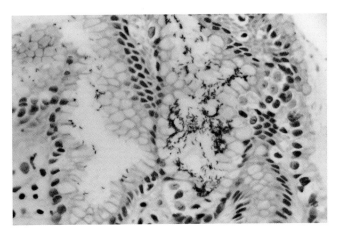

10. A 24-year-old wrestler with a recently acquired tattoo on his chest developed chest pain. A chest radiograph demonstrated an anterior mediastinal mass, which markedly increased in size during the following 2 weeks. A biopsy was inconclusive but suggested a fibromatosis. Surgery was performed. The mass involved the mediastinum, pericardium, lung, subcutaneous tissue, and sternum. Many histologic sections showed only fibrosis. Some sections showed abscesses around clumps of microorganisms, readily seen on hematoxylin-eosin staining. These microorganisms were better characterized by numerous special stains. Which of the following stains is NOT useful?
   a. Giemsa
   b. PAS
   c. Gomori methenamine silver (GMS)
   d. Gram
   e. Ziehl-Neelsen

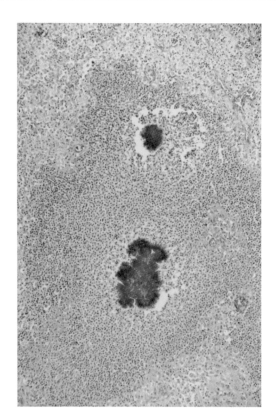

11. A U.S. tourist returned from Mexico with diarrhea and treated himself with antibiotics but did not get better. He saw a physician. Stool examination for ova and parasites was negative. At colonoscopy, colonic ulcers were seen, and a biopsy specimen was taken from the ulcer edge. The pathogens seen are:
   a. Cysts of *Entamoeba histolytica*
   b. Eggs of *E. histolytica*
   c. Trophozoites of *E. histolytica*
   d. *Balantidium coli*
   e. Intracellular bacteria

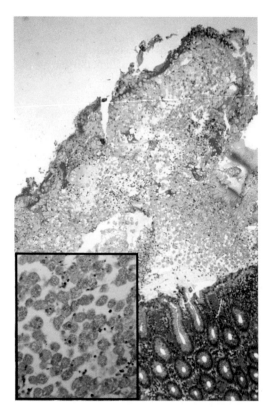

12. A patient with lung cancer developed pneumonia and empyema after a lobectomy. An open lung biopsy was performed and showed the lung tissue was partially necrotic. In the necrotic tissue, filamentous microorganisms were demonstrated on GMS stain only. Gram and acid-fast stains were negative. These organisms are:
    a. *Aspergillus*
    b. *Mucor*
    c. *Legionella*
    d. *Nocardia*
    e. *Actinomyces*

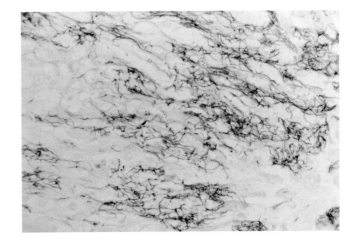

13. An Egyptian diplomat stated that he had had intermittent diarrhea for a long time, but recently it got worse. Colonoscopic findings suggested idiopathic inflammatory bowel disease (IBD). A biopsy specimen was taken from a nodular region in the sigmoid colon. Confluent nonnecrotizing granulomas were seen in the submucosa. Which of the following microorganisms would an acid-fast stain demonstrate?
    a. *Mycobacterium tuberculosis*
    b. *Mycobacterium intracellulare-avium* complex
    c. *Schistosoma mansoni*
    d. *Schistosoma haematobium*
    e. *Schistosoma intercalatum*

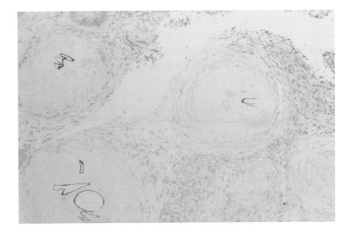

14. The image shows a section of lung from an autopsy of a patient with AIDS who died of renal failure. He had been treated for multiple infections, including *Pneumocystis jirovecii* pneumonia and *Mycobacterium avium-intracellulare* complex. Terminally, he developed skin nodules and central nervous system symptoms. The image shows which type of microorganism?
    a. *Streptococcus pneumoniae*
    b. *Cryptococcus neoformans*
    c. *Rhodococcus equi*
    d. *Histoplasma capsulatum*
    e. *P. jirovecii*

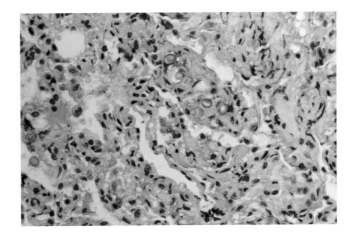

15. Which of the following statements BEST describes the parasite seen in this colonic biopsy specimen stained with Giemsa?
    a. It is an obligate intracellular protozoan parasite affecting immunocompromised patients exclusively.
    b. It is an intestinal parasite with a complex asexual and sexual life cycle, contracted primarily through drinking contaminated water.
    c. It is a frequent commensal, found mostly in the intestines of homosexuals.
    d. It is an obligate intracellular protozoan found exclusively in the colonic mucosa.
    e. This intestinal parasite accounts for a minority of cases of diarrhea in HIV-positive individuals.

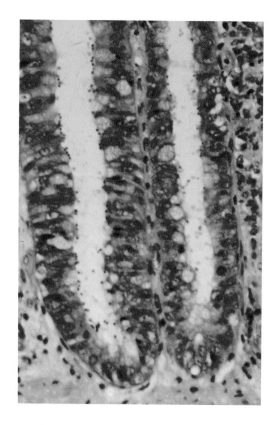

16. A patient with HIV infection had a recent episode of *Candida* esophagitis treated with fluconazole. Symptoms of pain and dysphagia persisted, and repeat endoscopy showed discrete ulcers in the distal esophagus and midesophagus. The biopsy diagnosis is:
    a. Cytomegalovirus (CMV) esophagitis
    b. Recurrent or persistent *Candida* esophagitis
    c. Nonspecific ulcer, possibly HIV-related
    d. Herpetic esophagitis
    e. Varicella esophagitis

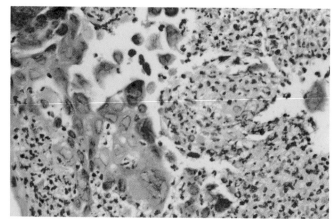

17. A healthy 60-year-old man underwent a routine colonoscopy, which disclosed several polyps that turned out to be adenomas. The colonic mucosa adjacent to the largest polyp showed filamentous organisms attached to the surface epithelium. The diagnosis is:
    a. Fungal infection
    b. Actinomycosis
    c. Cryptosporidiosis
    d. Enteroadherent *Escherichia coli*
    e. Intestinal spirochetosis

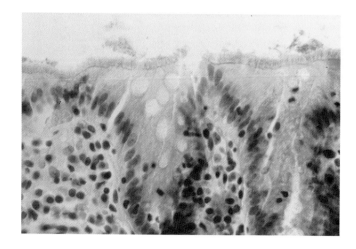

18. This lung biopsy was taken from a 70-year-old man with lymphoma and pneumonia, unresponsive to conventional antibiotic therapy. In his youth, he had been a cave explorer in South Africa. The organisms seen in macrophages stained positive with GMS. The most likely diagnosis is:

   a. Histoplasmosis
   b. Pneumocystosis
   c. Blastomycosis
   d. Toxoplasmosis
   e. Leishmaniasis

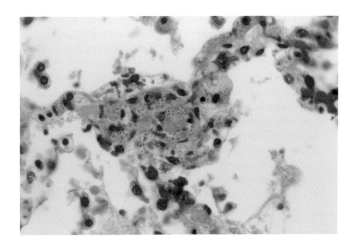

19. The infection demonstrated on this acid-fast stain of a small intestinal biopsy specimen from a patient with AIDS could be confused on PAS stain with which of the following conditions?

   a. Celiac disease
   b. CMV enteritis
   c. Fungal infection
   d. Whipple disease
   e. *R. equi* infection

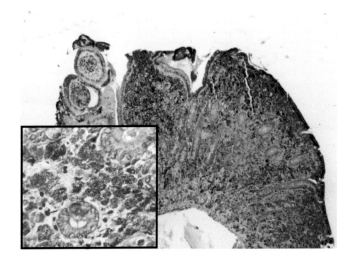

20. A renal transplant recipient developed an enlarging cavitating pulmonary lesion that did not respond to conventional antibiotic therapy. A tuberculin skin test was negative. A bronchoscopic biopsy was nondiagnostic. A lobectomy was performed. A section of the necrotic tissue surrounding the cavity was stained with GMS and disclosed fungal hyphae. All of the following statements about the infection are true EXCEPT:

   a. Blood vessel invasion is a characteristic feature.
   b. Infarction leads to cavitation.
   c. The fungus belongs to the class of Zygomycetes that includes *Rhizopus* and *Mucor*.
   d. Risk factors include immunosuppression, neutropenia, hematologic malignancies, and uncontrolled diabetes mellitus.
   e. The lung is the most commonly affected organ.

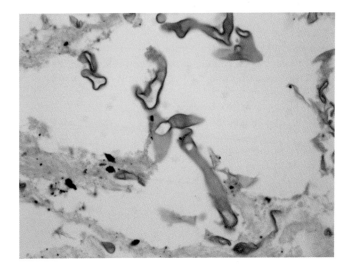

21. An immigrant from Sri Lanka complained of right lower abdominal pain and intermittent diarrhea. On endoscopy, the distal ileum, cecum, and adjacent right colon showed nodular, focally ulcerated mucosa. Biopsy specimens showed nonnecrotizing granulomas and shallow ulcers. Crohn disease was suspected. A tuberculin skin test was positive, and the pathologist was asked to do an acid-fast stain, which showed rare acid-fast organisms. Which of the following statements BEST summarizes what we can learn from this scenario?

  a. All gastrointestinal biopsy specimens with granulomas should be stained for acid-fast bacilli.

  b. Crohn disease may be caused by acid-fast bacilli.

  c. The absence of necrosis in a granuloma excludes tuberculosis.

  d. Finding an occasional acid-fast organism, especially in nonnecrotizing granulomas, is nonspecific.

  e. In developing countries, gastrointestinal tuberculosis is more common than Crohn disease, and in patients from such countries, acid-fast stains should be performed whenever granulomas are found.

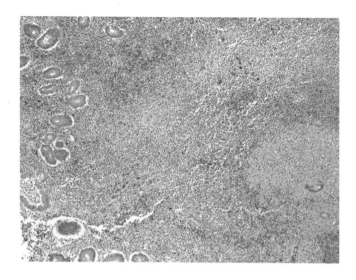

22. The image shows an acid-fast stain of a biopsy specimen of an intraabdominal mass in a patient with AIDS. The mass appeared mesenteric and was associated with enlarged mesenteric lymph nodes. The spindle cells in this mycobacterial pseudotumor stain positively with all of the following stains EXCEPT:

  a. GMS

  b. PAS

  c. Giemsa

  d. Antidesmin immunoperoxidase

  e. Antiactin immunoperoxidase

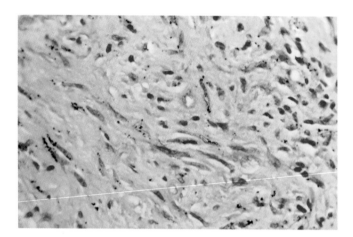

23. A jejunal biopsy specimen from a patient with AIDS and diarrhea, stained with the Brown-Brenn-Gram stain, showed numerous gram-positive intracytoplasmic microorganisms. The diagnosis is:

  a. Staphylococcal infection

  b. Cryptosporidiosis

  c. Enteroinvasive *E. coli* infection

  d. Microsporidiosis

  e. Isosporiasis

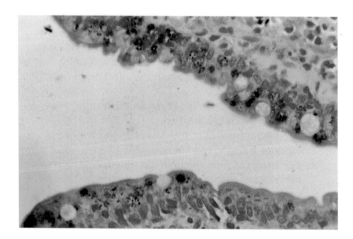

24. A 91-year-old man presented with nonbloody diarrhea. On physical examination, very poor hygiene was noted. Colonoscopy revealed worms in the colon. Which of the following options is NOT correct about this infection?

a. Female worms shed 3000 to 20,000 eggs per day.

b. Larvae will penetrate through the small intestinal wall and infect lungs.

c. The patient most likely acquired this infection through ingestion of eggs present in contaminated food or soiled hands.

d. Male parasites can be recognized by their curly-ended head.

e. Adult larvae can be found anywhere in the large bowel.

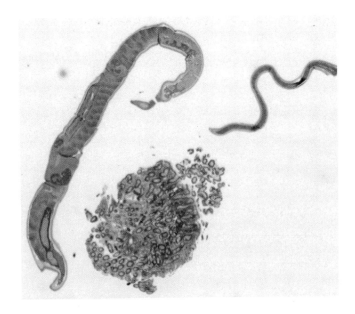

25. A 55-year-old woman with a history of cervical squamous cell carcinoma presented with sepsis, jaundice, and right upper quadrant abdominal pain. Imaging studies demonstrated a large mass in the hepatic hilar area, obstructing the left bile duct. Exploratory laparoscopy showed extensive involvement by squamous cell carcinoma from the hepatic hilum to the duodenum, which was adherent to the hilar plate. A left hepatectomy demonstrated metastatic squamous cell carcinoma. In addition, a 0.5-cm cavitary lesion was noted in the hepatic hilar area. A section of this area is shown in the image. What is the MOST likely cause of this process?

a. *E. histolytica*

b. *Aspergillus*

c. Hydatid cyst

d. *Candida*

e. *E. coli*

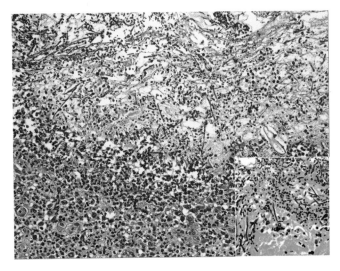

26. A 34-year-old pregnant woman presented with oral ulcers. Which of the following statements about this condition is TRUE?

   a. This condition is caused by a herpesvirus.

   b. There is a higher risk of neonatal disease if this patient acquired the disease in the third trimester of pregnancy.

   c. This condition occurs only in immunocompromised patients.

   d. Electron microscopy is commonly used in diagnosis of this disease.

   e. A large cytoplasmic basophilic inclusion with a clear halo is a diagnostic feature of this condition.

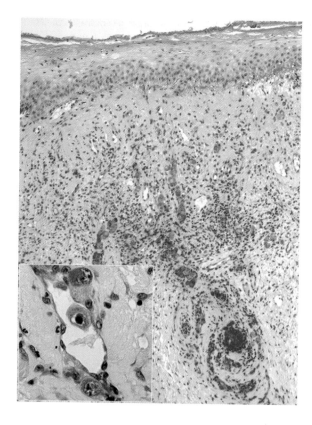

27. All of the following statements about this infection are true EXCEPT:

   a. Luxol fast blue stain can help in the diagnosis.

   b. The infectious agent is identified in oligodendrocytes only.

   c. No specific treatment option is currently available.

   d. This disease is caused by a virus.

   e. Immunosuppressed patients are most commonly affected by this infection.

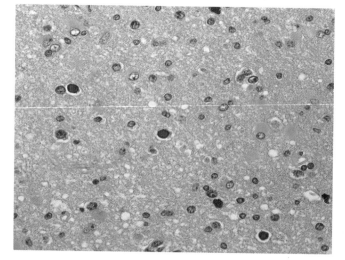

28. A 56-year-old HIV-positive patient presented with cough and was found to have bilateral nodular infiltrates in the lungs. A lung biopsy was performed, and the specimen is shown in the image. Which of the following statements is CORRECT?

   a. This infection is caused by a fungal organism.

   b. IgG-positive serologic test indicates current disease.

   c. Transmission rate during pregnancy is highest in the first trimester.

   d. The disease can be acquired through inhalation of cysts.

   e. Tachyzoites indicate acute infection.

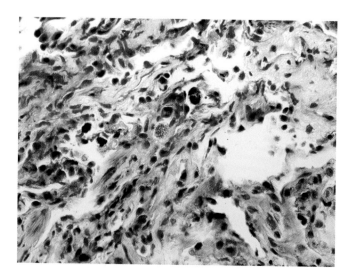

29. A 68-year-old woman with poorly controlled diabetes mellitus was admitted for worsening right lower lobe pneumonia despite antibiotic therapy. Subsequent sputum cultures demonstrated fungal organisms. Despite aggressive antifungal therapy, the patient developed severe hemoptysis and died. Which of the following BEST describes the organisms present in this case?

a. *Aspergillus* (90 degree–angle branching hyphae) and *Candida* (nonseptate hyphae and pseudohyphae)

b. *Candida* (mycelium) and *Aspergillus* (septate hyphae with acute-angle branching)

c. *Zygomycetes* (broad, nonseptate hyphae) and *Aspergillus* (thin, septate hyphae with acute-angle branching)

d. *Mucor* (broad septate hyphae with 90 degree–angle branching) and *Aspergillus* (nonseptate hyphae)

e. *Rhizopus* (spores and nonseptate hyphae) and *Candida* (hyphae and pseudohyphae)

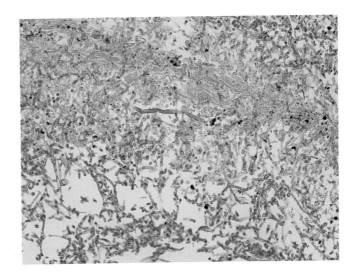

30. What organism is shown in the image?

a. *S. mansoni*

b. *S. intercalatum*

c. *S. haematobium*

d. *Schistosoma mekongi*

e. *Schistosoma japonicum*

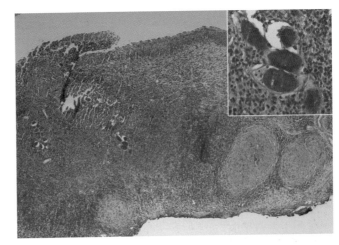

31. What is the BEST diagnosis in this case?

a. Isosporiasis

b. Histoplasmosis

c. Toxoplasmosis

d. Cryptosporidiosis

e. Amebiasis

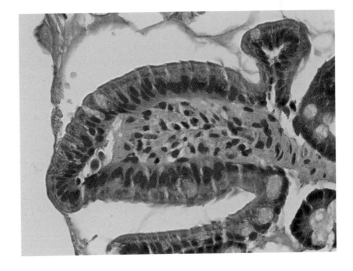

32. A 71-year-old woman with a history of ulcerative colitis presented to the emergency department with a 10-day history of fever, abdominal pain, and bloody diarrhea. Colonoscopy revealed edematous and hemorrhagic mucosa with ulcerations in the rectum and sigmoid colon. The findings of a sigmoid colon biopsy are most consistent with:
    a. Ulcerative colitis
    b. CMV enterocolitis
    c. Amebiasis
    d. Shigellosis
    e. Pseudomembranous colitis

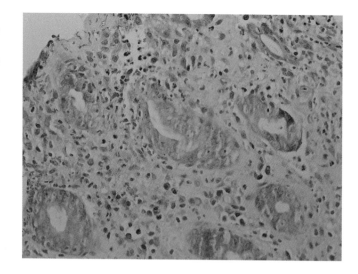

33. Epstein-Barr virus (EBV) was discovered in 1964 in cells cultured from a case of Burkitt lymphoma. Since then, EBV has been identified as the etiologic agent of various neoplastic and nonneoplastic conditions EXCEPT:
    a. Infectious mononucleosis
    b. Nasopharyngeal carcinoma
    c. Lymphoproliferative disease in patients with congenital or acquired immune deficiencies
    d. Thymoma
    e. Oral hairy leukoplakia

34. The association of *H. pylori* infection and gastric MALToma (mucosa-associated lymphoid tissue lymphoma) is well described. Which of the following statements BEST describes the pathogenesis?
    a. *H. pylori* gastritis may be complicated by atrophy and increased lymphocytosis, the precursor to lymphoma.
    b. *H. pylori* gastritis is typically associated with lymphoid hyperplasia, which, in combination with intestinal metaplasia, may lead to lymphoma.
    c. Specific strains of *H. pylori* predisposing to lymphoma have been isolated.
    d. *H. pylori* infection resistant to antibiotic treatment predisposes to lymphoma.
    e. *H. pylori* infection is associated with T cell–dependent B-cell proliferation. Certain genetic alterations in the proliferating B cell produce a neoplastic clone that remains responsive to antibiotic treatment in the early stages.

35. Primary infection with herpes simplex virus (HSV) 1 is usually asymptomatic. Rarely, symptomatic disease occurs and may manifest in a variety of ways EXCEPT:
    a. Gingivostomatitis
    b. Conjunctivitis
    c. Keratitis
    d. Encephalitis
    e. Hepatitis

36. The incidence of fungal infections in transplant recipients is 5% to 10%. Which of the following fungi are the MOST common causes?
    a. *Candida* and *Aspergillus*
    b. *Candida* and *Pneumocystis*
    c. *Aspergillus* and *Mucor*
    d. *Mucor* and *Candida*
    e. *Histoplasma* and *Candida*

37. Necrotizing fasciitis is a severe form of soft tissue infection, involving primarily the superficial fascia. If necrotizing fasciitis is not diagnosed early, the mortality rate is high. The pathologist first suggests the diagnosis. All of the following histologic findings are typical EXCEPT:
    a. Necrosis of superficial fascia
    b. Infiltration of dermis and fascia by polymorphonuclear leukocytes
    c. Large numbers of bacteria
    d. Muscle involvement
    e. Fibrin thrombi in arteries and veins

38. Cat-scratch disease is an infection with *Bartonella henselae*. Which of the following organs is MOST commonly involved?
    a. Bone
    b. Liver
    c. Lymph nodes
    d. Central nervous system
    e. Spleen

39. Gastrointestinal infection and diarrhea may be caused by various *E. coli* strains. Which of the following is associated with hemolytic uremic syndrome?
    a. Enteropathogenic *E. coli*
    b. Enteroaggregative *E. coli*
    c. Enteroinvasive *E. coli*
    d. Enterotoxigenic *E. coli*
    e. Enterohemorrhagic *E. coli*

40. Parvovirus B19 infection can manifest in various ways, including all of the following EXCEPT:
    a. Erythema infectiosum (fifth disease)
    b. "Gloves-and-socks syndrome"
    c. Arthritis
    d. Anemia
    e. Pneumonia

41. Which of the following statements about West Nile virus is CORRECT?
    a. West Nile virus is a flavivirus that causes seasonal outbreaks of diarrhea.

b. Only immunocompromised patients develop clinical symptoms.

c. West Nile virus is enzootic in Africa, Asia, and Europe and has recently become so in the United States as well, where outbreaks have occurred every winter.

d. West Nile virus infection should be considered in the differential diagnosis of all cases of encephalitis and viral meningitis during the summer months, especially in older patients with muscle weakness.

e. The mortality rate of symptomatic disease is greater than 50%.

42. Hantavirus pulmonary syndrome is an often fatal disease that was first described in the southwestern United States in 1993. Patients develop pulmonary edema, respiratory insufficiency, and shock. Autopsy findings include all of the following EXCEPT:
    a. Interstitial pneumonitis
    b. Hyaline membranes
    c. Diffuse alveolar damage
    d. Hantavirus antigens in endothelial cells
    e. Vasculitis

43. Human granulocytic ehrlichiosis is a tick-borne infection by pleomorphic coccobacilli. The diagnosis is made by serologic tests and demonstration of the microorganism in granulocytes. Besides granulocytes, which other cell types can be infected?
    a. Lymphocytes, monocytes, and macrophages
    b. Lymphocytes, megakaryocytes, and macrophages
    c. Lymphocytes, Kupffer cells, and macrophages
    d. Megakaryocytes, normoblasts, and macrophages
    e. Megakaryocytes, myeloblasts, and macrophages

44. Rabies is caused by RNA viruses in the family of Rhabdoviridae, genus *Lyssavirus*. Humans become infected after a bite by an infected animal; the virus travels by retrograde axoplasmic flow from the bite site to the central nervous system. At autopsy, the virus may be detected in practically any tissue. What is the PRIMARY site of replication?
    a. Endothelial cells
    b. Leukocytes
    c. Neurons
    d. Glial cells
    e. Salivary gland

45. Toxoplasmosis has a worldwide distribution. Nearly one third of humans have been exposed to this parasite. The prevalence of chronic (latent) toxoplasmosis is estimated to be 90% in Paris, France, and 50% in the United States. Reactivation of latent infection in patients with AIDS can produce severe illness and death. Which of the following is the MOST common presentation in this setting?
    a. Myocarditis
    b. Diffuse lymphadenopathy
    c. Encephalitis
    d. Pneumonia
    e. Hepatitis

46. Kaposi sarcoma–associated herpesvirus (KSHV), also known as human herpesvirus 8, has been causally linked to several neoplasms, including all of the following EXCEPT:
    a. Classic Kaposi sarcoma in elderly men of Eastern European or Mediterranean origin
    b. Endemic Kaposi sarcoma in African children and adults
    c. Kaposi sarcoma in organ transplant recipients and patients with AIDS

d. Burkitt lymphoma
e. Body cavity–related B-cell lymphoma

47. Which of the following statements about Whipple disease is FALSE?
    a. Whipple disease is a systemic bacterial infection.
    b. Whipple disease may produce diarrhea, lymphadenopathy, polyarthritis, myocarditis, and central nervous system lesions.
    c. The causative organism, *Tropheryma whipplei*, is easily grown in culture.
    d. Small bowel biopsy specimens show foamy macrophages that stain positively with PAS.
    e. Antimicrobial therapy is curative in most cases.

48. Nontuberculous mycobacteria (NTM) can cause various diseases, depending on the type of NTM, the mode of transmission, and the immune status of the host. Which of the following is LEAST likely caused by NTM?
    a. Hypersensitivity pneumonitis
    b. Keratitis
    c. Bronchiectasis
    d. Parenchymal lung disease
    e. Necrotizing skin ulcers

49. Cysticercosis is rare in the United States but is frequently diagnosed in immigrants from developing countries. Which of the following statements about cysticercosis is FALSE?
    a. Humans acquire the disease by ingesting eggs of *Taenia solium*.
    b. Larvae enter the bloodstream and encyst in tissues with cooler temperatures, preferably skin and soft tissue of extremities.
    c. Encystation progresses through three stages: (1) A fluid-filled bladder with inverted scolices is seen. (2) Rupture of the cyst results in local inflammation and pain. (3) The parasite is resorbed, and the cyst wall undergoes fibrosis and calcification.
    d. A definitive diagnosis requires histopathologic demonstration of the cysticercus.
    e. In most cases, multiple cysts are present.

50. A 30-year-old, previously healthy man developed pain, photophobia, and redness in both eyes. Visual acuity was decreased. He had worn contact lenses for many years and used tap water to clean them. Tissue scrapings of the cornea demonstrated pleomorphic organisms, 20 to 40 µm in size, with granular vacuolated cytoplasm and a large targetlike nucleolus surrounded by a halo. The diagnosis is:
    a. Herpetic keratitis
    b. Fungal keratitis
    c. Onchocerciasis
    d. *Acanthamoeba* infection
    e. Microsporidiosis

51. Lyme disease is the most common tick-borne disease in the United States. It is caused by *Borrelia burgdorferi*, which is transmitted via the bite of an *Ixodes* tick. At the site of the tick bite, the expanding macular rash of erythema migrans is the best clinical marker for early Lyme disease. If a biopsy specimen is obtained, what is the BEST special stain to visualize the organism?
    a. Gram stain
    b. Acid-fast stain

c. GMS stain
d. Giemsa stain
e. Steiner silver stain

52. All of the following methods can be used to detect fungal organisms in formalin-fixed tissue EXCEPT:
    a. GMS staining
    b. Dieterle staining
    c. Hematoxylin-eosin staining
    d. Fite-Faraco staining
    e. PAS staining

53. Which of the following infections can be transmitted through blood transfusions?
    a. Rabies
    b. Amebiasis

c. Leishmaniasis
d. Q fever
e. Echinococcosis

54. A 25-year-old man presented with a 2-week-history of chronic diarrhea and crampy right lower abdominal pain. He reported a recent trip to Mexico. Colonoscopy showed terminal ileum and periappendiceal nodularity. A biopsy specimen of the terminal ileum demonstrated granulomas, and fecal cultures grew *Yersinia enterocolitica*. This infection is associated with all of the following features EXCEPT:
    a. Pseudoappendicitis
    b. Hepatic abscess
    c. Caseating granulomas
    d. Arthritis
    e. Lymphadenitis

Answers

1. c. Echinococcal or hydatid cysts are caused by the dog tapeworm and have a characteristic cyst wall composed of a laminated membrane and a germinal layer. The laminated layer is no more than 1 mm thick and acellular. The germinal layer is 10 to 25 μm thick and contains nuclei that may be too degenerated to be seen clearly, as in this case. Scolices develop from the germinal layer (not seen on the image). They contain calcareous bodies, which can be seen free-floating in the degenerated cyst contents. Most cases of echinococcosis are caused by *Echinococcus granulosus*. Cysts develop mainly in the liver, but hematogenous dissemination may result in cysts in almost any anatomic location, especially lung, kidney, spleen, bone, and brain. Cyst rupture is described in approximately 25% of patients. Other complications include compression of the biliary tree, biliary fistulas, and anaphylactic shock.

Pedrosa I, Saíz A, Arrazola J, et al: Hydatid disease: radiologic and pathologic features and complications. *Radiographics* 2000; 20(3):795-817.
Raether W, Hänel H: Epidemiology, clinical manifestations and diagnosis of zoonotic cestode infections: an update. *Parasitol Res* 2003;91(5):412-438.

2. c. The slide shows *Helicobacter heilmannii* gastritis. *H. heilmannii* differs from *H. pylori* in bacterial size, shape, and number. *H. heilmannii* is larger, spiral rather than curved, and present in significantly smaller numbers, mainly in foveolar lumina, where it aggregates in clusters or stacks. *H. heilmannii* does not adhere to the epithelial cell surface, as does *H. pylori*. Evidence suggests that a unique lymphocytic pattern of inflammation, with the propensity to involve the foveolar lumen, is a distinctive histopathologic aspect of *H. heilmannii* chronic gastritis. Symptoms, treatment, and complications are identical to those of *H. pylori* gastritis. Immunohistochemical staining specific for *H. pylori* also reacts with *H. heilmannii*, indicating cross-reacting antigenic epitopes between both organisms.

Andersen LP: New *Helicobacter* species in humans. *Dig Dis* 2001; 19(2):112-115.
Singhal AV, Sepulveda AR: *Helicobacter heilmannii* gastritis: a case study with review of literature. *Am J Surg Pathol* 2005;29(11): 1537-1539.

3. a. The diagnosis is CMV appendicitis. Large mononuclear cells, probably endothelial, are seen under intact surface epithelium. Nuclei contain distinctive acidophilic inclusion bodies surrounded by a clear halo ("owl's eye" inclusion), and the cytoplasm contains smaller, granular, basophilic inclusions. A diagnosis of CMV infection can be made on purely morphologic grounds. Immunohistochemical staining can be performed if the diagnosis is in doubt. CMV infects primarily endothelial cells but can also be seen in smooth muscle cells, cardiac muscle cells, fibroblasts, histiocytes, ganglion cells, and glandular epithelial cells, including renal tubular cells but not squamous cells. This patient most likely also has CMV colitis. All reported cases of appendicitis have also had colonic infection. Although this infection may involve other sites, additional tests are not required. In patients with AIDS, the right colon is more commonly and more severely affected than the left colon. Although CMV appendicitis and colitis is typically secondary to reactivation of a latent infection in the setting of immunosuppression, it can also occur in an immunocompetent host as a primary infection. The presence of abnormal mucosa before CMV infection may increase the risk of this infection, such as in cases of IBD.

Unless CMV appendicitis is treated, disseminated disease may develop, and CMV inclusion bodies can be found in any organ at autopsy. Retina and gastrointestinal tract are the two most commonly involved sites. In the gastrointestinal tract, the colon is the prime target. CMV colitis can sometimes mimic ischemic colitis both grossly and microscopically.

Dieterich DT, Kim MH, McMeeding A, et al: Cytomegalovirus appendicitis in a patient with acquired immune deficiency syndrome. *Am J Gastroenterol* 1991;86(7):904-906.
Rafailidis PI, Mourtzoukou EG, Varbobitis IC, et al: Severe cytomegalovirus infection in apparently immunocompetent patients: a systematic review. *Virol J* 2008;5:47.
Siegal DS, Hamid N, Cunha BA: Cytomegalovirus colitis mimicking ischemic colitis in an immunocompetent host. *Heart Lung* 2005;34(4):291-294.

4. d. Cross sections of embryonated eggs are seen embedded within crypts. This patient was probably infected in

Vietnam, but the infection remained subclinical as long as his immunity was intact. *Strongyloides* has a remarkable ability to persist in a host virtually indefinitely through a process of autoinfection. The roundworm *S. stercoralis* can be present in numerous stages in the same specimen: eggs, rhabdoid and filariform larvae, and adult females.

Eggs measure approximately 30 μm × 50 μm, bordered by a thin cuticle, either in the morula or tadpole stages or with an embryo inside. The larvae have a cross-sectional diameter of 12 to 18 μm, and adult females have a cross-sectional diameter of 30 to 50 μm. In the stomach and duodenum, the parasites are commonly nested within gastric or duodenal glands, associated with a localized chronic inflammatory reaction that is nonspecific and consists of increased numbers of mononuclear cells. In hyperinfective strongyloidiasis, filariform larvae are seen in the wall of small and large intestine and may invade any organ. Strongyloidiasis must be considered as a possible cause of intestinal disease in immunocompromised patients, including transplant recipients and patients with AIDS who have traveled to endemic areas (tropical and temperate climates) at any time in their life.

Kishimoto K, Hokama A, Hirata T, et al: Endoscopic and histopathological study on the duodenum of *Strongyloides stercoralis* hyperinfection. *World J Gastroenterol* 2008; 14(11):1768-1773.

Rivasi F, Pampiglione S, Boldorini R, et al: Histopathology of gastric and duodenal *Strongyloides stercoralis* locations in fifteen immunocompromised subjects. *Arch Pathol Lab Med* 2006; 130(12):1792-1798.

5. c. The image shows *Pseudomonas aeruginosa* pneumonitis. *P. aeruginosa* is a gram-negative aerobic rod. Infection is often nosocomially acquired, particularly in intensive care units, in patients on ventilators, in elderly patients, and in patients with chronic lung disease or immunosuppression. Patients with cystic fibrosis or neutropenia are predisposed. In disseminated infections, endocarditis, pneumonia, and osteomyelitis are common. *P. aeruginosa* rarely affects healthy individuals; however, it has been associated with rapidly progressive pneumonia and a mortality rate of around 30% in this population.

Fujitani S, Sun HY, Yu VL, et al: Pneumonia due to *Pseudomonas aeruginosa*: part I: epidemiology, clinical diagnosis, and source. *Chest* 2011;139(4):909-919.

von Baum H, Welte T, Marre R, et al: Community-acquired pneumonia through *Enterobacteriaceae* and *Pseudomonas aeruginosa*: diagnosis, incidence and predictors. *Eur Respir J* 2010;35(3):598-605.

6. b. The image shows a typical case of pseudomembranous colitis following prolonged antibiotic treatment. The condition develops in about 4% of patients taking clindamycin or ampicillin, but the list of inciting antibiotics is long. Bacterial invasion occurs rarely and only in infants and patients with neutropenia. Tissue damage is due to a toxin. *C. difficile* is the most commonly identified cause. *C. difficile* can be isolated from the feces of 2% to 4% of healthy individuals and 10% to 20% of hospitalized patients without diarrhea. Disease results when *C. difficile* overgrows the normal gut flora and produces toxins (toxin A, an enterotoxin, and toxin B, a cytotoxin). Clinical findings range from an asymptomatic carrier state, to mild diarrhea

that may resolve when antibiotic therapy is stopped, to life-threatening diarrhea in older and debilitated patients. In the early stage of the disease, the mucosa is congested and edematous and only mildly inflamed. In the resolving phase, the mucosa shows subtle changes with occasional dilated crypts with regenerative epithelial changes and only a few luminal neutrophils. The diagnosis is made by a combination of histologic findings and identification of toxin B in feces.

Verma P, Makharia GK: *Clostridium difficile* associated diarrhea: new rules for an old game. *Trop Gastroenterol* 2011;32(1):15-24.

7. d. The biopsy specimen shows the typical "school of fish" arrangement of the trophozoites of the protozoan *Giardia lamblia*, aligned along the contour of a duodenal villus. Individual trophozoites are pear-shaped, but in sagittal sections they have a characteristic crescentic shape. There is only a mild increase in the number of plasma cells in the villous stroma but no villous atrophy. The inflammatory reaction to *Giardia* infection varies from none in asymptomatic carriers, to mild changes as in this case of mild infection, to villous atrophy in chronic infections of patients with weight loss and foul-smelling stools. Intestinal nodular lymphoid hyperplasia is found in patients with hypogammaglobulinemia and giardiasis. Hikers are frequently infected after drinking contaminated water. The diagnosis can be made by identification of the *Giardia* trophozoite or cyst forms in stool specimens; however, because of intermittent shedding, stools may be negative. Three stool specimens should be collected over several days.

Ankarklev J, Jerlström-Hultqvist J, Ringqvist E, et al: Behind the smile: cell biology and disease mechanisms of *Giardia* species. *Nat Rev Microbiol* 2010;8(6):413-422.

8. e. The Diff-Quik (Giemsa) touch preparation stains the nuclei of trophozoites and sporozoites of *P. jirovecii* organisms. The capsule of *Pneumocystis* stains with silver preparations. Diff-Quik (Giemsa staining) touch preparations allow for a rapid diagnosis and are often preferred over biopsy diagnoses, which take at least 24 hours. *P. jirovecii* pneumonia (previously known as *Pneumocystis carinii* pneumonia, or PCP) is one of the most prevalent opportunistic infections in HIV-positive patients. This patient turned out to be HIV positive, and PCP was her first AIDS indicator infection. All cell cycle stages occur in the lung. This organism cannot be cultured in artificial media. *P. jirovecii* pneumonia also occurs in other settings of immunodeficiency and has been described in patients without any underlying immunosuppression. Formerly known as *Pneumocystis carinii*, this organism was initially thought to be a protozoan, and for this reason its life cycle is described in zoologic terms. It is now reclassified as a fungus (see Question 58).

Huang L, Cattamanchi A, Davis JL, et al: HIV-associated *Pneumocystis* pneumonia. *Proc Am Thorac Soc* 2011;8(3):294-300.

Reid AB, Chen SC, Worth LJ: *Pneumocystis jirovecii* pneumonia in non-HIV-infected patients: new risks and diagnostic tools. *Curr Opin Infect Dis* 2011;24(6):534-544.

9. d. *H. pylori* is found extracellularly, mainly in the surface mucus and in foveolar lumina. Rarely, *H. pylori* can be seen in the cytoplasm of epithelial cells, especially parietal cells, but not in the lamina propria. *H. pylori* can be identified on hematoxylin-eosin–stained sections in most instances. If the number of organisms is small, special stains are helpful. Giemsa, Diff-Quik, various silver stains (Warthin-Starry, Steiner), and immunohistochemical staining are commonly used. The last-mentioned is most specific. Infection begins as a superficial gastritis, first acute (biopsy is not usually performed) and then chronic active (with neutrophils around gastric neck glands and increased plasma cells in the lamina propria), and, depending on the strain, host, and environmental factors, progresses to atrophic gastritis. In Western countries, where the infection is acquired late in life, antral gastritis is most common, and duodenal ulcer is the most frequent complication. In the developing world, where the infection is usually acquired in childhood, multifocal pangastritis is most common, and gastric ulcer and carcinoma are the most frequent complications.

Tan VP, Wong BC: *Helicobacter pylori* and gastritis: untangling a complex relationship 27 years on. *J Gastroenterol Hepatol* 2011;26(Suppl 1):42-45.
Versalovic J: *Helicobacter pylori*. Pathology and diagnostic strategies. *Am J Clin Pathol* 2003;119(3):403-412.

10. e. The microorganism shown is *Actinomyces*, a gram-positive, branched, filamentous bacterium that typically aggregates into granules, called sulfur granules because of their grossly recognizable yellow color. They stain positively with PAS, GMS, and Gram but are not acid-fast. Nonetheless, an acid-fast stain is useful to distinguish *Actinomyces* from *Nocardia*, which is partially acid-fast. The inflammatory reaction consists of abscesses, often interconnected via sinus tracts that may drain spontaneously to body surfaces; foamy macrophages; ill-defined granulomas; and fibrosis. The granules are often surrounded by refractile, intensely eosinophilic, clublike projections (Splendore-Hoeppli phenomenon). Such precipitates of antigen-antibody complexes are not unique to *Actinomyces* and can be seen around fungi, helminthic eggs and adult worms, and certain bacterial colonies. Clinically, the disease is classified into cervicofacial, thoracic, abdominal, and pelvic actinomycosis. Because of its mass effect, actinomycosis is often mistaken for a neoplasm.

Mabeza GF, Macfarlane J: Pulmonary actinomycosis. *Eur Respir J* 2003;21(3):545-551.
Wong VK, Turmezei TD, Weston VC: Actinomycosis. *BMJ* 2011;343:d6099.

11. c. Cysts of *E. histolytica* are present in contaminated water, and human ingestion causes the disease. Excystation occurs in the small intestine, and the cysts release trophozoites, which pass into the colon and produce proteinases that lyse host tissue. Cysts and trophozoites are excreted in the stool but disintegrate quickly and may be difficult to detect unless the stool specimen is fresh. In early infections, trophozoites are concentrated on the surface of the colonic mucosa; in later stages, they are concentrated in the ulcer craters. Studies suggest that cytotoxicity of *Entamoeba* is caused by induction of apoptosis in target cells. Trophozoites have a sharply outlined cell membrane; amphophilic cytoplasm containing vacuoles, ingested erythrocytes, and other cell debris; and small hypochromatic nuclei 2 to 3 μm in diameter. These features help to distinguish amebas from human cells, which have larger nuclei with more chromatin (and more genetic information) and less sharply outlined cell membranes.

Both trophozoite and cyst forms show a characteristic chromatin distribution, which confers a distinctive nuclear appearance, described as "ring and dot" nucleus.

Ralston KS, Petri WA Jr: Tissue destruction and invasion by *Entamoeba histolytica*. *Trends Parasitol* 2011;27(6):254-263.
Stanley SL Jr: Amoebiasis. *Lancet* 2003;361(9362):1025-1034.

12. d. *Nocardia* spp. are slender bacterial filaments, 1 μm wide (much smaller than any fungus), that branch at predominantly right angles and form tangled masses. On hematoxylin-eosin stains, they may appear as faintly basophilic tangles. Gram and GMS stains are the most sensitive methods for detection. Acid-fast stains are variably positive. Modified Gram (Brown and Brenn, Brown and Hopps) and modified acid-fast stains (Kinyoun, Coates-Fite, Fite-Faraco) are also useful. The most common species to cause pulmonary nocardiosis is *Nocardia asteroides*. Risk factors include immunocompromised state, corticosteroid therapy, and underlying pulmonary disease. Among patients with cancer, nocardiosis preferentially affects patients with hematologic malignancies. The most frequently infected organs are the lung and, if hematologic spread occurs, the brain.

Ambrosioni J, Lew D, Garbino J: Nocardiosis: updated clinical review and experience at a tertiary center. *Infection* 2010;38(2):89-97.
Minero MV, Marín M, Cercenado E, et al: Nocardiosis at the turn of the century. *Medicine (Baltimore)* 2009;88(4):250-261.

13. c. Eggs of *S. mansoni*, *S. japonicum*, and *S. intercalatum*, but not *S. haematobium*, are acid-fast positive. Intestinal schistosomiasis can be caused by any of these *Schistosoma* species, but most cases in Egypt are caused by *S. mansoni*. Submucosal granulomas with eggshells in the center are typical. Because eggshells tend to be broken, the characteristic lateral spine of *S. mansoni* or terminal spine of *S. haematobium* may not be visible. Colonic inflammatory polyps may be mistaken endoscopically for IBD. They occur mainly in the distal colon but in severe cases may involve the entire colon as well as small intestine. Appendicitis and pseudotumors are rare manifestations. Schistosomiasis affects more than 200 million people worldwide. An *S. mansoni* genome project was initiated by the World Health Organization in 1994 in an attempt to provide data for future vaccine development. The first draft of the genome was published more recently.

Berriman M, Haas BJ, LoVerde PT, et al: The genome of the blood fluke *Schistosoma mansoni*. *Nature* 2009;460(7253):352-358.
Vennervald BJ, Dunne DW: Morbidity in schistosomiasis: an update. *Curr Opin Infect Dis* 2004;17(5):439-447.

14. b. *C. neoformans* is an encapsulated yeastlike fungus that ranges in size from 2 to 20 μm but usually measures 4 to 10 μm in diameter. Yeasts are spherical, oval, or elliptical and bud. The capsule is a distinctive diagnostic marker and an important virulence factor. It is of variable thickness and appears as an optically clear halo on hematoxylin-eosin stains and a bright red halo on mucicarmine stains. The fungal cell wall stains well with GMS and PAS. The host reaction depends on the immunologic status of the patient. In anergic patients, there may be no reaction at all, and organisms multiply profusely and form "cystic" lesions with closely packed fungi with mucinous capsules that give the lesions a glistening appearance. In immunocompetent patients, the infection elicits a mixed suppurative and granulomatous reaction with varying degrees of necrosis. This case shows disseminated cryptococcosis with yeasts in alveolar septal capillaries. Cryptococcosis is the most common generalized fungal disease in patients with AIDS and ranks third (after candidiasis and aspergillosis) among invasive fungal infections in transplant recipients. In disseminated infection, the central nervous system, lung, and skin are the organs most frequently involved.

Hoang LM, Maguire JA, Doyle P, et al: *Cryptococcus neoformans* infections at Vancouver Hospital and Health Sciences Centre (1997-2002): epidemiology, microbiology, and histopathology. *J Med Microbiol* 2004;53(Pt 9):935-940.

Singh N, Dromer F, Perfect JR, et al: Cryptococcosis in solid organ transplant recipients: current state of the science. *Clin Infect Dis* 2008;47(10):1321-1327.

15. b. The image shows *Cryptosporidium*, spherical, 2 to 4 µm in diameter, protozoan parasites that attach to the luminal side of crypt and surface epithelium. Variation in size corresponds to the various developmental stages. Although on light microscopy these parasites seem to be outside the enterocyte, transmission electron microscopy shows them in parasitophorous vacuoles between the enterocyte cell membrane and cytoplasm, displacing the microvilli. This location provides sequestration from both the gut lumen and the cell cytoplasm and is believed to explain the resistance of the organism to chemotherapy. Although there is no direct epithelial cell damage, the organisms destroy microvilli causing malabsorption and profuse diarrhea.

Studies show that on entering the cell, *Cryptosporidium* organisms assemble a unique F-actin-based meshwork at the host-parasite interface, isolating themselves from the host cell cytoplasm. *Cryptosporidium* organisms are mainly found in small and large intestine but have also been described in bile ducts, gallbladder, and bronchi. First described in laboratory mice and thought to be animal pathogens only, *Cryptosporidium* organisms were found to be a major cause of diarrhea in patients with AIDS and are now recognized as one of the most common human enteric infectious agents in developed and developing countries in both immunodeficient and immunocompetent individuals.

O'Hara SP, Small AJ, Chen XM, et al: Host cell actin remodeling in response to *Cryptosporidium*. *Subcell Biochem* 2008;47:92-100.

Tzipori S, Ward H: Cryptosporidiosis: biology, pathogenesis and disease. *Microbes Infect* 2002;4(10):1047-1058.

16. d. The biopsy specimen shows typical changes of herpesvirus infection. The image shows multinucleated (squamous) giant cells with molded, ground-glass nuclei and a mononuclear epithelial cell with a red-staining Cowdry type A intranuclear inclusion body. The inflammatory exudate is rich in monocytoid histiocytes. Although herpetic esophagitis statistically is most likely due to HSV-1, HSV-1 cannot be distinguished morphologically from HSV-2 or varicella-zoster virus (also a herpesvirus). The appearance of discrete ulcers on endoscopy is consistent with either herpetic or CMV esophagitis. Coinfection with *Candida* and HSV is common, as is coinfection with *Candida* and CMV. The identification of one microorganism should lead to a meticulous search for a second (or third) organism.

Herpetic esophagitis occurs in both immunocompromised and immunocompetent individuals.

Itoh T, Takahashi T, Kusaka K, et al: Herpes simplex esophagitis from 1307 autopsy cases. *J Gastroenterol Hepatol* 2003;18(12):1407-1411.

17. e. Filamentous bacteria are attached to the apical cell membrane between microvilli of colonic and rectal epithelium, conferring a slightly basophilic fuzzy border on hematoxylin-eosin–stained sections. They must be distinguished from microvilli, which are shorter and eosinophilic. Intestinal spirochetes stain strongly positive with silver stains (Warthin-Starry). Filamentous bacteria are a heterogeneous group of bacteria. In humans, *Brachyspira aalborgi* and *Brachyspira pilosicoli* predominate. Colonization of the large intestinal mucosa is common in homosexuals and HIV-infected individuals but also occurs in patients with low intestinal transit time, in areas of relative stasis, such as proximal to stenosing lesions, which may be polyps, cancer, or diverticula. Filamentous bacteria are usually not associated with disease (other than the underlying predisposing condition). Spirochetal tissue invasion is extremely rare but may occur in severely immunosuppressed patients and produce diarrhea.

Tsinganou E, Gebbers JO: Human intestinal spirochetosis—a review. *Ger Med Sci* 2010;8:Doc01.

18. a. *H. capsulatum* is a dimorphic fungus. The characteristic features on hematoxylin-eosin–stained sections are intracellular location only in histiocytes, large number of organisms, basophilic cytoplasm of fungal yeasts, and size (3 to 6 µm). The natural habitat of *Histoplasma* is soil containing feces of chickens, other birds, and bats. Caves are frequently contaminated with *Histoplasma*. In the United States, highly endemic areas are the Ohio River valley and Mississippi River valley. Primary infection is usually asymptomatic but may remain dormant and reactivate as immunocompetence declines. Clinically, three forms of histoplasmosis can be distinguished: acute pulmonary, chronic pulmonary, and disseminated. Disseminated histoplasmosis occurs in severely immunocompromised patients, especially patients with hematologic malignancies, patients with AIDS, and transplant recipients. *Histoplasma* can manifest as a mass lesion and be mistaken for a neoplasm. *H. capsulatum* is the species most often seen in the United States. In Africa, *H. capsulatum* and *Histoplasma duboisii* are endemic.

Gupta N, Arora SK, Rajwanshi A, et al: Histoplasmosis: cytodiagnosis and review of literature with special emphasis on differential diagnosis on cytomorphology. *Cytopathology* 2010;21(4):240-244.

Knox KS, Hage CA: Histoplasmosis. *Proc Am Thorac Soc* 2010;7(3):169-172.

19. d. The image shows *Mycobacterium avium* complex (MAC) infection. MAC-infected histiocytes are PAS positive, similar to Whipple macrophages. MAC also stains weakly positive with silver stains, which may raise the question of fungal infection. However, fungi are much larger than the delicate rods of MAC and are not acid-fast. *R. equi* infection, similar to MAC, is characterized by an infiltrate of foamy histiocytes (mainly seen in the lung), but these are neither PAS positive nor acid-fast, and they are cocci and not rods. MAC infection is a common complication of late-stage HIV-1 infection, but the rate has markedly declined since the advent of highly active antiretroviral therapy (HAART), from 16% before 1996 to 4% after 1996. Risk factors for developing MAC infection include young age and no HAART.

Field AS: Light microscopic and electron microscopic diagnosis of gastrointestinal opportunistic infections in HIV-positive patients. *Pathology* 2002;34(1):21-35.

Karakousis PC, Moore RD, Chaisson RE: *Mycobacterium avium* complex in patients with HIV infection in the era of highly active antiretroviral therapy. *Lancet Infect Dis* 2004;4(9): 557-565.

20 e.   Most cases of mucormycosis affect the face, sinuses, or oropharyngeal cavity. *Mucor* is a broad, ribbonlike, pleomorphic hypha, branching at angles of between 45 and 90 degrees, with few or no septa (pauciseptate rather than aseptate). Most patients who develop this infection have an underlying disease; diabetes is the most common (36%). The most common clinical presentation in patients with diabetes is rhinocerebral mucormycosis (66%). In this population, pulmonary disease accounts for 16% of cases of mucormycosis. The inflammatory response may be neutrophilic (50%), predominantly granulomatous (5%), pyogranulomatous (25%), or absent (20%). Blood vessel invasion is said to be present in 100% of cases, and perineural invasion is present in 90%.

Frater JL, Hall GS, Procop GW: Histologic features of zygomycosis: emphasis on perineural invasion and fungal morphology. *Arch Pathol Lab Med* 2001;125(3):375-378.

Sun HY, Singh N: Mucormycosis: its contemporary face and management strategies. *Lancet Infect Dis* 2011;11(4):301-311.

21. e.   Tuberculosis is still common in developing countries; however, in the United States, intestinal tuberculosis is rare and is considered a diagnosis of exclusion. The finding of any acid-fast bacillus is significant and indicates infection; it is not a nonspecific finding. Although tuberculosis is characterized by necrotizing granulomas, nonnecrotizing granulomas are frequently present as well. The absence of necrosis does not rule out tuberculosis. Histologic features that are more frequently seen in tuberculosis cases include confluent granulomas, surrounding lymphoid cuff, submucosal location, and larger granulomas (>400 μm). Crohn disease more often manifests with small, poorly formed granulomas (<200 μm) that are more frequently located in the mucosa. Controversial evidence linked Crohn disease with *M. avium* subspecies *paratuberculosis*. *M. avium* subspecies *paratuberculosis* is cell wall deficient and cannot be identified on Ziehl-Neelsen stain; this is not the case in the present scenario.

Greenstein RJ: Is Crohn's disease caused by a *Mycobacterium*? Comparisons with leprosy, tuberculosis, and Johne's disease. *Lancet Infect Dis* 2003;3(8):507-514.

Pulimood AB, Amarapurkar DN, Ghoshal U, et al: Differentiation of Crohn's disease from intestinal tuberculosis in India in 2010. *World J Gastroenterol* 2011;17(4):433-443.

22. c.   Mycobacteria do not stain with Giemsa. Members of MAC, but not *M. tuberculosis*, may stain positively for desmin, actin, and cytokeratin. Lesions with this immunoprofile could potentially be misinterpreted as

smooth muscle tumors. Mycobacterial pseudotumors are a rare manifestation of tuberculosis and nontuberculous mycobacterial infection reported exclusively in immunosuppressed individuals, typically patients with AIDS. For this reason, acid-fast stains are essential in evaluation of any spindle cell lesion in patients with AIDS. Spindle cells typically stain positively for macrophage markers, such as CD68. Histologically, mycobacterial pseudotumors are spindle cell lesions that closely resemble mesenchymal tumors, especially Kaposi sarcoma. Proper distinction between these entities is of paramount importance because both therapy and prognosis are affected. Mycobacterial pseudotumors more commonly occur in lymph nodes but have also been described in the appendix, bone marrow, and brain.

Basilio-de-Oliveira C, Eyer-Silva WA, Valle HA, et al: Mycobacterial spindle cell pseudotumor of the appendix vermiformis in a patient with AIDS. *Braz J Infect Dis* 2001;5(2):98-100.

Morrison A, Gyure KA, Stone J, et al: Mycobacterial spindle cell pseudotumor of the brain: a case report and review of the literature. *Am J Surg Pathol* 1999;23:1294-1299.

Umlas J, Federman M, Crawford C, et al: Spindle cell pseudotumor due to *Mycobacterium avium*-intracellulare in patients with acquired immunodeficiency syndrome (AIDS). Positive staining of mycobacteria for cytoskeleton filaments. *Am J Surg Pathol* 1991;15(12):1181-1187.

23. d.   The order Microsporida comprises intracellular gram-positive spores ranging from 0.8 to 1.4 μm, as shown in the image. The modified Brown-Brenn stain is superior to other Gram stains. Spores of *Septata intestinalis* are stained more reliably and a darker blue than the smaller spores of *Enterocytozoon bieneusi*. Spores are characteristically birefringent, and birefringence is often better seen on Gram-stained sections than hematoxylin-eosin–stained sections. *S. intestinalis* infects enterocytes and macrophages, whereas *E. bieneusi* is restricted to enterocytes. Microsporida comprise a group of unicellular fungi that cause diarrheal disease in immunocompromised individuals. More than 10 species have been recognized as causes of human disease. The incidence of microsporidiosis in patients with AIDS has decreased markedly since the advent of new anti-HIV therapies; however, Microsporida organisms are increasingly seen in HIV-negative individuals.

Didier ES, Weiss LM: Microsporidiosis: not just in AIDS patients. *Curr Opin Infect Dis* 2011;24(5):490-495.

24. b.   *Trichuris trichiura*, a roundworm also known as human whipworm, causes a common parasitic infection most frequently associated with nonbloody diarrhea and abdominal pain. *Strongyloides*, not *Trichuris*, may invade the bloodstream through the intestinal wall and migrate to the lungs. Poor hygiene is a risk factor for infection. Children are most commonly affected. It is estimated that greater than 1 billion people are infected by *T. trichiura* worldwide. The life cycle involves ingestion of embryonated eggs that mature from larvae to young worms in the small intestine and migrate to the colon. Females start shedding eggs within 60 to 90 days of infection and can live 5 years. Once released, the deposited immature eggs mature in the soil within 2 to 3 weeks before becoming infective. Histologically, adult worms demonstrate a narrow head and a thicker posterior end. Eggs can be seen within the female parasite and have a distinctive barrel-shaped shell with two polar "caps." Females are larger than males, measuring up to 50 mm in length. Adult worms attach to the intestinal wall through their anterior ends and feed from mucosal secretions. Patients with severe infection can present with rectal prolapse, iron deficiency anemia, and vitamin A deficiency.

Bethony J, Brooker S, Albonico M, et al: Soil-transmitted helminth infections: ascariasis, trichuriasis, and hookworm. *Lancet* 2006;367(9521):1521-1532.

25. d. The image shows *Candida* organisms in both yeast and pseudohyphal forms. Liver abscesses are rare. Risk factors include obstructive biliary disease, systemic dissemination from other sources, immunosuppression, intraabdominal fistulas, postoperative status, and presence of tumors or ruptured cysts. The most common causes are (1) pyogenic abscesses (about 80% of cases), (2) amebic abscesses (about 10% of cases), and (3) fungal abscesses (<10% of cases). Fungal abscesses account for less than 10% of all liver abscesses. *Candida* is the most common causative organism and is frequently described in patients receiving prolonged antibiotic therapy and in immunocompromised patients. In the present case, the patient developed a fistula between duodenum and liver, most likely secondary to tumor infiltration, and an abscess ensued. Histologically, liver microabscesses and granulomas are the most common findings.

Pyogenic abscesses account for approximately 80% of all liver abscesses. Intestinal bacteria are the most common cause, and infections are often polymicrobial. Gram-negative aerobes such as *E. coli* and anaerobes such as *Bacteroides* spp. are often identified. Abscesses resulting from hematogenous spread can demonstrate different organisms. Hepatic amebic abscess is caused by *E. histolytica*. If recognized early, it is associated with a good prognosis with a good response to therapy. Risk factors include alcoholism and diabetes. Histologically, trophozoites are 50 μm, have a characteristic "ring and dot" nucleus, and commonly contain ingested red blood cells. Amebic abscesses have a distinctive appearance with a rim of fibrosis and little inflammation. They are filled with necrotic hepatocytes, debris, and trophozoites. The surrounding liver is normal. Studies showed that *Candida* infections trigger an interleukin 1β-driven Th17 response. This immune mechanism appears to be triggered by invasion of pseudohyphal tissue and not yeast proliferation, allowing for differentiation between colonization and invasion.

Cheng SC, van de Veerdonk FL, Lenardon M, et al: The dectin-1/inflammasome pathway is responsible for the induction of protective T-helper 17 responses that discriminate between yeasts and hyphae of *Candida albicans*. *J Leukoc Biol* 2011; 90(2):357-366.
Heneghan HM, Healy NA, Martin ST, et al: Modern management of pyogenic hepatic abscess: a case series and review of the literature. *BMC Res Notes* 2011;4:80.
Lewis JH, Patel HR, Zimmerman HJ: The spectrum of hepatic candidiasis. *Hepatology* 1982;2(4):479-487.

26. a. The image shows acutely inflamed buccal mucosa. The lower power image shows clusters of enlarged cells in the lamina propria; the *inset* shows that these cells are markedly enlarged endothelial cells with smudgy intracellular inclusions. CMV is part of the Herpesviridae group of viruses. CMV is ubiquitous among all human populations, and infection rates range from approximately 70% in the United States to nearly 100% in African countries. CMV manifests as a benign viral infection in most individuals and is often asymptomatic. Immunocompromised patients are at much higher risk for severe disease from both primary and reactivated latent infection. After primary infection, the virus remains dormant in the organism, but it can reactivate if the immune response is transiently or continually compromised. Humans shed CMV particles through blood, saliva, urine, feces, breast milk, and other body secretions, and CMV can be vertically transmitted. Congenital CMV occurs in 2% of newborns worldwide (0.7% in the United States); 80% of cases of congenital CMV remain asymptomatic. Histologically, infected cells are large and show both intranuclear and intracytoplasmic inclusions. The distinctive "owl's eye" inclusion is a basophilic intranuclear inclusion surrounded by a clear halo. Cytoplasmic inclusions are usually smaller and more acidophilic. Serologic tests cannot differentiate between prior infection and acute disease. Viral particles can be identified in body fluids (e.g., blood, saliva) by polymerase chain reaction or in tissue by immunohistochemistry.

Cannon MJ, Schmid DS, Hyde TB: Review of cytomegalovirus seroprevalence and demographic characteristics associated with infection. *Rev Med Virol* 2010;20:202-213.
Stagno S: Cytomegalovirus. In Remington JS, Klein JO (eds): *Infectious Diseases of the Fetus and Newborn Infant*, 3rd ed. Philadelphia: Saunders, 1990, pp 242-281.

27. b. Progressive multifocal leukoencephalopathy (PML) is a demyelinating disease caused by reactivation of JC virus (John Cunningham virus), a polyomavirus (DNA virus). JC virus infects mainly oligodendrocytes; however, viral particles can also be identified in a small proportion of astrocytes. Most individuals acquire the virus during childhood. The reactivated virus infects oligodendrocytes causing cell death and demyelination. PML is rare, and virtually all cases occur in the setting of immunosuppression. PML is a fatal disease if untreated. The diagnosis of PML can be established by immunohistochemical or in situ hybridization studies of a brain biopsy specimen. Polymerase chain reaction of a cerebrospinal fluid sample can also be used to detect JC viral DNA.

Histologically, infected oligodendrocytes show enlarged nuclei with a ground-glass appearance. Astrocytes can show marked reactive atypia with bizarre, enlarged nuclei. In later stages of infection, macrophages migrate to the affected areas to digest myelin debris. Although JC virus primarily infects oligodendrocytes, in situ hybridization studies detected viral DNA within a few reactive astrocytes. Electron microscopy failed to identify intact virion particles, suggesting an abortive infection secondary to incomplete or defective virion assembly. Studies have shown that JC virus enters oligodendrocytes through the serotonin receptor 5-hydroxytryptamine 2A. However, the use of serotonin blockers as a treatment option for PML remains experimental. BK virus and SV40 virus are also members of the polyomavirus group.

Aksamit AJ Jr: Progressive multifocal leukoencephalopathy: a review of the pathology and pathogenesis. *Microsc Res Tech* 1995;32(4):302-311.

Elphick GF, Querbes W, Jordan JA, et al: The human polyomavirus, JCV, uses serotonin receptors to infect cells. *Science* 2004; 306(5700):1380-1383.

Tan CS, Koralnik IJ: Progressive multifocal leukoencephalopathy and other disorders caused by JC virus: clinical features and pathogenesis. *Lancet Neurol* 2010;9(4):425-437.

28. e. *Toxoplasma gondii* is an obligate intracellular protozoan parasite that can be transmitted to humans through (1) ingestion of undercooked meat containing cysts, (2) ingestion of food or water contaminated by fecal oocytes, (3) vertical transmission, and (4) blood transfusion or organ transplantation. The ingested oocysts or cysts rupture and release parasites, which migrate through the intestinal epithelium and spread to other tissues. Tachyzoites are rapidly multiplying forms of *T. gondii* and can be seen in the acute phase of disease. The tachyzoites quickly multiply and kill host cells to be released and infect adjacent cells. When recognized by the immune system, parasites pass into a more quiescent stage in which bradyzoites slowly proliferate within cysts. Immunosuppression (e.g., AIDS, chemotherapy) allows for rupture of cysts and reemergence of active disease. Overall transmission rates during pregnancy are high—11% in the first trimester and about 90% in the third trimester. Tachyzoites are 4 to 8 μm long and crescent-shaped with a large nucleus. Bradyzoites are found within 5- to 50-μm spherical cysts. Giemsa staining is the preferred method for detecting *Toxoplasma* in tissue samples.

Hill D, Dubey JP: *Toxoplasma gondii*: transmission, diagnosis and prevention. *Clin Microbiol Infect* 2002;8(10):634-640.

Wilson M, Jones JL, McAuley JB: Toxoplasmosis. In Murray PR, Baron EJ, Jorgensen JH, et al (eds): *Manual of Clinical Microbiology*, 9th ed. Washington, DC: ASM Press, 2007, pp 2070-2081.

29. c. This case illustrates a polymicrobial fungal infection in a patient with deficient immune response secondary to uncontrolled diabetes. *Aspergillus* and Zygomycetes (*Mucor*) are saprophytic fungi that can colonize airways of healthy individuals. Immunocompromised patients can develop severe infections. In favorable environments, both fungi are prone to angioinvasion and systemic dissemination. In the lungs, infection can result in cavitation or rapidly progressive bronchopneumonia. Vascular invasion and necrosis can result in severe hemoptysis, which can be fatal. The Zygomycetes class of fungi includes *Mucor* and *Rhyzomucor* genera. Microscopically, they can be identified as ribbonlike and aseptate hyphae with 90-degree–angle branching. The broad hyphae (approximately 10 μm) have irregular contours and twist back on themselves. *Aspergillus* spp. can be recognized by their narrow hyphae (3 to 6 μm) with regular septation and acute-angle branching. Conidial heads are less commonly seen in human infections and are usually associated with severe disease. GMS and PAS stains can be used to highlight the organisms; however, Zygomycetes hyphae are better visualized with hematoxylin-eosin and PAS stains.

Richardson MD, Koukila-Kahkola P: *Rhizopus, Rhizomucor, Absidia*, and other agents of systemic and subcutaneous zygomycoses. In Murray PR, Baron EJ, Jorgensen JH, et al (eds): *Manual of Clinical Microbiology*, 9th ed. Washington, DC: ASM Press, 2007, pp 1839-1856.

Verweij PE, Brandt ME: *Aspergillus, Fusarium*, and other opportunistic moniliaceous fungi. In Murray PR, Baron EJ, Jorgensen JH, et al (eds): *Manual of Clinical Microbiology*, 9th ed. Washington, DC: ASM Press, 2007, pp 1802-1838.

Zhan HX, Lv Y, Zhang Y, et al: Hepatic and renal artery rupture due to *Aspergillus* and *Mucor* mixed infection after combined liver and kidney transplantation: a case report. *Transplant Proc* 2008;40(5):1771-1773.

30. c. The image shows *S. haematobium* ova, which can be recognized by their noticeable terminal spine. Schistosomiasis is a parasitic disease caused by *Schistosoma* spp. and is acquired by swimming in water contaminated by infected snails (intermediate hosts). *Schistosoma* cercaria penetrate human skin and circulate through various tissues finally to mature to adult worms in venules. Eggs of different species can be differentiated by their location (urine and bladder versus feces and intestines), size, and morphologic appearance. *S. mansoni* and *S. japonicum* are most commonly found in venules of the mesenteric plexus of the large and small bowel, respectively. *S. haematobium* is most commonly identified in venules of the venous plexus of the urinary bladder and rectum. *S. mansoni* infection causes obstruction of portal blood flow resulting in portal hypertension and cirrhosis. *S. haematobium* infection causes chronic cystitis and ureteritis, which can progress to malignancy. *S. mansoni* and *S. japonicum* can lodge in pulmonary venules and cause pulmonary hypertension.

Chitsulo L, Loverde P, Engels D: Schistosomiasis. *Nat Rev Microbiol* 2004;2(1):12-13.

Fried B, Reddy A, Mayer D: Helminths in human carcinogenesis. *Cancer Lett* 2011;305(2):239-249.

31. a. *Isospora belli* infects the intestinal epithelium. As shown in the image, the organisms are round-to-oval and located beneath the epithelium. *I. belli* is a protozoan known to infect only humans. Ingestion of contaminated food or water containing oocysts causes disease, which is usually self-limited in healthy individuals. *I. belli* infection is rare among immunocompetent individuals. Immunocompromised patients are susceptible to more severe infections. *Isospora* organisms have been detected in the stool of 0.2% to 3% of patients with AIDS. The differential diagnosis includes other protozoan infections, such as Microsporida and *Cryptosporidium*. Morphologic features are used to differentiate such organisms. Histologically, *Isospora* infection of the small bowel is characterized by mucosal atrophy with shortening of villi and crypt hypertrophy. Lamina propria eosinophilia is a distinct feature that is not usually present in other protozoan infections. *I. belli* organisms measure approximately 30 μm and are identified in and beneath enterocytes.

Field AS: Light microscopic and electron microscopic diagnosis of gastrointestinal opportunistic infections in HIV-positive patients. *Pathology* 2002;34(1):21-35.

Huppmann AR, Orenstein JM: Opportunistic disorders of the gastrointestinal tract in the age of highly active antiretroviral therapy. *Hum Pathol* 2010;41(12):1777-1787.

32. d. *Shigella* is a genus of rod-shaped, gram-negative invasive bacteria and can be seen within mucosal epithelial cells in the image. *Shigella* is a well-known cause of infectious diarrhea worldwide. Shigellosis is acquired by ingestion of contaminated food or water and causes fever, abdominal pain, and bloody diarrhea. Children, debilitated individuals, and individuals living in poor hygienic conditions are at higher risk of developing severe infections. The endoscopic and histologic changes caused by shigellosis mimic other infections as well as IBD. Organisms are infrequently identified in biopsy specimens, and cultures are recommended to diagnose shigellosis. Histologically, the changes are typical of acute infectious colitis. The colonic mucosa shows edema, a superficial neutrophilic infiltrate, and epithelial changes such as mucin depletion and cryptitis. Aphthoid ulcerations, a feature of Crohn disease, and pseudomembranes, as seen in *C. difficile* infections, are also described.

Carpenter HA, Talley NJ: The importance of clinicopathological correlation in the diagnosis of inflammatory conditions of the colon: histological patterns with clinical implications. *Am J Gastroenterol* 2000;95(4):878-896.

DuPont HL: Approach to the patient with infectious colitis. *Curr Opin Gastroenterol* 2012;28(1):39-46.

33. d. EBV is a member of the Herpesviridae family and infects B lymphocytes and epithelial cells. Infection occurs by contact with oral secretions containing viral particles shed from oropharyngeal epithelial cells. B cells are the site of persistent and latent EBV infection. Approximately 90% of humans are infected with EBV, and infection persists for life. The atypical lymphocytes characteristic of infectious mononucleosis are activated T cells responding to EBV-infected B cells. Burkitt lymphoma, a high-grade B-cell lymphoma, is associated with EBV in 90% of cases in Africa but in only 20% of cases in the United States. Patients with EBV-associated lymphoproliferative disease include patients with severe combined immunodeficiency, recipients of organ or bone marrow transplants, and patients with AIDS. EBV also may have a pathogenic role in Hodgkin disease, nasal T-cell lymphomas, lymphomatoid granulomatosis, angioimmunoblastic lymphadenopathy, central nervous system lymphomas in nonimmunocompromised patients, smooth muscle tumors in transplant recipients, and gastric carcinomas. Oral leukoplakia occurs in HIV-infected patients and transplant recipients and is characterized by EBV DNA and herpesvirus particles in keratinized epithelial cells.

Deyrup AT: Epstein-Barr virus-associated epithelial and mesenchymal neoplasms. *Hum Pathol* 2008;39(4):473-483.

Saha A, Robertson ES: Epstein-Barr virus-associated B-cell lymphomas: pathogenesis and clinical outcomes. *Clin Cancer Res* 2011;17(10):3056-3063.

34. e. Low-grade B-cell MALToma develops in the background of lymphoid follicular hyperplasia in a small percentage of patients infected with *H. pylori*. Certain genetic alterations within the proliferating B cells, such as chromosomal translocation t(11;18)(q21;q21) resulting in fusion of AP12 at 11q21 with a novel gene *MALT1* at 18q21, have been associated with unresponsiveness to *H. pylori* eradication treatment. Gastric MALTomas may be divided into three groups on the basis of molecular characteristics and responsiveness to antibiotics: (1) eradication responsive and fusion negative (63%), (2) eradication nonresponsive and fusion negative (19%), and (3) eradication nonresponsive

and fusion positive (18%). The nuclear factor κB pathway has been implicated in the pathogenesis of *H. pylori*–associated MALToma.

Inagaki H, Nakamura T, Li C, et al: Gastric MALT lymphomas are divided into three groups based on responsiveness to *Helicobacter pylori* eradication and detection of AP12-MALT1 fusion. *Am J Surg Pathol* 2005;28(12):1560-1567.

Nakamura T, Inagaki H, Seto M, et al: Gastric low grade B-cell MALT lymphoma: treatment response and genetic alteration. *J Gastroenterol* 2003;38(10):921-929.

Sagaert X, Van Cutsem E, De Hertogh G, et al: Gastric MALT lymphoma: a model of chronic inflammation-induced tumor development. *Nat Rev Gastroenterol Hepatol* 2010;7(6):336-346.

35. e. The most common manifestation of primary HSV-1 infection is gingivostomatitis, which is characterized by painful vesicular lesions of the oral mucosa. By comparison, conjunctivitis, keratitis, and encephalitis are rare. Herpetic hepatitis occurs only in reactivation disseminated disease, not as a primary manifestation. HSV-1 and HSV-2 are members of the Herpesviridae family, which are enveloped, double-stranded DNA viruses. About one third of individuals exposed to HSV develop latent infection in nerve cell ganglia proximal to the primary site of infection with orofacial (HSV-1) disease involving the trigeminal ganglia and genital (HSV-2) infections affecting the sacral nerve root ganglia. Both primary and secondary HSV-1 and HSV-2 infections can cause intrauterine or neonatal disease, often associated with cutaneous, ocular, and neurologic manifestations.

Ustacelebi S: Diagnosis of herpes simplex virus infection. *J Clin Virol* 2001;21(3):255-259.

36. a. Fungal infections tend to occur early after transplantation, usually within 2 months. *Candida* infections account for approximately 80% of fungal infections in transplant recipients, followed by *Aspergillus*, which cause 20% of these infections. *Candida* infection is a major complication in patients after intraabdominal solid organ transplantation because of surgical manipulation of the bowel. It is particularly prevalent among liver transplant recipients. In the posttransplantation setting, aspergillosis is associated with a nearly 100% mortality rate and more commonly infects the lungs and surgical wounds. Cryptococcal infections and *Pneumocystis* pneumonia are also important causes of morbidity in transplant recipients and have been reported in 3% to 10% of these patients.

Fishman JA, Issa NC: Infection in organ transplantation: risk factors and evolving patterns of infection. *Infect Dis Clin North Am* 2010;24(2):273-283.

37. d. Necrotizing fasciitis is usually caused by group A streptococci, but various other organisms (e.g., staphylococci, *Vibrio* spp.) have also been implicated. In the United States, necrotizing fasciitis is associated with a mortality rate of approximately 25%. Uncontrolled proliferation of bacteria is associated with bacterial invasion of blood vessels, followed by thrombosis and suppuration of blood vessels, as they course through the fascia, and progressive skin ischemia. Severe tissue damage results from a combination of bacteria-derived proteases and host-derived leukocytic enzymes. Multiple virulence factors explain the aggressiveness of this disease, including

Streptococcus pyogenes cell envelope protease, a bacterial protease that has the ability to inhibit key chemotactic agents such as interleukin 8 and prevent polymorphonuclear neutrophil influx and activity. Coagulopathy is a well-accepted mechanism of injury in necrotizing fasciitis. The virulence factors streptolysin O and M protein have been implicated in the prothrombotic state described in this disease.

O'Loughlin RE, Roberson A, Cieslak PR, et al: The epidemiology of invasive group A streptococcal infection and potential vaccine implications: United States, 2000-2004. *Clin Infect Dis* 2007;45(7):853-862.

Olsen RJ, Musser JM: Molecular pathogenesis of necrotizing fasciitis. *Annu Rev Pathol* 2010;5:1-31.

Wong CH, Wang YS: The diagnosis of necrotizing fasciitis. *Curr Opin Infect Dis* 2005;18(2):101-106.

38. c. Cat-scratch disease most often manifests as self-limiting, localized lymphadenitis in the draining site of a cat scratch; it typically affects children and young adults. Histologically, suppurative granulomas (stellate abscesses in epithelioid cell granulomas) are characteristic. The causative organism of cat-scratch disease, *B. henselae*, is also the cause of bacillary angiomatosis and bacillary peliosis, vascular diseases affecting the skin and the spleen, respectively. The initial site of infection is the skin, and patients may present with a papule. Disseminated disease develops in about 10% of infected patients. Liver, spleen, central nervous system, and bones have been reported to be involved.

Mogollon-Pasapera E, Otvos L Jr, Giordano A, et al: *Bartonella*: emerging pathogen or emerging awareness? *Int J Infect Dis* 2009;13(1):3-8.

Rolain JM, Chanet V, Laurichesse H, et al: Cat scratch disease with lymphadenitis, vertebral osteomyelitis, and spleen abscesses. *Ann N Y Acad Sci* 2003;990:397-403.

39. e. Enterohemorrhagic *E. coli*, serotype O157:H7, elaborates a Shiga-like toxin (verotoxin) that causes thrombocytopenia, hemolytic anemia, and nephropathy (hemolytic uremic syndrome) in approximately 15% of infected North American children. Colitis in this infection is predominantly right-sided. Biopsy specimens show either the typical features of an acute bacterial colitis with neutrophils and edema or superficial mucosal necrosis, resembling ischemic colitis or pseudomembranous colitis. Enteropathogenic *E. coli* is a major cause of seasonal and sporadic diarrhea, primarily in developing countries. It forms a choleralike toxin and is the main cause of traveler's diarrhea. Enteroaggregative *E. coli* causes acute and persistent pediatric diarrhea in both developing and developed countries, especially India. Enteroinvasive *E. coli* causes a dysenteric illness resembling shigellosis.

Pennington H: *Escherichia coli* O157. *Lancet* 2010;376(9750): 1428-1435.

40. e. Pneumonia is not a known presentation of parvovirus B19 infection. Most commonly, parvovirus B19 causes erythema infectiosum, also called "slapped cheek disease" because of its characteristic facial rash, or fifth disease, mainly in children. An erythematous rash of hands and feet, referred to as "gloves and socks syndrome," occurs in young adults. Arthritis caused by parvovirus B19 infection is more common in adults. The affinity of parvovirus B19 to

erythroid cells is the basis of hemolytic anemia and, in immunodeficient patients, of red blood cell aplasia. Parvovirus B19 is a single-stranded, nonenveloped DNA virus. Diagnostic intranuclear inclusion bodies can be seen in giant pronormoblasts in formalin-fixed and paraffin-embedded tissue sections but not in air-dried smears of bone marrow aspirates. Parvovirus B19–related hemophagocytic syndrome may occur in normal and immunodeficient individuals. Infection in pregnant women can lead to spontaneous abortion, hydrops fetalis, or stillbirth.

Krause JR, Penchansky L, Knisely AS: Morphologic diagnosis of parvovirus B19. A cytopathic effect easily recognized in air-dried, formalin-fixed bone marrow smears stained with hematoxylin-eosin or Wright-Giemsa. *Arch Pathol Lab Med* 1992;116(2):178-180.

Vafaie J, Schwartz RA: Parvovirus B19 infections. *Dermatology* 2004;43(10):747-749.

41. d. West Nile virus is a flavivirus that either causes subclinical disease or manifests as a febrile illness followed by changes in mental status. Overt disease is estimated to occur in 1 of 100 infected individuals. Clinical disease develops primarily in elderly patients, who also have an increased death rate compared with an overall mortality rate of 12% for all hospitalized patients. Animal reservoirs for the virus include wild and domestic birds. The vectors are mosquitoes. The virus is thought to have been introduced into the United States by an infected migratory or imported bird. In recent years, cases of blood transfusion–associated West Nile virus infection have prompted the implementation of routine polymerase chain reaction testing of all blood donors. Immunohistochemical studies can be used to demonstrate cells infected with West Nile virus.

Kilpatrick AM: Globalization, land use, and the invasion of West Nile virus. *Science* 2011;334(6054):323-327.

Tyler KL: West Nile virus encephalitis in America. *N Engl J Med* 2001;344(24):1858-1859.

42. e. *Hantavirus* infection has two distinct presentations: (1) hemorrhagic fever and renal syndrome, characteristically described in Europe and Asia, and (2) hantavirus pulmonary syndrome, originally described in the Americas but also reported in Europe. Vasculitis is not part of hantavirus pulmonary syndrome. The *Hantavirus* reservoir consists of rodents. The disease can be transmitted through inhalation of viral particles. *Hantavirus* antigens can be demonstrated by immunohistochemistry in microvasculature endothelial cells, follicular dendritic cells, macrophages, and lymphocytes. The disease generates a CD8$^+$ cytotoxic T-cell response. Histologically, endothelial cells may be swollen in hantavirus pulmonary syndrome, but the cells usually show no morphologic changes. Kupffer cells are hyperplastic and contain cellular debris. In particular, the number of immunoblasts is increased, and immunoblasts may be found in spleen, lymph nodes, and portal triads in the liver. The finding of immature lymphoid cells within vascular spaces is characteristic of hantavirus pulmonary syndrome.

Colby TV, Zaki SR, Feddersen RM, et al: Hantavirus pulmonary syndrome is distinguishable from acute interstitial pneumonia. *Arch Pathol Lab Med* 2000;124(10):1463-1466.

Snell NJ: Novel and re-emerging respiratory infections. *Expert Rev Anti Infect Ther* 2004;2(3):405-412.

Zaki SR, Greer PW, Coffield LM, et al: Hantavirus pulmonary syndrome. Pathogenesis of an emerging infectious disease. *Am J Pathol* 1995;146(3):552-579.

43. a. Ehrlichiosis is caused by tick-borne intracellular rickettsial bacteria, which infect primarily macrophages and granulocytes, but *Ehrlichia* organisms can also be identified within polymorphonuclear leukocytes, lymphocytes, and monocytes. Most cases occur in Texas and California during the summer season. Polymerase chain reaction and indirect fluorescent antibody tests can be used to diagnose ehrlichiosis. In tissue sections, the organism is best seen with Brown and Hopps stain. At autopsy, inflammatory infiltrates and morulae have been found in liver, spleen, kidney, heart, brain, and other organs. Infection occurs in immunocompetent and immunocompromised individuals—more frequently in the latter. Ehrlichiosis may coexist with other tick-borne diseases, such as Lyme disease and babesiosis.

Hamilton KS, Standaert SM, Kinney MC: Characteristic peripheral blood findings in human ehrlichiosis. *Mod Pathol* 2004;17(5): 512-517.
Rikihisa Y: *Anaplasma phagocytophilum* and *Ehrlichia chaffeensis*: subversive manipulators of host cells. *Nat Rev Microbiol* 2010; 8(5):328-339.

44. c. Rabies has decreased in incidence in the United States, and only one or two human cases are reported per year. Nonetheless, 15,000 to 40,000 people receive prophylaxis annually. In the United States, 29 confirmed human cases were reported during the period 2001 to 2011. In the United States, raccoons, skunks, bats, and foxes are primary reservoirs. Dogs remain the main reservoir in the developing world, where vaccination of dogs is rarely performed. In India and Sri Lanka, there are more than 3 cases of rabies per 100,000 persons per year. Cases of rabies transmitted through solid organ transplantation have been reported. When the virus reaches the brain, it can infect the cerebellum, Purkinje cells, hippocampus, and pontine nuclei. Histologically, characteristic viral inclusions in neuronal cells (Negri bodies) are a pathognomonic finding of rabies. After the virus reaches the central nervous system, it spreads in a centrifugal fashion to extraneural organs, such as salivary glands, gastrointestinal tract, and heart.

Blanton JD, Palmer D, Dyer J, et al: Rabies surveillance in the United States during 2010. *J Am Vet Med Assoc* 2011;239(6): 773-783.
Jackson AC, Ye H, Phelan CC, et al: Extraneural organ involvement in human rabies. *Lab Invest* 1999;79(8):945-951.
Rupprecht CE, Hanlon CA, Hemachudha T: Rabies re-examined. *Lancet Infect Dis* 2002;2(6):327-342.

45. c. Before the advent of HAART, toxoplasmic encephalitis affected 5% to 10% of U.S. patients with AIDS and about 25% of patients with AIDS in Europe, and although a significantly decreased incidence has been reported from many centers, it still occurs. The brain appears to be the first organ to lose immunity in patients with immunodeficiency of any kind. In disseminated infection, *T. gondii* may be demonstrated in virtually any organ. Preferential sites of infection besides the brain include retina, lungs, heart, and skeletal muscle. Lymphadenopathy, especially cervical lymphadenopathy, is the most common presentation of primary toxoplasmosis. It accounts for 3% to 7% of clinically significant lymphadenopathies. Neonatal toxoplasmosis may be acquired transplacentally from the infected mother; it manifests primarily in the brain and eyes.

Gray F, Chrétien F, Vallat-Decouvelaere AV, et al: The changing pattern of HIV neuropathology in the HAART era. *J Neuropathol Exp Neurol* 2003;62(5):429-440.
Innes EA: A brief history and overview of *Toxoplasma gondii*. *Zoonoses Public Health* 2010;57(1):1-7.
Kaye A: Toxoplasmosis: diagnosis, treatment, and prevention in congenitally exposed infants. *J Pediatr Health Care* 2011;25(6): 355-364.

46. d. KSHV is a member of the Herpesviridae family. This virus known to replicate in two different phases: latent and lytic phase. During the latent phase, the virus remains in episomes of Kaposi sarcoma cells for no more than 5 to 10 cell divisions. A small proportion of tumor cells enter the lytic phase, during which virion particles are produced and the virus is immortalized. During both latent and lytic phases, several viral proteins that are synthesized function as tumor promoters, resulting in cell division, inhibition of apoptosis, and angiogenesis. High KSHV viremia predicts a higher risk for the development of Kaposi sarcoma. In addition to Kaposi sarcoma and body cavity–related B-cell lymphoma, 50% of cases of the multicentric plasma cell type of Castleman disease are associated with KSHV. Most recently, an association with primary pulmonary hypertension has been reported. Burkitt lymphoma is related to EBV infection, not KSHV.

Cesarman E: Kaposi's sarcoma-associated herpesvirus—the high cost of viral survival. *N Engl J Med* 2003;349(12):1107-1109.
Gantt S, Casper C: Human herpesvirus 8-associated neoplasms: the roles of viral replication and antiviral treatment. *Curr Opin Infect Dis* 2011;24(4):295-301.

47. c. *T. whipplei*, the causative agent of Whipple disease, is a ubiquitous gram-positive bacterium that is classified as an actinomycete and is difficult to culture. Although Whipple disease was first described in 1907, it took almost 90 years to identify the causative organism. Identification was first accomplished by polymerase chain reaction; the organism was finally cultured in 2000. Whipple disease affects primarily white middle-aged men. Individuals who develop the disease are unable to degrade the bacterial organisms after they are phagocytized into macrophages. Defects in Th1-related immunity have been implicated in the susceptibility for the disease. Studies suggest that predisposed individuals express lower levels of interleukin 12 and interleukin 16.

Raoult D, Birg ML, La Scola B, et al: Cultivation of the bacillus of Whipple's disease. *N Engl J Med* 2000;342(2):620-625.
Schneider T, Moos V, Loddenkemper C, et al: Whipple's disease: new aspects of pathogenesis and treatment. *Lancet Infect Dis* 2008;8(3):179-190.

48. c. NTM are important environmental pathogens that can cause a broad spectrum of diseases. The number of infections and the number of new species as etiologic agents have markedly increased with the development of new diagnostic tools. In a study of granulomatous lesions, NTM accounted for 34% of mycobacteria identified by polymerase chain reaction. NTM is more commonly diagnosed in middle-aged and elderly women with or without a smoking history. Bronchiectasis is a known predisposing factor and is identified in a large subset of patients. NTM-induced hypersensitivity pneumonitis has been reported in patients with a previous diagnosis of lung disease and recent exposure to contaminated water sources (most commonly industrial reservoirs, hot tubs, and swimming pools). Three patterns of pulmonary disease have been described in NTM infections: (1) nodular disease, (2) patchy parenchymal consolidation, and (3) cavitary lesions. Pseudotumors and diarrhea secondary to intestinal infection were common in patients with AIDS before the advent of potent antiviral drugs. In recipients of solid organ transplants, the most common manifestations of NTM infection are cutaneous and pleuropulmonary diseases. NTM may also cause peritonitis in patients undergoing dialysis and pulmonary infections in patients with cystic fibrosis.

Beckett W, Kallay M, Sood A, et al: Hypersensitivity pneumonitis associated with environmental mycobacteria. *Environ Health Perspect* 2005;113(6):767-770.

Cook JL: Nontuberculous mycobacteria: opportunistic environmental pathogens for predisposed hosts. *Br Med Bull* 2010;96:45-59.

Schulz S, Cabras AD, Kremer M, et al: Species identification of mycobacteria in paraffin-embedded tissues: frequent detection of nontuberculous mycobacteria. *Mod Pathol* 2005;18(2):274-283.

49. b. Cysticercosis affects primarily the brain but can be found in various other locations including the orbit, spinal cord, and skeletal muscle. Cysticerci may remain viable for 10 years. Symptoms result from the mass effect or rupture of the cyst, evoking a brisk inflammatory response. At the time of diagnosis, the infection is usually several years old. The diagnosis of cysticercosis can be challenging, and guidelines suggesting the use of a combination of major and minor diagnostic criteria are available. The absolute criteria for the diagnosis of cysticercosis include identification of the parasite in tissue or direct funduscopic visualization of the parasite in the eye. The intensity of associated inflammation caused by the encysted cysticerci predicts the severity of symptoms. Taeniasis may be present in approximately 15% of patients with cysticercosis.

Hawk MW, Shahlaie K, Kim KD, et al: Neurocysticercosis. *Surg Neurol* 2005;63(2):123-132; discussion 132.

Sinha S, Sharma BS: Neurocysticercosis: a review of current status and management. *J Clin Neurosci* 2009;16(7):867-876.

50. d. *Acanthamoeba* trophozoites and cysts can be seen in corneal stroma, within phagocytic cells, or extracellularly. *Acanthamoeba* differ from other amebas by the marked variation in shape of trophozoites (round, pear-shaped, elongated) and the large (3 to 4 μm) targetlike nucleolus, also called a karyosome. The inflammatory reaction consists of mononuclear and multinucleated macrophages, few neutrophils and lymphocytes, and fibroblasts. *Acanthamoeba* can be isolated from water sources, including bottled water, dialysis machines, and air conditioning systems. These organisms are considered normal flora in some healthy individuals. Since the first case of *Acanthamoeba* keratitis was described in 1973, hundreds of cases have been diagnosed, mainly in contact lens users but also in patients with corneal trauma. Keratitis may be complicated by uveitis and meningoencephalitis.

Kaji Y, Hu B, Kawana K, et al: Swimming with soft contact lenses: danger of acanthamoeba keratitis. *Lancet Infect Dis* 2005;5(6):392.

51. e. *B. burgdorferi*, the causative agent of Lyme disease, is an elongated spirochete that stains best with silver stains, such as Steiner, Dieterle, and Warthin-Starry. The Steiner silver stain contains an additional incubation step with amylase, which allows for clearer delineation of organisms compared with other silver stains. The initial skin lesion of Lyme disease is a papule composed of a mixed inflammatory cell infiltrate, focal hemorrhage, and only rare spirochetes. Spirochetes are haphazardly distributed in the dermis, are mostly extracellular, and are often found around dermal blood vessels. Immunohistochemical studies are another diagnostic alternative for tissue samples that yield high sensitivity and specificity.

Aberer E, Duray PH: Morphology of *Borrelia burgdorferi*: structural patterns of cultured borreliae in relation to staining methods. *J Clin Microbiol* 1991;29(4):764-772.

Stanek G, Wormser GP, Gray J, et al: Lyme borreliosis. *Lancet* 2012;379(9814):461-473.

52. d. Fite-Faraco stain is a modified acid-fast stain first used to detect *Mycobacterium leprae* in tissues. It does not stain fungal organisms. Besides routine hematoxylin-eosin staining, the most commonly used methods to demonstrate fungal organisms are PAS and GMS, both of which stain the polysaccharide-rich fungal walls. A combination of PAS and GMS stains can be helpful in differentiating small budding yeast forms. Organisms showing weak PAS and strong GMS staining suggest a diagnosis of *Histoplasma* over *Candida* and *Blastomyces*, which show strong PAS positivity.

More specific methods can be used to stain a narrower number of organisms, such as alcian blue, which stains the mucoid capsule of *C. neoformans*. Gram stain is the most widely performed differential stain. It is based on chemical properties of cell walls of organisms. Gram-positive organisms have a thick peptidoglycan outer layer allowing for strong binding of crystal violet without removal by subsequent steps (gram-positive organisms stain dark blue or purple). Conversely, gram-negative organisms have a thin peptidoglycan layer covered by a lipopolysaccharide layer; in this case, crystal violet binds but is subsequently removed by the decolorizer and replaced by a counterstain dye (gram-negative organisms stain red or pink). Acid-fast stains detect long-chain fatty acids in the microorganism wall. These are present in only certain bacteria (e.g., most mycobacteria, *Legionella*, and *Nocardia*), protozoa (e.g., *Cryptosporidium*, *Isospora*), and the shell of some *Schistosoma* eggs (*S. mansoni* and *S. japonicum*). Warthin-Starry and Dieterle stains are silver-based methods used to identify spirochetes but are also known to stain some fungi, Donovan bodies, and *Legionella*.

Woods GL, Walker DH: Detection of infection or infectious agents by use of cytologic and histologic stains. *Clin Microbiol Rev* 1996;9(3):382-404.

53. c. Leishmaniasis is acquired through a sandfly bite. Organisms can be detected in peripheral blood monocytes and neutrophils and can potentially contaminate blood products. Transfusion-transmitted infections are most commonly viral (e.g., hepatitis A, B, and C; HIV; CMV). Infections with parasites (e.g., malaria, babesiosis, leishmaniasis) and cutaneous flora bacteria may also be transmitted through transfusions. Leishmaniasis is endemic along the Mediterranean shore and in West Africa, Mesopotamia, southern Russia, India, northern China, South and Central America, and Mexico.

Most leishmaniasis cases diagnosed in the United States result from increased traveling to endemic areas, either for tourism or for military missions. Numerous new cases have been reported among war veterans returning from Afghanistan and Iraq. Leishmaniasis can manifest in four forms: (1) cutaneous leishmaniasis, (2) visceral leishmaniasis, (3) mucocutaneous leishmaniasis, and (4) diffuse cutaneous leishmaniasis. Cutaneous leishmaniasis is the most common form. It is characterized by a large, hollow ulcer with raised borders. Localized disease can spread, especially in the head region, affecting mucosal surfaces (mucocutaneous leishmaniasis). Diffuse cutaneous leishmaniasis manifests as widespread skin nodules and occurs in individuals with a defective cell-mediated immune response to the *Leishmania* organisms, similarly to lepromatous leprosy. Leishmaniasis can also spread to multiple organs and cause visceral leishmaniasis, the most severe form of disease (kala-azar). Histologically, *Leishmania* amastigotes (known as Leishman-Donovan bodies) can be identified with Giemsa staining as multiple 2- to 4-μm round structures in the cytoplasm of macrophages or peripheral blood monocytes.

Berman JD: Human leishmaniasis: clinical, diagnostic, and chemotherapeutic developments in the last 10 years. *Clin Infect Dis* 1997;24(4):684-703.

Cardo LJ: *Leishmania*: risk to the blood supply. *Transfusion* 2006;46(9):1641-1645.

54. c. *Y. enterocolitica* are gram-negative coccobacilli associated with acute diarrhea. The disease is acquired through ingestion of contaminated water or food, most commonly pork, tofu, and milk. Most infections are centered in the terminal ileum and cecum. *Y. enterocolitica* infection is associated with suppurative, not caseating, granulomas. *Y. enterocolitica* replicate in the intestinal epithelium and may invade Peyer patches causing appendicitislike symptoms (pseudoappendicitis). It can also invade lymph nodes and rarely migrate to other organs. *Y. enterocolitica* are siderophilic bacteria. Individuals with iron overload, as seen in hereditary hemochromatosis, sickle cell anemia, and thalassemia, are at increased risk of infection. Histologically, *Y. enterocolitica* ileitis is characterized by lymphoplasmacytic inflammation and suppurative granulomas with multinucleated giant cells and neutrophilic microabscesses involving mainly the submucosa. *Yersinia* evades the immune system by inhibiting antigen presentation by dendritic cells. *Yersinia* injects its effector molecules within dendritic cells altering cells' actin cytoskeleton and the ability to phagocytize and present antigens.

Abdull Gaffar B: Granulomatous diseases and granulomas of the appendix. *Int J Surg Pathol* 2010;18(1):14-20.

Bedoui S, Kupz A, Wijburg OL, et al: Different bacterial pathogens, different strategies, yet the aim is the same: evasion of intestinal dendritic cell recognition. *J Immunol* 2010;184(5):2237-2242.

CHAPTER 20

PEDIATRIC AND PLACENTAL PATHOLOGY

Harsh M. Thaker and Jessica M. Comstock

Questions 1-21 refer to a photo or photomicrograph.

1. A 19-year-old gravida 0 woman presents to her obstetrician with vaginal bleeding. Her last menstrual period was 10 weeks ago. Pelvic examination reveals a 14-week-sized uterus. Ultrasound of the uterus shows cystic structures and no fetus. A dilatation and curettage is performed and a representative section is shown here. Ploidy analysis shows the submitted tissue to be diploid. All of the following are true in this condition EXCEPT:
   a. There is an increased risk of persistent or recurrent disease.
   b. There is an increased risk of malignant transformation.
   c. Molecular analysis typically reveals two sets of maternal chromosomes.
   d. Levels of a circulating gonadotropin are elevated.
   e. This condition is more prevalent in the Far East than in the United States.

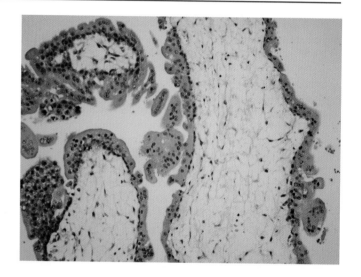

2. A 2-year-old boy presents with a solitary right testicular mass. The tumor is excised. On gross examination, a solid, soft tumor is identified that is 4 cm in the greatest dimension. A representative photograph is shown here. All of the following are true about this tumor EXCEPT:
   a. It is the most common testicular neoplasm in infants.
   b. Serum α-fetoprotein (AFP) levels are frequently elevated.
   c. Low-molecular-weight cytokeratin is frequently positive.
   d. Despite current therapies, the 5-year survival rate for children is less than 50%.
   e. Clinical stage is an important prognostic factor.

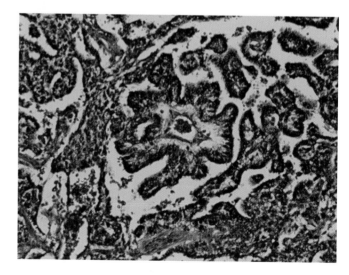

3. A 35-year-old gravida 4 para 3 woman presents with vaginal bleeding in the third trimester. A cesarean section is performed because of a disturbing fetal heart tracing. A gross photograph of the placenta is shown here. Which of the following is the diagnosis?
   a. Placenta previa
   b. Placental abruption
   c. Chorioamnionitis
   d. Placenta accreta
   e. Velamentous cord insertion

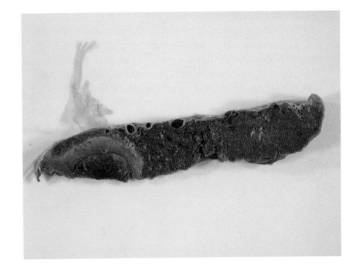

4. The condition depicted in this photomicrograph from the placental membranes of a 25-year-old patient is LEAST likely to be caused by which of the following organisms?
   a. Group B streptococcus
   b. *Escherichia coli*
   c. *Listeria*
   d. *Candida*
   e. *Cytomegalovirus* (CMV)

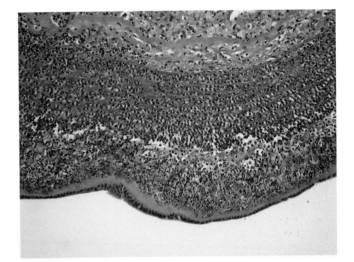

5. An 8-year-old girl presents to her physician with isosexual precocious puberty. Pelvic ultrasonography reveals a 10 × 6 × 6 cm mass in the right adnexa. A representative photomicrograph is shown here. All of the following are true about this entity EXCEPT:
   a. More than 75% of patients with this entity present with isosexual precocious puberty.
   b. In a small percentage of patients, this mass can rupture and cause hemoperitoneum.
   c. It is typically an aggressive and infiltrative lesion.
   d. It typically has a high cure rate.
   e. It is typically immunoreactive for inhibin.

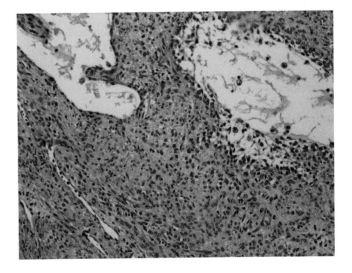

6. This photomicrograph is from a 12-year-old boy who presented with a diaphyseal mass of the left femur with extension into the surrounding soft tissue. The following immunostaining pattern was observed: positive for CD99 and FLI-1; negative for SMA, desmin, cytokeratin, WT1, and CD45. Which of the following is the MOST common translocation associated with this entity?
   a. t(x;18)
   b. t(11;22)
   c. t(21;22)
   d. t(2;13)
   e. t(1;13)

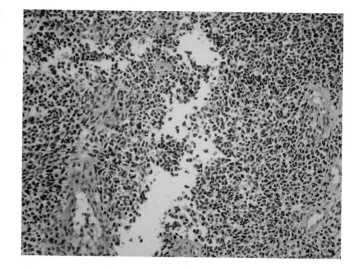

7. This photomicrograph is from a placenta of a 21-year-old woman with a neonate with intracranial calcification. Which of the following MOST likely caused this finding?
   a. Herpes simplex
   b. *Toxoplasma*
   c. CMV
   d. Varicella zoster
   e. *Treponema pallidum*

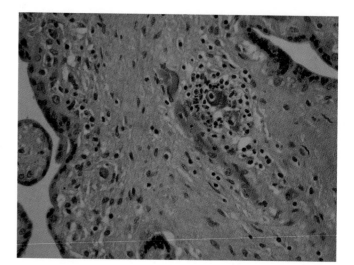

8. A 16-month-old infant is brought to her physician because her mother noticed an abdominal mass while bathing her. A computed tomography (CT) scan shows a large mass that compresses the upper pole of the right kidney. A biopsy of the mass is performed and a representative section is shown here. Which of the following statements is MOST characteristic of this tumor?
   a. *MYCN* gene amplification
   b. Translocation: t(11;22)
   c. WT-1 positivity
   d. Strap cells and myo-D1 positivity
   e. Translocation: t(X;18)

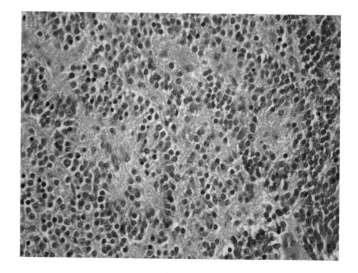

9. A 10-cm right-sided abdominal mass in a 2-year-old boy is resected. Grossly, a single, round mass is identified that is compressing the upper pole of the kidney. A representative section of the mass is shown here. Which of the following statements is TRUE?

   a. It has been reported to be bilateral in 50% of cases.
   b. The presence of diffuse anaplasia is not an important factor in predicting prognosis.
   c. Plasma levels of catecholamines and their metabolites are frequently elevated.
   d. It is associated with a t(12;15) translocation.
   e. WT-1 immunoreactivity is not required for the diagnosis.

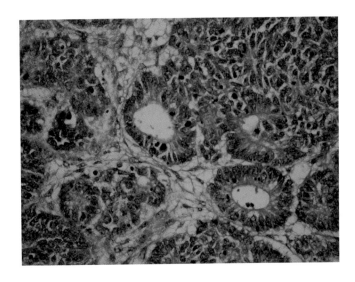

10. A polypoid mass arising from the vagina of a 3-year-old girl is resected. A desmin immunostain of a section of the mass with overlying vaginal mucosa is shown here. The cells are also positive for myo-D1. Cytogenetic analysis does not show a translocation involving the *FKHR* gene. Which of the following is TRUE about this entity?

   a. The prognosis is excellent with greater than 90% survival rate.
   b. S100 and HMB-45 immunostains are typically positive.
   c. Serum AFP is typically elevated.
   d. This entity is closely associated with diethylstilbestrol (DES) exposure in utero.
   e. Perineural invasion is common in this lesion.

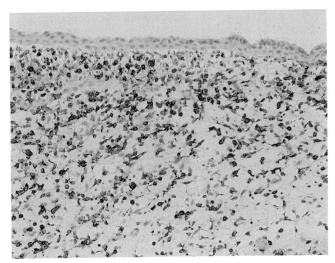

11. This gross photograph shows a placental lesion associated with a hydropic fetus. The diagnosis is:

   a. Choriocarcinoma
   b. Chorangioma
   c. Placental teratoma
   d. Placental infarct
   e. Intervillous thrombus

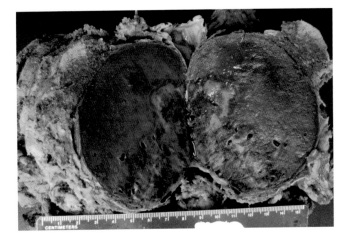

12. This gross photograph shows a right-sided view of a cardiac anomaly found in a 1-month-old child. The MOST likely cytogenetic abnormality in this child is:
   a. Autosomal trisomy
   b. Microdeletion on chromosome 22
   c. Monosomy X
   d. Unbalanced translocation
   e. Duplication of chromosome 22

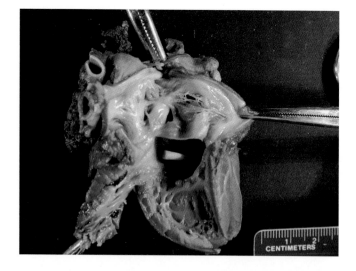

13. This photograph shows the fetal surface of a twin placenta in which the membrane separating the two sides has been stripped off to show the fused disk. Which of the following is LEAST likely to be true?
   a. The twins are discordant in size and hematocrit.
   b. The twins are concordant in size and hematocrit.
   c. The twins are discordant for gender.
   d. The twins are discordant for hydrops.
   e. The twins are the product of an in vitro fertilization (IVF) pregnancy.

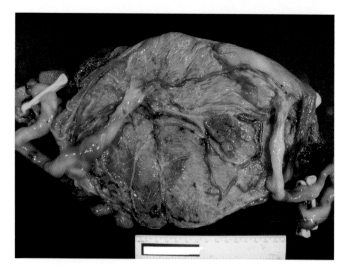

14. A 28-year-old gravida 3 para 2 mother presents with inevitable abortion at 18 weeks of gestation. This photograph shows a representative section of the placenta. Her serologic test is negative except for elevated *Toxoplasma* IgG titers. Which of the following is the MOST significant prior history in the acquisition of this infection?
   a. Recent exposure to a purified protein derivative (PPD)-positive individual
   b. Recent consumption of unpasteurized soft cheese
   c. Recent acquisition of two cats in the household
   d. Travel to endemic zones without malaria prophylaxis
   e. Drinking unfiltered water from a mountain stream

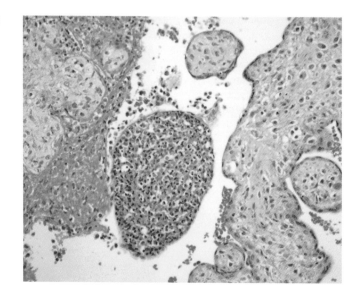

15. A 28-year-old gravida 3 para 2 mother presents with inevitable abortion at 18 weeks of gestation. A pale, hydropic fetus was delivered. This photograph shows a representative section of the placenta. The organism responsible for this abortion is:
   a. Polyomavirus
   b. Varicella zoster virus
   c. CMV
   d. Herpes simplex virus
   e. Parvovirus

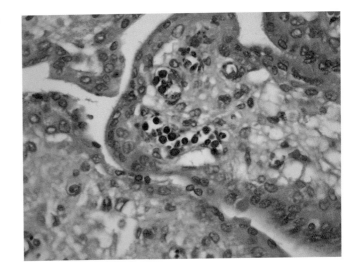

16. This photo shows INI-1 immunostain from a brain tumor in a 9-month-old infant. Which cytogenetic abnormality is associated with this tumor?
   a. Gain of chromosome 7 and loss of chromosome 10
   b. Isochromosome 17q
   c. Loss of 22q11.2
   d. Deletion of chromosome 22
   e. Hyperdiploidy

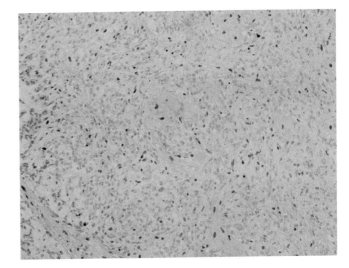

17. This photograph is from a liver mass in an 18-month-old child who was born large for gestational age with an omphalocele, and has macroglossia. Which of the following is TRUE?
   a. Cirrhosis is commonly seen with this tumor.
   b. Bone metastases are common.
   c. This tumor probably has loss of heterozygosity at 11p.
   d. Adenomatous polyposis coli (APC) screening should be performed on the child.
   e. Overall prognosis is poor.

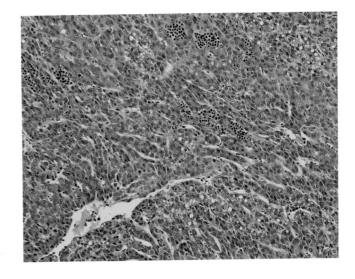

18. This picture is from an infant born near-term weighing 5630 g and with multiple anomalies, including cloacal dysgenesis. What is the MOST likely cause of these findings?
   a. Beckwith-Weidemann syndrome (BWS)
   b. Trisomy 21
   c. Eosinophilic leukemia
   d. Maternal diabetes
   e. Turner syndrome

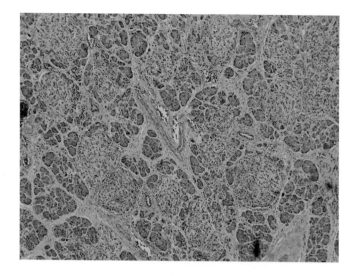

19. This photo is from the lung of a neonate born at 38 weeks' gestation. This finding is MOST consistent with:
   a. Intrauterine hypoxia
   b. Surfactant deficiency
   c. Acute pneumonia
   d. Multiple congenital anomalies
   e. Congenital cystic adenomatoid malformation

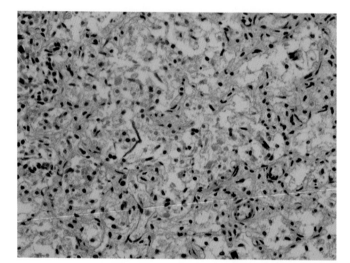

20. Which of the following is TRUE about this intraocular tumor?
   a. Patients with this tumor often develop second malignancies.
   b. The diagnosis is usually made histologically.
   c. Immunohistochemical staining is commonly performed.
   d. The most important prognostic indicator is the presence of metastases.
   e. Primary treatment is external beam radiation.

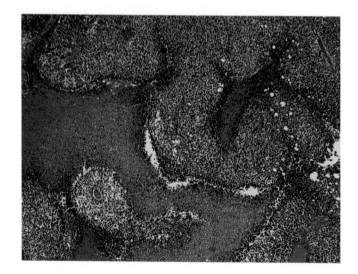

21. This 2-cm subcutaneous cystic mass in a 9-year-old boy is MOST likely a:
 a. Dermoid cyst
 b. Ruptured epidermal inclusion cyst
 c. Sebaceous adenoma
 d. Branchial cleft cyst
 e. Pilomatricoma

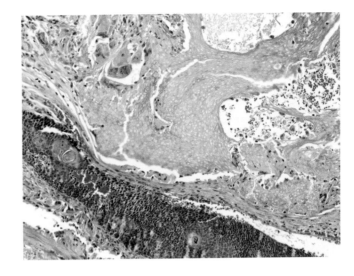

22. All of the following features favor the diagnosis of a partial rather than a complete hydatidiform mole EXCEPT:
 a. Presence of a malformed fetus
 b. Admixture of hydropic and nonhydropic villi
 c. Scalloped villous outlines and trophoblastic inclusions
 d. Nucleated red blood cells in villous vessels
 e. Diploid karyotype

23. The following statement is TRUE about choriocarcinoma:
 a. An intrauterine pregnancy is required for the development of this neoplasm.
 b. It arises from a hydatidiform mole in more than 90% of cases.
 c. It is characterized by malignant villi with anaplastic cytotrophoblast cells.
 d. It responds well to chemotherapy.
 e. Although it is locally invasive, distant metastasis is rare.

24. The MOST specific immunohistochemical marker to stain the Langerhans cell component of Langerhans histiocytosis is:
 a. S100
 b. CD45
 c. CD1a
 d. CD20
 e. CD68

25. Which of the following is FALSE about Hirschsprung disease?
 a. Obstruction is due to the absence of ganglion cells in the distal colon.
 b. 20% of infants with Hirschsprung disease have additional congenital anomalies.
 c. The disease occurs more frequently in men than in women.
 d. Contrast enema is diagnostic.
 e. Biopsy specimens should be taken at least 1.5 cm above the dentate line.

A NSWERS

1. c. This is a complete mole. Molecular analysis typically reveals two sets of paternal chromosomes (diploid). If incompletely removed there is a risk of recurrence, often as an invasive mole. There is a 2% risk of the development of choriocarcinoma with complete moles. Serum hCG (human chorionic gonadotropin) is typically markedly elevated and its levels are used in patient follow-up. For reasons that are unclear, complete moles are much more common in the Far East than in the United States.

Landolsi H, Missaoui N, Brahem S, et al: The usefulness of p57(KIP2) immunohistochemical staining and genotyping test in the diagnosis of the hydatidiform mole. *Pathol Res Pract* 2011;207(8):498-504.
Lurain JR: Gestational trophoblastic disease I: epidemiology, pathology, clinical presentation and diagnosis of gestational trophoblastic disease, and management of hydatidiform mole. *Am J Obstet Gynecol* 2010;203(6):531-539.
Pang YP, Rajesh H, Tan LK: Molar pregnancy with false negative urine hCG: the hook effect. *Singapore Med J* 2010;51(3):e58-61.

2. d. This picture shows a Schiller-Duval body seen in yolk sac tumor (YST). It is the most common testicular neoplasm in infants and children under 3 years of age. Serum AFP is

commonly elevated and a preoperative value is important to obtain in order to track disease progression, recurrence, and metastasis after treatment. YSTs are frequently strongly positive for low-molecular-weight cytokeratin and this feature can also help in the differential diagnosis. Clinical stage and degree of AFP elevation are prognostic indicators. Age at presentation is not as important a prognostic factor. The prognosis is generally favorable with current management, and the overall 5-year survival rate for children is around 90%.

Furtado LV, Leventaki V, Layfield LJ, et al: Yolk sac tumor of the thyroid gland: a case report. *Pediatr Dev Pathol* 2011;14(6): 475-479.
Maeda Y, Yoshikawa K, Kajiwara K, et al: Intracranial yolk sac tumor in a patient with Down syndrome. *J Neurosurg Pediatr* 2011;7(6):604-608.
Munghate GS, Agarwala S, Bhatnagar V: Primary yolk sac tumor of the common bile duct. *J Pediatr Surg* 2011;46(6):1271-1273.

3. b. The gross photograph shows a retroplacental blood clot with a surrounding area of infarction typical of placental abruption. Placental abruption should always be in the differential diagnosis of third trimester vaginal bleeding.

Typically it is associated with maternal abdominal pain and fetal distress. Maternal hypertension and preeclampsia are important predisposing factors. Placenta previa is an abnormally low implantation of the placenta, such that it impinges on the internal cervical os. Placenta accreta is a deficiency of decidua that results in an abnormally adherent placenta. Chorioamnionitis is an acute inflammation of the fetal membranes. Cord insertion is called velamentous when it attaches directly to the fetal membranes away from the placenta.

Aliyu MH, Salihu HM, Lynch O, et al: Placental abruption, offspring sex, and birth outcomes in a large cohort of mothers. *J Matern Fetal Neonatal Med* 2011;25(3):248-252.

Ananth CV, VanderWeele TJ: Placental abruption and perinatal mortality with preterm delivery as a mediator: disentangling direct and indirect effects. *Am J Epidemiol* 2011;174(1):99-108.

Melamed N, Aviram A, Silver M, et al: Pregnancy course and outcome following blunt trauma. *J Matern Fetal Neonatal Med* 2011;25(9):1612-1617.

4. e. This photo shows fetal membranes with a marked infiltrate of neurophils. The most important risk factor for the development of chorioamnionitis is prolonged rupture of membranes prior to delivery. Chorioamnionitis typically arises as an ascending infection, and the usual organisms are the ones present in the vagina. CMV, on the other hand, is a blood-borne infection that does not cause chorioamnionitis. Placental involvement with CMV may result in a histiocytic or plasmacytic villitis. *Listeria* is one organism that can infect the placenta via both the ascending and the hematogenous route.

Buhimschi IA, Buhimschi CS: Proteomics/diagnosis of chorioamnionitis and of relationships with the fetal exposome. *Semin Fetal Neonatal Med* 2012;17(1):36-45.

Dessardo NS, Mustać E, Dessardo S, et al: Chorioamnionitis and chronic lung disease of prematurity: a path analysis of causality. *Am J Perinatol* 2011;29(2):133-140.

Strunk T, Doherty D, Simmer K, et al: Histologic chorioamnionitis is associated with reduced risk of late-onset sepsis in preterm infants. *Pediatrics* 2012;129(1):e134-141.

5. c. The photomicrograph shows a juvenile granulose cell tumor (JGCT). These tumors typically present in females below the age of 30, and those who are prepubertal (50%) display isosexual precocious puberty in 80% of cases due to excess estrogen production by the tumor. Microscopically, this neoplasm consists of a solid population of granulosa cells and cystically dilated irregular immature follicles. These lesions typically have only rare Call-Exner bodies and rarely display nuclear grooving, in contrast to the adult-type granulosa cell tumor that commonly displays both of these features. Grossly, the lesion has areas of hemorrhage and necrosis, and in a small percentage of patients can rupture causing hemoperitoneum. JGCTs typically do not display aggressive or infiltrative behavior. They have a high cure rate and, when confined to the ovary, even those lesions with severe nuclear atypia and high mitotic rates have an excellent prognosis. Immunoreactivity for inhibin is typically positive.

Hashemipour M, Moaddab MH, Nazem M, et al: Granulosa cell tumor in a six-year-old girl presented as precocious puberty. *J Res Med Sci* 2010;15(4):240-242.

Oltmann SC, Fischer A, Barber R, et al: Pediatric ovarian malignancy presenting as ovarian torsion: incidence and relevance. *J Pediatr Surg* 2010;45(1):135-139.

Partalis N, Tzardi M, Barbagadakis S, Sakellaris G: Juvenile granulosa cell tumor arising from intra-abdominal testis in newborn: case report and review of the literature. *Urology* 2011; 79(5):1152-1154.

6. b. This photograph shows a cellular tumor composed of small round blue cells. The immunostaining pattern is most consistent with a Ewing sarcoma. The most common translocation associated with this entity is t(11;22), accounting for greater than 90% of Ewing sarcomas. This results in a fusion gene of EWS with FLI-1. The t(21;22) translocation is seen in a minority of Ewing sarcoma cases, resulting in a fusion gene of EWS with ERG. Of the other translocations, t(x;18) is seen in synovial sarcoma, and the two translocations involving chromosome 13—t(2;13) and t(1;13)—are associated with alveolar rhabdomyosarcoma.

Applebaum MA, Goldsby R, Neuhaus J, Dubois SG: Clinical features and outcomes in patients with Ewing sarcoma and regional lymph node involvement. *Pediatr Blood Cancer* 2011; 59(4):617-620.

Herrero-Martin D, Fourtouna A, Niedan S, et al: Factors affecting EWS-FLI1 activity in Ewing's sarcoma. *Sarcoma* 2011;2011: 352580.

Klijanienko J, Couturier J, Bourdeaut F, et al: Fine-needle aspiration as a diagnostic technique in 50 cases of primary Ewing sarcoma/ peripheral neuroectodermal tumor. Institut Curie's experience. *Diagn Cytopathol* 2012;40(1):19-25.

7. c. This photo shows a placental stem villous with a large cell containing a large, eosinophilic, cytoplasmic inclusion, with large intranuclear inclusion also. This is a characteristic CMV infection. Primary maternal infection in the first trimester can result in severe symptomatic infection in the fetus or neonate. There is almost no risk if primary infection occurs more than 6 months before contraception. The classic findings in the neonate with congenital CMV infection are chorioretinitis, microcephaly, and calcification of the cerebrum. However, most congenitally infected infants do not have any symptoms. CMV is one of the TORCH infections (along with toxoplasmosis, other agents, rubella, and herpes simplex virus [HSV]). Maternal primary CMV infection is often asymptomatic. CMV seropositivity in the United States is around 50%.

Din ES, Brown CJ, Grosse SD, et al: Attitudes toward newborn screening for cytomegalovirus infection. *Pediatrics* 2011; 128(6):e1434-1442.

Enders G, Daiminger A, Bäder U, et al: Intrauterine transmission and clinical outcome of 248 pregnancies with primary cytomegalovirus infection in relation to gestational age. *J Clin Virol* 2011;52(3):244-246.

Iwasenko JM, Howard J, Arbuckle S, et al: Human cytomegalovirus infection is detected frequently in stillbirths and is associated with fetal thrombotic vasculopathy. *J Infect Dis* 2011; 203(11):1526-1533.

8. a. The photomicrograph shows a neuroblastoma with small round blue cells arranged in typical Homer-Wright pseudorosettes, with fibrillary neuropil in the background. Although the clinical history might suggest a Wilms tumor, any abdominal mass that can grow to a large size in a small infant may be found this way. *MYCN* gene amplification is often seen in neuroblastoma, and imparts a poor prognosis when present. WT-1 positivity is typical for Wilms tumor and desmoplastic small round cell tumor, but is typically negative in neuroblastoma. Translocation t(11:22) is found in Ewing sarcoma, and t(X:18) is typical of synovial sarcoma. Strap cells and myo-D1 positivity are typical in rhabdomyosarcoma.

Okamatsu C, London WB, Naranjo A, et al: Clinicopathological characteristics of ganglioneuroma and ganglioneuroblastoma: a report from the CCG and COG. *Pediatr Blood Cancer* 2009; 53(4):563-569.

Shimada H: The international neuroblastoma pathology classification. *Pathologica* 2003;95(5):240-241.

Tornóczky T, Semjén D, Shimada H, Ambros IM: Pathology of peripheral neuroblastic tumors: significance of prominent nucleoli in undifferentiated/poorly differentiated neuroblastoma. *Pathol Oncol Res* 2007;13(4):269-275.

9. e. The photomicrograph shows a Wilms tumor, with all three characteristic components: blastema, tubules, and stroma. WT-1 is not expressed in all Wilms tumors and is not required to make the diagnosis. These tumors are bilateral in approximately 5% of patients. The presence of anaplasia, particularly when diffusely present, is an important predictor of prognosis, specifically the tumor's responsiveness to adjuvant therapy. Circulating catecholamines are elevated in patients with pheochromocytomas or neuroblastomas. The t(12;15) translocation is seen in mesoblastic nephroma.

Fernández-Pineda I, Cabello R, García-Cantón JA, et al: Fine-needle aspiration cytopathology in the diagnosis of Wilms tumor. *Clin Transl Oncol* 2011;13(11):809-811.

Hamilton TE, Shamberger RC: Wilms tumor: recent advances in clinical care and biology. *Semin Pediatr Surg* 2012;21(1):15-20.

Kieran K, Anderson JR, Dome JS, et al: Lymph node involvement in Wilms tumor: results from National Wilms Tumor Studies 4 and 5. *J Pediatr Surg* 2012;47(4):700-706.

10. a. Immunohistochemical stain for desmin shows positive cytoplasmic staining of tumor cells in this embryonal rhabdomyosarcoma. Note how there are more tumor cells just beneath the epithelium. The neoplasm arising in the vagina has an excellent prognosis (>90% survival rate). Embryonal rhabdomyosarcomas typically do not have translocations involving the *FKHR* gene; those are found in alveolar rhabdomyosarcoma. Option b is a feature of melanoma, option c of YST, and option d of clear cell carcinoma. Finally, option e is a feature of adenoid cystic carcinoma, which can arise from the Bartholin gland in this area.

Camboni M, Hammond S, Martin LT, Martin PT: Induction of a regenerative microenvironment in skeletal muscle is sufficient to induce embryonal rhabdomyosarcoma in p53-deficient mice. *J Pathol* 2012;226(1):40-49.

Jo VY, Mariño-Enríquez A, Fletcher CD: Epithelioid rhabdomyosarcoma: clinicopathologic analysis of 16 cases of a morphologically distinct variant of rhabdomyosarcoma. *Am J Surg Pathol* 2011;35(10):1523-1530.

Kikuchi K, Rubin BP, Keller C: Developmental origins of fusion-negative rhabdomyosarcomas. *Curr Top Dev Biol* 2011; 96:33-56.

11. b. The image shows a chorangioma. Histologically, this is essentially a hemangioma arising in the fetal villous blood vessels. Large chorangiomas, such as this, can cause significant fetal high-output cardiac failure and fetal hydrops, and can be seen on ultrasound. Small chorangiomas may be discovered as incidental findings during placental examination. They may be capillary, cavernous, cellular, angiomatous, degenerative, or atypical. Atypical chorangiomas are rare—characterized by increased cellularity and mitotic activity; variable nuclear atypia, necrosis, and solid areas—they may resemble sarcoma, but exhibit benign behavior.

Bagby C, Redline RW: Multifocal chorangiomatosis. *Pediatr Dev Pathol* 2011;14(1):38-44.

Gupta R, Nigam S, Arora P, et al: Clinico-pathological profile of 12 cases of chorangiosis. *Arch Gynecol Obstet* 2006; 274(1):50-53.

Mulliken JB, Bischoff J, Kozakewich HP: Multifocal rapidly involuting congenital hemangioma: a link to chorangioma. *Am J Med Genet A* 2007;143A(24):3038-3046.

12. a. The photograph shows a large, central septal defect that is composed of an atrial and a ventricular component. This is called an atrioventricular (AV) septal defect or an AV canal defect. Embryologically, this is a defect in the development of the "endocardial cushions." This is the characteristic cardiac defect seen in individuals with trisomy 21 (Down syndrome).

Monosomy X (Turner syndrome) is associated with left-sided obstructive lesions such as aortic coarctation. A chromosomal deletion on chromosome 22 (DiGeorge syndrome) is associated with conotruncal defects, such as tetralogy of Fallot. Unbalanced translocations can cause a variety of malformations. Chromosome 22 duplications are not associated with cardiac anomalies.

Jain R, Rentschler S, Epstein JA: Notch and cardiac outflow tract development. *Ann N Y Acad Sci* 2010;1188:184-190.

Lagendijk AK, Smith KA, Bakkers J: Genetics of congenital heart defects: a candidate gene approach. *Trends Cardiovasc Med* 2010;20(4):124-128.

Peal DS, Burns CG, Macrae CA, Milan D: Chondroitin sulfate expression is required for cardiac atrioventricular canal formation. *Dev Dyn* 2009;238(12):3103-3110.

13. c. The image shows a placenta composed on one large disk with two separate umbilical cords. The intervening membrane has been removed. Fetal plate vessels can be seen coursing directly from one umbilical cord insertion to the other. Barring rare exceptions, the presence of vascular anastomoses indicates that the placentation is monochorionic, which in turn almost always indicates that the twins are monozygotic, and, hence, they cannot be discordant for gender. When there are vascular anastomoses in a twin placenta, there is a risk of development of the "twin-twin transfusion syndrome" (TTTS), in which there is a net "transfusion" of blood from one twin to the other. The donor twin becomes pale and small, while the recipient twin becomes congested and may develop cardiac failure and hydrops; however, many vascular anastomoses are adequately balanced without a net transfusion of blood in either direction, and this can result in normal, concordant twins. The incidence of all twin gestations, including monochorionic twin gestations, is rising as a result of IVF.

Dias T, Contro E, Thilaganathan B, et al: Pregnancy outcome of monochorionic twins: does amnionicity matter? *Twin Res Hum Genet* 2011;14(6):586-592.

Morikawa M, Yamada T, Sato S, et al: Prospective risk of stillbirth: monochorionic diamniotic twins vs. dichorionic twins. *J Perinat Med* 2012;40(3):245-249.

Prats P, Rodríguez I, Nicolau J, Comas C: Early first-trimester free-β-hCG and PAPP-A serum distributions in monochorionic and dichorionic twins. *Prenat Diagn* 2012;32(1):64-69.

14. b. The photomicrograph shows severe acute villitis with villous destruction and microabscess formation in the placenta. These changes are typically seen in maternal *Listeria* infection, which is an important cause of second trimester abortion. It can also lead to premature delivery or stillbirth. The infection is often acquired by the mother from consumption of contaminated meat or unpasteurized dairy products. The placenta and fetus are infected via the hematogenous route. *Listeria* is most common in pregnant women, immunocompromised hosts, the elderly, and newborns.

Greenhow TL, Hung YY, Herz AM: Changing epidemiology of bacteremia in infants aged 1 week to 3 months. *Pediatrics* 2012;129(3):e590-596.

Lamont RF, Sobel J, Mazaki-Tovi S, et al: Listeriosis in human pregnancy: a systematic review. *J Perinat Med* 2011;39(3):227-236.

Pezdirc KB, Hure AJ, Blumfield ML, Collins CE: Listeria monocytogenes and diet during pregnancy; balancing nutrient intake adequacy v. adverse pregnancy outcomes. *Public Health Nutr* 2012;15(12):2202-2209.

15. e. Parvovirus infection, also known as fifth disease, or slapped-cheek syndrome due to the facial rash that develops, in a pregnant mother can result in transplacental infection of the fetus. The virus has a specific affinity for fetal erythroid precursors and results in severe fetal anemia, which can also cause hydrops. The placenta is usually very pale and edematous. Microscopic examination shows an increased number of intravillous nucleated red blood cells, many of which show characteristic glassy intranuclear viral inclusions. The appearance of these inclusions is reminiscent of the polyomavirus inclusions that are sometimes seen in urine cytologic specimens. About half of adults are parvovirus immune due to past infection.

Dijkmans AC, de Jong EP, Dijkmans BA, et al: Parvovirus B19 in pregnancy: prenatal diagnosis and management of fetal complications. *Curr Opin Obstet Gynecol* 2012;24(2):95-101.

Gervasi MT, Romero R, Bracalente G, et al: Viral invasion of the amniotic cavity (VIAC) in the midtrimester of pregnancy. *J Matern Fetal Neonatal Med* 2012;25(10):2002-2013.

Weiffenbach J, Bald R, Gloning KP, et al: Serological and virological analysis of maternal and fetal blood samples in prenatal human parvovirus b19 infection. *J Infect Dis* 2012;205(5):782-788.

16. c. Atypical teratoid/rhabdoid tumor (AT/RT) is a highly malignant tumor that affects infants and young children. It is uncommon in children over the age of 3 years. There is a male predominance. Median survival is less than 2 years. Loss of heterozygosity and mutation of the retained allele of a putative tumor suppressor gene *INI1(hSNF5/SMARCB1)* located on chromosome 22q11.2 is the defining molecular characteristic of AT/RT. AT/RT may be supratentorial or infratentorial. Histologically, AT/RT can mimic many different neoplasms. The rhabdoid cell should be seen, characterized by large nuclei with prominent nucleoli and eosinophilic cytoplasm. Because AT/RT can be histologically variable, it is a good idea to stain all brain tumors in young children with INI-1. The loss of nuclear reactivity for INI-1 is consistent with INI-1; however, it is not specific.

Loss of INI-1 can be seen in epithelioid sarcoma, renal medullary carcinoma, and some epithelioid MPNSTs. Luckily, these other tumors are not commonly in the differential diagnosis of AT/RT.

Bruggers CS, Bleyl SB, Pysher T, et al: Clinicopathologic comparison of familial versus sporadic atypical teratoid/rhabdoid tumors (AT/RT) of the central nervous system. *Pediatr Blood Cancer* 2011;56(7):1026-1031.

Hasselblatt M, Gesk S, Oyen F, et al: Nonsense mutation and inactivation of SMARCA4 (BRG1) in an atypical teratoid/rhabdoid tumor showing retained SMARCB1 (INI1) expression. *Am J Surg Pathol* 2011;35(6):933-935.

Schittenhelm J, Nagel C, Meyermann R, Beschorner R: Atypical teratoid/rhabdoid tumors may show morphological and immunohistochemical features seen in choroid plexus tumors. *Neuropathology* 2011;31(5):461-467.

17. c. Patients with familial adenomatous polyposis (FAP), a syndrome of early-onset colonic polyps and adenocarcinoma, frequently develop hepatoblastomas. It is estimated that 1 in 20 hepatoblastomas is probably associated with FAP. Loss of function mutations in APC lead to intracellular accumulation of the protooncogene β-catenin, an effector of Wnt signal transduction. β-Catenin mutations have been shown to be common in sporadic hepatoblastomas, occurring in as many as 67% of patients. Other components of the Wnt signaling pathway have also demonstrated a likely role for constitutive activation of this pathway in the cause of hepatoblastoma. Hepatoblastoma is usually diagnosed in children under the age of 3 years. It is very rare in adolescents or adults. Males are affected more often than females, and Caucasian children are most often affected. Patients with BWS should be screened for hepatoblastoma by having serum AFP tested every 3 months until at least 4 years of age. Also, AFP is a good marker for recurrence of disease. AFP testing should be interpreted with caution in neonates, who have a comparatively high AFP.

Krawczuk-Rybak M, Jakubiuk-Tomaszuk A, Skiba E, Plawski A: Hepatoblastoma in a 3-month-old infant with APC gene mutation—case report. *J Pediatr Gastroenterol Nutr* 2012;55(3):334-336.

Malogolowkin MH, Katzenstein HM, Meyers RL, et al: Complete surgical resection is curative for children with hepatoblastoma with pure fetal histology: a report from the Children's Oncology Group. *J Clin Oncol* 2011;29(24):3301-3306.

Meyers RL, Tiao GM, Dunn SP, Langham MR Jr: Liver transplantation in the management of unresectable hepatoblastoma in children. *Front Biosci* (Elite Ed) 2012;4:1293-1302.

18. d. Frequent findings in infants of diabetic mothers (IDMs) include nesidioblastosis (pictured), large for gestational age, and multiple congenital anomalies (of which cloacal dysgenesis is common). Three percent to 10% of all pregnancies are affected by abnormal glucose regulation (diabetes or impaired glucose tolerance). IDMs have an increased risk of growth abnormalities, respiratory distress, hypoglycemia, and congenital anomalies. If maternal blood glucose is tightly controlled, the risk of adverse events is markedly decreased (but is still increased over baseline). Nesidioblastosis generally refers to congenital hyperinsulinism with an abnormal microscopic appearance of the pancreas. If severe, near-total pancreatectomy may be needed (rare). Infants with BWS are large for gestation, but do not have nesidioblastosis. Infants with trisomy 21 are more likely to be small for gestational age and cloacal dysgenesis is an uncommon anomaly. Eosinophilic leukemia would be an incredibly rare diagnosis in a neonate. Infants with Turner syndrome do not get nesidioblastosis.

Delonlay P, Simon A, Galmiche-Rolland L, et al: Neonatal hyperinsulinism: clinicopathologic correlation. *Hum Pathol* 2007;38(3):387-399.

Rahier J, Guiot Y, Sempoux C: Morphologic analysis of focal and diffuse forms of congenital hyperinsulinism. *Semin Pediatr Surg* 2011;20(1):3-12.

Stanley CA: Hyperinsulinism in infants and children. *Pediatr Clin North Am* 1997;44(2):363-374.

19. a. This photo shows meconium and squamous cells in the airspaces. In utero meconium release is caused by fetal hypoxic stress. This stress can be caused by placental insufficiency, maternal hypertension or preeclampsia, maternal infection, oligohydramnios, maternal drug use, and other factors. Aspiration of meconium has four main effects: airway obstruction, surfactant dysfunction, chemical pneumonitis, and pulmonary hypertension. Meconium is composed of water, fetal intestinal epithelial cells, lanugos, mucus, and bile secretions. It is sterile, which differentiates it from stool. In utero meconium release is rare before 34 weeks of gestation. About 10% of infants born with meconium-stained amniotic fluid develop meconium aspiration syndrome. Meconium aspiration syndrome has a mortality rate of about 20%. Meconium reduces antibacterial activity of the amniotic fluid, increasing the risk of perinatal infection.

Fischer C, Rybakowski C, Ferdynus C, et al: A population-based study of meconium aspiration syndrome in neonates born between 37 and 43 weeks of gestation. *Int J Pediatr* 2012;2012:321545.

Jeng MJ, Soong WJ, Lee YS, et al: Meconium exposure dependent cell death and apoptosis in human alveolar epithelial cells. *Pediatr Pulmonol* 2010;45(8):816-823.

Vivian-Taylor J, Sheng J, Hadfield RM, et al: Trends in obstetric practices and meconium aspiration syndrome: a population-based study. *BJOG* 2011;118(13):1601-1607.

20. a. This photo shows a small round cell tumor with extensive necrosis, which is representative of retinoblastoma. Retinoblastoma is associated with the development of osteosarcoma, various soft tissue sarcomas, malignant melanoma, various carcinomas, leukemia and lymphoma, and various brain tumors. The diagnosis of retinoblastoma is most often made by radiologic examination and clinical presentation. An intraocular tumor with calcification is diagnostic. There is no specific immunohistochemical stain for retinoblastoma. Hematoxylin-eosin is all that is usually needed, though occasionally immunohistochemical stains may be helpful to rule out other tumors. In retinoblastoma, poor prognosis is indicated by extraocular extension, via growth directly through the sclera, or by extension through the optic nerve. Treatment with external beam radiation has numerous side effects, including midface hypoplasia and increased risk of second cancers. Currently, primary treatment is

chemotherapy, and surgical enucleation if there is no hope of preserving vision in the eye.

Chawla B, Sharma S, Sen S, et al: Correlation between clinical features, magnetic resonance imaging, and histopathologic findings in retinoblastoma: a prospective study. *Ophthalmology* 2012;119(4):850-856.

de Oliveira Reis AH, de Carvalho IN, de Sousa Damasceno PB, et al: Influence of MDM2 and MDM4 on development and survival in hereditary retinoblastoma. *Pediatr Blood Cancer* 2012;59(1):39-43.

Dommering CJ, Marees T, van der Hout AH, et al: RB1 mutations and second primary malignancies after hereditary retinoblastoma. *Fam Cancer* 2012;11(2):225-233.

21. e. The image shows pilomatricoma. Characteristic microscopic features of the lesion seen in this figure are blue "basaloid" cells with dark nuclei, pink "shadow" cells with no nuclei, keratin, and foreign body giant cells. The lesion can also show dystrophic calcification in varying amounts. There is a histologic resemblance to hair follicle and matrix, hence the name of this lesion. A dermoid cyst would show well-organized keratinizing squamous epithelium with dermal appendages. A ruptured epidermal inclusion cyst would have epidermis and keratin, but would lack the characteristic "shadow cells" seen here. The pale pink epithelium seen in this picture should not be confused with sebaceous differentiation. A branchial cleft cyst may take numerous forms depending on the site; those around the ear may have the appearance of epidermal or dermal inclusion cysts and, therefore, mimic this tumor.

Hamahata A, Kamei W, Ishikawa M, et al: Multiple pilomatricomas in Kabuki syndrome. *Pediatr Dermatol* 2013;30(2):253-255.

Price HN, Zaenglein AL: Diagnosis and management of benign lumps and bumps in childhood. *Curr Opin Pediatr* 2007;19(4):420-424.

Yencha MW: Head and neck pilomatricoma in the pediatric age group: a retrospective study and literature review. *Int J Pediatr Otorhinolaryngol* 2001;57(2):123-128.

22. e. Most partial hydatidiform moles are characterized by a triploid karyotype with two sets of chromosomes from the father and one set from the mother (e.g., 69, XXY). Most complete moles are diploid, with both sets of chromosomes of paternal origin. As a rule, a complete mole is not accompanied by a fetus. The presence of a fetus or evidence of fetal development (e.g., nucleated red blood cells) indicates a partial mole. Complete moles are characterized by diffuse, concentric, trophoblastic proliferation with central cisterns, but partial moles have polar trophoblastic proliferation that results in characteristic scalloped villous outlines and trophoblast (pseudo) inclusions. As the name suggests, a partial mole is typically composed of two populations of villi, with only some villi being "molar" (i.e., hydropic).

Murphy KM, Descipio C, Wagenfuehr J, et al: Tetraploid partial hydatidiform mole: a case report and review of the literature. *Int J Gynecol Pathol* 2012;31(1):73-79.

Sundari MS, Agarwal P, Mohan J: Triplet pregnancy with partial hydatiform mole. *J Indian Med Assoc* 2011;109(2):116-117.

Vang R, Gupta M, Wu LS, et al: Diagnostic reproducibility of hydatidiform moles: ancillary techniques (p57 immunohistochemistry and molecular genotyping) improve morphologic diagnosis. *Am J Surg Pathol* 2012;36(3):443-453.

23. d. Choriocarcinoma is a malignancy derived from trophoblastic cells. It has typical biphasic histologic appearance, with alternating sheets of malignant cytotrophoblast and syncitiotrophoblast cells; however, unlike hydatidiform moles, the trophoblast cells do not normally form villi. Choriocarcinoma is frequently associated with metastasis. It can arise in extrauterine sites in association with, or following, ectopic pregnancy. Serum β-hCG levels are typically very high. Only about half of all choriocarcinomas arise from hydatidiform moles; the rest are associated with nonmolar abortions or even normal pregnancies.

Goldstein DP, Berkowitz RS: Current management of gestational trophoblastic neoplasia. *Hematol Oncol Clin North Am* 2012; 26(1):111-131.

Hoffner L, Surti U: The genetics of gestational trophoblastic disease: a rare complication of pregnancy. *Cancer Genet* 2012;205(3):63-77.

Joneborg U, Papadogiannakis N, Lindell G, Marions L: Choriocarcinoma following ovarian hydatidiform mole: a case report. *J Reprod Med* 2011;56(11-12):511-514.

24. c. Langerhans cell histiocytosis (histiocytosis X, eosinophilic granuloma, Hand-Schuller-Christian disease, Letterer-Siwe disease) is clinically diverse and can have local or generalized symptoms. Histologically, the common feature is a proliferation of Langerhans-type histiocytes accompanied by a mixed inflammatory component. Approximately 85% of cases occur before age 30 and 60% occur before age 10. Prognosis is excellent for single-focus disease. Common sites include skin, bone, liver, and lung. CD1a positivity in the Langerhans cells is specific for this disorder. Although the Langerhans cells typically stain for S100 as well, it is not always positive and is not specific for this disorder. CD45 is a generalized lymphoid marker. CD20 is a B-cell marker.

CD68 is a histiocytic marker but is not specific for this entity.

Garabedian L, Struyf S, Opdenakker G, et al: Langerhans cell histiocytosis: a cytokine/chemokine-mediated disorder? *Eur Cytokine Netw* 2011;22(3):148-153.

Hawkes CP, Bourke JF, Fitzgibbon J, Dempsey EM: A disappearing neonatal skin lesion. *Eur J Pediatr* 2011;170(10):1353-1354.

Venkatramani R, Rosenberg S, Indramohan G, et al: An exploratory epidemiological study of Langerhans cell histiocytosis. *Pediatr Blood Cancer* 2012;59(7):1324-1326.

25. d. In patients with Hirschsprung disease ganglion cells are absent, leading to a marked increase in extrinsic intestinal innervation. This leads to contraction of the smooth muscle and functional obstruction. Approximately 20% of infants will have one or more associated abnormalities involving the neurologic, cardiovascular, urologic, or gastrointestinal system. Hirschsprung is also common in trisomy 21. The male-female ratio is approximately 4:1. Although contrast enema is useful, full-thickness rectal biopsy is the gold standard for diagnosis. Up to 25% of barium enemas will not show a transition zone. There is a physiologic aganglionic zone just proximal to the dentate line. Biopsies taken too low can produce a false-positive diagnosis of Hirschsprung disease.

Jia H, Zhang K, Chen Q, et al: Downregulation of Notch-1/ Jagged-2 in human colon tissues from Hirschsprung disease patients. *Int J Colorectal Dis* 2012;27(1):37-41.

Kapur RP, Reed RC, Finn LS, et al: Calretinin immunohistochemistry versus acetylcholinesterase histochemistry in the evaluation of suction rectal biopsies for Hirschsprung disease. *Pediatr Dev Pathol* 2009;12(1):6-15.

Yin H, Boyd T, Pacheco MC, et al: Rectal biopsy in children with Down syndrome and chronic constipation: Hirschsprung disease vs. non-Hirschsprung disease. *Pediatr Dev Pathol* 2012;15(2):87-95.

CHAPTER 21

FORENSIC PATHOLOGY

Jon J. Smith

QUESTIONS

Questions 1-38 refer to a photo or photomicrograph.

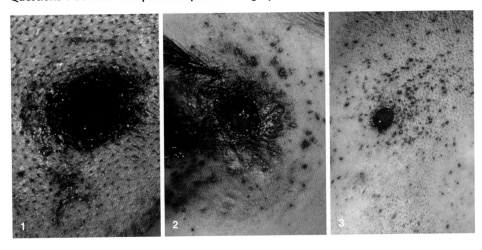

1. Match the entrance gunshot wounds shown in the image to the
   correct range of fire.
   a. 1, close; 2, contact; 3, intermediate
   b. 1, close; 2, intermediate; 3, distant
   c. 1, contact; 2, close; 3, intermediate
   d. 1, intermediate; 2, close; 3, distant
   e. 1, contact; 2, close; 3, distant

2. The gunshot wound shown in the image is BEST classified as:
   a. Contact
   b. Close range
   c. Intermediate range
   d. Distant range
   e. Exit

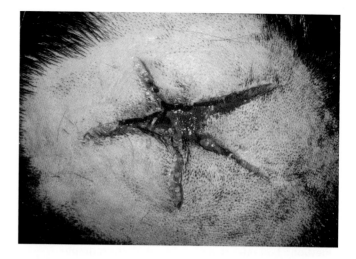

3. What is the range of fire of the shotgun wound shown in the image?
   a. Contact
   b. Less than 1 ft (30 cm)
   c. 2 to 3 ft (60 cm to 1 m)
   d. More than 9 to 10 ft (27 to 30 m)
   e. Cannot be determined

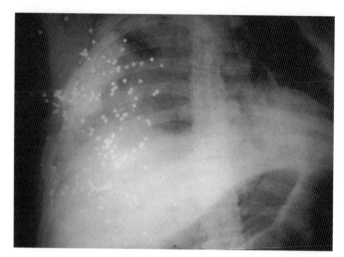

4. What type of injury is the scalp injury shown in the image?
   a. Laceration
   b. Stab
   c. Contusion
   d. Incision
   e. Abrasion

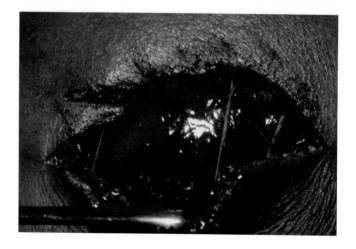

5. What type of injury is the chest wound depicted in the image?
   a. Laceration
   b. Stab wound
   c. Contusion
   d. Blunt force injury
   e. Abrasion

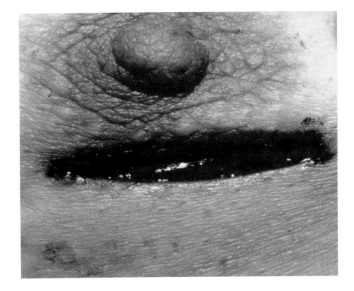

6. What is the manner of death shown in the image?
   a. Exsanguination owing to incisions
   b. Homicide
   c. Suicide
   d. Air embolism
   e. Therapeutic infection

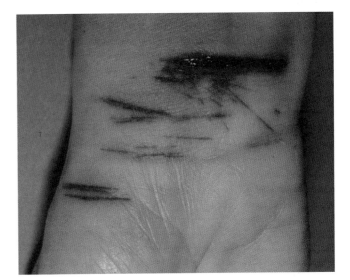

7. The findings depicted in the image are most consistent with:
   a. Descent from a height
   b. Pedestrian struck by a motor vehicle
   c. Torture
   d. Gunshot wounds
   e. Decomposition changes

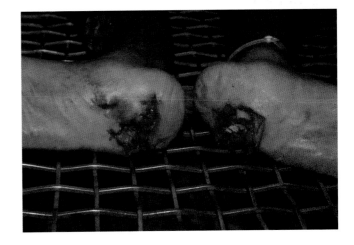

8. The hemorrhages shown in the image may be caused by all of the following EXCEPT:
   a. Manual strangulation
   b. Aggressive resuscitation
   c. Violently shaking an infant
   d. A neck ligature with only venous occlusion
   e. Vigorous Valsalva maneuver

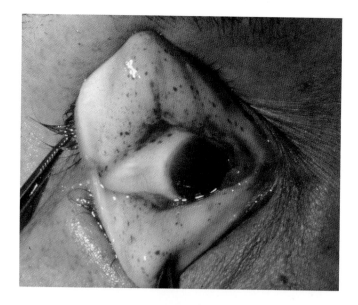

9. All of the following statements about the finding shown in the image are correct EXCEPT:
   a. In adults, it is never accidental.
   b. It may be consistent with ligature strangulation.
   c. The decedent probably has a history of depression.
   d. In young children, it is never accidental.
   e. It is consistent with hanging.

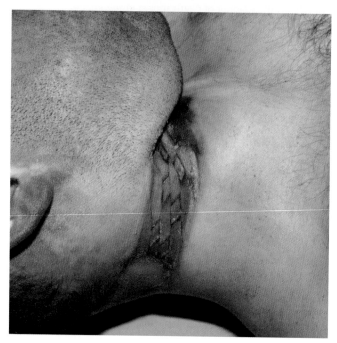

10. The abdominal radiograph shown was obtained from a person who was found dead in a motel room near JFK airport, New York. What is the MOST likely cause of death?
    a. Pulmonary embolism
    b. Diverticulitis
    c. Colon cancer
    d. Acute intoxication
    e. Accident

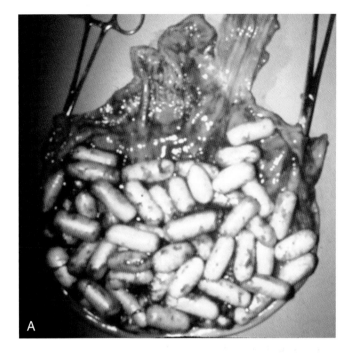

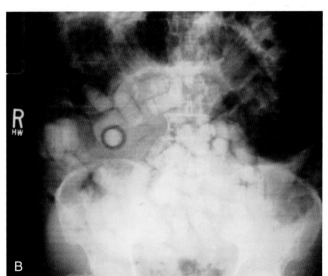

11. What does the photograph demonstrate?
    a. Algor mortis
    b. Rigor mortis
    c. Livor mortis
    d. Putrefaction
    e. First-degree thermal injury

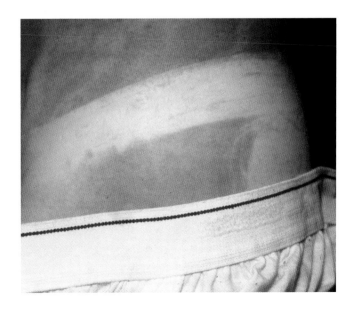

12. What is the postmortem change depicted in the image?
   a. Autolysis
   b. Adipocere formation
   c. Mummification
   d. Algor mortis
   e. Mold formation

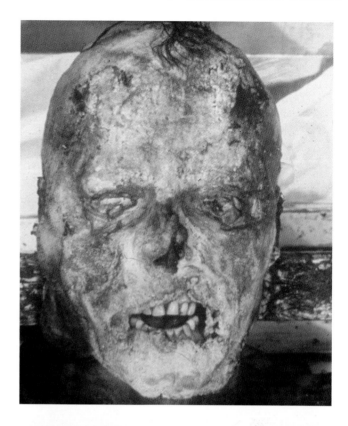

13. What is the diagnosis?
   a. Blunt impact of the eye ("black eye")
   b. Postmortem artifact (tache noire)
   c. Ocular melanoma in situ
   d. Acute thallium poisoning
   e. Neck compression

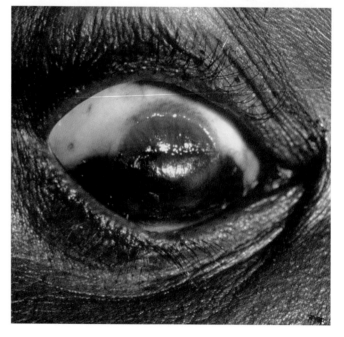

14. What is the diagnosis?
    a. Subarachnoid hemorrhage
    b. West Nile virus encephalitis
    c. Acute bacterial meningitis
    d. Putrefaction
    e. Cerebral anthrax

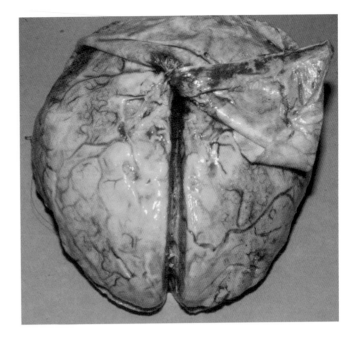

15. What caused the patterned injuries depicted in the image?
    a. Knife
    b. Rock
    c. Police baton
    d. Hammer
    e. Butt of a gun

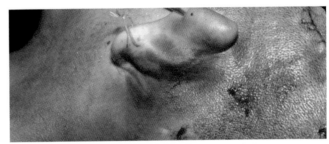

16. All of the following statements regarding the finding shown in the image are correct EXCEPT:
    a. This person was alive in a fire.
    b. This person typically would have an elevated carboxyhemoglobin.
    c. This is a sign of smoke inhalation.
    d. This person may have thermal injury.
    e. This person aspirated following a charcoal gastric lavage.

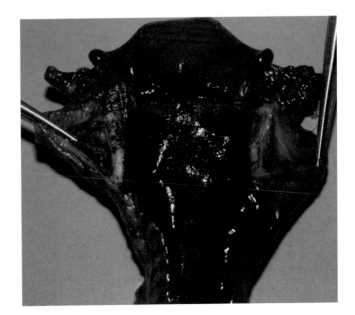

17. A 34-year-old man with a history of mitral valve prolapse was found dead in his living room. At autopsy, he was 6 ft 3 in (1.90 m) tall and weighed 182 lb (81 kg). He had a pectus excavatum, arachnodactyly, and moderate scoliosis. What is the diagnosis?

a. Ruptured myocardial infarct owing to atherosclerosis
b. Chordal rupture owing to mitral valve prolapse
c. Aortic dissection owing to fibrillin mutation
d. Ruptured myocardium owing to resuscitation artifact
e. Commotio cordis owing to blunt force injury of the chest

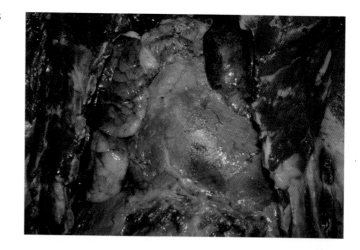

18. A 32-year-old man with a history of depression jumps off the Brooklyn Bridge in New York into the East River and submerges. At autopsy, no injuries are found; however, the photograph demonstrates one finding. His toxicology is positive for fluoxetine (an antidepressant medication). What is the manner of death?

a. Drowning
b. Accident
c. Suicide
d. Undetermined
e. Acute fluoxetine intoxication

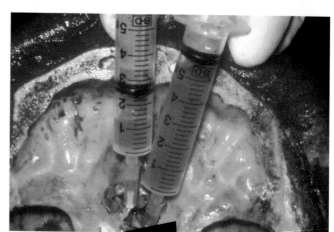

19. Immunohistochemical staining for β-amyloid precursor protein as shown in the image is used in the evaluation of:

a. Sudden cardiac death
b. Plasmacytomas
c. Myocarditis
d. Axonal injury
e. End-stage kidney disease

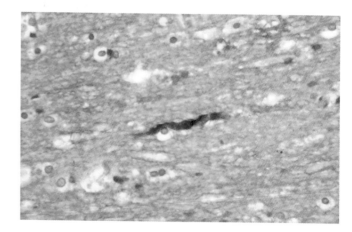

20. What is the range of fire?
    a. Cannot be determined because this is an exit wound
    b. Distant
    c. Intermediate
    d. Close
    e. Contact

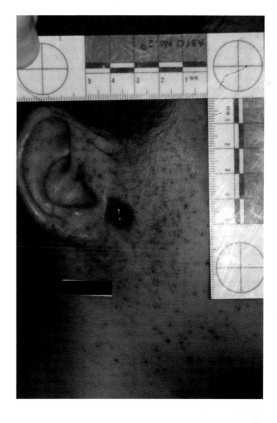

21. A 45-year-old man collapses in front of his wife, who immediately initiates cardiopulmonary resuscitation. Paramedics are summoned, and the man is transported to the hospital. After many attempts at resuscitation, the man dies within 1 hour of the onset of his symptoms owing to irreversible ventricular fibrillation. The photomicrograph is a representative section of the heart. Which one of the following conditions is associated with an acquired form of long QT syndrome?
    a. Liquid protein diets
    b. Atherosclerosis
    c. Wolff-Parkinson-White syndrome
    d. Jervell and Lange-Nielsen syndrome
    e. Romano-Ward syndrome

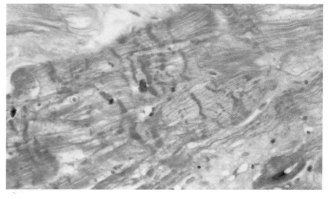

22. How would the lesion depicted in the photograph aid the
    pathologist?
    a. The lesion depicts a stab wound of the calvaria that could be
       used for tool mark identification.
    b. The lesion depicts an exit gunshot wound and would aid in
       projectile trajectory determination.
    c. The lesion depicts multiple fractures caused by a blunt force
       object impacting the head.
    d. The lesion depicts a cavity lesion associated with multiple
       myeloma.
    e. The lesion depicts an entrance gunshot wound and would
       aid in determining the projectile trajectory.

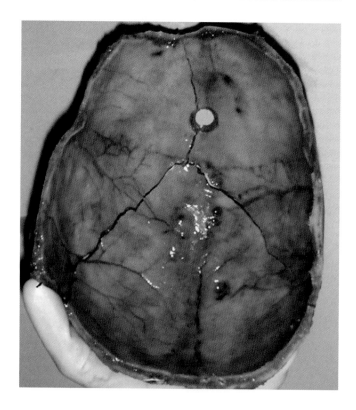

23. The photomicrograph of a representative area of the pyramidal
    neurons of the hippocampus is from a 29-year-old man who
    overdosed on heroin and died after several hours. What
    complication of the acute intoxication did this man
    experience?
    a. Hemorrhagic ischemic infarct
    b. Viral encephalitis
    c. Acute anoxic-ischemic encephalopathy
    d. État criblé
    e. État lacunaire

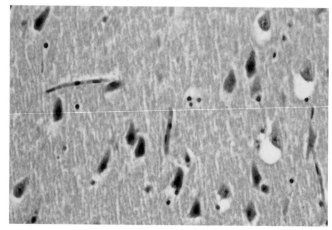

24. Two 21-year-old men were involved in a motor vehicle collision after being seen leaving a house party together in the same vehicle. The men were not wearing seatbelts, and both were ejected during a rollover collision that followed the loss of control of the speeding vehicle around a bend in the road. Both men were legally intoxicated with ethanol. The families of both men want to sue each other for wrongful death caused by driving under the influence. The photograph depicts a part of the face of one of the victims. What are you able to tell the family of this decedent?

- **a.** He was not driving the vehicle.
- **b.** He was driving the vehicle and caused the accident.
- **c.** He was driving the vehicle but did not cause the accident.
- **d.** He was not driving the vehicle, but he caused the accident.
- **e.** He was driving the vehicle.

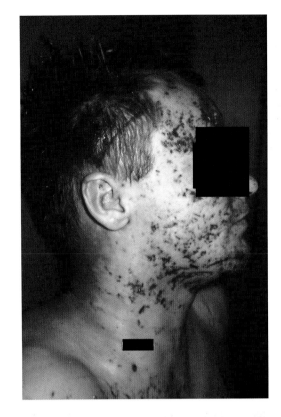

25. A 35-year-old man falls off a ladder while painting his house. He is taken to the hospital where a computed tomography (CT) scan of the head reveals subdural and subarachnoid hemorrhages without a skull fracture. The man does not regain consciousness and dies within hours of admission. At autopsy, a fracture of the skull base is identified. What type of fracture is demonstrated in the photograph?

- **a.** LeFort I
- **b.** LeFort II
- **c.** Hinge I
- **d.** Hinge II
- **e.** Hinge III

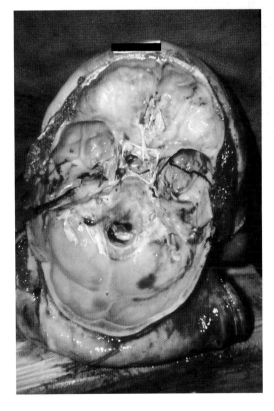

26. A 65-year-old woman with a known history of chronic alcoholism is found dead in her apartment. Her body was discovered after she had not been heard walking around for 1 day. At autopsy, her liver is yellow and waxy. No other pathologic process is identified that could explain her sudden death. A representative section of her liver is shown in the photomicrograph. What would her serum sodium level most likely be?

   a. 105 mEq/L
   b. 139 mEq/L
   c. 155 mEq/L
   d. Unable to determine because of the postmortem interval
   e. Unable to analyze postmortem blood for sodium levels

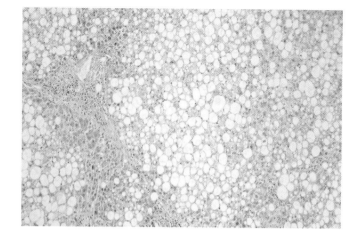

27. A full-term male infant was delivered to a 24-year-old woman, gravida 1, para 0, in the hospital. The infant was in significant distress and died 45 minutes after birth in his mother's arms with her husband and nurses present. A whole body radiograph of the infant is shown. What is the next most appropriate step to take after completion of the autopsy?

   a. Contact child protective services because physical abuse resulted in death
   b. Counsel the obstetrician to send the mother to a substance detoxification center because of substance abuse during pregnancy
   c. Counsel the family this is a nonheritable sporadic congenital deformation that will not affect future pregnancies
   d. Counsel the obstetrician to recommend sterilization of the father to prevent future paternal genetic malformations
   e. Contact the local police agency to investigate the physical abuse sustained by the mother during pregnancy that caused this malformation

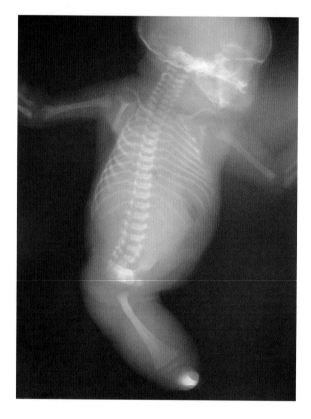

28. An 88-year-old woman was found dead in her bed. Positive findings at autopsy included significant atherosclerosis of the coronary arteries; a well-circumscribed, firm, 4-cm white mass within the left breast; right lung consolidation with expressible purulent yellow exudates from the bronchioles; diffuse nodularity of the fibrotic liver; moderate symmetric cerebral atrophy; and the lesion depicted in the photograph. What is the cause of death?
   a. Bilateral subdural hematomas
   b. Bacterial lobar pneumonia
   c. Hepatic cirrhosis
   d. Acute myocardial infarct
   e. Metastatic breast adenocarcinoma

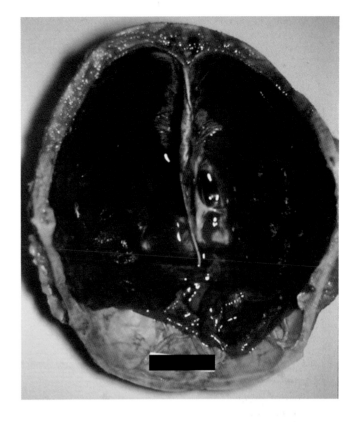

29. What is the MOST probable cause of the injury to the brain depicted in the photograph?
   a. *Taenia solium* infection
   b. Basilar skull fracture
   c. Incision
   d. Stab wound
   e. Gunshot wound

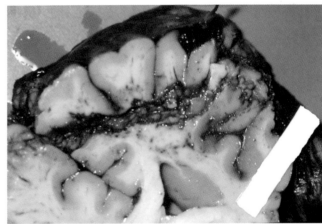

30. What is the manner of death depicted in the photograph?
   a. Homicide
   b. Suicide
   c. Accident
   d. Natural
   e. Undetermined

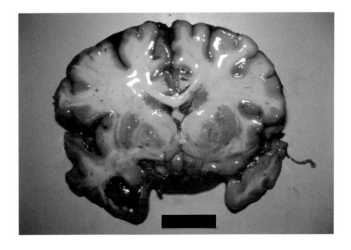

31. A 44-year-old woman was found dead at a friend's home after attending a party. Given the only significant finding photographed at autopsy of this woman, what is the MOST likely cause of death?
    a. Respiratory depression secondary to γ-hydroxybutyrate intoxication
    b. Pneumonia complicating long-term steroid use for atopy
    c. Electrolyte abnormalities secondary to bulimia
    d. Cardiac dysrhythmia secondary to acute cocaine intoxication
    e. Respiratory depression secondary to oxycodone intoxication

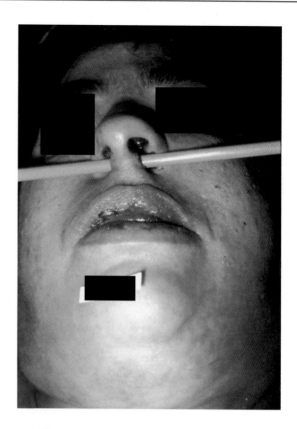

32. The lesion shown in the photograph is classic for which of the following?
    a. Cause of a bullet embolus
    b. Stab wound of the chest
    c. Motor vehicle collision
    d. Marfan syndrome
    e. Hanging

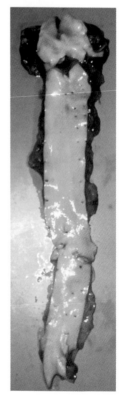

33. A 16-year-old girl developed nonsustained ventricular tachycardia and syncope. She was given beta blockers, and over the course of the next few years she developed left ventricular cardiomyopathy. At 19 years of age, she was found dead in her bed by her parents with whom she lived when she failed to get up for school. At autopsy, a multicystic tumor was noted within the cardiac conduction system, specifically in the area of the atrioventricular node. A representative section of the tumor is shown in the photomicrograph. Which of the following statements regarding this lesion is NOT correct?

    a. It may result in complete heart block.
    b. It is an embryologic malformation that occurs during atrioventricular node.
    c. It is an autosomal dominant genetic defect with incomplete penetrance.
    d. It is a pericardial remnant that migrates with the atrioventricular node following its invagination from the posterior wall of the heart in utero.
    e. Based on immunoperoxidase staining properties, it is not a true mesothelioma.

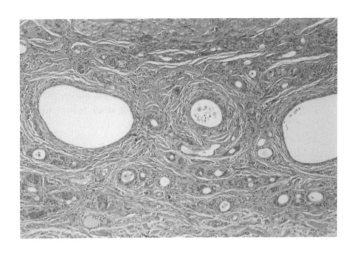

34. A 25-year-old man was found with an apparent self-inflicted gunshot wound of the head in the backyard of his home. All of the following questions would be pertinent for the investigation EXCEPT:

    a. Did he abuse illicit substances?
    b. Was he having relationship problems?
    c. Had he recently lost his job?
    d. Was he prescribed any medications?
    e. Was he right-handed or left-handed?

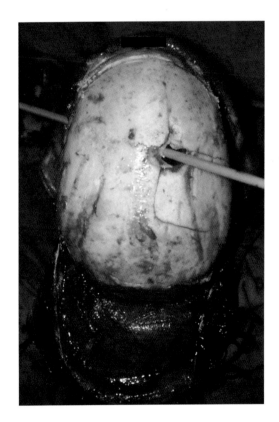

35. A 32-year-old man was scuba diving when an incident occurred while he was underwater. To extricate himself from the situation, he made a rapid ascent to the surface, yelled out, and became unconscious. His head remained above the water level, and he was emergently transported to the nearest hospital where he was declared dead after resuscitative efforts. An image from a CT scan of his head is shown. What is the cause of death?

    a. Drowning
    b. *Clostridium* infection
    c. Multiple jellyfish stings
    d. Extraalveolar air syndrome
    e. Acute intracerebral hemorrhage

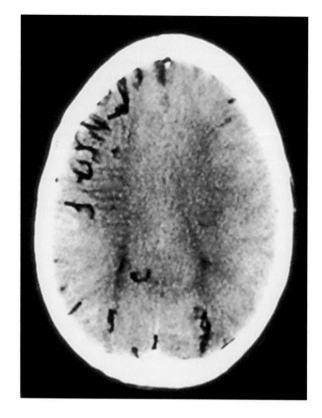

36. The process depicted in the photomicrograph is pathognomonic for what disease entity?

    a. Congestive heart failure
    b. Acute drug intoxication
    c. Drowning
    d. Thermal cutaneous injuries (burns)
    e. Not pathognomonic for any disease entity

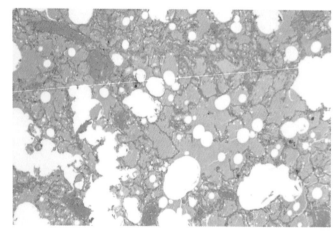

37. A 75-year-old woman who lives alone is found dead in a house fire that appeared to originate in the kitchen around the gas stove. The woman is found dead in her bed at the other end of the house without any thermal injuries. A representative section of the brain reveals the findings depicted in the photomicrograph. All of the following would be appropriate next steps EXCEPT:

    a. Request analysis for carbon monoxide
    b. Alert the police that this is a homicide because the woman is obviously paralyzed and would not be able to get to the kitchen to start the fire
    c. Ask the family about signs and symptoms of dementia
    d. Perform a ubiquitin immunoperoxidase stain
    e. Assess the body for cherry-red livor mortis

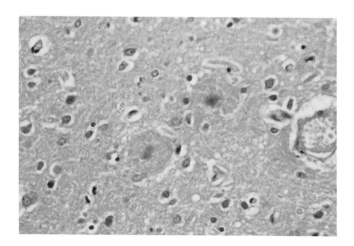

38. A 29-year-old man driving at a high rate of speed loses control of his truck and is involved in a head-on collision with a tree. The truck is an older model without air bags, and the driver was not wearing a seatbelt. During the external examination, the patterned contusion shown in the photograph is identified on his chest. All of the following injuries may be associated with this chest impact EXCEPT:

a. Cardiac contusion
b. Dicing injuries
c. Aortic transection
d. Sternal fracture
e. Rib fractures

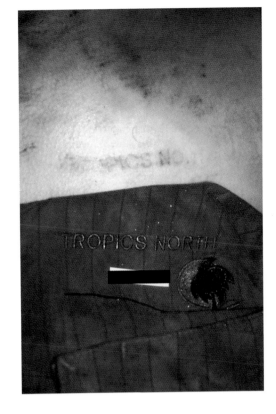

39. A 28-year-old investment banker is found dead in a secure office with a syringe in his arm. He has no natural disease at autopsy, but toxicology analysis detects morphine in his system. What is the cause of death?

a. Accident
b. Cardiopulmonary arrest
c. Asphyxia
d. Acute opiate intoxication
e. Natural

40. Which of the following is *not* a typical thermal artifact?

a. Pugilistic posture
b. Weight loss
c. Epidural hematoma
d. Subdural hematoma
e. Corneal clouding

41. All of the following statements about electrical injuries are correct EXCEPT:

a. All electrocutions leave visible burns on the body.
b. Lightning strikes may leave a skin pattern known as "ferning."
c. High-voltage electrocutions are usually defined as greater than 1000 V.
d. An examination of the suspected malfunctioning equipment is important in the investigation of electrocutions.
e. Deaths resulting from lightning are certified as accidents.

42. A thin, 66-year-old woman is found dead on the bedroom floor with a rectal temperature of 94° F (34° C) (room temperature 72° F [22° C]), moderate rigor mortis of arms and legs, and nonfixed purple lividity. How long has she been dead?

a. 1 hour
b. 4 hours
c. 12 hours

d. 24 hours
e. 36 hours

43. All of the following would affect the rate of decomposition EXCEPT:

a. Body size of the decedent
b. Ambient temperature of the scene
c. Medical health of the individual
d. Concentration of blood alcohol
e. Cause of death

44. At autopsy, the only way to determine definitively that a death is due to drowning is by:

a. The Gettler chloride test
b. Washerwoman skin changes
c. Pulmonary diatom detection
d. Hyperinflated, edematous, heavy lungs
e. Autopsy alone cannot be used to diagnose drowning

45. Which of the following statements regarding manual strangulation is CORRECT?

a. It is never suicidal.
b. It is always accompanied by petechiae and a fractured hyoid bone.
c. It is rarely seen along with sexual assault.
d. It is also known as burking.
e. It is also known as smothering.

46. All of the following statements regarding alcohol abuse are correct EXCEPT:

a. In a 70-kg man, 1 ounce of whisky increases the blood alcohol concentration by 0.02 g/dL.
b. Most ethanol is absorbed in the proximal small intestine.

c. The blood alcohol concentration in plasma is 1.2 times higher than in whole blood.

d. Ethanol may be produced after death during putrefaction by bacteria.

e. Most people with an alcoholic cardiomyopathy have cirrhosis.

47. All of the following statements regarding the pathology of traumatic diffuse axonal injury (DAI) are correct EXCEPT:

a. DAI is usually seen in the corpus callosum, paraventricular areas, and rostral pons.

b. DAI is usually caused by a rapid rotational acceleration-deceleration of the brain.

c. DAI may be detected with β-amyloid precursor protein.

d. DAI may have minimal gross cerebral findings.

e. DAI is never seen with retinal hemorrhages.

48. Sudden infant death syndrome (SIDS) is certified as the cause of death when:

a. A previously undiagnosed congenital heart abnormality is found at autopsy.

b. The postmortem toxicology is positive for benzoylecgonine.

c. There are no recent injuries to account for the infant's death.

d. There are no injuries or disease to account for the infant's death, all postmortem studies are negative, and a

thorough scene and clinical investigation reveals nothing suspicious.

e. No cause of death is detected at the autopsy.

49. Which of the following statements regarding commotio cordis is TRUE?

a. Commotio cordis refers to a fatal brain concussion.

b. Commotio cordis is the major cause of deaths in motor vehicle collisions.

c. Commotio cordis may be caused by a baseball striking the anterior chest over the sternum.

d. The presence of commotio cordis is evidence that a baby was born.

e. Commotio cordis is a known complication of lumbar puncture.

50. The body of a 32-year-old woman is discovered nude in the woods by hikers in the spring during 70° F weather. The woman was last known to be alive 2 days previously and appears to have been dead approximately 36 hours. What is the BEST area to swab for possible sperm collection?

a. Oral cavity

b. Vaginal pool

c. Rectum

d. a, b, and c

e. None of the above

ANSWERS

1. c. The range of fire of a gunshot wound is the distance from the muzzle of the gun to the target. When a loaded gun is fired, more than just the bullet comes out of the muzzle. Gas and burnt and unburnt powder grains are also discharged. Depending on how close the muzzle is to the target, some of this material may affect the wounding pattern or be deposited on or in the target. If gunshot residue is detected, an opinion about the range of fire may be offered. The classic ranges of fire are contact, close range, intermediate range, and distant (or indeterminate). Contact wounding occurs when the muzzle is in contact with the target. In contact wounds, the gas and gunshot residue are blasted into the wound, and there is no gunshot residue on the outside of the body. One may see a muzzle stamp in contact wounds from the skin and muzzle coming in contact during the discharge (Panel 1 of image). The terms *fouling* and *stippling* are used to describe the types of gunshot residue in close and intermediate range gunshot wounds. Fouling is the dustlike burnt powder grains that can be wiped off the body. Stippling (or tattooing) is from the unburnt powder striking the skin and causing a superficial injury. Gunpowder stippling cannot be wiped off and typically appears as numerous pinpoint abrasion-type injuries. A gunshot wound is classified as close range when there is fouling and stippling (Panel 2 of image). Typically for a handgun, close range is within about 6 inches (15 cm). Beyond 6 inches (15 cm), fouling does not reach the body, but stippling does (it may travel up to 30 inches); these wounds are classified as intermediate range (Panel 3 of image). No fouling or stippling is observed in distant gunshot wounds.

Many factors affect the range of fouling and stippling, including type of powder and length of the barrel. The "gold standard" for determining range of fire is to fire the same gun with the same ammunition at special targets from various distances in an attempt to reproduce the pattern (e.g., diameter of stippling) that was seen on the body.

DiMaio VJM: *Gunshot Wounds: Practical Aspects of Firearms, Ballistics, and Forensic Techniques*. Boca Raton: CRC Press, 1999.
Spitz WU: Injury by gunfire. In Spitz WU (ed): *Spitz and Fisher's Medicolegal Investigation of Death*. Springfield, IL: Charles C Thomas, 1993, pp 311-412.

2. a. The image shows a contact gunshot wound with stellate "blowback" lacerations caused by the rapid infusion of gas under the skin from the muzzle of the gun. This wound may be mistaken for an exit wound. One way to help distinguish these wounds is to look for a margin of abrasion or loss of skin tissue. If this were an exit wound, by reapproximating the wound edges, one would expect to see no margin of abrasion at the tips of the skin and complete closure of the wound. This is an entrance wound because there is a margin of abrasion at each inner tip of this gunshot wound. Inner table beveling of the skull or the detection of gunshot residue in the wound tract would be further evidence that this is an entrance wound.

DiMaio VJM: *Gunshot Wounds: Practical Aspects of Firearms, Ballistics, and Forensic Techniques*. Boca Raton: CRC Press, 1999.
Spitz WU: Injury by gunfire. In Spitz WU (ed): *Spitz and Fisher's Medicolegal Investigation of Death*. Springfield, IL: Charles C Thomas, 1993, pp 311-412.

3. e. One should not attempt to estimate the range of fire of a shotgun based on a radiograph of the pellets. A shotgun is a long gun with a smooth bore that typically fires small pellets (birdshot or buckshot). These pellets are held together in a plastic or cardboard wadding in the shotgun shell. The pellets (ranging from a few to many) and the wadding come out of the muzzle when the gun is fired. The pellets will begin to separate (to span out) as they travel from the muzzle. Owing to the billiard ball effect, shot spreads widely inside the body even though it may have entered the body through a single defect (i.e., from a 1-ft [30 cm] range). As the pellets in the front of the pack are slowed by striking the skin, the pellets collide with each other causing them to spread (similar to a cue ball hitting a rack of billiards).

DiMaio VJM: *Gunshot Wounds: Practical Aspects of Firearms, Ballistics, and Forensic Techniques.* Boca Raton: CRC Press, 1999.
Spitz WU: Injury by gunfire. In Spitz WU (ed): *Spitz and Fisher's Medicolegal Investigation of Death.* Springfield, IL: Charles C Thomas, 1993, pp 311-412.

4. a. There are four types of blunt force injury: contusions, abrasions, lacerations, and fractures. Neurovascular bridges have more tensile strength than adipose tissue and may remain intact to be visible traversing the wound depth. A laceration is an injury resulting from a blunt force impact. Fractures are technically lacerations of bone tissue. The term *laceration* is commonly misused in medicine to denote any skin injury that needs to be sutured.

Spitz WU: Blunt and sharp force injury. In Spitz WU (ed): *Spitz and Fisher's Medicolegal Investigation of Death.* Springfield, IL: Charles C Thomas, 1993, pp 199-252.

5. b. Sharp force injuries are a distinct type of injury and should be distinguished from blunt force injuries. Sharp injuries are caused by sharp objects (e.g., knives, broken glass, razor blades). There are two types of sharp force injury: stab wounds and incisions. Stab wounds have a longer depth of penetration into the body and a shorter cutaneous defect. Incisions have a shorter depth of penetration into the body and a longer cutaneous defect (e.g., surgical incision). Sharp injuries are characterized by smooth, straight edges with no tissue bridging.

Byard RW, Klitte A, Gilbert JD, et al: Clinicopathologic features of fatal self-inflicted incised and stab wounds: a 20-year study. *Am J Forensic Med Pathol* 2002;23:15-18.
Spitz WU: Blunt and sharp force injury. In Spitz WU (ed): *Spitz and Fisher's Medicolegal Investigation of Death.* Springfield, IL: Charles C Thomas, 1993, pp 199-252.

6. c. The cause and manner of death have distinct definitions in death certification. The cause of death is the disease or injury responsible for the fatality. Examples include atherosclerotic cardiovascular disease, lung carcinoma, and gunshot wound of the head. The manner of death is determined by the circumstances of the death. The manner of death may be certified as natural or unnatural. Homicide, suicide, and accident are unnatural manners of death. The cause of death in the image would be exsanguination owing to incisions of the wrist. Only Choices b and c are manners of death; the other choices are causes of death. The image demonstrates a deep incision of the wrist with multiple superficial epidermal incisions—so-called

hesitation wounds—which are self-inflicted sharp force injuries, so the manner of death is suicide.

Davis GG: Mind your manners. Part I: History of death certification and manner of death classification. *Am J Forensic Med Pathol* 1997;18(3):219-223.
Gill JR, Catanese C: Sharp injury fatalities in New York City. *J Forensic Sci* 2002;47(3):554-557.
Goodin J, Hanzlick R: Mind your manners. Part II: General results from the National Association of Medical Examiners Manner of Death Questionnaire, 1995. *Am J Forensic Med Pathol* 1997; 18(3):224-227.
Goodin J, Hanzlick R: Mind your manners. Part III: Individual scenario results and discussion of the National Association of Medical Examiners Manner of Death Questionnaire, 1995. *Am J Forensic Med Pathol* 1997;18(3):228-245.

7. a. The injuries shown in the image are lacerations associated with underlying fractures. They occur with a descent from a height with feet-first impacts. Other injuries seen with a feet-first type of impact include compression vertebral fractures, ring fractures of the base of the skull, acetabular fractures, and oblique symmetric inguinal lacerations. Pedestrians commonly have fractures of the lower legs from a horizontal impact with a vehicle (bumper fractures). The irregular pattern of the wounds, symmetry of the wounds, and location on the plantar feet exclude gunshot wounds. There is no evidence of decomposition; also, decomposition does not cause lacerations.

Gill JR: Fatal descent from height in New York City. *J Forensic Sci* 2001;46(5):1132-1137.

8. c. Petechiae are pinpoint hemorrhages that may be seen with neck or chest compression. Manual strangulation is the compression of the neck blood vessels by the hands. The struggling process during manual strangulation does not allow for constant occlusive pressure of the blood vessels, and the intravascular blood pressure fluctuates. Petechiae also may be a consequence of fluctuating intravascular blood pressure during cardiopulmonary resuscitation. Petechiae may be seen in a living person secondary to a Valsalva maneuver (e.g., vigorous coughing or vomiting or bearing down during labor and delivery). In these cases, the right side of the heart is volume overloaded resulting in an increased cephalic venous pressure. The hemorrhages shown in the image are not retinal hemorrhages (e.g., whiplash shaking of an infant), which occur in the back of the eye.

Ely SF, Hirsch CS: Asphyxial deaths and petechiae: a review. *J Forensic Sci* 2000;45(6):1274-1277.
Spitz WU: Asphyxia. In Spitz WU (ed): *Spitz and Fisher's Medicolegal Investigation of Death.* Springfield, IL: Charles C Thomas, 1993, pp 783-845.

9. d. In adolescents and adults, a ligature furrow of the neck is commonly seen with suicidal hangings. This furrow also may be due to homicidal ligature strangulation. The key difference between a hanging and a ligature strangulation is what causes the tightening of the ligature. In a hanging, the force that causes the tightening is the weight of the body owing to gravity. In a ligature strangulation, the force is caused by something other than gravity (usually another person). Fractures of the spine are rare in accidental and suicidal hangings. They are more common in judicial hangings (so-called drop hangings). The ligature furrow may be completely horizontal if the person hangs himself or herself while lying down. Complete suspension is not required to hang oneself. It can be done standing, sitting, or lying on the ground as long as the body relaxes to allow gravity to take over compressing the neck vasculature. Most ligature strangulations are homicides; however, it is possible to strangle oneself with a ligature (but not with one's own hands). Most ligature or hanging deaths in young children are accidental. For example, young children can become caught in curtain cords, or lanyard key chains around the neck can get hooked on bed posts. Rarely, adults may accidentally die from a hanging (e.g., autoerotic asphyxial deaths).

Denton JS: Fatal accidental hanging from a lanyard key chain in a 10-year-old boy. *J Forensic Sci* 2002;47(6):1345-1346.
Spitz WU: Asphyxia. In Spitz WU (ed): *Spitz and Fisher's Medicolegal Investigation of Death*. Springfield, IL: Charles C Thomas, 1993, pp 783-845.

10. d. The radiograph of the abdomen shows numerous, similarly shaped foreign bodies in the stomach and intestine. This is a case of a drug packer ("mule"), which refers to a person who swallows numerous small plastic containers, latex balloons, or condoms that are filled with cocaine or heroin. A gross disease specimen of the opened stomach with contents from autopsy would show containers with the drug. This person swallowed the containers with the drug in Colombia and flew to New York City. Once couriers clear customs, they typically unload their cargo at a nearby motel. If a balloon breaks, the courier may die from an acute intoxication (an overdose). The balloons also can cause death by intestinal obstruction or perforation. The manner of death would be an accident. A pulmonary embolism should always be considered in the differential diagnosis in a person who dies suddenly following a long airplane trip.

Gill JR, Graham SM: Ten years of "body packers" in New York City: 50 deaths. *J Forensic Sci* 2002;47(4):843-846.

11. c. Livor mortis is the settling of blood in dependent capillaries owing to gravity. Externally, it appears as a red, maroon, or purplish discoloration of the skin in the dependent areas. Tight clothing (e.g., elastic waist bands, bra straps) may prevent the settling of blood in certain areas. In this case, the elastic band prevented the settling of blood in the waistband region. Lividity becomes "fixed" after several hours; this means that the skin no longer blanches when pressure is applied, and the distribution of discoloration does not change if the position of the body changes. Lividity helps to demonstrate whether a body was moved sometime after death (i.e., the livor pattern is inappropriate for the position in which the body was found). Algor mortis is the temperature change of the body after death (equilibration with environmental temperature). Rigor mortis is the stiffening of the body after death. Putrefaction is a form of decomposition that is primarily driven by bacteria that normally reside in the body (intestines and skin). Because the immune system no longer functions after death, these bacteria proliferate creating many by-products including gas (which leads to bloating of the body). The body becomes green (usually starting over the abdomen), and the

superficial blood vessels are highlighted ("marbling effect"). Bleb formation and slippage of the epidermis occur. Temperature is a key factor in the rate of most postmortem changes. A first-degree burn is a typical sunburn and would not affect skin covered by clothing with sparing of the waistband area only.

Spitz WU: Time of death and changes after death. In Spitz WU (ed): *Spitz and Fisher's Medicolegal Investigation of Death*. Springfield, IL: Charles C Thomas, 1993, pp 14-70.

12. b. Adipocere is a postmortem change that occurs after prolonged exposure (>6 weeks) to very wet environments. It is commonly seen in remains at an exhumation if the coffin has been permeated by ground water. It is also known as "grave wax." It also may be seen in corpses submerged for weeks or months in bodies of water. Mummification, which is a leathery desiccation of the soft tissues of the body, occurs in dry environments. Autolysis is a form of decomposition in which the body is "digesting" itself. The pancreas is one the first organs of the body to undergo autolysis. Mold is a growth (of various colors including white) on the surface of the body.

Spitz WU: Time of death and changes after death. In Spitz WU (ed): *Spitz and Fisher's Medicolegal Investigation of Death*. Springfield, IL: Charles C Thomas, 1993, pp 14-70.

13. b. A postmortem artifact known as tache noire is shown. The "black spot" is due to desiccation of the surface of the eye because the eye remained opened after death. It should not be mistaken for a blunt injury. One may easily recognize tache noire by simply pulling up the eyelid. The part of the eye that was still covered by the lid has the typical white color. Melanoma would not respect this line of demarcation. Thallium poisoning may result in alopecia with sparing of the inner third of the eyebrow. Pinpoint hemorrhages of the conjunctiva or sclera (petechiae) may be seen with neck compression.

Spitz WU: Time of death and changes after death. In Spitz WU (ed): *Spitz and Fisher's Medicolegal Investigation of Death*. Springfield, IL: Charles C Thomas, 1993, pp 14-70.

14. c. In acute purulent bacterial meningitis, the surface of the brain is covered with pus. Subarachnoid hemorrhage is due to blood under the arachnoid membrane. West Nile virus infection causes encephalitis with inflammation of the brain parenchyma and lymphocytosis in the cerebrospinal fluid. Putrefaction is due to the postmortem proliferation of bacteria. In a dead body, there is no neutrophil response to bacteria and no pus. Anthrax typically involves the lungs and mediastinum, the gastrointestinal tract, or the skin.

Lundenberg R, Chason JL: Mechanical injuries of brain and meninges. In Spitz WU (ed): *Spitz and Fisher's Medicolegal Investigation of Death*. Springfield, IL: Charles C Thomas, 1993, pp 585-636.

15. d. A hammer can cause a variety of patterned injuries depending on how and where the hammer contacts the body. Curvilinear or crescent-shaped injuries are common from the head of the hammer and may be seen with other blunt objects with a rounded edge. The double claw of the hammer leaves distinctive paired rectangular puncture-type injuries. Long thin cylindrical objects (e.g., police batons) typically leave parallel linear contusions (tram-track patterns) separated by unremarkable uninjured skin.

Lundenberg R, Chason JL: Mechanical injuries of brain and meninges. In Spitz WU (ed): *Spitz and Fisher's Medicolegal Investigation of Death*. Springfield, IL: Charles C Thomas, 1993, pp 585-636.

16. e. Heavy black carbonaceous material in the airway is consistent with breathing in a smoky environment. The presence of this material indicates the person was alive during the fire. It is commonly seen in people who die of smoke inhalation. An elevated carboxyhemoglobin also would be expected with this finding. A person may die in a fire and have a normal carboxyhemoglobin saturation if there were resuscitation attempts before death or if there was a flash fire and the person died quickly. One would not expect this degree of carbonaceous material in the airway (or an elevated carboxyhemoglobin saturation) in a person who was dead before the fire or smoke started.

Adelson L: *Pathology of Homicide*. Springfield, IL: Charles C Thomas, 1974.

17. c. The image shows a hemopericardium (unopened) or "blue heart." From the history, the most likely cause would be an aortic dissection owing to Marfan syndrome. The decedent has many of the common findings of this syndrome. The genetic defect in Marfan syndrome is due to a mutation in an extracellular glycoprotein called fibrillin. Fibrillin is the major component of microfibrils in the extracellular matrix. Fibrillin is abundant in the aorta and has been mapped to chromosomes 15 and 5. Commotio cordis refers to damage to the heart resulting from a blow to the chest that frequently results in sudden death. Death is due to a cardiac electrical disturbance and not due to cardiac tamponade. Chordal rupture owing to a myocardial infarction may result in a myocardial perforation and a hemopericardium. Chordal rupture owing to mitral valve prolapse would not likely result in a hemopericardium. Chordal rupture from mitral valve prolapse would not likely result in a hemopericardium. Attempts at cardiopulmonary resuscitation may result in some blood in the pericardial sac but not to this extent.

Cotran RS, Kumar V, Collins T: Genetic disorders. In Cotran RS, Kumar V, Collins T (eds): *Robbins Pathologic Basis of Disease*, 8th ed. Philadelphia: Saunders, 1999, pp 148-149.

18. c. The scenario describes a classic suicide. The man committed an intentional act (jumping off a bridge) and has a history of depression (takes fluoxetine). The *cause* of death is drowning. Depending on the height of the bridge and the position of the body on impact, some people who jump from a bridge die as a result of blunt injuries or drowning (or both contribute to death). The autopsy in this case did not reveal a finding pathognomonic of drowning. However, some signs may be heavy edematous lungs, watery gastric contents, and watery sphenoid sinus fluid. The photograph depicts watery fluid being aspirated from the sphenoid sinus after exposure through the skull base.

DiMaio VJ, DiMaio DJ: Death by drowning. In DiMaio VJ, DiMaio DJ: *Forensic Pathology*, 2nd ed. Boca Raton: CRC Press, 2001, pp 400-407.

19. d. β-Amyloid precursor protein is a neuronal transmembrane glycoprotein that is transported by fast anterograde axoplasmic flow. Immunohistochemical stains are available to detect this protein in neurons. In an uninjured brain, the protein is diffusely distributed in the axons, and it is not detected by the stain. In traumatic axonal injury, tearing or stress causes damage to the neuronal cytoskeleton and interrupts axonal transport. With axonal injury, the protein accumulates focally and can be detected by immunohistochemical staining. Immunohistochemical stain can detect neuronal injury that has occurred 2 hours before death. Histochemical stains (e.g., silver stains) require survival intervals of approximately 12 hours or more to detect the morphologic changes of injured neurons. Ischemic injury or traumatic axonal injury may result in accumulation of the protein. The anatomic location of staining is important for the interpretation of the cause of the reactivity (ischemia versus trauma). Certain areas of the brain are more likely to be affected by traumatic DAI (e.g., tegmentum of the pons, corpus callosum) than by global ischemia/hypoxia.

Duhaime A, Christian C, Rorke L, et al: Nonaccidental head injury in infants—the "shaken-baby syndrome." *N Engl J Med* 1998;338(25):1822-1829.
Gleckman AM, Evans RJ, Bell MD, et al: Optic nerve damage in shaken baby syndrome: detection by beta-amyloid precursor protein immunohistochemistry. *Arch Pathol Lab Med* 2000; 124(2):251-256.

20. c. The image shows an entrance gunshot wound surrounded by stippling. Stippling is pathognomonic for an intermediate range of fire. The gunshot wound is well-circumscribed with a punched-out, "cookie-cutter" appearance, which is characteristic of an entrance-type gunshot wound. Exit wounds typically have a slitlike or stellate appearance in which the skin edges are easily reapproximated to close the defect. A distant range of fire would have a well-circumscribed entrance gunshot wound without soot deposition or gunpowder stippling on the skin surface. A close range of fire would have black soot deposition on the skin surface in conjunction with gunpowder particle stippling. A contact gunshot wound of the head would have a stellate entrance as a result of the gases that exit the barrel of the gun and collect between the skin and bony surfaces of the head. The gases subsequently have a retrograde release from the body around the gun barrel creating skin lacerations around the entrance wound and a stellate appearance.

DiMaio VJM: *Gunshot Wounds: Practical Aspects of Firearms, Ballistics, and Forensic Techniques*. Boca Raton: CRC Press, 1999.
Spitz WU: Injury by gunfire. In Spitz WU (ed): *Spitz and Fisher's Medicolegal Investigation of Death*. Springfield, IL: Charles C Thomas, 1993, pp 311-412.

21. a. Acquired forms of long QT syndrome are associated with drug intoxication, electrolyte abnormalities, toxic substances, hypothermia, anorexia nervosa, and liquid protein diets. Cardiac disease accounts for the greatest number of deaths in the United States. Sudden cardiac death accounts for the second highest number of deaths in the United States and is second only to the total number of deaths resulting from all cancers combined. Of people with underlying heart disease, 30% have an initial presentation characterized by sudden cardiac death. Sudden cardiac death is defined as death within 1 hour of the onset of symptoms outside the hospital setting. Sudden cardiac death accounts for 75% of all cardiac-related deaths in the 35- to 44-year-old age group. The most common dysrhythmia associated with sudden cardiac death is ventricular fibrillation. Prolonged QT interval, or long QT syndrome, is associated with the development of ventricular fibrillation. Contraction band necrosis, which is depicted in the photomicrograph, may be seen within the first hours of the onset of symptoms and is characterized by myocytes with a loss of cross-striations, nuclear karyorrhexis, and cytoplasmic hypereosinophilic wavy bands perpendicular to the orientation of the cells without inflammatory infiltrates. In the acquired forms of long QT syndrome, normal cardiac function resumes when the inciting factor is removed.

Davies MJ, Anderson RH, Becker AE: *The Conduction System of the Heart.* London: Butterworth, 1993, pp 301-323.
DiMaio VJ, DiMaio DJ: Death due to natural disease. In DiMaio VJ, DiMaio DJ: *Forensic Pathology,* 2nd ed. Boca Raton: CRC Press, 2001, pp 43-58.
Rodríguez-Sinovas A, Abdallah Y, Piper HM, et al: Reperfusion injury as a therapeutic challenge in patients with acute myocardial infarction. *Heart Fail Rev* 2007;12(3-4):207-216.

22. e. Being able to distinguish the entrance wound from the exit wound helps to orient positions of the victim and assailant at the time the injury was sustained. The lesion of the calvaria represents an entrance gunshot wound of the skull cap with multiple associated radiating fractures. If only skeletal remains are located, this trajectory analysis may help in the investigation of the case. When a projectile enters a flat bone such as a skull bone, the outer table defect is smaller in diameter than the inner table defect owing to the presence of internal (or inward) beveling of the bone similar to the appearance of beveled glass. As the projectile pushes through the bone to exit through the inner table, small fragments of the medullary bone and splinters of the inner table cortical bone fragment create the larger diameter of the inner surface. The opposite phenomenon is true for a projectile exiting the cranial vault when the projectile encounters the inner table first and subsequently exits the skull through the outer table of the bone. In this scenario, the inner table defect diameter would be smaller than the outer table defect diameter, and the defect would be associated with external (or outward) beveling of the bone similar to the appearance of beveled glass.

DiMaio VJM: *Gunshot Wounds: Practical Aspects of Firearms, Ballistics, and Forensic Techniques.* Boca Raton: CRC Press, 1999.
Spitz WU: Injury by gunfire. In Spitz WU (ed): *Spitz and Fisher's Medicolegal Investigation of Death.* Springfield, IL: Charles C Thomas, 1993, pp 311-412.

23. c. The photomicrograph depicts pyramidal neurons of the hippocampus with cytoplasmic hypereosinophilia and nuclear pyknosis with loss of nucleoli. This is anoxic-ischemic encephalopathy. Heroin overdose causes the respiratory center of the brain to shut down slowly and eventually causes a cessation of respiration as the drug levels increase in the brain over time. The pyramidal neurons of the hippocampus represent an area that is very sensitive to hypoxia and would be affected most severely initially.

A hemorrhagic infarct would have blood in the parenchyma with obliteration of the normal neuropil. Viral encephalitis would have evidence of inflammatory cells within the parenchyma associated with necrotic neurons possibly exhibiting viral cytopathic changes depending on the specific virus. État criblé is dilatation of the cerebral periarteriolar spaces within the basal ganglia and white matter in an elderly adult that is frequently identified by magnetic resonance imaging (MRI) and is associated with chronic vascular ischemia. État lacunaire is characterized by small cystic infarcts within the deep white matter structures of the brain in an elderly adult that are due to chronic ischemia and are associated clinically with repeated bouts of weakness, pseudobulbar palsy, gait disturbance, and incontinence.

Ellison D, Love S, Chimelli L, et al: Head and spinal injuries. In Ellison D, Love S (eds): *Neuropathology, A Reference Text of CNS Pathology,* 2nd ed. St. Louis: Mosby, 2004, pp 241-273.

24. a. The presence of the dicing injuries on the right side of the face allows one to determine that this decedent was in the front passenger seat of the vehicle and was not driving. Dicing injuries are caused by impact between the skin and the fragments of tempered glass from the side windows of vehicles. Dicing injuries and the presence of seatbelt marks (contusions or abrasions) allow the pathologist to determine the location of an individual within a vehicle when placement is unknown. Some authors describe dicing injuries as abrasions. However, glass is a sharp object, and dicing injuries are better described as superficial incisions and sometimes puncture wounds when the glass becomes embedded underneath the epidermis. The postmortem examination cannot prove or disprove who actually caused the accident. Many theories may be entertained including, but not limited to, the role of alcohol; the role of speeding; the role of passenger distraction; the role of sight aversion to distracting objects; and the role of the environment with regard to signage, weather conditions, and lighting.

Burke MP: Injuries sustained by motor vehicle occupants. In Burke MP: *Forensic Medical Investigation of Motor Vehicle Incidents.* Boca Raton: CRC Press, 2007, pp 61-87.

25. c. A hinge type I fracture extends between the middle cranial fossae. A hinge type II fracture extends from one anterior cranial fossa in an oblique angle to the contralateral posterior cranial fossa. A hinge type III fracture is a transverse fracture through bilateral anterior cranial fossae. LeFort fractures are fractures of the facial bones associated with facial instability. A LeFort type I fracture involves the jaw and nose, and a LeFort type II fracture involves the jaw, nose, and eyes.

DiMaio VJ, DiMaio DJ: Trauma to the skull and brain: craniocerebral injuries. In DiMaio VJ, DiMaio DJ: *Forensic Pathology,* 2nd ed. Boca Raton: CRC Press, 2001, pp 152-155.

26. a. The liver shows severe macrovesicular and microvesicular steatosis; this correlates with the gross finding of a yellow waxy liver. Chronic alcoholism or any process that causes hepatic steatosis can predispose to the development of low salt syndrome. Low salt syndrome is characterized by sodium levels below the normal range of

135 to 145 mEq/L. However, as a rule of thumb, sudden death associated with low salt syndrome does not occur until the sodium level is less than 125 mEq/L. Sodium is a very stable electrolyte in the postmortem state. Potassium and glucose are very unstable with a wide range of change independent of the postmortem time interval. Electrolytes are not analyzed in postmortem blood samples; the vitreous humor is a relatively stable environment for postmortem electrolyte analysis and is the appropriate sample to send for analysis. The vitreous electrolyte analysis would most closely resemble the antemortem electrolyte levels.

Crawford JM, Liu C: Liver and biliary tract. In Kumar V, Abbas A, Fausto N (eds): *Robbins and Cotran Pathologic Basis of Disease*, 7th ed. Philadelphia: Saunders, 2005, pp 904-908.
DiMaio VJ, DiMaio DJ: Topics in forensic pathology. In DiMaio VJ, DiMaio DJ: *Forensic Pathology*, 2nd ed. Boca Raton: CRC Press, 2001, pp 481-484.

27. c. Sirenomelia (mermaid syndrome) is a sporadic congenital malformation without a genetic inheritance and affects 1:60,000 to 1:100,000 newborn infants. It has the same rate as conjoined twins in the general population. Sirenomelia is a syndrome associated with a single umbilical artery. It occurs during the third week of gestation. In contrast to some other disorders associated with a single umbilical artery, sirenomelia is not linked to maternal diabetes. Common defects include renal agenesis or cystic dysgenesis, failed cleavage of the lower limb bud, sacral dysgenesis, imperforate anus, absent bladder, and Potter facies. Renal agenesis causes oligohydramnios secondary to the absence of urine production necessary for the production of amniotic fluid. Oligohydramnios causes pulmonary hypoplasia owing to decreased room for chest expansion and decreased amniotic fluid. When the infant is born, he or she immediately develops respiratory insufficiency and dies shortly after birth. Most affected fetuses die in utero. A whole body radiograph shows the malformed pelvic bones, the single rudimentary femur, and the malformed rudimentary tibia. The next most appropriate step following the autopsy would be to counsel the family this is a nonheritable sporadic congenital deformation that would not affect future pregnancies.

Kallen B, Castilla EE, Lancaster PA, et al: The cyclops and the mermaid: an epidemiological study of two types of rare malformation. *J Med Genet* 1992;29(1):30-35.
Oneije CI, Sherer DM, Handwerker S, et al: Caudal regression syndrome and sirenomelia in only one twin in two diabetic pregnancies. *Clin Exp Obstet Gynecol* 2004;31(2):151-153.
Rudolph AM, Kamei RK, Overby KJ: *Rudolph's Fundamentals of Pediatrics*. New York: McGraw-Hill, 2002.

28. b. Lobar pneumonia is typically caused by a bacterial infection, and elderly adults have an increased risk of developing fatal community-acquired pneumonia. The photograph depicts bilateral organizing subdural hematomas. The subdural hematomas appear thin without a significant space-occupying mass that would be associated with cerebral compression and subsequent herniation. Elderly adults are at risk for developing subdural hematomas even after minor head trauma owing to cerebral atrophy that often accompanies aging. As the brain atrophies, the bridging veins between the brain and the dura become

stretched. Even with minor trauma during a fall from standing height, these fragile blood vessels may become torn by the weight of the brain shifting within the cranial vault. Cerebral veins are under low pressure, so after a fall there may be a lucid interval of a day or more before the hematoma has enough volume to cause cerebral compression. Additionally, even thin noncompressive subdural hemorrhages have an increased risk for rebleeding during the organization phase when neovascularization creates thin, fragile blood vessels that are easily damaged. This condition is called acute-on-chronic subdural hematoma and can be visualized by its differences in density on CT scan.

DiMaio VJ, DiMaio DJ: Trauma to the skull and brain: craniocerebral injuries. In DiMaio VJ, DiMaio DJ: *Forensic Pathology*, 2nd ed. Boca Raton: CRC Press, 2001, pp 165-169.
Ellison D, Love S, Chimelli L, et al: Hemorrhage. In Prayson RA (ed): *Neuropathology, A Reference Text of CNS Pathology*, 2nd ed. Philadelphia: Mosby, 2004, pp 209-240.

29. e. The permanent pathway through the brain created by a projectile (bullet) is depicted in the photograph. *T. solium* infection causes cysticercosis, which has an appearance of circular, often calcified, cysts in the brain parenchyma and may be associated with seizure disorder, headaches, or mass effects. A basilar skull fracture may cause cortical lacerations of the adjacent brain but would not create perforating pathways through the brain. An incision of the head would not penetrate the skull and enter the brain. Stab wounds of the head rarely enter the brain. The most common occurrence is a stab wound to the squamous portion of the temporal bone because of the thin nature of the bone. Additionally, stab wounds of the brain do not leave gaping permanent cavities similar to projectiles.

Ellison D, Love S, Chimelli L, et al: Head and spinal injuries. In Prayson RA (ed): *Neuropathology, A Reference Text of CNS Pathology*, 2nd ed. Philadelphia: Mosby, 2004, pp 241-273.
King CH: Cestode infections. In Goldman L, Ausiello D (eds): *Cecil Medicine*, 23rd ed. Chap. 375. Philadelphia: Saunders, 2007.
Spitz WU: Injury by gunfire. In Spitz WU (ed): *Spitz and Fisher's Medicolegal Investigation of Death*. Springfield, IL: Charles C Thomas, 1993, pp 311-412.

30. e. There is not enough information to explain how the projectile entered the brain in this case. There are five manners of death: homicide, suicide, accident, natural, and undetermined. In its simplest definition, homicide is the death of an individual caused by another. Suicide is the intentional taking of one's life. An accident is an unintentional death either of oneself or another. Accidental deaths are also caused by inanimate objects, animals, and forces of nature. Natural deaths are related to pathologic processes. The term *undetermined* is used when a preponderance of evidence does not point to one specific manner, or there may be multiple manners that are equally valid, or there is not enough information to make a determination. If this individual was shot by another, the manner would be homicide. If this individual shot himself or herself, the manner would be suicide. If this individual was handling a gun without the intention to hurt himself or herself and the gun discharged, the manner would be an accident.

Davis GG: Mind your manners. Part I: History of death certification and manner of death classification. *Am J Forensic Med Pathol* 1997;18(3):219-223.

DiMaio VJM: *Gunshot Wounds: Practical Aspects of Firearms, Ballistics, and Forensic Techniques.* Boca Raton: CRC Press, 1999.

Goodin J, Hanzlick R: Mind your manners. Part II: General results from the National Association of Medical Examiners Manner of Death Questionnaire, 1995. *Am J Forensic Med Pathol* 1997; 18(3):224-227.

Goodin J, Hanzlick R: Mind your manners. Part III: Individual scenario results and discussion of the National Association of Medical Examiners Manner of Death Questionnaire, 1995. *Am J Forensic Med Pathol* 1997;18(3):228-245.

Spitz WU: Injury by gunfire. In Spitz WU (ed): *Spitz and Fisher's Medicolegal Investigation of Death.* Springfield, IL: Charles C Thomas, 1993, pp 311-412.

31. d. The photograph depicts a nasal septal perforation associated with chronic insufflation drug abuse. This lesion would be associated with chronic cocaine insufflation. Cocaine has both vasoconstrictive and anesthetic properties. The vasoconstriction is associated with tissue necrosis, and chronic repetitive use may cause complete destruction of the nasal septum owing to the small amount of highly vascular tissue in the area. Cocaine is a catecholamine, and most of its effects are on the heart and the conduction system. Cocaine use is associated with tachycardia and hypertension. As an anesthetic, cocaine is a sodium channel blocker, and it prevents the reuptake of neurotransmitters, which may be directly related to its cardiac-specific effects that lead to sudden death. The increased workload of the heart can cause cardiac cell death and arrhythmias as well as hypertensive cerebrovascular infarcts.

Stephens BG: Investigations of deaths from drug abuse. In Spitz WU (ed): *Spitz and Fisher's Medicolegal Investigation of Death.* Springfield, IL: Charles C Thomas, 2006, pp 1166-1217.

32. c. The ligamentum arteriosum is a remnant of the fetal circulation and creates a tethering point of the aorta. During rapid deceleration, as in a motor vehicle collision, the chest wall impacts an object, but the heart continues its forward motion inside the thoracic cavity. The weight of the forward-moving heart pulls and elongates the aorta at its tethering point stretching it beyond the elastic limit of the tissue; this creates tearing or a laceration of the tissue and when severe enough transects the aorta. The mechanism of death would be rapid exsanguination into the chest cavity.

Burke MP: Injuries sustained by motor vehicle occupants. In Burke MP: *Forensic Medical Investigation of Motor Vehicle Incidents.* Boca Raton: CRC Press, 2007, pp 61-87.

DiMaio VJ, DiMaio DJ: Bullet embolism: six cases and a review of the literature. *J Forensic Sci* 1972;17(3):394-398.

Kumar V, Abbas A, Fausto N (eds): *Robbins and Cotran Pathologic Basis of Disease,* 8th ed. Philadelphia: Saunders, 2010.

33. c. The lesion shown in the photomicrograph is a cystic tumor of the atrioventricular node; it has no genetic component. It previously was called a mesothelioma of the atrioventricular node because of the histologic appearance. Although these lesions tend to be small, the location in relation to the cardiac conduction system makes them significant with regard to symptoms. *Takeaway point:* Microscopic lesions of the cardiac conduction system may cause sudden unexpected death and should be considered during an autopsy.

Bharati S, Lev M: *The Cardiac Conduction System in Unexplained Sudden Death.* Mount Kisco, NY: Futura Publishing Company, 1990, pp 136-138.

Burke AP, Virmani R: Tumors and tumor-like conditions in the heart. In Silver MD, Gotlieb AI, Schoen FJ (eds): *Cardiovascular Pathology.* New York: Churchill Livingstone, 2001, pp 585-586.

Davies M: The investigation of sudden cardiac death. *Histopathology* 1999;34(2):93-98.

34. e. The photograph shows the projectile pathway through the skull with the entrance on the left side of the head and the exit on the vertex of the calvaria. The exit wound is identified by the external bevel of the outer table of the right parietal bone. The defect in the skull is consistent with a handgun type of ammunition with a "punched-out" osseous defect and lacking multiple comminuted skull fractures as would be expected with a rifle or shotgun wound to the head. Despite popular thought, knowing if someone is right-handed or left-handed is not useful information with regard to proving intention or ability to sustain a self-inflicted gunshot wound. Because not a lot of force is necessary to squeeze the trigger, some people use the dominant hand to steady the gun, especially in intraoral gunshot wounds.

Davis GG: Mind your manners. Part I: History of death certification and manner of death classification. *Am J Forensic Med Pathol* 1997;18(3):219-223.

DiMaio VJM: *Gunshot Wounds: Practical Aspects of Firearms, Ballistics, and Forensic Techniques.* Boca Raton: CRC Press, 1999.

Goodin J, Hanzlick R: Mind your manners. Part II: General results from the National Association of Medical Examiners Manner of Death Questionnaire, 1995. *Am J Forensic Med Pathol* 1997; 18(3):224-227.

Goodin J, Hanzlick R: Mind your manners. Part III: Individual scenario results and discussion of the National Association of Medical Examiners Manner of Death Questionnaire, 1995. *Am J Forensic Med Pathol* 1997;18(3):228-245.

Spitz WU: Injury by gunfire. In Spitz WU (ed): *Spitz and Fisher's Medicolegal Investigation of Death.* Springfield, IL: Charles C Thomas, 1993, pp 311-412.

35. d. The case scenario is a classic example of pulmonary barotrauma and the development of extraalveolar air syndrome. Some situation occurs underwater that causes the diver to panic, and the diver races to the surface forgetting to stop at periodic intervals for pressure equilibration. The most dangerous part of the dive is in the area between the water surface and approximately 5 ft in depth; this is the area where the partial pressure of the gas rapidly decreases and is associated with rapid expansion within the lung parenchyma causing alveolar rupture. In the classic scenario, the diver breaks the water surface and becomes unconscious with or without the head being submerged in water.

Caruso JL, Bell MD: The medicolegal investigation of recreational diving fatalities. Presented at the 54th annual meeting of the American Academy of Forensic Sciences, Atlanta, GA, Feb. 13-16, 2002.

Kindwall EP, Pellegrini J: Autopsy protocol for victims of scuba diving accidents. Appendix G. In 1990 Report on Diving Accidents and Fatalities. Divers Alert Network, 1990, pp 94-100.

36. e. Pulmonary edema is caused by increased vascular pressure in the alveolar capillaries and venules that allows for the extravasation of the fluid component of blood into the alveolar space. The fluid in the airspaces inhibits the normal transport of oxygen and carbon dioxide and can lead to a hypoxic death. Pulmonary edema is a mechanism of multiple disease entities and is not pathognomonic for any one disease or injury. All of the entities listed in the answer choices may be associated with pulmonary edema, and it is a common finding in people who have a protracted period of time between injurious insult and death.

Matthay MA, Martin TR: Pulmonary edema and acute lung injury. In Mason RJ, Broaddus VC, Martin TR, et al (eds): *Murray & Nadel's Textbook of Respiratory Medicine,* 5th ed. Philadelphia: Saunders, 2010, pp 1283-1325.

O'Brien JF, Falk JL: Heart failure. In Marx JA (ed): *Rosen's Emergency Medicine: Concepts and Clinical Practice,* 7th ed. Philadelphia: Mosby, 2009, pp 1075-1090.

37. b. The photomicrograph depicts two neuritic plaques within the cerebral cortex. The presence of neuritic plaques, neurofibrillary tangles, granulovacuolar degeneration, and Hirano bodies is diagnostic of Alzheimer disease. However, neuritic plaques (senile plaques) may be seen in brains of elderly adults without clinical evidence of dementia. The woman in this case had dementia and Alzheimer disease. Forgetfulness is associated with dementia. Demented individuals commonly leave the stove on, forget to eat or take medications, are unaware of their surroundings, and fail to take precautions to keep themselves safe. Individuals with dementia can become targets of abuse, so the pathologist must be aware of that potential and take action if necessary.

Burke MP: Medical factors in motor vehicle incidents. In Burke MP: *Forensic Medical Investigation of Motor Vehicle Incidents.* Boca Raton: CRC Press, 2007, pp 42-43.

Ellison D, Love S, Chimelli L, et al: Dementias. In Prayson RA: *Neuropathology, A Reference Text of CNS Pathology,* 2nd ed. Philadelphia: Mosby, 2004, pp 549-584.

38. b. The decedent in this case had to be driving at a high rate of speed to hit the steering wheel with enough force to cause the patterned chest contusion shown. Pulmonary and cardiac lacerations may occur with severe rib and sternal fractures. Dicing injuries are superficial incisions of the skin surface directly facing the exploding tempered glass of the vehicle side windows. In this case, dicing injuries would be expected on the left side of the face because the decedent was driving the vehicle. Dicing injuries would not be associated with a blunt force injury of the chest.

Burke MP: Injuries sustained by motor vehicle occupants. In Burke MP: *Forensic Medical Investigation of Motor Vehicle Incidents.* Boca Raton: CRC Press, 2007, pp 61-87.

39. d. The cause of death is acute opiate intoxication. The autopsy has ruled out other causes of death including natural disease. The drug of abuse was most likely heroin. Because of its short half-life, heroin (diacetylmorphine) is rarely detected in the blood. The metabolite of diacetylmorphine, 6-monoacetylmorphine, has a longer half-life and can be detected for a longer period in the vitreous humor or in the urine. By convention, the manner of death in acute drug intoxications from substance abuse is typically certified as accident. If an intoxication by any illicit drug of abuse contributes to a death, the death is *not* certified as natural.

Davis GG: Mind your manners. Part I: History of death certification and manner of death classification. *Am J Forensic Med Pathol* 1997;18(3):219-223.

Goodin J, Hanzlick R: Mind your manners. Part II: General results from the National Association of Medical Examiners Manner of Death Questionnaire, 1995. *Am J Forensic Med Pathol* 1997; 18(3):224-227.

Goodin J, Hanzlick R: Mind your manners. Part III: Individual scenario results and discussion of the National Association of Medical Examiners Manner of Death Questionnaire, 1995. *Am J Forensic Med Pathol* 1997;18(3):228-245.

Kircher T, Anderson R: Cause of death. Proper completion of death certificate. *JAMA* 1987;258(3):349-352.

40. d. Thermal skin injury usually does not cause immediate death. Typically, death results from the delayed complications of the burn with the resultant effects on the entire body (systemic inflammatory response) and the increased susceptibility to opportunistic infection. People who die in a fire or shortly afterward usually die of smoke inhalation. The extensive burns and charring seen on a dead body recovered after a fire are often postmortem occurrences. Common postmortem thermal artifacts can occur. The pugilistic posture is flexion of the arms (similar to a boxer pose) secondary to the heat that causes muscle contraction. The arms flex because the flexor muscles are usually "stronger" than the extensors. A subdural hematoma detected in a burned body occurred before death. A decrease in body weight (from loss of body water) and corneal clouding (from heat) are other common thermal artifacts.

DiMaio VJ, DiMaio DJ: Fire deaths. In DiMaio VJ, DiMaio DJ: *Forensic Pathology,* 2nd ed. Boca Raton: CRC Press, 2001, pp 367-387.

41. a. Most high-voltage electrocutions leave burns. High-voltage electrocutions may cause the clothing to explode into tattered shreds. Multiple objects on or near the body, such as jewelry, coins, and belt buckles, may brand the skin from thermal injury. Less than half of low-voltage (i.e., <1000 V) electrocutions involve burns. The examination of the scene is very important for the investigation of these deaths; this is one reason why workplace deaths are investigated by the medical examiner or coroner. For example, a carpenter who is electrocuted by a faulty drill remains conscious for 10 to 15 seconds after the heart was stopped by the electric current. The victim often shouts an expletive and then drops the drill. The victim may walk a few feet away from the work site and then collapse. The initial recognition of the possibility of these deaths and an examination of the tool are vital to prevent the next person from using the faulty drill. Lightning strikes result in a pathognomonic pink arborizing pattern of the skin (ferning) that fades with time. Ferning in a nonvascular distribution should not be confused with marbling from putrefaction in a vascular distribution or scarring from chronic injection drug abuse (track marks) in a vascular distribution.

Wetli CV: Keraunopathology: an analysis of 45 fatalities. *Am J Forensic Med Pathol* 1996;17(2):89-98.

Wright RK, Davis JH: The investigation of electrical deaths: a report of 220 fatalities. *J Forensic Sci* 1980;25(3):514-521.

42. b. These postmortem changes are consistent with a postmortem interval of 3 to 5 hours. In contrast to the forensic pathologists on popular television shows, forensic pathologists in real life are rarely able to tell the precise postmortem interval by evaluating rigor, livor, and algor mortis. Temperature (both the internal temperature of the body and the external temperature of the environment) plays a key role in the progression of postmortem changes. Rigor mortis is the stiffening of the body after death. It occurs gradually over several hours and usually reaches a peak ("full rigor") in about 12 hours. Over the next several hours, rigor mortis gradually disappears and typically is absent by 24 hours. Because rigor mortis is caused by chemical processes in the muscle (involving adenosine triphosphate), the rate of the changes may be affected by various intrinsic factors (some related to the cause of death—e.g., body habitus, muscular development, drug use, infection) and extrinsic factors (particularly the environmental temperature).

Algor mortis is the change in the temperature of the body after death. The body equilibrates with the environment, which usually means it cools down. If the person died in a one-room tenement apartment without air conditioning during a New York City heat wave in August with a room temperature of 103° F (39.4° C), the body temperature would increase. The body temperature usually cools at a rate of 1° to 2° F (~17° C) per hour; however, this depends on the environmental temperature, the body habitus, and amount of clothing. Livor mortis is the settling of blood in dependent capillaries owing to gravity.

The postmortem interval is unlikely to be 1 hour because the woman already is in moderate rigor mortis, and her temperature has decreased 4° to 5° F (2° C). It is unlikely to be 12 hours (or more) because her body temperature should have cooled more than 4° to 5° F (2° C). Another finding that may help differentiate the onset of rigor mortis from waning rigor mortis is the clarity of the corneas. The presence of moderate rigor mortis with cloudy corneas would favor waning rigor mortis. The corneas are more likely to be clear within a few hours of death as opposed to 24 hours.

Spitz WU: Time of death and changes after death. In Spitz WU (ed): *Spitz and Fisher's Medicolegal Investigation of Death.* Springfield, IL: Charles C Thomas, 1993, pp 14-70.

43. d. The concentration of ethanol in the blood would have no effect on the rate of decomposition. It does not provide any "preservative" effects on the body. A large body size (with plenty of insulating adipose tissue) retains body heat, which speeds up putrefaction. A thin body cools down more quickly and undergoes putrefaction at a slower rate. The bacteria responsible for putrefaction are sensitive to the temperature; warmth stimulates growth (bodies are refrigerated after death to slow down the putrefactive process, but refrigeration does not stop the process). The environmental temperature also affects the speed of putrefaction. A body in the trunk of a car in a Texas parking lot in the middle of August can become markedly putrefied in 24 hours, whereas a body in a cool Connecticut basement may not putrefy for several days. The cause of death as well as the health of the individual may play a role. A person who dies with sepsis already has a head start on putrefaction (bacteria are already in the blood and distributed

throughout the body), and the body putrefies more quickly. In addition, fever speeds the putrefactive process because of an increase in body temperature. *Sepsis* is a Greek word that means putrefaction. *Putrefaction* is from the Latin *putrefacio,* which means to "make rotten."

Spitz WU: Time of death and changes after death. In Spitz WU (ed): *Spitz and Fisher's Medicolegal Investigation of Death.* Springfield, IL: Charles C Thomas, 1993, pp 14-70.

44. e. There are no pathognomonic findings for drowning. Drowning is certified as the cause of death when the scene and clinical findings are consistent with it and there is no other reasonable cause at autopsy to account for the death. It is a diagnosis of exclusion. There are autopsy signs that are commonly seen in drowning. Foam from the mouth is due to pulmonary edema caused by the mixing of air and water within the lungs. Other signs include hyperinflated, edematous, heavy lungs; watery gastric contents; and watery sphenoid sinus fluid. However, none of these signs are diagnostic of drowning. "Dry" lungs are found in approximately 10% to 20% of cases of drowning. In addition, there are other causes of death (e.g., epilepsy, drug intoxications) that also have foam emanating from the mouth. Scientists have tried to find a way to diagnose drowning definitively. The Gettler chloride test was one attempt to diagnose drowning by comparing electrolyte concentrations in the right side and left side of the heart. It subsequently was demonstrated to be ineffective. The detection of diatoms (algae with a siliceous exoskeleton) has been used as an adjunctive test in suspected drownings. Because of the ubiquitous nature of diatoms, their detection is not conclusive of death by drowning. Washerwoman changes are a sign of submersion in water but not drowning.

Copeland AR: An assessment of lung weights in drowning cases. The Metro Dade County experience from 1978 to 1982. *Am J Forensic Med Pathol* 1985;6(4):301-304.

DiMaio VJ, DiMaio DJ: Death by drowning. In DiMaio VJ, DiMaio DJ: *Forensic Pathology,* 2nd ed. Boca Raton: CRC Press, 2001, pp 400-407.

45. a. Manual strangulation is compression of the neck with the hands. All manual strangulations are homicidal because a person who attempts to strangle himself or herself manually will become unconscious before death. When unconsciousness occurs, the self-applied manual compression of the neck will stop. The mechanism of death from neck compression is complex. Compression of the vasculature in the neck plays a major role in the pathophysiology of strangulation. It requires less force to compress the jugular veins and carotid arteries than the trachea. Compression of both carotid arteries usually causes unconsciousness in 10 to 14 seconds. If the pressure is then released, the person gradually regains consciousness. To cause death, this compression must continue for some time after the loss of consciousness. Burking is a combination of chest compression and smothering (see the Scottish "resurrectionists" Burke and Hare).

DiMaio VJ, DiMaio DJ: *Forensic Pathology.* Boca Raton: CRC Press, 2001, pp 243-244.

46. e. In a 70-kg man, 1 ounce of whiskey (100 proof), 4 ounces of wine, and 12 ounces of beer each would increase the blood alcohol by 0.02 g/dL. Because ethanol distributes in total body water, the same amount of ethanol would increase the blood alcohol by 0.04 g/dL in a 35-kg man and by 0.01 g/dL in a 140-kg man. Ethanol is metabolized at a rate of 0.015 g/dL per hour. Hospital laboratories often report the blood ethanol concentration as mg/dL (0.1 g/dL is equivalent to 100 mg/dL). Ethanol may be produced by bacteria in the body after death, which results in spurious ethanol concentrations (up to 0.2 g/dL). By testing the vitreous fluid (a relatively sequestered site), one can differentiate postmortem production from ingestion before death. If ethanol is not detected in the vitreous fluid but the blood has a concentration of 0.09 g/dL, the blood ethanol is consistent with postmortem production. One would expect to find ethanol in the vitreous fluid if the blood concentration was due to ingestion before death. Most people with an alcoholic cardiomyopathy do *not* have cirrhosis.

Adelson L: *Pathology of Homicide*. Springfield, IL: Charles C Thomas, 1974, pp 883-918.
Lefkowitch JH, Fenoglio JJ Jr: Liver disease in alcoholic cardiomyopathy: evidence against cirrhosis. *Hum Pathol* 1983;14(5):457-463.

47. e. The disease of traumatic DAI is usually seen in the corpus callosum, paraventricular areas, and rostral pons, although the gross cerebral findings may be minimal. The triad of gross findings of this syndrome includes retinal hemorrhages, small (noncompressive) subdural hemorrhage, and subarachnoid hemorrhage. The rapid rotational acceleration-deceleration of the brain causes shearing of the affected axons responsible for the subsequent neuronal changes of DAI. Axonal injury is considered to be the predominant mechanism for the neurotrauma seen with whiplash shaking (shaken baby syndrome).

Duhaime A, Christian C, Rorke L, et al: Nonaccidental head injury in infants—the "shaken-baby syndrome." *N Engl J Med* 1998;338(25):1822-1829.
Gleckman AM, Evans RJ, Bell MD, et al: Optic nerve damage in shaken baby syndrome: detection by beta-amyloid precursor protein immunohistochemistry. *Arch Pathol Lab Med* 2000;124(2):251-256.

48. d. SIDS is defined as the sudden unexpected death of an infant (<1 year old) that remains unexplained after a thorough investigation, including performance of a complete autopsy and review of the circumstances of death (clinical history). SIDS is a diagnosis of exclusion. Detection of drugs, a major cardiac anomaly, or a metabolic disorder would exclude SIDS as the cause of death. Benzoylecgonine is a metabolite of cocaine and would not be compatible with a diagnosis of SIDS. The absence of injury and the absence of a cause of death at autopsy are also insufficient by themselves to make the diagnosis of SIDS. Many causes of death (e.g., long QT syndrome, soft smothering) may have no autopsy findings. An investigation of the clinical history and circumstances must be conducted. Although the definition of SIDS includes infants up to 1 year of age, SIDS rarely occurs after 6 months of age. A medical examiner should be very hesitant to certify a death as due to SIDS in an infant older than 6 months (or <1 month) of age.

Krous HF, Beckwith JB, Byard RW, et al: Sudden infant death syndrome and unclassified sudden infant deaths: a definitional and diagnostic approach. *Pediatrics* 2004;114(1):234-238.

49. c. Commotio cordis refers to a sudden death that is due to a cardiac arrhythmia caused by a blunt impact to the anterior chest. It may occur during sporting activities when a baseball or hockey puck strikes the sternum. It also may occur during physical altercations from punches or kicks delivered to the sternum. The pathophysiology of commotio cordis has been experimentally produced using wooden balls striking the chest of baby pigs. It was found that if the impact occurred at a very specific, narrow part of the cardiac cycle (15 msec before the peak of the T wave), ventricular fibrillation resulted. These findings explain why not every chest impact is fatal. The impact must occur at a very narrow part of the cardiac cycle for the fatal arrhythmia to occur. It is possible for this mechanism of death to occur in a motor vehicle collision if the steering wheel impacts the chest; however, most deaths resulting from motor vehicle collisions are due to blunt force injuries of the head and trunk related to the rapid deceleration of the body impacting inanimate objects.

Link M, Wang P, Pandian N, et al: An experimental model of sudden death due to low-energy chest-wall impact (commotio cordis). *N Engl J Med* 1998;338(25):1805-1811.

50. b. The vaginal pool is the best possible area to swab because sperm may be retained on average 38 hours in the postmortem state. The oral cavity is a hostile environment for sperm; the sperm usually would be degraded within 6 hours. Sperm still may be present within the rectum an average of 28 hours after death. The best specimen for possible sperm detection is any dried stain that may be visualized on the clothing or skin with ultraviolet light. Sperm have been isolated from dried stains on clothing for 12 months or longer. In the absence of sperm, other tests may be used for the detection of the components of seminal fluid, glycoprotein p30 and acid phosphatase.

DiMaio VJ, DiMaio DJ: Rape. In DiMaio VJ, DiMaio DJ: *Forensic Pathology*, 2nd ed. Boca Raton: CRC Press, 2001, pp 435-444.
Spitz WU: Investigation of deaths in childhood. In Spitz WU (ed): *Spitz and Fisher's Medicolegal Investigation of Death*. Springfield, IL: Charles C Thomas, 2006, pp 406-408.

CHAPTER 22

IMMUNOPATHOLOGY
Matthias J. Szabolcs

QUESTIONS

Questions 1-20 refer to a photo or photomicrograph.

1. This is a section of a posterior mediastinal spindle cell neoplasm. Which of the following is the single MOST useful immunostain?
   a. S100
   b. CD34
   c. CD5
   d. Vimentin
   e. CD99

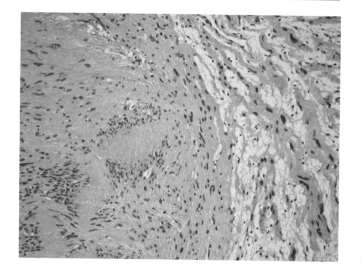

2. A woman presents with an erythematous, ulcerated lesion of the nipple. The following photomicrograph shows staining of neoplastic cells. These cells MOST likely demonstrate which of the following immunophenotypes?
   a. Cytokeratin 7 (CK7) positive, CEA (carcinoembryonic antigen) positive, HER-2/neu overexpressed, CAM5.2/B5BetaH11 positive
   b. CK5/6 positive, CK7 positive, CK20 positive, BerEp4 positive, B72.3 positive
   c. CEA positive, CK5/6 positive, CK7 negative, S100 negative, ER (estrogen receptor) positive, PR (progesterone receptor) positive
   d. CK7 positive, S100 positive, CK20 positive, EMA (epithelial membrane antigen) negative, HMB45 negative
   e. CK5/6 positive, S100 positive, CK20 positive, EMA negative, HMB45 negative

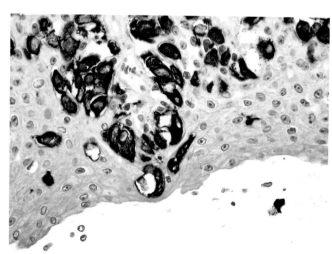

3. The following section of gastric mucosa shows an infiltrate of a mixture of centrocytelike and monocytoid cells infiltrating glandular epithelium ("lymphoepithelial" lesions). Lesional cells are CD20, CD79a, and CD43 positive. They are MOST likely to be:
   a. BCL2 positive
   b. CD10 positive
   c. BCL6 positive
   d. CD3 positive
   e. CD7 positive

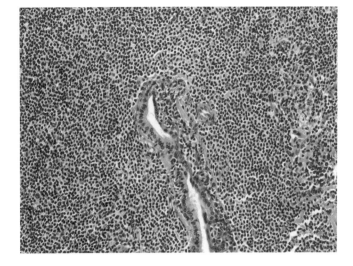

4. The adenocarcinoma seen in the following section of a liver biopsy taken from a woman with multiple liver nodules has the following immunostaining profile: CK7 positive, CK20 positive, CA19.9 positive, CEA positive, TTF-1 (thyroid transcription factor-1) negative, ER negative, PR negative, GCDFP15 negative, and weakly CDX2 positive. The MOST likely origin based on this profile is:
   a. Pancreas/bile ducts
   b. Breast
   c. Lung
   d. Colon
   e. Ovary

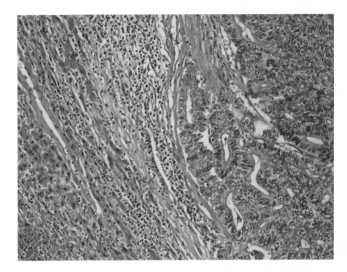

5. The following image shows intestinal tissue stained with an anticytomegalovirus (anti-CMV) antibody. Which of the following statements is TRUE?
   a. CMV immunostaining is more sensitive but less specific than culture.
   b. CMV immunostaining is less sensitive than direct histologic examination.
   c. CMV antigen is detectable only in cells with classic inclusions.
   d. In AIDS, CMV may be detected in cells, which do not show classic cytopathic alterations.
   e. None of the above

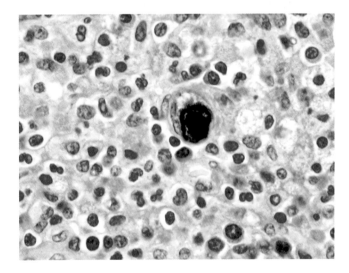

6. A 40-year-old man presented with an elevated mass on the back. Histologic examination showed a spindle cell neoplasm with storiform architecture at the dermal-subcutaneous interface with a high mitotic rate. The tumor is strongly positive for CD34. The MOST likely diagnosis is:

   a. Fibrous histiocytoma (FH)
   b. Atypical fibroxanthoma (AFX)
   c. Dermatofibrosarcoma protuberans (DFSP)
   d. Malignant fibrous histiocytoma (MFH)
   e. Dermatofibroma (DF)

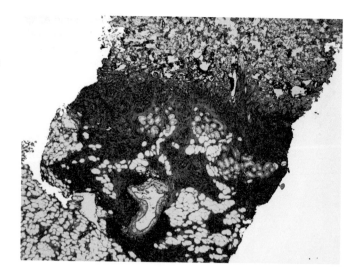

7. The following tumor, seen on the surface of the ovary, showed positive nuclear staining for WT1 and TP53. Which of the following statement(s) are TRUE?

   a. This staining profile is diagnostic of papillary serous carcinoma.
   b. This staining profile is diagnostic of surface papillary mesothelioma.
   c. This staining profile is diagnostic of malignant mesothelioma.
   d. All of the above
   e. None of the above

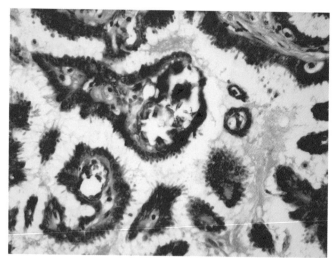

8. A 63-year-old woman presented with dysphagia and an esophageal ulcer. The following image shows a section stained with a polyclonal antibody to herpes simplex virus type 1 (HSV-1). Which of the following statements about HSV immunohistochemistry is TRUE?

   a. The section is not likely to stain with an anti-HSV-2 antibody because combined infection with HSV-1 and HSV-2 is uncommon.
   b. The section is likely to stain positively with an anti-HSV-2 antibody because combined HSV-1 and HSV-2 infection is common.
   c. Immunohistochemistry is more sensitive and specific than in situ hybridization for HSV-1 and HSV-2.
   d. The section is likely to react with anti-HSV-2 antibody because of cross-reactivity.
   e. HSV antibodies used in immunohistochemistry completely cross-react with varicella-zoster virus (VZV).

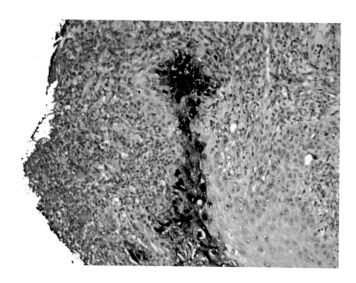

9. This tumor is positive for synaptophysin, chromogranin A, PAX5, CD99, and Fli-1 and negative for S100 and cytokeratin 7. The image following shows a cytokeratin 20 immunostained section of the tumor. This tumor MOST likely is:

   a. TTF-1 positive
   b. CD45 positive
   c. A metastatic small cell carcinoma of pulmonary origin
   d. A Merkel cell carcinoma
   e. A Ewing sarcoma/primitive neuroectodermal tumor (ES/PNET) family tumor

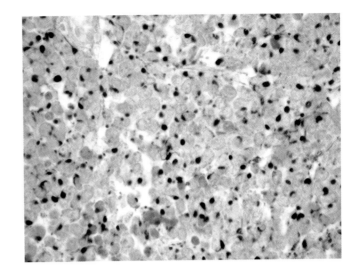

10. Which immunohistochemical stain would be MOST helpful to distinguish whether this cancer is a clear cell adenosquamous carcinoma or a squamous cell carcinoma with clear cell features?

    a. Antiestrogen receptor (anti-ER)
    b. Anti-PAX-2
    c. Anticarcinoembryonic antigen (anti-CEA)
    d. Anticytokeratin 5/6
    e. Anti-p16ink4a

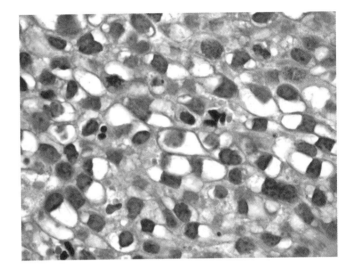

11. This 71-year-old woman presented with a 2.5-cm adrenal mass. A year earlier she underwent hysterectomy for endometrial carcinoma and pulmonary lobectomy for a primary adenocarcinoma of the lung, both with similar morphologic appearance but only the pulmonary carcinoma showed an activating mutation of the epidermal growth factor receptor (EGFR). Which combination of immunohistochemical stains can BEST help to identify the primary neoplasm of this adrenal metastasis?

    a. Antimelan A and anti-TTF-1
    b. Anti-TTF-1 and anti-PAX-8
    c. Antiinhibin and anti-PAX-2
    d. Antimelan A and antiinhibin
    e. Anti-CK7 and anti-PAX-8

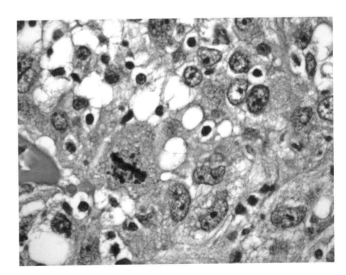

12. The metastatic adenocarcinoma (see also Question 11) of the adrenal gland shows strong nuclear staining for anti-PAX-8 suggestive of endometrial rather than pulmonary origin, which was confirmed by absence of an activating EGFR mutation previously detected in the pulmonary adenocarcinoma of the same patient. Which additional marker would BEST aid differentiating between pulmonary and endometrial adenocarcinoma?

   a. Anti-CEA
   b. Anti-PAX-5
   c. Anti-Napsin A
   d. Anti-CK5/6
   e. Antimucin 5A (anti-MUC5A)

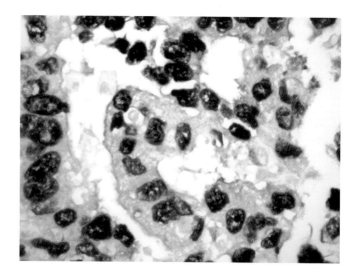

13. This 69-year-old man presented with restrictive heart disease, cardiac amyloidosis was detected by biopsy, and the amyloid subtype was identified by immunoassaying. Which of the following immunohistochemical stains will NOT help subclassify the amyloid type?

   a. Anti–serum amyloid A
   b. Antiimmunoglobulin light chain kappa or lambda
   c. Antiamyloid P
   d. Antiprealbumin
   e. Antitransthyretin

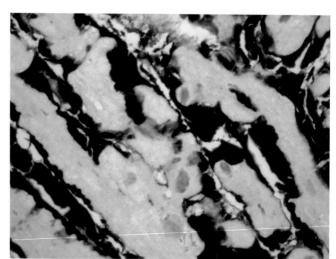

14. A 7.4-cm uterine mass was detected in this 79-year-old woman. It is a malignant mixed müllerian tumor with heterologous elements. Which panel of immunohistochemical stains will MOST likely confirm the diagnosis?

   a. Anticytokeratin (pan), antivimentin, anti–smooth muscle actin (anti-SMA), anti-S100
   b. Anti-CK7, anti-PAX-8, anti-CD10, anti-S100
   c. Anti-CK7, anti-PAX-8, anti-CD10, anti-SMA
   d. Anticytokeratin (pan), anti-PAX-2, anticollagen 2, antimyogenin
   e. Anticytokeratin (pan), antivimentin, anti-CD10, anti-S100

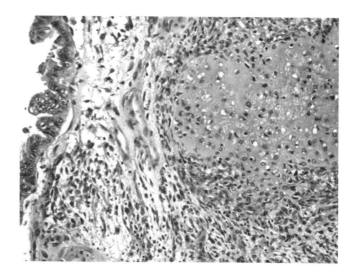

15. This lesion located on the scalp of a 5-month-old child is strongly positive for glucose transporter 1 (GLUT-1). What will the pathologist tell the physician regarding the growth dynamics of this lesion?

    a. This lesion commonly increases in size after birth and thereafter involutes slowly.

    b. This lesion involutes rapidly.

    c. This lesion neither will become larger nor will it regress.

    d. This lesion is commonly associated with cerebral hemangioblastomas.

    e. This lesion has to be considered malignant because GLUT-1 is a marker for malignant cells.

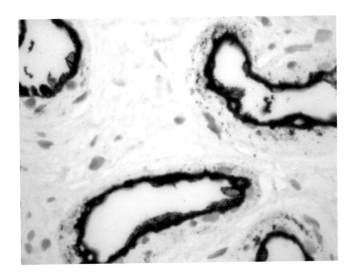

16. This 47-year-old woman had bilateral ovarian masses measuring 17 cm and 4.5 cm, respectively. The cancer cells are positive for anti-CDX-2, anti-CK7, anti-CK20, and anti-CA19.9 and negative for anti-PAX-8, anti-TTF-1, and anti-WT-1. Which of the following statements is CORRECT?

    a. The immunophenotype CDX-2 positive, PAX-8 negative favors a secondary malignancy over primary adenocarcinoma of müllerian origin.

    b. CA19.9 positive signet ring cells indicate that this is a variant of exocrine pancreatic cancer.

    c. The appendix is the most likely source of this carcinoma based on immunophenotype.

    d. A Herceptest (i.e., semiquantitative immunohistochemical study to evaluate amplification of HER-2/NEU) should be requested because it will aid differentiating between primary and secondary ovarian cancers.

    e. This type of cancer, if primary ovarian, will be strongly positive for p16ink4A.

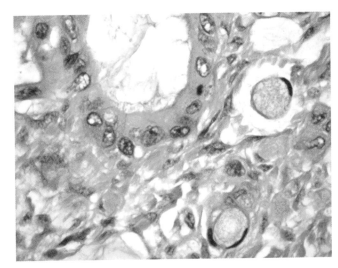

17. This bilateral ovarian neoplasm of a 25-year-old woman measured 12.5 cm in the left ovary and 4.5 cm in the right ovary. Which immunohistochemical stain will be CONSISTENTLY positive in this neoplasm?

    a. Anti-CD30

    b. Anti-Oct-4

    c. Anti-WT-1

    d. Anti-CD99

    e. Anti-CK7

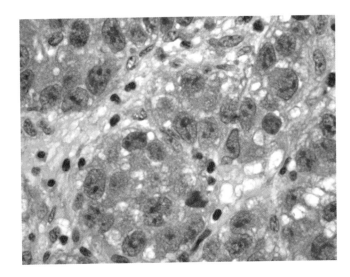

18. Which of the following neoplasms has NOT been reported to show prominent nuclear staining for β-catenin?
   a. Colorectal cancer
   b. Pancreas cancer
   c. Breast cancer
   d. Liver cancer
   e. Malignant melanoma

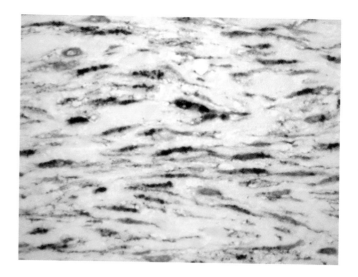

19. All neoplasms EXCEPT which one is commonly positive for the anti-HMB45?
   a. Hemangioblastoma
   b. Angiomyolipoma
   c. Junctional nevus (see figure)
   d. Lymphangiomyomatosis
   e. Perivascular epithelioid cell tumor (PEComa)

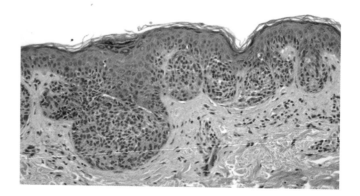

20. Which panel of immunohistochemical stains MOST likely will be diagnostic for this pleura-based spindle cell neoplasm?
   a. Anti-CD34, anti-CD117, anticytokeratin, anti-DOG1, anti-S100, antivimentin
   b. Anti-BCL2, anticalretinin, anti-CD117, anticytokeratin, antidesmin, anti-DOG1
   c. Anti-BCL2, anticalretinin, anti-CD34, anticytokeratin, anti-S100, anti-SMA
   d. Anticalretinin, anti-CD34, anti-CD117, anti-DOG1, S100, anti-SMA
   e. Anti-BCL2, anti-CD34, anticytokeratin, anti-S100, anti-SMA, anti-TTF-1

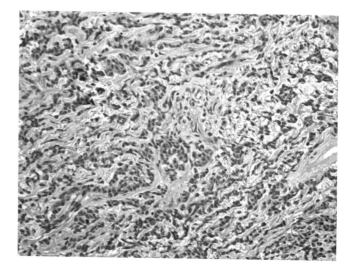

21. Which of the following is the MOST common immunophenotype of thymomas?
    a. CK positive, p63 positive, 34BetaE12 positive, Cam5.2 positive lesional cells, CD3 positive, CD1a positive, TdT and CD99 positive lymphocytes
    b. CK positive, CD5 positive, c-KIT positive lesional cells, CD3 positive, CD1a positive, TdT and CD99 positive lymphocytes
    c. CK positive, S100 positive, CD5 positive lesional cells with CD20 positive lymphocytes
    d. CK negative, CD20 positive lesional cells, CD3 positive lymphocytes
    e. CK positive, CD20 positive lesional cells, CD20 positive CD3 negative lymphocytes

22. A carcinoma presenting as a solitary abdominal wall skin lesion in a 75-year-old woman has the following profile: AE1/AE3 positive, Cam5.2 positive, CK7 negative, CK20 negative, vimentin positive, PAX2 positive, CEA negative, TTF-1 negative, and CDX2 negative. Which of the following is the MOST likely?
    a. Metastatic renal adenocarcinoma
    b. Metastatic pulmonary adenocarcinoma
    c. Adnexal carcinoma
    d. Metastatic thyroid carcinoma
    e. Metastatic colonic adenocarcinoma

23. A 70-year-old man with a history of resected colon cancer and chronic hepatitis C presents with a liver mass. Which of the following is the MOST likely immunophenotype of a primary hepatocellular carcinoma (HCC)?
    a. CK7 negative, CK20 negative, AE1/AE3 positive, Cam5.2 negative polyclonal (p) CEA cytoplasmic
    b. CK7 positive, CK20 negative, AE1/AE3 positive, Cam5.2 positive, pCEA membranous
    c. CK7 positive, CK20 positive, pCEA canalicular, Cam5.2 positive, AE1/AE3 positive, HepPar1 positive
    d. CK7 negative, CK20 negative, AE1/AE3 focal, Cam5.2 positive, pCEA canalicular, HepPar1 positive
    e. CK7 negative, CK20 positive, AE1/AE3 positive, Cam5.2 positive, pCEA canalicular, HepPar1 positive

24. Which of the following statements comparing monoclonal and polyclonal antibodies is TRUE?
    a. Monoclonal antibodies are mouse antibodies and polyclonal antibodies are rabbit antibodies.
    b. Monoclonal antibodies do not bind cross-reacting antigens.
    c. Affinity purification with the "correct" antigen or adsorption with cross-reacting antigens can reduce cross-reactivity of monoclonal antibodies.
    d. Monoclonal antibodies are always IgG and polyclonal antibodies are always IgM.
    e. Optimization of protocols using highly diluted polyclonal antibodies reduces the problem of cross-reactivity of polyclonal antibodies.

25. Which of the following statements about detection methods is TRUE?
    a. The avidin-biotin peroxidase method minimizes interference from endogenous biotin.
    b. When using the alkaline-phosphatase-antialkaline phosphatase (APAAP) method, the antialkaline phosphatase should be a mouse antibody when using a rabbit primary (and vice versa) to avoid cross-reactivity with the secondary antibody.
    c. Polymeric labeling methods, such as the Dako Envision-Plus (dextran-polymer linked, enzyme-labeled secondary antibody), incorporate secondary antibody and enzyme in the same step and avoid endogenous biotin but may suffer from steric effects limiting penetrative ability in the case of some antigens.
    d. Chromogens for alkaline phosphatase methods cannot be used for permanent cover slipping.
    e. None of the above

26. When evaluating HER2 overexpression in breast cancer, using the "Herceptest" immunostain, which of the following need to be considered?
    a. Overfixation, poor fixation, or delayed fixation can cause loss of signal and false-negative results.
    b. Excessive duration of antigen retrieval may cause false-positive or false-negative results.
    c. Crush artifacts and cracks may result in false-positive 2+ scores.
    d. Only approximately a third to one half of 2+ cases show gene amplification when tested by fluorescent in situ hybridization (FISH).
    e. All of the above

27. Which of the following statements about cytokeratin immunostaining of gliomas is TRUE?
    a. Gliomas never stain positively with AE1/AE3.
    b. Frozen, but not paraffin embedded, sections of gliomas stain positively with anticytokeratin antibodies.
    c. Gliomas do not stain with AE1/AE3, but stain positively with the more sensitive Cam5.2 antibody.
    d. Only glioblastomas (GBMs) stain with anticytokeratin antibodies.
    e. Gliomas are generally positive with AE1/AE3 antibody, but rarely stain with Cam5.2.

28. Which of the following statements about immunostaining of lung neoplasms is TRUE?
    a. Non–small cell carcinomas stain with TTF-1 more frequently than small cell carcinomas.
    b. TTF-1 stains most small cell carcinomas, pulmonary adenocarcinomas, squamous cell carcinomas, and carcinoids.
    c. Carcinomas of the lung are never positive for CDX2.
    d. TTF-1 stains most small cell lung carcinomas and the majority of pulmonary adenocarcinomas, and rarely stains pulmonary squamous cell carcinomas.
    e. The majority of pulmonary adenocarcinomas are CK7 negative, CK20 positive, TTF-1 positive, and CDX2 negative.

29. A patient presented with a small paratesticular tumor that histologically was composed of tubules lined by bland cuboidal to flattened cells. The tumor had the following immunoprofile: vimentin positive, CK positive, CK7 positive, EMA positive, Ber-EP4 negative, B72.3 negative, calretinin positive, CEA negative, inhibin negative, and LeuM1 negative. The MOST likely diagnosis is:
    a. Malignant mesothelioma
    b. Adenomatoid tumor
    c. Epithelioid hemangioma

d. Nephrogenic adenoma

e. Sex cord stromal tumor

30. Which of the following oncogenic mutations is NOT commonly monitored by immunohistochemistry?

a. Isocitrate dehydrogenase 1 (IDH1)

b. TP53

c. Integrase interactor 1 (INI-1)

d. *KRAS*

e. HER-2/NEU

31. Identify the tumor MOST likely to be negative for stem cell factor receptor (C-KIT).

a. Adenoid cystic carcinoma

b. Seminoma

c. Mast cell leukemia

d. Synovial sarcoma

e. Uterine leiomyosarcoma

32. Which panel of markers MOST likely will aid the differential diagnosis between PNET and neuroblastoma?

a. Anti-CD99, anti-Flt-1, antiperipherin

b. Anti-CD99, anti-Flt-1, antineuron specific enolase (anti-NSE)

c. Anti-Flt-1, antiperipherin, antisynaptophysin

d. Anti-CD99, anti-NSE, antivimentin

e. Anti-Flt-1, antineurofilament, anti-NSE

33. Which of the following markers is positive in Reed-Sternberg cells and negative in other lymphoid, plasma, and myeloid cells?

a. Anti-CD30

b. Anti-CD15

c. Antifascin

d. Anti-CD45RO

e. Antiepithelial membrane antigen (anti-EMA)

Answers

1. a. The photomicrograph shows a lesion with the characteristic appearance of a neurilemmoma (benign schwannoma). Neurilemmomas are diffusely and strongly positive for S100 protein. Although not specific for schwannoma, given this location and this histologic appearance, an S100 immunostain should suffice. This illustrates the importance of context in evaluating immunostaining results.

Marchevsky AM: Mediastinal tumors of peripheral nervous system origin. *Semin Diagn Pathol* 1999;16:65-78.

2. a. Paget disease of the nipple reflects the immunophenotype of the underlying breast cancer. It is most commonly positive for cytokeratin 7, low-molecular-weight cytokeratin, and CEA, as well as EMA. It usually overexpresses HER-2/neu. The majority of cases are S100 negative, and many are positive for ER and PR expression. Unlike extramammary Paget disease, which may be CK20 positive, Paget disease of the nipple is CK20 negative. Although CK7 is very sensitive for Paget disease of the nipple, Toker cells are also CK7 positive. CK5/6 would be negative in most cases of Paget disease or if positive would not distinguish between Paget disease and squamous cells.

Hitchcock A, Topham S, Bell J, et al: Routine diagnosis of mammary Paget's disease. A modern approach. *Am J Surg Pathol* 1992;16:58-61.

Smith KJ, Tuur S, Corvette D, et al: Cytokeratin 7 staining in mammary and extramammary Paget's disease. *Mod Pathol* 1997;10:1069-1074.

3. a. Low-grade lymphomas of mucosa-associated lymphoid tissue (MALT) are monocytoid B-cell lymphomas, which stain with CD20 and CD79a and demonstrate a marginal zone phenotype. They generally express surface immunoglobulin D (IgD), and are BCL2 positive, unlike germinal center cells. Only a minority of low-grade MALT lymphomas express CD43.

Arends JE, Bot FJ, Gisbertz IA, Schouten HC: Expression of CD10, CD75 and CD43 in MALT lymphoma and their usefulness in discriminating MALT lymphoma from follicular lymphoma and chronic gastritis. *Histopathology* 1999;35:209-215.

Dogan A, Bagdi E, Munson P, Isaacson PG: CD10 and BCL-6 expression in paraffin sections of normal lymphoid tissue and B-cell lymphomas. *Am J Surg Pathol* 2000;24:846-852.

4. a. Pancreatic/bile duct carcinomas are generally CK7 positive and often CK20 positive. They stain with anti-CEA antibodies and stain weakly or not at all with CDX2.

Lung and breast and ovarian tumors are generally CK7 positive, CK20 negative, and CDX2 negative. Colonic adenocarcinomas are usually CK7 negative, CK20 positive, and CDX2 positive.

Chu P, Wu E, Weiss LM: Cytokeratin 7 and cytokeratin 20 expression in epithelial neoplasms: a survey of 435 cases. *Mod Pathol* 2000;13:962-972.

Werling RW, Yaziji H, Bacchi CE, Gown AM: CDX2, a highly sensitive and specific marker of adenocarcinomas of intestinal origin: an immunohistochemical survey of 476 primary and metastatic carcinomas. *Am J Surg Pathol* 2003;27:303-310.

5. d. Immunostaining for CMV identifies tissue infection, and in most cases is more specific than culture. Although cytomegalic changes are generally easily identified, they may be obscured by inflammation (and in some settings, such as AIDS, may not be well developed), in which case immunostaining or in situ hybridization improves detection of CMV infection.

Francis ND, Boylston AW, Roberts AH, et al: Cytomegalovirus infection in gastrointestinal tracts of patients infected with HIV-1 or AIDS. *J Clin Pathol* 1989;42:1055-1064.

Schwartz DA, Wilcox CM: Atypical cytomegalovirus inclusions in gastrointestinal biopsy specimens from patients with the acquired immunodeficiency syndrome: diagnostic role of in situ nucleic acid hybridization. *Hum Pathol* 1992;23:1019-1026.

6. c. DFSP (a low-grade malignant tumor) consists of spindle cells arranged in a monotonous, storiform pattern. Occasionally, DFSP may contain areas of fibrosarcomatous transformation. Lesional cells exhibit diffuse and strong

CD34 expression. AFXs occur in the dermis of the sun-damaged skin of older individuals, are CD34 negative, and express myofibroblastic markers, such as SMA and HHF35. MFHs may be subcutaneous but are more pleomorphic than DFSP. Like AFXs, they express myofibroblastic markers. DFs (or FHs) have a more variegated appearance, containing foamy histiocytes, occasional multinucleated giant cells, and chronic inflammatory cells; characteristically entrap host collagen fibers at the edge of the lesion; and unlike DFSP, elicit a characteristic epidermal hyperplasia in the overlying epidermis. DFs are CD34 negative and express myofibroblastic markers. Other lesions that may be CD34 positive include desmoplastic melanoma and solitary fibrous tumor. The latter is a more deeply seated lesion, and the former is generally S100 positive.

Goldblum JR, Reith JD, Weiss SW: Sarcomas arising in dermatofibrosarcoma protuberans. A reappraisal of biologic behavior in eighteen cases treated by wide local excision with extended clinical follow up. *Am J Surg Pathol* 2000;24:1225-1230.

Horenstein MG, Prieto VG, Nuckols JD, et al: Indeterminate fibrohistiocytic lesions of the skin: is there a spectrum between dermatofibroma and dermatofibrosarcoma protuberans? *Am J Surg Pathol* 2000;24:996-1003.

7. e. Although positive immunostaining for TP53 and WT1 proteins is characteristic of papillary serous carcinoma, it is also seen in other tumors. Diffuse peritoneal malignant mesothelioma is characteristically WT1 positive and may express TP53. In this setting, calretinin, CK5/6, and thrombospondin may be used as mesothelial markers and BerEp4, CD15, CEA, and B72.3 as ovarian markers. Of the markers mentioned, calretinin is the most sensitive mesothelial marker and BerEp4 the most sensitive adenocarcinoma marker (when the differential diagnosis is limited to mesothelioma versus papillary serous carcinoma).

Acs G, Pasha T, Zhang PJ: WT1 is differentially expressed in serous, endometrioid, clear cell, and mucinous carcinomas of the peritoneum, fallopian tube, ovary, and endometrium. *Int J Gynecol Pathol* 2004;23:110-118.

Attanoos RL, Webb R, Dojcinov SD, Gibbs AR: Value of mesothelial and epithelial antibodies in distinguishing diffuse peritoneal mesothelioma in females from serous papillary carcinoma of the ovary and peritoneum. *Histopathology* 2002;40:237-244.

8. d. Immunohistochemistry is a useful adjunct in the diagnosis of HSV infection. Most antibodies stain both HSV-1 and HSV-2, precluding reliable identification of the specific HSV—in spite of some investigators' claims that HSV-1 antibodies stain HSV-2 less intensely, and vice versa. In situ hybridization allows distinction of HSV-1 and HSV-2 but is more labor intensive. Although some HSV antibodies may weakly cross-react with VZV, this is usually not a problem.

Martin JR, Holt RK, Langston C, et al: Type-specific identification of herpes simplex and varicella-zoster virus antigen in autopsy tissues. *Hum Pathol* 1991;22:75-80.

Nicoll JA, Love S, Burton PA, Berry PJ: Autopsy findings in two cases of neonatal herpes simplex virus infection: detection of virus by immunohistochemistry, in situ hybridization and the polymerase chain reaction. *Histopathology* 1994;24:257-264.

Strickler JG, Manivel JC, Copenhaver CM, Kubic VL: Comparison of in situ hybridization and immunohistochemistry for detection of cytomegalovirus and herpes simplex virus. *Hum Pathol* 1990;21(4):443-448.

9. d. Merkel cell carcinoma, a primary cutaneous or subcutaneous neuroendocrine carcinoma thought to arise from the Merkel cell found in the basal layer of the epidermis and hair-shaft, must be distinguished from the more aggressive metastatic small cell carcinoma. Merkel cell carcinomas, unlike pulmonary small cell carcinomas, are CK7 negative and show punctate, perinuclear positivity with CK20. Merkel cell carcinomas are negative for TTF-1, which stains the vast majority of small cell lung carcinomas, as well as a significant proportion of nonpulmonary small cell carcinomas. Merkel cell carcinomas are CD99 and Fli-1 positive, and their expression in an adult tumor is not indicative of EW/PNET, which affects younger individuals and is CK20 negative.

Dong HY, Liu W, Cohen P, et al: B-cell specific activation protein encoded by the PAX-5 gene is commonly expressed in Merkel cell carcinoma and small cell carcinomas. *Am J Surg Pathol* 2005;29:687-692.

Llombart B, Monteagudo C, Lopez-Guerrero JA, et al: Clinicopathological and immunohistochemical analysis of 20 cases of Merkel cell carcinoma in search of prognostic markers. *Histopathology* 2005;46:622-634.

10. c. The differential diagnosis for carcinomas with clear cells of the uterine cervix includes clear cell adenocarcinoma, clear cell adenosquamous carcinoma, and squamous cell carcinoma with clear cell features (i.e., glycogen-rich cytoplasm). In this case many clear cells were strongly positive for CEA, which favors endocervical glandular origin. Such cancers are commonly associated with HPV type 18. ER and PAX-2 are positive in endometrioid, serous, and mesonephric cancers, all of which may contain clear cells but are not able to distinguish between endocervical glandular and squamous cells. CK5/6 as a marker of squamous cells is expected to be positive in both squamous cell carcinoma and adenosquamous carcinoma.

P16ink4a can be positive in any form of HPV-related cervical cancer. Special stains to highlight mucin (e.g., mucicarmine) can be used to distinguish between clear cells derived from glandular (mucicarmine positive) or squamous (mucicarmine negative) epithelium.

Fujiwara H, Mitchell MF, Arseneau J, et al: Clear cell adenosquamous carcinoma of the cervix. An aggressive tumor associated with human papillomavirus-18. *Cancer* 1995;76:1591-1600.

Wells M, Brown LJ: Glandular lesions of the uterine cervix: the present state of our knowledge. *Histopathology* 1986;10:777-792.

11. b. PAX-2 and PAX-8 are paired box genes important for the development of mesonephric, metanephric, and paramesonephric structures. TTF-1 is positive in 80% to 90% of pulmonary adenocarcinomas. Melan A and inhibin are markers for adrenal cortical cells and, thus, will not aid distinguishing between endometrial and pulmonary primary neoplasms. CK7 is expected to be positive in both types of adenocarcinoma.

Johansson L: Histopathologic classification of lung cancer: relevance of cytokeratin and TTF-1 immunophenotyping. *Ann Diagn Pathol* 2004;8:259-267.

Tong GX, Devaraj K, Hamele-Bena D, et al: Pax8: a marker for carcinoma of Müllerian origin in serous effusions. *Diagn Cytopathol* 2011;39:567-574.

12. c. Napsin A is a pepsinlike protease present in type II alveolocytes and an additional marker for pulmonary adenocarcinoma, because TTF-1 can be positive in many nonpulmonary carcinomas. The combination of TTF-1 and Napsin A shows maximum sensitivity and specificity with respect to identifying pulmonary adenocarcinomas by immunohistochemistry. CEA is positive in pulmonary adenocarcinomas and endometrial carcinomas with mucinous metaplasia and thus is not an optimal marker. CK5/6 mark squamous elements, which can occur in both forms of adenocarcinomas. The glycoprotein MUC5A, though primarily present in the normal pulmonary and gastric mucosa, is detected immunohistochemically in 22% of endometrial and 14% of pulmonary adenocarcinomas, respectively.

Ye J, Findeis-Hosey J, Yang Q, et al: Combination of Napsin A and TTF-1 immunohistochemistry helps in differentiating primary lung adenocarcinoma from metastatic carcinoma in the lung. *Appl Immunohistochem Mol Morphol* 2011;19:313-317.
Ye J, Hameed O, Findeis-Hosey J, et al: Diagnostic utility of PAX8, TTF-1 and Napsin A for discriminating metastatic carcinoma from primary adenocarcinoma of the lung. *Biotech Histochem* 2012;87:30-34.

13. c. The three most common forms of cardiac amyloidosis are primary amyloidosis of the immunoglobulin (AL) light chain type, secondary cardiac amyloidosis of the amyloid A (AA) type, and senile cardiac amyloidosis of the prealbumin/transthyretin (ATTR) type, which is shown in the picture. Only amyloid P is a component of all types of amyloid and, thus, will not help to distinguish among subtypes of amyloid.

Kapoor P, Thenappan T, Singh E, et al: Cardiac amyloidosis: a practical approach to diagnosis and management. *Am J Med* 2011;124:1006-1015.
Yang GC, Gallo GR: Protein A-gold immunoelectron microscopic study of amyloid fibrils, granular deposits, and fibrillar luminal aggregates in renal amyloidosis. *Am J Pathol* 1990;137:1223-1231.

14. b. Anti-CK7 and anti-PAX-8 will consistently identify the epithelial elements of paramesonephric (müllerian) tumors, and CD10 is a marker for endometrial stroma. S100 is present in cartilage and, thus, capable of identifying the heterologous element shown in the figure. Antipancytokeratin (i.e., antibody cocktail to multiple cytokeratins) could be used in addition to anti-CK7 but not instead, because it will not distinguish endometrial carcinosarcomas from renal carcinosarcomas. The latter are also PAX-2, PAX-8, vimentin, and CD10 positive and both may contain heterologous elements. SMA is inferior to CD10 as a marker for endometrial stroma. Myogenin marks skeletal muscle rather than cartilage, which although commonly found in malignant mixed müllerian tumors is not present in the current neoplasm.

Ozcan A, Liles N, Coffey D, et al: PAX2 and PAX8 expression in primary and metastatic Müllerian epithelial tumors: a comprehensive comparison. *Am J Surg Pathol* 2011;35:1837-1847.
Vermeulen P, Hoekx L, Colpaert C, et al: Biphasic sarcomatoid carcinoma (carcinosarcoma) of the renal pelvis with heterologous chondrogenic differentiation. *Virchows Arch* 2000;437:194-197.

15. a. Commonly infantile capillary hemangiomas are GLUT-1 positive and grow rapidly after birth; thereafter, they regress slowly, usually by scar formation. They are not associated with hemangioblastomas. GLUT-1 negative capillary hemangiomas in small children are commonly congenital hemangiomas of either the rapidly involuting (RICH) or noninvoluting (NICH) type. Although GLUT-1 is a marker for malignant cells in many neoplasms, such as mesothelioma, this is not true for endothelial cell neoplasm, because it is rarely positive in angiosarcoma.

Monaco SE, Shuai Y, Bansal M, et al: The diagnostic utility of p16 FISH and GLUT-1 immunohistochemical analysis in mesothelial proliferations. *Am J Clin Pathol* 2011;135:619-627.
Picard A, Boscolo E, Khan ZA, et al: IGF-2 and FLT-1/VEGF-R1 mRNA levels reveal distinctions and similarities between congenital and common infantile hemangioma. *Pediatr Res* 2008;63:263-267.

16. a. A computed tomography (CT) scan showed a mass in the distal pancreas, which confirmed the diagnosis of metastatic signet ring cell carcinoma originating in the pancreas. It has been shown that only 21% of mucinous ovarian tumors express CDX-2, whereas CDX-2 is positive in nearly all gastrointestinal cancers with this morphologic appearance. Conversely, PAX-8 is positive in 79% of ovarian cancers but only 16% of pancreatic cancers, in which it preferentially stains those with neuroendocrine differentiation. Gastrointestinal cancers are essentially negative for PAX-8. The combination of CDX-2 positive and PAX-8 negative favors a secondary malignancy with signet ring cells (Krukenberg tumor) over an ovarian primary. Although the primary in this case arose from the pancreas, CA19.9 cannot distinguish between gastric and pancreatic origin.

Most mucinous appendiceal cancers would stain negative for CK7 and CA19.9.

HER-2/NEU amplification occurs in 8.3% of gastric cancers but rarely in cancers with signet ring cells or in pancreatic cancers. Amplification of this oncogene has also been found in 2.3% of ovarian cancers. WT-1 is positive in serous ovarian carcinomas rather than in mucinous ones; hence, this finding is unlikely to aid in distinguishing between primary and secondary neoplasm in this case.

Kim MJ: The usefulness of CDX-2 for differentiating primary and metastatic ovarian carcinoma: an immunohistochemical study using a tissue microarray. *J Korean Med Sci* 2005;20:643-648.
Tacha D, Zhou D, Cheng L: Expression of PAX8 in normal and neoplastic tissues: a comprehensive immunohistochemical study. *Appl Immunohistochem Mol Morphol* 2011;19:293-299.
Tapia C, Glatz K, Novotny H, et al: Close association between HER-2 amplification and overexpression in human tumors of non-breast origin. *Mod Pathol* 2007;20:192-198.

17. b. Dysgerminomas are neoplasms of undifferentiated germ cells and, thus, should stain for anti-Oct-4, antiplacental alkaline phosphatase (anti-PLAP), anti-CD117 (c-kit), antilactate dehydrogenase (anti-LDH), antivimentin, antiferritin, and anti-NY-ESO1 among others. Anti-CD30 is usually positive in embryonal carcinomas, anti-WT-1 in surface epithelial tumors of the serous type, and CD99 and antialpha inhibin in ovarian stromal cell neoplasm. Immature stromal and germ cell elements together suggest a gonadoblastoma, which may become overgrown by a dysgerminoma. Anti-CK7, like most other cytokeratins, is

usually negative in dysgerminoma, and positive staining would indicate a nondysgerminomatous component, which is important for treatment and prognosis.

Abiko K, Mandai M, Hamanishi J, et al: Oct4 expression in immature teratoma of the ovary: relevance to histologic grade and degree of differentiation. *Am J Surg Pathol* 2010;34: 1842-1848.

Cheng L, Thomas A, Roth LM, et al: OCT4: a novel biomarker for dysgerminoma of the ovary. *Am J Surg Pathol* 2004;28: 1341-1346.

Ulbright TM: Germ cell tumors of the gonads: a selective review emphasizing problems in differential diagnosis, newly appreciated, and controversial issues. *Mod Pathol* 2005; 18(Suppl 2):S61-79.

18. c. Nuclear accumulation of β-catenin is a consequence of mutations of the β-catenin gene, as is the case for HCC and solid pseudopapillary carcinoma of the pancreas, aberrant WNT/TGF-β signaling commonly found in melanomas, and adenomatous polyposis coli (APC) gene mutation, which is an early event in colorectal carcinomas. The APC gene product is responsible for β-catenin ubiquitination, which is instrumental for its degradation. Mutations of E-cadherin (CDH1) are a major feature of lobular breast cancer. It leads to loss of β-catenin along the cell surface but no nuclear accumulation because the mechanism for degradation (i.e., APC) is still intact.

Gough NR: Focus issue: Wnt and β-catenin signaling in development and disease. *Sci Signal* 2012;5(206):eg2.

Sarrió D, Moreno-Bueno G, Hardisson D, et al: Epigenetic and genetic alterations of APC and CDH1 genes in lobular breast cancer: relationships with abnormal E-cadherin and catenin expression and microsatellite instability. *Int J Cancer* 2003;106:208-215.

Wei Y, Van Nhieu JT, Prigent S, et al: Altered expression of E-cadherin in hepatocellular carcinoma: correlations with genetic alterations, beta-catenin expression, and clinical features. *Hepatology* 2002;36:692-701.

19. a. Hemangioblastomas are neoplasms commonly positive for mesenchymal and neural/neuroectodermal markers, such as anti-S100, anti-NSE, and anti-CD57. These tumors are consistently negative for endothelial markers and anti-HMB45. Central hemangioblastomas are commonly seen in von Hippel-Lindau disease, which in contrast to tuberous sclerosis is not associated with PEComas containing anti-HMB45 positive spindle cells. Angiomyolipoma and lymphangiomyomatosis are both characterized by anti-HMB45 positive smooth muscle cells, and junctional nevi contain anti-HMB45 positive melanocytes. PEComas may occur at any site of the body. The most common representatives are angiomyolipoma and lymphangiomyoma.

Walsh SN, Sangüeza OP: PEComas: a review with emphasis on cutaneous lesions. *Semin Diagn Pathol* 2009;26:123-130.

Xiong J, Chu SG, Wang Y, et al: Metastasis of renal cell carcinoma to a haemangioblastoma of the medulla oblongata in von Hippel-Lindau syndrome. *J Clin Neurosci* 2010;17:1213-1215.

20. c. This is a solitary fibrous tumor of the pleura (SFTP), which consistently is positive for anti-CD34 and anti-BCL2. SFTP has to be differentiated from mesothelioma by anticalretinin and anticytokeratin staining, nerve sheath tumors by anti-S100 staining and myofibroblastic and smooth muscle proliferations with smooth muscle markers. The pleural location essentially excludes any primary gastrointestinal stromal tumor, and thus, CD117 and DOG-1 staining are not a primary concern. Similarly, negative anticytokeratin staining excludes virtually all primary pulmonary carcinomas; thus, staining for anti-TTF-1 is a low priority. Antidesmin may be added to the panel to distinguish SFTP from other spindle cell neoplasms, but anti-SMA is a better choice because it covers both neoplastic and nonneoplastic smooth muscle and myofibroblastic proliferations. Both are negative in SFTP.

Robinson LA: Solitary fibrous tumor of the pleura. *Cancer Control* 2006;13:264-269.

21. a. The lesional cell of thymomas is the epithelial cell, which stains with various anticytokeratin antibodies, including antibodies to high-molecular-weight (34BetaE12) and low-molecular-weight (Cam5.2) cytokeratin. Most thymomas are p63 positive. Lymphocytes with a thymic phenotype (CD3 positive, CD1a positive, TdT positive, CD99 positive) are present in these tumors, even when they metastasize. CD5 and KIT are expressed by the majority of thymic carcinomas and only occasionally by thymomas. CD20 positive lymphocytes may predominate in micronodular thymomas with lymphoid hyperplasia, and CD20 also stains spindle-shaped thymoma cells, which are also CK positive.

Kornstein MJ, Rosai J: CD5 labeling of thymic carcinomas and other nonlymphoid neoplasms. *Am J Clin Pathol* 1998;109: 722-726.

Pan CC, Chen PC, Chiang H: KIT (CD117) is frequently overexpressed in thymic carcinomas but is absent in thymomas. *J Pathol* 2004;202:375-381.

22. a. This presentation is characteristic of metastatic renal cell carcinomas (RCCs). The most common type of RCC (clear cell or conventional) is typically CK7 negative, CK20 negative, and CAM5.2 positive, staining weakly with pancytokeratin antibodies. RCCs are generally vimentin positive and EMA positive. In addition, RCC and PAX2 are relatively specific markers of RCC, staining the conventional and papillary but not the chromophobe type. The latter stains with kidney-specific cadherin. Urothelial and pancreatic carcinomas are usually vimentin negative, CK7 positive, and CK20 positive/negative; adrenocortical carcinomas are only weakly positive or negative for cytokeratin and inhibin positive. Colon carcinomas are CK20 positive, and pulmonary adenocarcinomas are CK7 positive and may be TTF-1 positive. Both are PAX2 negative.

Chu PG, Weiss LM: Keratin expression in human tissues and neoplasms. *Histopathology* 2002;40:403-439.

Shen SS, Krishna B, Chirala R, et al: Kidney-specific cadherin, a specific marker for the distal portion of the nephron and related renal neoplasms. *Mod Pathol* 2005;18:933-940.

Wang HY, Mills SE: KIT and RCC are useful in distinguishing chromophobe renal cell carcinoma from the granular variant of clear cell renal cell carcinoma. *Am J Surg Pathol* 2005;29: 640-646.

23. d. HCCs only weakly express CK19, staining poorly with AE1/AE3, and express CK18, staining strongly with CAM5.2. They are generally CK7 negative, with the exception of the fibrolamellar variant. HCCs characteristically stain in a canalicular pattern with polyclonal CEA antibodies and fail to stain with most monoclonal anti-CEA antibodies. HepPar1 is a relatively specific HCC marker. Other relatively specific HCC markers are α-fetoprotein and α₁-antitrypsin. Colon cancer is usually diffusely AE1/AE3 and CK20 positive.

Goldstein NS, Silverman JF: Immunohistochemistry of the gastrointestinal tract, pancreas, bile ducts, gallbladder and liver. In Dabbs DJ (ed): *Diagnostic Immunohistochemistry.* New York: Churchill Livingstone, 2000, pp 333-406.
Maeda T, Kajiama K, Adachi E, et al: The expression of cytokeratins 7 and 20 in primary and metastatic carcinomas of the liver. *Mod Pathol* 1996;9:901-909.
Wang NP, Zee S, Zarbo RJ, et al: Coordinate expression of cytokeratins 7 and 20 defines unique subsets of carcinomas. *Appl Immunohistochem* 1995;3:99-107.

24. e. Monoclonal antibodies are obtained using hybridoma technologies. They bind to a single epitope on an antigen. If the antigen shares the epitope with other substances, cross-reactivity will be complete and cannot be reduced by affinity purification or adsorption. Polyclonal antibodies, which actually consist of a mixture of various antibodies, reactive against various epitopes on an antigen with varying affinities, can be made more specific by adsorption with cross-reacting antigen to remove cross-reacting antibodies and more avid by adsorption with the relevant antigen to select higher affinity antibodies. Although each monoclonal antibody is of a single type or isotype, both IgG and IgM antibodies are used. In recent years there has been increasing use of nonmurine monoclonal antibodies (e.g., AMACR is a rabbit monoclonal).

Taylor CR, Shi S-R, Barr NJ, Wu N: Techniques of immuno-histochemistry: principles, pitfalls, and standardization. In Dabbs DJ (ed): *Diagnostic Immunohistochemistry.* New York: Churchill Livingstone, 2002, pp 3-44.

25. c. The avidin-biotin peroxidase complex method, although highly sensitive, does cross-react with endogenous biotin. This reaction can be reduced by the use of avidin biotin block or a combination of egg white and skim milk powder. For routine diagnostic use, adoption of a polymer-linked, enzyme-labeled secondary antibody eliminates this problem and, by combining the secondary antibody and enzyme in the same step, speeds up the process. The three-dimensional branching structure of the dextran polymer may cause some steric effects with some antigens. The APAAP method utilizes the divalent nature of the secondary antibody to link the primary antibody to the APAAP complex; therefore, both the primary antibody and the anti-AP antibody should be of the *same* species. Chromogens, which can be used with permanent cover-slipping methods, are available and include nitroblue tetrazolium (NBT) and new fuchsin.

Taylor CR, Shi S-R, Barr NJ, Wu N: Techniques of immuno-histochemistry: principles, pitfalls, and standardization. In Dabbs DJ (ed): *Diagnostic Immunohistochemistry.* New York: Churchill Livingstone, 2002, pp 3-44.

26. e. When immunostaining breast cancer with the Herceptest kit, invasive carcinoma is scored as "0" (no staining, or fewer than 10% of cells showing any membranous staining), "1+" (faint staining of more than 10% of cells, without staining of the entire membrane), "2+" (weak to moderate staining of the entire membrane circumference of greater than 10% of cells), and "3+"(strong staining of the entire membrane circumference of greater than 10% of cells). Factors that can affect this semiquantitative test include delayed fixation, underfixation, or overfixation, leading to poor protein preservation. Excessive antigen retrieval can cause false-positive results, as can crush artifacts, and even small cracks in the section, as well as retraction artifacts around tumor cells. These technical factors lead to discordance with FISH results. Only about 30% to 50% of 2+ cases show gene amplification by FISH in various studies, with occasional 1+ cases being amplified and a small percentage of 3+ cases being nonamplified. Although the superior predictive value of FISH for trastuzumab responsiveness might have a biologic basis, technical factors are also significant.

Dowsett M, Bartlett J, Ellis IO, et al: Correlation between immunohistochemistry (HercepTest) and fluorescence in situ hybridization (FISH) for HER-2 in 426 breast carcinomas from 37 centres. *J Pathol* 2003;199:418-422.
Ellis CM, Dyson MJ, Stephenson TJ, Maltby EL: HER2 amplification status in breast cancer: a comparison between immunohistochemical staining and fluorescence in situ hybridisation using manual and automated quantitative image analysis scoring techniques. *J Clin Pathol* 2005;58:710-714.

27. e. Glial tissue and gliomas stain with AE1/AE3 but not with CAM5.2. This is thought to represent a cross-reaction between glial-fibrillary acidic protein (GFAP) and AE1/AE3. CAM5.2 does not stain glial tissue or gliomas, making the latter more useful for staining metastatic carcinomas in brain biopsies. Whereas most cytokeratin staining of normal brain tissue and gliomas is due to cross-reaction with noncytokeratin intermediate filaments, high-grade gliomas may also occasionally express cytokeratins, demonstrated by Northern or Western blotting.

Hirato J, Nakazato Y, Ogawa A: Expression of non-glial intermediate filament proteins in gliomas. *Clin Neuropathol* 1994;13:1-11.
Kriho VK, Yang HY, Moskal JR, Skalli O: Keratin expression in astrocytomas: an immunofluorescent and biochemical reassessment. *Virchows Arch* 1997;431(2):139-147.
Oh D, Prayson RA: Evaluation of epithelial and keratin markers in glioblastoma multiforme: an immunohistochemical study. *Arch Pathol Lab Med* 1999;123:917-920.

28. d. Carcinomas of the lung are generally CK7 positive and CK20 negative, with a variable proportion expressing TTF-1. Almost all small cell lung carcinomas are TTF-1 positive, a majority of adenocarcinomas are TTF-1 positive, and tumors with squamous differentiation are generally negative. Most lung carcinomas are CDX2 negative, except for mucinous pulmonary adenocarcinomas.

Chu PG, Weiss LM: Keratin expression in human tissues and neoplasms. *Histopathology* 2002;40:403-439.

29. b. Adenomatoid tumor, the most common benign paratesticular tumor, is of mesothelial derivation and characteristically stains for pancytokeratin, calretinin, EMA, and vimentin and is negative for adenocarcinoma markers. Mesothelioma has the same immunophenotype but tends to be larger, with more malignant cytologic appearance at presentation. Epithelioid hemangioma does occur in this area and may be keratin positive but is CD34 positive and calretinin negative. Nephrogenic adenoma (metaplasia) develops in the urinary tract and is characteristically AMACR and PAX2 positive. Sex cord stromal tumors, testicular neoplasms that may occur in the paratesticular region, contain abundant cytoplasmic lipofuscin, express inhibin, and may express calretinin but are CK7 negative and weakly CK positive or CK negative.

Gupta A, Wang HL, Policarpio-Nicolas ML: Expression of alpha-methylacyl-coenzime-A racemase in nephrogenic adenoma. *Am J Surg Pathol* 2004;28(9):1224-1229.

Ulbright TM, Amin MB, Young RH: Tumors of the testis, adnexa, spermatic cord, and scrotum. In *Atlas of Tumor Pathology*. Fascicle 25, 2nd series, Washington, DC: Armed Forces Institute of Pathology, 1999, pp 41-58.

30. d. The point mutation from arginine to histidine in codon 132 (R132H) of IDH1 is commonly found in astrogliomas and is not present in gliosis. The test can be performed with an antibody specific to the mutant IDH1. Mutations of TP53 commonly lead to a protein with a longer half-life than the short-lived wild-type p53 protein; thus, accumulation of this protein can be studied by immunohistochemistry. INI-1 is deleted in rhabdoid tumors and epithelioid sarcomas; thus, absence of the protein aids making the diagnosis of these entities. HER-2/NEU amplification is studied by Herceptest assessed according to the American Society of Clinical Oncology/College of American Pathologists (ASCO-CAP) or treatment of gastric cancer (ToG) guidelines for breast and gastric carcinoma, respectively. *KRAS* mutations are studied by rt-PCR techniques, because multiple activating point mutations are known and no suitable antibody exists to distinguish mutant from wild-type *KRAS*.

Camelo-Piragua S, Jansen M, Ganguly A, et al: Mutant IDH1-specific immunohistochemistry distinguishes diffuse astrocytoma from astrocytosis. *Acta Neuropathol* 2010;119: 509-511.

Sakharpe A, Lahat G, Gulamhusein T, et al: Epithelioid sarcoma and unclassified sarcoma with epithelioid features: clinicopathological variables, molecular markers, and a new experimental model. *Oncologist* 2011;16:512-522.

31. e. Smooth muscle neoplasms are likely negative for markers of gastrointestinal stromal tumors including anti-CD34, anti-CD117, and anti-DOG-1.

Dirnhofer S, Zimpfer A, Went P: The diagnostic and predictive role of kit (CD117). *Ther Umsch* 2006;63:273-278.

López-Guerrero JA, Navarro S, Noguera R, et al: Mutational analysis of the c-KIT AND PDGFRalpha in a series of molecularly well-characterized synovial sarcomas. *Diagn Mol Pathol* 2005;14:134-139.

Miettinen M, Lasota J: KIT (CD117): a review on expression in normal and neoplastic tissues, and mutations and their clinicopathologic correlation. *Appl Immunohistochem Mol Morphol* 2005;13:205-220.

32. a. Anti-CD99 and anti-Flt-1 (i.e., vascular endothelial growth factor receptor 1) are positive in PNETs and negative in neuroblastomas. PNETs carry the a reciprocal 11;22 (q24; q12) translocation with high levels of the EWS-FLT-1 fusion gene product. Conversely, neuroblastomas are positive for the class III intermediate filament peripherin, which is exclusively found in the peripheral nervous system and a subpopulation of neuroendocrine cells, whereas PNETs are negative for this marker. Anti-NSE, antineurofilament, antisynaptophysin, and antivimentin have been shown in both types of neoplasms and, thus, will not aid to distinguish neuroblastoma from PNET, although they may be useful to differentiate both from other small round blue cell neoplasms.

Willoughby V, Sonawala A, Werlang-Perurena A, Donner LR: A comparative immunohistochemical analysis of small round cell tumors of childhood: utility of peripherin and alpha-internexin as markers for neuroblastomas. *Appl Immunohistochem Mol Morphol* 2008;16:344-348.

33. c. Fascin is an actin bundling protein, which is upregulated in many transformed cells. Antifascin is a reliable marker for Reed-Sternberg cells and will not stain most other leukocytes, although it may stain other tumors, such as neuroendocrine lung tumors. Anti-CD15 is positive in myeloid cells and anti-CD30 in many activated lymphocytes (see Epstein-Barr virus [EBV] infection). Anti-CD15 and anti-CD30 label both cell membrane and the perinuclear Golgi area in Reed-Sternberg cells, a distribution distinct from that of other cell types. Anti-CD45RO is not a good marker for the purpose described earlier and anti-EMA is positive in plasma cells rather than Reed-Sternberg cells.

Adam P, Bonzheim I, Fend F, Quintanilla-Martínez L: Epstein-Barr virus-positive diffuse large B-cell lymphomas of the elderly. *Adv Anat Pathol* 2011;18:349-355.

Pinkus GS, Pinkus JL, Langhoff E, et al: Fascin, a sensitive new marker for Reed-Sternberg cells of Hodgkin's disease. Evidence for a dendritic or B cell derivation? *Am J Pathol* 1997;150:543-562.

CHAPTER 23

MOLECULAR PATHOLOGY DIAGNOSTICS

Mahesh M. Mansukhani

QUESTIONS

Questions 1-13 in this chapter refer to a photograph or photomicrograph.

1. The corresponding figure shows a karyotype of a CD20, CD10, PAX5, and BCL6 positive lymphoid neoplasm. Which of the following statements about this type of tumor is TRUE?
   a. This tumor harbors a t(14;18)(q32;q21) translocation, which causes overexpression of cyclin D1.
   b. Polymerase chain reaction (PCR) detects this translocation in a greater proportion of cases than does fluorescence in situ hybridization (FISH) or Southern blotting.
   c. Immunostaining for BCL2 in B cells is diagnostic of follicular lymphoma.
   d. Overexpression of BCL2 is associated with reduced apoptosis and resistance to chemotherapy.
   e. Detection of the BCL2 translocation by PCR is diagnostic of follicular lymphoma.

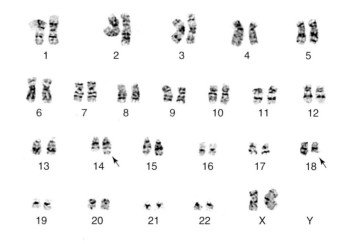

2. Which of the following regarding translocations in acute promyelocytic leukemia (APL) is TRUE?
   a. The most common translocation in APL, t(15;17)(q22; q21), results in fusion of portions of the *PML* gene from chromosome 17 and the retinoic acid receptor-alpha (RAR-α) gene (*RARA*) from chromosome 15.
   b. APL cases with t(11;17)(q23;q21) harboring the *ZBTB16-RARA* (*PLZF-RARA*) fusion are resistant to treatment with retinoic acid derivatives.
   c. The optimal method for demonstrating these translocations is DNA PCR.
   d. Treatment with retinoic acid derivatives consistently results in complete loss of detectable *PML-RARA* transcript in the blood.
   e. Real-time reverse transcription (RT)–PCR is not a reliable method for detecting fusion transcripts.

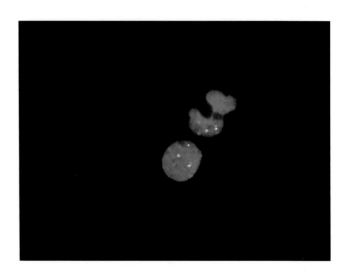

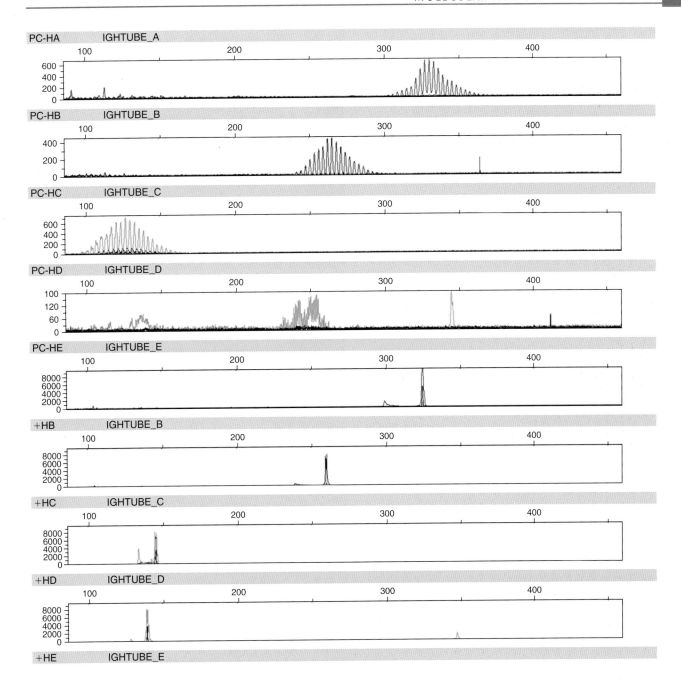

3. Which of the following statements about antigen receptor gene rearrangement analysis for detection of lymphoid clonality is TRUE?

a. PCR detects a larger proportion of rearrangements than does Southern blotting.

b. Unlike Southern blotting, which can be performed on paraffin-embedded tissue, PCR requires frozen tissue, because formalin inhibits DNA polymerases.

c. PCR is especially sensitive for the detection of clonal rearrangements among follicular lymphomas.

d. *IgH* and T-cell receptor (TCR) rearrangements are a better indicator of B- and T-cell lineage, respectively, than is immunohistochemical staining.

e. Southern blotting will show a clonal rearrangement in a significant proportion of PCR-negative follicular lymphomas.

4. The accompanying image of a renal neoplasm from a 61-year-old man demonstrates a t(X;1)(p11.2;q23) translocation. Which of the following statements regarding this type of tumor is TRUE?

   a. They are more common in older individuals.
   b. They are generally strongly positive for pancytokeratin, cytokeratin7, and the TFE3 protein.
   c. The presence of papillary areas with clear cells is diagnostic of this tumor.
   d. Staining with TFEB is diagnostic of this type of tumor.
   e. They share molecular similarities with alveolar soft part sarcoma (ASPS).

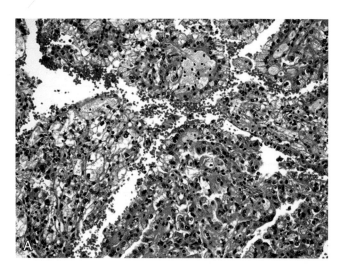

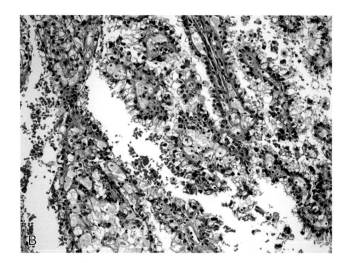

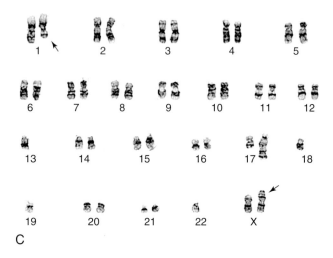

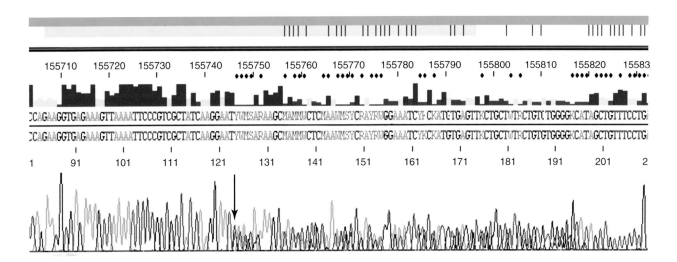

5. A 57-year-old nonsmoking woman with a lung nodule and enlarged mediastinal lymph nodes underwent endoscopic bronchial ultrasound that showed a TTF-1 positive adenocarcinoma. Sanger sequencing of a laser microdissected sample showed a deletion in exon 19. Which of the following statements regarding *EGFR* mutations in lung cancer is TRUE?

a. Frame-shift mutations of *EGFR*, such as those shown in the accompanying figure, are common in lung adenocarcinomas among female nonsmokers.

b. Inactivating exon 19 deletions, and the missense mutation "L858R" in exon 21, are the most common *EGFR* mutations in lung adenocarcinomas.

c. *EGFR* mutant tumors often have a cooperating mutation in the *KRAS* oncogene.

d. *EGFR* exon 20 mutations (e.g., "T790M") are associated with better response to the tyrosine kinase inhibitors (TKIs) gefitinib and erlotinib; exon 19 and 21 mutations are associated with resistance.

e. This patient is likely to benefit from treatment with erlotinib or gefitinib.

6. Which of the following statements regarding the tumor shown in the accompanying figure is TRUE?

   a. This tumor belongs to the Ewing sarcoma/primitive neuroectodermal tumor (ES/PNET) family of tumors.

   b. PCR performed on DNA extracted from paraffin embedded tissue will show an *EWSR1-FLI1* fusion.

   c. When cytogenetics cannot be performed, a negative result using a highly sensitive RT-PCR assay to include all *EWSR1/FLI1* variants rules out ES/PNET.

   d. FISH with break-apart probes, flanking the EWS breakpoint, is diagnostic of ES/PNET family tumors.

   e. Approximately 5% to 10% of desmoplastic small round cell tumors (DSRCT) show *EWSR1* translocations.

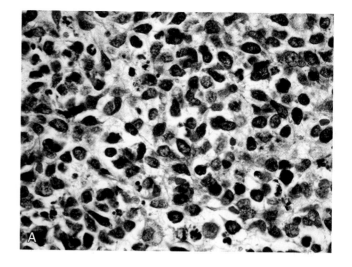

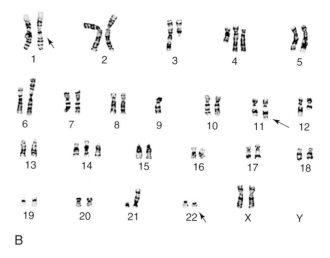

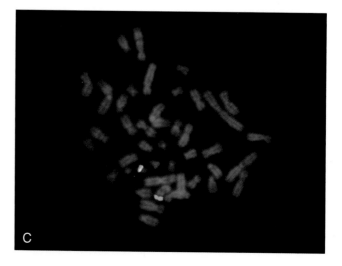

7. Which of the following statements regarding *MYCN* amplification in a neuroblastoma metastatic to the liver in an 11-month-old child is TRUE?
   a. This tumor is likely to have a hyperdiploid content and to be associated with a poor prognosis.
   b. This tumor is likely to show duplication of the short arm of chromosome 1 (1p), which is associated with a poor prognosis.
   c. This tumor is likely to express the TrkA neurotrophin receptor, which is associated with a poor prognosis.
   d. Amplification of the n-myc gene (*MYCN*) is not relevant in this case, because the patient has metastatic disease and is, therefore, a high-risk patient.
   e. MYCN amplification defines this patient as having high-risk disease.

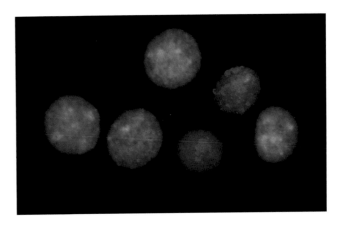

8. Which of the following statements regarding the tumor depicted in the image is TRUE?
   a. t(X;18)(p11;q11) is likely to be present in this tumor.
   b. The preceding translocation results in a fusion encoding a protein incorporating the transactivation domain of SYT encoded on the X chromosome and the carboxy-terminal portion of SSX1, SSX3, or SSX4 encoded on chromosome 18.
   c. Immunohistochemistry for SYT protein, although not diagnostic, can help in the diagnosis of tumors of this type.
   d. Cases with the different molecular forms (*SYT-SSX1*, *SYT-SSX2*, *SYT-SSX4*) are best distinguished by classic karyotyping and by FISH.
   e. *SYT-SSX1* is rarely seen in biphasic tumors of this type (tumors with distinct gland formation), and might be associated with a better prognosis.

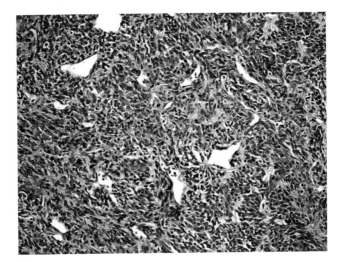

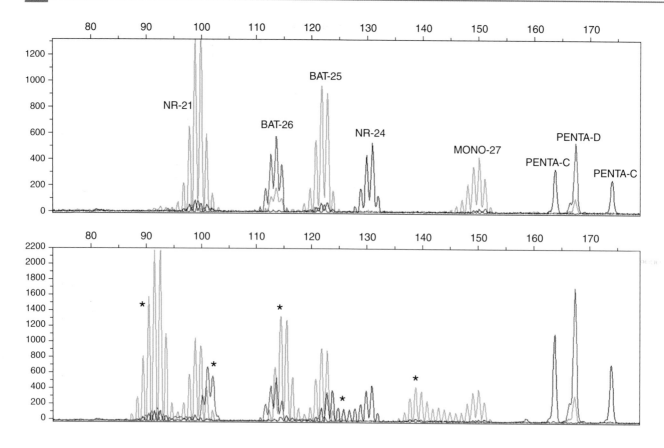

9. The accompanying capillary image shows results of analysis of a cecal carcinoma in a 40-year-old woman whose 43-year-old sister has endometrial carcinoma. Her mother had undergone a total abdominal hysterectomy and bilateral salpingo-oophorectomy in her 40s. On immunohistochemistry, the tumor stained strongly for MSH2 and MSH6, stained very weakly for PMS2, and was negative for MLH1 expression. Which of the following statements is TRUE?

a. Analysis of the tumor is likely to show a *BRAF* V600E mutation.

b. Germ line genetic testing will most likely show a gain of function mutation of *MSH6*.

c. Germ line testing will most likely show a loss of function mutation of *MSH2*.

d. Genetic testing will most likely show a loss of function mutation of *MLH1*.

e. Methylation analysis of tumor DNA will show hypermethylation of the *MLH1* promoter.

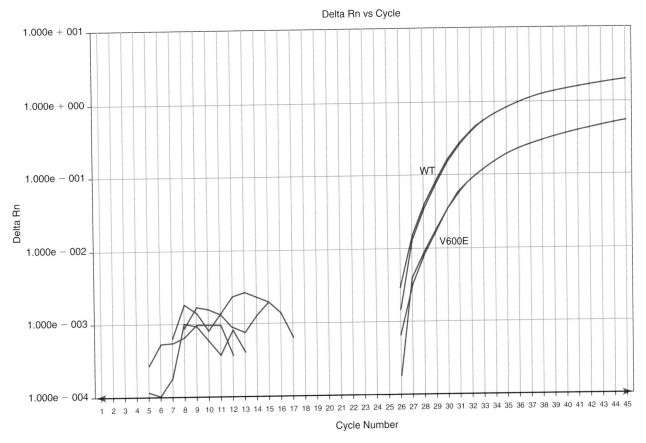

Delta Rn vs Cycle

Selected Detector: All
Document: PCR12D_76_BR_STUDY (ddCt Study)

10. Which of the following statements is TRUE?
   a. The mutant *BRAF* is strong evidence that this is a melanoma.
   b. If this is a melanoma, this tumor will respond to inhibitors of receptor tyrosine kinases, such as gefitinib or erlotinib.
   c. Given the ratio of wild type to mutant, the result is properly interpreted as a heterozygous mutation.
   d. Loss of function of BRAF is a good prognostic indicator in melanoma.
   e. If this patient has a metastatic melanoma, he/she may be a candidate for treatment with vemurafenib.

11. Which of the following statements regarding this tumor is TRUE?
   a. It is an embryonal rhabdomyosarcoma.
   b. RT-PCR is likely to show a fusion transcript involving the 5′ end of *PAX7* and the 3′ end of *FOXO1 (FKHR)*.
   c. A more common translocation in this tumor is the t(1;13)(p36;q14), which results in a *PAX3-FOXO1* fusion.
   d. The *PAX3-FOXO1* fusion is associated with a higher rate of bone marrow involvement than the *PAX7-FOXO1* fusion.
   e. The *PAX3-FOXO1* fusion is more likely to be amplified as double minutes (dmin).

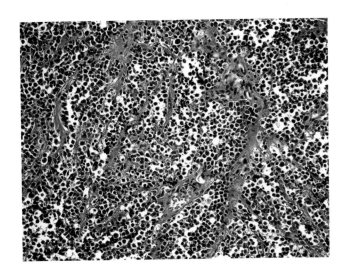

12. This is an image of a Southern blot using a probe to Epstein-Barr virus (EBV) termini. A single sharp band is seen. This indicates that:
    a. The individual is infected by a single strain of EBV, as different strains have termini of varying lengths.
    b. EBV is present as a provirus integrated into the host genome.
    c. The sample is a posttransplant B-cell lymphoma.
    d. The individual is acutely infected with EBV, and insufficient time has elapsed to develop variation in the length of the termini.
    e. The band represents EBV DNA from a clone of cells, indicating a single cellular infection event that occurred prior to clonal expansion.

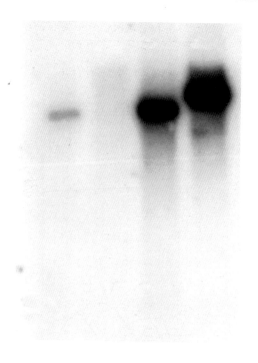

13. This tumor will MOST likely show:
    a. Negative immunostaining for cytokeratin 7
    b. Positive immunostaining for cytokeratin 20
    c. Negative staining for KIT
    d. Positive staining for PAX2
    e. A positive colloidal iron stain

14. Which of the following statements about *BCR-ABL1* translocations is TRUE?
    a. It may be seen in chronic myelomonocytic leukemia, and de novo acute lymphoblastic leukemia (ALL).
    b. The p190 fusion protein, resulting from a translocation within the major cluster region of *BCR*, is most often associated with ALL.
    c. The oncogenic properties of the fusion protein are the result of constitutive activation of the serine–threonine kinase activity of BCR.
    d. Imatinib mesylate, which inhibits ABL kinase activity of BCR-ABL1, is a specific treatment for chronic myelogenous leukemia.
    e. The *BCR-ABL* transcript becomes undetectable by RT-PCR within 6 months in most patients on imatinib treatment.

15. Amplification of HER2/neu (*ERBB2*) in breast cancer:
    a. Correlates with increased estrogen and progesterone receptor (ER/PR) expression
    b. Is not an independent predictor of prognosis, because it is related to ER/PR expression
    c. Is best detected by immunohistochemistry using monoclonal antibodies
    d. Results in increased ERBB2 protein expression, which helps tumors overcome the ERBB2 blocking effect of trastuzumab (Herceptin), causing resistance to this form of therapy
    e. Predicts response to treatment with trastuzumab

16. Which of the following statements regarding *KIT* and platelet-derived growth factor receptor-α (*PDGFRA*) mutations in gastrointestinal tumors is TRUE?
    a. Gastrointestinal stromal tumors (GISTs) characteristically contain mutations of exons 9, 11, 13, or 17 of *KIT*, and a cooperating mutation in exon 12 or 18 of *PDGFRA*.
    b. These mutations cause constitutive activation of the KIT or PDGFRA tyrosine kinases, produced by the preceding genes.
    c. Tumors with *PDGFRA* mutations tend to be negative for DOG-1 expression by immunohistochemistry.

d. All recurrent mutations of *KIT* and *PDGFRA*, in the absence of prior treatment of TKIs such as imatinib (Gleevec), show similar sensitivity to the drug.

e. The presence of a KIT mutation identifies a GIST as "high risk" or "malignant."

17. Which of the following statements regarding mutation testing of thyroid fine needle aspirates is TRUE?

a. A positive mutation for *BRAF* V600E mutation has a high positive predictive value for papillary thyroid carcinomas (greater than 90%).

b. Greater than 90% of follicular thyroid carcinomas harbor a *PAX8/PPARγ* translocation.

c. The finding of a *KRAS* mutation is strongly suggestive of a papillary thyroid carcinoma.

d. A normal result for *BRAF* V600E, *KRAS* codon 12 and 13 mutations, and *RET/PTC* translocations makes papillary thyroid carcinoma highly unlikely.

e. *RET/PTC* translocations and *RET* mutations are characteristic of radiation-associated papillary thyroid carcinomas.

18. Which of the following statements about cervical cancer screening is TRUE?

a. Testing of cervical specimens for high oncogenic risk human papillomavirus (HPV) types has both a high positive predictive value and a high negative predictive value for the development of cervical cancer.

b. HPV DNA testing of cervical specimens is approved only for cases with a diagnosis of atypical squamous cells of uncertain significance (ASCUS).

c. Among women over age 30, combined cervical cytologic test plus HPV DNA testing, or cervical cytologic test plus reflex HPV DNA, performed every 2 to 3 years, may be as effective as annual cytologic test in reducing cancer mortality rate, and more cost effective.

d. HPV DNA screening is recommended for both high oncogenic risk and low oncogenic risk viruses.

e. High oncogenic risk viruses include types 11, 16, 18, 31, and 33, among others.

19. Which of the following statements about gliomas is TRUE?

a. Oligodendrogliomas, especially pediatric oligodendrogliomas, are characterized by the loss of the short arm of chromosome 1 (1p) and the long arm of chromosome 19 (19q).

b. Oligodendrogliomas, especially pediatric oligodendrogliomas, are characterized by the loss of the long arm of chromosome 1 (1q) and the short arm of chromosome 19 (19p).

c. The characteristic deletion is associated with a higher rate of *IDH1* and *IDH2* mutations and a lower rate of *PTEN* deletions.

d. The characteristic deletion is associated with resistance to chemotherapy.

e. The chromosome 1 and 19 deletions are independent events and the chromosome 19 deletion precedes the chromosome 1 deletion.

20. Which of the following statements about anaplastic lymphoma kinase (ALK) in lung cancer is TRUE?

a. *ALK* point mutations are seen in approximately 5% to 15% of lung adenocarcinomas and indicate sensitivity to crizotinib.

b. A single RT-PCR reaction is the most sensitive method to detect *ALK* translocations in lung adenocarcinomas.

c. *ALK* translocations are more common among older individuals and smokers.

d. Disruption of the *ALK* gene, resulting from *ALK* translocations, results in loss of expression of ALK, a normally expressed protein in pneumocytes.

e. ALK translocation-positive lung carcinomas tend to be *EGFR* and *KRAS* wild type.

Answers

1. d. The hallmark translocation of follicular lymphomas, t(14;18)(q32;q21), places the *BCL2* gene—normally on chromosome 18—under the influence of the *IgH* enhancer on chromosome 14. The resultant overexpression of the antiapoptotic BCL2 protein is associated with resistance of follicular lymphomas to chemotherapy. This translocation may also be seen in up to 20% to 30% of de novo diffuse large B-cell lymphomas (DLBCL). The majority of these have a germinal center B-cell (GCB) phenotype, although it may rarely be seen in activated B-cell (ABC) phenotype DLBCL. Although nonneoplastic follicular center cells do not express BCL2 protein, normal mantle cells, B cells in hyperplastic marginal zones, and normal plasma cells express BCL2, as do normal T cells. In addition to follicular lymphomas, most MALT lymphomas, mantle cell lymphomas, chronic lymphocytic leukemias, and acute lymphoblastic leukemias express BCL2 protein. Cyclin D1 overexpression associated with t(11;14) is a hallmark of mantle cell lymphomas. Because of wide variability of chromosome 18 breakpoints, standard PCR—using primers that bind to the JH region, and recurrent breakpoints on chromosome 18 (major breakpoint region and minor cluster region)—detects the translocation

in only approximately 35% to 65% of cases in which it is demonstrable by FISH. Although the *BCL2/JH* translocation is believed to have oncogenic properties, the translocation is detectable at a low level in some reactive lymphoid proliferations. An interesting recent finding in follicular B-cell lymphomas has been the demonstration of activating mutations of the polycomb complex member histone methyltransferase *EZH2* in up to 20% of GCB-DLBCL, mainly those with BCL2 rearrangements. The mutation, which alters tyrosine 641 (Y641), results in increased activity in converting dimethylated to trimethylated H3K27. With wild type (WT) *EZH2* on the other allele, this leads to increased trimethylation of H3K27: a repressive modification of histones, with chromatin condensation and reduced gene expression. Wild type EZH2 is also increased in the remaining GCB-DLCBL. This presents a potential target for small molecule inhibitors of EZH2. Some B-cell lymphomas may harbor both *IgH-BCL2* and *MYC* rearrangements on 8q24 (with IgH or non-IgH partners). These "double-hit" lymphomas tend to behave in a more aggressive manner; however, in GCB-DLBCL, the presence of a BCL2 translocation identifies a group with poor treatment outcome with rituximab-CHOP treatment, independent of the MYC status.

Li S, Lin P, Fayad LE, et al: B-cell lymphomas with MYC/8q24 rearrangements and IGH@BCL2/t(14;18)(q32;q21): an aggressive disease with heterogeneous histology, germinal center B-cell immunophenotype and poor outcome. *Mod Pathol* 2012;25:145-156. Epub 2011 Oct 14.

Visco C, Tzankov A, Xu-Monette ZY, et al: Patients with diffuse large B cell lymphoma of germinal center origin with BCL2 translocations have poor outcome, irrespective of MYC status: a report from an International DLBCL rituximab-CHOP Consortium Program Study. *Haematologica* 2013;98:255-263. Epub 2012 Aug 28.

Seto M, Honma K, Nakagawa M: Diversity of genome profiles in malignant lymphoma. *Cancer Sci* 2010;101:573-578. Epub 2009 Nov 27.

2. b. The t(15;17)(q22;q21) translocation resulting in the *PML-RARA* fusion is the most common translocation seen in APL. Other translocations include t(11;17)(q23;q21) resulting in the *ZBTB16-RARA (PLZF-RARA)* fusion; t(5;17) (q35;q12-21) causing the *NPM1-RARA (NPM-RARA)* fusion; t(11;17)(q13;q21) with the *NUMA1-RARA (NuMA-RARA)* fusion; and der(17) effecting the *STAT5B-RARA* fusion (common/older terminology in parentheses). The *PML-RARA* fusion protein retains the DNA-binding and retinoic acid (RA)-binding domains of RAR-α, and the zinc finger and proline-rich domains of PML. In addition to inhibiting PML and RAR-α function, the fusion protein binds corepressors to recruit histone deacetylase (HDAC) to RA response genes, causing chromatin condensation and inhibiting transcription of these genes, resulting in differentiation arrest at the promyelocyte stage. Pharmacologic doses of all-trans retinoic acid (ATRA) inhibit this binding, and restore transcription of RA-responsive genes with differentiation and, ultimately, cell death. The PLZF (promyelocytic leukemia zinc finger)–RAR-α fusion protein contains a second, ATRA-resistant, corepressor binding site in the amino-terminal portion of PLZF, leading to resistance to treatment with ATRA. In addition, *PLZF* translocation positive cells are also resistant to arsenic trioxide (ATO), which is now used in conjunction with ATRA. In this setting, the use of HDAC inhibitors can partially reverse the resistance to ATRA and cause terminal differentiation. Because of the variability of chromosomal breakpoints, DNA PCR for this translocation is not practical; RT-PCR and FISH are used most often. Retinoic acid derivatives when used alone do not result in loss of detectable transcript, although following consolidation chemotherapy most responders become RT-PCR negative, and loss of transcript is predictive of long-term survival.

Wang ZY, Chen Z: Acute promyelocytic leukemia: from highly fatal to highly curable. *Blood* 2008;111(5):2505-2515.

Chendamarai E, Balasubramanian P, George B, et al: Role of minimal residual disease monitoring in acute promyelocytic leukemia treated with arsenic trioxide in frontline therapy. *Blood* 2012;119:3413-3419. Epub 2012 Feb 28.

3. e. Detection of clonal VDJ or VJ rearrangements of antigen receptor genes (especially immunoglobulin heavy chain, kappa light chain, TCR-β, and TCR-γ) by PCR amplification is increasingly popular because of its ease of performance, the ability to use small amounts of DNA, and, especially, fragmented DNA from paraffin-embedded tissue; however, because of somatic hypermutations, deletions, and failure of

"consensus" primers to amplify different V families with the same efficiency, individual PCR tests detect only 75% or even as low as 50% of all rearrangements detectable by Southern blotting. Primer sets developed by the BIOMED-2 consortium in an attempt to maximize detection still fail to detect 100% of all rearrangements detectable by Southern blotting. One additional benefit of PCR is the ability to detect minimal residual disease by sequencing the clonal product to identify the specific junctional sequence, and obtain a probe or primer specific for the rearranged allele. Ongoing rearrangements in ALL complicate this effort, necessitating the use of multiple targets to achieve acceptable sensitivity. Recently, high throughput sequencing has been used to detect clonality, somatic hypermutation (a prognostic feature in chronic lymphocytic leukemia [CLL]), and identify the junctional sequence specific to the malignant clone.

Logan AC, Gao H, Wang C, et al: High-throughput VDJ sequencing for quantification of minimal residual disease in chronic lymphocytic leukemia and immune reconstitution assessment. *Proc Natl Acad Sci USA* 2011;108(52):21194-21199. Epub 2011 Dec 12.

van Dongen JJ, Langerak AW, Bruggemann M, et al: Design and standardization of PCR primers and protocols for detection of clonal immunoglobulin and T-cell receptor gene recombinations in suspect lymphoproliferations: report of the BIOMED-2 Concerted Action BMH4-CT98-3936. *Leukemia* 2003;17:2257-2317.

4. e. Tumors with Xp11.2 translocations are a recently recognized category of renal cortical tumors found more commonly among children and adolescents, although they may also be seen in adults. Translocations, which involve the gene *TFE3* on Xp11.2, include t(X;1)(p11.2;q21) (*PRCC-TFE3*); t(X;1)(p11.2;p34) (*TFE3-SFPQ*); inv(X)(p11.2;q12) (*NONO-TFE3*); t(X;17)(p11.2;q25) *ASPCR1-TFE3*; and t(X;17) (p11.2;q23) (*CLTC-TFE3*). In addition, tumors with t(6;11) (p21;q12) and a resulting α-TFEB gene fusion share some similarities with this group of tumors. These tumor share features of mixed papillary and nested architecture irregular cytokeratin staining (negative for TFEB tumors), and positive nuclear staining with antibodies to either TFE3 (Xp11.2 tumors) or TFEB (6p21 tumors), both members of the MiTF/TFE3 family of transcription factors. *TFEB* tumors and *CTLC-TFE3* tumors also stain with melan-A and HMB-45. *PRCC-TFE3* carcinomas are said to show a more solid, compact architecture, less frequent psammoma bodies, and less prominent nucleoli than *ASPCR-TFE3* tumors; they also have a fibrous pseudocapsule. The *ASPCR-TFE3* (formerly *ASPL-TFE3*) fusion product is also seen in ASPS.

Armah HB, Parwani AV: Xp11.2 translocation renal cell carcinoma. *Arch Pathol Lab Med* 2010;134:124-129.

Bruder E, Passera O, Harms D, et al: Morphologic and molecular characterization of renal cell carcinoma in children and young adults. *Am J Surg Pathol* 2004;28(9):1117-1132.

Argani P, Ladanyi M: Recent advances in pediatric renal neoplasia. *Adv Anat Pathol* 2003;10:243-260.

5. e. Activating *EGFR* mutations are seen in approximately 15% to 20% of all lung adenocarcinomas, and in up to 75% of East Asian female never smokers with the condition. EGFR, a receptor tyrosine kinase, activates downstream pathways that promote cell cycle progression and cell survival, following ligand binding. Activating mutations in lung adenocarcinomas (and occasionally in other non–small cell carcinomas) result in ligand independent signaling. One of the downstream pathways is through the RAS-RAF-mitogen-activated protein kinase (MAPK) pathway. Thus, activating *KRAS* and *EGFR* mutations rarely occur together in the same tumor. Most *EGFR* mutations in lung adenocarcinomas are in-frame exon 19 deletions, or a missense mutation in exon 21 (c.2573 T > G; p.L858R). Exons 18 and 20 each account for approximately 5% of detected mutations. Mutations in exons 19 and 21 are associated with sensitivity to inhibition by the TKIs gefitinib and erlotinib; small deletions in exon 20 and the missense mutation "T790M" are associated with resistance to these drugs. Small exon 20 insertions also tend to be resistant to these TKIs. Sensitivity of exon 18 mutations is intermediate between these. In patients with exon 19 or exon 21 mutation-positive lung carcinomas, treatment with a TKI is associated with improved progression-free and overall survival, when compared to chemotherapy. Patients with *EGFR* wild type tumors do better with chemotherapy; therefore testing for these mutations is now standard. Laboratories may test for *EGFR* either by Sanger sequencing *or* by testing for specific mutations. The latter may use allele-specific primers ("Amplification Resistant Mutation Screen") to amplify specific mutations with a detection limit of 1% mutant allele in normal; PCR with minisequencing using specific extension primers (e.g., "Sequenom," which uses mass spectrometry to distinguish alleles, and the "SnapShot" assay, which uses fluorescent dyes) with a detection limit of 5% to 10% mutant allele in normal; or real-time PCR with "melting curve" or allele-specific probes. Sanger sequencing can potentially detect any mutation in the targeted region, but requires approximately 15% to 25% mutant allele in normal and the sample must be enriched for tumor, e.g., by microdissection. Next generation sequencing technologies should be able to reliably detect at least as low as 5% mutant in normal. Most patients who initially respond to TKIs develop secondary resistance (defined as systemic progression following initial response to a single agent TKI, of a tumor known to harbor a TKI sensitive *EGFR* mutation, while on continuous treatment with the TKI). Up to 50% of these patients will show a "T790M" mutation on the same allele as the sensitizing mutation; up to 20% show amplification of the *MET* oncogene (HGF receptor). The mechanism of resistance in up to 40% of tumors with neither is unclear; some of the relapsed tumors have had a small cell histologic appearance, although still carrying the sensitizing *EGFR* mutation.

Pao W, Chmielecki J: Rational, biologically based treatment of EGFR-mutant non-small-cell lung cancer. *Nat Rev Cancer* 2010;10:760-774.

Cheng L, Alexander RE, Maclennan GT, et al: Molecular pathology of lung cancer: key to personalized medicine. *Mod Pathol* 2012;25:347-369. Epub 2012 Jan 27.

6. a. The morphologic appearance, immunophenotypic profile, and cytogenetics of this tumor are those of ES/PNET. Chromosomal translocations that interrupt the EWSR1 gene and create a fusion with a member of the ETS (erythroblastosis virus transforming sequence) family of transcription factors characterize ES/PNET. FLI1 on chromosome 11q24 accounts for 85% of cases and ERG at 21q22 for approximately 10%. Rare cases involve ETV1 on 7p22, ETV4 on 17q21, FEV on 2q33, NFATC2 on 20q13.2, PATZ1 (alias ZNF278) on 22q12.2, or even FUS-FEV and FUS-ERG translocations; therefore, negative EWS-FLI1, or EWS-ERG negative RT-PCR, does not exclude ES/PNET. FISH with a "break-apart" probe, spanning the chromosome 22q12 breakpoint, to demonstrate "split" signals should be positive regardless of the fusion partner, and support a diagnosis of ES/PNET, although it is not diagnostic. The specificity of this break-apart probe is limited by the involvement of EWSR1 translocations in other sarcomas, including: DSRCT (fusion partner WT1 on 11p13); malignant melanoma ("clear cell sarcoma of soft parts," fusion partner ATF1 on 12q13, or CREB1 on 2q34); extraskeletal myxoid chondrosarcoma (fusion partner NR4A3 [formerly "CHN"] on 9q22); a minority of cases of myxoid liposarcoma; and some bone sarcomas and soft tissue myoepithelial neoplasms/hidradenomas (partners POU5F1 on 6p21.31; PBX1 on 1q23; or ZNF444 on19q13.43). EWSR1, FUS, and TAF15 belong to a family of RNA binding factors that may occasionally substitute for each other in translocations with the partner gene defining the tumor phenotype (e.g., although the vast majority of myxoid liposarcomas carry an FUS-DDIT3 translocation, they may rarely harbor an EWSR1-DDIT3 fusion); similarly TAF15 or EWS can partner with NR4A3 in extraskeletal myxoid chondrosarcomas. Germ line FUS mutations are seen in occasional cases of amyotrophic lateral sclerosis (fALS); and cytoplasmic inclusions of FUS are seen in fALS and in cases of frontotemporal degeneration.

Szuhai K, Cleton-Jansen AM, Hogendoorn PC, Bovée JV: Molecular pathology and its diagnostic use in bone tumors. *Cancer Genet* 2012;205(5):193-204.

Bovée JV, Hogendoorn PC: Molecular pathology of sarcomas: concepts and clinical implications. *Virchows Arch* 2010; 456(2):193-199. Epub 2009 Sep 29.

7. e. Neuroblastomas are a heterogeneous group of tumors with a highly variable outcome ranging from spontaneous regression to death of the patient. Good prognosis tumors tend to have a hyperdiploid DNA content, with gains of whole chromosomes, without structural chromosomal abnormalities, and expression of the TrkA neurotrophin receptor. Unfavorable tumors, on the other hand, have a diploid DNA content with structural chromosomal alterations including deletions of 1p and 11q, gain of 17q, and MYCN amplification. They tend to express the TrkB neurotrophin receptor and BDNF. Children below 1 year of age tend to have a better prognosis, even with disseminated disease, especially when disseminated disease is confined to the liver, skin, or bone marrow (stage 4S); however, with MYCN amplification, the 3-year event-free survival rate in infants with metastatic disease drops from 93% to around 10%; therefore, along with age, stage, and "Shimada" histologic appearance, MYCN amplification and DNA ploidy are used to classify tumors into low-, intermediate-, or high-risk groups. The international consensus for neuroblastoma diagnostics in 2009 included MYCN status, 11q23 losses, and ploidy as obligatory markers to be used for therapy stratification, and started prospective evaluation of losses on 1p, 3p, 4p, and 11q, and gains on 1q, 2p, and 17q. Activating ALK mutations are seen in approximately 5% to 7% of neuroblastomas, with two hot spots. Copy number gains of the ALK locus may be associated with a poor prognosis.

Ambros PF, Ambros IM, Brodeur GM, et al: International consensus for neuroblastoma molecular diagnostics: report from the International Neuroblastoma Risk Group (INRG) Biology Committee. *Br J Cancer* 2009;100:1471-1482.

Brodeur GM: Neuroblastoma: biological insights into a clinical enigma. *Nat Rev Cancer* 2003;3:203-216.

Maris JM: The biologic basis for neuroblastoma heterogeneity and risk stratification. *Curr Opin Pediatr* 2005;17:7-13.

8. a. The t(X;18)(p11;q11) translocation, which results in the fusion of most of the 5′ end of the *SYT* gene on chromosome 18 with the 3′ end of either the *SSX1*, *SSX2*, or *SSX4* gene on chromosome Xp11 (and encodes a protein that contains most of the amino-terminal portion of SYT, and the carboxy-terminal end portion of the SSX), is the hallmark of synovial sarcoma. Because SYT is ubiquitously expressed, immunohistochemistry for this protein is of little value. Although immunohistochemistry for SSX has been used, SSX proteins are among the "cancer/testis" antigens expressed in a number of cancers, and their detection is of limited diagnostic value. Like most translocations that express a fusion transcript, this translocation can be detected with classic cytogenetics, FISH, RT-PCR, or Southern blotting, although the latter is of little value in routine practice. Because all SSX genes are near each other on the X chromosome, tumors harboring the different molecular fusion forms appear identical on cytogenetics. RT-PCR can distinguish these, using either sequence-specific primers or consensus primers followed by specific probes, restriction enzymes, or sequencing. Distinguishing the major molecular forms may be of some clinical value, as *SYT-SSX2*, which is rarely seen in biphasic tumors, may be associated with a better prognosis, although available data are conflicting. The association of *SSX2* with a better prognosis has not been shown to be independent of histologic grade or tumor size. Monophasic synovial sarcomas may be difficult to distinguish from malignant peripheral nerve sheath tumors (and occasionally even diagnosed as benign nerve sheath tumors). In addition to epithelial membrane antigen and cytokeratin staining, molecular testing can be of significant value in distinguishing these tumors.

Fisher C: Soft tissue sarcomas with non-EWS translocations: molecular genetic features and pathologic and clinical correlations. *Virchows Arch* 2010;456:153-166. Epub 2009 Apr 28.

Ladanyi M, Antonescu CR, Leung DH, et al: Impact of SYT–SSX fusion type on the clinical behavior of synovial sarcoma: a multi-institutional retrospective study of 243 patients. *Cancer Res* 2002;62:135-140.

Scheithauer BW, Amrami KK, Folpe AL, et al: Synovial sarcoma of nerve. *Hum Pathol* 2011;42(4):568-577. Epub 2011 Feb 4.

9. d. Lynch syndrome (formerly called hereditary nonpolyposis colon cancer, or HNPCC) is associated with germ line mutations of mismatch repair genes, including *MLH1*, *MSH2*, *MSH6*, *PMS2*, and *MLH3*, most often the first two. Tumors in this familial cancer syndrome include colonic, endometrial, urothelial, small intestinal, stomach, and hepatobiliary carcinomas, and demonstrate microsatellite instability (MSI). Molecular diagnosis is indicated to help design special screening protocols for those

at risk. Because of the impracticality of testing all colon tumors, various guidelines specify which tumors should be screened for MSI. The modified Bethesda criteria, meant to maximize sensitivity at the expense of specificity, include testing of all colorectal cancers (CRCs) before the age of 50. (Other criteria include CRC with MSI histologic appearance before age 60; any synchronous or metachronous HNPCC-associated tumors; at least one HNPCC-associated tumor before age 50, in any first-degree relative; and CRC with two or more first- or second-degree relatives with any HNPCC-associated tumor.) Recent reviews recommend eschewing family history and testing all CRC cases that meet certain criteria (e.g., age) or even all CRC cases. Not all cancers with MSI are associated with HNPCC. Some are due to somatic silencing of mismatch repair genes. BRAF mutations, when present in MLH1 deficient colon cancer, almost always indicate sporadic, non-Lynch associated tumors. In the absence of chemotherapy, patients with high MSI appear to have a better overall survival. In recent years, MSI has emerged as a predictor of response to chemotherapy. Testing strategies for detecting Lynch syndrome include MSI testing and immunohistochemistry. Microsatellites are tandem repeats of nucleotides, usually one to four nucleotides. During DNA replication these are subject to "slippage" and repaired by the mismatch repair system. Loss of function of one of the enzymes results in daughter cells with repeat-numbers that differ from the germ line. This phenomenon is called "microsatellite instability." The image shows a test with five mononucleotide repeat markers to test for MSI and two polymorphic pentanucleotide repeat markers to test for patient identity (to ensure that tumor and normal are from the same patient). Alteration of 40% or more of markers is generally considered MSI-high (MSI-H); tumors with alteration of fewer than 40% of markers are considered "MSI-low," and those with no alteration are considered MSS. (These numbers make most sense when using 10 markers.) Mononcleotide markers have been shown to be more sensitive, and will detect a large percentage of Lynch cases with just five markers; however, no test is 100% sensitive, and immunohistochemistry for loss of expression of mismatch repair genes in the tumor will detect some cases missed by MSI testing (and vice versa).

Palomaki GE, McClain MR, Melillo S, et al: EGAPP supplementary evidence review. DNA testing strategies aimed at reducing morbidity and mortality from Lynch syndrome. *Genet Med* 2009;11:42-65.

Evaluation of Genomic Applications in Practice and Prevention (EGAPP) Working Group: Recommendations from the EGAPP Working Group: genetic testing strategies in newly diagnosed individuals with colorectal cancer aimed at reducing morbidity and mortality from Lynch syndrome in relatives. *Genet Med* 2009;11(1):35-41.

Bertagnolli MM, Niedzwiecki D, Compton CC, et al: Microsatellite instability predicts improved response to adjuvant therapy with irinotecan, fluorouracil, and leucovorin in stage III colon cancer: Cancer and Leukemia Group B Protocol 89803. *J Clin Oncol* 2009;27:1814-1821. Epub 2009 Mar 9.

10. e. BRAF is one of the serine threonine kinase isoforms that activates MEK following RAS activation. Melanomas have activating mutations of the RAS pathway, most commonly *BRAF* (50%) and *NRAS* (20%). Approximately 1% have an activating mutation of the KIT receptor tyrosine kinase upstream of NRAS. *BRAF* mutations are even more common among nevi; therefore, a *BRAF* mutation is NOT diagnostic of melanoma. *BRAF* mutations, however, are an important target for treatment with vemurafenib, a BRAF inhibitor. Vemurafenib is selective for mutated BRAF, and will not inhibit the pathway in the absence of *BRAF* mutations. Greater than 90% of BRAF mutations in melanomas involve Valine 600, and the vast majority of these are "V600E" (valine to glutamine) mutations resulting from a 1799 T > A transversion. Uveal melanomas, blue nevi, and central nervous system melanocytic lesions activate the MAP kinase pathway by activating mutations of the G protein alpha subunits, *GNA11* and *GNAQ*.

Flaherty KT, Fisher DE: New strategies in metastatic melanoma: oncogene-defined taxonomy leads to therapeutic advances. *Clin Cancer Res* 2011;17:4922-4928. Epub 2011 Jun 13.

Van Raamsdonk CD, Bezrookove V, Green G, et al: Frequent somatic mutations of GNAQ in uveal melanoma and blue naevi. *Nature* 2009;457:599-602. Epub 2008 Dec 10.

Van Raamsdonk CD, Griewank KG, Crosby MB, et al: Mutations in GNA11 in uveal melanoma. *N Engl J Med* 2010;363:2191-2199. Epub 2010 Nov 17.

11. d. Approximately 55% of patients with alveolar rhabomyosarcoma (ARMS) in reports from the Intergroup Rhabdomyosarcoma Study IV (IRS-IV) harbor RT-PCR-detectable *PAX3-FOXOA1* transcripts [from t(2;13)(q35; q14)], 22% have *PAX7-FOXOA1* transcripts [from t(1;13) (p36;q14)], and the remainder have neither fusion transcript. The *PAX7-FOXOA1* occurs more often in younger patients, in tumors from the extremities, and in localized tumors. Metastases, when present, in *PAX7-FOXOA1* tumors often involve only bone or lymph nodes, whereas those in PAX3 fusion tumors more often involve multiple metastatic sites, including bone marrow. Furthermore, patients with metastases and *PAX7* fusions have a 75% 4-year overall survival rate (approximately equal to that in patients with locoregional disease), with an 8% overall survival rate among *PAX3*-harboring patients with metastatic disease. Amplification of the fusion gene in the form of dmin commonly occurs in tumors with the PAX7-FOXO1 fusion. Some alveolar rhabdomyosarcomas may have a solid histologic appearance and require detection of the translocation for diagnosis. ARMS cases with RT-PCR-undetectable *PAX3-FOXO1* or *PAX7-FOXO1* transcripts constitute a heterogeneous group with an intermediate prognosis. Some cases may have the translocation but express RNA at a level that cannot be detected. Others may harbor alternate translocations, such as *AFX75* or *NCOA1*.

Parham DM, Alaggio R, Coffin CM: Myogenic tumors in children and adolescents. *Pediatr Dev Pathol* 2012;15(1 Suppl):211-238.

Barr FG: Gene fusions involving PAX and FOX family members in alveolar rhabdomyosarcoma. *Oncogene* 2001;20:5736-5746.

Barr FG, Qualman SJ, Macris MH, et al: Genetic heterogeneity in the alveolar rhabdomyosarcoma subset without typical gene fusions. *Cancer Res* 2002;62:4704-4710.

12. e. EBV infections of B cells are characterized by latency with long-term persistence in these cells. Each cell is infected once. During infection the virus forms a circular episome, incorporating a variable number of terminal repeats. EBV DNA in progeny cells has the same number of repeats as the "parent" cell. Southern blotting, following BamH1 digestion to cut sequences flanking the termini, using a probe that

binds to the terminal repeats, reveals multiple bands in polyclonal populations of cells with separate circularization events, and a single band in DNA from clonal B-cell samples. Length of termini is not an indication of strain, or of duration of infection. Although clonal EBV infection is characteristic of posttransplant B-cell lymphomas, it is seen in other lymphomas, including endemic Burkitt's lymphoma, immunoblastic B-cell lymphomas in acquired immunodeficiency syndrome, EVB-associated T/NK cell lymphomas, and, rarely, posttransplant T-cell lymphomas. Southern blotting is no longer widely used for diagnosis of EBV-associated conditions; however, in situ hybridization for Epstein-Barr virus early RNA (*EBER*) and viral load testing for EBV DNA are now widely used in diagnosis of EBV-associated lesions and management of patients in the posttransplant setting.

Piccaluga PP, Gazzola A, Agostinelli C, et al: Pathobiology of Epstein-Barr virus-driven peripheral T-cell lymphomas. *Semin Diagn Pathol* 2011;28:234-244.

Gulley ML, Tang W: Laboratory assays for Epstein-Barr virus-related disease. *J Mol Diagn* 2008;10:279-292. Epub 2008 Jun 13.

Gulley ML: Molecular diagnosis of Epstein–Barr virus-related diseases. *J Mol Diagn* 2001;3:1-10.

13. e. The tumor shows 38 chromosomes, with losses of chromosomes 1, 2, 5, 6, 10, 13, 17, 21, and Y. This karyotype with loss of multiple chromosomes is characteristic of chromophobe cell renal cell carcinoma. These tumors characteristically express cytokeratin 7 and KIT, and are negative for PAX2 and cytokeratin 20. They are also characteristically positive for colloidal iron. Other characteristic changes in renal tumors include deletions of chromosome 3p25 in conventional RCC, trisomy 7, and trisomy 17, and loss of the Y chromosome in papillary renal cell carcinoma, losses of chromosomes 1 and Y in some oncocytomas, and chromosome 11p13 translocations in other oncocytomas. Strong CK-7 staining can help distinguish eosinophilic chromophobe RCC from oncocytoma in difficult cases. When karyotyping is not possible, copy number microarrays or genome wide SNP microarrays can detect characteristic changes.

Shen SS, Truong LD, Scarpelli M, Lopez-Beltran A: Role of immunohistochemistry in diagnosing renal neoplasms: when is it really useful? *Arch Pathol Lab Med* 2012;136(4):410-417.

Maher ER: Genomics and epigenomics of renal cell carcinoma. *Semin Cancer Biol* 2013;23(1):10-17. Epub 2012 Jun 28.

Meloni-Ehrig AM: Renal cancer: cytogenetic and molecular genetic aspects. *Am J Med Genet* 2002;115:164-172.

14. d. The *BCR-ABL1* fusion transcript with its fusion protein with a constitutively active ABL1 tyrosine kinase is the pathogenic mechanism of chronic myelogenous leukemia and "Philadelphia-positive" acute lymphoid leukemia (Ph-positive ALL). The t(9;22)(q34;q11) translocation causes a fusion between the ABL gene on the long arm of chromosome 9 and the BCR gene on chromosome 22. The breakpoint on chromosome 9 always occurs in a 300-kb region between the 5'-UTR and intron 1b of the ABL1 gene, preserving exon 2 of ABL1. The breakpoints on chromosome 22 are either in a 4.8Kb; a major breakpoint region between exons 11 and 14 (M-bcr) responsible for the p210BCR-ABL protein that characterizes CML; a 55-kb minor breakpoint region between exons 2' and 2 of the BCR gene (m-BCR) responsible for the p190BCR-ABL protein that characterizes most cases of Ph-positive ALL; or a small region in intron 19 BCR (μBCR) that is responsible for p230 gene product seen in chronic neutrophilic leukemia. The tyrosine kinase is a target for the TKI imatinib. Thus, monitoring of response to the treatment is of clinical value. Monitoring can be performed by following complete blood count, by classic karyotyping to detect the Philadelphia chromosome, by FISH, and by RT-PCR. A complete hematologic response refers to normalization of the complete blood count and differential, which can be seen even in the presence of significant disease; a complete cytogenetic response refers to 0% Ph+metaphases, which probably has a sensitivity of 1 tumor cell in 100; a major molecular response (MMR) refers to a three log reduction in transcript relative to a control gene. Because of the many factors that affect quantitation with RT-PCR, it is considered best to measure the level of BCR-ABL1 as a ratio to a "housekeeping" gene. Measurement is done using real-time methods, usually with hydrolysis ("Taqman") probes or dual hybridization FRET ("Light Cycler") probes, although other types of probes exist. The Ct or the fractional cycle number at which the signal rises above a threshold—with 100% efficient PCR—varies inversely with the $\log_2$ of the starting copy number of the target in the reaction. Results vary by up to 10-fold between laboratories, even when the laboratories themselves have a high precision; therefore, the use of absolute calibrators and an international scale are needed. In the meanwhile, results within each laboratory should be compared with the initial sample. Because of the kinetics of response, the significance of a specific value depends on the duration since start of imatinib treatment. At 18 months approximately 76% develop a complete cytogenetic response on imatinib, with a 7-year event-free survival rate of 81% and a 93% progression-free survival rate; at 12 months, individuals who have a transcript level that is greater than 10% of baseline have a 68% overall survival rate at 7 years versus 90% of those with a lower level; individuals with an MMR have a 99% PFS at 7 years compared with 90% for those with a higher transcript level. Secondary resistance to imatinib can develop, due to ABL-kinase mutations. When this happens, there is an increase in transcript levels above the nadir. NCCN guidelines recommend testing for mutations when there is a one log increase in transcript levels, although a twofold increase in levels has been shown to correlate with detection of ABL1 mutations. Control RNAs that are used include ABL1, GUSB (β-D-glucuronidase), and β2-microglobulin.

Akard LP, Wang YL: Translating trial-based molecular monitoring into clinical practice: importance of international standards and practical considerations for community practitioners. *Clin Lymphoma Myeloma Leuk* 2011;11(5):385-395.

Hughes T, Deininger M, Hochhaus A, et al: Monitoring CML patients responding to treatment with tyrosine kinase inhibitors: review and recommendations for harmonizing current methodology for detecting BCR-ABL transcripts and kinase domain mutations and for expressing results. *Blood* 2006;108(1):28-37. Epub 2006 Mar 7.

15. e. Amplification of the HER2/Neu (ERBB2) gene, with associated HER2 protein overexpression and constitutive activation of its tyrosine kinase activity, is more frequent in ER/PR-negative breast cancers and is an independent indicator of poor prognosis. More importantly, ERBB2 is a target of, and ERBB2 amplification is a marker of, sensitivity to treatment with trastuzumab (Herceptin). In addition, the small TKI lapatinib, and the new anti-HER2 antibody, pertuzumab, which targets a different HER2 epitope, have been shown to be effective in HER2 amplified breast cancer. The latter has been shown to improve progression-free survival rate by almost 50% in patients with advanced breast cancer, when added to docetaxel and trastuzumab. Although semiquantitative immunohistochemical tests for protein expression, such as Herceptest, are convenient, variability of antigen preservation and retrieval, as well as interobserver variability in interpretation, make immunohistochemistry a less reliable predictor of response than FISH. The American Society of Clinical Oncology and College of American Pathologists have issued guidelines for evaluating the HER2 status of breast tumors. Resistance to trastuzumab is poorly understood, and many mechanisms may be involved, including loss of the ERBB2 external domain, overexpression of MUC4, increased transcription of ERBB2, and bypassing EGFR signaling by activation of downstream pathways, especially the PI3-kinase/mTOR pathway, including activating PIK3CA mutations and loss of PTEN. One means of overcoming resistance is treatment with mTOR pathway inhibitors, such as everolimus. Although modest responses have been shown in pretreated patients, clinical trials to evaluate the drug in combination with chemotherapy and trastuzumab are under way. Trastuzumab has also been shown to be active in HER2 amplified/overexpressing adenocarcinoma of the stomach and distal esophagus. The criteria for immunohistochemical and FISH evaluation from the trastuzumab for gastric cancer (ToGA) trial that show this benefit differed from the College of American Pathologists/American Society for Clinical Oncology (CAP/ASCO) criteria, although a recent publication from Memorial Sloan Kettering shows that the CAP/ASCO criteria may be adequate.

Wolff AC, Hammond ME, Schwartz JN, et al: American Society of Clinical Oncology/College of American Pathologists guideline recommendations for human epidermal grown factor receptor 2 testing in breast cancer. *Arch Pathol Lab Med* 2007;131(1):18-43.

Murphy CG, Morris PG: Recent advances in novel targeted therapies for HER2-positive breast cancer. *Anticancer Drugs* 2012;23(8):765-776.

Tafe LJ, Janjigian YY, Zaidinski M, et al: Human epidermal growth factor receptor 2 testing in gastroesophageal cancer: correlation between immunohistochemistry and fluorescence in situ hybridization. *Arch Pathol Lab Med* 2011;135:1460-1465.

16. b. The majority (70% to 85%) of GISTs have detectable activating mutations of the KIT tyrosine kinase. Many of the remaining have PDGFRA mutations. These mutations involve the juxtamembrane domain (exon 11, 60% to 65%, mainly small in-frame deletions and insertions, and occasional point mutations), the extracellular domain (exon 9, 10% to 20%, duplication insertion of Ala-Tyr 501-502, or of Phe-Ala-Phe 506-508), the kinase 1 (TK1) domain (exon 13, approximately 1%, Lys642Glu), and the activation loop (exon 17 < 1%, Asn822Lys or Asp820Tyr). When sensitive methods and frozen tissue are used to identify *KIT* mutations, they are found at a similar frequency among high-risk ("malignant") and very low-risk ("benign") GISTs.

PDGFRA mutations are associated with negative staining for KIT by IHC, and have been detected in its juxtamembrane domain (exon 12) and activation loop (exon 18). KIT exon 11 mutations have been associated with the greatest response rates to treatment with imatinib, with partial response rates of greater than 80%, but other tumors have response rates ranging between 23% and 45%. One PDGFRA activation loop mutation (Asp842Val) has been associated with poor response to imatinib. Other mutations have been associated with good responses. Tumors that progress following an initial response to imatinib show new mutations in the KIT TK1 domain (especially V654A and T670I); gene amplification with increased KIT or PDGFRA protein expression; or loss of expression—and presumably loss of dependence on kinase activity—of KIT/PDGFRA. Newer TKIs, such as sunitinib, sorafenib, and others, may inhibit some of the imatinib-resistant variants, and clinical trials are awaited. GISTs in neurofibromatosis 1 and Carney triad do not harbor mutations of either gene.

Lasota J, Miettinen M: KIT and PDGFRA mutations in gastrointestinal stromal tumors (GISTs). *Semin Diagn Pathol* 2006;23(2):91-102.
Cassier PA, Fumagalli E, Rutkowski P, et al: Outcome of patients with platelet-derived growth factor receptor alpha-mutated gastrointestinal stromal tumors in the tyrosine kinase inhibitor era. *Clin Cancer Res* 2012;18:4458-4464. Epub 2012 Jun 20.
Corless CL, Fletcher JA, Heinrich MC: Biology of gastrointestinal stromal tumors. *J Clin Oncol* 2004;22:3813-3825.

17. a. Genetic alterations that activate the MAPK pathway are common in papillary thyroid carcinomas. These include point mutations of *BRAF* (40% to 50%; mainly BRAF V600E) and *RAS* genes (10% to 20%; mainly *HRAS* and *NRAS* codon 61 mutations); *RET/PTC* translocations (10% to 20%; fusions of *RET* with 11 different partners, mainly *RET/PTC1* [fusion partner CCDC6] and *RET/PTC3* [fusion partner NCOA4]); and *TRK* translocations (uncommon; <5%) (Nikiforov 2011). BRAF V600E mutations in papillary thyroid carcinomas are associated with classical and tall cell histologic appearance and predict more aggressive behavior even in pT1 tumors. They are seen in only 10% of follicular variant tumors. *RAS* mutations are seen mainly in the follicular variant of papillary thyroid carcinoma. *RET/PTC* translocations are associated with classical histologic appearance, a younger age at diagnosis, lymph node metastasis, and radiation exposure. In the latter setting, the *RET/PTC2* translocations are most common. *RAS* (*HRAS* and *NRAS* codon 61) mutations are seen in up to 50% of follicular thyroid carcinomas and *PAX8/PPAR* gamma translocations in another *30% to 35%*. *RAS* mutations can also be seen in follicular adenomas, although these might be the precursors of follicular carcinomas. Activating *RET* mutations are seen in medullary thyroid carcinoma. Germ line mutations are seen in greater than 95% of familial cases (MEN 2 or familial medullary thyroid carcinoma). Testing of thyroid fine needle aspirates for *BRAF V600E* mutations, *NRAS* and *HRAS* codon 61 mutations, and *RET/PTC* translocations helps manage thyroid nodules. A positive BRAF V600E mutation, or RET/PTC translocation has a high positive predictive value for malignancy, provided the limit of detection of the test is below 1% mutant in normal or 1% lesional cell in normal. A positive *RAS* mutation is indicative of a neoplasm. A positive *PAX8-PPAR* gamma translocation, although not diagnostic of invasive carcinoma, is strongly associated with invasion in a follicular neoplasm. In specimens with indeterminate cytologic findings, the finding of one of the preceding mutations was associated with an 88%, 87%, and 95% risk of malignancy in the Bethesda categories, follicular lesion of uncertain significance, follicular neoplasm, and suspicious for malignancy, respectively, versus 6%, 14%, and 28% in the mutation negative cases. Thus, although a negative result does not exclude malignancy, the high positive predictive values can allow total thyroidectomy instead of thyroid lobectomy in positive cases.

Nikiforov YE: Molecular diagnostics of thyroid tumors. *Arch Pathol Lab Med* 2011;135:569-577.
Bose S, Walts AE: Thyroid fine needle aspirate: a post-Bethesda update. *Adv Anat Pathol* 2012;19:160-169.
Eszlinger M, Krogdahl A, Münz S, et al: Impact of molecular screening for point mutations and rearrangements in routine air-dried fine-needle aspiration samples of thyroid nodules. *Thyroid* 2014;24(2):305-313. Epub 2013 Oct 29.

18. c. Although cytologic testing has been extremely effective in reducing cervical cancer fatality, continued occurrence of cervical cancer in screened populations has led to DNA testing for high oncogenic risk HPVs. These viruses include HPV 16, 18, 31, and 33, among others. HPV-11 is a low oncogenic risk virus. HPV DNA testing may be performed either as reflex testing of ASCUS (atypical squamous cells of uncertain significance) or as a combined DNA/liquid cytologic screen. HPV DNA testing is more sensitive and less specific than cytologic testing, with a high negative predictive value and a low positive predictive value. There is no logical indication to test for low oncogenic risk viruses in a screening program. Mathematical models, using known costs, sensitivity, and specificity of the various tests, and age-specific incidence of cervical cancer, have shown that biennial or triennial testing consisting of cytologic testing plus DNA testing (either dual screen or reflex testing) is more cost effective in women more than 30 years of age, with no reduction in cancer prevention when compared to annual screening strategies. Because the majority of cancers show HPV 16 or 18, genotyping for these may play a role in the management of cytologic negative HPV positive cases; however, with vaccination for HPV 16 and 18 now standard, this may change.

Mandelblatt JS, Lawrence WF, Womack SM, et al: Benefits and costs of using HPV testing to screen for cervical cancer. *JAMA* 2002;287:2372-2381.
Wright TC Jr, Cox JT, Massad LS, et al: ASCCP-Sponsored Consensus Conference. 2001 Consensus Guidelines for the management of women with cervical cytological abnormalities. *JAMA* 2002;287:2120-2129.

19. c. The codeletion of 1p and 19q is a favorable prognostic marker in ologodendrogliomas. It results from an unbalanced translocation between chromosomes 1 and 19, with loss of the derivative that contains the long arm of chromosome 1 and the short arm of chromosome 19. The deletion 1p and 19q is evaluated either by FISH using 1p36 and 19q13 probes, with control probes on the long and short arms of chromosomes 1 and 19, respectively, or by LOH analysis using polymorphic microsatellite markers on the chromosomes 1p and 19q. Although the codeletion is virtually diagnostic of oligodendrogliomas, not all oligodendrogliomas harbor these deletions. They are rarely, if ever, seen in pediatric oligodendrogliomas. 1p and 19q deletions are associated with *MGMT* promoter methylation and *IDH1* or *IDH2* mutations. *IDH1* or *IDH2* mutations are seen in 70% to 80% of grades II and III astrocytomas and oligodendrogliomas, and virtually all 1p/19q deleted oligodendrogliomas. They are also seen in glioblastomas that arose from low-grade gliomas, but virtually never in de novo glioblastomas. IDH1/2 mutated gliomas are either 1p/19q deleted or carry p53 mutations. MGMT is a DNA repair enzyme that removes alkyl groups from DNA. Promoter hypermethylation of *MGMT* is associated with loss of expression of MGMT and sensitivity of gliomas to alklylating agents.

Ichimura K: Molecular pathogenesis of IDH mutations in gliomas. *Brain Tumor Pathol* 2012;29:131-139. Epub 2012 Mar 8.

Horbinski C, Nikiforova MN, Hobbs J, et al: The importance of 10q status in an outcomes-based comparison between 1p/19q fluorescence in situ hybridization and polymerase chain reaction-based microsatellite loss of heterozygosity analysis of oligodendrogliomas. *J Neuropathol Exp Neurol* 2012;71(1):73-82.

20. e. An inversion in the short arm of chromosome 2 results in an echinoderm microtubule-associated protein like 4-anaplastic lymphoma kinase (EML4-ALK) fusion protein with tyrosine kinase activity. At least 11 variants have been described that fuse various 5′ portions of *EML4* to exon 20 of *ALK*; the most common variants involve exons 13 (variant 1) and exons 6a/b (variants 3a/b) of EML4. In addition, TFG and KIF5B have been identified as additional partners. ALK translocations are seen in approximately 3% to 13% of patients with adenocarcinomas, and can occur with various histologic patterns, although they have been described to be more common in patients with a signet ring morphologic appearance or an acinar growth pattern. Squamous and adenosquamous carcinomas also may rarely harbor a mutation. Patients tend to be younger, be of Asian origin, present at an advanced stage, and be nonsmokers. ALK positive lung cancers can be detected by RT-PCR, FISH, and immunohistochemistry for ALK. RT-PCR to detect the fusion gene requires multiple different primers, including primers for *TFG* and *KIF5B* to detect all variants. FISH using "break-apart" probes flanking the ALK breakpoints (with red and green signals overlapping in the normal state, and separated when there is a rearrangement) should theoretically detect all variants; however, with variant 1, because of the small separation of signal, there is low interobserver agreement by FISH. Immuno-histochemistry, which works well for anaplastic large cell lymphoma, is not as sensitive for lung tumors because of the low level of expression, especially for variant 1; however, recent, more sensitive antibodies have improved the situation. The best approach may be to combine RT-PCR with a FISH or immunohistochemical test. ALK translocations render tumors sensitive to the kinase inhibitor crizotinib, and ALK translocation positive tumors show response rates of more than 50% and a disease control rate (response or stable disease) of almost 80%. Germ line ALK activating point mutations are seen in hereditary neuroblastoma.

Cheng L, Alexander RE, Maclennan GT, et al: Molecular pathology of lung cancer: key to personalized medicine. *Mod Pathol* 2012;25:347-369. Epub 2012 Jan 27.

Sasaki T, Rodig SJ, Chirieac LR, Jänne PA: The biology and treatment of EML4-ALK non-small cell lung cancer. *Eur J Cancer* 2010;46:1773-1780. Epub 2010 Apr 24.

Wallander ML, Geiersbach KB, Tripp SR, Layfield LJ: Comparison of reverse transcription-polymerase chain reaction, immunohistochemistry, and fluorescence in situ hybridization methodologies for detection of echinoderm microtubule-associated protein like 4-anaplastic lymphoma kinase fusion-positive non-small cell lung carcinoma: implications for optimal clinical testing. *Arch Pathol Lab Med* 2012;136:796-803.

CHAPTER 24

CYTOPATHOLOGY

Diane Hamele-Bena, Xiao-Jun Wei, and Samer N. Khader

UESTIONS

Questions 1-65 refer to a photo or photomicrograph.

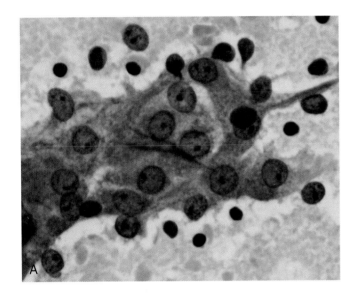

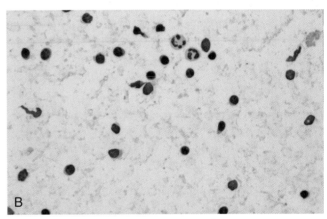

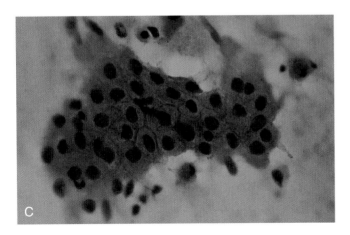

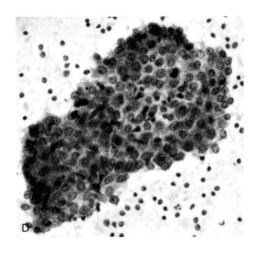

1. Which of the following features of this salivary gland lesion is TRUE?
   a. Derived from neuroendocrine cells entrapped during embryologic development in the parotid gland
   b. Almost always occurs in the submandibular gland
   c. Most often presents as bilateral masses
   d. Higher prevalence in smokers
   e. Often regresses following treatment with antibiotics

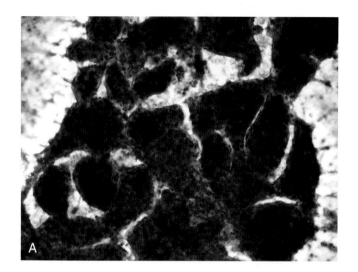

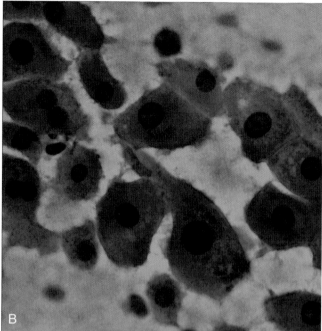

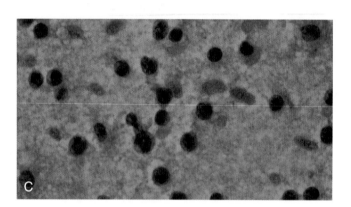

2. These photomicrographs represent computed tomography (CT)-guided fine needle aspiration (FNA) biopsy findings of a hepatic mass in a 60-year-old man. Which of the following statements BEST describes a pathologic characteristic of this lesion?

a. Abundant bile ducts and normal hepatocytes are important diagnostic features.

b. Reticulin stain may accentuate the trabecular and anastomosing pattern in cell blocks.

c. Binucleated cells and intranuclear pseudoinclusions are important clues to malignancy.

d. Malignant cells are commonly seen in ascitic fluid from patients with this lesion.

e. Absence of bile production by tumor cells is a helpful clue to the diagnosis.

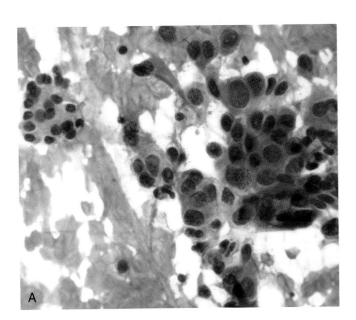

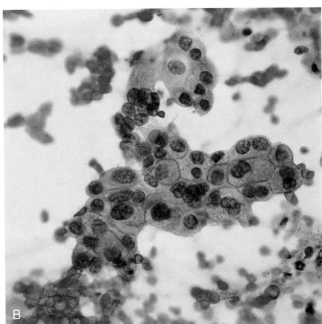

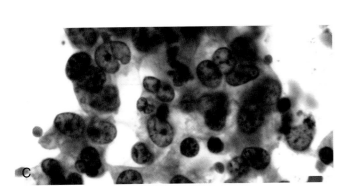

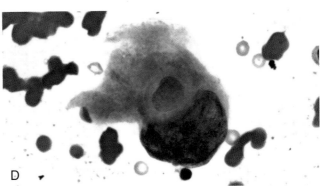

3. These photomicrographs are from an endoscopic ultrasound (EUS)-guided FNA of a pancreatic mass in a 72-year-old man. Which of the statements regarding this lesion is the MOST accurate?

   a. This lesion represents a complication of acute and chronic pancreatitis.

   b. An increased level of serum α-fetoprotein (AFP) is noted in some patients with this lesion.

   c. The 5-year survival rate of patients with this lesion is around 50%.

   d. This lesion characteristically arises in the head, neck, or body of the pancreas in young women.

   e. Molecular analysis can show mutation of *SMAD4* and *KRAS* genes.

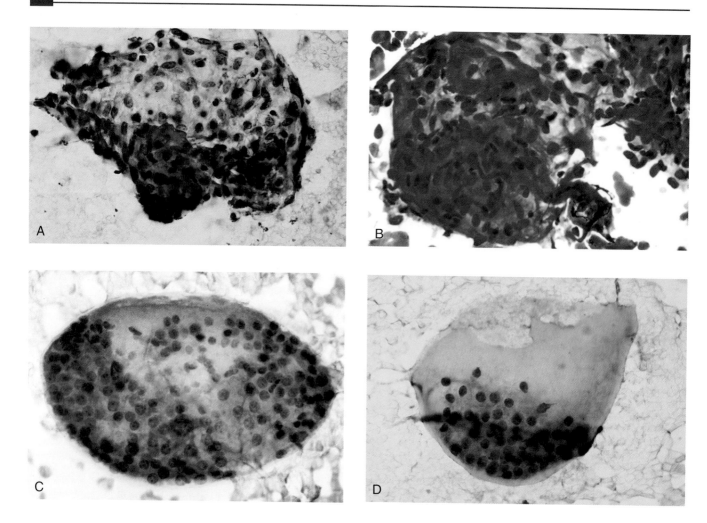

4. Which is the BEST diagnosis for this FNA biopsy of a painful,
   diffusely enlarged thyroid gland in a 45-year-old woman?
   a. Benign nodular goiter
   b. Papillary thyroid carcinoma (PTC)
   c. Follicular neoplasm
   d. Subacute (de Quervain) thyroiditis
   e. Riedel disease

5. An FNA of a firm, 3-cm thyroid mass from a 27-year-old woman yielded the smears depicted in the photos. Among the cytologic features that are helpful in diagnosing this depicted lesion, which is the MOST specific for this entity?
   a. Enlarged nuclei
   b. Nuclear grooves
   c. Multinucleated histiocytes
   d. Papillary configuration
   e. Intranuclear cytoplasmic inclusions

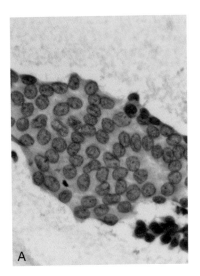

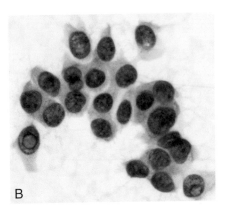

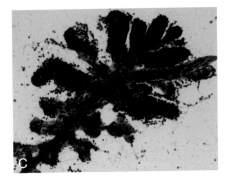

6. An FNA biopsy of a liver mass in a 65-year-old man yielded the cells in the photomicrographs. The cells appear positive with an immunocytochemical stain for CDX2 and negative for thyroid transcription factor-1 (TTF-1). The MOST likely diagnosis is:

a. Metastatic colonic adenocarcinoma
b. Hepatocellular carcinoma (HCC)
c. Metastatic melanoma
d. Metastatic bronchogenic adenocarcinoma
e. Metastatic renal cell carcinoma (RCC)

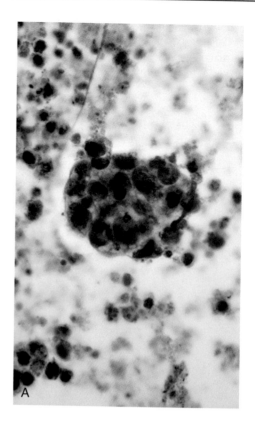

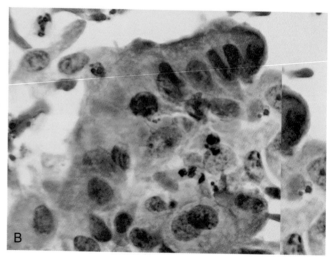

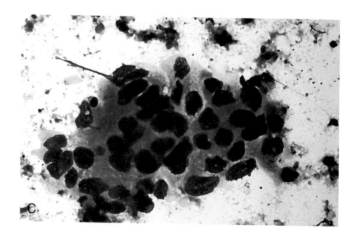

7. These photomicrographs are from an EUS-guided FNA biopsy of a well-circumscribed tumor in the tail of the pancreas in a 50-year-old woman. Which of the following statements MOST accurately describes a pathologic finding of this neoplasm?

   a. Pancreatic intraepithelial neoplasia (PanIN) is a precursor lesion for this neoplasm.

   b. Cyst fluid analysis of this tumor is helpful in making an accurate diagnosis.

   c. Significant nuclear pleomorphism suggests malignancy.

   d. The cell of origin of this neoplasm is the acinar cell of the pancreas.

   e. The majority of these tumors are nonfunctional.

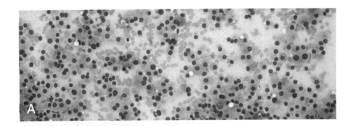

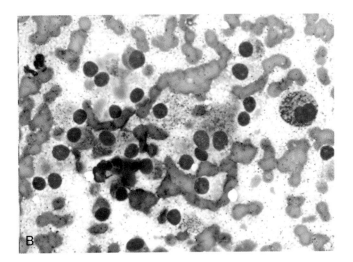

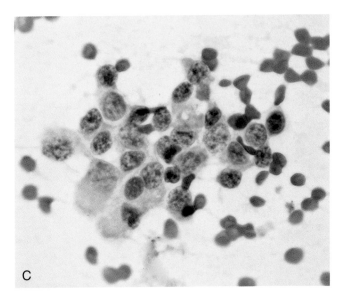

8. These photomicrographs are of a voided urine specimen from a
73-year-old man. What is the MOST likely diagnosis?
   a. High-grade urothelial carcinoma
   b. Human papillomavirus (HPV) infection
   c. Cytomegalovirus (CMV) infection
   d. Herpes infection
   e. Human polyomavirus infection

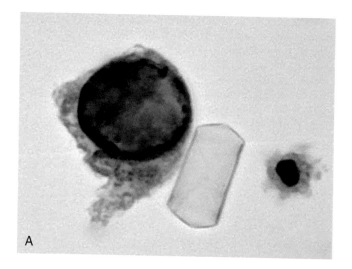

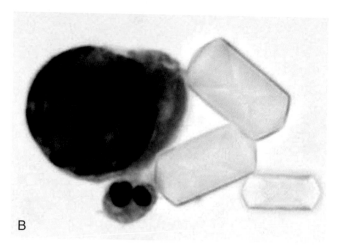

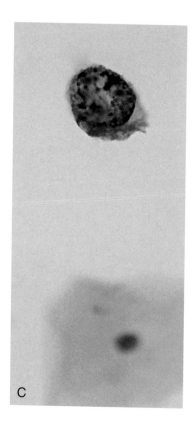

9. Which of the following statements regarding the organisms in this lymph node FNA is TRUE?
   a. They are the most common fungal infection detected in central nervous system (CNS) specimens.
   b. Broad-based budding is typical in this fungal infection.
   c. Nonseptate hyphae with irregular branching are common in respiratory specimens.
   d. Dimorphism is helpful in identification of this fungus.
   e. This fungus can develop fruiting heads in aerobic conditions.

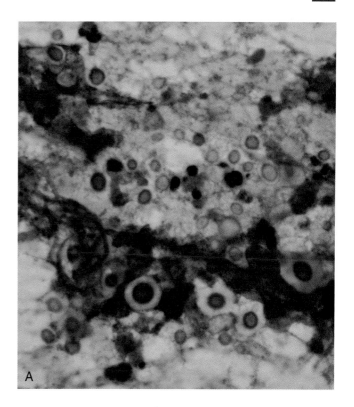

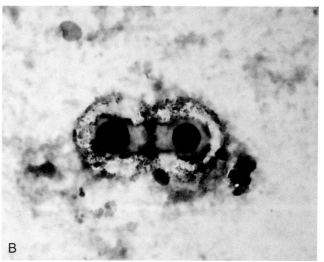

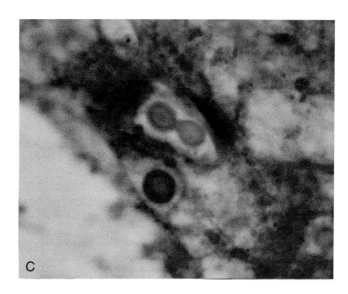

10. The photomicrographs represent FNA material from a mass in the tail of the pancreas of a 23-year-old woman. Which of the following is the MOST likely diagnosis?

   a. Solid pseudopapillary tumor (SPPT)
   b. Pancreatic endocrine neoplasm (PEN)
   c. Acinar cell carcinoma (ACC)
   d. Well-differentiated pancreatic adenocarcinoma
   e. Intraductal papillary mucinous neoplasm (IPMN)

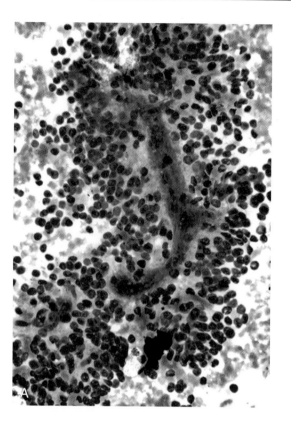

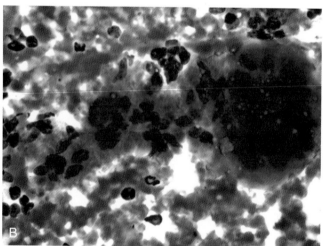

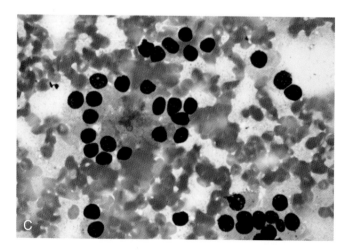

11. Which of the following statements is MOST likely to be true regarding the cells in this cerebrospinal fluid (CSF) specimen?

a. The presence of pigmented cells representing hemosiderin-containing macrophages and red blood cells is consistent with a diagnosis of meningeal endometriosis.

b. These cells likely represent a previous hemorrhagic event.

c. The cells would likely be positive with stains for S100 and tyrosinase.

d. These bone marrow cells probably were derived from the lumbar puncture needle inadvertently entering a vertebral body during sampling.

e. The cells would likely be positive with immunocytochemical stains for hepatocyte paraffin (Hep Par 1) and polyclonal carcinoembryonic antigen (CEA).

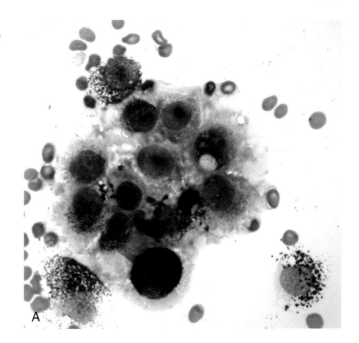

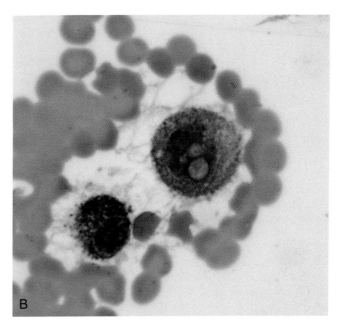

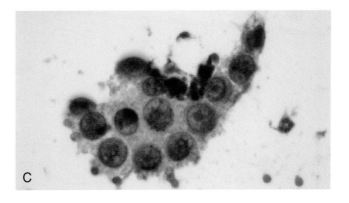

12. These photomicrographs depict an FNA biopsy of an anterior neck mass. What is the MOST common molecular abnormality associated with this tumor?

a. RET/PTC1 and PTC3 rearrangements on chromosome 10 (10q11.2)

b. PAX8/PPAR gamma rearrangement, a translocation (2;3)(q13;p25)

c. TRK rearrangement of the *NTRK1* gene of chromosome 1q22

d. Point mutation in the *RAS* gene (HRAS, KRAS, and NRAS codon-specific nucleotide substitutions)

e. Point mutation in the *BRAF* gene at codon 600 (BRAFT1799A [V600E])

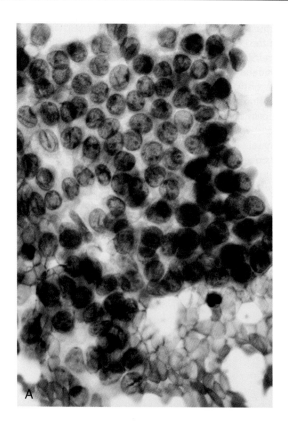

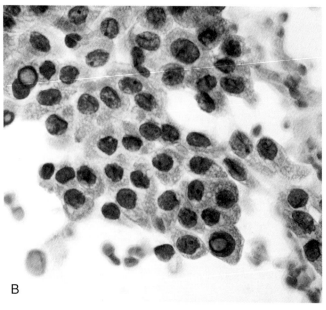

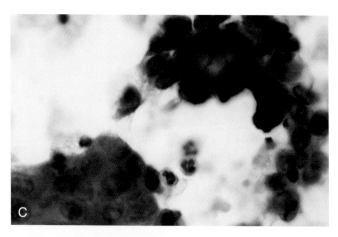

13. Consider these photomicrographs of a transbronchial FNA of a lung lesion in a 70-year-old male smoker. Which of the following statements is TRUE?

   a. Crush artifact often is present in smears of this lesion.

   b. Activating mutations in epidermal growth factor receptor (EGFR) commonly are found in these lesions.

   c. By definition, necrosis must not be present.

   d. TTF-1 and CD45 positivity confirm the diagnosis.

   e. Occasional macronucleoli are not unusual.

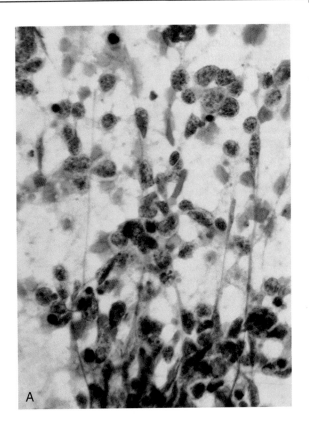

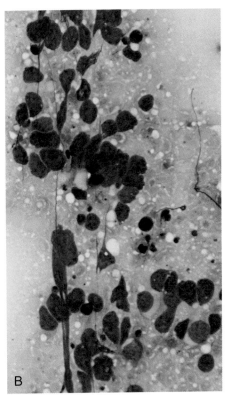

14. The cytologic finding depicted in this photomicrograph is MOST frequently found in FNA biopsies of lymph nodes containing which of the following metastatic tumors?
   a. Small cell carcinoma
   b. Adenocarcinoma of lung
   c. Melanoma
   d. Squamous cell carcinoma
   e. Lobular carcinoma of the breast

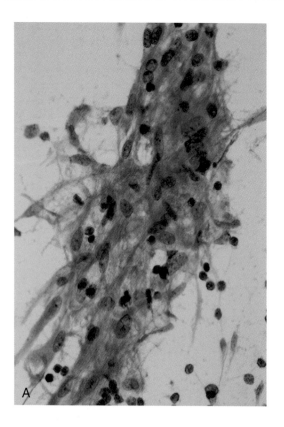

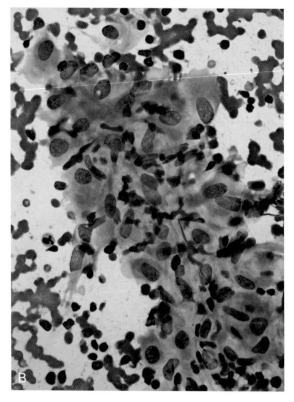

15. The photomicrographs depict an FNA biopsy sample from an incidentally discovered renal mass in a 60-year-old woman. What is the MOST likely diagnosis?

a. Papillary renal cell carcinoma (PRCC)
b. Conventional RCC
c. Chromophobe RCC
d. Adrenal neuroblastoma
e. Oncocytoma

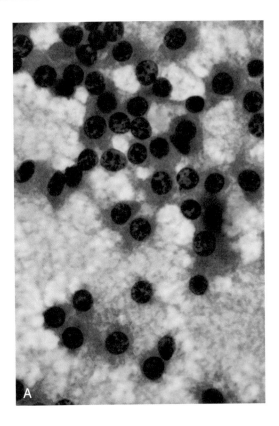

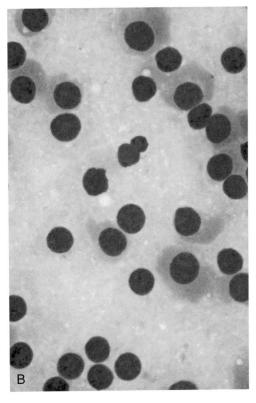

16. Which of the statements regarding the depicted findings in a bronchoalveolar lavage (BAL) specimen is TRUE?

a. This Gomori methenamine silver (GMS)-positive organism formerly was classified as a protozoan, but now is considered to be a fungus.

b. GMS highlights trophozoites inside cysts.

c. Confirmatory special stains are necessary when this entity is suspected on Papanicolaou (Pap) stain.

d. This organism commonly results in pulmonary abscess formation.

e. The gold standard for the diagnosis is microbiologic culture, although the organism often is identifiable with special stains.

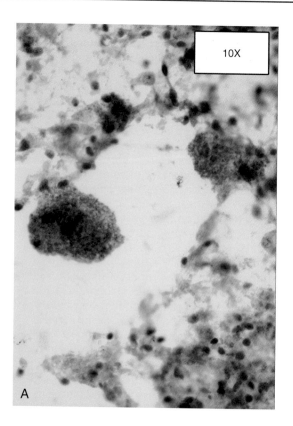

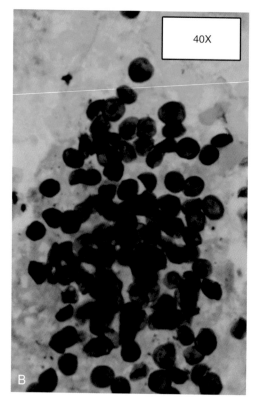

17. A 20-year-old woman presents with vesicular lesions of the cervix and inguinal adenopathy. Cytologic examination reveals the findings depicted in the photomicrographs. Which of the following is TRUE?

    a. Primary infection often is followed by multiple recurrences.

    b. The most diagnostic cytologic abnormalities are evident in the chronic phase.

    c. Large nuclear inclusions often are accompanied by basophilic cytoplasmic inclusions.

    d. Infection characteristically is accompanied by cytoplasmic eosinophilia and narrow perinuclear halos.

    e. Infection is associated with follicular cervicitis.

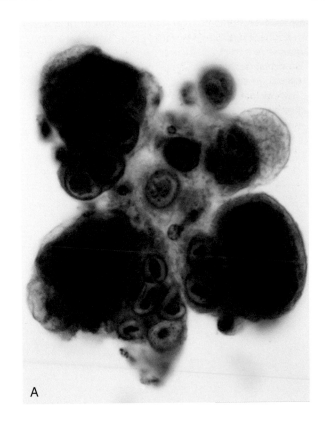

A

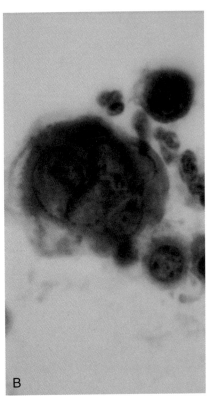

B

18. These cells were present in an FNA biopsy specimen of a posterior neck mass in a 41-year-old man. What is the BEST diagnosis?

    a. Branchial cleft cyst
    b. Metastatic squamous cell carcinoma
    c. Thyroglossal duct cyst
    d. Pilomatricoma
    e. Infundibular cyst

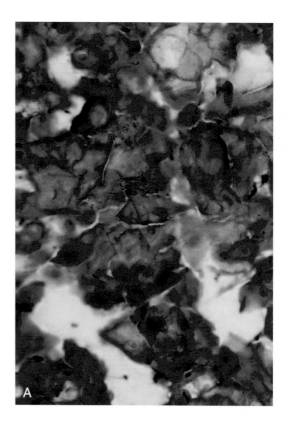

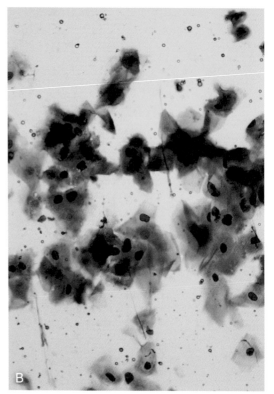

19. Which of the following immunocytochemical staining patterns is MOST consistent with these photomicrographs of a liquid-based preparation of an FNA biopsy of a retroperitoneal lesion?

   a. RCC positive, CD10 positive, CK7 negative, CD117 negative, AMACR negative, E-cadherin negative

   b. RCC negative, CD10 negative, CK7 positive (strong), CD117 positive, AMACR negative, E-cadherin positive

   c. RCC positive, CD10 negative, CK7 positive, CD117 negative, AMACR positive, E-cadherin negative

   d. RCC negative, CD10 negative, CK7 positive (weak), CD117 positive, AMACR negative, E-cadherin positive

   e. RCC negative, CD10 negative, CK7 negative, CD117 negative, AMACR positive, E-cadherin negative

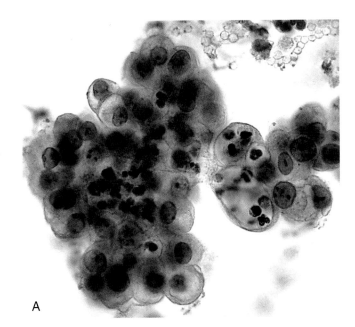

A

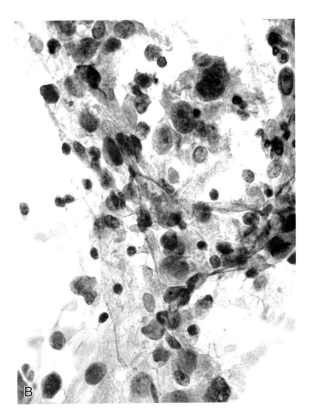

B

20. The photomicrograph represents a CT-guided FNA biopsy of a cystic anterior mediastinal mass in a 35-year-old man. Grossly, the aspirate yielded slimy, semitransparent, viscous material. What is the MOST likely diagnosis?
   a. Malignant lymphoma with large cell transformation
   b. Germinoma
   c. Mature cystic teratoma
   d. Metastatic mucinous adenocarcinoma
   e. Thymic carcinoma

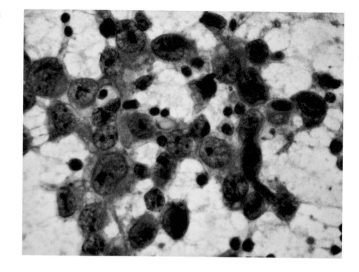

21. The depicted cells are from an FNA of a thyroid lesion in the upper pole of the left thyroid lobe of a 60-year-old man. These cells MOST likely are positive for:
   a. Thyroglobulin
   b. Calcitonin
   c. Glial fibrillary acidic protein (GFAP)
   d. Congo red
   e. Crystal violet

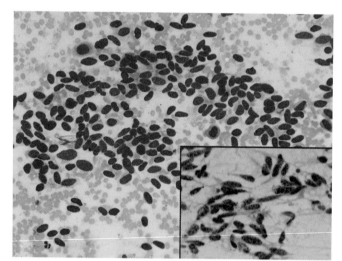

22. This FNA specimen is from a dominant 1.5-cm echogenic nodule in an enlarged, painless thyroid of a 40-year-old woman. Ultrasound examination of the thyroid appeared heterogeneously echogenic. The lesion depicted is MOST often associated with which of the following:
   a. Lack of antimicrosomal antibody
   b. Increased incidence of sarcoma
   c. Hypothyroidism
   d. Infectious cause
   e. Squamous cell metaplasia

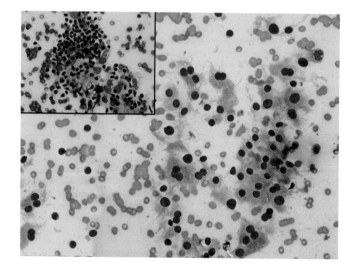

23. An FNA biopsy of a dominant, well-circumscribed, anechogenic thyroid nodule in a 30-year-old woman with multiple thyroid nodules was performed. A satisfactory specimen was obtained, and a representative area is shown in this photomicrograph. What is the BEST diagnosis?
   a. Colloid nodule
   b. Hashimoto thyroiditis
   c. Follicular carcinoma
   d. Thyroglossal duct cyst
   e. Parathyroid cyst

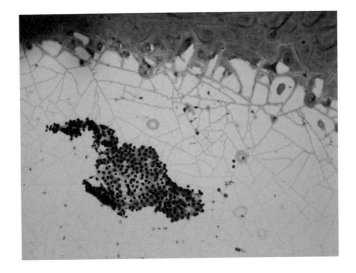

24. This photomicrograph depicts an FNA smear from a 4-cm solitary nodule in the right lobe of the thyroid in a 47-year-old man. Sparse colloid was present. What is the BEST diagnosis?
   a. Papillary thyroid carcinoma
   b. Hürthle cell tumor
   c. Nodular goiter
   d. Follicular neoplasm
   e. Hashimoto thyroiditis

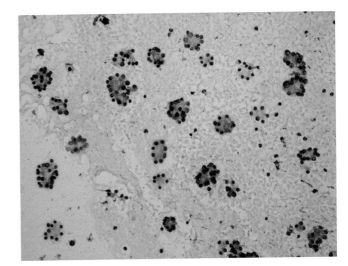

25. A Diff-Quik-stained FNA smear from a 3-cm parotid mass is shown in the photomicrograph. Which of the following is TRUE?
   a. Excision of most of the tumor nodule often is sufficient treatment, because small amounts of residual tumor spontaneously regress.
   b. In the parotid, it usually presents as a painless, slowly growing nodule in the deep lobe.
   c. It is commonly seen in the parotid gland but has not been reported to occur in minor salivary glands.
   d. It is associated with "daisy head" crystals that stain orangeophilic on Pap stain.
   e. When malignant transformation occurs, the malignant component is usually sarcomatous.

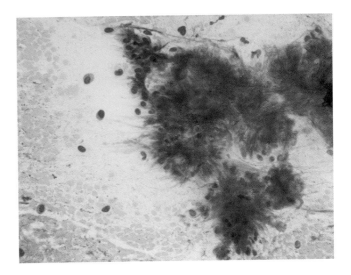

26. What is the MOST likely diagnosis of this painful salivary gland mass?
   a. Pleomorphic adenoma
   b. Acinic cell carcinoma
   c. Mucoepidermoid carcinoma
   d. Metastatic thyroid follicular carcinoma
   e. Adenoid cystic carcinoma

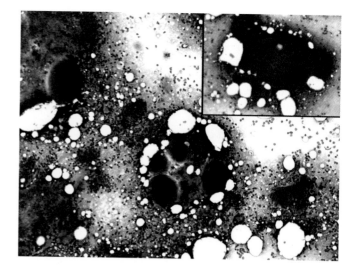

27. The cells in the photomicrograph are from ascites fluid from a 57-year-old woman with bilateral ovarian masses. They MOST likely represent:
   a. Mucinous cystadenocarcinoma of ovary
   b. Endometrial adenocarcinoma
   c. Benign hepatocytes
   d. Endometriosis
   e. Benign mesothelial cells

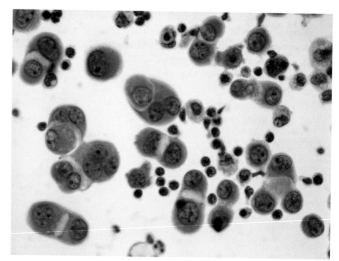

28. This low-power photomicrograph depicts a pleural fluid from a 55-year-old woman. The MOST likely diagnosis is:
   a. Colonic adenocarcinoma
   b. Small cell carcinoma of the lung
   c. Breast carcinoma
   d. Lymphoma
   e. Mesothelioma

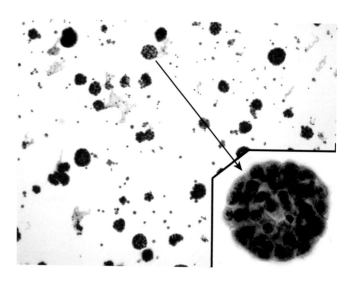

29. The photomicrographs show FNA findings from a well-circumscribed breast mass in a 30-year-old woman. The findings are MOST suggestive of:

   a. Phyllodes tumor

   b. Fibroadenoma

   c. Papillary neoplasm

   d. Colloid carcinoma

   e. Lactating adenoma

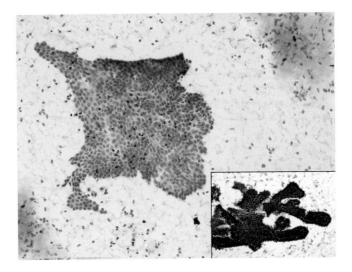

30. This photomicrograph displaying FNA findings from a palpable breast mass in a 40-year-old woman reveals:

   a. Apocrine metaplasia associated with fibrocystic change

   b. Foam cells associated with fibrocystic change

   c. Paget cells in ductal adenocarcinoma

   d. Adipocytes as part of a lipoma

   e. Hemosiderin-laden macrophages in fat necrosis

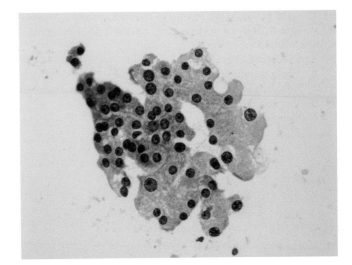

31. The photomicrograph depicts an FNA from a firm mass in the breast of a 60-year-old woman. The BEST diagnosis is:

   a. Colloid carcinoma

   b. Ductal carcinoma

   c. Medullary carcinoma

   d. Tubular carcinoma

   e. Comedocarcinoma

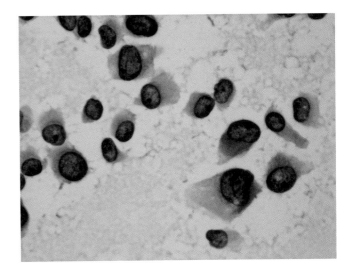

32. An aspirate from a breast mass in a 70-year-old woman yielded sparsely cellular smears containing the cells in the photomicrograph. Which of the following statements regarding this lesion is TRUE?

    a. It is a common source of false-negative diagnoses in breast FNA.

    b. Lymphoglandular bodies are common.

    c. Intracytoplasmic lumina and single file arrangement are diagnostic.

    d. It is thought to be of neural origin and related to Schwann cells.

    e. It is the most common type of mammary carcinoma in males.

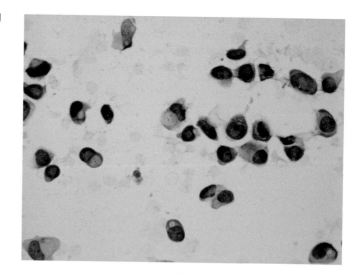

33. This photomicrograph represents FNA biopsy findings from a painless mass in the lateral anterior neck of a 22-year-old man. The MOST likely diagnosis is:

    a. Parathyroid cyst

    b. Nodular goiter with cystic degeneration

    c. Branchial cleft cyst

    d. Dermoid cyst

    e. Paraganglioma

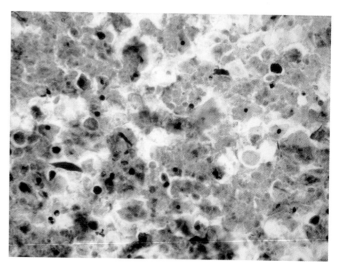

34. This photomicrograph shows cells derived from a CT-guided aspirate of a right kidney mass. They MOST likely represent:

    a. Mesothelial cells

    b. Benign hepatocytes

    c. Lymph node germinal center cells

    d. Pheochromocytoma

    e. RCC

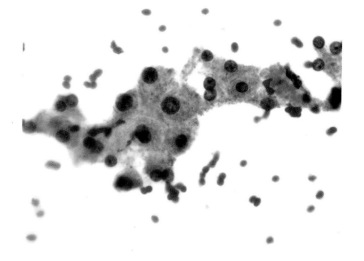

35. These photomicrographs depict material obtained from an
EUS-guided FNA biopsy of a mass in the head of the pancreas in
a 74-year-old man. They MOST likely represent:
   a. Well-differentiated pancreatic adenocarcinoma
   b. Benign gastric epithelium
   c. Benign small intestinal epithelium
   d. Low-grade mucinous cystic neoplasm (MCN)
   e. Benign pancreatic ductal epithelium

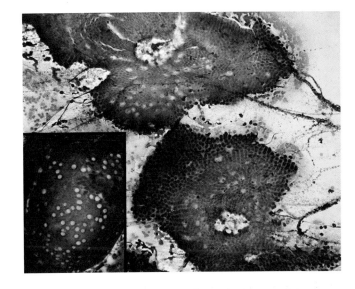

36. This photomicrograph depicts a Pap-stained smear of a gastric
brushing specimen from a 65-year-old man with a gastric ulcer.
What is the BEST diagnosis?
   a. Herpes infection
   b. Granulomatous gastritis
   c. Intestinal metaplasia
   d. Reactive change
   e. Well-differentiated adenocarcinoma

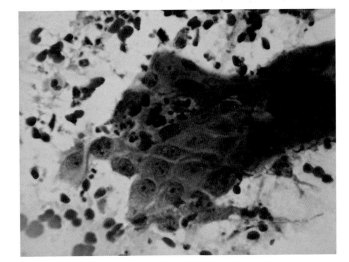

37. The cells noted in this photomicrograph were present in a
CSF sample from a 45-year-old woman. Which statement
regarding these cells is the MOST accurate?
   a. The cells are leukocyte common antigen (LCA) positive.
   b. The cells are reactive with PAS with diastase predigestion
   (PAS-D).
   c. They most likely represent a primary CNS tumor.
   d. These cells represent monocytes of "Mollaret" meningitis.
   e. The cells suggest bacterial meningitis.

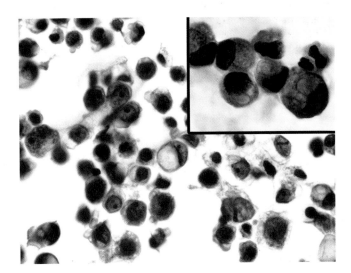

38. A 60-year-old man presented with a 1-month history of hematuria. A voided urine specimen is represented in the photomicrograph. What is the MOST likely diagnosis?
   a. High-grade urothelial carcinoma
   b. Low-grade urothelial carcinoma
   c. Small cell carcinoma
   d. Lymphoma
   e. Adenocarcinoma

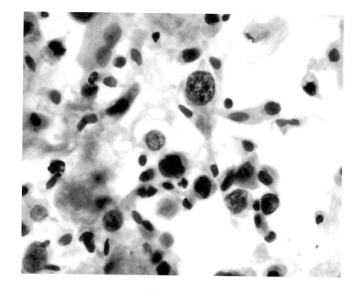

39. Which one of following statements regarding the two large cells in this photomicrograph of a lymph node FNA is the MOST accurate?
   a. This finding is specific for lymphoid hyperplasia.
   b. They may be seen in lymph nodes with metastatic carcinoma.
   c. They usually are present in low-grade lymphomas.
   d. These cells are reactive for CD1a immunostain.
   e. These cells are diagnostic of Hodgkin lymphoma.

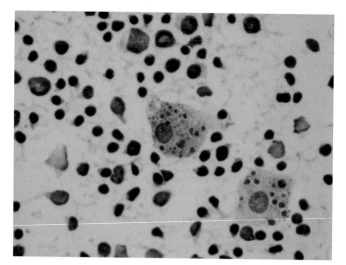

40. The MOST likely immunocytochemical staining profile of these large cells in a cervical lymph node FNA biopsy of a 62-year-old man is:
   a. LCA positive, CD15 positive, CD30 positive, epithelial membrane antigen (EMA) positive
   b. LCA positive, CD15 positive, CD30 positive, EMA positive
   c. LCA positive, CD15 negative, CD30 positive, EMA positive
   d. LCA negative, CD15 positive, CD30 positive, EMA negative
   e. LCA positive, CD15 negative, CD30 negative, EMA positive

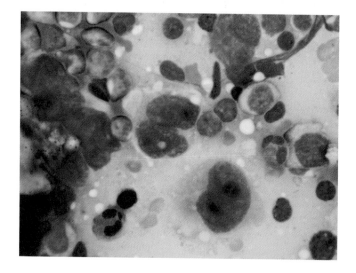

41. This photomicrograph is from an FNA biopsy of a 3.0-cm soft tissue mass in the thigh near the knee in a 19-year-old woman. The neoplastic cells are diffusely positive for CD99. Reverse transcriptase polymerase chain reaction (RT-PCR) revealed a (11;22)(q24;q12) translocation. What is the MOST likely diagnosis?
   a. Synovial sarcoma
   b. Small cell osteogenic sarcoma
   c. Alveolar soft part sarcoma
   d. Ewing sarcoma/primitive neuroectodermal tumor (ES/PNET)
   e. Alveolar rhabdomyosarcoma

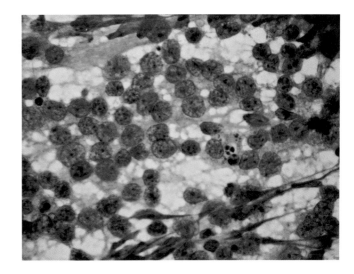

42. A sputum specimen from a 32-year-old man with hemoptysis revealed the findings depicted in the photomicrograph. Which organism is MOST likely?
   a. *Strongyloides*
   b. *Ascaris*
   c. *Trichuris*
   d. *Echinococcus*
   e. *Enterobius*

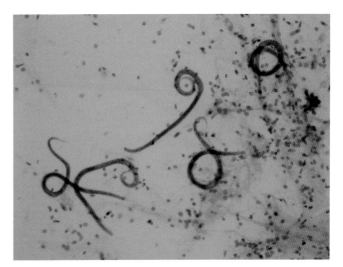

43. This photomicrograph is from a CT-guided FNA biopsy of a 10-cm mass in the kidney of a 5-year-old girl. In addition to the findings depicted in the photomicrograph, smears showed larger cells with abundant cytoplasm in gland and tubular arrangements as well as spindle cells in metachromatic stroma. What is the MOST likely diagnosis?
   a. Wilms tumor (nephroblastoma)
   b. Neuroblastoma
   c. Lymphoma
   d. Ewing sarcoma
   e. Mesoblastic nephroma

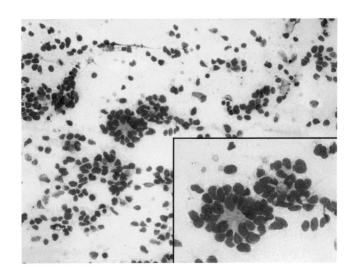

44. The lesion in this cervical smear is MOST likely associated with which of the following viral types?

 a. HPV type 16
 b. HPV type 18
 c. HPV type 11
 d. Herpes simplex virus (HSV) type II
 e. HIV 2

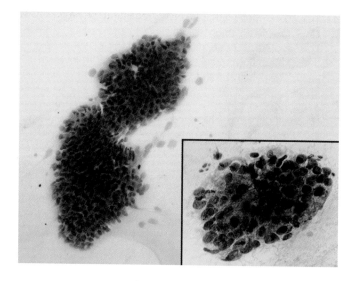

45. The cells depicted here were present in a liquid-based cervicovaginal cytologic preparation from a 50-year-old woman at an annual routine examination. How should this finding be reported?

 a. Reactive cellular changes associated with radiation
 b. Atrophy
 c. Endometrial cells present in a woman 40 or more years of age
 d. Atypical squamous cells of undetermined significance (ASC-US)
 e. Atypical endocervical cells, favor neoplasia.

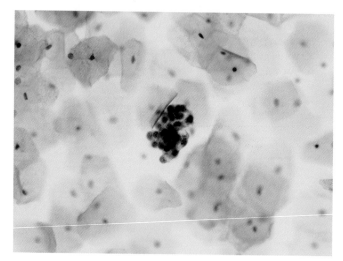

46. Which of the following statements regarding the organisms depicted in the photomicrograph is TRUE?

 a. Glycogen-rich superficial cells are the principal target, leading to cytolysis.
 b. They contribute to normal vaginal pH.
 c. They are encapsulated gram-negative bacilli.
 d. They are most commonly found in advanced atrophy in postmenopausal women.
 e. They have been associated with toxic shock syndrome in women wearing tampons.

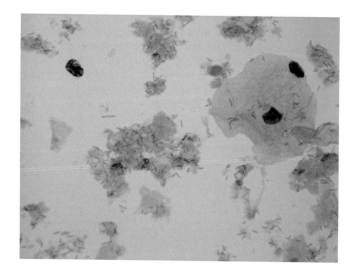

47. Which of the following statements regarding the organisms in the photomicrograph is CORRECT?
   a. Adding potassium hydroxide (KOH) to the thin, homogeneous discharge caused by these organisms generates a fishy amine odor.
   b. They are commonly present in association with *Leptothrix*.
   c. The presence of flagella is necessary for diagnosis.
   d. These organisms are often found in the vagina/cervix under acidic (low pH) conditions.
   e. These organisms typically are acquired from contaminated drinking water.

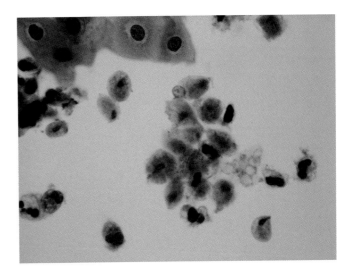

48. The photomicrograph depicts findings from a vaginal cytology specimen from a patient who underwent a hysterectomy for endometrial carcinoma. Which of the following statements regarding the findings is TRUE?
   a. The findings are suspicious for recurrent carcinoma.
   b. Topical estrogen should be followed by repeat sampling.
   c. Precise diagnostic confirmation requires culture.
   d. The features are consistent with repair.
   e. The features are diagnostic of radiation effect.

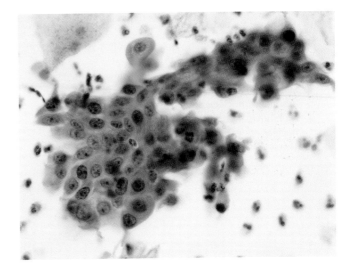

49. A cervicovaginal specimen yields the cells depicted in the photomicrograph. Which is the MOST likely diagnosis?
   a. Low-grade squamous intraepithelial lesion (LSIL)
   b. High-grade squamous intraepithelial lesion (HSIL)
   c. Parakeratosis
   d. Squamous cell carcinoma
   e. Metastatic carcinoma

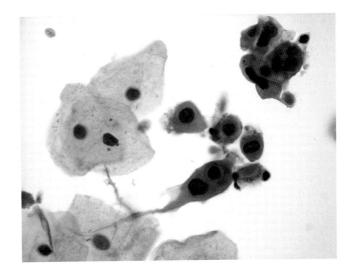

50. Which of the following statements regarding this finding in a cervicovaginal specimen is TRUE?

   a. It is frequently associated with inguinal adenopathy.

   b. It may be associated with *Chlamydia trachomatis* infection.

   c. A monotonous population of lymphoid cells favors a benign process.

   d. It is frequently associated with *Trichomonas vaginalis* infection.

   e. Endometrial sampling is warranted.

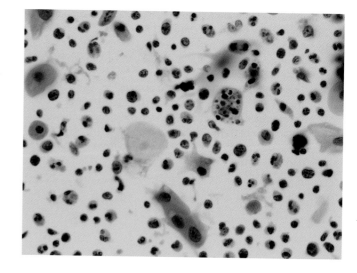

51. Which of the following statements regarding the cells in the photomicrograph is TRUE?

   a. Biopsy will reveal a high-grade lesion in 15% to 25% of patients with this finding.

   b. Cytoplasmic characteristics typically include marked keratinization and bizarre shapes.

   c. Prominent nucleoli are a common finding.

   d. Multinucleation, nuclear molding, and a ground-glass nuclear appearance are characteristic.

   e. These lesions infrequently regress.

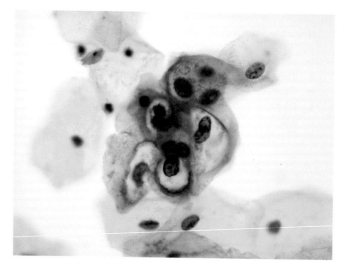

52. What is the BEST diagnosis for the cells in the photomicrograph?

   a. HSIL

   b. Degenerated endocervical cells

   c. Carcinoma, favor metastatic

   d. LSIL

   e. Benign histiocytes

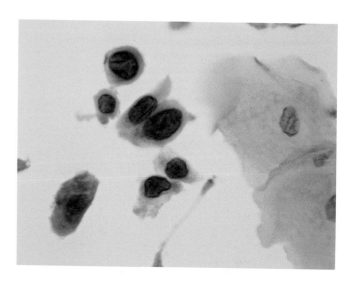

53. The photomicrograph represents a right-sided pleural effusion from a 53-year-old man with arthritis. Which of the following statements is TRUE?
    a. The spindle cells most likely represent keratinizing squamous cell carcinoma.
    b. Multinucleated giant cells and necrosis are suggestive of tuberculosis in an immunocompromised patient.
    c. The spindle cells are negative with an immunohistochemical stain for cytokeratin.
    d. The effusion most likely is bilateral.
    e. The pleural effusion is likely to be associated with ascites showing similar cytologic findings.

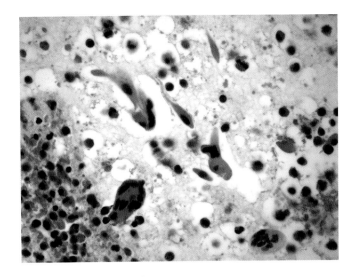

54. What is the MOST likely cause of the findings in this voided urine specimen from a 75-year-old man?
    a. Sarcoidosis
    b. Xanthogranulomatous pyelonephritis
    c. Fungal infection
    d. Bacillus Calmette-Guérin (BCG) treatment
    e. Multinucleated umbrella cells in normal urine

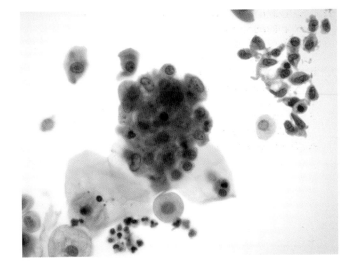

55. Which of the following statements regarding this urine sample obtained during cystoscopy of a 55-year-old man with renal calculi is TRUE?
    a. It would be highly unlikely that similar clusters would be seen in a voided sample from this patient prior to cystoscopy.
    b. Even if single malignant cells do not accompany the urothelial clusters, the cystoscopist can often detect the presence of urothelial carcinoma in situ by visual inspection of the urinary bladder mucosa.
    c. The presence of papillary clusters in a patient with renal calculi suggests a concurrent papillary urothelial neoplasm and warrants additional investigation of the upper urinary tract.
    d. The presence of papillary clusters may be due to instrumentation effect, a papillary urothelial neoplasm, or renal calculi in this patient.
    e. Renal calculi often yield single highly atypical cells and chronic inflammatory cells, but are not commonly associated with papillary clusters.

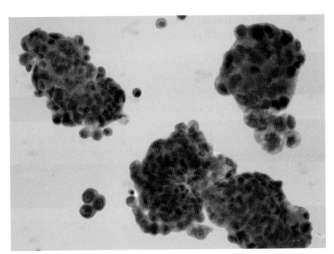

56. What is the significance of the cells present in this urine sample from a 67-year-old man with a history of urothelial carcinoma?
- **a.** The granular background suggests recurrent carcinoma that is invasive.
- **b.** The presence of abundant histiocytes is consistent with a history of radiation therapy.
- **c.** The lack of readily identifiable urothelial cells and the background of histiocytes and debris suggest the presence of prostatitis.
- **d.** They are degenerated epithelial cells.
- **e.** The presence of bacteria indicates an infection that should be cultured and treated.

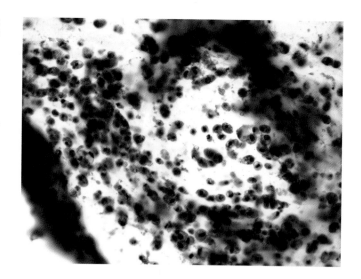

57. What is depicted in this photomicrograph of a liquid-based cervical Pap test from a 54-year-old woman?
- **a.** HSV
- **b.** Carpet beetle part
- **c.** *Alternaria* organisms
- **d.** Vegetable matter
- **e.** Arrowwood contaminant

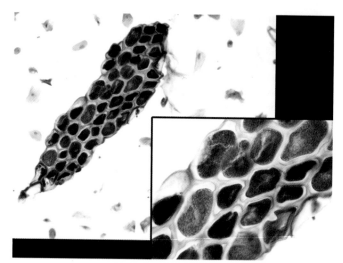

58. Which of the following statements regarding the cells in the photomicrograph in a pleural effusion fluid is MOST likely to be true?
- **a.** They are found with equal frequency in pleural, peritoneal, and pericardial effusion fluids.
- **b.** They usually are found in fluids that are transudates.
- **c.** The most likely cause is an underlying malignancy.
- **d.** Their presence likely indicates parasitic infection.
- **e.** In many cases, the cause of these cells in an effusion is idiopathic.

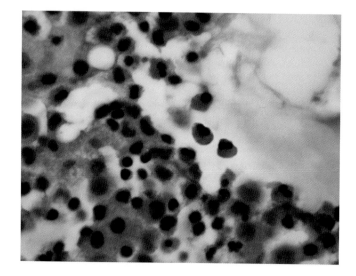

59. A 35-year-old woman did not have a menstrual period for 3 weeks. A home pregnancy test was positive. A cervical cytology test was taken in a local hospital, and the findings are shown in this picture. What is the next management step?
   a. A follow-up/repeat cervical cytologic test in 6 months
   b. Immediate colposcopy
   c. Immediate colposcopy with endocervical curettage to rule out glandular involvement
   d. Immediate loop electrosurgical excision procedure (LEEP)
   e. Nothing should be done now. A follow-up/repeat cervical cytology test should be performed immediately after term delivery.

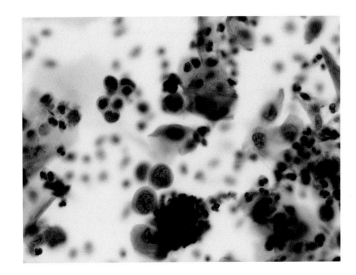

60. A 62-year-old woman with a history of sigmoid colon cancer that was treated a few years prior had the Pap test findings in the photomicrograph. What is the MOST likely diagnosis?
   a. ASC-US
   b. Reparative change; negative for intraepithelial lesion
   c. Cellular changes consistent with radiation effect; negative for intraepithelial lesion
   d. Atypical glandular cells (AGCs), suspicious for recurrent adenocarcinoma
   e. Cellular changes consistent with HSV infection

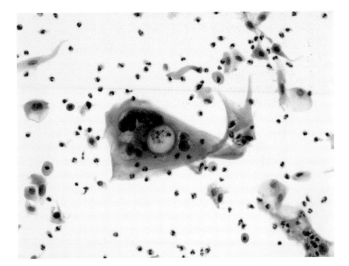

61. The picture depicted is a liquid-based cervical cytology sample taken from a 38-year-old woman whose last menstrual period was 27 days prior. According to the American Society for Colposcopy and Cervical Pathology (ASCCP), what is the recommended management for this woman?
   a. Repeat cytologic test and high-risk HPV testing in 6 months
   b. Colposcopy and a diagnostic excisional procedure
   c. Endometrial curettage
   d. Total hysterectomy
   e. Radiation therapy

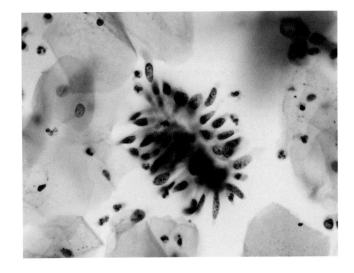

62. A 16-year-old girl underwent her first cervical Pap test. The findings are depicted in the figure. What is the appropriate management for her?
    a. Immediate colposcopy
    b. Reflex high-risk HPV DNA testing
    c. Repeat cervical cytologic testing at 12 months as follow-up
    d. Confirmatory cervical biopsy
    e. HPV vaccine administration, which is curative

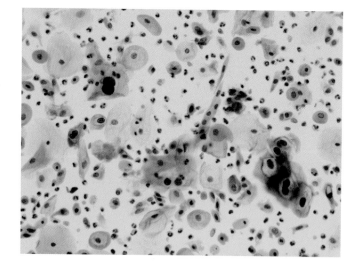

63. A 70-year-old woman underwent a cervical Pap test during a preoperative work-up for an ovarian mass. Which one of the statements about the findings in the photomicrograph is CORRECT?
    a. It shows HSIL.
    b. HPV DNA testing is likely to be positive.
    c. The findings are likely to be the result of estrogen replacement therapy in a postmenopausal woman.
    d. A Ki-67 immunostain performed on a corresponding cervical biopsy would likely show a high mitotic index.
    e. Topical estrogen application may be helpful to confirm the diagnosis.

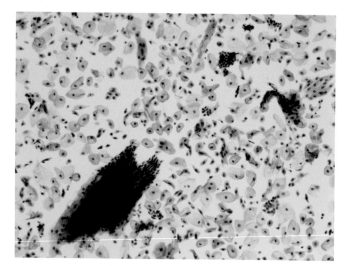

64. What is the MOST likely diagnosis for this Diff-Quik-stained CSF specimen from a 16-year-old patient with an abdominal mass?
    a. Burkitt lymphoma
    b. Anaplastic large cell lymphoma
    c. Precursor B- or T-cell lymphoblastic lymphoma
    d. Diffuse large B-cell lymphoma (DLBCL)
    e. Small lymphocytic lymphoma

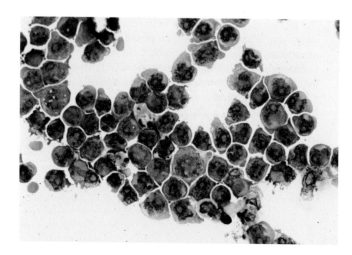

65. Which of the following is the BEST diagnosis for this ultrasound-guided FNA biopsy of a 3-cm partially cystic parotid mass in a 31-year-old man?
    a. Necrotizing sialometaplasia
    b. Salivary duct carcinoma
    c. Acinic cell carcinoma
    d. Polymorphous low-grade adenocarcinoma
    e. Mucoepidermoid carcinoma

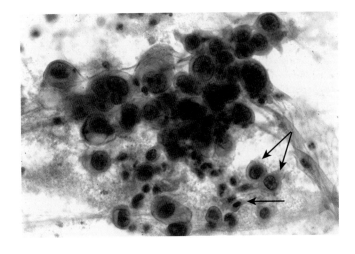

66. A percutaneous FNA of a peripherally located pleura-based lung lesion from a 60-year-old nonsmoking female patient is hypercellular and contains numerous monolayer sheets and cohesive cell balls along with some single epithelial cells. A few papillary structures are present. The cells are polygonal and fairly well spaced with uniform, regular, centrally located oval/round nuclei with finely granular chromatin. Nucleoli are conspicuous in some of the nuclei. Occasional binucleated cells are seen. The cells at the outer rims of the clusters appear "hobnailed." The background is clean. What is the MOST likely diagnosis?
    a. Reactive respiratory epithelial cells
    b. Mesothelial cells
    c. Well-differentiated adenocarcinoma with bronchioloalveolar features
    d. Carcinoid tumor
    e. Metastatic papillary thyroid carcinoma

67. Which of the following statements MOST accurately describes Schaumann bodies?
    a. Yellow-brown structures of unknown significance associated with histiocytes, and resembling fungi
    b. Eosinophilic inclusion bodies with radiating lines in the cytoplasm of multinucleated giant cells
    c. Birefringent calcium oxalate and calcium carbonate microcalcifications
    d. Calcium and protein inclusions inside multinucleated giant cells that may be found in several granulomatous conditions
    e. Concentrically laminated small calcifications most commonly seen in papillary neoplasms

68. "Koilocytes" in gynecologic Pap tests are found in association with which of following conditions?
    a. HPV infection
    b. *T. vaginalis* infection
    c. *Chlamydia* infection
    d. Pregnancy
    e. Estrogen replacement therapy

69. Which of the following cytologic features favors LSIL over HSIL?
    a. Smaller cells
    b. Higher nucleus-to-cytoplasm (N:C) ratios
    c. Greater irregularities of nuclear outlines
    d. Coarser chromatin and chromatin clumping
    e. Larger nuclear volume

70. In a cervicovaginal Pap test showing HSIL, which feature is MOST suggestive of microinvasion?
    a. Hyperchromatic crowded groups (HCGs)
    b. Naked nuclei
    c. Coarser chromatin
    d. Increased N:C ratios
    e. Nucleoli

71. The differential diagnosis of hyperchromatic crowded groups of small cells in gynecologic Pap tests includes which of the following entities?
    a. Atrophy
    b. HSIL
    c. Endometrial cells
    d. Adenocarcinoma
    e. All of the above

72. What is the MOST appropriate management for a 30-year-old woman with a recent gynecologic Pap test showing: "Atypical squamous cells, cannot exclude high-grade squamous intraepithelial lesion (ASC-H)"?
    a. High-risk HPV test
    b. Colposcopy
    c. Repeat Pap test in 4 to 6 months
    d. Immediate LEEP
    e. Repeat Pap smear after topical estrogen treatment

73. Which of the following statements regarding HPV is TRUE?
    a. It is a large, linear, double-stranded, nonenveloped DNA virus that replicates entirely in the cytoplasm of infected cells.
    b. Its coding regions contain early and late genes.
    c. E1 and E2 are encoding proteins that play a role in host cell transformation.
    d. HPV first infects the superficial layer of squamous epithelium, therefore causing the cytopathic change of "koilocytes."
    e. The locations of the viral genome integration sites in the host genome are consistent.

74. Which of the following statements regarding cytologic patterns in gynecologic Pap tests in pregnancy is TRUE?
    a. There is a shift in maturation toward a predominance of superficial squamous cells.
    b. Marked cytolysis may occur owing to *Leptothrix*.
    c. An atrophic pattern may be an indication of intrauterine fetal demise.

d. The presence of navicular cells is diagnostic for pregnancy.

e. An atrophic pattern occurs in the postpartum period in virtually all mothers.

75. According to the 2001 Bethesda System, which one of the following statements regarding adequacy of the squamous cell component in liquid-based cervical cytologic preparations is CORRECT?

a. An estimated minimum of 2000 well-visualized/well-preserved squamous cells is required for a specimen to be considered adequate.

b. An estimated minimum of 8000 well-visualized/well-preserved squamous cells is required for a specimen to be considered adequate.

c. An estimated minimum of 2500 well-visualized/well-preserved squamous cells is required for a specimen to be considered adequate.

d. An estimated minimum of 5000 well-visualized/well-preserved squamous cells is required for a specimen to be considered adequate.

e. An estimated minimum of 12,000 well-visualized/well-preserved squamous cells is required for a specimen to be considered adequate.

Answers

1. d. Smears from Warthin tumors contain oncocytic cells, lymphocytes, and cystic debris (granular background). They arise from ducts entrapped during embryologic development of lymph nodes and occur almost exclusively in the lower pole of the parotid gland, but sometimes arise in periparotid lymph nodes. Warthin tumors are multifocal or bilateral in approximately 10% of patients. Smokers have a higher risk of developing Warthin tumors. Surgical resection with preservation of facial nerve is the usual treatment.

Ballo MS, Shin HJ, Sneige N: Sources of diagnostic error in the fine-needle aspiration diagnosis of Warthin's tumor and clues to a correct diagnosis. *Diagn Cytopathol* 1997;17(3):230-234.

Klijanienko J, Vielh P: Fine-needle sampling of salivary gland lesions. II. Cytology and histology correlation of 71 cases of Warthin's tumor (adenolymphoma). *Diagn Cytopathol* 1997; 16(3):221-225.

2. b. The malignant cells in this well-differentiated hepatocellular carcinoma (HCC) resemble normal hepatocytes (Fig. 24-2B). A helpful diagnostic feature is the presence of clusters of liver cells surrounded by a layer of endothelial cells in HCC (Fig. 24-2A and D). Naked hepatocyte nuclei (Fig. 24-2C) may occur in benign conditions, but are more numerous in HCC. HCC lacks bile duct cells. Poorly differentiated tumors show marked nuclear pleomorphism, high N:C ratios, spindle cells, atypical mitoses, and tumor giant cells. Thickened plates of hepatocytes surrounded by sinusoidal vessels are best seen in cell block preparations and are highlighted by reticulin staining showing an abnormal, decreased, or absent reticulin framework. Binucleated cells and intranuclear pseudoinclusions may be seen in both HCC and benign hepatocytes. Although ascites frequently accompanies HCC, the presence of malignant cells in these effusions is rare. The presence of bile pigment in the cytoplasm of malignant cells is an important diagnostic characteristic of HCC.

Kuo FY, Chen WJ, Lu SN, et al: Fine needle aspiration cytodiagnosis of liver tumors. *Acta Cytol* 2004;48(2):142-148.

Wee A: Fine-needle aspiration biopsy of hepatocellular carcinoma and related hepatocellular nodular lesions in cirrhosis: controversies, challenges, and expectations. *Pathol Res Int* 2011;2011:587936. Epub 2011 Jun 30.

3. e. The photomicrographs depict pancreatic adenocarcinoma. Figure 24-3A shows a cluster of malignant epithelial cells with nuclei that are enlarged compared to the small cluster of benign epithelial cells in the upper left of the photo. Figure 24-3B displays a "drunken honeycomb" pattern of disorganization, with nuclear overlapping and variation in nuclear sizes (anisonucleosis). Figure 24-3C shows malignant cells with irregular nuclear contours, prominent nucleoli, and anisonucleosis. In Figure 24-3D there is a single large malignant epithelial cell (note size compared to red blood cells). Pancreatic pseudocyst is a complication of acute and chronic pancreatitis. Pseudocysts lack an epithelial lining. Patients with pancreatoblastoma and ACC may have elevated levels of AFP, but patients with pancreatic adenocarcinoma usually do not. The 5-year survival rate of patients with pancreatic adenocarcinoma is less than 10%. SPPT of the pancreas characteristically arises in the pancreas in young women. More than 90% of SPPTs behave in a benign fashion. *KRAS* mutations are present in 95% of pancreatic adenocarcinomas. Mutation of SMAD4 (DPC4) also is seen.

Bardales RH, Stelow EB, Mallery S, et al: Review of endoscopic ultrasound-guided fine-needle aspiration cytology. *Diagn Cytopathol* 2006;34(2):140-175.

Lin F, Staerkel G: Cytologic criteria for well differentiated adenocarcinoma of the pancreas in fine-needle aspiration biopsy specimens. *Cancer* 2003;99(1):44-50.

4. d. FNA of the thyroid is painful in subacute (de Quervain) thyroiditis. Smears usually are of low to moderate cellularity, with few reactive follicular cells (Fig. 24-4A); large, multinucleated giant cells (Fig. 24-4C and D) that may contain more than 100 nuclei; granulomas composed of loosely cohesive epithelioid histiocytes (Fig. 24-4B); and a mixed inflammatory infiltrate. Smears of nodular goiter show orderly sheets and macrofollicles composed of uniform, small follicular cells with dark (not pale) chromatin in a background of abundant colloid. Smears from PTC show crowded sheets of abnormal, enlarged follicular cells with fine, powdery chromatin; irregular nuclear contours; nuclear grooves; and pseudoinclusions. A microfollicular pattern may be indicative of the follicular variant of papillary carcinoma. Smears from follicular neoplasms typically are cellular, show a predominant microfollicular pattern, and contain small, crowded clusters of follicular cells with enlarged, overlapping nuclei. Riedel disease presents as a diffusely enlarged, painless, and very firm thyroid. The thyroid is fibrotic, hence aspirates are scanty and often nondiagnostic. Giant cells usually are not present. Reactive mesenchymal cells (myofibroblasts) with abundant cytoplasm and enlarged nuclei and a mixed inflammatory infiltrate (lymphocytes, neutrophils, histiocytes, and eosinophils) are commonly seen.

Harigopal M, Sahoo S, Recant WM, DeMay RM: Fine-needle aspiration of Riedel's disease: report of a case and review of the literature. *Diagn Cytopathol* 2004;30(3):193-197.

Shabb NS, Salti I: Subacute thyroiditis: fine-needle aspiration cytology of 14 cases presenting with thyroid nodules. *Diagn Cytopathol* 2006;34(1):18-23.

5. e.   All of the features listed are characteristic of papillary thyroid carcinoma (PTC); however, among these, intranuclear cytoplasmic invaginations (pseudoinclusions) are the most reliable diagnostic feature. They may be seen with Diff-Quik and Pap stains. Pseudoinclusions must have sharp borders and should occupy at least 50% of the nuclear area; they are visible in Figure 24-5B. The nuclei of papillary carcinoma cells generally are larger than those of nonneoplastic follicular cells, but the N:C ratio is not altered. Figure 24-5A shows a sheet of follicular cells with enlarged nuclei and nuclear grooves. Nuclear folds or grooves are a characteristic, but not specific, feature of PTC. Multinucleated histiocytes are a common finding in PTC, but they may be seen in other conditions, such as subacute thyroiditis, lymphocytic thyroiditis, and cystic nodular goiter. Complex papillary clusters (Fig. 24-5C) may be seen in classic PTC. However, in the follicular variant of papillary carcinoma, the most common subtype of PTC, the appearance is that of a follicular neoplasm with the nuclear features of papillary carcinoma; true well-formed papillae are not present.

Cibas ES, Ali SZ: The Bethesda system for reporting thyroid cytopathology. *Thyroid* 2009;19(11):1159-1165.

Nikiforov YE: Molecular analysis of thyroid tumors. *Mod Pathol* 2011;24(Suppl 2):S34-43.

6. a.   The photomicrographs show metastatic colonic adenocarcinoma with necrosis. In Figure 24-6A, there is a cluster of malignant cells with hyperchromatic nuclei in a background of "dirty" necrosis. Cytologic clues to the diagnosis include malignant cells displaying columnar shapes, a palisading picket fence arrangement (Fig. 24-6B), and necrosis. Mucin production, CDX2 positivity, and TTF-1 negativity support the diagnosis. Malignant cells in HCC may have some features of normal hepatocytes; however, poorly differentiated HCC may be difficult to distinguish from metastatic adenocarcinoma. TTF-1 demonstrates a granular cytoplasmic staining pattern in HCC. The cytomorphologic appearance of melanoma includes single large cells with abundant cytoplasm, round to oval nuclei, intranuclear pseudoinclusions, and prominent large nucleoli. Fine, granular melanin pigment may be seen. Melanoma cells stain with S100, HMB45, MART-1, melan-A, and tyrosinase. CDX2 positivity and TTF-1 negativity support a colonic primary over a pulmonary primary. A pattern of positive reactivity for CK7 and TTF-1 and lack of staining for CK20 would favor a bronchogenic origin. Smears from conventional (clear) RCC usually are bloody and demonstrate large groups of cells with abundant vacuolated cytoplasm. The cells usually are CK7, CK20, Hep Par 1, and TTF-1 negative, but are positive for PAX8, CD10, EMA, and RCC.

Granados R, Aramburu JA, Murillo N, et al: Fine-needle aspiration biopsy of liver masses: diagnostic value and reproducibility of cytological criteria. *Diagn Cytopathol* 2001;25(6):365-375.

Kuo FY, Chen WJ, Lu SN, et al: Fine needle aspiration cytodiagnosis of liver tumors. *Acta Cytol* 2004;48(2):142-148.

7. e.   This cellular aspirate from a pancreatic endocrine neoplasm (PEN) contains a monotonous population of neoplastic cells that are single and in loose sheets. Rosettes may be seen, and tumor cells may be anchored on branching capillaries. The neoplastic cells are round, oval, or polygonal, with uniform nuclei that may be eccentrically located, imparting a plasmacytoid appearance to the cells. Figure 24-7C shows characteristic "salt and pepper" chromatin (Pap stain), and metachromatic granules are evident with a Diff-Quik stain in Figure 24-7B. The majority of PENs do not secrete endocrine hormones, that is, they are nonfunctional tumors. "Functional" PENs secrete endocrine hormones, including (in descending order of frequency) insulin, gastrin, glucagon, vasoactive intestinal polypeptide, and somatostatin. PanIN lesions are precursors to ductal adenocarcinoma, not PEN, and they usually are too small to form discrete detectable masses by standard imaging techniques. They usually are seen in association with carcinoma. Most (95%) cases of PEN are solid rather than cystic, and cyst fluid analysis usually is not helpful in the evaluation of these neoplasms. Significant pleomorphism in occasional cells is not an indicator of malignancy in PEN. Mitoses, necrosis, and vascular invasion suggest malignancy; however, the best indicator of malignancy is distant metastases. The cell of origin of PEN is the islet cell. Acinar cell carcinoma is derived from acinar cells (Table 24-1).

Chang F, Chandra A, Culora G, et al: Cytologic diagnosis of pancreatic endocrine tumors by endoscopic ultrasound-guided fine-needle aspiration: a review. *Diagn Cytopathol* 2006;34(9):649-658.

Jhala NC, Jhala DN, Chhieng DC, et al: Endoscopic ultrasound-guided fine-needle aspiration. A cytopathologist's perspective. *Am J Clin Pathol* 2003;120(3):351-367.

Klimstra DS: Nonductal neoplasms of the pancreas. *Mod Pathol* 2007;20(Suppl 1):S94-112.

Stelow EB, Bardales RH, Shami VM, et al: Cytology of pancreatic acinar cell carcinoma. *Diagn Cytopathol* 2006;34(5):367-372.

8. e.   The cells depicted in the figure are so-called decoy cells resulting from human polyomavirus infection. Decoy cells are approximately twice the size of basal urothelial cells. They appear singly and have scant, degenerated cytoplasm; enlarged nuclei; and high N:C ratios. These features may result in a misdiagnosis of urothelial carcinoma, hence the term *decoy cell*. The most important feature differentiating these cells from malignant cells is the presence of homogeneous, smudged, and sometimes washed-out chromatin in the polyomavirus-infected cells (intranuclear viral inclusions). Urine from high-grade urothelial carcinoma usually is cellular and shows single and clustered large urothelial cells with obvious atypical features, including increased N:C ratios, coarse and hyperchromatic chromatin, irregular nuclear membranes, and sometimes prominent nucleoli. HPV-infected cells in the urine are similar in appearance to those of cervical origin. Both low-grade (koilocytes) and high-grade cells may be present in urine. Most HPV-infected cells in the urine of women originate from the cervix. CMV-affected cells are large and typically have a single, dark, basophilic nuclear inclusion surrounded by a halo, with multiple small, basophilic cytoplasmic inclusions. Herpes-infected cells are large and multinucleated with glassy chromatin, nuclear molding, eosinophilic inclusions, and peripheral condensation (margination) of chromatin. In some cases the cells have large, eosinophilic nuclear (Cowdry type A) inclusions.

Herawi M, Parwani AV, Chan T, et al: Polyoma virus-associated cellular changes in the urine and bladder biopsy samples: a cytohistologic correlation. *Am J Surg Pathol* 2006;30(3): 345-350.

Koss LG, Melamed MR: *Koss' Diagnostic Cytology and Its Histopathologic Bases*, 5th ed. Philadelphia: Lippincott Williams & Wilkins, 2006, pp 757-761.

Thiryayi SA, Rana DN: Urine cytopathology: challenges, pitfalls, and mimics. *Diagn Cytopathol* 2012;40(11):1019-1034.

9. a. *Cryptococcus* is the most common cause of fungal meningitis and can be detected in CSF specimens. The yeasts vary from 5 to 15 μm in diameter and have thick mucopolysaccharide capsules and refractile centers. They demonstrate a single, narrow, teardrop-shaped budding pattern (Fig. 24-9C) that helps to distinguish them from other budding yeasts. Yeasts of *Blastomyces* demonstrate single, broad-based budding; measure 8 to 15 μm; and have thick, refractile walls. Hyphae are not present. *Blastomyces* may cause a marked pneumonic process, including microabscess and granuloma formation. Phycomycosis (mucormycosis) appears as nonseptate branching hyphae displaying variable widths. They may cause hemorrhagic pulmonary infections. Definitive identification requires culture. *Coccidioides* is a dimorphic fungus that usually causes self-limited infection except in immunocompromised patients. Thick-walled fungal spherules measure 20 to 60 μm and contain endospores measuring 1 to 5 μm in size. Endospores do not bud, and hyphae usually are not present. *Aspergillus* forms fruiting heads in aerobic conditions. It is characterized by septate hyphae with 45-degree branching. Calcium oxalate crystals, when present, are a useful clue to the presence of *Aspergillus*.

Koo V, Lioe TF, Spence RA: Fine needle aspiration cytology (FNAC) in the diagnosis of granulomatous lymphadenitis. *Ulster Med J* 2006;75(1):59-64.

Srinivasan R, Gupta N, Shifa R, et al: Cryptococcal lymphadenitis diagnosed by fine needle aspiration cytology: a review of 15 cases. *Acta Cytol* 2010;54(1):1-4.

10. a. SPPT of the pancreas is a rare neoplasm of low malignant potential and often indolent behavior that occurs predominantly in adolescent girls and young women. It usually arises in the body or tail of the pancreas. Complete surgical excision generally is curative. Aspirates from SPPT usually are highly cellular and contain branching, delicate papillary fronds containing central fibrovascular stalks covered by one or more layers of neoplastic cells (Fig. 24-10A). The tumor cells are relatively monotonous and possess variable amounts of pale, poorly defined cytoplasm. In Figure 24-10C, bland, monotonous, small tumor cells are arranged in a pseudorosette. The nuclei commonly display grooves and have been described as being coffee bean–shaped. Hyaline globules (Fig. 24-10B) are present both intracellularly and extracellularly, often are surrounded by tumor cells, appear metachromatic with the Diff-Quik stain, and are PAS positive and diastase resistant. In some cases, the neoplastic cells may be difficult to distinguish from PEN and ACC. Aspirates from SPPT, PEN, and ACC have some overlapping cytologic features. Aspirates from all three entities usually are very cellular. The correct diagnosis in most cases rests upon the results of immunocytochemical staining. The cytoplasm of adenocarcinoma cells is vacuolated and often abundant. Sheets of adenocarcinoma cells have a "drunken honeycomb" appearance in which the nuclei are distributed unevenly within the sheets. Irregular nuclear contours are present in almost all cases, and at least some of the nuclei should appear enlarged. Single cells with malignant features are present in most cases, although there may be very few in well-differentiated carcinomas. IPMNs and MCNs are pancreatic tumors that yield thick, glistening, viscid mucus when aspirated. In contrast to "contaminant" mucin obtained from the gastrointestinal tract in endoscopic ultrasound-guided aspiration biopsy procedures, the mucus derived from these mucinous neoplasms is thicker and difficult to smear. Low-grade IPMNs frequently are lined by gastric or pancreatobiliary-type epithelium that may be indistinguishable from normal gastric epithelium or pancreatic ductal cells. In higher-grade lesions, nuclear abnormalities are more common and cells with goblet cell features may be noted (Table 24-1).

TABLE 24-1 Summary of Immunocytochemical Staining for Solid Pancreatic Tumors

	Pancreatic Adenocarcinoma	PEN	SPPT	ACC
Pan CK	+	+ (CAM5.2)	or +/-(focal)	+
Synaptophysin	–	+	or +/-(focal)	–
Chromogranin	–	+		–
Vimentin	–	May be +	+	
Trypsin	–	–	–	+
Lipase	–	–	–	+
NSE		+	+	
Progesterone receptor			+	
β-Catenin		May see membranous and cytoplasmic staining	+ (nuclear and cytoplasmic)	May see membranous staining
α₁-Antitrypsin	–	–	+	+
α₁-antichymotrypsin	–	–	+	+
CD10		–	+	
CD56		+	+	
Chymotrypsin	–	–	+	–
E-cadherin	+	+	–	

Note: Exceptions to these may occur, but these are the most common staining profiles.
ACC, acinar cell carcinoma; CK, cytokeratin; NSE, neuron specific enolase; PEN, pancreatic endocrine neoplasm; SPPT, solid pseudopapillary tumor.

Bardales RH, Centeno B, Mallery JS, et al: Endoscopic ultrasound-guided fine-needle aspiration cytology diagnosis of solid-pseudopapillary tumor of the pancreas: a rare neoplasm of elusive origin but characteristic cytomorphologic features. *Am J Clin Pathol* 2004;121(5):654-662.

Bardales RH, Stelow EB, Mallery S, et al: Review of endoscopic ultrasound-guided fine-needle aspiration cytology. *Diagn Cytopathol* 2006;34(2):140-175.

Stelow EB, Bardales RH, Shami VM, et al: Cytology of pancreatic acinar cell carcinoma. *Diagn Cytopathol* 2006;34(5):367-372.

11. c. The malignant cells in the photos have features consistent with melanoma. They display large nucleoli and cytoplasmic pigment, and one cell in Figure 24-11B contains a prominent intranuclear cytoplasmic inclusion. Immunocytochemical stains for HMB45, S100, tyrosinase, and MART-1 are helpful in confirming the diagnosis of malignant melanoma. The presence of hemosiderin-laden macrophages would be consistent with a previous hemorrhagic event; however, the cells in the photomicrographs are not benign. If the nature of the pigment in cells is in question, an iron stain may be helpful in documenting the presence of hemosiderin. Cells from vertebral bone marrow unintentionally may be obtained during a lumbar puncture. Megakaryocytes and nucleated red blood cells are clues to this occurrence. Care must be taken not to mistake megakaryocytes for malignant cells. The combination of Hep Par 1 and polyclonal CEA positivity is consistent with HCC, not melanoma. Brain metastases from HCC are rare; however, recent evidence suggests that, with the prolongation of survival of patients with advanced HCC, the incidence of brain metastases may have increased.

Koss L, Melamed MR: *Koss's Diagnostic Cytopathology*, 5th ed. Philadelphia: Lippincott Williams & Wilkins, 2006.

Walts AE: Cerebrospinal fluid cytology: selected issues. *Diagn Cytopathol* 1992;8(4):394-408.

12. e. The photomicrographs display characteristic cytologic features of papillary thyroid carcinoma (PTC). Figure 24-12A and B show flat sheets of round to oval follicular cells with pale powdery chromatin, nuclear grooves, intranuclear cytoplasmic invaginations (pseudoinclusions), and small nucleoli. Figure 24-12C shows a psammoma body. BRAF mutations are the most commonly detected abnormality in PTC, present in around 45% of adult cases. Ninety percent of these mutations show valine to glutamate point mutation BRAFT1799A (V600E). RET/PTC1 and PTC3 rearrangements on chromosome 10 (10q11.2) represent the second most common molecular abnormality seen in PTC, present in approximately 20% of cases. PAX8/PPAR gamma rearrangement, a translocation (2;3)(q13;p25), is the second most common mutation found in follicular carcinomas, present in approximately 30% of follicular carcinomas and approximately 5% of oncocytic (Hürthle cell) carcinomas. TRK rearrangement of the *NTRK 1* gene of chromosome 1q22 is found in less than 5% of PTCs. Point mutations in the *RAS* gene (HRAS, KRAS, and NRAS codon-specific nucleotide substitutions) are the most common somatic mutations found in follicular thyroid carcinoma.

Hassell LA, Gillies EM, Dunn ST: Cytologic and molecular diagnosis of thyroid cancers: is it time for routine reflex testing? *Cancer Cytopathol* 2012;120(1):7-17.

Ohori NP, Nikiforova MN, Schoedel KE, et al: Contribution of molecular testing to thyroid fine-needle aspiration cytology of "follicular lesion of undetermined significance/atypia of undetermined significance." *Cancer Cytopathol* 2010; 118(1):17-23.

Theoharis C, Roman S, Sosa JA: The molecular diagnosis and management of thyroid neoplasms. *Curr Opin Oncol* 2012; 24(1):35-41.

13. a. The depicted lesion is small cell carcinoma. The smears show clusters and single small blue cells with scant or no cytoplasm. The cells may be round, oval, or spindle-shaped. They tend to cluster together with close contact—"molding"—that is more prominent on smears than in cytospin or liquid-based cytologic preparations. The chromatin characteristically has a stippled "salt and pepper" appearance on the Pap stain (Fig. 24-13A). The typical size of small cell carcinoma cells is about the size of neutrophils; however, size alone should never be the sole diagnostic criterion. Better-preserved tumor cells may be larger, especially in FNA samples, and some nuclei may be as large as four times the size of lymphocytes. Cytoplasmic globules, also called paranuclear blue inclusions, may be seen. The fragility of the nuclei results in characteristic crush and streaking artifacts in smears (Fig. 24-13A and B). Crush artifact is commonly seen in both small cell carcinoma and lymphoid cells (benign and malignant); therefore, it can be used as supporting evidence for small cell carcinoma, but is not specific for it. Activating mutations in EGFR are found in pulmonary non–small cell carcinoma (usually adenocarcinoma), not in small cell carcinoma. Necrosis and apoptosis are common in small cell carcinoma. Hyperchromatic or pyknotic nuclei, representing the necrotic component of the tumor, are seen along with viable tumor cells with vesicular nuclei lacking nucleoli. The differential diagnosis of small cell carcinoma includes other small blue cell tumors, such as basaloid squamous cell carcinoma, pulmonary blastoma, adenoid cystic carcinoma, PNET, and lymphoma. Clinical data and immunocytochemical studies are very important. TTF-1 is positive in small cell carcinoma; however, CD45 (LCA) is positive in benign lymphocytes and many non-Hodgkin lymphomas, but is negative in the malignant cells of small cell carcinoma. Nucleoli are inconspicuous in small cell carcinoma.

Billah S, Stewart J, Staerkel G, et al: EGFR and KRAS mutations in lung carcinoma: molecular testing by using cytology specimens. *Cancer Cytopathol* 2011;119(2):111-117.

Siddiqui MT: Pulmonary neuroendocrine neoplasms: a review of clinicopathologic and cytologic features. *Diagn Cytopathol* 2010;38(8):607-617.

14. d. The photomicrographs show granulomas, that is, collections of epithelioid histiocytes with indistinct cell borders and elongated, spindle-shaped and carrot-shaped nuclei with pale chromatin and small nucleoli. Squamous cell carcinoma, seminoma, and thymoma are the most common metastatic tumors associated with granuloma formation in lymph nodes. Granulomas may also be found in lymph nodes harboring primary or secondary malignant diseases, including Hodgkin lymphoma and T-cell non-Hodgkin lymphoma. The other malignancies listed are not usually associated with granuloma formation.

Khurana KK, Stanley MW, Powers CN, Pitman MB: Aspiration cytology of malignant neoplasms associated with granulomas and granuloma-like features: diagnostic dilemmas. *Cancer* 1998;84:84-91.

15. e. The photomicrographs show smears from an FNA biopsy of a renal oncocytoma. The neoplastic cells are present singly and in small, loose clusters. They are relatively uniform cells with round nuclei and granular cytoplasm with distinct cellular borders. Occasional larger cells with hyperchromatic nuclei may be present. Nucleoli often are prominent. PRCC is divided morphologically into two types: 1 (low grade) and 2 (high grade). Smears from PRCC show clusters of cells with a papillary or tubular architecture demonstrating fibrovascular cores and foamy macrophages. Tumor cells in type 1 are uniform and small to medium in size, sometimes with nuclear grooves and intracytoplasmic hemosiderin. Psammoma bodies are seen in some cases. Tumor cells in type 2 are tall and large, with abundant eosinophilic cytoplasm and prominent nucleoli. Neoplastic cells with abundant clear cytoplasm, prominent nucleoli, and a rich vascular network would favor a diagnosis of clear (conventional) RCC. The neoplastic cells from chromophobe RCCs may appear granular, similar to oncocytoma cells; however, cells from chromophobe carcinoma also display characteristic prominent cell borders, wrinkled nuclei, occasional binucleation, and perinuclear halos (koilocytic appearance). Intranuclear inclusions may be present. Hale's colloidal iron staining is positive in chromophobe RCC but not in oncocytoma. Smears from adrenal neuroblastomas are cellular, showing numerous dyscohesive, small, oval, poorly differentiated malignant cells with scanty cytoplasm, hyperchromatic, granular nuclei, and small nucleoli (small, round blue cell tumor). Occasional Homer-Wright rosettes may be seen.

Strojan Fležar M, Gutnik H, Jeruc J, Kirbiš IS: Typing of renal tumors by morphological and immunocytochemical evaluation of fine needle aspirates. *Virchows Arch* 2011; 459(6):607-614.

Volpe A, Kachura JR, Geddie WR, et al: Techniques, safety and accuracy of sampling of renal tumors by fine needle aspiration and core biopsy. *J Urol* 2007;178(2):379-386.

16. a. Figure 24-16A is a Pap-stained slide of a BAL specimen demonstrating clustered cystic forms of *Pneumocystis* in foamy alveolar casts (pink in the photo) that have a honeycomb appearance. They also may be seen with the GMS stain (Fig 24-16B). With the GMS stain, some of the cysts may appear cup-shaped and may contain dotlike structures. Although *Pneumocystis* was previously believed to be a protozoan, DNA studies have revealed it to be a fungus. GMS stains the cyst walls, but not the trophozoites inside of the cysts. Although confirmatory stains such as GMS are commonly utilized, the diagnosis of *Pneumocystis* almost always can be made with Pap or Giemsa stains, due to its characteristic appearance in BAL specimens. In immunocompromised patients, *Pneumocystis* infection commonly elicits very little inflammatory reaction. The background in BAL specimens typically is clean. *Pneumocystis* cannot be cultured, and bronchoscopy with BAL is the gold standard procedure for diagnosis at this time.

Chabé M, Aliouat-Denis CM, Delhaes L, et al: Pneumocystis: from a doubtful unique entity to a group of highly diversified fungal species. *FEMS Yeast Res* 2011;11(1):2-17.

Nassar A, Zapata M, Little JV, Siddiqui MT: Utility of reflex Gomori methenamine silver staining for Pneumocystis jirovecii on bronchoalveolar lavage cytologic specimens: a review. *Diagn Cytopathol* 2006;34(11):719-723.

17. a. Cytologic features characteristic of Herpes simplex virus (HSV) infection occur in the acute phase, and include nuclear enlargement and multinucleation. Nuclei display a ground-glass, opaque appearance and nuclear membranes appear thickened, with margination of chromatin around the periphery of the nucleus. The nuclei appear molded against each other. (Note the three Ms: multinucleation, margination, molding.) Eosinophilic intranuclear (Cowdry type A) inclusions surrounded by clear zones are evident in Figure 24-17A. Primary genital herpes infection may be accompanied by systemic symptoms, such as fever and malaise, or may be asymptomatic. Multiple recurrences are common. Cytoplasmic inclusions are not a feature of HSV infection. Cells infected with CMV display eosinophilic intranuclear inclusions surrounded by halos that sometimes are accompanied by basophilic cytoplasmic inclusions. Cytoplasmic eosinophilia and narrow perinuclear halos in squamous cells are reactive features that are often, though not always, related to *Trichomonas* or *Candida* infection. Follicular cervicitis has been associated with *Chlamydia trachomatis* infection.

Koss L, Melamed MR: *Koss's Diagnostic Cytopathology*, 5th ed. Philadelphia: Lippincott Williams & Wilkins, 2006.

Solomon D, Nayar R: *The Bethesda System for Reporting Cervical Cytology*, 2nd ed. New York: Springer-Verlag, 2004.

18. e. An infundibular cyst also is referred to as an "epidermal inclusion cyst" (EIC) or keratinous cyst. Aspirate material contains both anucleated and nucleated squamous cells. This common benign skin cyst may be intradermal or subcutaneous and presents as a superficial swelling. It results from cystic dilatation of the hair follicle when the orifice is obstructed. The most common sites are the face, neck, scalp, and trunk. Infected or ruptured epidermal inclusion cysts typically have a "dirty" background containing degenerated cells and inflammatory debris, inflammatory cells, and multinucleated giant cells. Aspirates yield white, pasty, smelly material that is keratin, not sebum; hence, the term *sebaceous cyst* is a misnomer. Aspirates from branchial cleft cysts may reveal nucleated mature squamous cells, anucleated squames, and columnar cells in a background of inflammatory cells (lymphocytes and histiocytes), cholesterol clefts, and amorphous debris. Aspirates from squamous cell carcinoma usually show pleomorphic, keratinized cells with dark hyperchromatic nuclei in a necrotic background. Nonkeratinized malignant cells may also be present. Anucleated squames and keratinous debris also may be seen. The cytologic picture of a thyroglossal duct cyst may resemble that of a branchial cleft cyst. The aspirate may show columnar ciliated respiratory cells, mucous cells, mature squamous cells, follicular cells, histiocytes, lymphocytes, and some colloid. Not uncommonly, however, they may contain only histiocytes with no or very few epithelial cells. Branchial cleft cysts and thyroglossal duct cysts are recognized by their lateral and midline neck locations, respectively. Aspirates of pilomatricoma show degenerated cells (ghost cells, shadow cells) and keratinized clusters of squamous and basaloid cells with calcification and inflammation. This lesion is more common in children and adolescents.

Handa U, Chhabra S, Mohan H: Epidermal inclusion cyst: cytomorphological features and differential diagnosis. *Diagn Cytopathol* 2008;36(12):861-863.

Pérez-Guillermo M, García Solano J, Acosta Ortega J: Pilomatrixoma: a diagnostic pitfall in fine-needle aspiration biopsies. A review from a small county hospital. *Ann Diagn Pathol* 2005;9(3):182-183.

19. a. The malignant cells with abundant vacuolated or clear cytoplasm and prominent nucleoli in the photomicrographs are cytomorphologically consistent with clear cell RCC. The immunocytochemical staining pattern in Choice a (RCC positive, CD10 positive, CK7 negative, CD117 negative, AMACR negative, E-cadherin negative) is typical for conventional (clear cell) RCC.

In Choice b the immunocytochemical staining pattern (RCC negative, CD10 negative, CK7 positive [strong], CD117 positive, AMACR negative, E-cadherin positive) is most consistent with chromophobe RCC. Cells from chromophobe RCC display characteristic prominent cell borders and perinuclear halos.

In Choice c the immunocytochemical staining pattern (RCC positive, CD10 negative, CK7 positive, CD117 negative, AMACR positive, E-cadherin negative) is most consistent with papillary RCC. Smears from papillary RCC show clusters of cells with a papillary or tubular architecture demonstrating fibrovascular cores and foamy macrophages.

In Choice d the immunocytochemical staining pattern (RCC negative, CD10 negative, CK7 positive (weak), CD117 positive, AMACR negative, E-cadherin positive) is most consistent with renal oncocytoma. Oncocytomas are composed of relatively uniform cells with moderate to abundant granular cytoplasm and distinct cellular borders.

Finally, in Choice e the immunocytochemical staining pattern (RCC negative, CD10 negative, CK7 negative, CD117 negative, AMACR positive, E-cadherin negative) is suggestive of metastatic prostate adenocarcinoma. Smears from FNAs of metastatic prostatic adenocarcinoma typically are hypercellular, with numerous small to medium-sized cohesive cells in acini, solid groups, and cribriform microacinar arrangements as well as scattered single cells and stripped nuclei. The neoplastic cells may be relatively bland, with round to oval nuclei, and possess prominent nucleoli.

Hammerich AH, Ayala GE, Wheeler TM: Application of immunohistochemistry to the genitourinary system (prostate, urinary bladder, testis, and kidney). *Arch Pathol Lab Med* 2008;132:432-440.

Skinnider BF, Amin MB: An immunohistochemical approach to the differential diagnosis of renal tumors. *Semin Diagn Pathol* 2005;22(1):51-68.

Zhou M, Roma A, Magi-Galluzzi C: The usefulness of immunohistochemical markers in the differential diagnosis of renal neoplasms. *Clin Lab Med* 2005;25(2):247-257.

20. b. The typical aspirate from a germinoma grossly appears slimy and viscous. The Diff-Quik-stained smear shows large, round and polygonal, poorly cohesive cells with a moderate amount of pale delicate cytoplasm, and distinct cell membranes. The cells have relatively round nuclei and prominent nucleoli. Inflammatory cells, with a predominance of lymphocytes, are noted. The background has a characteristic lacy and foamy "tigroid" appearance on Diff-Quik-stained smears that corresponds to the viscous appearance of the aspirate. The granular background is likely composed of cytoplasmic remnants. Lymphocytes and lymphoglandular bodies usually are present, and granulomas and syncytiotrophoblast-like multinucleated giant cells may be observed. Immunostaining in germinomas includes cytoplasmic staining for placental alkaline phosphatase (PLAP) and membrane staining for c-kit in neoplastic cells. The cytoplasm is PAS positive due to its glycogen-rich nature. Aspirates from normal lymph nodes or non-Hodgkin lymphoma grossly appear as whitish or blood-tinged, thick, granular material. The microscopic presence of a "tigroid" background and epithelial cells rather than only lymphoglandular bodies favors a diagnosis of germinoma. If non-Hodgkin lymphoma is a diagnostic consideration, a portion of the sample should be sent for flow cytometry. Mature cystic teratoma of the mediastinum usually is seen in children and adolescents. Aspirates of a mature cystic teratoma usually are scanty and composed of cells representing multiple tissue elements, such as skin (mature squamous cells), skin appendages (sebaceous cells and hair), gastrointestinal epithelium, or pancreatic cells. Granulomas may also be noted. Adenocarcinoma usually is easy to distinguish from germinoma; however, the distinction may be difficult in cases of poorly differentiated adenocarcinoma. Immunocytochemical stains may be helpful. *Thymic carcinoma* is a term used for a number of malignant epithelial neoplasms that show unequivocal cytologic atypia. This diverse group includes squamous cell carcinoma, basaloid carcinoma, mucoepidermoid carcinoma, lymphoepitheliomalike carcinoma, sarcomatoid carcinoma, clear cell carcinoma, adenocarcinoma, and poorly differentiated/undifferentiated carcinomas.

Chhieng DC, Lin O, Moran CA, et al: Fine-needle aspiration biopsy of nonteratomatous germ cell tumors of the mediastinum. *Am J Clin Pathol* 2002;118:418-424.

Gupta R, Mathur SR, Arora VK, Sharma SG: Cytologic features of extragonadal germ cell tumors: a study of 88 cases with aspiration cytology. *Cancer* 2008;114(6):504-511.

Wakely PE Jr: Cytopathology-histopathology of the mediastinum: epithelial, lymphoproliferative, and germ cell neoplasms. *Ann Diagn Pathol* 2002;6(1):30-43. Review.

21. b. The lesion depicted is medullary thyroid carcinoma (MTC). The neoplastic cells are dispersed or, as in these photomicrographs, form loose clusters. They rarely form microfollicles or papillae. In the main photo, a Diff-Quik-stained smear, the neoplastic cells mostly appear oval. In the inset photo of a Pap-stained smear, the tumor cells have a spindly appearance. However, they also may have plasmacytoid, polygonal, oncocytic, or giant cell appearances; may demonstrate mild pleomorphism; and may be bi- or multinucleated. The nuclei often have a "salt and pepper" or "speckled" chromatin pattern on Pap-stained smears (inset photo). Small nucleoli may be seen, but are usually inconspicuous. Mitotic figures are present in 15% of cases. On Diff-Quik staining, red cytoplasmic granules, corresponding to neurosecretory granules containing calcitonin, may be seen. The neoplastic cells of medullary carcinoma appear positive with immunocytochemical staining for calcitonin and generally are also positive for CEA, chromogranin, synaptophysin, and TTF-1. MTC generally does not stain for thyroglobulin. Although amyloid may be present in the stroma of MTC, it is often absent in aspirated specimens. When present, extracellular amyloid is positive with Congo red and crystal violet stains. Glial fibrillary acidic protein (GFAP) is an intermediate filament protein found in glial cells, such as astrocytes and ependymal cells. In the peripheral nervous system, GFAP has been demonstrated in Schwann cells, enteric glial cells, and satellite cells of human sensory ganglia. In neoplastic tissues, this antibody is useful for the identification of astrocytomas and ependymomas.

Bhanot P, Yang J, Schnadig VJ, Logroño R: Role of FNA cytology and immunochemistry in the diagnosis and management of medullary thyroid carcinoma: report of six cases and review of the literature. *Diagn Cytopathol* 2007;35(5):285-292.

22. c.   The depicted findings are characteristic of Hashimoto thyroiditis. Smears typically show a combination of oncocytic (Hürthle) cells and lymphocytes, hence the alternate term *lymphocytic thyroiditis with oxyphilia*. Hürthle cells, shown in the main photomicrograph, are metaplastic, oncocytic epithelial cells with abundant, finely granular cytoplasm and enlarged, variably sized, typically round nuclei that may display prominent nucleoli. The second component in Hashimoto thyroiditis is a polymorphous lymphoplasmacytic infiltrate, often with germinal center formation. Lymphoid tangles, lymphohistiocytic aggregates (inset), tingible body macrophages (TBMs), and background lymphoglandular bodies may be the overwhelming findings on the smears. Multinucleated histiocytes also may be seen. The classic sonographic appearance of the thyroid in patients with Hashimoto thyroiditis is that of a diffusely heterogeneous gland that is hypoechoic relative to the normal thyroid. Thyroid function may be reduced, elevated, or normal; however, most patients progress to hypothyroidism, although the time course of this progression is variable. Hashimoto thyroiditis is an autoimmune disease. In more than 80% of patients, serologic tests are positive for antithyroid antibody or antimicrosomal antibody. Hashimoto thyroiditis is associated with an increased incidence of lymphoma, usually high-grade B-cell type, but not sarcoma. Granulomatous thyroiditis may have a viral cause. Squamous metaplasia is not a feature of Hashimoto thyroiditis.

Kumarasinghe MP, De Silva S: Pitfalls in cytological diagnosis of autoimmune thyroiditis. *Pathology* 1999;31(1):1-7.
Nikiforova MN, Caudill CM, Biddinger P, Nikiforov YE: Prevalence of RET/PTC rearrangements in Hashimoto's thyroiditis and papillary thyroid carcinomas. *Int J Surg Pathol* 2002;10(1):15-22.

23. a.   The photomicrograph contains a flat sheet of follicular cells in a honeycomb arrangement in a case of nodular goiter. The follicular cell nuclei are round and uniform and are evenly spaced. Abundant colloid displaying cracking artifact is present above. Material aspirated from a colloid nodule typically appears as a thin film of shiny fluid when smeared on slides. Follicular cells in nodular goiter vary in size within a nodule, but generally range from 7 to 10 μm in diameter (red blood cells measure ~7 μm in diameter). Small groups of spindle cells with fairly ample cytoplasm, indicative of cyst wall lining, and histiocytes may also be seen. Hürthle cell (oncocytic) metaplasia and lymphoplasmacytic infiltration, neither of which is seen in the photomicrograph, are typical of Hashimoto thyroiditis. Follicular carcinoma usually yields hypercellular smears composed of uniformly enlarged and overlapping follicular cells forming mainly microfollicles. Mitotic figures may also be present. The presence of abundant colloid reduces, but does not exclude, the likelihood of neoplasia. It may be impossible to differentiate follicular carcinoma from adenoma or adenomatous hyperplasia cytologically, without histologic confirmation. Thyroglossal duct cysts typically are midline neck lesions anterior to the trachea that move vertically upon swallowing. Aspiration of thyroglossal duct cysts produces clear mucoid fluid and the smears show predominantly proteinaceous material containing respiratory epithelial or squamous cells, cholesterol crystals, and a variable number of inflammatory cells. Rarely, colloid and thyroid follicular cells may be seen in thyroglossal duct cysts. Parathyroid cysts are usually large cysts and aspiration characteristically yields clear watery fluid that is grossly different from colloid. The fluid is usually paucicellular with a few nondescript epithelial cells that may resemble thyroid follicular cells and are not particularly diagnostic. Immunocytochemical staining for parathyroid hormone (PTH), lack of staining for thyroglobulin, and a PTH level performed on a portion of the fluid may be diagnostically useful.

Clark P, Faquin WC: *Thyroid Cytopathology (Essentials in Cytopathology)*, 2nd ed. New York: Springer, 2010.
Koss L, Melamed MR: *Koss's Diagnostic Cytopathology*, 5th ed. Philadelphia: Lippincott Williams & Wilkins, 2006.

24. d.   The photomicrograph shows a highly cellular specimen containing follicular cells arranged in a microfollicular pattern. This appearance combined with finding scanty or no colloid is suggestive of a follicular neoplasm. Rosettelike microfollicles may not appear as well formed as those in the photomicrograph. Clusters or small, tight aggregates of follicular cells may be seen. The follicular cell nuclei are enlarged and often are overlapping. Single naked nuclei (lacking cytoplasm) also are common. Inspissated colloid may be present within the clusters. Differentiating follicular adenoma from well-differentiated follicular carcinoma often is impossible based on cytomorphologic appearance alone. In well-differentiated follicular carcinoma, especially, only minimal cytologic atypia may be present. Surgical excision with histologic examination is necessary for reliable distinction between follicular adenoma and follicular carcinoma. Although a papillary architecture is absent in the follicular variant of PTC, the nuclear features of this neoplasm are present. Hürthle cell tumors are composed almost exclusively of a relatively monotonous population of oncocytic (Hürthle) cells present singly and in clusters. Differentiating follicular neoplasia from adenomatous hyperplasia (in nodular goiter) sometimes may be challenging. Large flat sheets of follicular cells, focal oncocytic (Hürthle cell) metaplasia, and abundant colloid favor the latter diagnosis. FNA biopsy of Hashimoto thyroiditis yields oncocytic (Hürthle) cells and a lymphoplasmacytic infiltrate.

DeMay RM: Follicular lesions of the thyroid. Whither follicular carcinoma? *Am J Clin Pathol* 2000;114(5):681-683.

Nikiforov YE: Molecular diagnostics of thyroid tumors. *Arch Pathol Lab Med* 2011;135(5):569-577.

25. d. The photomicrograph demonstrates a pleomorphic adenoma, also called benign mixed tumor (BMT). Aspirates of BMT contain a combination of stroma, sheets and clusters of epithelial cells, and spindle mesenchymal (myoepithelial) cells. The chondromyxoid stroma, often containing blood vessels, is critical in making the diagnosis. It appears gray-green with the Pap stain and red or magenta with the Diff-Quik stain (as in the figure). The stroma is believed to be produced by myoepithelial cells. "Hyaline cells" are modified myoepithelial cells that appear plasmacytoid, with dense, glassy cytoplasm. They tend to present singly and may also be embedded within the fibrillary chondromyxoid stroma, and their presence is quite characteristic of BMT. Tyrosine-rich crystals with radiating, flower-shaped or "daisy head" appearances stain orangeophilic on Pap stain and are not pathognomonic but, when present, support the diagnosis of BMT. They are detectable in less than 10% of BMTs. Other types of crystals have been reported. BMT has an excellent prognosis following complete surgical excision; however, incomplete removal may result in local recurrences that may be difficult to treat. In the parotid, 90% of these tumors arise as painless, slowly growing masses in the superficial lobe. BMT is the most common type of salivary gland tumor, especially in the parotid, and it constitutes 40% to 70% of minor salivary gland tumors (e.g., in the lip and palate). The most common type of malignant transformation ("carcinoma ex pleomorphic adenoma") is adenocarcinoma. Demonstration of infiltrative growth is required for the diagnosis of ex pleomorphic adenoma. The presence of malignant cytologic features, mitoses, and necrosis are not sufficient for the diagnosis.

Handa U, Dhingra N, Chopra R, Mohan H: Pleomorphic adenoma: cytologic variations and potential diagnostic pitfalls. *Diagn Cytopathol* 2009;37(1):11-15.

Klijanienko J, Vielh P: Fine-needle sampling of salivary gland lesions. I. Cytology and histology correlation of 412 cases of pleomorphic adenoma. *Diagn Cytopathol* 1996;14(3):195-200.

26. e. The classic cytologic appearance of adenoid cystic carcinoma is that of small, bland-looking epithelial cells surrounding acellular spherical globules of metachromatic hyaline material. In the photomicrograph, the balls of magenta hyaline basement membrane material are surrounded by clusters of epithelial cells. The central acellular cores are seen better with polychrome stains (e.g., Diff-Quik and Giemsa) than with the Pap stain. The epithelial cells have a basaloid appearance, with scanty cytoplasm. Adenoid cystic carcinoma typically presents as a slowly enlarging, painful mass due to frequent involvement of the facial nerve. Aspirates of pleomorphic adenoma (BMT) contain a combination of chondromyxoid stroma, sheets and clusters of epithelial cells, and mesenchymal cells. Acinic cell carcinoma is a slowly growing, low-grade malignant salivary gland tumor most often arising in the parotid. It is the most common malignant salivary gland

tumor in children. Aspirates are usually very cellular, yielding many sheets and clusters of tumor cells that are larger than normal acinic cells, varying markedly in size and shape. Nuclei are small and eccentric and the cytoplasm may be pale or granular, and many round, naked nuclei also commonly are present. Mucoepidermoid carcinoma is the most common malignant salivary gland tumor in adults. Low-grade tumors consist of sparsely cellular, thick, mucoid material containing a combination of intermediate cells with small nuclei and larger mucus-producing cells with clear cytoplasm. High-grade tumors usually yield specimens that are more cellular, containing malignant squamous cells, with a scant mucinous component. Squamous cells usually are not keratinized. Intermediate-grade tumors may contain squamous cells that appear deceptively benign, in addition to occasional mucus-producing and intermediate cells. Metastatic thyroid follicular carcinoma may display rosettelike microfollicles and would not have the acellular, spherical globules of metachromatic hyaline material shown in the photomicrograph.

Hunt JL: An update on molecular diagnostics of squamous and salivary gland tumors of the head and neck. *Arch Pathol Lab Med* 2011;135(5):602-609.

Klijanienko J, Vielh P: Fine-needle sampling of salivary gland lesions. III. Cytologic and histologic correlation of 75 cases of adenoid cystic carcinoma: review and experience at the Institut Curie with emphasis on cytologic pitfalls. *Diagn Cytopathol* 1997;17(1):36-41.

Saqi A, Mercado CL, Hamele-Bena D: Adenoid cystic carcinoma of the breast diagnosed by fine-needle aspiration. *Diagn Cytopathol* 2004;30(4):271-274.

27. e. The larger cells in the photomicrograph are benign mesothelial cells with dense cytoplasm and relatively uniform nuclei. Typically, the cytoplasm appears more dense centrally (endoplasm) and more pale toward the periphery (ectoplasm). Benign mesothelial cells may vary from small to large, and binucleated and multinucleated forms ("tête-à-tête arrangements") are common. The nuclei also may be variably sized, and high N:C ratios may be seen in benign cells. Nucleoli may be prominent, especially in reactive mesothelial cells. A characteristic finding is the presence of a space or "window" between adjacent mesothelial cells, due to long microvilli on their surfaces. Intercellular windows are evident in the photomicrograph and are an important clue to the identification of mesothelial cells. In fluids, mesothelial cells may appear in flat sheets, singly, or in clusters. The key feature in establishing a diagnosis of carcinoma in a fluid is identifying a separate population of cells that is distinct from the mesothelial cell population. In the photomicrograph, only mesothelial cells, lymphocytes, red blood cells, and a few histiocytes are present. Carcinoma cells usually appear distinctly different from the background population of mesothelial cells. In ovarian carcinoma, malignant features, such as pleomorphism, enlarged and abnormally shaped nuclei, large nucleoli, and irregular nuclear contours, likely would be present and would be helpful in establishing a malignant diagnosis. Benign hepatocytes very rarely may be seen in abdominal fluid specimens. These cells have well-defined borders, granular cytoplasm, and centrally placed round, smooth nuclei. The cytoplasm may contain pigment (e.g., lipofuscin). Intercellular windows are not a typical feature. Endometriosis may be suspected in a fluid if the characteristic triad of small endometrial cells, endometrial stromal cells, and hemosiderin-laden macrophages are seen; however, all three of these findings are uncommonly present, and the diagnosis is difficult to make based on fluid cytologic findings alone.

DeMay RM: *The Art and Science of Cytopathology*, 2nd ed. Chicago: American Society for Clinical Pathology, 2011.

Saleh HA, El-Fakharany M, Makki H, et al: Differentiating reactive mesothelial cells from metastatic adenocarcinoma in serous effusions: the utility of immunocytochemical panel in the differential diagnosis. *Diagn Cytopathol* 2009;37(5): 324-332.

Tong GX, Devaraj K, Hamele-Bena D, et al: Pax8: a marker for carcinoma of Müllerian origin in serous effusions. *Diagn Cytopathol* 2011;39(8):567-574.

Westfall DE, Fan X, Marchevsky AM: Evidence-based guidelines to optimize the selection of antibody panels in cytopathology: pleural effusions with malignant epithelioid cells. *Diagn Cytopathol* 2010;38(1):9-14.

28. c. Metastatic breast carcinoma has a few characteristic patterns in fluid cytology, one of which is depicted in this photomicrograph, which was taken at very low power. Each of the round structures represents a large so-called morule (also called "proliferation sphere") that also is referred to as a "cannonball" because of this low-power appearance. Cannonballs are large, tightly cohesive balls of relatively uniform, neoplastic epithelial cells; a high-power view of one of the cannonballs in the photomicrograph is shown in the inset. Very few single malignant epithelial cells may be present (notice the relatively very small single cells in the background in the figure). Although cannonballs are suggestive of breast origin, they also occasionally may be seen in carcinomas from other sites. Malignant fluids from metastatic colorectal carcinomas characteristically contain clusters of obviously malignant cells, and the presence of some cells demonstrating a palisading or columnar appearance provides a clue to the diagnosis. Small cell carcinoma cells appear as small malignant cells that may be round to spindle-shaped. Cytoplasm is scanty or absent and nuclear chromatin is coarse. Nucleoli may be more evident in fluids than in bronchial specimens. The malignant cells may be single or in small clusters, and nuclear molding is characteristic. Single file arrangements may also be present. Malignant lymphoma cells appear singly and nuclear membrane irregularities may be prominent. N:C ratios are often high, with scanty cytoplasm; however, large cell lymphoma cells may display more abundant cytoplasm. Massive karyorrhexis in a fluid displaying a single cell pattern of neoplastic cells is highly suggestive of lymphoma. On Diff-Quik staining, lymphoglandular bodies, which are small blue fragments of the cytoplasm of lymphoid cells, may be evident. Immunocytochemistry and flow cytometry may be helpful in establishing a specific diagnosis.

Mesothelioma often produces very large groups containing many neoplastic cells. In addition, single neoplastic cells are present and display a spectrum of cytologic atypia, with cells ranging from benign-appearing mesothelial cells to malignant cells, many of which retain mesothelial features (Table 24-2).

TABLE 24-2 Cytologic Patterns in Fluids

If you see ...	Consider these possibilities (among others) ...
Papillary clusters	Ovary, mesothelial hyperplasia, mesothelioma, colon, lung, pancreatobiliary
Psammoma bodies	Ovary, mesothelial hyperplasia, mesothelioma, thyroid, endosalpingiosis
Cannonballs	Breast, lung, ovary, gastrointestinal
Single cell pattern	Lymphoma/leukemia, small cell carcinoma, breast, stomach
Linear, single files	Breast (especially lobular), small cell carcinoma
Single large malignant cells	Squamous cell carcinoma of lung, melanoma, sarcoma
Signet ring	Lobular breast carcinoma, gastric carcinoma

DeMay RM: *The Art and Science of Cytopathology*, 2nd ed. Chicago: American Society for Clinical Pathology, 2011.

Pereira TC, Saad RS, Liu Y, Silverman JF: The diagnosis of malignancy in effusion cytology: a pattern recognition approach. *Adv Anat Pathol* 2006;13(4):174-184.

29. b. The photomicrographs demonstrate the diagnostic components of a fibroadenoma. The main photograph shows a flat, honeycomb sheet of benign ductal epithelial cells. The darker nuclei scattered within this sheet are myoepithelial cells. Scattered in the background are single, naked, bipolar/oval nuclei that are of myoepithelial or stromal origin. In the upper right and lower left corners of this photo, there are pale blue-gray stromal fragments. Stromal fragments often are easier to see with a Diff-Quik stain, where they appear magenta. The inset photo demonstrates a cohesive cluster of ductal epithelial cells in an antlerlike arrangement, another common finding in fibroadenomas. Single naked myoepithelial/stromal nuclei are present in the background. The three diagnostic components of a fibroadenoma include flat sheets of benign ductal epithelial cells; single, naked oval nuclei of myoepithelial or stromal origin; and stromal fragments. In contrast to fibroadenomas, which characteristically appear during the patient's 20s or early 30s and are the most common breast mass in adolescent girls, the usual age of presentation of phyllodes tumors is the 40s and 50s. Phyllodes tumors may present with a history of rapid enlargement. Although most phyllodes tumors behave in a benign fashion, these tumors may recur locally and may metastasize. Aspirates of phyllodes tumors typically contain the same triad of features as fibroadenomas, and the epithelial component is usually indistinguishable from fibroadenoma. The main differentiating diagnostic feature is the stromal component: large, highly cellular, stromal fragments; single, intact mesenchymal cells; stromal cell atypia; and mitotic activity in stromal cells are features that favor phyllodes tumor over fibroadenoma. The surgical treatment of phyllodes tumors differs from that of fibroadenomas; in the former, there is a risk of local recurrence, and complete excision is necessary. Papillary neoplasms, including benign papillomas and invasive and noninvasive papillary carcinomas, may clinically mimic fibroadenomas. A subareolar location and nipple discharge favor a papillary neoplasm. FNAs from papillary neoplasms may be similar to those of fibroadenomas; however, complex, branching, three-dimensional clusters containing fibrovascular cores are a feature of papillary neoplasms and not of fibroadenomas. The background may contain cyst fluid and macrophages. In addition, the stromal component is usually sparse or absent in papillary neoplasms. Tall, columnar, epithelial cells are characteristic of papillary neoplasms, but may be seen in fibroadenomas, as well. Distinguishing benign papilloma from papillary carcinoma on the basis of cytomorphologic appearance alone can be difficult if not impossible. Clinically, colloid carcinoma (also termed *mucinous carcinoma*) may mimic fibroadenoma, but colloid carcinoma usually occurs in older patients. Although a diagnosis of colloid carcinoma may be suggested based on FNA findings, histologic examination of the entire tumor is required for an accurate diagnosis of pure colloid carcinoma. This distinction is important, because a diagnosis of pure colloid carcinoma suggests a relatively good prognosis, but mixed colloid/ductal carcinoma has the same prognosis as usual ductal carcinoma. FNA of colloid carcinoma yields epithelial cells in balls, sheets, and singly, in a background of mucin. Branching capillaries may be present within the mucus. The neoplastic epithelial cells are relatively monomorphic and may appear quite bland. Occasionally, an aspirate of colloid carcinoma yields only mucus, with few or no tumor cells. Benign papillomas, fibroadenomas with myxoid degeneration, and mucocele-like lesions may also yield relatively bland epithelial cells in a mucinous background or mucus alone. Lactating adenomas usually are round and mobile, similar to fibroadenomas. Aspirates typically are cellular and are characterized by large, cohesive, intact lobular clusters; flat sheets of epithelial cells; dispersed round naked epithelial cell nuclei; and some naked, bipolar nuclei. The single epithelial cells and those in the clusters display prominent nucleoli. The epithelial cell cytoplasm is vacuolated and wispy due to milk secretions. Cytoplasmic debris and proteinaceous and fatty secretions result in a granular, "dirty" background.

Benoit JL, Kara R, McGregor SE, Duggan MA: Fibroadenoma of the breast: diagnostic pitfalls of fine-needle aspiration. *Diagn Cytopathol* 1992;8(6):643-647; discussion 647-648.
Simsir A, Cangiarella J: Challenging breast lesions: pitfalls and limitations of fine-needle aspiration and the role of core biopsy in specific lesions. *J Diagn Cytopathol* 2012;40(3):262-272.

30. a. The photomicrograph contains a sheet of apocrine metaplastic cells. Apocrine cells have abundant, finely granular cytoplasm and well-defined cell borders. The nuclei are round and some display a prominent nucleolus. The N:C ratios are low, and the nuclear borders are smooth. Note the slight variation in nuclear size. The presence of occasional larger nuclei is a common feature in apocrine cells and does not necessarily indicate true atypia or malignancy. Apocrine cells are a common finding in benign breast aspirates in conditions such as fibrocystic change. Foam cells are another common component of fibrocystic change. They have abundant, foamy, vacuolated cytoplasm (in contrast to apocrine cells) and round to oval nuclei. Cytoplasmic pigment or inclusions may be present. Nucleoli may be prominent, and cells may be binucleated or multinucleated. Paget cells are carcinoma cells involving nipple ducts. They usually are large cells with abnormal nuclei, prominent nucleoli, and abundant cytoplasm that may contain mucin. FNAs of lipomas may be virtually acellular, containing only

oily material, or mature adipocytes may be present singly or in fibrofatty tissue fragments. Adipocytes possess a single vacuole containing lipid that almost completely fills the cytoplasm, flattening the nucleus to the periphery. Branching capillaries may be present. Adipose tissue from a lipoma is indistinguishable from normal fat on FNA; therefore, it is important to be certain that the needle obtained material representative of the targeted mass. Aspirates of fat necrosis typically contain foamy macrophages in a dirty, granular background. Hemosiderin, a golden brown, refractile pigment indicating old bleeding, may be present within the cytoplasm of macrophages. Multinucleated macrophages and epithelioid histiocytes are common. Epithelial cells usually are scanty and may display atypia.

Sneige N: Fine-needle aspiration of the breast: a review of 1,995 cases with emphasis on diagnostic pitfalls. *Diagn Cytopathol* 1993;9(1):106-112.

31. b. In the photomicrograph, the presence of pleomorphic, single malignant epithelial cells with ample cytoplasm points to the diagnosis of ductal carcinoma. Malignant cells of classic lobular carcinoma typically do not have abundant cytoplasm and such a range of nuclear sizes. FNA of colloid carcinoma yields epithelial cells in balls, sheets, and singly in a background of mucin. Branching capillaries may be present within the mucus. The neoplastic epithelial cells are relatively monomorphic and may appear quite bland. Occasionally, an aspirate of colloid carcinoma yields only mucus with few or no tumor cells. The differential diagnosis in these cases includes mucocele-like lesions. Occasionally, myxoid fibroadenoma may enter the differential diagnosis as well. Aspirates of mammary medullary carcinoma contain pleomorphic, obviously malignant epithelial cells with irregular nuclear contours, coarse chromatin, and prominent nucleoli. The malignant cells are present singly and in syncytia-like aggregates in which the epithelial cells have indistinct cell borders. Lymphocytes and plasma cells also are present and, thus, lymphoglandular bodies may be seen. FNAs of tubular carcinoma contain cohesive clusters of cells; single epithelial cells are a less common feature than in usual ductal carcinoma. A characteristic feature is the presence of rigid, tubular structures that may appear angulated. The epithelial cells are relatively bland, and cytologic atypia may be minimal. Naked, bipolar nuclei are usually sparse or absent, but may be prominent in some cases. Stromal fragments are common. Colloid, medullary, and tubular carcinomas are subtypes of mammary carcinomas, the diagnoses of which cannot be reliably established on cytomorphologic findings alone. Aspirates of comedo-type carcinoma show large, pleomorphic, obviously malignant, epithelial cells in a background of necrosis. Microcalcifications may be evident. In the photomicrograph, proteinaceous material is present in the background, but true necrosis would have the appearance of thicker, more granular debris.

Khirwadkar N, Clark AH: Fine needle aspiration cytology of tubular carcinoma of the breast. *Acta Cytol* 2005;49(3):344-345.
Racz MM, Pommier RF, Troxell ML: Fine-needle aspiration cytology of medullary breast carcinoma: report of two cases and review of the literature with emphasis on differential diagnosis. *Diagn Cytopathol* 2007;35(6):313-318.

Ventura K, Cangiarella J, Lee I, et al: Aspiration biopsy of mammary lesions with abundant extracellular mucinous material. Review of 43 cases with surgical follow-up. *Am J Clin Pathol* 2003;120(2):194-202.

32. a. The photomicrograph shows relatively small single malignant epithelial cells with cytoplasm containing intracytoplasmic lumina with sharply defined borders—features that are typical of lobular-type breast carcinoma. The intracytoplasmic lumina frequently contain a mucin droplet (mucicarmine positive). The cells usually are present singly and in small, loose groups, and may be arranged in single file. The single malignant cells may appear deceptively bland. However, closer inspection reveals some cells with irregular nuclear contours. Aspirates of lobular carcinoma may be sparsely cellular; this feature, along with the relatively small size and bland appearance of the malignant cells, account for the fact that lobular carcinoma is the most common source of false-negative diagnoses in breast aspirates. Lymphoglandular bodies are fragments of cytoplasm derived from lymphoid cells. They may be seen in benign and malignant lymphoid proliferations. Lymphocytes are not associated with lobular carcinoma.

When prominent, the presence of intracytoplasmic lumina and single file arrangements are suggestive of lobular carcinoma; however, these features are not specific, and may also be seen in ductal carcinoma. Granular cell tumors are thought to be of neural origin, and they may arise in the breast. FNA of granular cell tumors yields cells containing PAS-positive cytoplasmic granules, abundant granular cytoplasm, and bland, regular, small nuclei that often display prominent nucleoli. The most common type of breast carcinoma in males is ductal carcinoma. Lobular carcinoma is rare in males.

Hwang S, Ioffe O, Lee I, et al: Cytologic diagnosis of invasive lobular carcinoma: factors associated with negative and equivocal diagnoses. *Diagn Cytopathol* 2004;31(2):87-93.

Rajesh L, Dey P, Joshi K: Fine needle aspiration cytology of lobular breast carcinoma. Comparison with other breast lesions. *Acta Cytol* 2003;47(2):177-182.

Rosen PP: *Rosen's Breast Pathology*, 3rd ed. Philadelphia: Lippincott Williams & Wilkins, 2009.

33. c. The photomicrographs show nucleated and anucleated squamous cells and proteinaceous debris, findings characteristic of a branchial cleft cyst. FNAs of branchial cleft cysts yield turbid material composed of proteinaceous material; histiocytes; and nucleated and anucleated squamous cells, which may be sparse or numerous. FNAs of inflamed branchial cleft cysts contain squamous cells that may display significant cytologic atypia in a background of inflammatory cells. The differential diagnosis in this setting includes metastatic squamous cell carcinoma, especially in older patients. These cysts usually arise in the lateral neck, anterior to the sternocleidomastoid muscle. They may be seen at any age, but more commonly are detected in young patients. Aspirates of parathyroid cysts characteristically yield thin, clear, watery fluid. Epithelial cells are typically sparse, relatively uniform, and bland, resembling thyroid follicular cells. Immunocytochemical staining for PTH and analysis of cyst fluid for PTH may be diagnostically helpful. Aspirates of cysts in nodular goiter typically reveal histiocytes and colloid and follicular epithelial cells. Aspirates of dermoid cysts and epidermoid (keratinous) cysts produce cheesy, keratinous material. Numerous squamous cells are present in a background of keratinous debris. Dermoid cysts usually arise in the *midline* of the neck or in the area of the mouth, eye, or nose. In contrast to epidermoid cysts, which contain only squamous epithelial cells, aspirates of dermoid cysts may contain elements from skin appendages, including sebaceous cells and hair. Aspirates from paragangliomas (carotid body tumor; glomus jugulare) may yield cells displaying a range of appearances, from relatively bland to markedly pleomorphic. The nuclear chromatin has a "salt and pepper" appearance. Intranuclear cytoplasmic invaginations and rosette arrangements may occur. Red cytoplasmic granules may be seen on Diff-Quik and Giemsa stains. On palpation, paragangliomas may be pulsating, and a bruit may be heard.

Firat P, Ersoz C, Uguz A, Onder S: Cystic lesions of the head and neck: cytohistological correlation in 63 cases. *Cytopathology* 2007;18(3):184-190.

Lieu D: Cytopathologist-performed ultrasound-guided fine-needle aspiration of parathyroid lesions. *Diagn Cytopathol* 2010;38(5):327-332.

34. b. These polygonal cells with well-defined cell borders; abundant, granular cytoplasm; low N:C ratios; and central nuclei are hepatocytes. Normal hepatocytes may appear in aspirates of abdominal organs if the needle inadvertently enters the liver. Hepatocytes may display binucleation and multinucleation, and cytoplasmic pigments, especially lipofuscin, may be evident. Mesothelial cells can show a wide cytomorphologic spectrum. In reactive conditions, mesothelial cells can be pleomorphic, showing irregular nuclear contours and nuclear hyperchromasia with prominent nucleoli. Mesothelial cells are often separated from each other by a narrow space or "window." Germinal center aspirates usually are cellular and show a heterogeneous population of single small lymphocytes (around 8 μm, with dense, coarse chromatin), centrocytes (intermediate-sized B cells that measure around 10 μm and have scant, weakly staining basophilic cytoplasm, fine chromatin, and irregularly shaped nuclei that may be cleaved), centroblasts (larger than centrocytes, with round, vesicular nuclei with several marginal nucleoli and scant basophilic cytoplasm that may be vacuolated), and immunoblasts (the largest of the lymphoid cells, measuring 20 to 30 μm, with round, often peripherally placed nuclei, fine chromatin, 1 to 2 strongly basophilic macronucleoli, and scant basophilic cytoplasm) in a background of "lymphoglandular bodies." Tingible body macrophages, capillaries, and aggregates of dendritic cells usually also are present. Smears from pheochromocytomas are highly cellular and bloody and contain pleomorphic cells present singly and in dyscohesive cell clusters with indistinct cell borders. The nuclei are irregular in contour. Large, bizarre nuclei may be seen with binucleated and multinucleated forms, prominent nucleoli, and intranuclear cytoplasmic pseudoinclusions. Aspirates from conventional (clear cell) RCC contain malignant cells with round, slightly irregular nuclei; abundant vacuolated or granular cytoplasm; and low N:C ratios. Small or large nucleoli may be seen, depending on the grade of the carcinoma.

Volpe A, Kachura JR, Geddie WR, et al: Techniques, safety and accuracy of sampling of renal tumors by fine needle aspiration and core biopsy. A review. *J Urol* 2007;178(2):379-386. Epub 2007 Jun 11.

35. c. Cells derived from small intestinal epithelium usually appear as flat sheets of cohesive, uniform cells in a honeycomb arrangement. Small intestinal epithelium may be recognized by the presence of goblet cells, as depicted in the photomicrograph. In contrast, cytomorphologic features of aspirates of pancreatic adenocarcinoma include increased cellularity; sheets of disorganized cells ("drunken" honeycomb) with overlapping, pleomorphic nuclei with irregular nuclear membranes; coarse and irregular chromatin; and increased N:C ratios. Three-dimensional clusters, single malignant cells, and mitotic figures may also be present. Gastric epithelium may be virtually indistinguishable from benign pancreatic ductal epithelium. Goblet cells usually are not seen. Smears from low-grade MCNs are grossly gelatinous and usually hypocellular and show flat, usually organized, sheets of bland mucinous epithelium in a background of abundant thick mucin. The cells are columnar, with mucin-filled cytoplasmic vacuoles and basally located nuclei. Differentiating benign gastric and intestinal mucosal epithelial cells from mucinous neoplasms can be difficult. One helpful feature is the presence of thicker and more abundant mucin in association with MCN. Benign intestinal epithelium may be very similar to benign pancreatic ductal epithelium; however, pancreatic ductal epithelium has no goblet cells.

Mitsuhashi T, Ghafari S, Chang CY, Gu M: Endoscopic ultrasound-guided fine needle aspiration of the pancreas: cytomorphological evaluation with emphasis on adequacy assessment, diagnostic criteria and contamination from the gastrointestinal tract. *Cytopathology* 2006;17(1):34-41.
Moparty B, Logroño R, Nealon WH, et al: The role of endoscopic ultrasound and endoscopic ultrasound-guided fine-needle aspiration in distinguishing pancreatic cystic lesions. *Diagn Cytopathol* 2007;35(1):18-25.

36. d. This photomicrograph shows typical reactive/reparative epithelial changes. Reactive/reparative features typically include flat, cohesive sheets of epithelial cells that may appear to be stretched, with nuclear streaming. Epithelial atypia may be mild or marked. Some nuclei may be enlarged, but N:C ratios usually are maintained. Nucleoli may be multiple and quite enlarged. Frequently, inflammatory cells are interspersed among epithelial cells and are present in the background. An important clue to the benign nature of these cells is cellular cohesion, fine chromatin, and lack of single, highly atypical epithelial cells. In the photo, the reactive changes are present in the context of gastritis and ulceration, and *Candida* organisms are present in the lower right. Herpesvirus may be evident in cytologic specimens of the oral cavity and esophagus. Typical findings include multinucleated cells with molded, ground-glass nuclei. Eosinophilic intranuclear inclusions may also be observed. Cytologic findings in granulomatous gastritis (including Crohn disease, tuberculosis, sarcoid and fungal infection) may include epithelioid histiocytes and multinucleated giant cells. Intestinal metaplasia appears in brushings as sheets of orderly glandular cells containing scattered goblet

cells with secretory vacuoles. Goblet cells may also appear singly. Single and clustered epithelial cells displaying obvious malignant features, high N:C ratios, irregular nuclear membranes, and hyperchromasia are necessary for a diagnosis of gastric adenocarcinoma.

Geramizadeh B, Shafiee A, Saberfirruzi M, et al: Brush cytology of gastric malignancies. *Acta Cytol* 2002;46(4):693-696.
Vidyavathi K, Harendrakumar ML, Lakshmana Kumar YC: Correlation of endoscopic brush cytology with biopsy in diagnosis of upper gastrointestinal neoplasms. *Indian J Pathol Microbiol* 2008;51(4):489-492.

37. b. Small malignant cells with signet ring configurations, such as those in the photomicrograph, are suggestive of adenocarcinoma. PAS-D and mucicarmine positivity support this diagnosis. LCA stains lymphocytes in malignant lymphoma, viral meningitis, and other conditions. Malignant lymphoma cells and activated lymphocytes in CSF are almost always present singly, without clustering. This is also true in other fluids. Nuclei often have irregular nuclear contours. In large cell types of lymphoma, nucleoli often are quite large, irregularly shaped, and multiple, and the cytoplasm is usually scanty. Lymphomas composed of smaller cells may be more difficult to recognize. Massive karyorrhexis suggests a diagnosis of lymphoma. Large cell lymphomas may be difficult to distinguish from metastatic carcinoma. Immunocytochemical stains, including LCA and cytokeratin, may be helpful. Cells from primary CNS tumors are infrequently present in CSF specimens derived from lumbar punctures, and usually represent spread of a known tumor. Malignant cells from CNS tumors frequently appear relatively monotonous, with hyperchromatic nuclei, scanty cytoplasm, and prominent nucleoli. Mollaret meningitis is a rare form of recurrent aseptic meningitis in which the CSF contains large, monocytoid cells with abundant cytoplasm and characteristic footprint-shaped nuclei. Neutrophils, monocytes, plasma cells, and lymphocytes also occur. This diagnosis should be considered following exclusion of other forms of inflammatory meningitis. Acute bacterial meningitis is characterized by neutrophils, and a polymorphous population of activated lymphocytes is present in viral meningitis.

Chan TY, Parwani AV, Levi AW, Ali SZ: Mollaret's meningitis: cytopathologic analysis of fourteen cases. *Diagn Cytopathol* 2003;28(5):227-231.
Chhieng DC, Elgert P, Cohen JM, et al: Cytology of primary central nervous system neoplasms in cerebrospinal fluid specimens. *Diagn Cytopathol* 2002;26(4):209-212.
Enting RH: Leptomeningeal neoplasia: epidemiology, clinical presentation, CSF analysis and diagnostic imaging. A review. *Cancer Treat Res* 2005;125:17-30.

38. a. Urine from high-grade urothelial carcinoma usually is cellular, and shows single and clustered large urothelial cells with increased N:C ratios, large nucleoli, and hyperchromatic and coarse chromatin, in a background of degenerated cells and tumor diathesis. Urine from low-grade urothelial carcinoma usually is cellular and shows clusters of mildly atypical, crowded urothelial cells with increased N:C ratios, homogeneous cytoplasm, slightly irregular nuclear membranes, granular chromatin, and inconspicuous nucleoli. The presence of true papillary fragments with fibrovascular cores is highly suggestive of papillary urothelial carcinoma. In small cell carcinoma of the urinary bladder, urine contains numerous small cells (twice the size of lymphocytes) with occasional larger cells, displaying hyperchromatic and finely granular nuclei, nuclear molding, scant cytoplasm, and inconspicuous nucleoli, in a necrotic background. Mitoses and pyknotic bodies are abundant. Primary lymphoma of the urinary bladder is rare. The urine contains abundant single neoplastic lymphoid cells. Most lymphoma types have been described in the urinary bladder, but diffuse large B-cell lymphoma is the most common type. In the urine, most adenocarcinomas appear as small clusters and single epithelial cells with enlarged, eccentric nuclei, hyperchromatic chromatin, prominent nucleoli, and a moderate amount of amphophilic, finely vacuolated cytoplasm. Glandular differentiation of urothelial carcinoma can occur.

El-Fakharany M, Mazzara P: Cytologic features of urothelial carcinoma in catheterized urine with cellular fragments. *Acta Cytol* 2006;50(3):312-316.

Thiryayi SA, Rana DN: Urine cytopathology: challenges, pitfalls, and mimics. *Diagn Cytopathol* 2012;40(11):1019-1034.

39. b. Tingible body macrophages (TBMs) are large, specialized histiocytes containing engulfed cellular debris in their abundant cytoplasm. They have round nuclei with smooth nuclear membranes and small nucleoli and usually reside in reactive germinal centers. TBMs are seen most commonly in reactive lymphoid hyperplasia, but they are not specific, and may be present in high-grade lymphomas, Hodgkin lymphoma, and lymph nodes containing metastatic carcinoma. High numbers of TBMs in lymph node aspirates indicate rapid cellular turnover, proliferation, and apoptosis. Smears from high-grade lymphomas such as anaplastic large cell lymphoma, diffuse large B-cell lymphoma, and acute lymphoblastic leukemia usually have many TBMs; however, TBMs are not usually present in low-grade lymphomas. TBMs are positive for CD68, but are negative for CD1a. Langerhans cells are positive for CD1a. The cytologic hallmark of Hodgkin lymphoma is the Reed-Sternberg cell, which is a large, mononuclear or multinucleated cell with irregular nuclei and huge, inclusion-like nucleoli. Reed-Sternberg cells do not have engulfed debris in their cytoplasm.

Nasuti JF, Yu G, Boudousquie A, Gupta P: Diagnostic value of lymph node fine needle aspiration cytology: an institutional experience of 387 cases observed over a 5-year period. *Cytopathology* 2000;11(1):18-31.

Stani J: Cytologic diagnosis of reactive lymphadenopathy in fine needle aspiration biopsy specimens. *Acta Cytol* 1987; 31(1):8-13.

40. d. The cells depicted are examples of classic Hodgkin cells characteristic of classic Hodgkin lymphoma. These cells are large, and, in the photomicrograph, one is mononucleated and the other is binucleated. Both cells display prominent, inclusion-like nucleoli. The binucleated cell, also called a Reed-Sternberg cell, has a "mirror image" or "owl's eye" appearance. The background shows mixed inflammatory cells, including neutrophils, small lymphocytes, and eosinophils. The immunohistochemical staining pattern

(LCA negative, CD15 positive, CD30 positive, EMA negative) is diagnostic of classic Hodgkin cells (classic Reed-Sternberg cells). LCA positive, CD15 negative, CD30 negative, EMA positive is the immunophenotypic pattern of lymphocytic and histiocytic cells (L&H cells). They are diagnostic of nodular lymphocyte predominant Hodgkin lymphoma. The immunophenotypic pattern (LCA positive, CD15 positive, CD30 positive, EMA positive) may be seen in a minority of cases of peripheral T-cell lymphoma. The immunophenotypic pattern (LCA positive, CD15 negative, CD30 positive, EMA positive) is consistent with anaplastic large cell lymphoma (Ki-1 lymphoma). The immunophenotypic pattern (LCA negative, CD15 positive, CD30 positive, EMA positive) is not typical but can be seen in a minority of cases of classic Hodgkin lymphoma.

Das DK, Francis IM, Sharma PN, et al: Hodgkin's lymphoma: diagnostic difficulties in fine-needle aspiration cytology. *Diagn Cytopathol* 2009;37(8):564-573.

Dey P, Amir T, Al Jassar A, et al: Combined applications of fine needle aspiration cytology and flow cytometric immunophenotyping for diagnosis and classification of non Hodgkin lymphoma. *CytoJournal* 2006;3:24.

Zhang JR, Raza AS, Greaves TS, Cobb CJ: Fine-needle aspiration diagnosis of Hodgkin lymphoma using current WHO classification—re-evaluation of cases from 1999-2004 with new proposals. *Diagn Cytopathol* 2006;34(6):397-402.

41. d. This photomicrograph shows a case of ES/PNET that is highly cellular, with small, relatively uniform, dispersed malignant cells with scant to moderate pale cytoplasm; some have fine cytoplasmic vacuoles. The nuclei are oval or round, with finely granular chromatin. Occasional nucleoli are present. A few apoptotic cells and crush artifact also are present. The cells may also form small clusters with occasional pseudorosette or rosette formations. Two populations of cells, darker and lighter, may be noted. CD99 is diffusely positive in almost all cases. Mitotic activity is usually brisk and necrosis is common. More than 95% of ES/PNETs show t(11;22), which results in the fusion of the *EWS* gene with *FLI* or *ERG* genes.

Synovial sarcomas may be monophasic or biphasic, with epithelial and sarcomatous components. Smears usually are highly cellular. The mesenchymal component usually is composed of small spindle cells with scanty cytoplasm. Occasionally, a glandular component may be identified. Monophasic types may yield round cells causing diagnostic difficulty with ES/PNET. Immunocytochemical stains for cytokeratin are positive in the epithelial component and sometimes in the spindle cell component; however, ES/PNET cells may also be positive for low-molecular-weight cytokeratin. A significant proportion of cases of synovial sarcoma are positive for CD99 (O13, MIC2). More than 90% of cases show t(x;18). Small cell extraskeletal osteogenic sarcoma usually occurs in young adults and is composed of small cells that are cytomorphologically difficult to distinguish from ES/PNET. The presence of osteoid is a key distinguishing feature. The tumor cells may be positive for CD99; however, the t(11;22) translocation of ES/PNET is not present. Alveolar soft part sarcoma most commonly involves the thighs of young women. Smears are usually bloody and very cellular. The cytologic appearance is different from ES/PNET: the neoplastic cells are large and fairly uniform. They are mostly single, but may form loose aggregates. The nuclei are large, with single macronucleoli. Occasional intranuclear cytoplasmic inclusions may be seen. Cytoplasm is ample, finely granular, and PAS/PAS-D positive. The cytoplasmic granules correspond to rhomboid crystals evident on electron microscopy. Alveolar rhabdomyosarcoma is another round cell tumor involving the extremities of young patients. FNA smears typically are highly cellular, containing predominantly round cells with large, irregular nuclei, very prominent nucleoli, and coarse chromatin. Cytoplasm may be scanty. Myogenic differentiation is evidenced by positive staining for myogenin, myo-D1, desmin, and other muscle markers. A majority of cases show t(2;13) or t(1;13).

Pohar-Marinsek Z: Difficulties in diagnosing small round cell tumours of childhood from fine needle aspiration cytology samples. *Cytopathology* 2008;19(2):67-79.

Rajwanshi A, Srinivas R, Upasana G: Malignant small round cell tumors. *J Cytol* 2009;26(1):1-10.

42. a. These larvae are morphologically consistent with *Strongyloides stercoralis*. They are large, round, thick, coiled, rhabditiform worms with short buccal cavities. The larvae measure 400 to 500 μm and have pointed, slightly notched tails and closed gullets. Ascariasis is caused by the roundworm *Ascaris lumbricoides*. They affect the gastrointestinal tract, but their life cycle includes migration through the lung. They are yellow-brown and are characterized by their large size, reaching up to 35 cm in length and measuring around 50 μm in diameter. The eggs can be seen in fecal examination. Trichuriasis is caused by the nematode *Trichuris trichiura* (whipworm). These worms are smaller than *Ascaris*, measuring 35 to 45 mm. Each worm has a scolex and four suckers. They may be seen as contaminants from feces/perianal skin in vaginal smears/preparations. *T. trichiura* eggs are brown and barrel-shaped, with polar prominences. Echinococcosis (hydatid disease) is caused by the tapeworm *Echinococcus granulosus*. It has three segments and four suckers and forms cysts in the liver. FNA cytologic findings may reveal scolices and hooklets. *Enterobius vermicularis* (pinworm) is a nematode that also may be seen as contaminants from feces/perianal skin in vaginal smears/preparations. *E. vermicularis* can be indentified by its ovoid eggs with double-walled shells that appear flattened on one side. The eggs measure 30 to 60 μm. Rarely, larvae may be seen.

Avant CC, Hitchcock T, Colello CJ, Hoda RS: Strongyloides stercoralis in a bronchoalveolar lavage processed as ThinPrep. *Diagn Cytopathol* 2007;35(8):503-504.

Kuzucu A: Parasitic diseases of the respiratory tract. *Curr Opin Pulm Med* 2006;12(3):212-221.

43. a. Wilms tumor, also known as nephroblastoma, is the most common malignant renal tumor in pediatric patients. Classic Wilms tumor is a triphasic neoplasm with variable amounts of blastema, epithelial, and stromal components. The photomicrograph shows the blastema component of a Wilms tumor, characterized by small blue cells with fine chromatin, inconspicuous nucleoli, and very scanty cytoplasm. The blastema cells may form rosettes, as depicted in the photomicrograph, which may suggest an erroneous diagnosis of neuroblastoma. Although epithelial and stromal components are useful clues to the diagnosis of Wilms tumor, they are not always evident in FNA material. Epithelial cells are larger and have more abundant cytoplasm than blastema cells. They can form nests, glands, tubules, and glomeruloid bodies. Neuroblastoma frequently occurs in the adrenal medulla or retroperitoneal space adjacent to the kidney and is composed of monotonous small blue cells. Rosettes are a characteristic feature but, as depicted in the photomicrograph, may also be present in Wilms tumors. Tubule formation, present in some cases of Wilms tumors, is not a feature of neuroblastoma. In contrast to Wilms tumors, neuroblastomas demonstrate neuronal differentiation that may be evident in the form of tangled fibrillar material (neuropil) or axonal processes. The stromal and epithelial elements of Wilms tumors are not present in neuroblastomas. Lymphoma in children usually is large B-cell or blastic type. Smears show relatively uniform single cells. Lymphoglandular bodies are a helpful cytologic feature. Positive staining for LCA (CD45) helps to confirm the diagnosis. Ewing sarcoma consists of small groups or sheets of uniform, small, round, undifferentiated cells. Rosettes may be seen in some cases. An important differentiating cytologic feature is the presence of glycogen-containing cytoplasmic vacuoles. Mesoblastic nephroma is the most common benign renal tumor in newborns and infants. FNA material is generally paucicellular, containing mildly atypical spindle cells. The blastema, epithelial, and tubular elements characteristic of Wilms tumor are not present.

Fernández-Pineda I, Cabello R, García-Cantón JA, et al: Fine-needle aspiration cytopathology in the diagnosis of Wilms tumor. *Clin Transl Oncol* 2011;13(11):809-811.

Ravindra S, Kini U: Cytomorphology and morphometry of small round-cell tumors in the region of the kidney. *Diagn Cytopathol* 2005;32(4):211-216.

44. b. The photomicrograph depicts endocervical adenocarcinoma in situ (AIS). It shows neoplastic endocervical cells in cohesive, three-dimensional crowded clusters. The nuclear chromatin is hyperchromatic and coarsely granular in comparison to normal or reactive endocervical cells. The cells and nuclei are stratified, and palisading at the edges of the cellular clusters creates an appearance referred to as "feathering." There is an association between HPV infection and glandular neoplasia. HPV-18 is more commonly encountered in cervical glandular cancers than HPV-16. HPV type 16 is more frequently observed in high-grade squamous dysplasia and invasive squamous cell carcinoma than HPV type 18. Types 6 and 11 usually cause genital warts/condylomata or LSIL, many of which regress. HSV type 2 is the cause of genital herpes. HSV can induce chromosomal alterations, and evidence of concomitant infection of HSV2 and HPV in cervical cells has been observed; however, there is no definitive evidence of its direct association with cervicovaginal intraepithelial lesions. HIV 2 is less pathogenic than HIV 1. HIV infection can increase the risk of HPV infection, presumably due to its ability to compromise the immune system (Table 24-3).

TABLE 24-3 Features of Glandular Cells in Gyn Pap Tests

Endocervical cells	Reactive changes	AIS	Invasive adenocarcinoma
Cellularity	Low to moderate	Moderate	High
Clustering	++	++	+
Rosettes	–	++	+
Single cells	Few	Few	Frequent
Feathering	–	++	+/–
Nuclei	Enlarged, round, well spaced, and pale	Elongated, overlapping, and	Enlarged and overlapping
	Fine chromatin	hyperchromatic	Coarse chromatin
Nucleoli	Prominent	Inconspicuous	Enlarged and prominent
Nuclear membrane	Regular and smooth	Regular and smooth	Irregular
Nuclear variability	++	+/–	+++
N:C ratio	Normal	Slightly increased	Markedly increased
Mitosis	+/–	+	++
Inflammation	++	+/–	+/–
Normal endocervical cells	+++	+	+/–
Tumor diathesis	–	–	+

AIS, adenocarcinoma in situ; N:C ratio, nucleus-to-cytoplasm ratio.

Gray W, McKee GT: *Diagnostic Cytopathology*, 2nd ed. London: Churchill Livingstone, 2003.

Koss L, Melamed MR: *Koss's Diagnostic Cytopathology*, 5th ed. Philadelphia: Lippincott Williams & Wilkins, 2006.

45. c. This is a cluster of normal endometrial cells. Exfoliated endometrial cells usually form tight clusters. The cells are small and have high N:C ratios and bland, dark nuclei with fine chromatin and occasional grooves. The nuclei are the same size as the nuclei of intermediate squamous cells. The presence of central crowded/collapsed stromal cells in a cell ball is a helpful finding indicating endometrial origin (not depicted in photo). Normally, exfoliated endometrial cells are seen in cervicovaginal cytologic specimens during the first half of the menstrual cycle. They should not be seen in the latter half of the cycle or in postmenopausal women. The presence of exfoliated endometrial cells in women aged 40 or older should be reported. Because an individual woman's risk factors for endometrial carcinoma, clinical symptoms, menstrual history, hormone therapy history, and menopausal status are often not provided to the laboratory, the 2001 Bethesda System created a category called "Other" for reporting the presence of exfoliated endometrial cells in all women aged 40 or older. Radiation changes include marked cellular and nuclear enlargement with maintained N:C ratios (cytomegaly); irregular nuclear contours; open, smudged chromatin; and visible nucleoli. Cytoplasmic and nuclear vacuolation and multinucleation also may be observed. A history of radiation to the area is essential. In atrophy, the entire cellular population appears blue (with Pap stain) owing to lack of squamous cell maturation resulting in an absence of pink, flat superficial squamous cells. The main cellular component is parabasal squamous cells with oval nuclei, present in clusters or as isolated cells. Aggregates of naked parabasal cell nuclei, inflammation, and degenerated cells with large smudged nuclei known as "blue blobs" also may be present. Compared to exfoliated endometrial cells, endocervical cells usually are larger in size, with polarized nuclei and lower N:C ratios, and often occur as flat sheets rather than spherical clusters.

Solomon D, Nayar R: *The Bethesda System for Reporting Cervical Cytology*, 2nd ed. New York: Springer-Verlag, 2004.

46. b. The photomicrograph shows rod-shaped bacterial organisms called "lactobacilli" or "Döderlein's bacilli," a naked nucleus, fragments of cytoplasm from partially disintegrated intermediate squamous cells, and a single intact intermediate squamous cell. *Lactobacillus* is the most common organism composing normal vaginal flora. Lactobacilli are nonencapsulated gram-positive, rod-shaped bacteria that utilize the glycogen present in glycogen-rich intermediate squamous cells, resulting in cytolysis. Glycogen fermentation results in lactic acid production, contributing to the normal pH of the vagina. These organisms physiologically maintain the vaginal pH value at around 4.5. The principal target of lactobacilli is glycogen-rich intermediate squamous cells; parabasal squamous cells and mature superficial squamous cells containing much less glycogen usually are spared. Lactobacilli are most numerous when intermediate cells predominate, including during pregnancy, the latter half of the menstrual cycle, progesterone-containing contraceptive drug use, the premenopausal phase, and the early menopausal phase, as well as in diabetic menopausal women. They are rarely present before puberty or in atrophic postmenopausal smears. *Staphylococcus aureus* is the pathogen that has been associated with toxic shock in women using vaginal tampons.

Gray W, McKee GT: *Diagnostic Cytopathology*, 2nd ed. London: Churchill Livingstone, 2003.

Koss L, Melamed MR: *Koss's Diagnostic Cytopathology*, 5th ed. Philadelphia: Lippincott Williams & Wilkins, 2006.

47. b. *Trichomonas vaginalis* organisms appear as round, elliptical, or pear-shaped gray-green structures. Sizes are variable, ranging from 8 to 20 μm. Small, eccentric, round or elliptical nuclei are typically seen, but are not evident in all of the organisms. Occasionally, red cytoplasmic granules and flagella may be seen, but the identification of flagella is not required for diagnosis. Squamous cell changes associated with *Trichomonas* infestation include marked cytoplasmic eosinophilia of normally basophilic intermediate and parabasal cells and narrow perinuclear halos. The increase of vaginal and cervical pH that occurs prior to and during the menstrual period promotes the growth of *Trichomonas*. *Trichomonas* infection is typically obtained via sexual contact. The filamentous bacteria *Leptothrix* often coexist with trichomonad organisms. In bacterial vaginitis, adding KOH to the thin, homogeneous discharge caused by *Gardnerella vaginalis* generates a fishy amine odor.

Gray W, McKee GT: *Diagnostic Cytopathology*, 2nd ed. London: Churchill Livingstone, 2003.
Koss L, Melamed MR: *Koss's Diagnostic Cytopathology*, 5th ed. Philadelphia: Lippincott Williams & Wilkins, 2006.

48. d. Typical features of reparative epithelial changes are flat sheets of epithelial cells with enlarged, vesicular nuclei with regular nuclear contours, smooth chromatin and prominent nucleoli, and nuclear "streaming." Although the nuclei are enlarged, the N:C ratios are still maintained. Nucleoli may be multiple, and mitotic figures may be present. The cellular sheets or clusters often are infiltrated by neutrophils. Changes of repair can be associated with many conditions, such as trauma; surgical procedures; vaginal delivery; endocervical polyps; foreign objects, such as intrauterine devices (IUDs); and inflammation. Endometrial carcinoma cells have enlarged, atypical nuclei with coarse chromatin, irregular nuclear contours, and significant nuclear crowding. Many mitoses, including atypical forms, and necrosis may be seen. These features are not observed in the photomicrograph. Topical estrogen followed by repeat sampling may be used in cases in which the distinction between atrophic changes and dysplasia is difficult. Topical estrogen application promotes maturation of the squamous cells; if the findings concerning for dysplasia resolve following estrogen application, then the findings were likely due to atrophy alone. Reparative/reactive atypia may follow radiation treatment. Cells displaying radiation changes are characteristically cytomegalic (macrocytosis), and thus the nuclei and cytoplasm both appear enlarged, so that a relatively normal N:C ratio is maintained. Other features suggestive of radiation include bizarre cellular configurations, "smudged" nuclei, polychromatic or two-tone cytoplasmic staining, and nuclear and cytoplasmic vacuolization. Binucleation and multinucleation are common.

Koss L, Melamed MR: *Koss's Diagnostic Cytopathology*, 5th ed. Philadelphia: Lippincott Williams & Wilkins, 2006.
Solomon D, Nayar R: *The Bethesda System for Reporting Cervical Cytology*, 2nd ed. New York: Springer-Verlag, 2004.

49. d. The lesion depicted in the photomicrograph is squamous cell carcinoma. There are variably sized keratinized and nonkeratinized dysplastic cells with bizarre shapes, including a so-called tadpole cell with an elongated cytoplasmic process. Chromatin is coarse or clumped. The malignant cells possess dense, orangeophilic cytoplasmic keratin. Anucleate keratin fragments also are present. Compared to HSIL, squamous cell carcinoma cells show increased cytologic pleomorphism, orangeophilic cytoplasm with tadpole cytoplasmic processes, and more vesicular nuclei with clumped chromatin and prominent nucleoli. A tumor diathesis is suggestive of invasive squamous cell carcinoma. Cytologic changes of LSIL include koilocytes displaying cellular enlargement with abundant, well-defined dense cytoplasm; nuclear enlargement with

coarse, dark chromatin; irregular nuclear contours; frequent binucleation or multinucleation; and distinct perinuclear halos. Nucleoli are inconspicuous or absent. Cells in HSIL present singly, in sheets, or in syncytial clusters. They have increased N:C ratios and hyperchromatic nuclei, often with nuclear membrane irregularities. Nucleoli are inconspicuous. The cellular and nuclear sizes usually are smaller than those in LSIL. The volume of cytoplasm is significantly reduced. Parakeratotic cells are small, keratinized, superficial squamous cells with dense, orangeophilic or eosinophilic cytoplasm and small pyknotic nuclei. These cells usually have low N:C ratios and lack nuclear atypia. Squamous cell carcinoma in a cervical cytologic preparation most likely represents a cancer arising in a cervicovaginal location. Metastatic carcinomas occur, but are uncommon. Colorectal cancers or urinary bladder carcinomas with squamous differentiation may directly invade into the cervix or vagina, yielding abnormal Pap tests, but this also is not common.

Solomon D, Nayar R: *The Bethesda System for Reporting Cervical Cytology*, 2nd ed. New York: Springer-Verlag, 2004.

50. b. The process depicted in this photomicrograph is follicular cervicitis, an inflammatory/reactive process, with TBMs; a polymorphous population of lymphocytes, including small, medium, and large lymphocytes; and a few squamous cells. Follicular cervicitis is an uncommon chronic cervicitis often seen in menopausal woman as an incidental finding. It usually is asymptomatic. However, in younger women, it may be associated with *C. trachomatis* infection, and inguinal lymphadenopathy may present in those cases. When the lymphoid cells appear monotonous, non-Hodgkin lymphoma should be excluded. *Trichomonas* infection is often associated with acute inflammation, not chronic lymphocytic inflammation. Follicular cervicitis is a chronic lymphocytic inflammatory process primarily involving the submucosal layer of the uterine cervix, not the endometrial cavity. It may be seen on cervical cytologic sampling if there is an ulceration or following vigorous sampling.

Gray W, McKee GT: *Diagnostic Cytopathology*, 2nd ed. London: Churchill Livingstone, 2003.
Koss L, Melamed MR: *Koss's Diagnostic Cytopathology*, 5th ed. Philadelphia: Lippincott Williams & Wilkins, 2006.
Solomon D, Nayar R: *The Bethesda System for Reporting Cervical Cytology*, 2nd ed. New York: Springer-Verlag, 2004.

51. a. A cluster of koilocytes from a case of LSIL is shown. Koilocytes are superficial or intermediate squamous cells with enlarged, hyperchromatic and sometimes multiple nuclei. Nucleoli usually are not present. A sharply demarcated, clear cytoplasmic halo with a dense rim surrounds the atypical nucleus. Koilocytes may occur singly or in clusters. They are pathognomonic of HPV infection. Upon further evaluation, 15% to 25% of women with LSIL on cervicovaginal cytologic examination are found to have histologic cervical intraepithelial neoplasia (CIN2 and CIN3). Cytoplasmic characteristics seen in squamous cell carcinoma typically include marked keratinization and bizarre shapes; these are not seen in LSIL. Koilocytes, the cells with characteristic features seen in LSILs, usually have inconspicuous nucleoli. Prominent nucleoli may be seen in reactive squamous cells as well as in invasive squamous cell carcinoma, along with other relevant cytologic features. Multinucleation, nuclear molding, and a ground-glass nuclear appearance are characteristic of HSV-infected squamous cells. The majority of LSILs undergo spontaneous regression.

Solomon D, Nayar R: *The Bethesda System for Reporting Cervical Cytology*, 2nd ed. New York: Springer-Verlag, 2004.

52. a. The picture shows a few isolated and loosely grouped variably sized cells with high N:C ratios. The nuclei are hyperchromatic and have irregular nuclear contours. They have inconspicuous nucleoli and delicate cytoplasm. Although the N:C ratios are high, the overall cell sizes are small. These cells represent HSIL. Keratinized forms of HSIL display thick, orange or yellow cytoplasm. Degenerated endocervical cells often remain in a group and may have diminished cytoplasm, but they usually have bland-appearing nuclei, open chromatin, smooth nuclear contours, and small or prominent nucleoli. Although the cytoplasm of the cells may be degenerated, the polarity of the nuclei still can be appreciated. The morphologic features of the cells in the photo do not meet the criteria for diagnosing a carcinoma. Cells of LSIL are large, with enlarged nuclei, irregular and coarse chromatin, and low N:C ratios. Binucleation or multinucleation and "koilocytes" are features of LSIL. Histiocytes may be seen in Pap tests, particularly during and immediately after menstruation. Histiocytes have low N:C ratios and bland, small, oval or kidney bean–shaped pale nuclei lacking nuclear hyperchromasia and irregularity. They tend to be present singly. The cytoplasm may contain engulfed particles or vacuoles, or may appear degenerated.

Solomon D, Nayar R: *The Bethesda System for Reporting Cervical Cytology*, 2nd ed. New York: Springer-Verlag, 2004.

53. c. The photomicrograph shows three characteristic features seen in rheumatoid effusions: necrotic debris and degenerated cells (lower left portion of photo); multinucleated giant cells; and elongated, spindle-shaped or carrot-shaped epithelioid cells that are histiocytes and thus are cytokeratin negative. The slender epithelioid histiocytes may resemble so-called snake cells seen in squamous cell carcinoma. Squamous carcinomas occasionally involve serous surfaces, and they can shed single tadpole-shaped cells. Usually, malignant cells in clusters also are present. The clinical history combined with the triad of necrotic material, epithelioid spindle cells, and multinucleated giant cells favor a rheumatoid effusion. Immunocytochemical staining may be helpful for diagnostic confirmation, and correlation with clinical laboratory findings is also important. Necrosis and multinucleated giant cells are uncommon findings in tuberculous effusions. Tuberculous effusions typically contain numerous lymphocytes and rare or no mesothelial cells. Rheumatoid effusions are almost always unilateral and are almost always pleural. Pericardial and peritoneal rheumatoid effusions are rare.

De las Casas LE, Morales AM, Boman DA, et al: Laparoscopic aspiration cytology in rheumatoid ascites: a case report. *Acta Cytol* 2010;54(6):1123-1126.

DeMay RM: *The Art and Science of Cytopathology*, 2nd ed. Chicago: American Society for Clinical Pathology, 2011.

54. d. The photomicrograph contains two collections (one tight cluster and one relatively loose) of epithelioid histiocytes demonstrating nuclei with several different shapes, including indented (bean-shaped), oval, elongated, and tapered (carrot-shaped). A few lymphocytes also are present. These findings are consistent with a granulomatous process. Intravesical bacillus Calmette-Guérin (BCG) is a form of immunotherapy that often is used to treat and prevent recurrence of superficial urothelial carcinomas of the urinary bladder. There frequently is a granulomatous response in the wall of the urinary bladder, and granulomas may be evident in the urine in the form of loose aggregates of epithelioid histiocytes, sometimes accompanied by multinucleated giant cells of Langhans type. Morphologic evidence of granulomas is important in the work-up and diagnosis of patients with sarcoidosis; however, direct urinary bladder involvement by sarcoidosis is extremely rare. Cytologic findings do have an unequivocal role in the diagnostic work-up of patients with sarcoidosis, especially with the recent use of FNA endobronchial ultrasound-guided transbronchial needle aspiration in evaluating patients with sarcoidosis involving lung and mediastinal and hilar lymph nodes, organs that are involved in the majority of patients with sarcoidosis. Xanthogranulomatous pyelonephritis is an uncommon chronic destructive granulomatous process of renal parenchyma. There are few reports of FNA biopsy findings of this uncommon condition. If there is communication with the renal pelvis, urine examination may show inflammatory cells, but the findings are nonspecific. By far, the most common fungus affecting the urinary bladder is *Candida*. Other, much less common fungal infections that have been reported in urine specimens include *Blastomyces*, *Aspergillus*, *Curvularia*, and *Histoplasma*. Although fungal organisms may be seen in urine specimens, they are not typically accompanied by granulomas. Multinucleated giant cells must be differentiated from multinucleated umbrella cells. Multinucleated umbrella cells are urothelial cells that may be quite large, and the number of nuclei may be anywhere from 3 to 50 or even more. They are not commonly seen in normal voided urine specimens, but they are especially common in washings or brushings of the bladder or ureters. Their shape is polygonal and their borders are scalloped. In contrast, multinucleated histiocytes have smooth borders and the nuclei often form a circle or semicircle at the periphery of the cell (Langhans type). They often are accompanied by granulomas (collections of epithelioid histiocytes).

Arora SK, Gupta N, Nijhawan R, Mandal AK: Epithelioid cell granulomas in urine cytology smears: same cause, different implications. *Diagn Cytopathol* 2010;38(10):765-767.

Koss LG: *Diagnostic Cytology of the Urinary Tract with Histopathologic and Clinical Correlations*. Philadelphia: Lippincott-Raven, 1996.

Mehrotra R, Dhingra V: Cytological diagnosis of sarcoidosis revisited: a state of the art review. *Diagn Cytopathol* 2011; 39(7):541-548.

55. d. In this photomicrograph of a urine sample obtained during a cystoscopic procedure, there are several three-dimensional crowded "papillaroid" clusters of urothelial cells. Clusters such as these may be a result of reactive changes due to calculi, inflammation, or instrumentation (e.g., catheterization, cystoscopy), and care must be taken not to misinterpret them as a papillary neoplasm. Calculi act as abrasive, cutting objects; therefore, the cytologic features in voided urine specimens may resemble those seen as a result of instrumentation: numerous, large clusters of urothelial cells may be seen, and may be impossible to distinguish from low-grade papillary urothelial tumors. Urothelial carcinoma in situ does not form a tumor mass. In many cases, no visible lesion can be detected cystoscopically. In other cases, an area of erythema or "cobblestoning" similar to that found in cases of inflammation may be seen in foci of in situ carcinoma. Papillary clusters may be seen in urine specimens as a result of calculi in the absence of neoplasia; however, patients with renal calculi are at increased risk for the development of urothelial carcinoma, especially carcinoma in situ. If single cells with features of carcinoma in situ are identified in a urine sample from a patient with calculi, further investigation to locate their source is warranted.

Koss LG: *Diagnostic Cytology of the Urinary Tract with Histopathologic and Clinical Correlations*. Philadelphia: Lippincott-Raven, 1996.

Layfield LJ, Elsheikh TM, Fili A, et al: Review of the state of the art and recommendations of the Papanicolaou Society of Cytopathology for urinary cytology procedures and reporting: the Papanicolaou Society of Cytopathology Practice Guidelines Task Force. Papanicolaou Society of Cytopathology. *Diagn Cytopathol* 2004;30(1):24-30.

56. d. These degenerated cells with pyknotic nuclei resemble histiocytes, but are degenerated ileal glandular epithelial cells in ileal urine. They usually lack a columnar appearance because epithelial cells tend to "round up" in fluid, and they frequently resemble macrophages. Ileal urine commonly has a granular background containing bacteria, cellular debris, and inflammatory cells. This background debris may make it difficult to identify neoplastic cells from a recurrent or metachronous tumor; however, the malignant cells actually may be better preserved than the degenerated intestinal cells, and will show cytologic features characteristic of malignant urothelial cells. Cytologic changes due to radiation of urothelium are similar to its effects on other types of epithelial cells; features include marked cell enlargement (cytomegaly; enlargement of both the nucleus and the cell itself), vacuolization of the cytoplasm and nucleus, "smudged" nuclei, and polychromatic or two-tone cytoplasmic staining. Radiation changes may persist for years following treatment. Examination of voided urine is not a primary method of diagnosing prostatic diseases. In fact, it is very uncommon to find normal prostatic cells or evidence of benign disorders of the prostate in voided urine. Neutrophils, lymphocytes, and histiocytes almost always are present in ileal urine specimens and do not necessarily indicate an infectious process.

Ajit D, Dighe SB, Desai SB: Cytology of ileal conduit urine in bladder cancer patients: diagnostic utility and pitfalls. *Acta Cytol* 2006;50(1):70-73.

Koss LG: *Diagnostic Cytology of the Urinary Tract with Histopathologic and Clinical Correlations*. Philadelphia: Lippincott-Raven, 1996.

Thiryayi SA, Rana DN: Urine cytopathology: challenges, pitfalls, and mimics. *Diagn Cytopathol* 2012;40(11):1019-1034.

57. d. The photomicrograph demonstrates a sheet of large, rectangular, thick-walled plant cells with distinct edges, in a honeycomb, palisaded arrangement. Vegetable cells can be seen in several cytologic samples, including sputum, bronchial washes, and anal Pap smears. The presence of fecal material in cervical samples usually is related to contamination but rarely can be due to a rectovaginal fistula. HSV infection in a cervical sample may present as a single enlarged nucleus or, more commonly, as multinucleated cells that demonstrate thickened nuclear membranes and nuclear molding. Margination of chromatin to the periphery or beneath the nuclear envelope leaves a homogeneous, ground-glass appearance in the rest of the nucleus. Carpet beetle parts in cervical samples usually are introduced during the process of sampling and preparation. They often originate from cotton swabs and gauze pads, but they may also originate from the introduction of organisms or their parts into the vagina by tampons or incontinence pads. They are elongated structures with arrow-shaped heads. *Alternaria* species are easily identified by their brown, septated conidia that have a snowshoelike appearance. Arrowwood contaminants are derived from the arrowwood (*Viburnum dentatum*) plant. They are large star-shaped (stellate) or treelike structures with thick, transparent walls and stain a golden pink color with Pap stain.

Bechtold E, Staunton CE, and Katz SS: Carpet beetle larval parts in cervical cytology specimens. *Acta Cytol* 1985;29:345-352.

Demay RM: *The Art and Science of Cytopathology*, 2nd ed. Chicago: American Society for Clinical Pathology, 2012.

Farkas TA: Images in clinical medicine. Arrowwood contaminant in Pap smear. *N Engl J Med* 2005;352(21):e20.

Quiroga-Garza G, Nassar D, Khalbuss WE, et al: Vegetable cell contaminants in urinary bladder diversion cytology specimens. *Acta Cytol* 2012;56(3):271-276. Epub 2012 Apr 26.

58. e. Most commonly, eosinophilic effusions are idiopathic, and an underlying cause is not found. Eosinophils occur most commonly in pleural fluid. They are much less commonly seen in peritoneal fluid and are rarely seen in pericardial fluids. Eosinophilic effusions are exudates. Although an eosinophilic effusion may be associated with an underlying malignancy, most eosinophilic effusions are not associated with malignancy. Parasitic infection (e.g., hydatid disease) should be included in the differential diagnosis of an eosinophilic pleural effusion that is accompanied by peripheral eosinophilia.

DeMay RM: *The Art and Science of Cytopathology*, 2nd ed. Chicago: American Society for Clinical Pathology, 2011.

Matthai SM, Kini U: Diagnostic value of eosinophils in pleural effusion: a prospective study of 26 cases. *Diagn Cytopathol* 2003;28(2):96-99.

59. b. The photomocrograph shows atypical squamous cells with hyperchromatic nuclei, high N:C ratios, irregular/ "raisinoid" nuclei with coarse chromatin, inconspicuous nucleoli, and scant cytoplasm; these are features of HSIL. Colposcopy is recommended for all women—pregnant, nonpregnant, and adolescent—with HSIL detected by cytologic testing. If no CIN2 or CIN3 lesion is detected, follow-up cytologic testing and colposcopy are recommended, but no sooner than 6 weeks postpartum. Endocervical curettage is not advisable in pregnant women with HSIL. Immediate LEEP is not an acceptable next step in a pregnant woman with HSIL.

Wright TC Jr, Massad LS, Dunton CJ, et al: 2006 consensus guidelines for the management of women with abnormal cervical cancer screening tests. 2006 American Society for Colposcopy and Cervical Pathology–sponsored Consensus Conference. *Am J Obstet Gynecol* 2007;197(4):346-355.

60. c. Marked enlargement of cellular and nuclear sizes with maintained N:C ratios (cytomegaly), fine chromatin, small or inconspicuous nucleoli, multinucleation, and nuclear and cytoplasmic vacuoles are classic features of radiation effect. Reparative changes usually present as tight, flat sheets of cells with cellular "stretching" and nuclear "streaming"; large, vesicular nuclei; smooth or slightly coarse chromatin; prominent nucleoli; and smooth nuclear contours. A neutrophilic infiltrate is commonly present in the cellular clusters. Marked cytomegaly, multinucleation, and nuclear and cytoplasmic vacuolization are not typical findings in reparative changes. Although the cells in the picture are pleomorphic, they lack typical malignant features, such as markedly irregular nuclei, coarse chromatin, prominent nucleoli, nuclear crowding, and mitoses. In addition, the cell in the photograph is a squamous, not glandular, cell. The multinucleation seen as a result of radiation therapy may be confused with HSV cytopathic changes; however, the multinucleated cells in the latter condition usually contain tightly packed nuclei with "molding," a ground-glass chromatin appearance and chromatin margination, absence of nucleoli, and occasional eosinophilic intranuclear inclusions.

Gray W, McKee GT: *Diagnostic Cytopathology*, 2nd ed. London: Churchill Livingstone, 2003.
Solomon D, Nayar R: *The Bethesda System for Reporting Cervical Cytology*, 2nd ed. New York: Springer-Verlag, 2004.

61. b. The cytologic features depicted in the photomicrograph are those of adenocarcinoma in situ (AIS). There is an abnormal cellular cluster containing cells with a columnar appearance. The nuclei are enlarged, variably sized, oval, and elongated, with nuclear palisading or stratification ("feathering"). The nuclei are hyperchromatic and have coarse chromatin. Nucleoli are inconspicuous. The background is relatively clean. If a cervical Pap test shows AIS, colposcopy is indicated. If no invasive disease is detected, a diagnostic excisional procedure is recommended. For an initial cytologic diagnosis of "atypical glandular cells, favor neoplasia" or "AIS," neither HPV testing nor repeat cervical Pap testing is an appropriate next step. Endometrial sampling is recommended in women 35 years and older, but in conjunction with colposcopy and endocervical sampling. Hysterectomy may be warranted, but the decision to proceed with this surgery should take into account many factors, including endocervical excisional biopsy findings, additional testing to evaluate the extent of disease, and the desire to preserve reproductive ability. If AIS is confirmed on diagnostic excisional biopsy, a hysterectomy is the preferred treatment. If conservative treatment is desired, then a negative surgical margin of excisional biopsy should be achieved, and close long-term follow-up might be an appropriate approach. Radiation therapy is not the standard treatment for AIS. Whether radiation therapy is needed depends on the subsequent endocervical excisional biopsy result (evaluating the presence of invasion) and further work-up to evaluate the extent and stage of the disease.

Wright TC Jr, Massad LS, Dunton CJ, et al: 2006 consensus guidelines for the management of women with cervical intraepithelial neoplasia or adenocarcinoma in situ. 2006 American Society for Colposcopy and Cervical Pathology–sponsored Consensus Conference. *Am J Obstet Gynecol* 2007;197(4):340-345.
Wright TC Jr, Massad LS, Dunton CJ, et al: 2006 consensus guidelines for the management of women with abnormal cervical cancer screening tests. 2006 American Society for Colposcopy and Cervical Pathology–sponsored Consensus Conference. *Am J Obstet Gynecol* 2007;197(4): 346-355.

62. c. The abnormal squamous cells in the photomicrograph are koilocytes and are a typical cytologic feature of LSIL. Repeat cervical Pap testing at 12 months as follow-up is the recommended management for adolescents with LSIL on a cervical Pap test. For adult premenopausal woman, pregnant adult women, and postmenopausal women who are found to have LSIL on a Pap test, the recommended management is colposcopy. HPV DNA testing and tissue biopsy are not recommended for adolescents with LSIL. The currently available HPV vaccines cover only two types of high-risk HPV, types 16 and 18. The HPV vaccine is a preventive method to protect women from these types of HPV infections, but it does not treat existing HPV infections.

Centers for Disease Control and Prevention: HPV vaccination. Available at http://www.cdc.gov/vaccines/vpd-vac/hpv/.
Wright TC Jr, Massad LS, Dunton CJ, et al: 2006 consensus guidelines for the management of women with abnormal cervical cancer screening tests. 2006 American Society for Colposcopy and Cervical Pathology–sponsored Consensus Conference. *Am J Obstet Gynecol* 2007;197(4):346-355.

63. e. The photomicrograph shows features associated with advanced atrophy, in which the predominant cell type is parabasal cells, with minimal maturation. Parabasal and basal cells are present singly as well as in syncytium-like aggregates or hyperchromatic crowded groups. Aggregates of naked, oval nuclei and occasional dark, smudged cells also may be seen (not demonstrated in photo). In cases in which it is difficult to distinguish between atrophy and HSIL, treating the patient with topical estrogen may promote the maturation of atrophic squamous cells, whereas true HSIL cells will not be affected. The latter will persist in a background of mature squamous cells on a follow-up cervicovaginal Pap test. Although atrophy may mimic syncytical HSIL due to the presence of highly cellular clusters in both, the cells in atrophy lack HSIL features, such as hyperchromatic and irregular nuclei, coarse chromatin, and nuclear disarray and overlapping. Atrophy is unrelated to HPV infection. In cases in which it is difficult to distinguish between atrophy and HSIL in an atrophic background, Ki-67 and p16 immunostains may be helpful. The Ki-67 stain will show increased mitotic activity going up into the intermediate and superficial layers in tissue biopsies of HSIL; p16 typically is diffusely positive in HSIL, but not in atrophy.

Solomon D, Nayar R: *The Bethesda System for Reporting Cervical Cytology*, 2nd ed. New York: Springer-Verlag, 2004.

Wright TC Jr, Massad LS, Dunton CJ, et al: 2006 consensus guidelines for the management of women with abnormal cervical cancer screening tests. 2006 American Society for Colposcopy and Cervical Pathology–sponsored Consensus Conference. *Am J Obstet Gynecol* 2007;197(4):346-355.

64. a. Burkitt lymphoma commonly presents with an abdominal mass. CSF is involved in approximately one third of cases. The photomicrograph shows medium-sized (15 to 25 µm) lymphoid cells with round, dark nuclei, several (2 to 5) small nucleoli, and deeply blue, vacuolated cytoplasm. Apoptotic bodies and abundant mitotic figures usually are also present. Burkitt lymphoma expresses the following germinal center markers: CD19, CD20, CD10, and bcl-6, and IgM. It is bcl-2 negative (in contrast to other germinal center lymphomas). Burkitt lymphoma is associated with translocations of the *c-MYC* gene on chromosome 8. The t(8;14) translocation involving the immunoglobulin (Ig) heavy chain locus is the most common. Rearrangement of c-MYC is diagnostically important. Anaplastic large cell lymphoma cells are not usually seen in CSF. The malignant cells are large (rather than medium-sized) and display irregular mononuclear and multinuclear forms. Horseshoe-shaped nuclei—"hallmark" cells—that may resemble Reed-Sternberg cells may also be noted. Precursor lymphoblastic lymphomas are much more common in children, who present with mediastinal lymphadenopathy or skin lesions. Lymphoblasts are uniform intermediate cells (10 to 25 µm) with scant cytoplasm, round nuclei, finely granular chromatin, and inconspicuous nucleoli. Mitotic figures and nuclear molding may be seen. Malignant cells in DLCBL are predominantly large cells (25 to 50 µm), with irregular nuclear contours, vesicular chromatin, prominent nucleoli, and a moderate amount of cytoplasm. Several morphologic variants are present: immunoblastic, centroblastic, T-cell rich, and anaplastic. This malignancy may affect any age group, but it is more common in older patients. Most patients with small lymphocytic lymphoma are older than 60. Hepatosplenomegaly is common. The neoplastic cells appear uniform and small, with clumped chromatin, some irregularity of the nuclear membrane, inconspicuous nucleoli, and scant cytoplasm. A small number of larger cells (prolymphocytes) also is present.

Caraway NP: Strategies to diagnose lymphoproliferative disorders by fine-needle aspiration by using ancillary studies. *Cancer* 2005;105(6):432-442.

Roma AA, Garcia A, Avagnina A, et al: Lymphoid and myeloid neoplasms involving cerebrospinal fluid: comparison of morphologic examination and immunophenotyping by flow cytometry. *Diagn Cytopathol* 2002;27(5):271-275.

Wu JM, Georgy MF, Burroughs FH, et al: Lymphoma, leukemia, and pleiocytosis in cerebrospinal fluid: is accurate cytopathologic diagnosis possible based on morphology alone? *Diagn Cytopathol* 2009;37(11):820-824.

65. e. The photomicrograph represents a Pap-stained smear from an FNA of a mucoepidermoid carcinoma of the parotid gland. The smear shows single and loose pleomorphic glandular cells with obvious malignant features, including irregular nuclear contours, coarse and clumped chromatin, and very prominent nucleoli. The single arrow indicates a smaller cell with squamous features (hyperchromatic nucleus and dense, orange cytoplasm) and the double arrow shows intermediate cells (bland, smaller cells with less cytoplasm). The background contains mucin. Necrotizing sialometaplasia usually occurs in the minor salivary glands. The smears are hypocellular and show squamous metaplastic cells and atypical epithelial cells in a background of fibrous and necrotic material. Ductal and acinar salivary gland epithelial cells usually are also noted. Smears of salivary duct carcinoma show sheets and clusters of large, polygonal epithelial cells with obvious malignant features, including irregular nuclear contours, abundant vacuolated cytoplasm, and prominent nucleoli. Necrosis is present. This tumor is more common in older men. FNAs of acinic cell carcinoma yield cellular smears composed of loosely cohesive, bland-appearing cells in a background of denuded nuclei and lymphocytes. The cells have abundant, granular cytoplasm with indistinct cell borders, round to oval nuclei, and small nucleoli. Blood vessels may be seen in some clusters. Polymorphous low-grade adenocarcinoma is a difficult diagnosis to make on FNA biopsy. This tumor occurs mainly in minor salivary glands of older adults. Smears show clusters, tubules, and cords of uniform cells with fine chromatin. Hyaline globules similar to those in adenoid cystic carcinoma may be seen.

Mukunyadzi P: Review of fine-needle aspiration cytology of salivary gland neoplasms, with emphasis on differential diagnosis. *Am J Clin Pathol* 2002;118(Suppl):S100-115.

Rajwanshi A, Gupta K, Gupta N, et al: Fine-needle aspiration cytology of salivary glands: diagnostic pitfalls-revisited. *Diagn Cytopathol* 2006;34(8):580-584.

66. c. The best choice is well-differentiated adenocarcinoma with bronchioloalveolar carcinoma (BAC) features. The FNA biopsy specimens of classic BAC show abundant large and small clusters, sheets, or papillae of bland and orderly glandular cells without cilia. The nuclei are uniform and round or oval, with some nuclear overlap, mild nuclear membrane irregularities, and finely granular chromatin. Nuclear clearing and macronucleoli may be seen. Intranuclear cytoplasmic inclusions and grooves are a helpful diagnostic clue but are not pathognomonic. The neoplastic cells of BAC can be very similar to hyperplastic type II pneumocytes. Helpful differentiating features include the hypercellularity of smears containing these seemingly "reactive"-appearing epithelial cells, lack of cilia, and a clean background in BAC. The cellularity of a specimen containing only reactive bronchial cells is usually less than that containing adenocarcinoma. Benign clusters are flat and orderly and most of the cells have scant cytoplasm, bland nuclei, and small nucleoli. They demonstrate cilia and terminal bars. The background often shows inflammation. Mesothelial cells picked up by the aspiration needle may mimic well-differentiated adenocarcinoma. Mesothelial cells usually present as a few sheets of polygonal cells with well-defined, evenly spaced nuclei and cell-to-cell windows. Neuroendocrine tumors, particularly carcinoid tumor with plasmacytoid features, sometimes can mimic less differentiated adenocarcinomas that have more single cells. Cohesive epithelial groups and the chromatin pattern are useful distinguishing features. Metastatic PTC may also resemble BAC. Nuclear membrane irregularities are usually much more prominent in PTC. Knowledge of clinical history is important, and immunocytochemical studies may be very helpful (Table 24-4).

TABLE 24-4 Cytologic Features of Bronchioloalveolar-type Adenocarcinoma

	Reactive	Nonmucinous BAC	Mucinous BAC
Cellularity	Low	High	High
Clusters	Small and flat, orderly	Large and small, flat, +/- orderly	Large and small, flat and 3-D, +/- orderly
Cytoplasm	Very scant	Scant	Ample
Nuclei	Bland/mild atypical	Atypical	Bland/atypical
Nucleoli	Smaller	Larger	Larger
N:C ratio	Low	High	Low
Cilia	+	−	−
Terminal structures	++	−	+/−
Background	Inflammation	Clean	Mucinous

BAC, bronchioloalveolar carcinoma; N:C ratio, nucleus-to-cytoplasm ratio.

MacDonald LL, Yazdi HM: Fine-needle aspiration biopsy of bronchioloalveolar carcinoma. *Cancer* 2001;93(1): 29-34.

Travis WD: Pathology of lung cancer. *Clin Chest Med* 2011; 32(4):669-692.

Travis WD, Brambilla E, Noguchi M, et al: International Association for the Study of Lung Cancer/American Thoracic Society/European Respiratory Society International Multidisciplinary Classification of Lung Adenocarcinoma. *J Thorac Oncol* 2011;6:244-285.

67. d. Schaumann bodies are calcium and protein inclusions inside multinucleated giant cells and may be found in several granulomatous conditions. Hamazaki-Wesenberg bodies are yellow-brown structures of unknown significance associated with histiocytes; they resemble fungi. Asteroid bodies are eosinophilic inclusion bodies with radiating lines in the cytoplasm of multinucleated giant cells. Birefringent calcium oxalate and calcium carbonate microcalcifications may be found in sarcoidosis. Psammoma bodies are concentrically laminated small calcifications most commonly seen in papillary neoplasms. They may be seen in papillary neoplasms of the endometrium, ovary, peritoneum, and thyroid, as well as meningioma. They may also occur in association with benign mesothelial hyperplasia.

Mehrotra R, Dhingra V: Cytological diagnosis of sarcoidosis revisited: a state of the art review. *Diagn Cytopathol* 2011; 39(7):541-548.

68. a. Koilocytes are HPV-infected mature squamous or intermediate cells with clear, well-defined cytoplasmic vacuoles or halos with condensation of peripheral cytoplasm. "Koilocyte" is a morphologic description that is specific for HPV infection-related changes in squamous cells. In *Trichomonas* infection, the squamous cells display reactive changes, including "pseudokoilocytosis," in which a thin perinuclear halo is seen without associated nuclear changes. Parabasal and intermediate squamous cells, which normally have basophilic cytoplasm, display cytoplasmic eosinophilia. When these changes are seen, *T. vaginalis* organisms often are detected. Although columnar epithelial cells and metaplastic cells in the female genitoreproductive tract are the primary target of *Chlamydia* infection, the squamous cells often show reactive changes such as "pseudokoilocytosis." Under progesterone influence, particularly during pregnancy, squamous cells mature into intermediate cells with increased glycogen content that

results in cytoplasmic clearing with a light yellowish hue (navicular cells). These cells may be mistaken for koilocytes. Estrogen replacement therapy results in maturation of cervical squamous epithelial cells and the presence of superficial cells. It does not cause significant perinuclear halos.

Koss L, Melamed MR: *Koss's Diagnostic Cytopathology*, 5th ed. Philadelphia: Lippincott Williams & Wilkins, 2006.

Solomon D, Nayar R: *The Bethesda System for Reporting Cervical Cytology*, 2nd ed. New York: Springer-Verlag, 2004.

69. e. In LSIL, the overall cell size is larger than normal superficial squamous cells, the nuclei are more than three times larger than normal intermediate cells, and the N:C ratios are low. Compared with LSIL cells, HSIL cells are smaller and more uniform, with reduced volume of cytoplasm and reduced nuclear size. In high-grade dysplastic squamous cells, the reduction of cytoplasmic volume is more significant than reduction of nuclear size; therefore, the overall N:C ratio is significantly increased. The nuclear features of high-grade dysplastic squamous cells are more pronounced owing to more condensed nuclei and more significant nuclear irregularities. As part of an increase in dysplastic features, HSIL cell nuclear chromatin is coarser and clumped, but in LSIL, the nuclei are hyperchromatic and the chromatin is often evenly distributed, smudged, or densely opaque.

Solomon D, Nayar R: *The Bethesda System for Reporting Cervical Cytology*, 2nd ed. New York: Springer-Verlag, 2004.

70. e. Nucleoli often are not visible in LSIL and HSIL, but they become visible and prominent when the lesion becomes invasive (microinvasive squamous cell carcinoma or invasive squamous cell carcinoma). HCGs may be seen in both HSIL and invasive squamous cell carcinoma. The presence of naked nuclei is a nonspecific finding and may be seen in both HSIL and invasive carcinoma. Coarse chromatin can be seen in HSIL as well as invasive squamous cell carcinoma. As dysplasia progresses, increased N:C ratios become more pronounced, but this occurrence does not differentiate between HSIL and invasion. Moderate to well-differentiated squamous cell carcinomas may have lower N:C ratios than HSIL cells.

Koss L, Melamed MR: *Koss's Diagnostic Cytopathology*, 5th ed. Philadelphia: Lippincott Williams & Wilkins, 2006.

Solomon D, Nayar R: *The Bethesda System for Reporting Cervical Cytology*, 2nd ed. New York: Springer-Verlag, 2004.

71. e. Atrophy, HSIL, endometrial cells, and adenocarcinoma can give rise to HCGs, which can make diagnosis and differential diagnosis very challenging. Atrophy may present in cervicovaginal Pap tests as syncytial clusters of densely packed parabasal cells with small oval nuclei and minimal cytoplasm, with an appearance of hyperchromatic clusters. In HSIL, the dysplastic cells tend to be small, with high N:C ratios, and, when in highly packed clusters, have an appearance of HCGs of cells. Endometrial cells exfoliated during menstruation appear as dense clusters of highly packed, hyperchromatic cells with minimal cytoplasm. The cellular density is exaggerated due to the presence of condensed stromal cells in the central cores. In both poorly differentiated squamous cell carcinoma and adenocarcinoma, tumor cell clusters may appear as hyperchromatic groups of cells. Features suggesting malignancy include loss of cell polarity; coarse, hyperchromatic chromatin; and mitoses.

Koss L, Melamed MR: *Koss's Diagnostic Cytopathology*, 5th ed. Philadelphia: Lippincott Williams & Wilkins, 2006.
Solomon D, Nayar R: *The Bethesda System for Reporting Cervical Cytology*, 2nd ed. New York: Springer-Verlag, 2004.

72. b. Currently, the recommended management of ASC-H is referral for colposcopy. If CIN2 or CIN3 is not detected, follow-up with cervical Pap testing at 6 months and 12 months or follow-up HPV testing at 12 months is an acceptable recommendation. Immediate LEEP is not the management for patients following a diagnosis of ASC-H, but it is one of the management choices following an unequivocal diagnosis of HSIL on Pap testing; however, this recommendation does not apply to pregnant women or adolescents. High-risk HPV testing is recommended when ASC-US is detected on cervicovaginal Pap screening tests in women over the age of 20. Repeat Pap smear after topical estrogen treatment sometimes is used when atrophic cells raise the concern of HSIL due to similar patterns shared by both. In this case, application of topical estrogen may produce sufficient maturation to allow definitive diagnosis on follow-up cytologic testing.

Solomon D, Nayar R: *The Bethesda System for Reporting Cervical Cytology*, 2nd ed. New York: Springer-Verlag, 2004.
Wright TC Jr, Massad LS, Dunton CJ, et al: 2006 consensus guidelines for the management of women with abnormal cervical cancer screening tests. 2006 American Society for Colposcopy and Cervical Pathology–sponsored Consensus Conference. *Am J Obstet Gynecol* 2007;197(4):346-355.

73. b. HPV is a small, circular, double-stranded, 7900 base-paired, nonenveloped DNA virus that replicates in the nucleus of infected host cells. The coding regions of HPV viruses contain seven early genes (E) and two late genes (L) or "open reading frames" that encode viral gene products (proteins) to permit viral replication and infection and induce host cell proliferation and transformation. E1 and E2 proteins are necessary for viral replication. E6 and E7 are oncoproteins that play roles in host cell transformation. HPVs initially infect the basal cells of squamous epithelium, and then complete their maturation in the superficial squamous layer. The integration sites of HPV genomic material in the host genome are random.

Gray W, McKee GT: *Diagnostic Cytopathology*, 2nd ed. London: Churchill Livingstone, 2003.
Koss L, Melamed MR: *Koss's Diagnostic Cytopathology*, 5th ed. Philadelphia: Lippincott Williams & Wilkins, 2006.
Robboy S, Anderson M, Russell P: *Pathology of the Female Reproductive Tract*. London: Churchill Livingstone, 2002.

74. c. In pregnancy, a shift toward lower maturation (i.e., an atrophic pattern) suggests progesterone deficiency and may indicate intrauterine fetal demise. However, infection also may result in changes in the usual maturation patterns. The corpus luteum of pregnancy and the placenta produce progesterone, resulting in a predominance of intermediate squamous cells. Cytolysis may be marked during pregnancy, but it is due to lactobacilli, not *Leptothrix*. "Navicular" cells are boat-shaped intermediate cells containing abundant glycogen. This is not a specific finding in pregnancy. Navicular cells also may be seen during administration of progesterone or androgen-containing hormones. Postpartum smears show a predominantly atrophic pattern in approximately one third of nonlactating mothers and two thirds of lactating mothers.

Gray W, McKee GT: *Diagnostic Cytopathology*, 2nd ed. London: Churchill Livingstone, 2003.
Koss L, Melamed MR: *Koss's Diagnostic Cytopathology*, 5th ed. Philadelphia: Lippincott Williams & Wilkins, 2006.

75. d. In a *conventional* Pap smear preparation, an estimated minimum of 8000 to 12,000 well-preserved and well-visualized squamous epithelial cells should be present for the sample to be considered adequate. An adequate liquid-based preparation should have an estimated minimum of 5000 well-preserved, well-visualized squamous cells. In the satisfactory category, one also needs to assess and state the presence or absence of an endocervical/transformation zone component and other quality indicators such as obscuring blood or inflammation. The unsatisfactory category includes processed and fully evaluated specimens with inadequate well-preserved/well-visualized squamous components due to factors such as low cellularity or obscuring blood as well as specimens rejected (specimens not processed) because of lack of or erroneous labeling, slide breakage, or similar problems. Any specimen with abnormal cells, such as ASC-US, AGC, or a more severe abnormality, should be considered satisfactory regardless of the number of squamous cells present. The presence of normal endometrial cells or microorganisms in a specimen containing less than an estimated 5000 well-preserved, well-visualized squamous cells without any atypia does not make the specimen a satisfactory specimen. However, these findings should be indicated in the report as a comment under the main category "unsatisfactory for evaluation."

Solomon D, Nayar R: *The Bethesda System for Reporting Cervical Cytology*, 2nd ed. New York: Springer-Verlag, 2004.

ACKNOWLEDGMENT

The authors wish to acknowledge Guo Xia Tong, MD, who contributed questions to the first edition of this book, some of which, in part, have been retained in this edition.

INDEX

Note: Page numbers followed by *f* indicate figures, *b* indicate boxes and *t* indicate tables.